Pediatric Clinical Practice Guidelines & Policies

A Compendium of Evidence-based Research for Pediatric Practice

26th Edition

American Academy of Pediatrics
345 Park Blvd
Itasca, IL 60143
www.aap.org

**AMERICAN ACADEMY OF PEDIATRICS
PUBLISHING STAFF**

Mark Grimes
Vice President, Publishing

Jeff Mahony
Senior Director, Professional and Consumer Publishing

Jennifer McDonald
Senior Editor, Digital Publishing

Soraya Alem
Manager, Digital Publishing

Leesa Levin-Doroba
Production Manager, Practice Management

Peg Mulcahy
Manager, Art Direction and Production

Linda Smessaert, MSIMC
Director, Marketing

Mary Louise Carr
Marketing Manager, Clinical Publications

Published by the American Academy of Pediatrics
345 Park Blvd
Itasca, IL 60143
Telephone: 630/626-6000
Facsimile: 847/434-8000
www.aap.org

The American Academy of Pediatrics is an organization of 67,000 primary care pediatricians, pediatric medical subspecialists, and pediatric surgical specialists dedicated to the health, safety, and well-being of all infants, children, adolescents, and young adults.

The recommendations in this publication do not indicate an exclusive course of treatment or serve as a standard of medical care. Variations, taking into account individual circumstances, may be appropriate.

Any websites, brand names, products, or manufacturers are mentioned for informational and identification purposes only and do not imply an endorsement by the American Academy of Pediatrics (AAP). The AAP is not responsible for the content of external resources. Information was current at the time of publication.

This publication has been developed by the American Academy of Pediatrics. The authors, editors, and contributors are expert authorities in the field of pediatrics. No commercial involvement of any kind has been solicited or accepted in the development of the content of this publication.

Every effort has been made to ensure that the drug selection and dosage set forth in this publication are in accordance with the current recommendations and practice at the time of publication. It is the responsibility of the health care professional to check the package insert of each drug for any change in indications and dosage and for added warnings and precautions.

Please visit www.aap.org/errata for an up-to-date list of any applicable errata for this publication.

Special discounts are available for bulk purchases of this publication. Email Special Sales at nationalaccounts@aap.org for more information.

Printed in the United States of America

9-5/0925 1 2 3 4 5 6 7 8 9 10
MA1224
ISBN: 978-1-61002-885-1
eBook: 978-1-61002-886-8
ISSN: 1942-2024

INTRODUCTION TO
PEDIATRIC CLINICAL PRACTICE GUIDELINES & POLICIES: A COMPENDIUM OF EVIDENCE-BASED RESEARCH FOR PEDIATRIC PRACTICE

Clinical practice guidelines have long provided physicians with evidence-based decision-making tools for managing common pediatric conditions. Policy statements issued and endorsed by the American Academy of Pediatrics (AAP) are developed to provide physicians with a quick reference guide to the AAP position on child health care issues. We have combined these 2 authoritative resources into 1 comprehensive manual/eBook resource to provide easy access to important clinical and policy information.

This manual contains

- Abstracts and Key Action Statements for current AAP clinical practice guidelines
- Clinical practice guidelines endorsed by the AAP, including abstracts where applicable
- Full text of all 2025 AAP policy statements, clinical reports, and technical reports
- Policy statements, clinical reports, and technical reports issued or endorsed through December 2025, including abstracts where applicable

The eBook, which is available via the code on the inside cover of this manual, builds on content of the manual and points to the full text of all AAP

- Clinical practice guidelines
- Policy statements
- Clinical reports
- Technical reports

For easy reference within this publication, dates when AAP clinical practice guidelines, policy statements, clinical reports, and technical reports first appeared in the AAP journal *Pediatrics* are provided. In 2009, the online version of *Pediatrics* at https://publications.aap.org/pediatrics became the official journal of record; therefore, date of online publication is given for policies from 2010 to present.

Additional information about AAP policy can be found in a variety of professional publications such as

Pediatric Nutrition, 9th Edition

Red Book®, 33rd Edition, and *Red Book*® *Online* (https://publications.aap.org/redbook)

Equitable and Inclusive Care in Pediatrics: A Compendium of AAP Clinical Practice Guidelines and Policies

Pediatric Pulmonology, 2nd Edition

Neonatal Care: A Compendium of AAP Clinical Practice Guidelines and Policies, 2nd Edition

Breastfeeding Handbook for Physicians, 3rd Edition

To order these and other pediatric resources, please call 866/843-2271 or visit https://aap.org/shopaap-books.

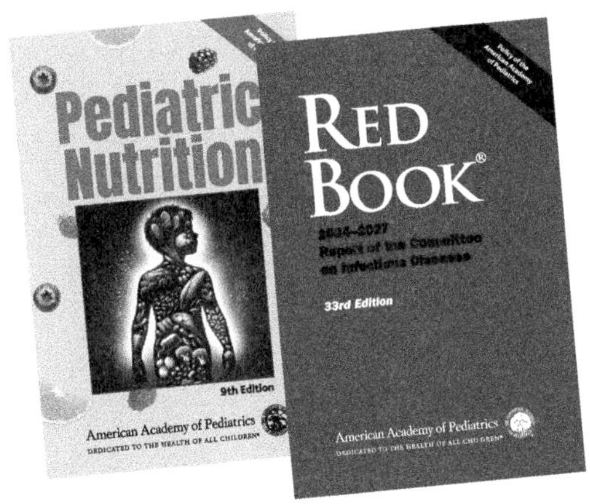

All policy statements, clinical reports, and technical reports from the American Academy of Pediatrics automatically expire 5 years after publication unless reaffirmed, revised, or retired at or before that time. Please check the American Academy of Pediatrics website at www.aap.org for up-to-date reaffirmations, revisions, and retirements.

AMERICAN ACADEMY OF PEDIATRICS

The American Academy of Pediatrics (AAP) and its member pediatricians dedicate their efforts and resources to the health, safety, and well-being of infants, children, adolescents, and young adults. The AAP has approximately 67,000 members in the United States, Canada, and Latin America. Members include pediatricians, pediatric medical subspecialists, and pediatric surgical specialists.

Core Values. *We believe*

- In the inherent worth of all children; they are our most enduring and vulnerable legacy.
- Children deserve optimal health and the highest quality health care.
- Pediatricians, pediatric medical subspecialists, and pediatric surgical specialists are the best qualified to provide child health care.
- Multidisciplinary teams including patients and families are integral to delivering the highest quality health care.

The AAP is the organization to advance child health and well-being and the profession of pediatrics.

Vision. Children have optimal health and well-being and are valued by society. American Academy of Pediatrics members practice the highest quality health care and experience professional satisfaction and personal well-being.

Mission. The mission of the AAP is to attain optimal physical, mental, and social health and well-being for all infants, children, adolescents, and young adults. To accomplish this mission, the AAP shall support the professional needs of its members.

EQUITY, DIVERSITY, AND INCLUSION STATEMENT

The American Academy of Pediatrics is committed to principles of equity, diversity, and inclusion in its publishing program. Editorial boards, author selections, and author transitions (publication succession plans) are designed to include diverse voices that reflect society as a whole. Editor and author teams are encouraged to actively seek out diverse authors and reviewers at all stages of the editorial process. Publishing staff are committed to promoting equity, diversity, and inclusion in all aspects of publication writing, review, and production.

Table of Contents

SECTION 4

CURRENT POLICIES FROM THE AMERICAN ACADEMY OF PEDIATRICS

American Academy of Pediatrics
DEDICATED TO THE HEALTH OF ALL CHILDREN®
AAP Partnership for Policy Implementation

See Appendix 1

American Academy of Pediatrics
DEDICATED TO THE HEALTH OF ALL CHILDREN®
AAP Partnership for Policy Implementation

See Appendix 1

American Academy of Pediatrics
DEDICATED TO THE HEALTH OF ALL CHILDREN®
AAP Partnership for Policy Implementation

See Appendix 1

SECTION 5

ENDORSED POLICIES

SECTION 1

Clinical Practice Guidelines

From the American Academy of Pediatrics

- *Clinical Practice Guidelines*
  EVIDENCE-BASED DECISION-MAKING TOOLS FOR MANAGING COMMON PEDIATRIC CONDITIONS

FOREWORD

To promote the practice of evidence-based medicine and to improve the health outcomes of children, the American Academy of Pediatrics (AAP) provides physicians with evidence-based guidelines for managing common pediatric conditions. The AAP has established an organizational process and methodology for the development, implementation, and improvement of these clinical practice guidelines.

The evidence-based approach to developing clinical practice guidelines begins by systematically reviewing and synthesizing the literature to provide the scientific basis for guideline recommendations. Clinical practice guideline teams with stakeholder representation systematically develop recommendations by carefully considering the evidence, risk, benefits, patient and caregiver preferences, and effect on equity, diversity, and inclusion. Each clinical practice guideline undergoes a thorough peer-review process before publication. Beginning in 2025, all new American Academy of Pediatrics clinical practice guidelines and accompanying systematic reviews will adhere to the GRADE (Grading of Recommendations Assessment, Development and Evaluation) approach. The AAP supports efforts to implement the recommendations into practice and to evaluate whether they are leading to improved outcomes. Every 5 years, each clinical practice guideline and the scientific literature are ideally reevaluated by the subcommittee to ensure that the recommendations are based on the most up-to-date science.

American Academy of Pediatrics clinical practice guidelines are designed to provide physicians with an analytic framework for evaluating and treating common pediatric conditions and are not intended as an exclusive course of treatment or standard of care. The AAP recognizes circumstances in which there is a lack of definitive data and relies on expert consensus in cases in which data do not exist. American Academy of Pediatrics clinical practice guidelines allow for flexibility and adaptability at the local and patient levels to address unique circumstances and should not replace sound clinical judgment.

If you have any questions about current or future clinical practice guidelines, please contact Carolyn McCarty, PhD, senior manager of clinical guideline methodology and operations at the AAP (cmccarty@aap.org).

Ulfat Shaikh, MD, MPH, MS, FAAP
Chairperson, Council on Quality Improvement and Patient Safety

Clinical Practice Guideline Revision: Management of Hyperbilirubinemia in the Newborn Infant 35 or More Weeks of Gestation

- *Clinical Practice Guideline (available at https://doi.org/10.1542/peds.2022-058859)*
  - *Abstract*
  - *Key Action Statements*
  - *PPI: AAP Partnership for Policy Implementation See Appendix 1 for more information.*

American Academy of Pediatrics
DEDICATED TO THE HEALTH OF ALL CHILDREN®

AAP Partnership for Policy Implementation

CLINICAL PRACTICE GUIDELINE Guidance for the Clinician in Rendering Pediatric Care

American Academy of Pediatrics

DEDICATED TO THE HEALTH OF ALL CHILDREN™

Clinical Practice Guideline Revision: Management of Hyperbilirubinemia in the Newborn Infant 35 or More Weeks of Gestation

Alex R. Kemper, MD, MPH, MS, FAAP,[a] Thomas B. Newman, MD, MPH, FAAP,[b] Jonathan L. Slaughter, MD, MPH, FAAP,[c] M. Jeffrey Maisels, MB BCh, DSc, FAAP,[d] Jon F. Watchko, MD, FAAP,[e] Stephen M. Downs, MD, MS,[f] Randall W. Grout, MD, MS, FAAP,[g] David G. Bundy, MD, MPH, FAAP,[h] Ann R. Stark, MD, FAAP,[i] Debra L. Bogen, MD, FAAP,[j] Alison Volpe Holmes, MD, MPH, FAAP,[k] Lori B. Feldman-Winter, MD, MPH, FAAP,[l] Vinod K. Bhutani, MD,[m] Steven R. Brown, MD, FAAFP,[n] Gabriela M. Maradiaga Panayotti, MD, FAAP,[o] Kymika Okechukwu, MPA,[p] Peter D. Rappo, MD, FAAP,[q] Terri L. Russell, DNP, APN, NNP-BC[r]

More than 80% of newborn infants will have some degree of jaundice.[1,2] Careful monitoring of all newborn infants and the application of appropriate treatments are essential, because high bilirubin concentrations can cause acute bilirubin encephalopathy and kernicterus.[3] Kernicterus is a permanent disabling neurologic condition characterized by some or all of the following: choreoathetoid cerebral palsy, upward gaze paresis, enamel dysplasia of deciduous teeth, sensorineural hearing loss or auditory neuropathy or dyssynchrony spectrum disorder, and characteristic findings on brain MRI.[4] A description of kernicterus nomenclature is provided in Appendix A. Central to this guideline is having systems in place including policies in hospitals and other types of birthing locations to provide the care necessary to minimize the risk of kernicterus.

This article updates and replaces the 2004 American Academy of Pediatrics (AAP) clinical practice guideline for the management and prevention of hyperbilirubinemia in the newborn infant ≥35 weeks' gestation.[3] This clinical practice guideline, like the previous one, addresses issues of prevention, risk assessment, monitoring, and treatment.

[a]Division of Primary Care Pediatrics, Nationwide Children's Hospital, Columbus, Ohio; [b]Departments of Epidemiology & Biostatistics and Pediatrics, School of Medicine, University of California, San Francisco, San Francisco, California; [c]Center for Perinatal Research, Nationwide Children's Hospital, Columbus, Ohio; [d]Department of Pediatrics, Oakland University William Beaumont School of Medicine, Rochester, Michigan; [e]Department of Pediatrics, University of Pittsburgh School of Medicine, Pittsburgh, Pennsylvania; [f]Department of Pediatrics, Wake Forest University, Winston-Salem, North Carolina; [g]Children's Health Services Research, Indiana University School of Medicine, Indianapolis, Indiana; [h]Medical University of South Carolina, Charleston, South Carolina; [i]Department of Neonatology, Beth Israel Deaconess Medical Center, Boston, Massachusetts; [j]Allegheny County Health Department, Pittsburgh, Pennsylvania; [k]Geisel School of Medicine at Dartmouth, Children's Hospital at Dartmouth-Hitchcock, Lebanon, New Hampshire; [l]Department of Pediatrics, Division of Adolescent Medicine, Cooper Medical School of Rowan University, Camden, New Jersey; [m]Department of Pediatrics, Neonatal and Developmental Medicine Stanford University School of Medicine, Stanford, California; [n]University of Arizona College of Medicine – Phoenix Family Medicine Residency, Phoenix, Arizona; [o]Division of Primary Care, Duke Children's Hospital and Health Center, Duke University Medical Center, Durham, North Carolina; [p]Department of Quality, American Academy of Pediatrics, Itasca, Illinois; [q]South Shore Hospital, South Weymouth, Massachusetts; and [r]National Association of Neonatal Nurses, Chicago, Illinois

To cite: Kemper AR, Newman TB, Slaughter JL, et al. Clinical Practice Guideline Revision: Management of Hyperbilirubinemia in the Newborn Infant 35 or More Weeks of Gestation. *Pediatrics.* 2022;150(3):e2022058859

Hyperbilirubinemia Clinical Practice Guideline Key Action Statements

Action Statement Summary

Clinical Practice Guideline Revision: Management of Hyperbilirubinemia in the Newborn Infant 35 or More Weeks of Gestation

Key Action Statement 1

If the maternal antibody screen is positive or unknown because the mother did not have prenatal antibody screening, the infant should have a direct antiglobulin test (DAT) and the infant's blood type should be determined as soon as possible using either cord or peripheral blood. (Aggregate Evidence Quality Grade B, Recommendation)

Key Action Statement 2

Oral supplementation with water or dextrose water should not be provided to prevent hyperbilirubinemia or decrease bilirubin concentrations. (Aggregate Evidence Quality Grade B, Strong Recommendation)

Key Action Statement 3

Use TSB as the definitive test to guide phototherapy and escalation-of-care decisions, including exchange transfusion. (Aggregate Evidence Quality Grade X, Recommendation)

Key Action Statement 4

All infants should be visually assessed for jaundice at least every 12 hours following delivery until discharge. TSB or TcB should be measured as soon as possible for infants noted to be jaundiced <24 hours after birth. (Aggregate Evidence Quality Grade X, Strong Recommendation)

Key Action Statement 5

The TcB or TSB should be measured between 24 and 48 hours after birth or before discharge if that occurs earlier. (Aggregate Evidence Quality Grade C, Recommendation)

Key Action Statement 6

TSB should be measured if the TcB exceeds or is within 3 mg/dL of the phototherapy treatment threshold or if the TcB is ≥15 mg/dL. (Aggregate Evidence Quality Grade C, Recommendation)

Key Action Statement 7

If more than 1 TcB or TSB measure is available, the rate of increase may be used to identify infants at higher risk of subsequent hyperbilirubinemia. A rapid rate of increase (≥0.3 mg/dL per hour in the first 24 hours or ≥0.2 mg/dL per hour thereafter) is exceptional and suggests hemolysis. In this case, perform a DAT if not previously done. (Aggregate Evidence Quality Grade D, Option)

Key Action Statement 8

If appropriate follow-up cannot be arranged for an infant recommended to have an outpatient follow-up bilirubin measure, discharge may be delayed. (Aggregate Evidence Quality Grade D, Option)

Key Action Statement 9

For breastfed infants who are still jaundiced at 3 to 4 weeks of age, and for formula-fed infants who are still jaundiced at 2 weeks of age, the total and direct reacting (or conjugated) bilirubin concentrations should be measured to identify possible pathologic cholestasis. (Aggregate Evidence Quality Grade X, Recommendation)

Key Action Statement 10

Intensive phototherapy is recommended at the total serum bilirubin thresholds in Fig 2 (Supplemental Table 1 and Supplemental Fig 1) or Fig 3 (Supplemental Table 2 and Supplemental Fig 2) on the basis of gestational age, hyperbilirubinemia neurotoxicity risk factors, and age of the infant in hours. (Aggregate Evidence Quality Grade X, Recommendation)

Key Action Statement 11

For newborn infants who have already been discharged and then develop a TSB above the phototherapy threshold, treatment with a home LED-based phototherapy device rather than readmission to the hospital is an option for infants who meet the following criteria: gestational age ≥38 weeks, ≥48 hours old, clinically well with adequate feeding, no known hyperbilirubinemia neurotoxicity risk factors (Table 2), no previous phototherapy, TSB concentration no more than 1 mg/dL above the phototherapy treatment threshold (Fig 2, Supplemental Table 1, Supplemental Fig 1), an LED-based phototherapy device will be available in the home without delay, and TSB can be measured daily. (Aggregate Evidence Quality Grade D, Option)

Key Action Statement 12

For hospitalized infants, TSB should be measured within 12 hours after starting phototherapy. The timing of the initial TSB measure after starting phototherapy and the frequency of TSB monitoring during phototherapy should be guided by the age of the child, the presence of hyperbilirubinemia neurotoxicity risk factors, the TSB concentration, and the TSB trajectory. (Aggregate Evidence Quality Grade X, Recommendation)

Key Action Statement 13

For infants receiving home phototherapy, the TSB should be measured daily. Infants should be admitted for inpatient phototherapy if the TSB increases and the difference between the TSB and the phototherapy threshold narrows or the TSB is ≥1 mg/dL above the phototherapy threshold. (Aggregate Evidence Quality Grade X, Recommendation)

Key Action Statement 14

For infants requiring phototherapy, measure the hemoglobin concentration, hematocrit, or complete blood count to assess for the presence of anemia and to provide a baseline in case subsequent anemia develops. Evaluate the underlying cause or causes of hyperbilirubinemia in infants who require phototherapy by obtaining a DAT in infants whose mother had a positive antibody screen or whose mother is blood group O regardless of Rh(D) status or whose mother is Rh(D)–G6PD activity should be measured in any infant with jaundice of unknown cause whose TSB increases despite intensive phototherapy, whose TSB increases suddenly or increases after an initial decline, or who requires escalation of care. (Aggregate Evidence Quality Grade X, Recommendation)

Key Action Statement 15

Discontinuing phototherapy is an option when the TSB has decreased by at least 2 mg/dL below the hour-specific threshold at the initiation of phototherapy. A longer period of phototherapy is an option if there are risk factors for rebound hyperbilirubinemia (eg, gestational age <38 weeks, age <48 hours at the start of phototherapy, hemolytic disease). (Aggregate Evidence Quality Grade C, Option)

Key Action Statement 16

Repeat bilirubin measurement after phototherapy is based on the risk of rebound hyperbilirubinemia. It is an option to measure TcB instead of TSB if it has been at least 24 hours since phototherapy was stopped. (Aggregate Evidence Quality Grade X, Recommendation)

Key Action Statement 17

Care should be escalated when an infant's TSB reaches or exceeds the escalation-of-care threshold, defined as 2 mg/dL below the exchange transfusion threshold, as detailed in Fig 5 (infants with no known hyperbilirubinemia neurotoxicity risk factors; Supplemental Table 3 and Supplemental Fig 3) or Fig 6 (infants whose TSB is increasing despite phototherapy or infants with at least 1 recognized hyperbilirubinemia neurotoxicity risk factor; Supplemental Table 4 and Supplemental Fig 4). (Aggregate Evidence Quality Grade X, Recommendation)

Key Action Statement 18

For infants requiring escalation of care, blood should be sent STAT for total and direct reacting serum bilirubin, a complete blood count, serum albumin, serum chemistries, and type and crossmatch. (Aggregate Evidence Quality Grade X, Recommendation)

Key Action Statement 19

Infants requiring escalation of care should receive intravenous hydration and emergent intensive phototherapy. A neonatologist should be consulted about urgent transfer to a NICU that can perform an exchange transfusion. (Aggregate Evidence Quality Grade C, Recommendation)

Key Action Statement 20

TSB should be measured at least every 2 hours from the start of the escalation-of-care period until the escalation-of-care period ends. Once the TSB is lower than the escalation-of-care threshold, management should proceed according to the section "C. Monitoring Infants Receiving Phototherapy." (Aggregate Evidence Quality Grade X, Recommendation)

Key Action Statement 21

Intravenous immune globulin (IVIG; 0.5 to 1 g/kg) over 2 hours may be provided to infants with isoimmune hemolytic disease (ie, positive DAT) whose TSB reaches or exceeds escalation of care threshold. The dose can be repeated in 12 hours. (Aggregate Evidence Quality Grade C, Option)

Key Action Statement 22

An urgent exchange transfusion should be performed for infants with signs of intermediate or advanced stages of acute bilirubin encephalopathy (eg, hypertonia, arching, retrocollis, opisthotonos, high-pitched cry, or recurrent apnea). (Aggregate Evidence Quality Grade C, Recommendation)

Key Action Statement 23

An urgent exchange transfusion should be performed for infants if the TSB is at or above the exchange transfusion threshold. If, while preparing for the exchange transfusion but before starting the exchange transfusion, a TSB concentration is below the exchange transfusion threshold and the infant does not show signs of intermediate or advanced stages of acute bilirubin encephalopathy, then the exchange transfusion may be deferred while continuing intensive phototherapy and following the TSB every 2 hours until the TSB is below the escalation of care threshold. (Aggregate Evidence Quality Grade C, Recommendation)

Key Action Statement 24

Beginning at least 12 hours after birth, if discharge is being considered, the difference between the bilirubin concentration measured closest to discharge and the phototherapy threshold at the time of the bilirubin measurement should be calculated and used to guide follow-up, as detailed in Fig 7. (Aggregate Evidence Quality Grade C, Recommendation)

Key Action Statement 25

Before discharge, all families should receive written and verbal education about neonatal jaundice. Parents should be provided written information to facilitate postdischarge care, including the date, time, and place of the follow-up appointment and, when necessary, a prescription and appointment for a follow-up TcB or TSB. Birth hospitalization information, including the last TcB or TSB and the age at which it was measured, and DAT results (if any) should be transmitted to the primary care provider who will see the infant at follow-up. If there is uncertainty about who will provide the follow-up care, this information should also be provided to families. (Aggregate Evidence Quality Grade X, Strong Recommendation)

Clinical Practice Guideline for the Evaluation and Treatment of Children and Adolescents With Obesity

- *Clinical Practice Guideline (available at https://doi.org/10.1542/peds.2022-060640)*
  - *Greetings*
  - *Key Action Statements*
  - *PPI: AAP Partnership for Policy Implementation*
    See Appendix 1 for more information.

American Academy of Pediatrics
DEDICATED TO THE HEALTH OF ALL CHILDREN®

AAP Partnership for Policy Implementation

CLINICAL PRACTICE GUIDELINE Guidance for the Clinician in Rendering Pediatric Care

American Academy of Pediatrics

DEDICATED TO THE HEALTH OF ALL CHILDREN™

Clinical Practice Guideline for the Evaluation and Treatment of Children and Adolescents With Obesity

Sarah E. Hampl, MD, FAAP,[a] Sandra G. Hassink, MD, FAAP,[b] Asheley C. Skinner, PhD,[c] Sarah C. Armstrong, MD, FAAP,[d] Sarah E. Barlow, MD, MPH, FAAP,[e] Christopher F. Bolling, MD, FAAP,[f] Kimberly C. Avila Edwards, MD, FAAP,[g] Ihuoma Eneli, MD, MS, FAAP,[h] Robin Hamre, MPH,[i] Madeline M. Joseph, MD, FAAP,[j] Doug Lunsford, MEd,[k] Eneida Mendonca, MD, PhD, FAAP,[l] Marc P. Michalsky, MD, MBA, FAAP,[m] Nazrat Mirza, MD, ScD, FAAP,[n] Eduardo R. Ochoa, Jr, MD, FAAP,[o] Mona Sharifi, MD, MPH, FAAP,[p] Amanda E. Staiano, PhD, MPP,[q] Ashley E. Weedn, MD, MPH, FAAP,[r] Susan K. Flinn, MA,[s] Jeanne Lindros, MPH,[t] Kymika Okechukwu, MPA[u]

[a]Children's Mercy Kansas City Center for Children's Healthy Lifestyles & Nutrition, University of Missouri-Kansas City School of Medicine, Kansas City, Missouri; [b]Medical Director, American Academy of Pediatrics, Institute for Healthy Childhood Weight, Wilmington, Delaware; [c]Department of Population Health Sciences, Duke University School of Medicine, Durham, North Carolina; [d]Departments of Pediatrics and Population Health Sciences, Duke Clinical Research Institute, Duke University, Durham, North Carolina; [e]Department of Pediatrics, University of Texas Southwestern Medical Center, Children's Medical Center of Dallas, Dallas, Texas; [f]Department of Pediatrics, University of Cincinnati College of Medicine, Cincinnati, Ohio; [g]Children's Health Policy & Advocacy, Ascension; Department of Pediatrics, Dell Medical School at The University of Texas at Austin, Austin, Texas; [h]Department of Pediatrics, The Ohio State University, Center for Healthy Weight and Nutrition, Nationwide Children's Hospital, Columbus, Ohio; [i]Centers for Disease Control and Prevention; Atlanta, Georgia; [j]Division of Pediatric Emergency Medicine, Department of Emergency Medicine, University of Florida College of Medicine–Jacksonville, University of Florida Health Sciences Center–Jacksonville, Jacksonville, Florida; [k]Family Representative; [l]Departments of Pediatrics and Biostatistics & Health Data Science, Indiana University School of Medicine, Indianapolis, Indiana; [m]Department of Pediatric Surgery, The Ohio State University, College of Medicine, Nationwide Children's Hospital, Columbus, Ohio; [n]Children's National Hospital, George Washington University, Washington, DC; [o]Department of Pediatrics, University of Arkansas for Medical Sciences, Arkansas Children's Hospital, Little Rock, Arkansas; [p]Department of Pediatrics, Yale School of Medicine, New Haven, Connecticut; [q]Louisiana State University Pennington Biomedical Research Center, Baton Rouge, Louisiana; [r]Department of Pediatrics, University of Oklahoma Health Sciences Center, Oklahoma City, Oklahoma; [s]Medical Writer/Consultant, Washington, DC; [t]American Academy of Pediatrics, Itasca, Illinois; and [u]American Academy of Pediatrics, Itasca, Illinois

To cite: Hampl SE, Hassink SG, Skinner AC, et al. Clinical Practice Guideline for the Evaluation and Treatment of Children and Adolescents With Obesity. *Pediatrics.* 2023;151(2): e2022060640

Greetings

You have in your hands, or at your fingertips, the first edition of the American Academy of Pediatrics clinical practice guideline for evaluation and management of children and adolescents with overweight and obesity. Putting together this guideline was no small task, and the Academy is grateful to the efforts of all the professionals who contributed to the production of this document. This work is a true testament to their passion and dedication to combatting childhood and adolescent overweight and obesity.

The Subcommittee responsible for developing this guideline comprises a diverse group of professionals from a variety of disciplines representing both governmental entities and private institutions. Experts all, they are united by a common desire to provide the finest, most effective care and treatment to children and adolescents with overweight and obesity. Over the course of several months, the members of the Subcommittee reviewed the technical reports produced from the study review, then worked in concert to develop the Key Action Statements and Expert Consensus Recommendations contained within this guideline. These were crafted with meticulous care by the Subcommittee members, to align with current literature and to place appropriate emphasis on each statement.

While representing such a broad spectrum of perspectives, the members of this committee are all keenly aware of the multitude of barriers to treatment that patients and their families face. These barriers impact not only their access to treatment, but their ability to follow prescribed treatment plans. Whereas some patients are able to adopt the lifestyle changes and habitualize elements of their prescribed treatment plans, so many others struggle to do so for a wide variety of reasons. The members of the Subcommittee understand all of this. To assist with optimizing health equity and overcoming these barriers, guidance on a number of multilevel factors related to barriers to treatment have been included in this guideline. During the course of their work, members of the Subcommittee acknowledged that, although so much has been learned to advance the treatment of children and adolescents with overweight and obesity, there is still so much we have yet to discover. The Subcommittee recognizes the importance that future studies will play in advancing our knowledge and understanding of this chronic disease, knowledge and understanding that will lead to the development of new and more effective treatments. Specific discussion about the needs for future research are included in the guideline.

It is the fervent hope of every member of the Subcommittee that this guideline and the resources that accompany it will provide you with a more complete understanding of the issues, factors, and needs of patients combating overweight and obesity, as well as successful treatment options to assist them in their battle. This guideline and the resources that accompany it are not only for you, they are because of you, and all that you do to care for each and every patient as if they were the most important one. Because, as we all know, they are.

Be well,

Doug Lunsford, Family Representative

Obesity Clinical Practice Guideline Key Action Statements

Action Statement Summary

Clinical Practice Guideline for the Evaluation and Treatment of Children and Adolescents With Obesity

Key Action Statement 1

Pediatricians and other PHCPs should measure height and wt, calculate BMI, and assess BMI percentile using age- and sex-specific CDC growth charts or growth charts for children with severe obesity at least annually for all children 2 to 18 y of age to screen for overweight (BMI ≥ 85th percentile to <95th percentile), obesity (BMI ≥ 95th percentile), and severe obesity (BMI ≥ 120% of the 95th percentile for age and sex). (Grade B. Moderate recommendation.)

Key Action Statement 2

Pediatricians and other PHCPs should evaluate children 2 to 18 y of age with overweight (BMI ≥ 85th percentile to <95th percentile) and obesity (BMI ≥ 95th percentile) for obesity-related comorbidities by using a comprehensive patient history, mental and behavioral health screening, SDoH evaluation, physical examination, and diagnostic studies. (Grade B. Strong recommendation.)

Key Action Statement 3

In children 10 y and older, pediatricians and other PHCPs should evaluate for lipid abnormalities, abnormal glucose metabolism, and abnormal liver function in children and adolescents with obesity (BMI ≥ 95th percentile) and for lipid abnormalities in children and adolescents with overweight (BMI ≥ 85th percentile to <95th percentile). (Grade B. Strong recommendation.)

Key Action Statement 3.1

In children 10 y and older with overweight (BMI ≥ 85th percentile to <95th percentile), pediatricians and other PHCPs may evaluate for abnormal glucose metabolism and liver function in the presence of risk factors for T2DM or NAFLD. In children 2 to 9 y of age with obesity (BMI ≥ 95th percentile), pediatricians and other PHCPs may evaluate for lipid abnormalities. (Grade C. Moderate recommendation.)

Key Action Statement 4

Pediatricians and other PHCPs should treat children and adolescents for overweight (BMI ≥ 85th percentile to <95th percentile) or obesity (BMI ≥ 95th percentile) and comorbidities concurrently. (Grade A. Strong recommendation.)

Key Action Statement 5

Pediatricians and other PHCPs should evaluate for dyslipidemia by obtaining a fasting lipid panel in children 10 y and older with overweight (BMI ≥ 85th percentile to <95th percentile) and obesity (BMI ≥ 95th percentile) and may evaluate for dyslipidemia in children 2 through 9 y of age with obesity. (Grade B [children ≥10 y with obesity]. Strong recommendation.) (Grade C [children 2–9 y]. Moderate recommendation.)

Key Action Statement 6

Pediatricians and other PHCPs should evaluate for prediabetes and/or diabetes mellitus with fasting plasma glucose, 2-h plasma glucose after 75-g oral glucose tolerance test (OGTT), or glycosylated hemoglobin (HbA1c).[a] (Grade B. Moderate recommendation.)

[a]Per KAS 3 and 3.1: Pediatricians and other PHCPs should evaluate children 10 y and older with obesity (BMI ≥ 95th percentile) for abnormal glucose metabolism and may evaluate children 10 y and older with overweight (BMI ≥ 85th percentile to <95th percentile) with risk factors for T2DM or NAFLD for abnormal glucose metabolism. (Refer to evidence tables for KAS 3 and 3.1.)

Key Action Statement 7

Pediatricians and other PHCPs should evaluate for NAFLD by obtaining an alanine transaminase (ALT) test.[b] (Grade A. Strong recommendation.)

[b]Per KAS 3 and 3.1: Pediatricians and other PHCPs should evaluate children 10 y and older with obesity (BMI ≥ 95th percentile) for abnormal liver function and may evaluate children 10 y and older with overweight (BMI ≥ 85th percentile to <95th percentile) with risk factors for TD2M or NAFLD for abnormal liver function. (Refer to evidence tables for KAS 3 and 3.1.)

Key Action Statement 8

Pediatricians and other PHCPs should evaluate for hypertension by measuring blood pressure at every visit starting at 3 y of age in children and adolescents with overweight (BMI ≥ 85 to <95th percentile) and obesity (BMI ≥ 95th percentile). (Grade C. Moderate recommendation.)

Key Action Statement 9

Pediatricians and other PHCPs should treat overweight (BMI ≥ 85th percentile to <95th percentile) and obesity (BMI ≥ 95th percentile) in children and adolescents, following the principles of the medical home and the chronic care model, using a family-centered and nonstigmatizing approach that acknowledges obesity's biologic, social, and structural drivers. (Grade B. Strong recommendation.)

Key Action Statement 10

Pediatricians and other PHCPs should use motivational interviewing (MI) to engage patients and families in treating overweight (BMI ≥ 85th percentile to <95th percentile) and obesity (BMI ≥ 95th percentile). (Grade B. Moderate recommendation.)

Key Action Statement 11

Pediatricians and other PHCPs should provide or refer children 6 y and older (Grade B) and may provide or refer children 2 through 5 y of age (Grade C) with overweight (BMI ≥ 85th percentile to <95th percentile) and obesity (BMI ≥ 95th percentile) to intensive health behavior and lifestyle treatment. Health behavior and lifestyle treatment is more effective with greater contact hours; the most effective treatment includes 26 or more hours of face-to-face, family-based, multicomponent treatment over a 3- to 12-mo period. (Grade B [ages 6 y and older]. Moderate recommendation.) (Grade C [ages 2–5 y]. Moderate recommendation.)

Key Action Statement 12

Pediatricians and other PHCPs should offer adolescents 12 y and older with obesity (BMI ≥ 95th percentile) weight loss pharmacotherapy, according to medication indications, risks, and benefits, as an adjunct to health behavior and lifestyle treatment. (Grade B. Moderate recommendation.)

Key Action Statement 13

Pediatricians and other PHCPs should offer referral for adolescents 13 y and older with severe obesity (BMI ≥ 120% of the 95th percentile for age and sex) for evaluation for metabolic and bariatric surgery to local or regional comprehensive multidisciplinary pediatric metabolic and bariatric surgery centers. (Grade C[c]. Moderate recommendation.)

[c]This KAS was given a Grade C recommendation, as available evidence is from observational and case-controlled studies. As described in the methods section for the evidence review, only randomized and comparative effectiveness studies were included for the CPG. The Evidence Review Panel made the decision to include observational and case-control studies specifically for surgical interventions only, because of ethical considerations and practical challenges to randomization.

Opioid Prescribing for Acute Pain Management in Children and Adolescents in Outpatient Settings

- *Clinical Practice Guideline (available at https://doi.org/10.1542/peds.2024-068752)*
  - *Clinical Practice Guideline*
  - *Key Action Statements*
  - *PPI: AAP Partnership for Policy Implementation*
    See Appendix 1 for more information.

American Academy of Pediatrics
DEDICATED TO THE HEALTH OF ALL CHILDREN®

AAP Partnership for Policy Implementation

CLINICAL PRACTICE GUIDELINE Guidance for the Clinician in Rendering Pediatric Care

American Academy of Pediatrics

DEDICATED TO THE HEALTH OF ALL CHILDREN™

Opioid Prescribing for Acute Pain Management in Children and Adolescents in Outpatient Settings: Clinical Practice Guideline

Scott E. Hadland, MD, MPH, MS, FAAP,[a] Rita Agarwal, MD, FAAP, FASA,[b] Sudha R. Raman, PhD,[c] Michael J. Smith, MD, MSCE,[d] Amy Bryl, MD, FAAP,[e] Jeremy Michel, MD, MHS, FAAP,[f] Lorraine I. Kelley-Quon, MD, MSHS, FACS, FAAP,[g] Mehul V. Raval, MD, MS, FAAP,[h] Madeline H. Renny, MD, MS, FAAP,[i] Beth Larson-Steckler,[j] Scott Wexelblatt, MD, FAAP,[k] Robert T. Wilder, MD, PhD, FAAP,[l] Susan K. Flinn, MA[m]

abstract

This is the first clinical practice guideline (CPG) from the American Academy of Pediatrics outlining evidence-based approaches to safely prescribing opioids for acute pain in outpatient settings. The central goal is to aid clinicians in understanding when opioids may be indicated to treat acute pain in children and adolescents and how to minimize risks (including opioid use disorder, poisoning, and overdose). The document also seeks to alleviate disparate pain treatment of Black, Hispanic, and American Indian/Alaska Native children and adolescents, who receive pain management that is less adequate and less timely than that provided to white individuals. There may also be disparities in pain treatment based on language, socioeconomic status, geographic location, and other factors, which are discussed.

The document recommends that clinicians treat acute pain using a multimodal approach that includes the appropriate use of nonpharmacologic therapies, nonopioid medications, and, when needed, opioid medications. Opioids should not be prescribed as monotherapy for children or adolescents who have acute pain. When using opioids for acute pain management, clinicians should prescribe immediate-release opioid formulations, start with the lowest age- and weight-appropriate doses, and provide an initial supply of 5 or fewer days, unless the pain is related to trauma or surgery with expected duration of pain longer than 5 days. Clinicians should not prescribe codeine or tramadol for patients younger than 12 years; adolescents 12 to 18 years of age who have obesity, obstructive sleep apnea, or severe lung disease; to treat postsurgical pain after tonsillectomy or adenoidectomy in patients younger than 18 years; or for any breastfeeding patient.

[a]Mass General for Children; Harvard Medical School, Boston, Massachusetts; [b]Stanford University School of Medicine, Stanford, California; Departments of [c]Population Health Sciences and [d]Pediatrics, Duke University School of Medicine, Durham, North Carolina; [e]Division of Emergency Medicine, Rady Children's Hospital San Diego and Department of Pediatrics, University of California San Diego, San Diego, California; [f]Department of Pediatrics, Perelman School of Medicine, University of Pennsylvania and Department of Biomedical Informatics, Children's Hospital of Philadelphia, Philadelphia, Pennsylvania; [g]Division of Pediatric Surgery, Children's Hospital Los Angeles and Departments of Surgery and Population and Public Health Sciences, Keck School of Medicine, University of Southern California, Los Angeles, California; [h]Division of Pediatric Surgery, Department of Surgery, Northwestern University Feinberg School of Medicine, Ann & Robert H. Lurie Children's Hospital of Chicago, Chicago, Illinois; [i]Departments of Emergency Medicine, Pediatrics, and Population Health Science and Policy, Icahn School of Medicine at Mount Sinai, New York, New York; [j]Childhood Pancreatitis Foundation, Minot, North Dakota; [k]Department of Pediatrics, University of Cincinnati College of Medicine, Cincinnati Children's Hospital Medical Center Perinatal Institute, Cincinnati, Ohio; [l]Mayo Clinic Alix School of Medicine, Rochester, Minnesota; and [m]Medical Writer

To cite: Hadland SE, Agarwal R, Raman SR, et al. American Academy of Pediatrics. Opioid Prescribing for Acute Pain Management in Children and Adolescents in Outpatient Settings: Clinical Practice Guideline. *Pediatrics.* 2024;154(5): e2024068752

The CPG recommends providing opioids when appropriate for treating acutely worsened pain in children and adolescents who have a history of chronic pain; clinicians should partner with other opioid-prescribing clinicians involved in the patient's care and/or a specialist in chronic pain or palliative care to determine an appropriate treatment plan. Caution should be used when treating acute pain in those who are taking sedating medications. The CPG describes potential harms of discontinuing or rapidly tapering opioids in individuals who have been on stable, long-term opioids to treat chronic pain.

The guideline also recommends providing naloxone and information on naloxone, safe storage and disposal of opioids, and direct observation of medication administration. Clinicians are encouraged to help caregivers develop a plan for safe disposal. The CPG contains 12 key action statements based on evidence from randomized controlled trials, high-quality observational studies, and, when studies are lacking or could not feasibly or ethically be conducted, from expert opinion. Each key action statement includes a level of evidence, the benefit-harm relationship, and the strength of recommendation.

Opioid Prescribing Clinical Practice Guideline Key Action Statements

Action Statement Summary

Opioid Prescribing for Acute Pain Management in Children and Adolescents in Outpatient Settings: Clinical Practice Guideline

Key Action Statement 1

Pediatricians and other pediatric health care providers (PHCPs) should treat acute pain using a multimodal approach that includes the appropriate use of nonpharmacologic therapies, nonopioid medications, and, when needed, opioid medications. (Evidence quality: B; recommendation strength: Strong recommendation)

Key Action Statement 2

Pediatricians and other PHCPs should NOT prescribe opioids as monotherapy for children and adolescents who have acute pain. (Evidence quality: B; recommendation strength: Strong recommendation)

Key Action Statement 3

When prescribing opioids for acute pain in children and adolescents, PHCPs should provide immediate-release opioid formulations, start with the lowest age- and weight-appropriate doses, and provide an initial supply of 5 days or fewer, unless the pain is related to trauma or surgery with an expected duration of pain of more than 5 days. (Evidence quality: C; recommendation strength: Recommendation)

Key Action Statement 4.1

When treating acute pain in children and adolescents younger than 12 years, pediatricians and other PHCPs should NOT prescribe codeine or tramadol. (Evidence quality: X; recommendation strength: Strong recommendation)

Key Action Statement 4.2

When treating acute pain in adolescents 12–18 years of age who have obesity, obstructive sleep apnea, or severe lung disease, pediatricians and other PHCPs should NOT prescribe codeine or tramadol. (Evidence quality: X; recommendation strength: Strong recommendation)

Key Action Statement 4.3

When treating postsurgical pain after tonsillectomy or adenoidectomy in children and adolescents younger than 18 years, pediatricians and other PHCPs should NOT prescribe codeine or tramadol. (Evidence quality: X; recommendation strength: Strong recommendation)

Key Action Statement 4.4

When treating acute pain in people of any age who are breastfeeding, pediatricians and other PHCPS should NOT prescribe codeine or tramadol. (Evidence quality: X; recommendation strength: Strong recommendation)

Key Action Statement 5

When treating acute pain in children or adolescents who are taking sedating medications, such as benzodiazepines, pediatricians and other PHCPs should use caution when prescribing opioids. (Evidence quality: X; recommendation strength: Strong recommendation)

Key Action Statement 6

When prescribing opioids, pediatricians and other PHCPs should provide naloxone and counsel patients and families on the signs of opioid overdose and on how to respond to an overdose. (Evidence quality: X; recommendation strength: Recommendation)

Key Action Statement 7

When prescribing opioids, pediatricians and other PHCPs should educate caregivers about safe storage and directly observed administration of medications to children and adolescents. (Evidence quality: D; recommendation strength: Option)

Key Action Statement 8

When prescribing opioids, pediatricians and other PHCPs should educate caregivers about safe disposal of unused medications, help caregivers develop a plan to safely dispose of unused medications, and, if possible, offer safe disposal in their practice setting. (Evidence quality: A; recommendation strength: Strong recommendation)

Key Action Statement 9

When treating acute, worsened pain in children and adolescents with preexisting chronic pain, pediatricians and other PHCPs should prescribe opioids when indicated and partner with any other opioid-prescribing clinicians involved in the patient's care and with specialists in chronic pain, palliative care, and/or other opioid stewardship programs to determine an appropriate treatment plan. (Evidence quality: D; recommendation strength: Option)

Evaluation and Management of Well-Appearing Febrile Infants 8 to 60 Days Old

- *Clinical Practice Guideline (available at https://doi.org/10.1542/peds.2021-052228)*
  - *Abstract*
  - *Key Action Statements*
  - *PPI: AAP Partnership for Policy Implementation See Appendix 1 for more information.*

American Academy of Pediatrics
DEDICATED TO THE HEALTH OF ALL CHILDREN®

AAP Partnership for Policy Implementation

CLINICAL PRACTICE GUIDELINE

American Academy of Pediatrics

DEDICATED TO THE HEALTH OF ALL CHILDREN™

Clinical Practice Guideline: Evaluation and Management of Well-Appearing Febrile Infants 8 to 60 Days Old

Robert H. Pantell, MD, FAAP,[a] Kenneth B. Roberts, MD, FAAP,[b] William G. Adams, MD, FAAP,[c] Benard P. Dreyer, MD, FAAP,[d] Nathan Kuppermann, MD, MPH, FAAP, FACEP,[e] Sean T. O'Leary, MD, MPH, FAAP,[f] Kymika Okechukwu, MPA,[g] Charles R. Woods Jr, MD, MS, FAAP[h] SUBCOMMITTEE ON FEBRILE INFANTS

This guideline addresses the evaluation and management of well-appearing, term infants, 8 to 60 days of age, with fever ≥38.0°C. Exclusions are noted. After a commissioned evidence-based review by the Agency for Healthcare Research and Quality, an additional extensive and ongoing review of the literature, and supplemental data from published, peer-reviewed studies provided by active investigators, 21 key action statements were derived. For each key action statement, the quality of evidence and benefit-harm relationship were assessed and graded to determine the strength of recommendations. When appropriate, parents' values and preferences should be incorporated as part of shared decision-making. For diagnostic testing, the committee has attempted to develop numbers needed to test, and for antimicrobial administration, the committee provided numbers needed to treat. Three algorithms summarize the recommendations for infants 8 to 21 days of age, 22 to 28 days of age, and 29 to 60 days of age. The recommendations in this guideline do not indicate an exclusive course of treatment or serve as a standard of medical care. Variations, taking into account individual circumstances, may be appropriate.

abstract

[a]Department of Pediatrics, School of Medicine, University of California San Francisco, San Francisco, California; [b]Department of Pediatrics, School of Medicine, University of North Carolina at Chapel Hill, Chapel Hill, North Carolina; [c]Boston Medical Center/Boston University School of Medicine, Deparment of Pediatrics, Boston, Massachusetts; [d]Department of Pediatrics, NYU Grossman School of Medicine, New York, New York; [e]Departments of Emergency Medicine and Pediatrics, School of Medicine, University of California, Davis School of Medicine, Sacramento, California; [f]Department of Pediatrics, University of Colorado Anschutz Medical Campus, Aurora, Colorado; [g]American Academy of Pediatrics, Itasca, Illinois; and [h]Department of Pediatrics, Children's Hospital at Erlanger and College of Medicine, The University of Tennessee at Chattanooga, Chattanooga, Tennessee

The recommendations in this guideline do not indicate an exclusive course of treatment or serve as a standard of medical care. Variations, taking into account individual circumstances, may be appropriate.

All clinical practice guidelines from the American Academy of Pediatrics automatically expire 5 years after publication unless reaffirmed, revised, or retired at or before that time.

DOI: https://doi.org/10.1542/peds.2021-052228

Address correspondence to Robert H. Pantell, MD. E-mail: Robert.Pantell@UCSF.edu

PEDIATRICS (ISSN Numbers: Print, 0031-4005; Online, 1098-4275).

To cite: Pantell RH, Roberts KB, Adams WG, et al. Clinical Practice Guideline: Evaluation and Management of Well-Appearing Febrile Infants 8 to 60 Days Old. *Pediatrics.* 2021;148(2):e2021052228

Well-Appearing Febrile Infants Clinical Practice Guideline Key Action Statements

Action Statement Summary

Evaluation and Management of Well-Appearing Febrile Infants 8 to 60 Days Old

Infants 8 to 21 d of age (Key Action Statements 1–7): Clinicians...

Key Action Statement 1

Should obtain urine specimen by catheterization or suprapubic aspiration (SPA) of bladder for urinalysis and, if urinalysis result is positive, for culture. (Grade: A; Strong Recommendation)

Key Action Statement 2

Should obtain a blood culture. (Grade: A; Strong Recommendation)

Key Action Statement 3

May assess inflammatory markers (IMs). (Grade: B; Weak Recommendation)

Key Action Statement 4

Should obtain cerebrospinal fluid (CSF) for analysis (white blood cell [WBC], protein, glucose, Gram stain) and culture for bacteria. See notes for viral testing. (Grade: A; Strong Recommendation)

Key Action Statement 5

Should initiate parenteral antimicrobial therapy. (Grade: A; Strong Recommendation)

Key Action Statement 6

Should actively monitor infants while awaiting results of bacterial cultures in a hospital setting with nurses and staff experienced in the care of neonates/young infants. (Grade: B; Moderate Recommendation)

Key Action Statement 7a

Should discontinue parenteral antimicrobial agents and discharge hospitalized patients when all of the following criteria are met: (1) culture results are negative for 24–36 h or only positive for contaminants; (2) the infant continues to appear clinically well or is improving (eg, fever, feeding); (3) there are no other reasons for hospitalization. (Grade: B; Strong Recommendation)

Key Action Statement 7b

Should treat infants' positive bacterial pathogens in urine, blood, or CSF with targeted antimicrobial therapy for the duration of time consistent with the nature of the disease, responsible organism, and response of the infant to treatment. (Grade: A; Strong Recommendation)

Infants 22 to 28 d of age (KASs 8–14): Clinicians...

Key Action Statement 8

Should obtain urine specimen by catheterization or SPA of bladder for urinalysis and, if urinalysis result is positive, for culture. (Grade: A; Strong Recommendation)

OR

Should obtain urine specimen by bag, spontaneous void, or stimulated void for urinalysis and, if urinalysis result is positive, obtain a catheterization or SPA specimen for culture. (Grade: A; Strong Recommendation)

Key Action Statement 9

Should obtain a blood culture. (Grade: A; Strong Recommendation)

Key Action Statement 10

Should assess IMs. (Grade: B; Strong Recommendation)

Key Action Statement 11a

May obtain a CSF analysis on infants 22–28 d of age even if all of the following criteria are met: (1) urinalysis result is negative or positive; (2) no IM obtained is abnormal; (3) blood and urine cultures have been obtained; (4) infant is hospitalized. (Grade: C; Moderate Recommendation)

Key Action Statement 11b

Should obtain CSF for analysis (WBC, protein, glucose, Gram stain), and bacterial culture if any IM obtained is positive. (Grade: B; Moderate Recommendation)

Key Action Statement 12a

Should administer parenteral antimicrobial therapy in a hospital if either of the following apply: (1) CSF analysis suggests bacterial meningitis; (2) urinalysis result is positive. (Grade: A; Strong Recommendation)

Key Action Statement 12b

May administer parenteral antimicrobial therapy in a hospital if ALL of the following apply: (1) CSF analysis is normal; (2) urinalysis is normal; (3) any IM obtained is abnormal. (Grade: B; Moderate Recommendation)

Key Action Statement 12c

May administer parenteral antimicrobial therapy to hospitalized infants even if ALL of the following are met: (1) urinalysis is normal; (2) no IM obtained is abnormal; (3) CSF analysis is normal or enterovirus-positive. (Grade: B; Weak Recommendation)

Key Action Statement 12d

Should administer parenteral antimicrobial therapy for infants who will be managed at home even if ALL of the following are met: (1) urinalysis is normal; (2) no IM obtained is abnormal; (3) CSF analysis is normal. (Grade: C; Moderate Recommendation)

Key Action Statement 13a

May manage infants at home if all of the following criteria are met: (1) urinalysis is normal; (2) no IM obtained is abnormal. (3) CSF analysis is normal or enterovirus-positive. (4) verbal teaching and written instructions have been provided for monitoring throughout the period of time at home. (5) follow-up plans for reevaluation in 24 h have been developed and are in place. (6) plans have been developed and are in place in case of change in clinical status, including means of communication between family and providers and access to emergency medical care. (Grade: B; Moderate Recommendation)

Key Action Statement 13b

Should hospitalize infants in a facility with nurses and staff experienced in the care of neonates/young infants when CSF is not obtained or is uninterpretable. (Grade: B; Weak Recommendation)

Key Action Statement 14a

Should discontinue antimicrobial agents and discharge hospitalized infants after 24 to 36 h of negative culture results if both of the following are met: (1) the infant is clinically well or improving (eg, fever, feeding); (2) there are no other reasons for hospitalization. (Grade: B; Strong Recommendation)

Key Action Statement 14b

Should discontinue antimicrobial agents on infants managed at home when all of the following criteria are met: (1) infant is clinically well or improving (eg, fever, feeding) at time of reassessment; (2) all culture results are negative at 24–36 h; (3) there is no other infection requiring treatment (eg, otitis media). (Grade: B; Strong Recommendation)

Key Action Statement 14c

Should treat infants' positive bacterial pathogens in urine, blood, or CSF with targeted antimicrobial therapy for the duration of time consistent with the nature of the disease, responsible organism, and response of the infant to treatment. (Grade: A; Strong Recommendation)

Infants 29 to 60 d of age (KASs 15–21): Clinicians...
Key Action Statement 15

Should obtain urine specimen by bag, spontaneous void, or stimulated void for urinalysis and, if urinalysis result is positive, obtain a catheterization or SPA specimen for culture. (Grade: A; Strong Recommendation)

OR

Should obtain urine specimen by catheterization or SPA of bladder for urinalysis and, if result is positive, for culture. (Grade: A; Strong Recommendation)

Key Action Statement 16

Should obtain a blood culture. (Grade: B; Moderate Recommendation)

Key Action Statement 17

Should assess IMs. (Grade: B; Moderate Recommendation)

Key Action Statement 18a

May obtain CSF for analysis (WBC, differential, protein, glucose, Gram stain), culture for bacteria, and test for enterovirus when CSF pleocytosis is detected or during enterovirus season if any IM is abnormal. (Grade: C; Weak Recommendation)

Key Action Statement 18b

Need not obtain CSF for analysis and culture if all IMs obtained are normal. (Grade: B; Moderate Recommendation)

Key Action Statement 19a

Should use parenteral antimicrobial therapy if CSF analysis suggests bacterial meningitis. (Grade: A; Strong Recommendation)

Key Action Statement 19b

May use parenteral antimicrobial therapy if both of the following apply: (1) CSF analysis (if CSF obtained) is normal; (2) any IM obtained is abnormal. (Grade: B; Moderate Recommendation)

Key Action Statement 19c

Should initiate oral antimicrobial therapy if all of the following apply: (1) CSF analysis (if CSF obtained) is normal; (2) urinalysis result is positive; (3) no IM obtained is abnormal. (Grade: B; Strong Recommendation)

Key Action Statement 19d

Need not use antimicrobial therapy while awaiting bacterial culture results if all of the following are met: (1) CSF analysis, if obtained, or normal or enterovirus-positive; (2) urinalysis result is negative; (3) no IM obtained is abnormal. (Grade: B; Moderate Recommendation)

Key Action Statement 20a

Should hospitalize infants in a unit with nurses and staff experienced in the care of 29- to 60-d-old infants if CSF analysis, if obtained, is abnormal. (Grade: A; Strong Recommendation)

Key Action Statement 20b

May hospitalize infants in a unit with nurses and staff experienced in the care of 29- to 60-d-old infants if any IM obtained is abnormal. (Grade: B; Moderate Recommendation)

Key Action Statement 20c

Should manage patients at home if all of the following criteria are met: (1) CSF analysis, if CSF obtained, is normal; (2) urinalysis result is negative; (3) all IMs obtained are normal; (4) appropriate parental education has been provided; (5) follow-up plans for reevaluation in 24 h have been developed and are in place; (6) plans have been developed and are in place in case of change in clinical status, including means of communication between family and providers and access to emergency medical care. (Grade: B; Moderate Recommendation)

Key Action Statement 20d

May manage infants without antimicrobial treatment at home without having obtained interpretable CSF if all of the following are met: (1) urinalysis result is negative; (2) all IMs obtained are normal; (3) parents can return promptly if there is a change in infant condition and agree to follow-up in 24 to 36 h. Infants monitored at home should be reassessed in the following 24 h. (Grade: B; Moderate Recommendation)

Key Action Statement 20e

Need not treat with antimicrobial therapy if all of the following apply: (1) CSF analysis (if CSF obtained) is normal; (2) urinalysis result is negative; (3) no IM obtained is abnormal. (Grade: C; Moderate Recommendation)

Key Action Statement 21a

Should discontinue antimicrobial agents when all of the following are met: (1) all bacterial culture results are negative at 24–36 h; (2) infant is clinically well or improving (eg, fever, feeding); (3) there is no other infection requiring treatment (eg, otitis media). (Grade: B; Strong Recommendation)

Key Action Statement 21b

Should discharge hospitalized patients with positive urine culture results if all of the following are met: (1) blood culture result is negative; (2) result of CSF culture, if obtained, is negative; (3) infant is clinically well or improving (eg, fever, feeding); (4) there are no other reasons for hospitalization. (Grade: B; Strong Recommendation)

Key Action Statement 21c

Should discontinue parenteral antibiotics (if started) and begin or continue oral antimicrobial for infants with urinary tract infections managed at home when all of the following are met: (1) urine culture result is positive; (2) all other bacterial culture results are negative at 24–36 h; (3) infant is clinically well or improving (eg, fever, feeding). (Grade: B; Strong Recommendation)

Key Action Statement 21d

Should treat infants' positive bacterial pathogens in urine, blood, or CSF with targeted antimicrobial therapy for the duration of time consistent with the nature of the disease, responsible organism, and response of the infant to treatment. (Grade: A; Strong Recommendation)

SECTION 2

Endorsed Clinical Practice Guidelines

The American Academy of Pediatrics endorses and accepts as its policy the following guidelines from other organizations.

BRAIN DEATH

Pediatric and Adult Brain Death/Death by Neurologic Criteria Consensus Guideline

David M. Greer, MD, MA; Matthew P. Kirschen, MD, PhD; Ariane Lewis, MD; Gary S. Gronseth, MD; Alexander Rae-Grant, MD; Stephen Ashwal, MD; Maya A. Babu, MD, MBA; David F. Bauer, MD, MPH; Lori Billinghurst, MD, MSc; Amanda Corey, MD; Sonia Partap, MD, MS; Michael A. Rubin, MD, MA; Lori Shutter, MD; Courtney Takahashi, MD; Robert C. Tasker, MBBS, MD; Panayiotis Nicolaou Varelas, MD, PhD; Eelco Wijdicks, MD, PhD; Amy Bennett, JD; Scott R. Wessels, MPS, ELS; and John J. Halperin, MD

ABSTRACT. ***Background and Objectives.*** The purpose of this guideline is to update the 2010 American Academy of Neurology (AAN) brain death/death by neurologic criteria (BD/DNC) guideline for adults and the 2011 American Academy of Pediatrics, Child Neurology Society, and Society of Critical Care Medicine guideline for infants and children and to clarify the BD/DNC determination process by integrating guidance for adults and children into a single guideline. Updates in this guideline include guidance related to conducting the BD/DNC evaluation in the context of extracorporeal membrane oxygenation, targeted temperature management, and primary infratentorial injury.

Methods. A panel of experts from multiple medical societies developed BD/DNC recommendations. Because of the lack of high-quality evidence on the subject, a novel, evidence-informed formal consensus process was used. This process relied on the panel experts' review and detailed knowledge of the literature surrounding BD/DNC to guide the development of preliminary recommendations. Recommendations were formulated and voted on, using a modified Delphi process, according to the 2017 AAN Clinical Practice Guideline Process Manual.

Major Recommendations. Eighty-five recommendations were developed on the following: (1) general principles for the BD/DNC evaluation, (2) qualifications to perform BD/DNC evaluations, (3) prerequisites for BD/DNC determination, (4) components of the BD/DNC neurologic examination, (5) apnea testing as part of the BD/DNC evaluation, (6) ancillary testing as part of the BD/DNC evaluation, and (7) special considerations for BD/DNC determination. (10/23)

CARDIOPULMINARY RESUSCITATION AND COVID-19

Guidance for Cardiopulmonary Resuscitation of Children With Suspected or Confirmed COVID-19

Ryan W. Morgan, MD, MTR; Dianne L. Atkins, MD; Antony Hsu, MD; Beena D. Kamath-Rayne, MD, MPH; Khalid Aziz, BA, MA, Med (IT); Robert A. Berg, MD; Farhan Bhanji, MD; Melissa Chan, MD; Adam Cheng, MD; Kathleen Chiotos, MD, MSCE; Allan de Caen, MD; Jonathan P. Duff, MD, Med; Susan Fuchs, MD; Benny L. Joyner, Jr., MD, MPH; Monica Kleinman, MD; Javier J. Lasa, MD; Henry C. Lee, MD; Rebecca E. Lehotzky, PhD; Arielle Levy, MD, MEd; Mary E. McBride, MD, MEd; Garth Meckler, MD, MSHS; Vinay Nadkarni, MD, MS; Tia Raymond, MD; Kathryn Roberts, MSN, RN, CCRN-K, CCNS; Stephen M. Schexnayder, MD; Robert M. Sutton, MD, MSCE; Mark Terry, MPA; Brian Walsh, PhD, RRT; Carolyn M. Zelop, MD; Comilla Sasson, MD, PhD; Alexis Topjian, MD, MSCE; on behalf of the American Heart Association Emergency Cardiovascular Committee and Get with the Guidelines-Resuscitation Pediatric Task Force in Collaboration with the American Academy of Pediatrics, American Association for Respiratory Care, and American Society of Anesthesiologists

ABSTRACT. This article aims to provide guidance to health care workers for the provision of basic and advanced life support to children and neonates with suspected or confirmed coronavirus disease 2019 (COVID-19). It aligns with the 2020 American Heart Association Guidelines for Cardiopulmonary Resuscitation (CPR) and Emergency Cardiovascular care while providing strategies for reducing risk of transmission of severe acute respiratory syndrome coronavirus 2 to health care providers. Patients with suspected or confirmed COVID-19 and cardiac arrest should receive chest compressions and defibrillation, when indicated, as soon as possible. Because of the importance of ventilation during pediatric and neonatal resuscitation, oxygenation and ventilation should be prioritized. All CPR events should therefore be considered aerosol-generating procedures. Thus, personal protective equipment (PPE) appropriate for aerosol-generating procedures (including N95 respirators or an equivalent) should be donned before resuscitation, and high-efficiency particulate air filters should be used. Any personnel without appropriate PPE should be immediately excused by providers wearing appropriate PPE. Neonatal resuscitation guidance is unchanged from standard algorithms, except for specific attention to infection prevention and control. In summary, health care personnel should continue to reduce the risk of severe acute respiratory syndrome coronavirus 2 transmission through vaccination and use of appropriate PPE during pediatric resuscitations. Health care organizations should ensure the availability and appropriate use of PPE. Because delays or withheld CPR increases the risk to patients for poor clinical outcomes, children and neonates with suspected or confirmed COVID-19 should receive prompt, high-quality CPR in accordance with evidence-based guidelines. (8/22)

SECTION 3

2025 Policies

From the American Academy of Pediatrics

- *Policy Statements*
  ORGANIZATIONAL PRINCIPLES TO GUIDE AND DEFINE THE CHILD HEALTH CARE SYSTEM AND TO IMPROVE THE HEALTH OF ALL CHILDREN

- *Clinical Reports*
  GUIDANCE FOR THE CLINICIAN IN RENDERING PEDIATRIC CARE

- *Technical Reports*
  BACKGROUND INFORMATION TO SUPPORT AMERICAN ACADEMY OF PEDIATRICS POLICY

Includes policy statements, clinical reports, and technical reports published between January 1, 2025, and December 31, 2025

INTRODUCTION

This section of ***Pediatric Clinical Practice Guidelines & Policies: A Compendium of Evidence-based Research for Pediatric Practice*** is composed of policy statements, clinical reports, and technical reports issued by the American Academy of Pediatrics (AAP) and is designed as a quick reference tool for AAP members, AAP staff, and other interested parties. Section 3 includes the full text of all AAP policies published in 2025. Section 4 is a compilation of all active AAP policies (through December 31, 2025) arranged alphabetically, with abstracts where applicable. A subject index is also available. These materials should help answer questions that arise about the AAP position on child health care issues. **However, remember that AAP policy statements, clinical reports, and technical reports do not indicate an exclusive course of treatment or serve as a standard of medical care. Variations, taking into account individual circumstances, may be appropriate.**

Policy statements have been written by AAP committees, councils, sections, or task forces and approved by the AAP Board of Directors. Most of these statements have appeared previously in ***Pediatrics*** or *AAP News*.

This section does not contain all AAP policies. It does not include
- Press releases.
- Motions and resolutions that were approved by the Board of Directors. These can be found in the Board of Directors' minutes.
- Policies in manuals, pamphlets, booklets, or other AAP publications. These items can be ordered through the AAP. To order, visit http://shop.aap.org/books or call 866/843-2271.
- Testimony before Congress or government agencies.

All policy statements, clinical reports, and technical reports from the American Academy of Pediatrics automatically expire 5 years after publication unless reaffirmed, revised, or retired at or before that time. Please check the American Academy of Pediatrics website at www.aap.org for up-to-date reaffirmations, revisions, and retirements.

2025 Recommendations for Preventive Pediatric Health Care

- *Policy Statement*

POLICY STATEMENT Organizational Principles to Guide and Define the Child Health Care System and/or Improve the Health of All Children

American Academy of Pediatrics

DEDICATED TO THE HEALTH OF ALL CHILDREN™

2025 Recommendations for Preventive Pediatric Health Care: Policy Statement

Committee on Practice and Ambulatory Medicine

The 2025 Recommendations for Preventive Pediatric Health Care (Periodicity Schedule) has been approved by the American Academy of Pediatrics (AAP). Each child and family is unique; therefore, these recommendations are designed for the care of children who are receiving nurturing parenting, have no manifestations of any important health problems, and are growing and developing in a satisfactory fashion. Developmental, psychosocial, and chronic disease issues for children and adolescents may require more frequent counseling and treatment visits separate from preventive care visits. Additional visits also may become necessary if circumstances suggest concerns. The AAP continues to emphasize the great importance of continuity of care in comprehensive health supervision and the need to avoid fragmentation of care.[1]

To ensure that health care professionals have the most current recommendations, the Periodicity Schedule is not published in *Pediatrics* but is posted on the American Academy of Pediatrics website (www.aap.org/periodicityschedule). This webpage includes the most recent version of the Periodicity Schedule and the full set of footnotes. The Periodicity Schedule is reviewed and revised annually to reflect current evidence and recommendations. This review process did not identify sufficient evidence to support updates to the 2025 Periodicity Schedule. The approved 2025 Periodicity Schedule remains unchanged from the 2024 Periodicity Schedule.

COMMITTEE ON PRACTICE AND AMBULATORY MEDICINE, 2024–2025

Robin M. Warner, MD, FAAP, Chairperson
Carolyn Cleary, MD, FAAP
Mona Doss Roberts, MD, FAAP
Elizabeth Hawse, MD, FAAP
Cailly Howell-McLean, MD, FAAP
Lisa M. Kafer, MD, FAAP
Seth D. Kaplan, MD, FAAP – *Section on Administration and Practice Management Liaison*

https://doi.org/10.1542/peds.2025-071066

To cite: American Academy of Pediatrics, Committee on Practice and Ambulatory Medicine. 2025 Recommendations for Preventive Pediatric Health Care: Policy Statement. *Pediatrics.* 2025;155(5):e2025071066

Tomitra Latimer, MD, FAAP
Robert H. Wiskind, MD, FAAP

COMMITTEE ON PRACTICE AND AMBULATORY MEDICINE, 2023–2024

Jesse M. Hackell, MD, FAAP, Chairperson
Yvette M. Almendarez, MD, FAAP
Patricia E. Cantrell, MD, FAAP
Carolyn Cleary, MD, FAAP
Elizabeth Hawse, MD, FAAP
Lisa M. Kafer, MD, FAAP
Seth D. Kaplan, MD, FAAP – *Section on Administration and Practice Management Liaison*
Tomitra Latimer, MD, FAAP
Alisa Skatrud, MPA – Family Liaison
Robert H. Wiskind, MD, FAAP

STAFF

Lauren Barone, MPH
Maureen Cooney, MPH
Mackenzie Magnus, MBA, MPH
Bailey Sone, PhD, CCC-SLP

REFERENCES

1. Hagan JF, Shaw JS, Duncan PM, eds. *Bright Futures: Guidelines for Health Supervision of Infants, Children, and Adolescents.* 4th ed. American Academy of Pediatrics; 2017.

Abusive Head Trauma in Infants and Children (Technical Report)

- *Technical Report*

TECHNICAL REPORT

American Academy of Pediatrics
DEDICATED TO THE HEALTH OF ALL CHILDREN™

Abusive Head Trauma in Infants and Children: Technical Report

Sandeep K. Narang, MD, JD, FAAP,[1] Suzanne Haney, MD, MS, FAAP,[2] Ann-Christine Duhaime, MD, FAAP,[3] Jonathan Martin, MD, FAANS, FACS, FAAP,[4] Gil Binenbaum, MD, MSCE FAAP,[5] Alejandra G. de Alba Campomanes, MD, MPH, FAAP,[6] Rich Barth, MD, FAAP,[7] Gina Bertocci, PhD,[8] Margarite Care, MD,[9] Declan McGuone, MD,[10] COUNCIL ON CHILD ABUSE AND NEGLECT; SECTION ON OPHTHALMOLOGY, SECTION ON RADIOLOGY, AND SECTION ON NEUROLOGICAL SURGERY; SOCIETY FOR PEDIATRIC RADIOLOGY; AMERICAN ASSOCIATION OF CERTIFIED ORTHOPTISTS; AMERICAN ASSOCIATION FOR PEDIATRIC OPHTHALMOLOGY AND STRABISMUS; and AMERICAN ACADEMY OF OPHTHALMOLOGY

INTRODUCTION

Abusive head trauma (AHT) in infants and children is a complex and challenging clinical diagnosis. Because of its clinical, social, and legal implications, few pediatric diagnoses evoke as much cognitive difficulty and emotional distress as AHT. Over the past several decades, considerable literature has been published on various aspects of the AHT diagnosis including epidemiology, historical features, clinical findings, biomechanics, differential diagnoses, outcomes, and prevention. The volume and critical analysis of the published literature can be daunting to even the most motivated pediatric provider.

To date, the American Academy of Pediatrics (AAP) has not promulgated, in the form of a technical report, a comprehensive review of the evidence-based literature surrounding AHT. Although the AAP has addressed the subject matter in other treatises, a scientific review in the form of a technical report offers the benefit of openly available, readily accessible, and more frequently updatable scientific information.[1,2] Additionally, as the diagnosis has engendered some media and legal controversy, which then spills into a clinical venue, a technical report can assist the pediatric provider in communicating the scientific information to interdisciplinary colleagues such as child welfare agencies and courts.

With respect to the methodology used for this technical report, the authors recognize that properly conducted formal systematic review methods provide a standardized, relatively objective compilation of strength-graded evidence on a specific focused topic of inquiry. However, the broad topic of AHT, in which evidence comes from a wide variety of sources, fields, and disciplines using many different methods to approach a range of related areas of focus, is not a topic that easily lends itself to a formal systematic review process. Instead, in each area of this technical report, authors or groups of authors performed a wide review

[1]*Professor of Pediatrics, Medical College of Wisconsin; Chief, Section of Child Advocacy and Protection, Child Advocacy and Protection Services, Children's Wisconsin, Milwaukee, Wisconsin;* [2]*Children's Nebraska and University of Nebraska Medical Center, Omaha, Nebraska;* [3]*Department of Neurosurgery, Massachusetts General Hospital and Harvard Medical School, Boston, Massachusetts;* [4]*Division Head, Neurosurgery, Connecticut Children's; Professor, Surgery and Pediatrics, UConn School of Medicine, Farmington, Connecticut;* [5]*Division of Ophthalmology at Children's Hospital of Philadelphia; Perelman School of Medicine at the University of Pennsylvania, Philadelphia, Pennsylvania;* [6]*Department of Ophthalmology, University of California San Francisco, San Francisco, California;* [7]*Department of Radiology, Lucile Packard Children's Hospital, Stanford University, Stanford, California;* [8]*Department of Bioengineering, University of Louisville, Louisville, Kentucky;* [9]*Department of Radiology and Medical Imaging, Cincinnati Children's Hospital Medical Center; Department of Radiology, University of Cincinnati College of Medicine, Cincinnati, Ohio; and* [10]*Department of Pathology, Yale School of Medicine; Associate Medical Examiner, Connecticut Office of the Chief Medical Examiner, New Haven, Connecticut*

All authors wrote one or more sections, critically reviewed and revised the entire manuscript, approved the final manuscript and agree to be accountable for all aspects of the work.

To cite: Narang SK, Haney S, Duhaime A-C, et al; American Academy of Pediatrics, Council on Child Abuse and Neglect; Section on Ophthalmology, Section on Radiology, and Section on Neurological Surgery; Society for Pediatric Radiology; American Association of Certified Orthoptists; American Association for Pediatric Ophthalmology and Strabismus; and American Academy of Ophthalmology. Abusive Head Trauma in Infants and Children: Technical Report. *Pediatrics.* 2025; 155(3):e2024070457

of peer-reviewed publications within each subtopic (generally limited to articles published in English), emphasizing those sources with the highest quality of evidence but not eliminating sources for which descriptive methods nonetheless provide useful and relevant information. The overall manuscript was reviewed several times by multiple participants with source documents reviewed for content when appropriate. References are provided for statements and conclusions so that the reader can access the sources directly.

Additionally, there are various medical terms utilized in this technical report that are commonly encountered in the AHT diagnosis (ie, acute subdural hematoma/hemorrhage, chronic subdural hematoma/hemorrhage, short distance fall, subdural hygroma, etc) but may have some variance in definition throughout the medical literature. For transparency and to promote a common understanding of these terms, there is an Appendix of definitions at the conclusion of this report. Many of the definitions for the pathoanatomic entities were from the National Institutes of Health Common Data Elements for Traumatic Brain Injury.[3] Some other definitions, such as those within the biomechanics section, are described/defined in more detail in the relevant sections.

DEFINITION

AHT has been known by multiple terms in the past and is referenced by other terms currently in some other countries.[4] Aside from the challenges and confusion that multiple terminologies represent, more challenging has been the lack of consistent case definition amongst clinical and research sectors.

In 2008, the Centers for Disease Control and Prevention (CDC) convened an expert panel group of "pediatricians, child maltreatment experts, abusive head trauma experts, injury surveillance experts, ICD coding experts, and experienced state health department personnel" with the aim of identifying a common set of codes (ICD-9-CM and ICD-10) "that could be uniformly implemented to define abusive head trauma among children under 5 years of age."[5] Through an iterative process, the expert panel group arrived at the following definition of AHT:

> "an injury to the skull or intracranial contents of an infant or young child (<5 years of age) due to inflicted blunt impact and/or violent shaking."

Although this definition was engineered to facilitate consistency in "public health surveillance and research," the breadth of the definition also provides a practical framework for clinical application. It is noteworthy that this definition is intentionally broad (ie, not confined to exclusively intracranial findings or findings indicative of particular mechanisms of injury). The breadth of the definition offers the benefit of reducing heuristic application of certain variables to the AHT diagnosis, thereby minimizing concerns for circularity in research.

EPIDEMIOLOGY

Incidence

AHT is the third leading cause of head injury in children younger than 5 years, only surpassed by motor vehicle collisions and falls.[5] It is also the leading cause of severe head injury in infancy.[5] The mortality rate of AHT ranges from 10% to 20%.[6–9] The current incidence of AHT in the United States is estimated at 25 to 35 children per 100 000 annually younger than 1 year of age.[6,8,10] Some researchers have found an incidence as high as 40 children per 100 000 annually using more rigorous research methods as defined by the CDC.[5,11] Most studies find a peak in incidence at around 2 months of age with a median of 4 months of age; however, some additional studies have noted a second, smaller peak that occurs at 8 months of age.[6,9] After infancy, the incidence drops steeply with an incidence as low as 3.8 per 100 000 for children between 1 and 2 years of age and few cases noted after 5 years of age.[12]

There is geographic variation in the incidence of AHT. A number of researchers have noted that the incidence of AHT varies based on US region: the highest incidences are reported in the Midwest and the lowest in the Northeast.[7,11] At this time, there has been no clear reason found for this regional variation; however, there does appear to be an increased risk of AHT in rural populations, which are more prevalent in the Midwest.[13] The United States appears to have one of the highest reported national incidences of AHT, with Scotland reporting 24.6 per 100 000 infants annually and New Zealand reporting 14.7 to 19.6 per 100 000 infants.[14,15]

TAKEAWAY POINTS

1. AHT is the third leading cause of head trauma in children younger than 5 years.
2. Mortality rate ranges from 10% to 20%.
3. The current incidence of AHT in the United States is estimated at 25 to 35 children per 100 000 annually younger than 1 year of age.
4. Peak incidence is around 2 months of age; the median is at 4 months of age, with decreasing incidence after infancy.

DISPARITIES IN AHT DIAGNOSIS

Children who have experienced AHT are have been reported disproportionately as male, Black, or American Indian/Alaska Native.[6,10,11,15,16] This broad statement impugns race per se as an associated risk factor for AHT in children. Importantly, this overarching statement does not reflect rigorous statistical adjustment for social drivers of health (SDOHs), which are similarly associated with the incidence of AHT. This is heralded by the findings of Wood et al (2016) demonstrating an increase in the incidence of AHT during the 2007–2009 US recession. Taken together, the data to date suggest considerable confounding affects any assertion of race per se as a risk factor for AHT and instead elevates the probability that AHT may reflect yet another racial disparity (defined as a difference in outcomes not attributable to biology but rather due to social circumstances or structural or implicit bias).[17]

Implicit bias may affect one's ability to appropriately diagnose AHT and likely affects certain groups disproportionately—that is, in overreporting).[18–20] In the converse, Jenny et al (1999) identified an underreporting or lesser likelihood to diagnose AHT in white and intact families. This is juxtaposed with the findings of Lane et al (2002) indicating that Black, Hispanic, and Indigenous children were more likely to be evaluated for abuse.[21,22] Luken et al (2021) used exploratory mapping in the National Child Abuse and Neglect Data System (NCANDS) data to find that there was a 15 times greater rate of reporting abuse in Black communities than in white communities.[23] Regional variations in reporting highlight policy and practice concerns that further identify the importance of place and social/policy circumstances affecting the diagnosis of AHT in minorities.[23] Finally, other risk factors such as poverty and financial stress consistent with known SDOHs are more prevalent in communities of color, present challenges in quantitative assessment, and likely serve as candidate root causes for the observed disparities.[15]

TAKEAWAY POINTS

1. There is an overrepresentation of Black, Hispanic, and American Indian/Alaska Native children having experienced AHT, with the associations potentially and largely influenced by the confounders of social circumstances and bias of reporters. Future study of AHT requires more rigorous assessment of socioeconomic status, SDOHs, and other drivers of AHT.
2. Bias in reporting can also adversely affect nonminoritized communities through underreporting (positive implicit bias), in addition to the previously acknowledged concerns for overreporting in minoritized communities (negative implicit bias).

RISK FACTORS

Risk factors are identified when one group (with the risk factor) is more likely than another (without the risk factor) to experience abuse. Risk factors can be effective in prevention strategies (and public policies) as they can help target interventions[24] but should not be used for individual diagnostic decision making.[25,26]

The reported perpetrators are most commonly male caregivers (father, stepfather, or mother's boyfriend), followed by female babysitters.[27,28] Mothers are the perpetrator in 13% to 16% of cases.[27,28] Other risk factors for AHT include young age of the mother, late prenatal care, low birth weight, and multiple births.[6,12] Kelly and colleagues (2017) found that prematurity was a stronger risk factor than low birth weight and multiple births.[29]

Crying is frequently reported as a trigger for an abusive event.[30] Barr and colleagues (2006) have noted that the normal crying curve is paralleled by the incidence in AHT in infancy, with peak incidence of the normal crying curve occurring at 5 to 6 weeks of age and the peak incidence of AHT hospitalization rates occurring approximately 4 weeks later.[31] The absence of the aforementioned risk factors does not preclude the diagnosis. In fact, AHT has been diagnosed many times in the absence of these risk factors.

TAKEAWAY POINTS

1. The full assortment of risk factors for AHT remains under investigation but includes poverty, maternal factors (eg, young maternal age), low birth weight, multiparity, and a male caregiver.
2. Known risk factors are insufficient to serve as a screening tool for children at risk for AHT, as AHT can occur in the absence of known risk factors.
3. Addressing known risk factors may be effective in developing prevention strategies, including public policy objectives.

CLINICAL PRESENTATION

History

Introduction

A key component in the evaluation of suspected AHT is whether the reported history is consistent with the child's clinical presentation.[32,33] This inconsistency with the history is a cornerstone of the maltreatment diagnosis in general and no different with AHT. Therefore, gathering a detailed history is highly important in the evaluation of suspected abuse, as it is in all of medicine. Detailed components of the trauma history include what and when symptoms were noted by the caregiver, when the child was last observed by the caregiver to have been acting "normally" in the caregiver's estimation (and for what period that normalcy existed), a detailed account of any traumatic events, the child's behavior and symptoms after the traumatic event, and the caregiver's response for medical assistance, if any.[33] When attaining history from a caregiver, interviewing each caregiver independently, if feasible, and asking questions in a nonleading, inquisitive, and nonjudgmental manner assists in attaining the most reliable historical information.[34]

Historical "red flags" have long been taught as cornerstone markers for suspicion of AHT.[35] Over the past couple of decades, several historical features have been studied more systematically to investigate their association with the AHT diagnosis.

An Absent Trauma History

An absent trauma history, in light of traumatic findings, has been considered a key associative feature of abuse/AHT.[32,36] In 2003, Hettler and Greenes performed a retrospective review of 163 children, aged 0 to 3 years, including patients admitted from 1993–2000 with acute traumatic intracranial injury.[37] The authors classified cases as either "definite abuse" or "not definite abuse" on the basis of radiologic, ophthalmologic, and physical examination findings, without regard to the presenting history. Forty-nine of the cases (30%) were classified as "definite abuse" and 114 (70%) were classified as "not definite abuse." These authors found that an absent history of trauma, in patients with a clear traumatic injury, had a 97% specificity and 92% positive predictive value (PPV) for AHT.[37]

In 2020, Hymel et al published a study that sought to replicate Hettler and Greenes' retrospective analysis on a cross-sectional dataset containing prospective data.[38] Similar to Hettler and Greenes, cases were categorized a priori as "definite" or "not definite" AHT solely on the basis of patients' clinical and radiologic findings unrelated to history. Hymel et al found that a caregiver's specific denial of any trauma had a 90% specificity (95% confidence interval [CI], 0.84–0.94), 81% PPV (95% CI, 0.71–0.88), and a positive likelihood ratio of 4.83 (95% CI, 3.07–7.61) for definite AHT.[38]

An Evolving or Changing Trauma History

The longstanding clinical adage is that "accidental histories don't change."[33] It is uncommon for the history of an accidental injury scenario to vary substantively from provider to provider. It can, however, be difficult to determine what constitutes a "substantive" variance in the trauma history.

There are primarily 2 studies that provide reliable data on this historical variable: Hettler and Greenes (2003) and Hymel et al (2020). In Hettler and Greenes' cohort, only 6% of all cases had an evolving or changing history.[37] *All* of those were in the "definite abuse" cohort (9/49 [18%]). There were no cases (0/114) in the "not definite abuse" cohort that had evolving or changing histories. However, Hettler and Greenes did not operationalize a definition for what constituted a "change" to or "evolution" of the initial history and instead relied on the judgment of the providers as documented in the records.

The Pediatric Brain Injury Network (PediBIRN) data set used by Hymel et al also did not define what constituted a "substantive" change but instead relied on the investigators to determine whether they thought the history had "changed substantively with repetition over time."[38] In their prospective dataset of 346 patients, 248 patients provided an accidental trauma history—81 in the "definite abuse" cohort, and 167 in the "not definite abuse" cohort. Hymel et al found 41 cases in which the history "changed substantively with repetition over time." Of the "definite abuse" cases, 31 of 81 (38%) had "changed" histories. Additionally, of the "not definite abuse" cases, 10 of 167 (6%) had "changed" histories. Hymel et al found a "changed" history to have 94% specificity (95% CI, 0.89–0.97), a 76% PPV (95% CI, 0.59–0.87), and a 6.39 positive likelihood ratio (95% CI, 3.30–12.38) for the "definite abuse" cohort.

Thus, although there is currently no explicit operational definition in the evidence-based literature on what constitutes a "substantive" change in caregiver trauma history, there is some evidence that indicates a substantive change to be much more strongly associated with abuse than accident.

A History That Is Inconsistent With the Child's Developmental Capabilities

There are multiple potential scenarios in which a child's developmental abilities could be inconsistent with a given trauma history. One commonly cited example among AHT scenarios is the history of a 1- or 2-month-old infant "rolling" off an elevated surface (such as a couch or a bed), before the developmental capability of rolling from back-to-front or front-to-back is achieved. But, similar to the earlier discussion on changing histories, there are a limited number of studies that have empirically assessed the association of an inconsistency with the reported developmental capabilities of a child and the abuse diagnosis.[38,39]

In the PediBIRN data set of 346 patients used by Hymel et al, an accidental trauma history was provided in 248 cases (72%).[38] Of those, 22 of 248 cases (9%) had a caregiver accident history that was deemed inconsistent with the child's known or expected gross motor skills. In the a priori "definite AHT" and "not definite AHT" groups, developmental inconsistency with the trauma history had a specificity of 95% (95% CI, 0.90–0.98), a 64% PPV (95% CI, 0.41–0.82), and a 3.61 positive likelihood ratio (95% CI, 1.58–8.25) for the definite abuse cohort.

Although a limited evidence base supports the assertion that incongruence of reported developmental capabilities and abuse are linked, other authors have cautioned providers about overreliance on the normative ranges of developmental capabilities in infants and toddlers in suspected abuse cases.[34]

A Delay in Seeking Medical Care

There are several studies that have addressed the historical variable of delay in seeking medical care in suspected AHT. Vinchon et al offer one of the few studies to provide data surrounding the time range of what constitutes a "delay" in abusive and nonabusive head trauma.[40] In their cohort of 45 confessed abuse cases and 39 witnessed accidents, the authors found that the mean and median times from injury to referral for care were shorter in the accidental group than the abusive group (21 vs 57 hours mean and 3.5 vs 12 hours median, respectively), but these findings did not reach statistical significance. Similarly, Hettler and Greenes did not find a statistically significant difference of delay in seeking care between their definite and not definite abuse groups. [37]

In distinction to the studies by Vinchon et al and Hettler and Greenes, Kennedy et al did find a statistically significant difference between AHT and non-AHT (nAHT) groups with regard to delay in seeking care.[41] Kennedy et al retrospectively reviewed charts of children younger than 6 years who had acute head injury and were admitted to the pediatric intensive care unit at a pediatric hospital from 2013 to 2017. The authors defined a "delay in seeking care" as waiting approximately 30 minutes or more from severe symptom onset (which was defined as when a caregiver identified that the child was clearly ill). Patients who had AHT were significantly more likely to have a delayed presentation to care than those who had accidental head trauma (61.8% vs 20.0%; $P = .0017$). In a secondary analysis of the AHT group ($n = 34$), a delay in presentation to care was not significantly associated with age, sex, race, Medicaid insurance status, length of stay, or discharge disposition.

Vadivelu et al sought to evaluate "delay in seeking care" from another perspective—the effect on overall patient neurologic outcome at discharge.[42] In their 10-year retrospective review at a single institution, the authors included only those AHT cases in which a perpetrator was identified by data in the New York State Central Register and predefined "delay" criteria were applied (ie, 0–6 hours = "no delay"; 6–12 hours = "moderate delay"; and >12 hours = "severe delay") based on parallel definition in the stroke literature. The authors identified 28 children who met inclusion criteria and reviewed those charts to assess the association of delay, if any, with neurologic outcomes. They found the majority of patients with AHT (61%) presented with either moderate or severe delay; the majority (61%) had an admission Glasgow coma score (GCS) of less than 7; additionally, the majority of those with a GCS of less than 7 presented with either no or moderate delay.

Vadivelu et al also found that patients presenting to medical care 6 to 12 hours after AHT (moderate delay) appeared to have worse outcomes than those presenting with no delay ($P < .0426$). Interestingly, however, the authors found that those patients presenting with severe delay did not have worse outcomes than those presenting with no delay or moderate delay. The authors attributed this aberrance to be secondary to higher GCSs in the children with severe delay.[42]

TAKEAWAY POINTS

1. An absent trauma history, in the presence of traumatic findings, has high specificity and positive predictive values for AHT.
2. A "substantive" change in a caregiver's trauma history also holds high specificity and positive predictive values for AHT, but what constitutes a "substantive" change is an area needing further research.
3. There is some literature support to indicate that inconsistency between the caregiver's history and the child's developmental capabilities is more strongly associated with AHT than nAHT; this is also an area needing further research.
4. The current evidence base is unclear on whether there is a strong association between "delay" in seeking medical care and AHT. Additionally, further research is needed on what constitutes a "delay" in seeking medical care in cases of suspected AHT.

Symptoms

Introduction

The neurologic presentation of the infant and toddler with AHT varies widely, ranging from the neurologically asymptomatic patient commonly presenting with macrocephaly to the patient in acute cardiopulmonary arrest with profound neurologic impairment.[43] Frequently, symptoms in the infant are nonspecific; symptoms including vomiting, irritability, and lethargy overlap with medical diagnoses such as viral illness and undernutrition/growth impairment, leading to challenges in injury detection.[15] Jenny and colleagues conducted a 5-year retrospective single center review of children younger than 3 years seen by an institutional child advocacy and protection team.[21] Of the 173 children in whom AHT was eventually diagnosed, 54 (31%) were initially unrecognized with regard to the cause of their symptoms. Children presenting with coma, respiratory compromise, or seizures were more likely to have a diagnosis of head injury, while those presenting with irritability or vomiting were less likely to be identified.

Additionally, it can be challenging for the provider performing the evaluation to describe the degree of neurologic impairment. Pediatric variants of the GCS remain the most commonly used scales for describing the neurologic status of the injured child, despite their reliance on motor and verbal skills (which may be more difficult to determine in young children). [23] There is a paucity of data available on the predictive abilities of the GCS in pediatric neurologic injury.[10] One interesting observation regarding the limited value of neurologic symptoms informing the clinician regarding the diagnosis of AHT is the lack of reliance on neurologic symptoms in AHT clinical decision rules (Pittsburgh Infant Brain Injury Score [PIBIS] and PediBIRN).[44–46]

Factors including the mechanism of injury and magnitude of force applied influence both patient presentation and outcome.[47] On the basis of parallels with accidental trauma, children with high-force inertial injuries can be expected to be more neurologically impaired. As described by Oluigbo and colleagues in a single institutional retrospective study of 37 children undergoing decompressive craniectomy, 14 (38%) children had experienced AHT and presented with acute encephalopathy and a mean GCS of 4.5.[48] Less severe injuries presented with less profound acute symptoms or, in some cases, presented with a delay in time from the initial traumatic event. In contrast to acutely severe presentations, Klimo et al performed a single institutional retrospective study of 26 children presenting for treatment of chronic subdural collections. Twenty-four (92%) children in this cohort who had experienced AHT presented with "global findings" to include macrocephaly, seizure, sun-setting eyes (persistent downward deviation of gaze), lethargy, and irritability. Sixty-two percent of patients presented with occipitofrontal circumference exceeding the 90th percentile, suggesting the collections temporally evolve from an acute hemorrhage or tear in the arachnoid mater and that symptoms likely were not severe at the time of injury but only evolved as the chronic collection enlarged gradually. Mortality in this series was only 4.2%.[49]

Apnea and Seizures

Piteau et al performed a systematic review of clinical characteristics associated with AHT over nAHT in a hospitalized population of children 6 years or younger.[50] Although the authors were challenged by a lack of consistent reporting of variables in the included studies, their meta-analysis determined odds ratios (ORs) for 11 radiographic and 8 clinical variables. Among neurologic signs and symptoms, seizure (OR, 7.25; 95% CI, 3.04–17.27; P <.001) and apnea (OR, 5.31; 95% CI, 2.34–12.05; P <.001) achieved ORs >1.0, suggesting a higher likelihood of a diagnosis of AHT. Similarly, Maguire and colleagues reviewed data from 6 studies in children younger than 3 years, pooling data on 1053 children, among whom 348 (33%) had experienced AHT. Multilevel logistic regression analysis revealed seizure (OR, 5.075) and apnea (OR, 6.948) as neurologic symptoms more highly associated with AHT in this study.[51]

Irritability, Vomiting, or Developmental Delay

Although symptoms such as irritability, vomiting, and developmental delay are commonly present in children with AHT, these symptoms are of limited utility in discriminating AHT from other common childhood disease.[52] Feldman et al conducted a 5-year retrospective multicenter study of children with AHT and subdural hemorrhage.[53] Although the majority (80%) of patients in this study were symptomatic, 40.7% presented with nonspecific neurologic and somatic symptoms including lethargy and vomiting. Ten percent presented with no neurologic symptoms, and 3% presented with asymptomatic macrocephaly alone.

Timing of Clinical Symptoms

Forensically, a key issue that arises in AHT cases is the timing of onset of clinical symptoms. Because the manifesting symptoms in AHT are variable and often subtle to the lay caregiver, it is important to gather medical and forensic information relating to the last time the child was noted to be "normal" (ie, symptom-free) in the eyes of caregivers.

One forensic issue that arises in the setting of fatal AHT is the topic of a "lucid interval" prior to neurologic decline. The term "lucid interval" classically has been described in the setting of a contact injury to the skull with subsequent expanding extra-axial hemorrhage (epidural hemorrhage) in verbal pediatric or adult patients.[54] De Leeuw reported the presence of lucid interval following confessed AHT only in the setting of contact injuries to the skull.[55]

Arbogast and coauthors illustrated challenges with the study of lucid intervals in patients with AHT in their analysis of fatal head injuries within the Pennsylvania Trauma System Outcome database.[56] Of the 37% of injuries classified as AHT, 6.8% were reported as having a GCS >7 at presentation. Patients younger than 24 months with AHT were 10 times more likely to present with moderate GCSs than those in motor vehicle crashes. The authors acknowledged the methodologic problems inherent in the retrospective nature of their study: "Whether [our results are] because of differences in pathologic injury, neurologic responses unique to the infant brain, or limitations of the bedside methods used to assess neurologic function in young children cannot be determined by this study."

Most cases of fatal AHT are a result of inertial brain injury with acute subdural hemorrhage and brain swelling.[57] Among patients analyzed in their series, Duhaime et al observed "...there is no evidence of a prolonged interval of lucidity between the injury and the onset of symptoms in children with acute subdural hemorrhage and brain swelling."[58] However, in the infant or preverbal child, even the definition of lucidity is problematic, particularly in the setting of AHT, in which the report of the caregiver may be unreliable. "...It is not clear what is meant by a lucid state in an infant, and who should verify whether this is present or not."[59]

Studies of fatal nAHT in this age group represent one means of reducing concerns for bias present in the study of AHT patients. Willman et al examined 95 fatal head injuries in pediatric patients with nAHT and identified only 2 patients with reliable reports of a lucid interval prior to death. Both occurred in the setting of epidural hemorrhage.[60]

TAKEAWAY POINTS

1. Symptoms of AHT are frequently nonspecific and include vomiting, irritability, and lethargy.
2. Seizure and apnea are neurologic signs highly, but not exclusively, associated with AHT.
3. Determination of "lucidity" in the infant is challenging; reliance on this aspect of patient history for the timing of injuries can be problematic.
4. In cases of severe head injury (cerebral edema with acute subdural bleeding), it is unlikely that there is a prolonged period of wellness between the injury and symptom onset.

Physical Findings

Introduction

Much like symptomology, physical examination findings indicative of AHT can be variable and subtle and are often missed.[21,61] Research has identified bruising as a key sentinel injury in infants (ie, younger than 12 months), and its recognition is vital to the prevention of more severe abuse such as AHT. Sheets et al identified sentinel injuries in over 28% of subsequently identified "definite" abuse cases and bruising as the sentinel finding that was missed or underappreciated in 80% of those cases.[62] The physical findings discussed immediately below are those in the clinical literature of nonfatal AHT cases. Epidemiologic and clinical features of fatal AHT cases are discussed in the "Pathology" section of this technical report.

a) Macrocephaly

Macrocephaly is defined operationally as an occipitofrontal circumference greater than 2 standard deviations above mean or above the 97th percentile as measured from the glabella to the most prominent portion of the occiput. Macrocephaly can also be relative, when the head is large out of proportion to the length and weight of the child. The differential diagnosis for macrocephaly is broad and includes conditions resulting in enlargement of the extra-axial spaces, the ventricular system, and brain parenchyma itself.[63] The majority of infants with macrocephaly do not harbor pathologic conditions that warrant diagnostic imaging or evaluations by a neurosurgeon.[64] Haws et al examined 466 patients with benign macrocephaly diagnosed by ultrasonography, none of which required surgical intervention.[65] The relative frequency of macrocephaly led editors reviewing the work of Haws et al to advocate for close observation with a tape measure in the child with isolated macrocephaly and no neurologic findings.[66]

Despite the benign implications of macrocephaly in most infants, AHT is often associated with fluid collections in the extra-axial compartment, more specifically in the subdural space, leading to macrocephaly in some patients.

Repetitive episodes of AHT are well described in the literature, and either repetitive or single injuries with venous and/or arachnoid tears may lead to the formation of subdural collections and macrocephaly.[30] Increasing head circumference is a useful sign that a hemorrhagic subdural collection may be related to a previous subdural hemorrhage and, therefore, to a previous episode of trauma.[67] Hobbs and colleagues reported on 186 children with a diagnosis of subdural hemorrhage collected from a national registry in Great Britain from 1998–1999.[68] Thirty-eight children (20%) were noted to have macrocephaly at presentation.

b) Soft Tissue Injuries

Soft tissue findings in AHT can include scalp swelling, scalp contusions/hematomas, subgaleal hematomas, intra-oral injuries (including frenular contusions/tears, intra-oral mucosal contusions, tooth injuries, and palatal/pharyngeal injuries), subconjunctival hemorrhage, and bruises to the face, ear, neck, or torso. Although many cases of AHT will have no visible soft tissue manifestations about the head, bruising to the head and neck is reported in 29% to 54% of cases of AHT and is the most common site of bruising in children who have been abused.[69,70] However, bruising to the head is also common in nAHT.

Meta-analysis has shown that bruising about the head, *in general*, in a child younger than 3 years with intracranial injury is *not* a discriminating factor between AHT and nAHT (PPV for AHT was 37%; OR, 0.8; $P > .2$).[71,72] However, clinical distinctions between nAHT and AHT bruising can emerge depending on a child's age and the distribution of bruising on certain areas of the head.

Pierce et al found bruising in any region of the body in children 4 months and younger as suggestive of abusive versus accidental bruising.[73,74] Larger systematic reviews have focused more on a child's mobility (rather than a specific age) in correlation to susceptibility to abusive or accidental bruising.[69,75] Accidental bruising is rare (0–1.3%) in premobile infants (ie, those who do not yet crawl, cruise, or ambulate).[76–80] Thus, any bruising in premobile infants will raise concerns for physical abuse/AHT, and thus, an appropriate evaluation is warranted.

With regard to distribution of bruising, large meta-analyses have identified certain body regions that are more characteristic of accidental bruising.[69,75] In mobile children, these include the shins, knees, and bony prominences. When the face is involved, accidental bruising characteristically follows a "T" distribution (ie, the forehead, nose, upper lip, and chin). Even in mobile children, accidental bruising to certain body regions—the soft tissue of the cheek, ears, neck, abdomen, buttocks, and genitalia—is extremely uncommon.[75]

However, abusive bruising tends to appear in a different body distribution and a more nuanced distribution about the head.[69,73,74,77,81–83] In a prospective, multicenter study, Pierce et al validated a clinical decision rule that was designed to distinguish abusive from nonabusive bruising.

They found that bruising in the "TEN-4-FACESp" regions (described as any bruising in an infant 4 months or younger; bruising to the torso, ear, or neck in a child younger than 4 years; and bruising to the frenulum, angle of jaw, cheeks, eyelids, subconjunctiva, or patterned bruising) had a 96% sensitivity and 87% specificity for identifying abusive injury.[73] Two other comparative studies of cohorts of children who were abused and not abused found similar results—that bruising to the ear, face, neck, torso, and buttocks was significantly more common in children who were abused (P <.001).[82,83] Thus, although in general, bruising about the head is not, in itself, a discriminating feature, certain regions of the head (ears, fleshy cheek, angle of jaw, and neck) assist in discriminating between the likelihood of AHT and nAHT.

The number of bruises may also assist in distinguishing AHT from nAHT.[73,74,76,77,79] Although the number of bruises children sustain through normal activity increases as they get older and their level of independent mobility increases, children experiencing accidents have a mean of 1 to 3 and a median of 1 to 5 bruises per child, with a range of 1 to 16.[73,77] Children who have been abused have a median of 3 to 11 bruises per child, with larger medians at each developmental stage.[73]

It is noteworthy that the current clinical practice of assessing a suspected bruise is based on both optics (eg, color perception) and pattern matching. Clinical detection and assessment of bruising in children with darker skin tones can be particularly challenging because of the difficulty in visualizing these injuries in some cases.[84,85] Visualization of bruising may be aided with appropriate lighting. It is important to note that some cultural and nontraditional medical practices, such as cupping and coining, can be misdiagnosed as abusive injury, so it is prudent for providers to be aware of how these appear.[86]

Finally, as bleeding disorders are often a diagnostic consideration in children with suspected AHT, a limited number of studies have examined the location, pattern, and number of bruises in children with known bleeding disorders.[87,88] One study looked specifically at the characteristics of bruising in preschool children with inherited bleeding disorders.[88] In this study, there were 5613 bruises recorded from children with inherited bleeding disorders and 3523 bruises from children without a bleeding disorder. Children with severe bleeding disorders had more and larger bruises than children without bleeding disorder at all developmental stages. However, even children with bleeding disorders rarely had bruises on the ears, neck, cheeks, eyes, or genitalia.

Takeaway Points

1. Sentinel injury research has identified bruising as a key sentinel finding in infants, occurring in upwards of 28% of "definite" abuse cases.
2. Although not specific for AHT, and typically benign in many infants, macrocephaly can be an initial finding in children with AHT who have chronic subdural collections.
3. Bruising that is more likely to occur in AHT versus nAHT can be distinguished on the basis of a child's age, developmental abilities, and distribution of bruising.
4. Bruising in nonmobile children has a strong association with abuse over accident.
5. Bruising in the TEN-4-FACESp distribution has high sensitivity and specificity for abusive injury. Thus, in general, bruising in such locations, absent a clear and consistent accidental history, warrants an evaluation for possible abuse.
6. Children with severe, inherited bleeding disorders have more and larger bruises than children without a bleeding disorder; however, even children with inherited bleeding disorders rarely bruise on the ears, neck, fleshy cheeks, eyes, or genitalia.

c) Intracranial Hemorrhage/Hematoma

Subdural hemorrhage has been reported to be the most common intracranial manifestation of AHT, occurring in more than 80% in some series.[89–92] In comparative studies, including a 2011 systematic review by Kemp et al, subdural hemorrhage more commonly occurs following abusive rather than accidental head injury.[50,93–101] Duhaime et al found 13 of 16 cases (81%) of subdural hemorrhage resulted from abusive injury in 100 consecutively hospitalized infants and young children younger than 2 years.[96] Reece et al found subdural hemorrhage in 46% (25/54) of definite AHT cases compared with 10% (23/233) in infants and young children with accidental causes.[98] Feldman et al found 76% of subdural hemorrhage that occurred without a readily identifiable cause occurred as a result of abuse. In contrast, epidural hemorrhage more commonly occurs from nAHT. [94–96,99,100] Subarachnoid hemorrhage, which is common in many types of trauma, is reported as not being a distinguishing feature of AHT versus nAHT in several series.[94–96,100,102]

In AHT, subdural hemorrhage is often multifocal, may be both supratentorial and infratentorial in location, but is frequently located over the cerebral convexities or vertex location, and posteriorly along the tentorium and parieto-occipital locations. [92,95,97,103–106] An association between interhemispheric location and abusive head trauma has been shown in multiple studies.[95] The subdural hemorrhage found in AHT may be small in volume, often with a more severe parenchymal insult, although, it also can be larger in volume, requiring emergent surgical decompression.[107]

Traumatic subdural hemorrhage most often results from bridging vein injury, although nontraumatic etiologies also exist.[108–110] Small, localized vertex clots on imaging, typically centered along parasagittal bridging veins, are thought to represent focal vein injury and were reported in over 80% (45/55) of abusive head trauma patients compared with only 36.4% (8/22) with accidental causes.[111–113] In one series, concurrent findings of retinal and subdural hemorrhages with parasagittal vertex clots significantly increased the odds of a patient having abusive injuries.[111] However, no vertex clots were present in 88 controls who presented with accidental trauma and had no subdural hemorrhage on computed tomography (CT).

d) Edema, Hypoxic Injury, and Cortical Injury

Patterns of cytotoxic edema and hypoxic-ischemic injury are observed much more frequently following abusive head injuries and strongly contribute to the significant morbidity and mortality seen in this population.[95,107,114–116] In a comparative study, patterns of restricted diffusion indicating cytotoxic edema and/or hypoxic-ischemic injury occurred in 37% (11/30) of abusive cases versus 9% (2/22) of those with accidental trauma undergoing brain magnetic resonance imaging (MRI).[107] Of those with abuse, a pattern of diffuse, bilateral hypoxic-ischemic injury predominated, a pattern also described in several other series.[114,115,117,118] However, asymmetric cortical involvement and unilateral hemispheric involvement also may be observed.[116,119] This diffuse pattern of injury/insult is not in a typical vascular distribution and likely has multifactorial causes, including apnea, hypoperfusion, craniocervical injury, and/or excitatory or metabolic cascades resulting in permanent neuronal injury. [120–123] Although parenchymal findings may be subtle on initial CT, changes occurring as early as 72 minutes following the traumatic insult have been described, becoming more conspicuous over the initial 24-hour period.[90]

Parenchymal contusions, lacerations, and traumatic axonal injury also may be seen following abusive head injury, but these traumatic lesions are infrequent.[107,114,124] Parenchymal contusions, when present, often coexist with other traumatic lesions such as skull fractures or adjacent/overlying extra-axial hemorrhage.[107,114,116,117] Slit-like tears or clefts near the cortical-white matter junction, predominantly in the anterior temporal and frontal lobes, occur in young infants and appear as small fluid-like clefts with layering hemorrhage.[109,125] They may occur from inflicted head injuries, but also are described in the perinatal period following instrument-assisted deliveries.[125,126]

e) Spinal Injury

Spinal injuries occur in abusive and accidental trauma and may involve the vertebral column, ligamentous structures, and intraspinal contents.[121,127–131] Cervical ligamentous injury is more common in abusive (78% or 52/67 cases) compared with cases of accidental trauma (46% or 21/46 cases) undergoing spinal MRI.[121] Abused patients with a diffuse pattern of hypoxic-ischemic brain injury increasingly have been shown to have a significant association with MRI findings of cervical spine injuries, occurring in just over 80% of cases in one series.[129] However, spinal injuries are missed on initial clinical evaluation in over 50% of cases, as they may be clinically silent and/or difficult to detect because of coexistent, devastating brain injuries.[128,131]

Spinal subdural hemorrhage was observed in 60% of children with AHT undergoing spinal MRI but was infrequently observed in cases of accidental injury.[128] It may result from tracking of intracranial hemorrhage into the spine rather than from direct spinal trauma.[109]

Unlike ligamentous injuries in abuse, which more commonly occur in the cervical or craniocervical junction locations, spinal fractures from abuse are more commonly located in older children in the thoracic and lumbar spine, with 22 of 25 being spinal thoracic and lumbar compression deformities in a series by Kleinman et al.[127,130–133] Overall, vertebral fractures are uncommon relative to other skeletal injuries in child physical abuse, accounting for between 0.4% and 2.7% of fractures on skeletal surveys in several series. [127,130,131,134–136] However, spinal fractures may be the only additional finding on a skeletal survey to suggest abuse.[136]

f) Ocular Findings

1. Anatomy. The retina is a multilayered structure that forms the inner lining of the eye. It extends from the posterior pole of the eye anteriorly to the front third of the eye (ie, toward the iris). The retina is composed of 10 layers. The innermost layer, the internal limiting membrane (ILM), is the structural interface between the retina and the vitreous, which in young children is a gelatinous structure filling the posterior segment of the eye, and the retinal pigment epithelium is the outermost layer adjacent to the choroid, which is the layer of tissue between the sclera and the retina. The retinal vasculature is a complex network of vessels and capillaries that permeate the inner retina. Retinal hemorrhages most commonly occur within the retinal layers.[137] The posterior pole encompasses the optic nerve and the macula. The region around the optic nerve is called the peripapillary region. The macula is defined clinically as the region between the major temporal vascular arcades. Anteriorly, the ora serrata is the peripheral termination of the retina at its junction with the ciliary body (the part of the eye that connects the iris to the choroid). The retina between the macula posteriorly and the ciliary body anteriorly is referred to as the peripheral retina, which may be subdivided into the near, mid, and far peripheries, where the near periphery is adjacent to the macula and the far periphery is adjacent to the ciliary body.

Blood that has entered the potential space between the vitreous and the retina is referred to as preretinal or subhyaloid hemorrhage, the hyaloid surface being the outer surface of the vitreous. Such hemorrhages may obscure the underlying retinal structures and appear denser on examination. Hemorrhages found under the retina between the retina and choroid are called subretinal hemorrhages; they commonly appear slightly fainter and partially obscured by overlying structures, such as the retinal vasculature. Mechanical injury to the retina from inertial forces causing traction between the vitreous and the retina results in extravascular leakage of blood that may be trapped in and between the different retinal layers (intraretinal hemorrhage), under the retina (subretinal), or above the retina but under the vitreous (preretinal).[138,139]

The clinical appearance of intraretinal hemorrhage varies depending on the location of the hemorrhage within the retinal layers. Superficial blood within the nerve fiber layer is flame or splinter shaped because of the orientation of fibers, and hemorrhages in the deeper layers of the retina have a dot or blot configuration because of the configuration of cells in those layers. When there is retinoschisis, or splitting of the retinal layers, hemorrhage may collect in the potential space of the retinoschisis cavity and appear as a blister-like cavity. Traumatic retinoschisis in AHT is often between the ILM and the other layers of the retina but may occur between other layers as well.

2. Findings. Although also seen in nAHT, retinal hemorrhages are the most frequent and most sensitive acute sign of AHT. In a systematic review of 20 observational studies (level II-III evidence) that included eye examinations of 973 children who had experienced AHT, retinal hemorrhages were seen in about 80% of children, with a mean sensitivity of 75% for AHT.[137] The extent, distribution, and pattern of retinal hemorrhages and other associated ophthalmic findings determine their specificity, which can be as high as 94% for abuse.[137]

In addition to retinal and vitreous hemorrhages, the ocular findings of AHT may include retinal folds, retinoschisis, papilledema, and optic nerve sheath and orbital fat hemorrhage on autopsy. Vitreoretinal findings of trauma not visible with indirect ophthalmoscopy, such as vitreoretinal traction, vitreous separation, and subclinical retinoschisis, may require specialized retinal imaging (ie, optical coherence tomography) to identify and may be seen on autopsy in fatal injuries.[140–142] Poor vision on presentation, decreased pupillary response, papilledema, and severe retinal hemorrhages and retinal folds are ophthalmologic findings of AHT associated with increased mortality.[143–146] Longer-term sequelae associated with AHT include optic nerve atrophy and retinal scarring.

Retinal folds appear as arcuate or circular hypopigmented ridges or lines, usually around the macula and less commonly in the more peripheral retina. They may be found at the edges of an area of traumatic retinoschisis but may also occur in the absence of a clinically evident schisis cavity.[147–149] Retinal folds may be unilateral or bilateral. They occur in about 3% of clinical cases of AHT, but the incidence increases to 23% to 42% in severe or fatal cases of AHT.[137,147]

Retinal folds or lines around the schisis cavity may help differentiate it from subhyaloid blood. A "hemorrhagic macular cyst" is a dense macular schisis hemorrhage, sometimes with a meniscal interface between red blood cells and serum.

Papilledema, a term referring to optic disc swelling specifically attributable to raised intracranial pressure, is found in less than 10% of patients with AHT.[150] It usually takes a minimum of 12 to 24 hours to develop in patients with increased intracranial pressure following head injury; therefore, if noted on initial presentation, it may suggest delay in seeking care after the injury occurred. Papilledema is an ominous finding associated with high mortality.[143,151]

3. Mechanism. Retinal hemorrhages arising from head trauma may be caused by one or multiple mechanisms. Vitreoretinal traction from head and ocular acceleration/deceleration injury, as would be caused by shaking and/or head impact, is the leading mechanism, supported by clinical, imaging, and animal study evidence.[140,141] The vitreous is attached to the retina throughout the interface between the 2 structures, but there are areas of particularly strong attachment, which are directly perceptible by surgeons at the time of vitreoretinal surgery. These areas include the posterior pole, especially around the optic nerve head and along the major vascular arcades, and anteriorly at the vitreous base, which straddles the ora serrata and attaches to both the far peripheral retina and the adjacent ciliary body. Retinal hemorrhages in abusive head trauma often appear predominantly in these areas, sometimes producing a pattern in which hemorrhages are in the posterior pole and in the far retinal periphery but relatively sparce in the mid-peripheral retina.[152]

The mechanism of traumatic retinoschisis in AHT is vitreoretinal traction generated by firm adhesions between the vitreous and the posterior retina as the child's head is submitted to acceleration-deceleration forces. This phenomenon results in in splitting of the retinal layers.[140] Most commonly, this split is between the ILM and underlying retinal layers. Damage to blood vessels traversing the split layers may result in blood filling the schisis cavity. Perimacular retinal folds likewise occur in an area of strong vitreoretinal attachment. The resulting retinoschisis results from traction, and optical coherence tomography provides direct visualization and evidence of vitreoretinal traction.[140–142] Animal studies of inertial injury also demonstrate ocular hemorrhages in areas of strong vitreoretinal attachment in the animals, posteriorly and anteriorly at the vitreous base.[153]

Birth-related retinal hemorrhages occur in patterns often resembling those of AHT or nAHT.[154–156] The mechanism of these hemorrhages is not established. However, vitreoretinal traction may be one cause if direct eye compression causes distortion and lengthening along a single axis. Other proposed mechanisms include ocular compression with prolonged highly raised intraocular pressure and subsequent decompression retinopathy, which is known to cause retinal hemorrhage in patients with glaucoma with acutely lowered intraocular pressure following glaucoma surgery, and release of leukotrienes or other vasoactive factors resulting in increased retinal vessel permeability.

Central retinal venous occlusion, which is a common cause of retinal hemorrhage in adults, is another possible contributing cause in AHT. However, central retinal vein occlusion produces a characteristic radiating pattern of retinal hemorrhages that is usually absent in head trauma and is accompanied by retinal venous tortuosity and optic disc swelling, which also are not commonly present in head trauma.[151] Branch retinal venous occlusion produces a sectoral pattern not reported in head trauma. Increased intracranial pressure, whether acute or subacute, does not produce retinal hemorrhage in patterns seen in AHT and is discussed below.

4. Incidence. As stated earlier, retinal hemorrhages are seen in about 80% (45%–100%) of children with AHT.[137] The prevalence of retinal hemorrhages in healthy children (ie, without trauma or other medical cause) is estimated at less than 0.1%.[157] A study of 7758 retinal examination of children between 1 and 24 months of age suggests that retinal hemorrhage does not spontaneously occur in healthy children after the postnatal period; even a single hemorrhage should be considered of medical significance and a plausible etiology sought.

Retinal hemorrhages in AHT occur along a spectrum of severity, ranging from mild to severe. Hemorrhages are usually bilateral, although they can be asymmetric or completely unilateral in up to 30% of cases.[137] In approximately two-thirds of cases of AHT, the hemorrhages are too numerous to count, are multilayered, and extend into the retinal periphery, often to the ora serrata.[143] Patients may have vitreous hemorrhage that can obscure the underlying retinal hemorrhages. However, retinal hemorrhages associated with AHT can also be few in number, exclusively intraretinal, and confined to the posterior pole.[58,150–152,158–160]

Retinal hemorrhages are rare in young children with normal neuroimaging and no evidence of head trauma on physical examination.[159,161,162] In one study of 190 children evaluated for AHT, all 15 children with retinal hemorrhages had positive neuroimaging, and none of 85 children with negative neuroimaging had retinal hemorrhages.[162] In a larger study of 353 children without traumatic brain injury (TBI) on neuroimaging, retinal hemorrhages were found in only 2 children (0.6%; 95% CI, 0.1–2.0).[163] Similarly, in one study of 78 infants with isolated long-bone fractures and dilated fundus examinations, none had retinal hemorrhages.[164] This evidence supports the conclusion that dedicated retinal examinations are not needed in children without evidence of traumatic head injury.

5. Signs and symptoms. Children with AHT commonly show no externally visible ocular sign or symptom.[143,165] Signs of external eye trauma, such as periorbital ecchymosis, eyelid edema, or subconjunctival hemorrhage, usually indicate direct trauma to the face or eye, as opposed to inertial or impact injury to the head.[166,167] Corneal injuries, hyphema (blood in the anterior chamber), secondary glaucoma, lens subluxation, traumatic cataract, and pupillary abnormalities have all been reported as a result of child physical abuse. Anterior segment injuries, when present, are rarely isolated and tend to be associated with severe trauma and a poor prognosis.

6. Description. The term "multilayered retinal hemorrhages" refers to hemorrhages that are present at multiple locations (intra, preretinal, and/or subretinal).[151] Hemorrhage within the vitreous (vitreous hemorrhage) may appear as more indistinct localized globules of hemorrhage or sometimes appears as diffuse dispersed hemorrhage. Retinal hemorrhages are detected and characterized with examination of the retina and vitreous best performed through a dilated pupil using an indirect ophthalmoscope, which provides a binocular, 3-dimensional view of the posterior segment of the eye and permits appreciation of the physical locations and morphologic characterization of these different types of hemorrhages. Vitreous hemorrhage, when present, may partially or fully obscure a view of retinal hemorrhages or the retina itself. Specification of these various configurations and locations within the posterior pole is important, because it helps to describe the geographic distribution and patterns of retinal hemorrhage associated with different causes. Of note, some patients may have "white-centered" retinal hemorrhages.[168] Such hemorrhages are not diagnostic of septic emboli or of an infectious origin. White-centered retinal hemorrhages, in fact, are nonspecific and may be caused by central clearing of the blood within any intraretinal hemorrhage from any cause, or artifactual light reflection from an ophthalmoscope or retinal camera. Thus, describing such findings as "Roth spots," a historical eponym associated with endocarditis and septic emboli, can be misleading.

7. Differential diagnosis of RHs. i) Trauma. Although many systemic and ocular conditions may result in retinal hemorrhages in children, the most common cause of retinal hemorrhage in infants and young children is trauma, birth-related in the first month of life; AHT after the first month; and less commonly, nAHT.[137,155,156,169–171]

The pattern and distribution of the hemorrhages, presence of other retinal findings, clinical history, nonocular physical examination, and laboratory tests help to distinguish traumatic from nontraumatic causes of retinal hemorrhage. Vitreous hemorrhage may also be present in AHT but is less commonly seen than retinal hemorrhage. Retinoschisis and retinal folds are also less common but are highly specific for severe trauma, including AHT.[137] Apart from their diagnostic significance, retinoschisis and retinal folds are indictors of poor prognosis and associated with severe neurologic injury and mortality.[143,144] Retinal detachment is another less common sign and may signify a late presentation.[172]

Generally, increased severity of retinal hemorrhages correlates with increased severity of head trauma.[150,173] Extensive hemorrhages that are "too numerous to count," found at multiple layers, and extend to the peripheral ora serrata are highly specific for severe head trauma, including AHT and unambiguous severe nAHT.[40,174,175] However, the features of multilayered or peripheral RHs in isolation do not define a level of severity and, in and of themselves, are not diagnostic of AHT; the number and geographic distribution must also be considered.[158] Retinal hemorrhages are less common in AHT characterized only by blunt impact, similar to the low incidence observed in accidental falls.[137,151] Retinal hemorrhages occasionally occur from witnessed accidental "household" falls (ie, typically representing low-height or short-distance falls), but in this setting typically are sparse and not in the pattern more specific to AHT.[93,96,175] Retinal hemorrhages tend to occur more frequently in children who have died versus unimpaired survivors.[143,150,151,176,177]

A systematic review of 20 observational studies comprised ocular findings in 1948 children, including 242 children with nAHT and 973 children with AHT as determined by perpetrator confession, third-party witness, legal decision, autopsy findings, or multidisciplinary assessment.[137] This review found that intraocular hemorrhage was present in 44% to 100% of children with AHT but in less than 10% of children with nonabusive head injury. It should be noted that the children with accidental trauma in most comparative series typically have different types of intracranial injuries than do children with AHT, only infrequently having subdural hemorrhages. However, with this caveat in mind, the sensitivity of intraocular hemorrhages for AHT was 75%; the specificity for AHT was 94%. The specificity for AHT was highest for intraocular hemorrhage that was bilateral, multilayered (preretinal in addition to intraretinal), extended beyond the posterior pole, and of moderate to severe number/extent.

In addition to the multilayered, numerous in number, and extending to the periphery retinal hemorrhages, retinal folds and retinoschisis are also highly specific for severe head trauma, most commonly AHT.[178–180] They also have been reported after unequivocal severe accidental head injury, such as fatal motor vehicle crashes, head crush injury, and high-elevation (eg, 10 m) falls, and more rarely in association with certain established medical diagnoses, including a ruptured intracranial aneurysm and leukemia.[152,181] Thus, when macular retinoschisis or perimacular retinal folds are present in a child without a history of major accidental head trauma, the likelihood of AHT is very high. The presence of retinal folds typically implies severe injury that often results in death or neurologic sequelae, although some surviving patients may experience good visual recovery.[143,144]

ii) Increased intracranial pressure. Raised intracranial pressure causes specific patterns of retinal hemorrhages that are different from head trauma. Raised intracranial pressure is associated with superficial intraretinal hemorrhages on or adjacent to a clearly swollen optic nerve head and, therefore, are in a peripapillary distribution.[182] Current evidence and extensive clinical experience with patients with raised intracranial pressure unrelated to trauma does not support raised intracranial pressure as a cause of widespread or multilayered retinal hemorrhages.[183,184] A very rapid elevation of intracranial pressure resulting from intracranial hemorrhage can cause intraocular hemorrhage in a condition referred to as Terson syndrome.[185–190] The pattern of hemorrhages in Terson syndrome is mainly of vitreous and preretinal hemorrhage adjacent to the optic nerve head or in the posterior pole with no or few intraretinal hemorrhages. Terson syndrome is uncommon in infants and children and does not refer to a specific cause, such as a ruptured arteriovenous malformation.[151,191,192]

iii) Other systemic illness. Patients with severe coagulopathies may rarely be found to have retinal hemorrhages, which are usually few in number and confined to the posterior pole; although they may be more widespread in children with leukemia.[193] It is not clear to what degree coagulopathy might worsen the severity of retinal hemorrhage attributable to head trauma, but even coagulopathy is not known to cause spontaneous extensive retinal hemorrhages.[194] Sepsis, meningitis, and endocarditis may be associated with hemorrhages that are typically intraretinal and confined to the posterior pole but can also be more extensive.[195–197] In a prospective case series of 159 critically ill children without abusive head injury receiving ophthalmologic evaluation within 48 to 72 hours of admission, the prevalence of retinal hemorrhages was 15% (95% CI, 9.5%–21%).[193] Most of these children had fewer than 5 single-layered retinal hemorrhages, but 6 children (3.7%) were found to have more numerous or multilayered hemorrhages and had diagnoses of fatal nonabusive traumatic brain injury, severe coagulopathy, and/or sepsis associated with leukemia.[193] In retinitis attributable to cytomegalovirus, retinopathy of prematurity, and hypertensive retinopathy, retinal hemorrhages are accompanied by characteristic retinal lesions such as cotton wool spots, white retinal patches, lipid exudates, and neovascular tissue.[151] Generally, in medical causes of retinal hemorrhages, accompanying diagnostic clinical history, examination, and laboratory findings are present.

iv) Cardiopulmonary resuscitation. Cardiopulmonary resuscitation (CPR) uncommonly causes retinal hemorrhages in children, with a reported prevalence of approximately 3%.[193,198–201] In these cases, the retinal hemorrhages are few in number, single-layered, and confined to the posterior pole. In most instances there is an associated coagulopathy. Severe and abrupt increases in intrathoracic pressure may cause Purtscher retinopathy, which is characterized by white retinal patches and retinal edema most commonly around the optic disc, with retinal hemorrhages as a minor feature, and not the pattern strongly associated with AHT.[202]

v) Seizures, coughing, vomiting, and others. In multiple studies, severe coughing, forceful vomiting, and seizures have not been found to cause retinal hemorrhages.[203–207] Vaccinations also have not been found to cause retinal hemorrhages.[157] Diabetic retinopathy, a common cause of intraretinal hemorrhages in adults, does not occur in children at this age.[208] Glutaric acidemia type 1 (GA1) is an organic acidemia caused by biallelic pathogenic variants in the GCDH gene that is sometimes associated with retinal hemorrhages.[161] Case reports describing retinal hemorrhages in this disease entity mention few pre- or intraretinal hemorrhage confined to the posterior pole.[161] Neurosurgical procedures that might result in sudden changes in intracranial or intravascular pressure have not been found to be associated with retinal hemorrhages and are unlikely to confound the interpretation of retinal findings in children being evaluated for AHT who recently underwent neurosurgery.[209]

8. Dating retinal hemorrhages. Retinal hemorrhages cannot be accurately dated to determine the precise timing of the traumatic event. However, some conclusions can be drawn on the basis of the known rates of resolution of hemorrhages, depending on the type, size, location, and number of hemorrhages. Resolution timing ranges from less than 24 hours for some intraretinal hemorrhages to several months for nonclearing vitreous hemorrhage.[145] The resolution of retinal hemorrhages has been studied both in newborn infants and in children with nAHT or AHT, with identical findings in both settings with regard to the rate of resolution. General characteristics are as follows:

- Intraretinal hemorrhages resolve very quickly, starting within 24 to 48 hours, with numerous hemorrhages clearing within just days, significantly fewer hemorrhages remaining at 1 week, and nearly all hemorrhages clearing within 2 weeks. Isolated (single) dense intraretinal hemorrhages can persist longer, up to 2 months. On the basis of these findings, the presence of too-numerous-to-count intraretinal hemorrhages suggests an injury that has occurred recently, typically in the previous few days.[156,210]
- Preretinal hemorrhages can take considerably longer to clear, on the order of weeks or months.
- Intraretinal hemorrhages are uniformly present to some degree at presentation when retinal hemorrhages are present. Therefore, initially, preretinal hemorrhages in AHT are always accompanied by intraretinal hemorrhages. However, because they take longer to clear, the presence of preretinal hemorrhages with few or no intraretinal hemorrhages suggests a more chronic injury.[210]
- Because of variability in rate of resolution, the presence of bright red hemorrhages along with fading hemorrhages does not necessarily imply separate traumatic events.
- Blood in a schisis cavity and subretinal hemorrhage resolves more slowly; vitreous hemorrhage is the slowest to resolve.
- It takes time for retinal scars and optic atrophy to develop, so their presence suggests a distant previous injury.

TAKEAWAY POINTS

1. Retinal hemorrhages do not spontaneously occur in healthy children after the postnatal period.
2. Retinal hemorrhages are the most frequent and most sensitive acute ocular sign of AHT; they can be bilaterally symmetric, bilaterally asymmetric, or unilateral.
3. Retinal hemorrhages that are numerous, present in multiple layers of the retina, and extend peripherally beyond the posterior pole are highly specific (94%) for severe head trauma and particularly AHT.
4. Retinal hemorrhages cannot be accurately dated to determine the precise timing of the traumatic event, but the rate of resolution of different types of retinal hemorrhage can sometimes provide general guidance as to injury timing.
5. Retinal hemorrhages are rare in the absence of neuroimaging findings or other evidence of head trauma; thus, dedicated retinal examinations are not needed in children evaluated for physical abuse in whom there is an absence of neuroimaging findings or other evidence of head trauma.
6. Other ocular clinical findings may include vitreous hemorrhage, retinal folds, retinoschisis, and papilledema. Autopsy findings may also include optic nerve sheath

hemorrhage and orbital fat hemorrhage. With specialized retinal imaging (OCT), vitreoretinal traction, vitreous separation, and subclinical retinoschisis can also be identified.
7. Papilledema occurs infrequently in AHT (less than 10%).
8. Nontraumatic causes of retinal hemorrhages usually occur in patterns different from head trauma.

g) Skeletal findings. 1. Skull fractures. Like bruising, skull fractures are commonly seen in both AHT and nAHT. Skull fractures are identified in 25% to 40% of AHT cases.[90,94,211] In nAHT cases, skull fractures are most commonly linear and involve the parietal bone.[212] Isolated skull fractures, in general, while indicative of trauma, are not differentiating features between AHT and nAHT.[12,93,213–217]

Skull fractures may not be associated with major signs or symptoms at the time of the traumatic event, and although scalp swelling is common, not all skull fractures are associated with scalp swelling. Approximately 10% of children with skull fractures have no clinically appreciable or radiographic evidence of scalp or facial soft tissue swelling at the time of presentation.[218] It should be noted, however, that because scalp swelling itself can be an indication for imaging, the true incidence of skull fractures without associated scalp swelling remains unknown.[219–221]

Linear skull fractures may be associated with delayed onset of apparent scalp "swelling" as scalp hematomas liquefy and become more protuberant. This can occur days to several weeks after fracture with a median of 3 days, and is sometimes the only sign associated with a recent fracture. Absent scalp swelling does not necessarily imply a delay in seeking care, especially in active toddlers who may fall frequently with minimal or transient symptoms.[222–224]

It is unclear whether skull fractures in conjunction with intracranial hemorrhage are differentiating features of accidental versus AHT etiologies. Piteau et al found skull fractures plus intracranial injury to have an OR for abuse of 7.76 (95% CI, 1.06–57.08) in children 6 years or younger.[50] Yet, Maguire et al found that skull fracture and intracranial injury in children younger than 3 years had a PPV for AHT of 44% (95% CI, 22%–68%) and an OR of 0.8 (95% CI, 0.3–2.3).[71] Large comparative studies seem to indicate that it is not the fracture itself that is discriminatory but the presence and severity of intracranial injury that was associated with AHT (OR, 2.38; 95% CI, 2.09–2.70).[225]

It is well known that short-distance falls can rarely result in linear, parietal skull fractures with a small underlying extra-axial (most commonly epidural) hemorrhage or focal parenchymal contusion. However, nonfocal (ie, not underlying the skull fracture site) hemorrhage and/or more severe brain injury is an uncommon finding in short-distance falls and other minor accidental trauma.[226,227]

Finally, some older studies suggested that certain features of skull fractures—multiple skull fractures, depressed skull fractures, or skull fractures crossing the suture lines—are more strongly associated with or specific for AHT.[68,228] However, other studies have not confirmed these findings as differentiating features.[212]

2. Rib fractures. The incidence of rib fractures in AHT cases is less well-studied, but can occur in up to 28% of cases.[12,229] Multiple studies have found a strong association of rib fractures with AHT over nAHT.[12,50,51,68,71,217,230,231] Two separate meta-analyses concluded that in a child with intracranial injury and rib fracture, the ORs for AHT were in the range of 3 to 10.[50,71] Another meta-analysis on distinguishing abusive from accidental fractures in all children younger than 48 months (not just confined to AHT cohorts) concluded that, "in those aged less than 18 months with rib fractures the odds ratio (OR) for abuse was 23.7 (95% CI, 9.5, 59.2)" and "the positive predictive value for rib fractures in relation to suspected or confirmed abuse is 66% (95% CI, 42.5–89.7)."[232] Limitations to the larger meta-analyses include small numbers of rib fractures recorded in some studies and use of an imputation strategy to account for the fact that not all cases of nAHT had skeletal surveys.

Rib fractures associated with AHT can occur along the entire anatomic rib arc—anteriorly, anterolaterally, posterolaterally, and posteriorly.[233] The mechanism for rib fractures is predominantly anteroposterior compression of the thoracic cavity.[234] Although not exclusively specific for AHT, posterior fractures at the costovertebral junction have a high specificity for abuse and are thought to result from a squeezing injury leveraging the posteromedial rib over the spinal transverse process.[235] In a review of 1463 fractures in 141 infants who were abused, costovertebral junction rib fractures were the single most common site for a rib fracture; however, the majority of rib fractures were in a location other than the costovertebral junction.[236] Costovertebral junction fractures are much less common in nonabuse cases. When rib fractures occur unilaterally and are located either anteriorly or laterally, then blunt trauma to the chest can also be considered. Finite element modeling studies have further supported the anteroposterior compression mechanism because of their demonstration of stress profiles consistent with fracture locations seen in AHT cases.[212]

Birth trauma and CPR are potential differential diagnostic considerations in suspected AHT cases. In both circumstances, rib fractures are an extremely uncommon occurrence.[237–240] In CPR, rib fractures are almost always anterolateral. Although some evidence argues that 2-handed techniques of CPR may increase the risk of posterior rib fractures, the occurrence of multiple posterior fractures remains rare.[236,240–243]

3. Long bone fractures. Long bone fractures occur in approximately 17% to 36% of AHT cases.[12,120,217] A large meta-analysis aiming to distinguish abusive from nonabusive fractures in children younger than 15 years (and not specifically in AHT cohorts) found that age and fracture locations can be discriminatory features between patients who have been abused and those who have not.[232] Fractures were much more common in children younger than 18 months who were abused than in those who were not.

In children younger than 18 months, tibia/fibular fractures had an OR of 12.8 (95% CI, 5.1, 32.6) for abuse.[232] And radial/ulnar fractures had an OR of 5.8 (95% CI, 2.4, 14.3) for abuse in those younger than 4 years. Abusive femoral fractures are more likely to occur in children who are not yet walking, and spiral or oblique humeral fractures in children younger than 5 years more commonly occur in abused children. However, supracondylar humeral fractures in children are more associated with accidental injury. Finally, metaphyseal fractures, or classic metaphyseal lesions, are more commonly described in abuse than in accidents.[232]

The aggregate of these data demonstrates that in a child with intracranial injury and long bone fracture, the positive predictive value for AHT was 59% (95% CI, 48%–69%) and OR 1.7 (95% CI, 0.8–3.6).[72] However, as with rib fractures, these larger meta-analyses are limited by small numbers of long bone fractures recorded in some studies and the imputation strategy used to account for the fact that not all cases of nAHT had skeletal surveys.

TAKEAWAY POINTS

1. Isolated skull fractures, in general, while indicative of trauma, are not differentiating features between AHT and nAHT.
2. No skull fracture type is pathognomonic for AHT, and short-distance household falls frequently present with linear skull fractures, with parietal location most common.
3. Two separate meta-analyses have concluded that, in a child with intracranial injury and rib fracture, there are significant ORs for AHT (in the range of 3 to 10).
4. The primary mechanism for rib fractures is anteroposterior chest compression, and rib fractures associated with AHT can occur along the entire anatomic rib arc.
5. Although a diagnostic consideration, rib fractures related to birth and CPR are an extremely uncommon occurrence.
6. In a child younger than 18 months, femoral, humeral, radius/ulna, and tibia/fibula fractures are much more common in children who have been abused than those who have not.

BIOMECHANICS

Introduction

Determining whether injuries are attributable to accident or abuse in children requires a multidisciplinary team; *if available,* engineers with appropriate expertise can play an important role on this team. Although engineers with injury biomechanics expertise can aid in determining whether a child's head injuries could have been caused by the caregiver-provided history, they are uncommonly involved with daily clinical pediatrics. When available, these engineers should have expertise in pediatric injury biomechanics that includes experience with children who have had injuries attributable to accidental causes, as well as experience with children who have been injured from abuse. It is important for engineers to be knowledgeable of the types of injuries that can result from accidental causes (eg, household falls) in children to be able to effectively differentiate them from abusive injuries.

The Importance of Biomechanical Compatibility of Injury With History

An engineer's role is to determine *biomechanical compatibility* between the caregiver-stated cause and the *constellation of injuries.*[244,245] In the presence of a short-distance fall history, determining biomechanical compatibility rests on answering whether the single fall described by the caregiver biomechanically accounts for *all* of the child's injuries. A comprehensive evaluation of biomechanical compatibility will account for *all injuries* and not just the severe or fatal head injuries.

To determine biomechanical compatibility between the stated cause of injury and the constellation of injuries, a comprehensive biomechanical assessment that includes evaluating biodynamic compatibility and a quantitative biomechanical assessment is needed.[244] For example, if a short-distance fall history is provided, the biodynamic compatibility evaluation must determine whether the fall dynamics (how a child's body falls from their initial pre-fall position to their final post-fall resting position) can account for all of the child's injuries (including all bruises, lacerations excepting those associated with medical intervention) and the evidence of impact to the body. Soft tissue injuries and fractures (in most cases) are indicative of impact and provide a roadmap of the child's exposure to forces. Unless a child impacts an object during a fall descent, evidence of impact (eg, bruise, fracture) typically is limited to 1 or 2 adjoining planes of the body.[246–248] For example, if an infant fell from a bed directly onto a hardwood floor landing in a prone position, evidence of impact would be expected to be limited to the anterior plane of the body. If the child was found to have bruising on 3 or 4 planes of the body, the bed fall history would be biomechanically incompatible with these injuries.

When a quantitative biomechanical assessment is warranted, engineers attempt to reconstruct the fall to estimate levels of acceleration, velocity, and forces applied to the body and head using physics-based calculations, anthropomorphic test device (ATD; test dummy) experiments, and/or computer simulations. These estimates of biomechanical measures can then be compared to pediatric head injury thresholds and corroborated or video-recorded events with documented head acceleration/velocity/forces and known injuries to estimate the likelihood of injury. However, it is important to remember various techniques used to estimate biomechanical measures have advantages/disadvantages, and limitations must be considered.[244]

Lastly, a critical review of the evidenced-based injury biomechanics and clinical scientific literature will assist in determining whether the assessment of likelihood of injury is consistent. Combining findings from their biodynamic compatibility and quantitative biomechanical assessments, along with review of the evidenced-based scientific literature, will enable engineers to formulate an opinion as to the *biomechanical compatibility* of the constellation of injuries and caregiver history. This opinion is best framed as either *biomechanically compatible, likely biomechanically compatible, indeterminate biomechanical compatibility, unlikely biomechanical compatibility, or biomechanically incompatible.*

Types of Injury Biomechanics Studies Used to Investigate AHT

Various types of injury biomechanics studies are used to investigate injury risk, to evaluate the effectiveness of safety devices, and to study how injuries may occur, how the human body responds to accelerations/forces, and which factors may influence injury risk. These studies can be categorized as in-depth event investigation and/or reconstruction, human surrogate experiments, computational models and simulations, animal injury models, and postmortem human subject (PMHS) experiments.[249–251] It is important to remember, like all scientific studies, biomechanical studies have limitations, each of which must be carefully considered when drawing conclusions regarding likelihood of injury.

In-Depth Event Investigations and/or Dynamic Reconstructions

In-depth event investigations and/or dynamic reconstructions can provide an improved understanding of injuries resulting from a specific event and injury causation. Identification of environmental or human factors related to injury causation are often the goal of in-depth investigations. Reconstructions of event dynamics (eg, fall dynamics) can be accomplished using physics-based software or manual physics-based calculations to estimate key biomechanical measures (eg, head acceleration) associated with the event.[226]

Human Surrogate Experiments

A brief summary of human surrogate studies is provided in Table 1. Human surrogate experiments utilize ATDs or surrogates to represent a specific population (eg, age, mass percentile). Surrogates are a mechanical analogue of a human and provide opportunities to measure mechanical quantities such forces, strains, and accelerations during exposure to impact, accelerations, or other potentially injurious conditions using onboard instrumentation (eg, accelerometers, force sensors). ATDs are designed to represent the anthropometrics (geometry), mass, and mass distribution of the target human. It is extremely important they be as *biofidelic* (human-like) as possible in their response. The reliability and accuracy of biomechanical measures obtained from surrogate experiments are highly dependent on their biofidelity.

Although human surrogate studies have advanced our understanding of pediatric head biomechanics in shaking, forceful impact, and falls involving infants and children, some limitations exist and can influence interpretation of findings. It is important to note that differences in surrogate design can yield substantial differences in outcomes.

Biofidelity of the human surrogate is critical to the accurate prediction of injury probability, regardless of the mechanism (eg, falls, shaking, etc) being investigated.[252] Biomechanical properties of the neck and spine (ie, stiffness or flexibility) are particularly important when investigating head injury risk. A flexible and multisegmented neck and spine are key to achieving infant and child-like kinematics (motion of the body). Slight changes in surrogate design (eg, neck properties) can result in different biomechanical outcomes and thus, differing predictions of head injury risk.[253,254] Limitations related to surrogate biofidelity can influence findings from surrogate experiments.[252,255] Although considerable progress has been made to account for more of the details of these properties in infants of different ages, the exact biomechanical properties of the cervical spine of infants during maturation and with different characteristics remain incompletely understood. For this reason, although models can "bracket" the likely range of possibilities, it is not yet known with complete certainty how to create an exact biofidelic model for children of a specific age or to model a specific injury scenario.

The level of surrogate biofidelity attainable is dependent on the availability of biomechanical properties (ie, how the body responds to dynamic loading) of infants and young children, along with our ability to design mechanical analogues matching those properties.[255]

Surrogate studies cannot predict the injurious effects of repeated or ongoing cumulative trauma that may occur in AHT. Nor can they predict the independent injurious effects

TABLE 1. Human Surrogate Studies

1st Author, Date	Title	Age	Surrogate Design	Mechanism Investigated	Findings	Limitations
Duhaime, 1987	The shaken baby syndrome. A clinical, pathological, and biomechanical study.	1 mo	Just Born Doll with weighted thorax, modified head, neck and skull. Head was filled with cotton and water to achieve desired mass. 3 different neck designs (flexible rubber, stiff rubber, hinged) and thermoplastic skull vs no skull were evaluated.	Shaking, forceful impacts	Accelerations due to impact were approximately 50 times greater than those associated with shaking. SBS, at least in its most severe form, is not usually caused by shaking alone. Although shaking may be a part of the process, it is more likely that such infants experience blunt impact.	Unknown surrogate mass distribution, anthropometrics, neck properties, thorax properties, and joint properties. Extremities had negligible mass. Unclear whether chin-to-chest or occiput-to-back contact occurred.
Cory, 2003	Can shaking alone cause fatal brain injury? A biomechanical assessment of the Duhaime shaken baby syndrome model.	1 mo	Just Born Doll (same as used by Duhaime, 1987) with adjustable design parameters. Investigated varying head-neck joint location (ie, occipital condyle location), neck construction (rubber neck vs hinged neck), torso padding (cotton wool vs silicone), and location of the surrogate center of gravity (CG).	Shaking	Altering certain surrogate design parameters led to increased head accelerations that exceeded those measured by Duhaime et al (1987). Chin-to-chest and occiput-to-back contacts exceeded impact thresholds. Cannot categorically be stated 'pure shaking' cannot cause fatal head injuries in infant. "There must now be sufficient doubt in the reliability of the Duhaime et al (1987) study to warrant the exclusion of such testimony in cases of suspected shaken baby syndrome."	Unknown surrogate mass distribution, anthropometrics, neck properties, thorax properties, and joint properties.
Prange, 2003	Anthropomorphic simulations of falls, shakes, and inflicted impacts in infants.	1.5 mo	Custom-designed surrogate included torso, hinged neck, and head. Head from a toy doll (La Baby) with polypropylene skull and rubber scalp. Extremities were not represented. Mass of arms and legs incorporated into the torso. Torso was constructed of single wooden block.	Shaking, forceful impact, falls	Angular accelerations and velocities associated with shaking were not sufficient to cause trauma to an infant. Inflicted impacts against hard surfaces are more likely to be associated with inertial brain injuries than falls from a height of <1.5 m or from shaking. There are no data demonstrating that the angular acceleration and angular velocity experienced during shaking and impact against a padded surface … cause SDH or TAI in infants. Vigorous shakes produced rotational responses similar to those resulting from minor falls, but inflicted impacts produced responses that were significantly higher.	Surrogate torso was rigid and lacked any spine flexibility, which led to unrealistic kinematics. Extremities were not included in surrogate. Neck motion was limited to the sagittal plane.

(Continued on next page)

TABLE 1. Human Surrogate Studies (Continued)

1st Author, Date	Title	Age	Surrogate Design	Mechanism Investigated	Findings	Limitations
Lloyd, 2011	Biomechanical evaluation of head kinematics during infant shaking versus pediatric activities of daily living.	12 mo	CRABI-12 and National Center for SBS doll 7-month-old child	Shaking, activities of play	Aggressive shaking and resuscitative shaking are not likely to be the primary cause of DAI, primary RH, or SDH in a healthy infant. Rotational accelerations during shaking of ATD were indistinguishable from the accelerations endured by a 7-month-old boy at play.	CRABI-12 ATD designed for evaluating injury risk in seated posture in high-energy events (motor vehicle crashes). CRABI-12 ATD neck is overly stiff compared with an infant's neck. CRABI-12 ATD does not have a segmented spine and is overly stiff. Overall kinematics of shaking CRABI-12 ATD differ greatly from those expected in a child due to overly stiff neck and spine.
Miyazaki, 2015	The mechanism of shaken baby syndrome based on the visualization of intracranial brain motion.	12 mo	CRABI-12 with modified head, including transparent skull, deformable brain, CSF, falx, tentorium - reconstructed from CT images.	Shaking, falls	Relative displacement between skull and cerebrum were measured. Displacement of brain with respect to skull exceeded bridging vein (BV) rupture thresholds during shaking. Potential mechanism for brain injury is reverse rotation of brain relative to skull following chin-to-chest or occiput-to-torso contact. Peak BV stretch occurred just following maximum extension of head/neck when skull reverses direction of rotation. Relative brain motion associated with falls (0.4 m to 1.2 m height) generated BV stretch below thresholds.	CRABI-12 ATD neck is overly stiff compared with an infant's neck. CRABI-12 ATD does not have a segmented spine and is overly stiff. Overly stiff neck and spine led to unrealistic kinematics. Uncertainty regarding mechanical properties of the brain and its subregions.
Jenny, 2017	Biomechanical response of the infant head to shaking: An experimental investigation.	5th percentile Japanese newborn	Aprica 2.5 - custom designed 12 segment surrogate, including flexible 2-segment spine (thoracic and lumbar regions). Mechanical properties of surrogate documented using standardized ATD testing procedures - documented elsewhere.	Shaking	Angular head accelerations and velocities exceeded those measured by Duhaime et al and Prange et al. Maximum angular head accelerations and velocities occurred during chin-to-chest contact and suggest higher potential for injury in shaking than previously reported.	Mechanical properties of thorax not reported but available in other related publications. Mechanical properties of mandible not reported.

ATD indicates anthropomorphic test device; CSF, cerebrospinal fluid; CT, computed tomography; DAI, diffuse axonal injury; SBS, shaken baby syndrome; SDH, subdural hemorrhage; TAI, traumatic axonal injury.

of a combination of mechanisms (ie, shaking combined with forceful impacts or throwing a child). Cumulative deleterious effects associated with multiple mechanisms cannot currently be assessed using human surrogates.

To predict likelihood of brain injury from surrogate experiments, biomechanical outcomes such as head angular and translational accelerations are compared with available injury thresholds.[255,256] Unfortunately, published pediatric brain injury thresholds vary widely, depending on the injury model (eg, adult primates or immature swine or other animals), the techniques used to scale from adult brain size to child brain size (eg, mass, strain, geometry), the test conditions used to arrive at thresholds (eg, impact, indirect loading), and the injury type (eg, subdural hemorrhage, cerebral concussion).[257] Scaling from adult injury models may fail to capture anatomical differences of the immature skull (eg, open fontanelle) and brain (eg, composition, extent of myelination).[258,259] Additionally, the physiological response of an immature brain to dynamic loading has also been shown to differ from that of an adult brain, further undermining injury predictions based on scaled adult thresholds.[260]

Computational Models and Simulations

Computer models incorporating 3-dimensional (3D) digital humans or body segments (eg, head) in a virtual environment (eg, fall environment, motor vehicle crash) can be used to simulate potentially injurious events such as falls.[261–264] Anatomic accuracy and biofidelic response are key in the development of 3D digital human models. Similar to surrogates, 3D human models may be equipped with virtual sensors to predict biomechanical measures. The motion and response of human models are governed by user-defined body characteristics and the laws of physics; they are not animations.

Animal Injury Models

Animal models have been used to gain further understanding of injury mechanisms and injury thresholds since this information is otherwise not attainable using human subjects. Ensuring translatable outcomes to humans and animal welfare are key to animal injury models. The animal or animal specimen must represent the equivalent human structure and function with appropriate scaling for differences in mass, maturation, or material properties, and the animal's biologic response should parallel that of the human population as much as possible.

Animal models of inflicted injury have been used in a number of contexts, with most studies focusing on 2 main research areas. The first category employs animal models to gain insights into possible mechanisms of injury. Such studies reflect the premise that by subjecting an animal to similar mechanical phenomena (eg, forces, accelerations) that an infant or child might experience during an abusive event, the resultant injuries potentially reflect injuries that may happen in humans and, thus, enable investigators to better understand injury mechanisms. Such models might also advance our understanding of predictors of outcome or response to interventions.

The second main use of animal models is to facilitate the study of factors influencing pathophysiology and evolution of injury. Such factors might include maturational stage, specific types of insults, or stressors that might exacerbate damage. This approach applies a specific insult or combination of insults thought to be part of abusive head trauma and evaluates the effects of relevant controlled variables to assess the comparative evolution of injury and, in some instances, to investigate prognostic variables or response to treatment. Specific models are described in more detail below.

Postmortem Human Subject Experiments

PMHS experiments simulating potentially injurious events can provide insight into injury mechanisms, injury types resulting from exposure to mechanical phenomena such as acceleration or force, and injury thresholds. PMHS studies have the advantage of accurate anatomic representation and biomechanical response of the targeted human population. However, the lack of PMHS vascular perfusion and respiratory inflation, the presence of rigor mortis, and the use of preservation techniques could alter biomechanical response compared with living humans.

What Can We Learn From Biomechanical Studies Focused on AHT?

As discussed earlier, different types of biomechanical studies have been used to address questions related to pediatric head injury. These studies have investigated pediatric head injury risk related to forceful impact and shaking mechanisms.[250,251] It is important to note that this is not an exhaustive review of the biomechanics scientific literature related to pediatric head trauma.

Diffuse brain injuries and/or focal brain injuries can occur in AHT. These distinct types of injuries are caused by exposure to different physical phenomena. When a child is subjected to violence, the forces and accelerations they are exposed to are likely complex in nature and may include a combination of direct and indirect forces, along with angular and linear accelerations.

Biomechanical studies have demonstrated that direct or indirect forces applied to the body leading to rotation of the head and angular head acceleration can cause diffuse brain injuries, such as diffuse axonal injury, concussion, or a subdural/subarachnoid hemorrhage that often is in a more widespread distribution rather than being very focal.[265–268] Conversely, forces applied to the body that generate linear motion of the head and translational head acceleration can cause focal brain injuries, such as brain contusions or focal subdural hemorrhage. Impact forces applied directly to the head can also lead scalp contusions, subgaleal hemorrhage, and/or skull fractures as well as intracranial contusions and focal intracranial hemorrhages.

Forceful impacts onto hard surfaces are likely to cause skull fractures and focal brain injuries (eg, brain contusion, epidural hemorrhages, focal subarachnoid or subdural hemorrhage), but sudden deceleration against even a softer surface may also generate rotational accelerations at levels capable of producing diffuse brain injuries (eg, concussion, subdural hemorrhage, diffuse axonal injury).[269,270]

With the exception of one study, surrogate experiments focused on head injury risk typically measure global head accelerations and velocities.[271] Although early animal studies have shown that brain injury risk correlates with angular and translational head accelerations, the prediction of some brain injuries may be better correlated to other measures paralleling their specific anatomic mechanism/etiology of injury. For example, many subdural hemorrhages occur through tearing of bridging veins that accompanies rotational motion of the brain relative to the skull. Thus, measuring bridging vein strain (ie, stretch) and/or brain motion relative to the skull could provide an improved prediction of subdural hemorrhages risk related to rotation. Future surrogates incorporating anatomical detail with high biofidelity that enables investigation of physiologically relevant brain injury mechanisms are needed.[271]

a) Can shaking alone cause severe brain injury or fatality in infants?. Findings from biomechanical studies investigating shaking are mixed as to whether shaking alone can cause severe brain injury or fatality in infants. Studies have used animal models, surrogate models, postmortem tissue studies, and wearable instrumentation from human subjects to approach this question.[253,254,268–283] From a biomechanics perspective, a challenge to answering this question is the threshold at which specific brain injuries occur in infants and young children, as most pediatric brain injury thresholds are derived from adult humans or immature animals and may not account for differences in the infant brain composition or the infant physiological response to trauma.[284]

1. Surrogate studies. Surrogate studies investigating shaking alone as a mechanism of brain injury have mixed findings. Some studies have concluded that severe brain injury is unlikely to be caused by shaking alone, while others concluded that shaking is potentially injurious.[253,254,269–271,278,283] The latter studies identified chin-to-chest and/or occiput-to-back contact/impact as a potential mechanism of injury in the surrogate scenario, generating the highest levels of head acceleration during a shaking cycle, thus combining shaking and impact mechanisms.

It has been shown using several surrogate models that shaking generates lower angular head velocity/angular head acceleration than certain types of impact, but other surrogate models have yielded much higher levels of angular, tangential or centripetal acceleration associated with shaking with some attributable to chin-to-chest and/or occiput-to-back impact.[253,254,269,270,278,283] These latter studies reported head accelerations that exceeded published pediatric brain injury thresholds, but uncertainty remains as to the risk of fatal injury or whether the head-to-torso contact predicted in surrogate shaking is representative of a "shaking" event in infants.

Differences in findings across surrogate studies are primarily attributable to differences in surrogate design and their level of biofidelity. Surrogates that incorporate a flexible spine and neck better approximate the expected motion of an infant during shaking but may include elements of chin-to-chest and/or occiput-to-back contact. Models that capture such events also may not be fully "biofidelic" in that they may not incorporate the compressibility of these structures in living human children, which likely would slow deceleration. Another surrogate model, developed to investigate the mechanism of subdural hemorrhages, generated displacements of the brain relative to the skull during shaking that were consistent with tearing of bridging veins associated with subdural hemorrhages.[271] Despite these findings, the roles of cervical injury, apnea, physiologic and/or electrophysiologic responses, and other factors remain incompletely understood in AHT and more generally, in infant brain injury.[100,285–287]

2. Animal studies. To test the theory that children may be injured by violent shaking, a number of animal models have investigated shaking animals in various ways and then studying the resulting injuries. Although what constitutes "shaking" varies across models, most include a repetitive cyclic motion of some type. Smith et al subjected 6-day old rats suspended upside down in a 2-inch diameter tube to repetitive back and forth movement of the tube and found scattered subarachnoid hemorrhage and cortical atrophy that was not blocked by administration of an aminosteroid antioxidant.[288] Bonnier and colleagues used a similar unrestrained head device and found no subdural hemorrhages but delayed scattered microscopic injury that was decreased by pretreatment with a glutamate antagonist (MK801).[289] Wang and colleagues used an elastic-and-spring device to deliver repeated head flexion-extension forces to young mice. They found a reduction in blood flow and subarachnoid hemorrhage but no mortality.[290] Kawamata and colleagues subjected rat pups to axially oriented shaking (head to tail cyclic motion on a customized laboratory shaker device.[291] Mice behaved normally and did not develop subdural hemorrhages but had very small microhemorrhages visible on microscopy and MRI.

There have been several challenges to this approach. First, the type and magnitude of mechanical force to which human infants and children are subjected during nonaccidental trauma remain incompletely understood. The range of injuries and histories, when available, including from confessions reflect the fact that injuries and their mechanisms vary among patients.[30,50,89,292] Secondly, concepts of what constitutes a specific mechanism may vary among individuals. For instance, what research subjects demonstrate or are instructed when asked to perform "vigorous shaking" of a child surrogate is variable.[254,270,278] Thus, reproducing "shaking" comparable to what human children may experience can be challenging. More importantly, the specific tissue strains resulting from angular acceleration/deceleration are heavily dependent on the direction of motion, center of rotation, and, most notably, the mass of the brain.[293,294] Therefore, creating sufficient angular acceleration in the very small brain of rodents to mimic what the large human brain experiences is especially challenging.

The biomechanical challenges of scaling angular acceleration and inertial forces are more easily met with large animal models, but even here the magnitudes needed to create similar forces are significant because of the much smaller brain size. For instance, 1-month-old human infants have brain weights of approximately 500 g, while infant Yorkshire piglets and lambs have brains approximately 1/10th that weight.[269,295,296]

Manual shaking of anesthetized lambs by humans has been used to assess the role of shaking on the immature brain. Variations in shaking kinematics were found, in part related to subject body weight and variable motion of the unrestrained head.[297] At 6 hours postinjury, small focal subdural or subarachnoid hemorrhages were seen in a subset of subjects, and more widespread amyloid precursor protein reactivity and albumin extravasation was found, but the larger subdural hemorrhages and diffuse brain swelling seen in severe cases of human injury were not produced by this mechanism. Some of the smaller animals died, but the exact cause of death was not clearly defined.[275,298]

Immature swine at 5 days and 1 month of age have been subjected to single rapid angular rotations in the horizontal plane at different magnitudes, with physiologic and neuropathologic response noted. Variable degrees of subarachnoid hemorrhage, beta-amyloid precursor protein (APP) and neurofilament-68 staining were found, which was related both to the age of the subjects and the magnitude of angular acceleration. The data also suggested that the younger subjects showed increased susceptibility to injury even accounting for traditional brain weight scaling.[273] To investigate the effects of repetitive rather than single-event rotational forces, Coats et al. scaled the forces created by manual shaking of anthropomorphic models to the infant piglet. Multiple cyclic events separated over time showed only modest injury detected by beta-APP, and animals did not sustain significant subdural hemorrhages, brain swelling, or demonstrate major acute neurologic symptoms.[272]

Large animal models have been used in an attempt to recreate some of the pathologic and clinical findings seen in severe inflicted injuries. By adding various insults, including mechanical trauma, subdural hemorrhage, apnea, and seizures, the combination of insults required to create the widespread hemispheric damage seen in children can be studied. This approach has shown that neither mechanical trauma nor subdural hemorrhage alone can create the widespread injury seen, that younger subjects tend to have more bilateral damage, and that older subjects with a combination of synergistic insults have more widespread injury preferentially on the side of the subdural hemorrhage.[295,299,300] Moreover, the degree of damage correlates with the duration of seizures, similar to human children.[301] Although these animal models may provide some insights, as yet there is no animal model that can reproduce all the feature seen in human abusive head trauma.

Together, these experiments demonstrate that animals can be injured by a variety of mechanisms, but the attempt to "match" the mechanics of human infants and young children to what is experienced by animal surrogates remains challenging. For this reason, firm conclusions about required mechanisms of injury to cause the clinical picture seen in human patients remain elusive.

The role of repetition also remains unclear; does each successive repetition lower the threshold for brain injury? A series of studies using an infant animal model found that cyclic repetitions increase the risk of brain injury compared to a single head rotation, but that multiple repetitions across different intervals still did not cause severe injury.[272] However, AHT may involve multiple exposures including to both shaking and impact; shaking is a common part of the history in many but not all case series, and, on that basis, that repetitive cyclic events seem likely to play a role in some injury consequences. Additionally, there is no evidence (biomechanical or clinical) to support the notion that rocking in an infant swing, normal play, or typical care activities cause fatal subdural hemorrhages in healthy children. Thus, in most cases, whether or not shaking can cause fatal injury is less relevant to the determination of inflicted versus accidental etiology than is the pattern of injuries in the context of a specific history.

b) Can short-distance falls lead to severe head injury or fatality in children?. Numerous studies have focused on describing injuries associated with short-distance falls involving children. To gain an objective understanding of injuries that can result from short-distance falls involving children, one must consider the level of evidence and study design. Short-distance fall studies can be categorized as epidemiologic, clinical-retrospective medical record or autopsy review, clinical with in-depth fall investigation, clinical-corroborated falls, and biomechanical.[219,226,270,302–327]

Biomechanical studies investigating head injury risk associated with short-distance falls can be further divided into those using human surrogates, PMHS studies, computational simulations, and in situ video-recorded falls with wearable sensors.[261,262,264,270,279–282,302–309] Findings from PMHS studies utilizing drop testing have found that linear skull fractures occurred in infants from a fall height of 82 cm (32 in) onto stone, carpet, and linoleum.[279,280] Studies including video-recorded falls, falls corroborated by noncaregivers, and in-hospital falls provide a high level of evidence and typically offer greater fall detail and reduced concern that abuse has been erroneously included in the sample (Table 2). These studies can be summarized as follows:

- A total of 4060 short-distance falls are included across 7 studies providing the highest level of evidence.[302,324–330] These falls were either video recorded, occurred in-hospital, or were corroborated by a second noncaregiver. Studies including corroborated falls included a rigorous method to rule out abuse.
- The maximum fall height was approximately 1.5 m.
- 1 fatality occurred when a 16-month-old child was struck by another child who was pushed into her. The child fell rearward onto cobblestone pavement impacting the occipital region of her head.
- Serious or fatal head injuries occurred in 0.12% (n = 5) of falls. Amongst studies providing a high level of evidence, 3 cases with subdural hemorrhages (including 1 fatality) were associated with occipital impacts from rearward falls where children were unable to brace themselves[328]; 2 of these falls involved the child being pushed with impact onto concrete and cobblestone. (All falls [n = 3] were witnessed by noncaregivers.)
- Skull fractures occurred in 10 falls (0.24%). When skull fractures occurred as a result of short-distance falls, they typically were nondisplaced, narrow, linear, or curvilinear fractures. Minimally depressed skull fractures occurred in falls with head impact onto edged or cornered surfaces.

TAKEAWAY POINTS

1. Biomechanical compatibility between provided history and presenting injuries is an important factor when determining whether a child's injuries are the result of abuse or an accident.
2. Various types of biomechanical studies have been conducted to investigate the potential for head injury when children are exposed to short-distance falls, inflicted impact to the head, and shaking. These studies include in-depth event investigation and/or reconstruction, human surrogate experiments, computational models and simulations, animal injury models, and PMHS experiments.
3. Biomechanical studies have demonstrated that angular head acceleration/deceleration of sufficient magnitude can cause diffuse brain injuries, such as concussion, subdural hemorrhage, and/or diffuse axonal injury. Forces applied to the body that generate linear or rotational motion of the head and translational or angular head acceleration can cause focal brain injuries, such as brain contusions or focal subdural hemorrhage, as well as more diffuse injury patterns.
4. Findings from biomechanical studies investigating shaking are mixed as to whether shaking alone can cause severe brain injury or fatality in infants.
5. Head impacts onto surfaces causing forces of sufficient magnitude may cause skull fractures and/or focal brain injuries but may also generate rotational head accelerations at levels capable of producing diffuse brain injuries or subdural and subarachnoid hemorrhage, depending on the magnitude of acceleration/deceleration and other factors. Many head injuries in the clinical setting are the result of both direct impact and inertial (brain motion) forces and acceleration.
6. Short-distance falls rarely result in fatality in children. There is a low incidence of serious head injuries in short-distance falls, but they most frequently occur when there is momentum from concomitant activities (eg, play equipment, a child is pushed), in rearward falls onto hard surfaces when children are unable to brace themselves, or from expanding intracranial hemorrhages and/or contusional swelling from contact events. It is important to note that "short-distance" fall heights are measured as head-to-ground height rather than feet-to-ground height or height of support surface, which can lead to underestimating the forces/accelerations imparted to the head.

EVALUATION

Introduction

Children with abusive head trauma may present with clear signs/symptoms of either abuse (unexplained bruising or fractures) or head trauma (seizures, loss of consciousness). However, many children also present with nonspecific symptoms such as vomiting and excessive fussiness.[21] A thorough physical examination including head circumference, the entire skin, oral cavity, and ears can assist in determining which patients would benefit from a more detailed evaluation for abuse.[73]

When children present with clear concerns for trauma, the American College of Surgeons developed widely accepted methodology for the initial evaluation and stabilization of the trauma patient, to include children with AHT. The Advanced Trauma Life Support (ATLS) Program was introduced in 1980 and currently is in its 10th edition.[331] By ATLS methodology, all trauma patients undergo an initial primary survey including assessment of airway, breathing, circulation, neurologic disability, and exposure with immobilization and stabilization of the cervical spine.[331] The neurologic assessment includes pupillary response, GCS, and notation of any lateralization or pattern of neurologic disability such as hemiplegia or paraplegia. Relevant to the patient with suspected or proven AHT, a more detailed secondary survey includes inspection and palpation of the entire head and face, repeat assessment of pupillary response and GCS, and examination of the cervical spine. Specific guidance regarding the evaluation and management of the pediatric trauma patient to include age-based vital sign ranges, modifications of the GCS verbal score, and appropriate modifications of neutral positioning of the cervical spine are also presented. For offices or facilities lacking appropriate clinical and diagnostic resources, rapid transfer to an appropriate facility is suggested. Institutions with a dedicated trauma team and neurosurgical support prioritize the initial diagnostic evaluation based on the clinical needs of the patient. Although a comprehensive child abuse evaluation[33] might involve a variety of radiologic examinations to include a skeletal survey, the risk of transporting the patient outside of the emergency department or ICU setting needs to be considered.[332]

Laboratory

Occult, nonobvious injuries can occur in the setting of physical abuse, especially in young children who are nonverbal or children who cannot localize pain for various reasons. Given the co-occurrence of head and abdominal trauma in young infants, laboratory evaluation to assess for occult abdominal trauma, which includes hepatic transaminases, is reasonable.[333] If these transaminases are significantly elevated (greater than 80 IU/L), then further abdominal imaging may be required.[333] Renal injuries can manifest with abnormalities in creatinine and/or blood urea nitrogen levels, or they may be evidenced by the presence of blood or other abnormalities on a urinalysis.

The evidence base for bleeding disorder evaluation in the context of suspected AHT has been addressed previously in the AAP clinical report by Anderst et al.[334] It stated that an initial evaluation for bleeding disorders in the context of intracranial hemorrhage should include: a complete blood cell count (CBC), prothrombin time (PT), and activated partial thromboplastin time (aPTT).[334] Mild, transient elevations in PT and aPTT may be seen in the setting of parenchymal injury, but these do not lead to severe, life-threatening bleeding.[105,335,336] A panel for disseminated intravascular coagulation (DIC) may be needed for clinical care if the child is severely ill. Further testing for mild factor deficiencies such as factor VIII or factor IX may be needed if there is a history of trauma causing the intracranial hemorrhage. However, in the setting of other abusive injuries, such as fractures or burns, there may be no need to do the extensive factor testing.[334] Von Willebrand disease, although relatively common, is rarely associated with intracranial bleeding, and testing is only necessary in the setting of a child with intracranial bleeding who returns to neurologic baseline or if there is a clear family or medical history suggestive of such a condition.[334]

Although some rare metabolic conditions can mimic AHT, these diagnoses may be considered on the differential when other clinical indicia of the metabolic condition are present. A review of the newborn screen can assess for many metabolic conditions, and one should consider evaluating for the presence of glutaric aciduria type 1 (GA1) with serum amino acid levels and urine organic acid levels if there are clinical indications such as preexisting developmental delay.[33]

Berger and colleagues have evaluated the ability of serum biomarkers to identify pediatrics traumatic brain injury. They have derived and validated a multivariable mode (using three serum biomarkers and serum hemoglobin) to identify intracranial hemorrhage in children with suspected AHT. To date, this biomarker research has not yet been able to differentiate abusive from nAHT.[337]

Imaging

Neuroimaging

Currently, CT is the imaging modality of choice in acute pediatric head trauma[338] and is indicated in the infant or young child presenting with neurologic findings and suspicions for abusive injury.[339,340] The American College of Radiology Appropriateness Criteria for imaging the child with suspected physical abuse provides additional guidance and stratification of imaging studies for different ages and clinical scenarios in this population.[340] Routine use of multiplanar and 3D reconstructions is helpful and can be generated without additional imaging.[338] These 3D reconstructions provide increased ability to identify convexity and posterior fossa hemorrhages as well as more detailed evaluation of fractures and developmental skull anomalies.[341–343]

Frequently requiring sedation, MRI is often used in the nonacute setting to further evaluate brain parenchymal abnormalities, hemorrhages, and coexistent spinal injuries in the child presenting with injuries suspicious for child physical abuse and concurrent neurologic symptoms.[339,340] Diffusion-weighted imaging is invaluable for the detection of cytotoxic edema and hypoxic-ischemic brain injury and should be included in all suspected abusive head injury magnetic resonance (MR) protocols.[339,340] Gradient echo or susceptibility-weighted sequences, to evaluate for blood products, are also routinely utilized, in addition to standard T1- and T2-weighted sequences, which provide excellent anatomic detail.[340]

Rapid MRI protocols may provide a feasible alternative to CT imaging in the initial assessment of patients with macrocephaly and those at high risk for abuse, potentially reducing exposure to unnecessary radiation and sedation.[344–349] Flom et al proposed a screening MR protocol, using a reduced number of typical MR sequences, to potentially replace CT in the initial screening of infants and found it was highly sensitive in the detection of intracranial hemorrhage in both the study and control cases.[347] More recently, this protocol was tweaked and included the addition of a

Table 2. Short Distance Falls in Children: Studies with High Level of Evidence

1st Author, Date	Title	Study Design	Age	Sample Size	Findings/Injuries
Bertocci, 2020	Injuries and biomechanics of falls involving young children in a child care setting.	Prospective, observational; video recorded falls in a child care center with wearable biometric devices.	12–36 months	3255	- no fatalities, no serious head injuries - no children had multiple injuries - 4 minor (AIS 1) injuries to soft tissue (3 lacerations; 1 nosebleed) - 0.12% of falls resulted in minor injury - max fall height 1.2 m (measured to head COM)
Williams, 1991	Injuries in infants and small children resulting from witnessed and corroborated free falls.	Retrospective; witnessed by 2nd person other than caregiver.	< 3 years	106	- 3 serious (non-life threatening) injuries in falls between 4–5 ft (1.2–1.5 m); small depressed skull fractures without loss of consciousness from falling against edged surfaces - 1 fatality from 70 ft (21.3 m) - not short distance fall - fall heights were estimated
Helfer, 1977	Injuries resulting when small children fall out of bed.	Retrospective; review of hospital incident reports; in hospital falls.	< 6 years	85	- 57 falls: no injury - 37 falls: minor injury - 1 fall: skull fracture w no sequelae (fall from ED bed) - approx. 0.9 m fall height
Nimityongskul, 1987	The likelihood of injuries when children fall out of bed.	Retrospective; review of hospital safety records; in hospital falls.	< 16 years (75% 1–5 years)	76	- 1 nondisplaced skull fracture in 1-year-old child w no ICH – no treatment required - 1 tibia fracture in patient with OI - 74 children had minor or no injuries; 4 required sutures - approx 1–3 ft (0.3–0.9 m) fall height
Levene, 1991	Accidents in hospital wards.	Retrospective; in-hospital incidents.	< 16 years	328	- 42% of incidents involved falls from heights - 2 limb fractures (3 m fall and unspecified fall) - 2 skull fractures (fall from bed and fall from chair); no treatment required
Lyons, 1993	Falling out of bed: a relatively benign occurrence.	Retrospective; review of hospital incident reports; in-hospital falls.	< 7 years	207	- 31 injuries: 29 "trivial" injuries (no sutures), 1 simple linear skull fracture with no neurologic signs (10-month-old, fall from crib), 1 clavicle fracture (21-month-old) - no children had multiple injuries - approx 25–54 in (0.6–1.3 m) fall height
Atkinson, 2018	Childhood falls with occipital impacts.	Retrospective; survey of child abuse physicians requesting occipital impacts from falls w SDH ± RH; child abuse team ruled out abuse.	7–16 months	3 directly witnessed - noncaregiver/ nonrelative witnesses	- Fall 1: pushed by 3-year-old and fell rearward onto concrete from standing: unilateral small to moderate SDH w mass effect; bilateral RHs (multiple) - Fall 2: standing on couch, fell rearward impacting head on wooden table and then floor: unilateral SDH w midline shift required surgical evacuation; bilateral RH (numerous) - Fall 3: fatality (16-month-old) – one child pushed by another child who fell into child who died; child who died fell rearward from standing impacting head on cobblestone pavement (multiple witnesses): unilateral SDH overlying frontal, parietal and temporal lobes; diffuse edema; SAH; unilateral few RH + optic nerve sheath hemorrhage - no skull fracture or other fractures - all developed immediate symptoms - median 4.5-day hospital stay; 2 survivors returned to baseline on discharge
			TOTAL	**4060**	

AIS indicates Abbreviated Injury Scale; COM, center of mass; ED, emergency department; ICH, intracranial hemorrhage; OI, osteogenesis imperfecta (a metabolic bone disorder); RH, retinal hemorrhage; SDH, subdural hemorrhage; SAH, subarachnoid hemorrhage.

more rapid T2-acquisition, a single-shot T2 fast spin echo sequence, and diffusion-weighted sequences.[346] The authors concluded this protocol had the potential to significantly reduce head CT imaging in high-risk infants. Limited MR studies, either using limited numbers of sequences or more rapid sequences, may be used for follow-up to assess parenchymal volume loss, ventricular sizes, and subdural hemorrhages or collections in pediatric trauma patients. Limitations, however, include limited availability for 24-hour MR coverage in many institutions, more motion artifact, more complex to perform than CT in critically injured patients, and less sensitivity in the detection of skull fractures and small hemorrhages.[346,347,350]

Radiographic images of the spine for fracture detection are an important part of the routine skeletal survey in cases of suspected abuse and include both dedicated anterior/posterior and lateral views.[340] Cervical spine MRI is valuable in cases with high clinical concerns of spinal injury or in cases of spinal injury identified on other imaging modalities and has been shown to be superior to CT assessing injury to the pediatric cervical spine.[340,351] On the basis of the increased detection of spinal injuries described earlier in this report, it is prudent to strongly consider spinal MRI in cases of abusive head injury in which spinal injury would be difficult to exclude clinically or by plain radiography.[131] MRI is especially important in infants and young children with diffuse bilateral hypoxic-ischemic brain injury, which has been shown to have a high association with cervical ligamentous injuries.[129] MRI of the entire spine also may be valuable to evaluate for additional sites of spinal injury or spinal subdural hemorrhage.[128,340]

Spine MR protocols include multiplanar T1- and T2-weighted sequences to provide anatomic detail, as well as either STIR (short tau inversion recovery) or fat-saturated T2-weighted sequences, which optimize evaluation of soft tissue and marrow edema and, thus, aid in assessing for ligamentous or vertebral injures.[340,352]

a) Dating intracranial hemorrhage. Aging or dating subdural hemorrhage strictly on the imaging appearance may be challenging, as the imaging appearance depends on the stage and composition of the blood products and potential admixture of cerebrospinal fluid in the subdural compartment.[43,53,90,353–360] Dating intracranial hemorrhage based on neuroimaging is estimative. In children with suspected abuse, serial CT and/or MRI may provide an increased ability to estimate the acuity or chronicity of imaging findings and intracranial hemorrhage, especially when correlated with a multidisciplinary child protection team discussion.[90,91]

High-attenuation subdural hemorrhage on CT typically represents an "acute" hemorrhage, indicating that the hemorrhage occurred within approximately 7 days of the date of the CT.[358,361] "Subacute" hemorrhage gradually becomes lower in attenuation on CT over a period of several days up to 2 to 3 weeks from the date of the CT.[358,361] A "chronic" subdural hemorrhage contains aging blood products, may contain neomembranes and be compartmentalized, is low in attenuation on CT, is generally present beyond 2 to 3 weeks of the date of the CT, and often is well demonstrated on MRI.[354,355,358] However, a subdural hygroma is a term occasionally used to refer to a low-attenuation subdural containing fluid attenuation on CT or signal on MRI without the presence of membranes. Hematohygroma is a subdural collection containing both blood and fluid (either cerebrospinal fluid or serum) and may be used to describe a mixed-attenuation subdural hemorrhage.[353] Both a subdural hygroma and hematohygroma may present acutely after trauma, again emphasizing that dating solely on the basis of the appearance of the subdural may be challenging.[353]

In AHT, up to 67% of cases of subdural hemorrhage may demonstrate mixed attenuation on the initial CT study,[102] whereas the majority of nAHT cases presented with more uniformly high-attenuation subdural hemorrhage.[90,95]

Mixed-attenuation subdural hemorrhages may exist in several scenarios.[53,90,354–356,362] It may be the result of differing stages or components of hemorrhage, such as clotted and unclotted blood or serum in an acute and hyperacute subdural hemorrhage or clotted subdural hemorrhage mixing with serum in an acute subdural hemorrhage.[354,355] It may also represent acute hemorrhage mixing with cerebrospinal fluid resulting from traumatic injury to the arachnoid.[353] Finally, it may represent acute bleeding or rebleeding into a preexisting chronic subdural hemorrhage.[53,90,354,355,362]

1. Skeletal surveys. Skeletal surveys are recommended in children younger than 2 years when there are concerns for physical abuse.[33,340] Duffy and colleagues found that skeletal surveys found almost 11% of children with suspected abuse had a positive skeletal survey.[363] Skeletal surveys should be performed by an institution with experience in caring for and imaging children, following the American College of Radiology (ACR)-Society of Pediatric Radiology (SPR) "Practice Parameter for the Performance and Interpretation of Skeletal Surveys in Children."[364] This document, as well as the ACR Appropriateness Criteria, provide guidance regarding the skeletal images that are recommended, relative radiation levels for the imaging modalities, and additional guidance for radiation safety and imaging techniques as this skeletal imaging uses ionizing radiation.[340,364] Skeletal surveys may consist of over 22 images detailing each area of the body with some imaged in multiple planes. Despite the number of images, the radiation risk of a skeletal survey has been estimated to be low, ~0.2 mSv, and the risk of not performing a skeletal survey and missing a case of child physical abuse must be weighed against the potential low radiation risk associated with skeletal imaging.[365]

ACR Appropriateness Criteria indicates that, in children younger than 24 months of age with a high clinical suspicion for abuse and a negative initial skeletal survey, a repeat follow-up skeletal survey performed 2 to 3 weeks after the initial examination may add diagnostic information.[340] Abusive fractures may not be visible on initial skeletal surveys and prospective studies have shown that repeat skeletal imaging increases the number of skeletal fractures diagnosed in more than 25% of children who were abused. According to a meta-analysis by Maguire et al, new fractures were found by repeating the skeletal survey in 8.4% to 37.6% of cases and repeat skeletal surveys added new information that influenced child protection procedures.[366] The addition of further injury findings on repeat skeletal surveys can improve diagnostic specificity and sensitivity for abuse.[33,367,368]

2. Other studies (literature on abdominal CT, etc). There is limited literature specific to evaluation of abdominal trauma in the setting of suspected or confirmed AHT.[369] However, a child with suspected abuse and concern for thoracic or abdominal injuries should have a skeletal survey.[340] The investigation of suspected abdominal and thoracic injuries in suspected physical abuse should be the same imaging used for accidental trauma with body CT as the imaging modality of choice.[370]

3. Postmortem imaging. Postmortem skeletal surveys can provide important information regarding the presence and chronicity of extremity fracures that may not be documented at autopsy. McGraw and colleagues reported postmortem skeletal findings in 14 children who were abused including 11 with blunt force injuries to the cranium.[371] In 6 (43%) of these 14 patients, radiography detected 26 extremity fractures not detected at autopsy. All fractures carried a high index of suspicion for abuse.

Whole-body post-mortem computed tomography (PMCT) also may detect relevant findings that can explain sudden unexpected death and can be extremely valuable for detecting non-accidental injuries. Proisy and colleauges reported high concordance of PMCT and autopsy in 15 of 18 children with unexplained death.[372]

Ophthalmologic Evaluation

Consultation with an ophthalmologist is extremely important for any child suspected to have sustained AHT.[373] Ideally, this examination takes place within 24 to 36 hours after the patient presents for medical care, because retinal hemorrhage patterns may change quickly. The number of intraretinal hemorrhages can decrease noticeably within even 48 hours, and preretinal hemorrhage can spread into the vitreous and prevent a view of the retina, so whenever possible, the ophthalmologic assessment should be performed within that time window, regardless of whether or not the pupils can be pharmacologically dilated.[183,374]

It is important that an ophthalmologist with experience and tools to identify, describe, and manage retinal hemorrhage in children perform the evaluation.[373,375] An indirect ophthalmoscope (a head-mounted unit used with a hand-held lens) provides a 3-dimensional wide-angle view of the retina and is used as the primary technique for the assessment of the retina. Sometimes an eyelid speculum and scleral depression, a technique in which the sclera is indented to bring into view the farther peripheral retina and ora serrata, are necessary. It is important that the presence, number, types, and locations of hemorrhages be documented in a detailed written description for each eye, as well as the presence or absence of retinal folds, retinoschisis, optic disc swelling, or other retinal findings, such as white lesions or lipid exudates.[375] Although nonophthalmologists may identify if retinal hemorrhages are present using a direct ophthalmoscope, there is a high false-negative rate and a direct ophthalmoscope provides a small field of view, inadequate to examine wide areas of retina or to clearly see the details of the pattern of retinal hemorrhage.[376] Similarly, ocular ultrasonography and radiographic studies are inadequate for discerning the details of the pattern of hemorrhage.

Pupillary dilation facilitates the best view of the retina, whether by pharmacologic dilation or pathologic dilation, and the examination is best when conducted through dilated pupils. However, the initial examination can be performed as soon as possible and not delayed because of inability to administer eye drops. In patients whose pupils are being closely monitored for signs of extreme intracranial hypertension, short-acting drops (dilation for 2–3 hours) and/or dilation of 1 eye at a time may be an option. In addition to fundoscopy, a complete bedside ophthalmologic examination includes assessment of visual function, keeping in mind that normal visual behavior does not preclude the presence of intraocular injury, pupillary reactivity, gaze preference and ocular motility, and external examination of the ocular adnexa and ocular anterior segment to assess for signs of direct ocular or orbital trauma. Retinal photography with a digital fundus camera can help to document retinal findings. However, photography is not obligatory.[375] The ophthalmologist's detailed written description is sufficient.

Evaluation of Contacts

Siblings, or other children in the same environment of a child identified as having experienced abuse, are also at risk for being abused. When siblings were evaluated, Alexander and colleagues found abuse or neglect in siblings of 33% of their AHT cases.[377] In a similar vein, Sinal and Ball's case series of children who had experienced AHT revealed 2 suspicious deaths in siblings of children who were abused.[378]

In the multicenter ExSTRA study (Examining Siblings To Recognize Abuse), conducted in 2010–2011, skeletal surveys identified at least 1 abusive fracture in 16 of 134 contacts (11.9%; 95% CI, 7.5–18.5) <24 months of age.[379] The prevalence of a fracture or other abusive injury was greater for the younger children.

Twins have a substantially increased risk of abuse. Groothuis and colleagues found that child maltreatment was more prevalent in families with twins, and Hansen described a case in which the twin of a child with AHT was also found to have indications of being injured.[380,381] The ExSTRA study found that twins were at substantially increased risk of fracture relative to nontwin contacts (OR, 20.1; 95% CI, 5.8–69.9).[379]

In 2023, an international consensus statement addressed the screening of contact children in the setting of suspected child physical abuse, as uniformly established guidelines are lacking.[382] This statement and imaging recommendations were based on expert consensus and suggests that contact children younger than 1 year undergo a dedicated skeketal survey and cross-sectional imaging of the brain, ideally MRI imaging of the brain utilizing both routine anatomic and advanced techniques to detect brain insult and intracranial hemorrhage. Head CT with pediatric dose techniques and multiplanar reconstructions could be considered, if MRI is not available. Screening sagittal spine MRI is also recommended, if the brain imaging is abnormal in the contact child. A skeletal survey without dedicated neuroimaging is recommended in a contact child 1 to 2 years of age, with no imaging specifically recommended in contacts 2 years or older.

TAKE AWAY POINTS

1. The initial work up of children with suspected abuse includes an evaluation for medical causes for the child's condition as well as evaluating for other abusive injuries.
2. Laboratory evaluation may include assessment for bleeding disorders, genetic conditions, and other organ injuries including the liver and kidney.
3. A head CT is the current imaging modality of choice for detection of cranial and intracranial injury in children presenting with acute head injury or neurologic symptoms and concerns for abuse. MRI is playing an increasing role as well.
4. A skeletal survey looking for occult skeletal injuries is performed in a child 2 years or younger with concerns of abuse. In addition, a follow-up skeletal survey at 2 to 3 weeks after presentation is also considered, as this will allow detection of now healing fractures that were occult or subtle on the initial skeletal survey.
5. Postmortem skeletal surveys can provide important additional information regarding the extent and chronicity of extremity fractures that may not be documented at autopsy.
6. Siblings of children with suspected abuse are also at risk; the literature supports that their health and safety be considered during a child abuse evaluation.

DIFFERENTIAL DIAGNOSIS

Accidental Trauma

Introduction

When children present with an apparent traumatic injury in which AHT is considered to be in the differential diagnosis, accidental trauma often is one of the primary diagnostic considerations. To determine whether an injury is likely to have been caused by accidental mechanisms, the clinician needs to analyze the history provided including developmental abilities of the child and the clinical presentation in the context of the physical examination and radiologic findings, to determine whether the pattern fits with known data on accidental injury.[310] The certainty with which a specific patient can be determined to have a nonaccidental versus an accidental etiology varies among patients and injury constellations.[94,383] In this section, the most relevant elements of the history and presentation that the provider can obtain to facilitate comparison to what is known about accidental injury mechanisms are reviewed.

Obtaining an Optimal History to Help Differentiate Accidental Trauma From AHT

There are few quantitative studies regarding the most reliable way to elicit a history from caregivers to obtain accurate data regarding reported mechanism of injury and/or clinical appearance of the child before, during, and after a presumed traumatic event, to attempt to differentiate accidental trauma from AHT. However, some methods, including those adapted from biomechanical reconstruction questionnaires, have been suggested. These include gathering details relevant to known data on accidental and nonaccidental head injury mechanisms provided by both clinical series and biomechanical studies.[33,47,96,226,316] Suggested methods for data-gathering from caregivers include facilitating an initial uninterrupted narrative of the history.[33] Gathering specific details of the history from the last time the child was seen well, through the events surrounding the injury or onset of symptoms, and up until presentation to medical care, has been recommended, including how the child was positioned or held, what anatomic structures sustained impacts against what types of surfaces, and from what height the child fell.[47,384]

Most standard furniture dimensions in the United States include couches and other seating heights about 18 to 20 inches, beds 1 to 3 feet, and changing tables and countertops 2.5 to 3 feet.[37,314,316,327,385] Children held by parents, while in a standing position, at the parent's shoulder level, typically have head-to-ground falls of approximately 4 to 5 feet.[96,386] Biomechanical scene reconstructions have shown that most caregivers overestimate fall height when providing a history.[226] Because different authors define "low height," "short height," or "household" falls differently, more exact measurements of head-to-ground distance are more accurate than using these more general terms; however, most papers define low-height or short-distance falls as under 3 to 4 feet.[37,96,226,310,316]

In addition to the reported mechanism of injury or, alternatively, a description of the events surrounding the presentation when no history of trauma is provided, a number of authors have advocated that providers elicit details in the history including a description of the level of consciousness, degree of eye opening, movements of extremities, behaviors that might represent seizures, and breathing status, since clinical features such as apnea and seizures have been associated with a higher likelihood of AHT compared with accidental trauma.[14,50,93,387,388] (Additional data on other features of the history in AHT can be found in the History section of this report.)

Besides the history of the event itself, in order to help differentiate accidental injury from AHT, some authors have pointed out the importance of gathering information about the child's past medical history, including typical normal behaviors and capacities, such as whether the child sits, rolls, crawls, or cruises.[33]

a) General characteristics of the history associated with accidental trauma compared with AHT. Most often, in the setting of accidental trauma, caregivers are able to give a clear, consistent description of events surrounding the injury and presentation.[96,389] In contrast, a history describing a possible accidental mechanism in which caregivers are unable to describe events, the description of events changes in major ways over time, or the description is clearly developmentally implausible have been noted as characteristics occurring more often in AHT compared with accidental trauma.[50] Some accidental injuries will happen when children are unsupervised, and guidance has been offered to help differentiate this from neglect or abuse, depending on the overall clinical context.[96,390]

In one study of children younger than 2 years with accidental injuries and AHT serious enough to lead to hospitalization in an intensive care or monitored unit or who died, 75% of the accidental injuries were witnessed by caregivers, while witnesses were reported in 2.5% of children with AHT.[387] For children younger than 3 years with subdural hemorrhages, Feldman et al found that parents are not always present when an accidental injury occurred, especially when children are mobile (crawling, walking) or are supervised by older children or other caregivers.[94] A history of a child who falls, cries, and is readily consoled, with the injury only becoming apparent later, is common in low-height/short-distance falls in accidental trauma, most often in the setting of liquefaction of a scalp hematoma associated with a linear skull fracture, as will be discussed further in the next section.[222–224]

In contrast, in various clinical series, approximately 85% to 95% of children judged to have AHT present with either a) no history of trauma, with presentation because of signs or symptoms (range 43%–72% of children); or b) a description of an accidental traumatic mechanism, usually of a minor nature, such as a fall less than 3 feet (25%–42% of children). The remainder present with various other descriptions of potential traumatic events.[37,50,89,94,387] In a series from New Zealand, about 14% of cases determined to stem from assault had an associated admission (confession) of injury causation, but this was age dependent, with a higher percentage of assault admissions in children older than 2 years. Variable injury mechanisms were described in the younger children with admitted AHT, while all children older than 2 years who had been assaulted had blunt impacts reported.[89]

b) Associations between history, clinical, and radiologic findings in accidental trauma. Data linking the history, physical examination, and imaging findings assists in assessing whether the injury pattern is typically associated with the accidental mechanism described, or, when the event is unwitnessed, is likely in the developmental context of the child. Several lines of research have investigated these associations. As mentioned earlier, "low-height falls" or "short-distance falls" have been defined variably in the literature but generally include free-fall translational forces under about 3 to 4 feet (head to ground), as noted below. Some of the relevant studies and findings are summarized below.

- Low-height/short-distance falls can cause linear skull fractures, especially in infants.[328,386]
- Bilateral skull fractures can occur from a single impact event, typically in the occipital or frontal region.[391] These fractures may be separate and noncontiguous, can cross over the suture, and generally depict contiguous fracture planes.[392]
- Epidural hemorrhages, which can be life-threatening, most often occur from low-height/short-distance falls in young children and most often are associated with skull fractures but are uncommonly associated with abuse.[220,393,394]
- Thin, crescent-shaped hemorrhagic collections underlying skull fractures often represent venous epidural hemorrhages from the fracture itself and can be misread as subdural hemorrhages on CT scan.[47]
- Subdural hemorrhages occur in both AHT and accidental trauma but are much more common in infants and young children in the setting of child abuse.[92]
- Low-height occipital impacts and other contact mechanisms have been reported to be associated with subdural and/or subarachnoid hemorrhage, but these are usually clinically benign.[328,389]
- Falls involving higher head-to-ground heights, additional velocity (such as being pushed, or on moving equipment), or greater angular forces can be associated with more significant injuries, including contusions and subdural and subarachnoid hemorrhages.[219,328] Falls from playground equipment have been associated very rarely with subdural hemorrhage, contusion, brain swelling, and death; however, these have included children from 1 to 13 years of age and in some cases involved head-to-ground heights over 3 to 4 feet and/or additional forces such as falls from moving equipment or while being pushed.[311]
- As noted earlier, free falls with head-to-ground height under about 3 feet are uncommonly associated with

serious injury except for skull fractures and epidural hemorrhage. In contrast, inflicted impacts (throwing the subject down onto a surface) using instrumented anthropomorphic models are associated with significantly greater angular deceleration forces than low-height/short-distance falls, with magnitudes in the range predicted to cause injuries such as concussion and subdural hemorrhage.[270,307] (More on biomechanics studies can be found in the Biomechanics section.)

c) Deaths from short-distance falls. Most head injuries in infants and children younger than 24 months occur as a result of falls.[96] Typical, short-distance falls are not life threatening, often with little to no neurologic symptoms.[96,314,325,327] Other than in the setting of epidural hemorrhage, low-height/short-distance falls rarely, if ever, cause severe injuries or death.[98,219,226,310,316,395]

However, some literature has suggested that fatal or significant intracranial injuries may result from short-distance falls.[311,317] Plunkett described 18 children sustaining fatal head injuries from reported falls off playground equipment from more than 75,000 cases in the United States Consumer Product Safety Commission database.[311] Some limitations of this study are that 6 of 18 were witnessed only by a single caretaker; only 5 were younger than 24 months, and none were infants. Additionally, these numbers do not include all of the children who might have sustained insignificant injuries after falling off playground equipment but who were never reported or taken for medical treatment.

Hall et al reviewed pediatric fall fatalities seen at the Cook County Medical Examiner's office.[317] Nearly 41% (18/44 cases) had isolated intracranial injuries associated with short-distance falls ≤3 feet, several with a delay in seeking care. The authors acknowledged that some of these injuries might have been the result of abuse, because significant injuries from these types of short-distance falls are exceedingly rare and should raise suspicions of child physical abuse.

Numerous case series in the medical literature find very few, if any, significant or fatal head injuries occurring as a result of witnessed and corroborated, short-distance falls or falls occurring in a hospital setting.[314,324,325,327,396] However, presenting histories in children in whom abusive head injuries are diagnosed are not infrequently short-distance falls.[89]

Chadwick et al estimated the potential mortality rate from a short-distance fall for infants and young children to be much less than 1 fatality per 1 million young children per year.[310] This is based on an extensive review of the available literature as well as several public database reviews and supports the conclusion that a fatal head injury resulting from a short-distance fall is exceedingly rare.

TAKEAWAY POINTS

1. Accidental trauma is a primary differential consideration in children suspected of experiencing abuse. Detailed history of the child and reported trauma is essential in attempting to differentiate the cause of the child's injuries.
2. Accidental household falls of low height/short distance occur frequently in this population and may result in skull fractures with small volume adjacent intracranial hemorrhage, often venous epidural blood that may be misinterpreted on imaging as subdural hemorrhage.
3. Epidural hemorrhage is common following accidental trauma but is uncommon in abusive head injury.
4. Deaths or clinically significant intracranial injury from low-height/short-distance, household falls are exceedingly rare.

Bleeding Disorders

Unlike some alternative medical explanations, bleeding disorders are known causes of intracranial hemorrhage (ICH) and retinal hemorrhage (RH) and are a heterogeneous group of conditions that vary in etiology, presenting symptoms, and prevalence. When considering bleeding disorders as the potential etiology for the hemorrhagic findings seen in AHT, the AAP has previously suggested, in addition to detailed symptom and family history gathering, a testing strategy for evaluating a possible bleeding disorder that incorporates the probability of an ICH occurring in a child with a given congenital bleeding disorder.[334,397] For example, the probability of an individual in the general population having an ICH because of factor XIII deficiency can be calculated by using the estimated prevalence of the condition (1 in 2 million people) and the prevalence of intracranial hemorrhage within the population with the condition (33%), or 1 in 6 million [(1 in 2 million) × (1/3)].[397]

Within this testing strategy, it is helpful for the pediatric provider to know where the data for prevalence of ICH within a particular congenital bleeding disorder population is derived. A primary source of data for symptoms in children with bleeding disorders is the Universal Data Collection (UDC) database of the Centers for Disease Control and Prevention. The UDC contains specific information on intracranial hemorrhage and subdural hemorrhage in subjects with congenital bleeding disorders. Thus, on the basis of these data and prevalence of conditions, the AAP clinical report on bleeding disorders provided a table of "Probabilities for Congenital Coagulopathies Causing Intracranial Hemorrhage," which may be helpful to the pediatric provider.[334] The essential takeaway point of this table is that the probability of a congenital coagulopathy to cause ICH ranges from "low" to "1 in 50 million," depending on the coagulopathy.

To further evaluate these probabilities, Anderst and Carpenter reviewed the UDC in subjects <4 years of age to "characterize the prevalence and calculate the probabilities of any intracranial hemorrhage, traumatic intracranial hemorrhage, and nontraumatic intracranial hemorrhage in children with congenital bleeding disorders."[398] The authors found that of 3717 subjects, 255 (6.9%) had any intracranial hemorrhage and 206 (5.5%) had nontraumatic intracranial hemorrhage. The highest prevalence of intracranial hemorrhage was in severe hemophilia A (9.1%) and B (10.7%). Of the 1233 subjects <2 years of age in which the specific location of any ICH was known, 13 (1.1%) had spontaneous subdural hemorrhage (12 with severe hemophilia; 1 with type 1 von Willebrand disease). The authors concluded that "In congenital bleeding disorders, nontraumatic intracranial hemorrhage occurs most commonly in severe hemophilia. In this study, von Willebrand disease is not supported as a 'mimic' of AHT."

With regard to the prevalence and probability of RHs in congenital coagulopathies, a systematic review by Thau et al sought to identify whether coagulopathies have been reported with RH similar to those of AHT.[194] Of 61 articles that met inclusion criteria, the authors found that there were only 32 children within the AHT age range (younger than 5 years) who had RH and concomitant coagulopathy. RH has not been reported in congenital factor II, VII, X, XII, or XIII deficiencies. More extensive RH (with extension to the periphery) has been reported in hemophilia A and B, and mild von Willebrand disease, albeit rare in these entities as well. Of the 32 children, only 5 of those cases could be confused for abuse. Of those 5 cases, none had retinoschisis or retinal folds. The authors concluded that disorders of coagulopathy rarely result in RH in children.

TAKEAWAY POINTS

1. Most bleeding disorders are rare.
2. The more common bleeding disorders typically are mild.
3. Intracranial hemorrhage resulting from bleeding disorders is a rare complication of the more severe bleeding diatheses.
4. When bleeding disorders are a reasonable clinical consideration (based on parental concern of bleeding/bruising symptoms and/or family history), it is prudent to obtain a hematology subspecialty consultation.

Birth Trauma

Injuries common to both birth trauma and AHT include scalp hematoma, skull fracture, intracranial hemorrhage, and retinal hemorrhage. Although much of birth-related injury is clinically asymptomatic, presentation varies depending on the severity of the injury.

Intracranial Hemorrhage

Acute subdural hemorrhage has been a reported finding following vaginal and cesarean deliveries.[399–403] The prevalence of birth-related subdural hemorrhage ranges from 7% to 50%.[399,400,402,404,405] The precise mechanisms of birth-related ICH remain unknown. Multiple mechanisms have been proposed, including mechanical deformation of the cranium with consequent disruption of the dural border cell layer, mechanical deformation resulting in bridging vein rupture, and increased intracranial pressure.

Birth-related subdural hemorrhages can be either supratentorial or infratentorial.[399,400,404,406] Although more commonly located in the posterior fossa, birth-related subdural hemorrhages can also be located along the frontal, parietal, and interhemispheric regions.[399,400,404,406] Thus, the location of subdural hemorrhage alone is not specific enough to distinguish AHT from birth-related intracranial injury.

Most birth-related subdural hemorrhages are asymptomatic.[399,400,402,407] However, when symptomatic, the severity of presenting symptoms correlates to the presence of underlying parenchymal injury.[406,408,409] The majority of clinical symptoms present within the first 24 hours of life but can present as late as 11 days postnatally.[399,406,410] Delayed symptoms (weeks to months from birth) have not been reported outside the context of birth-related intracranial injury complications (eg, anoxic brain injury, hydrocephalus, etc).

The vast majority (greater than 94%) of birth-related subdural hemorrhages resolve by 4 weeks of age.[399,402] Current literature involving longitudinal radiologic evaluation of birth-related subdural hemorrhage has not documented the persistence of birth-related subdural hemorrhage beyond 3 months of age.[399,400,402] Rebleeding of birth-related subdural hemorrhage (in association with significant neurologic sequelae) is discussed herein below in the "alternative medical theories" section.

The outcomes of asymptomatic infants with birth-related subdural hemorrhage (and no concurrent parenchymal injury) are relatively benign. Rooks et al analyzed 2-year clinical follow-up of 43 of 46 infants with birth-related subdural hemorrhage, and none had gross motor delay; 6 (14%) children were noted to have speech delay.[399] Zamora et al showed similar cognitive and neurodevelopmental outcomes at age 24 months between normal controls and those with asymptomatic birth-related subdural hemorrhage.[411]

Retinal Hemorrhages

RHs are a relatively common finding with parturition. Several well-conducted studies have placed the incidence of birth-related RHs at approximately 20% to 35%.[154,155,412–415] Birth-related hemorrhages occur in 20% to 30% of infants in the first 24 hours of life, decreasing to

10% to 15% when infants are examined in the first 72 hours of life.[151,415,416] They can occur with any type of delivery, including cesarean section (6% incidence rate), but they are more common in spontaneous vaginal (25.6%) or vacuum-assisted deliveries (42.6%). A systematic review of 13 clinical studies representing 1777 infants revealed that birth-related retinal hemorrhages are commonly bilateral (59%), predominantly intraretinal, and localized in the posterior pole but rarely can be numerous and extend to the periphery.[156] Preretinal hemorrhages may also occur, but subretinal hemorrhages are rare.[177] Despite extensive incidence and descriptive studies referenced earlier, to date, retinoschisis has not been a reported feature of parturition.[154,155,412–415]

The rate of disappearance of birth-related retinal hemorrhage depends on the size and type of hemorrhage. The majority of intraretinal hemorrhages (85%) resolve within 14 days.[415] Dense isolated intraretinal hemorrhages may persist past 3 weeks of age, with the longest reported being 58 days, but numerous intraretinal hemorrhages do not.[415,417] Preretinal and vitreous hemorrhage may last significantly longer than intraretinal hemorrhage. This evidence implies that on the basis of the pattern of resolution, the presence of numerous intraretinal hemorrhages after 3 weeks of age, or single or few intra-RHs after 8 weeks of age, cannot be ascribed to birth.

The mechanism of birth-related RHs is incompletely understood. However, vitreoretinal traction may be one cause if direct eye compression causes distortion and lengthening along a single axis.[155,415] Other proposed mechanisms include ocular compression with prolonged highly raised intraocular pressure and subsequent decompression retinopathy, and release of leukotrienes or other vasoactive factors resulting in increased retinal vessel permeability. Finally, some literature indicates that poor visual outcomes are much more common in AHT than in birth-related retinal hemorrhages.[418–421]

TAKEAWAY POINTS

1. Birth-related subdural hemorrhages are common, often asymptomatic, and can occur in similar locations as those in AHT cases.
2. The vast majority of birth-related subdural hemorrhages resolve by 4 weeks of age, with current literature not documenting the persistence of birth-related subdural hemorrhage beyond 3 months of age.
3. The outcomes of asymptomatic infants with birth-related subdural hemorrhage (and no concurrent parenchymal injury) are relatively benign.
4. Birth-related RHs are common and can be bilateral, involving multiple layers; however, unlike AHT, they uncommonly are numerous or extend to the retinal periphery.
5. Additional distinguishing features between birth-related RHs and retinal findings seen in AHT are the lack of retinoschisis documented in parturition, the lack of persistence of birth-related RHs beyond 2 months of age, and a stronger association of severe retinal findings and poor visual outcomes with AHT.

Benign Enlargement of the Subarachnoid Spaces

Infants and young children often have more prominent subarachnoid spaces than older children and young adults.[422,423] Some hypothesize that the presence of these enlarged subarachnoid spaces predispose a young infant to the development of subdural hemorrhages with little or no trauma, thus potentially causing confusion and a misdiagnosis of abusive head injury.[424–431] Most of these are small series or case reports without clear methodology, and it has been demonstrated that subdural hemorrhages are not a common finding following pediatric minor head injury.[96]

Several studies have evaluated infants and young children with enlarged subarachnoid spaces and macrocephaly.[432–435] Each found a small percentage of patients that might have developed subdural collections/hemorrhage with little to no trauma. Importantly, each patient had little to no clinical symptoms, and each article discusses the importance of considering inflicted injury. Greiner et al found no subdural collections in asymptomatic patients with macrocrania and normal subarachnoid spaces.[432] Tucker et al found the prevalence of subdural collections was higher in patients with a larger degree of expansion of the subarachnoid spaces.[434] Holste et al found that in 480 patients with enlargement of the subarachnoid spaces, 8.1% developed spontaneous subdural hemorrhages and in those with any subdural hemorrhage in their study, only 15.5% required surgical intervention.[435]

Hansen et al studied 149 children younger than 2 years who were evaluated by the child protection team and presented with a subdural hemorrhage.[436] Forty-three were either asymptomatic at presentation or had very mild symptoms attributable to a small subdural. These were compared with 106 severely injured patients. Benign enlargement of the subarachnoid spaces was present in 34 of the total cohort (22.8%), half in each category. The presence of enlarged subarachnoid spaces was associated with a lower occurrence of other suspicious injuries. However, over one-third of patients presenting with a subdural and mild associated symptoms in the presence of enlarged subarachnoid spaces also had other concerning abusive injuries.

In conclusion, it has been shown that a small percentage of patients with benign enlargement of the subarachnoid spaces (BESS) may present with small, asymptomatic subdural collections with little to no reported trauma. However, the authors in each of these articles stress the need to consider abuse as a potential etiology in each case and not simply dismiss the presence of the subdural as a result of the enlarged subarachnoid spaces.

TAKEAWAY POINTS

1. Enlargement of the subarachnoid spaces in common in infants and young children.
2. Infrequently, enlarged subarachnoid spaces may predispose to the development of small, asymptomatic subdural collections with little or no head trauma.
3. Each case of unexpected subdural collection or hemorrhage needs thoughtful consideration as to potential of abuse and not simply dismissed as being attributable to the enlarged subarachnoid spaces.

Alternative Medical Hypotheses Lacking Evidence-Based Research

Hypoxic-Ischemic Injury

Some authors suggest that subdural hemorrhage in infants and young children may result from hypoxic-ischemic injury or hypoxic-ischemic encephalopathy in the perinatal period.[437–439] Several studies, however, have found no such causal association.[440–443] Hurley et al, in analyzing 50 infants with nontraumatic cardiorespiratory collapse, found no extra-axial hemorrhage in the 24 infants with brain imaging and no macroscopic subdural hemorrhage in 39 of 40 with a postmortem examination.[441] One infant had a very small clot adjacent to the dura that was determined to be birth related. Byard et al, evaluating a potential causal relationship of hypoxic ischemic injury and subdural hemorrhage, investigated 82 fetuses, infants, and young children and found no cases of macroscopic subdural hemorrhage on postmortem examinations.[440] Rafaat et al looked at CT findings in 156 young children experiencing near drowning events and found no intra-axial or extra-axial hemorrhage on initial or follow-up imaging in any patients who presented with abnormal initial CT imaging or in those who had normal initial but subsequent abnormal follow-up CT imaging.[444]

Paroxysmal Coughing and Dysphagic Choking

Some authors suggest that rapid, repetitive episodes of elevated intrathoracic pressure, such as paroxysmal coughing or choking on feeds, may result in elevated intracranial venous pressure from venous backflow causing the thin film subdural and retinal hemorrhages that might be seen in cases of suspected AHT.[437,439,445,446]

However, Goldman et al found no retinal hemorrhages in 100 infants and young children presenting with severe coughing episodes requiring hospitalization.[203] Herr et al found no retinal hemorrhages in 100 infants undergoing surgery for hypertrophic pyloric stenosis, 89% being described as having multiple episodes of projectile vomiting.[207] Multiple authors have demonstrated that retinal hemorrhages in the setting of an apparent life-threatening event are exceedingly rare, but when present, should raise concerns for AHT.[447–449]

Hansen et al studied 170 patients younger than 2 years presenting with subdural hemorrhage, 64 presenting with a reported apparent life-threatening event (ALTE) (now described as a brief, resolved, unexplained event [BRUE]) and subdural bleeding.[436] Those with an ALTE-associated subdural hemorrhage were more likely to have a fatal outcome, have permanent neurologic injury, and were 5 times more likely to have at least 1 extracranial injury that was suspicious for inflicted trauma. Ten patients presenting with an ATLE-associated subdural hemorrhage and a dysphagic/choking history witnessed only by 1 caregiver all had evidence of at least 1 other suspicious extracranial injury.

Cerebral Sinovenous Thrombosis

Intracranial or cerebral sinovenous thrombosis (CSVT) historically has a reported incidence between 0.67 and 1.58 cases per 100,000 pediatric patients per year.[450,451] However, the incidence rate in young infants, especially in the neonatal period, is much higher.[450–452] Underlying risk factors for the development of CSVT are present in the majority of pediatric patients and vary with patient age.[450–453] Neonatal CSVT usually occurs from perinatal complications.[450] In the older infant and child, etiologies are often multifactorial and may include dehydration, head and neck infections, underlying malignancies and chronic disease states, prothrombotic factors, and trauma.[451–456]

Some physicians and investigators have suggested that spontaneous or nontraumatic CSVT is a potential source of subdural hemorrhage, thus mimicking the imaging findings of abusive head injury.[437,445,446,457,458]

Outside of the perinatal period, except in rare case reports in the medical literature, subdural hemorrhage is not a frequent finding in nontraumatic cases of pediatric CSVT.[450,455] The Canadian Pediatric Stroke Registry described 9% of patients as having extra-parenchymal hemorrhage on imaging in their report.[450] Subsequently, it has been reported by McLean et al that the registry patients were imaged during the neonatal period, a time when small subdural hemorrhages can be found routinely.[399,400,402,455] This more recent study found no subdural hemorrhage in 36 patients with nontraumatic CSVT, even in the patients with extensive, intracranial thrombosis.[455]

Rebleeding of Intracranial Hemorrhage With Severe Neurologic Sequelae and/or Death

Some authors have suggested that spontaneous rebleeding into preexisting subdural hemorrhage, including birth-related hemorrhage, may lead to the acute compromise of the child.[457,459,460] Several authors have shown that many cases of mixed-attenuation subdural hemorrhages found during an AHT evaluation do not necessarily represent new hemorrhage into "chronic subdural hemorrhages."[53,90,362,461] Many occur without acute clinical symptoms and suspicious extracranial injuries and represent acute, low-attenuation subdural fluid mixing with different components of blood (hematohygroma), not necessarily different episodes or ages of injuries.[353–356,362]

Datta et al studied 74 children younger than 2 years with either subdural hemorrhage or effusions on neuroimaging.[461] Twenty-six had mixed-attenuation subdural hemorrhages. However, 20 of 26 had extracranial findings of prior abuse and signs of elevated intracranial pressure or acute mental status changes suggesting repeated episodes of abuse, not simple rebleeding. No spontaneous bleeding occurred in postinfectious subdural collections.

Bradford et al found evidence of rebleeding into a preexisting subdural hemorrhage in 16% of 105 cases of abusive head injury, all rebleeds being small and asymptomatic at the time of imaging.[90]

Feldman et al performed a multicenter retrospective review of 383 abused infants and children with suspected acute (291/383) and reported mixed acute/chronic (92/383) subdural hemorrhage.[53] Nearly 80% of each group presented with acute neurologic symptoms and other injuries concerning for abuse, suggesting each likely experienced an acute or repeated inflicted injury, not spontaneous rebleeding.

Wright et al studied 85 children younger than 3 years with a subdural hemorrhage, diagnosis of AHT, and both initial and follow-up imaging.[362] Almost 64% (54/85) had imaging evidence of rebleeding within 1 year. This was significantly associated with parenchymal volume loss, ventricular enlargement, large subdural depth, and macrocephaly, but not new brain injury at follow-up. Most rebleeding was found on routine follow-up imaging and was in the original subdural location in 94.4% (51/54) of cases. All rebleeding was asymptomatic and occurred into preexisting low-attenuation subdural collections. None had acute neurologic compromise or new concerning abusive injuries, and none occurred in a previously resolved subdural hemorrhage.

Feldman et al and Wright et al specifically mention an association of asymptomatic rebleeding in patients with preexisting subdurals and macrocephaly.[53,362] In both of these studies, the rebleeding was isolated to the location of the prior subdural supporting that rebleeding could occur with little or no additional trauma in children with chronic subdurals.[108] However, the neovascularity in the chronic subdural hemorrhage would not result in rebleeding in other distinct locations.

TAKEAWAY POINTS

1. The correlation between hypoxic-ischemic injury and the development of subdural hemorrhages lacks evidence base.
2. Paroxysmal coughing and choking are not associated with the development of RHs and/or subdural hemorrhage.
3. Isolated subdural hemorrhage has not been demonstrated to occur as a result of CSVT. However, in pediatric patients, CSVT often has an underlying risk factor and can occur as a complication of traumatic head injury.
4. Rebleeding into preexisting subdural hemorrhage or collections is common in patients having experienced prior abusive head injury. However, it is almost always asymptomatic and does not result in acute, significant neurologic compromise in the child.

DIAGNOSIS

As discussed earlier, the diagnosis of AHT is made in the context of a complete history, physical examination, and medical evaluation using the same process as in any other medical diagnosis: the differential diagnosis.[52] In addition, many providers have the advantage of a multidisciplinary hospital child protection team.[462] Such a team can help to minimize the risk of individual error that may occur from judgment heuristics or cognitive bias.[463] Throughout the diagnostic differentiation process, the pediatric provider will have to manage various uncertainties until the individual threshold of diagnostic sufficiency is reached.[464]

Prediction Rules and Pooled Analyses

Assisting providers in reaching a diagnosis are recently published prediction rules and pooled analyses. "Clinical decision rules," and "clinical prediction rules" are evidence-based tools that combine clinical features to assist clinicians in probabilistic determinations of clinical diagnosis, prognosis, or response to therapy.[465] Several of these tools—the PredAHT tool, the PEDIBIRN clinical decision rule, and Maguire's pooled analysis—have been discussed earlier.[51,466,467] The value of these tools is that they offer clinicians a meta-analysis of the import of these collective variables and, thereby, minimize inherent risks of individual biases, cognitive errors, and local circumstances.

Communicating the AHT Diagnosis in Court and Other Medicolegal Considerations

With regard to the differential diagnosis methodology, courts have varied in their interpretation and understanding of it. Some courts have interpreted it to be the methodology for arriving at causation by "ruling out" alternative causes.[468] Others have interpreted it to require both a "ruling out" and "ruling in" process for arriving at causation.[469] And others have even created legal concepts, such as "differential etiology," declaring it to be different from "differential diagnosis."

Most courts have found the differential diagnosis methodology to be "a well-recognized and widely used technique in the medical community to identify and isolate causes of disease and death." [Gunderson, 279 S.W.3d at 107 (citing Globetti v. Sandoz Pharms. Corp., 111 F.Supp.2d 1174, 1177 (N.D. Ala. 2000)); State v. Edwards, 2011 WL 1378927 (Ohio Ct. App. April 13, 2011); State v. Carr, 2010 WL 2473337 (Ohio Ct. App. June 18, 2010)] However, some courts have questioned its reliability.[470]

Tangent to this misunderstanding has been the prevalent issue of referring to the AHT diagnosis as a "triad" (ie, diagnosed if the child has subdural hemorrhages, RHs, and cerebral edema).[471] It is this relegation to heuristic application of the 3 more common findings of the diagnosis that has fostered legal misunderstanding of the aforementioned complex diagnostic process. The pediatric provider will need to be prepared to explain to courts that the evolution of diagnostic understanding of AHT has broadened to try and capture, in definition, the myriad of ways inflicted injury to a child's head can occur and manifest. This understanding, again, may be fostered by current clinical prediction rules and pooled analyses, showing how variable combinations of clinical features can hold extremely high odds for the AHT diagnosis and not just the "triad."[51]

Finally, and probably most importantly, has been the prevalent issue of ethical expert testimony in AHT cases. Some authors have asserted that AHT cases have been a minefield of irresponsible expert testimony.[472,473] In a medicolegal analysis of overturned shaken baby syndrome (SBS)/AHT convictions in the US appellate system over a 10-year period, Narang et al found that: 1) medical evidence-related themes raised on appeal seldom reflected new scientific or clinical discoveries but rather were alternative or differing medical opinions from those offered at the original trial; and 2) that their review of over 1400 appellate cases over a 10-year period "tended to support the concerns of other authors regarding irresponsible communication of medical information in AHT/SBS cases."[473] Thus, the pediatric provider should be prepared to educate the legal system not only about what is sound science in AHT, but also what is junk science. To complete this task, it will be important for the pediatric provider to be versed in the principles of ethical expert testimony espoused by the AAP.[474]

MANAGEMENT

Introduction

Although AHT comprises a significant fraction of head injuries requiring hospitalization in children younger than 5 years, no evidence-based guidelines for the management of the child with AHT currently exist.[98] Guidance regarding the medical and surgical treatment may be abstracted from a combination of existing literature on the management of pediatric and adult head injury as well as a small volume of literature specific to AHT.

Medical Treatment

Guidelines for the management of pediatric severe traumatic brain injury were initially developed in 2003 by a panel of experts in traumatic brain injury during the fifth Annual Aspen Neurobehavioral Conference.[475,476] The guidelines were updated most recently by the Brain Trauma Foundation in 2019.[477] Current guidelines present evidence-based recommendations on 3 broad categories: monitoring (3 topics), thresholds for treatment (2 topics), and treatment (10 topics). These guidelines are not specific to the infant population or to the child with AHT. In 2 topics covered by the guidelines, additional literature specific to the infant or child with AHT mandates special consideration of this patient population:

- Intracranial pressure monitoring: The 2019 Guidelines for the Management of Pediatric Severe Traumatic Brain Injury suggest the use of intracranial pressure monitoring as an option capable of improving overall neurologic outcomes in pediatric patients. However, the guidelines clarify that "(b)ecause there are no imaging or other biomarkers that indicate a patient with intracranial hypertension, it is recommended that ICP is measured to determine if intracranial hypertension is present" and that "studies support the association of successful ICP monitor–based management of intracranial hypertension with improved survival and neurologic outcome."[477] Furthermore, as suggested treatment thresholds are based on measurements, a lack of intracranial pressure monitoring in the setting of intracranial hypertension limits management.
- Thresholds for Treatment: The 2019 Guidelines for the Management of Pediatric Severe Traumatic Brain Injury suggest the treatment of intracranial pressure (ICP) targeting a threshold of <20 mm Hg as "mortality is often due to refractory sustained increases in ICP." Thus, "preventing intracranial hypertension is central to current neurocritical care of these children."[477] In addition, thee 2019 guideline further suggests treatment to maintain CPP (cerebral perfusion pressure) at a minimum of 40 mm Hg using a range from 40 to 50 mm Hg, "with infants at the lower end and adolescents at or above the upper end of this range."[477]
- Treatment Topics: The 2019 Guidelines for the Management of Pediatrics Severe Traumatic Brain Injury further identified the following recommendations[477]:
  - Bolus hypertonic saline (3%) is recommended in patients with intracranial hypertension. Recommended effective doses for acute use range from 2 to 5 mL/kg over 10 to 20 minutes.
  - Continuous infusion hypertonic saline is suggested in patients with intracranial hypertension. Suggested effective doses as a continuous infusion of 3% saline range from 0.1 to 1.0 mL/kg of body weight per hour,

administered on a sliding scale. The minimum dose needed to maintain ICP <20 mm Hg is suggested.
  - Bolus of 23.4% hypertonic saline is suggested for refractory ICP. The suggested dose is 0.5 mL/kg with a maximum of 30 mL. (Level II Evidence)
  - With use of multiple ICP-related therapies as well as appropriate use of analgesia and sedation in routine intensive care, avoiding bolus administration of midazolam and/or fentanyl during ICP crises is suggested because of risks of cerebral hypoperfusion.
  - Cerebrospinal fluid drainage through an external ventricular drain is suggested to manage increased ICP.
  - Prophylactic severe hyperventilation to a partial pressure of arterial carbon dioxide <30 mm Hg in the initial 48 hours after injury is not suggested.
  - If hyperventilation is used in the management of refractory intracranial hypertension, advanced neuromonitoring for evaluation of cerebral ischemia is suggested.
  - Prophylactic moderate (32°–33°C) hypothermia is not recommended over normothermia to improve overall outcomes.
  - Moderate (32°–33°C) hypothermia is suggested for ICP control.
  - High-dose barbiturate therapy is suggested in hemodynamically stable patients with refractory intracranial hypertension despite maximal medical and surgical management.
  - Decompressive craniectomy is suggested to treat neurologic deterioration, herniation, or intracranial hypertension refractory to medical management.
  - Use of an immune-modulating diet is not recommended.
  - Initiation of early enteral nutritional support (within 72 hours from injury) is suggested to decrease mortality and improve outcomes.
  - The use of corticosteroids is not suggested to improve outcome or reduce ICP.
- Treatment of the patient with severe traumatic brain injury patient is complex, and the recommendations are often difficult to translate into bedside management. Kochanek et al in 2019 established an algorithm for first- and second-tier therapies, in part utilizing the recommendations from the 2019 Guidelines for the Management of Pediatric Severe Traumatic Brain Injury and supplementing with consensus when evidence was insufficient to fully formulate an evidence-based approach.[478] Although the first-tier pathway distinguishes a linear ICP, CPP, brain tissue oxygen (if monitoring), and herniation pathways, the paper specifically noted that treatments may warrant a rapid and nonlinear approach.[478]
- Evaluation and management of post-traumatic seizures: The 2019 Guidelines for the Management of Pediatric Severe Traumatic Brain Injury suggest the use of prophylactic treatment for the first 7 days post-TBI to reduce the occurrence of early post-traumatic seizures in pediatric patients. References cited in the guidelines include authors citing rates of 2.4% and 17% of early post-traumatic seizures in the pediatric population studied.[479,480] However, the incidence of clinical and nonconvulsive seizures is significantly higher in the patients with AHT with a seizure incidence ranging from 51% to 77%, providing additional evidence for the use of anticonvulsant use in this pediatric subgroup.[480–482] Hasbani et al performed a retrospective study reviewing use of continuous encephalogram (EEG) monitoring in AHT patients at their intensive care unit.[388] Of 32 children admitted during the periods studied, 21 (66%) were monitored with seizures noted in 12 (37.5%) and status epilepticus in 8 (25%). Two-thirds of children never had clinical signs associated with their electrographic seizures; thus, EEG monitoring is required to diagnose and guide acute seizure management. In a larger study performed by O'Neill et al, age less than 2.4 years and AHT mechanism was strongly associated with the presence of seizures (OR, 8.7 and 6.0, respectively).[483] In a prospective study of patients with consecutive moderate to severe TBI admitted to the intensive care unit at 2 institutions, AHT mechanism was a significant risk factor for seizures, with 17 of 22 (77.3%) experiencing seizures.[482] AHT was also a significant risk factor for electrographic-only seizures.

Surgical Management

A significant number of children presenting with AHT require surgical intervention. In a 5-year review of children presenting to Le Bonheur Children's Hospital, 58 of 213 children with AHT required surgical intervention. Unfortunately, no evidence-based guidelines exist to guide the selection of surgical strategies for the management of the patient with AHT. Case series and pathology-specific literature can guide providers in the care of these patients.[9]

- Skull fractures and epidural hemorrhage: Literature-based guidance regarding the management of depressed skull fractures and epidural hemorrhage is limited. The Brain Trauma Foundation sponsored a "rigorous literature-based" review to provide recommendations for the surgical management of patients with post-traumatic intracranial mass lesions.[462,463] The document provided indications for elevation of open and closed fractures as well as evacuation of epidural hemorrhage on the basis of size and neurologic status of the patient.[484,485]
- Subdural hemorrhage: Fluid collections are common in the subdural space of children who have experienced AHT. Subdural hemorrhagic collections have variable physical properties depending on factors to include the age of blood in the fluid present and include jelly-like

collections of clotted blood, pink-tinged mixtures of spinal fluid and blood, and clear yellow or thick motor oil consistency fluid. In addition to influencing the selection of surgical technique used for management, the heterogeneity of these collections can lead to inconsistent use of terminology and resultant confusion among those reading diagnostic reports.[354]

At the time of this publication, no established guidelines for the management of subdural fluid collections in AHT have been established. Options to include simple transfontanelle tap, irrigation/closed drainage, irrigation/open drainage, minicraniotomy, and subdural peritoneal shunt placement have been described on the basis of anecdotal experience and provider preference.[49,486,487] For subdural hemorrhages with mass effect, standard craniotomy and sometimes decompression is undertaken. In children requiring surgery for solid clots with mass effect or those failing maximal medical management, decompressive craniectomy has been advocated, although the mortality and complication rates of this procedure are significant in the infant and toddler. Oluigbo et al described their experience with this population, with a reported mortality rate of 35.7%.[48]

- Cerebral infarction: The most severe injuries sustained by children with AHT result in regional ischemia/infarction; the mechanisms of these injuries are incompletely understood, but they affect up to 30% of patients with AHT with an estimated mortality of 25%.[118]

Team Approach to Management of the Child With AHT

Several organizations have cited the value of a multidisciplinary team approach to the evaluation and treatment of the child with AHT.[31,466] Essential team members include the trauma surgeon, neurosurgeon, pediatrician (ideally, a child abuse pediatrician), and a social worker.[488] The expertise of additional medical and surgical subspecialists to include orthopedics, ophthalmology, critical care, neurology, hematology, radiology, and others may be required in individual cases. Additional resources to include nursing, behavioral health, physical and occupational therapy, child life, child protective services, and law enforcement. All parties strive to ensure the timely collection of clinical information affecting both medical decision-making and forensic analysis of the patient's presentation. Excellent communication between neurosurgeons, intensivists, and ophthalmologists can allow for safe diagnostic eye evaluations without effect on patient monitoring.[373] Additional radiographic evaluations and interviews between child abuse pediatricians, social workers, and families can provide critical information regarding timing and mechanism of injury.

Community Management

Individual clinicians are responsible for the assessment of their own capabilities and those of their place of practice. There is currently no literature that establishes which patients can be safely evaluated and/or cared for by whom and in what setting. Likewise, no literature exists that provides guidance regarding which patient requires transfer for specialized care and by what means. However, materials are available relevant to the consideration of this topic. The consequences of missed injuries are well established; in a review of 54 children seen by physicians for symptoms related to AHT, Jenny et al reported a reinjury rate of 27.8% and a mortality of 7.4%.[21] The American College of Surgeons (ACS) established "Best Practice Guidelines for Trauma Center Recognition" that establish the challenges and extensive resource requirements for certification by their organization regarding the diagnosis and treatment of abusive head trauma.[488] This same organization provides instruction on the initial evaluation of the trauma patient that establishes the referring health care provider as responsible for selecting and initiating the appropriate mode of transfer for the patient.[331] Finally, the potential for conflict of interest influencing family decision making regarding self-transport has been recognized in prior research examining the selection of transport means for pediatric patients seen at a level 1 trauma center.[489] Cost of transport was a recognized driver of decision making, suggesting that factors other than patient well-being may influence family decisions. The referring provider may strongly consider the patient's safety in their selection of a mode of transport for a patient with known or suspected AHT.

TAKEAWAY POINTS

1. Medical guidelines for the management of pediatric severe closed head injury are not specific to AHT.
2. Existing literature points to low utilization of ICP monitoring and high rates of subclinical status epilepticus in patients with AHT.
3. Treatment options for chronic/liquid subdural hemorrhage include observation, transfontanelle tap, irrigation with open or closed drainage, craniotomy, and subdural peritoneal shunt placement; management of acute hemorrhage with mass effect follows similar principles for older children including consideration of decompression.
4. AHT with cerebral infarction caries significant mortality.
5. Children with AHT have the potential for multisystem medical disease and require evaluation and treatment that is optimally provided through multidisciplinary collaborative care.
6. Physicians may strongly consider the patient's safety when referring/transporting a patient from either an

outpatient facility or small hospital with limited resources.

PATHOLOGY

Introduction

The National Association of Medical Examiners (NAME) and the AAP endorse universal forensic autopsies for all unexplained infant deaths.[490] All unexpected pediatric deaths are investigated by a medicolegal death investigation system consisting of a mixture of physician medical examiners and lay coroners spread over approximately 2000 autonomous jurisdictions; autopsies are usually performed by forensic pathologists certified by the American Board of Pathology.[491] Forensic pathologists routinely serve as panel members on regional child death/fatality review committees.[492–494]

The medicolegal autopsy aims to understand the cause, manner, and mechanism of death, each of which has a specific connotation when used in this context.[495–497] The *cause* of death refers to the injury or disease process that initiated the lethal sequence of events (eg, traumatic head injury) while the *manner* considers the circumstances.[495] The *mechanism* of death refers to the terminal pathophysiologic derangement that ended in death (eg, seizure, hypoxic-ischemic encephalopathy, cardiac arrythmia, etc) and is usually not etiologically specific.[498]

The potential causes of sudden unexpected death in early childhood are numerous and span a spectrum from rare natural diseases to inflicted injuries. To accurately catalog the cause of pediatric demise, death investigation is a dynamic and comprehensive process that integrates pathoanatomic findings at autopsy with available history, imaging data, circumstances of the death, and the results of ancillary studies that include but are not limited to histology, toxicology, microbiology, metabolic, and molecular studies, among others.[499,500]

As mentioned earlier in this report, the literature on physical findings was derived primarily from the clinical literature of non-fatal AHT cases. Epidemiologic and clinical features of fatal AHT cases are discussed in the section below.

Autopsy in Suspected AHT

Although as many as one-third of AHT cases have a lethal outcome and require an autopsy, determination of the cause of death may be challenging, because a history of trauma is often not easily forthcoming and external signs of injury may be subtle or absent.[500,501] Published reports and guidelines from professional societies assist forensic pathologists in the investigation and certification of sudden pediatric death.[490,502–506] The National Association of Medical Examiners currently has no formal recommendations for suspected head trauma in infants and young children, the 2014 position paper having sunsetted per the society's routine 5-year limitation policy; however, this resource is still informally referenced by many pathologists for guidance on autopsy procedures, interpretation, and documentation of findings.[500,501,507]

An autopsy in suspected AHT is, thus, a specific and large independent dataset with core data elements that include digital photography, radiologic skeletal survey comprising full-body plain radiography, with comprehensive external and internal examination, and ancillary studies to document injury and exclude significant natural disease.[500] These findings are interpreted in the context of history from medical records and other agencies including law enforcement.[500,508] A forum has addressed some of the challenges and controversies faced by forensic pathologists in the autopsy investigation and analysis of childhood death.[509–516]

Limitations of Autopsy Data

Autopsy data are an endpoint with published descriptions of AHT findings generally consisting of small descriptive series. These data are often limited by small sample sizes; incomplete and variable data; selection bias; small numbers of adequate controls; varied survival intervals; confounding variables, such as secondary changes from life-saving interventions instituted during life or artifacts of maintenance on artificial ventilation before death in children with hypoxic-ischemic brain injury; inconsistent inclusion of histopathologic descriptions; and noncontemporaneous methodology to assess axonal pathology in older series limiting comparisons across datasets.[122,133,269,286,517–528]

Even though specialized autopsy techniques for examination of the central nervous system and related structures are described, some of these procedures require technical expertise and are variably implemented by forensic pathologists.[529–535] In addition, AHT fatalities are typically investigated as discrete individual events, such that robust study designs including blinding are almost never feasible. The situation is further strained by an underresourced, understaffed, and nonstandardized death investigation system.[536,537] Despite these limitations, autopsy observations continue to inform the pathobiology and classification of pathologic mechanisms of AHT and represent the bedrock of forensic investigation in sudden and unexplained childhood death.

The most common neuropathologic findings reported across AHT autopsy series include subdural hemorrhage (90%–100%), subarachnoid hemorrhage (60%–100%), RH (20%–100%), cerebral edema (28%–100%), global hypoxic-ischemic injury (37%–78%), traumatic axonal injury (less than 6%), and contusions (7%–67%).[109,122,133,269,501,517–520,522,523,527,538–542] It should be noted that these broad ranges are derived primarily from small qualitative studies, many of which had low numbers (less than 20 cases), missing datapoints, or nonspecified diagnostic criteria. In isolation, none of these findings is specific to inflicted trauma. However, the constellation of these findings in a pattern not explained by the available history, or combined with unexplained extracranial injuries, alerts the pathologist to the potential of inflicted trauma.[543] These findings are, in turn, modulated by developmental host responses to injury, which are subject to age-dependent maturational differences of the developing brain.[544–546] Importantly, neuropathologic examination serves also to exclude other potential nAHT pathologic processes, such as infection or a ruptured vascular malformation that could account for unexpected death.

FINDINGS AT AUTOPSY

External Findings

The proportion of AHT cases with external contact injuries of the head or facial region varies markedly across autopsy series, with contact injury found in 16% to 100% of cases, although many series are again limited by low case numbers.[133,269,517,519,522,523,527,528,540,547] However, not all fatally injured children have an impact site despite careful examination.[133,521,522,548] This absence of external contact findings could support the inference that injury in these children relates to violent shaking or head impact with deceleration against a padded surface.[133,269,501,522,540] Case selection criteria influence reported skull fracture frequency across autopsy series with reported proportions ranging from 17% to 64% and a propensity for the posterior parietal or occipital bone.[269,517,518,523,540,549] Nondisplaced skull fractures may be difficult to detect at autopsy, and microscopic confirmation of a suspected fracture site stage of healing might be necessary.[500]

Acute Subdural Hemorrhage

Acute subdural hemorrhage (SDH) is observed in more than 90% of AHT autopsies, typically as a thin film of hemorrhage, (<5–10 mL), along the posterior interhemispheric fissure or convexity surfaces of the posterior cerebrum.[90,106,109,501,517,539,550] Although considered a marker for the amount of force transmitted through the brain and underlying brain injury, it is rarely a space-occupying lesion in infants.[109,539] The pathogenesis includes laceration of bridging veins extending from the cerebral surface to the dural sinuses as a consequence of acceleration-deceleration of the head, and less frequently laceration of a dural venous sinus from displaced skull bone fragments.[68,92,109,110,112,551–555] Nontraumatic causes including coagulation disorders, neurosurgical intervention, ruptured vascular malformations, neoplastic and metabolic disease, among others, are rare and can be distinguished with assistance of a complete autopsy and ancillary studies as indicated.[556]

Chronic SDH

The pathogenesis of chronic SDH is complex and poorly understood but includes extravasation of blood and cerebrospinal fluid into the subdural space following border cell layer disruption resulting in fibroproliferative and chronic inflammatory responses with neomembrane formation, angiogenesis, and localized coagulopathy.[557,558] Estimating the timeframe of these pathologic processes by microscopic examination is imprecise and potentially error prone.[559] Gradual enlargement of a chronic subdural hemorrhage may result from microhemorrhage associated with neovascularization.[109] Prospective imaging studies have demonstrated that acute rebleeding within chronic SDH is uncommon and usually minor and asymptomatic when it occurs.[90,362]

Subarachnoid Hemorrhage

Acute subarachnoid hemorrhage (SAH) is common in traumatic brain injury, with a propensity for parasagittal surfaces of the cerebrum, often in a patchy distribution. Although not a distinguishing feature between AHT and nAHT in clinical studies of live children, SAHs are reported in 60% to 100% of fatal AHT cases.[109,269,501,517,519,520,523,540,547] Nontraumatic causes of SAHs, such as ruptured vascular malformation or venous sinus thrombosis, are usually readily distinguished from traumatic causes on examination of the brain at autopsy.

Epidural Hemorrhages

Intracranial epidural hemorrhage (EDH) of arterial or venous origin is uncommon in AHT autopsy series and is rare without associated skull fracture.[517,523,560–563] The dura in infants is more tightly adherent to the skull than later in life, which may be one reason why EDHs are less common in children. Arterial EDHs typically result from laceration of the middle meningeal artery; venous EDHs are associated with skull fractures and lacerated diploic veins, particularly in the posterior fossa.[564] EDHs are relatively infrequently described in autopsy series, reflecting amenability to surgical intervention and an overall favorable prognosis, although some may spontaneously resolve.[565,566]

Cerebral Edema

Rapidly progressive cerebral edema leading to diffuse brain swelling is a prominent autopsy finding in children with fatal head injury.[567,568] Although limited data exist for AHT, several nAHT series report a high prevalence of cerebral edema associated with ischemia and traumatic axonal injury following head injury in young children.[569–573] The pathogenesis of rapid cerebral edema following brain trauma remains poorly understood and is likely multifactorial with cellular and vascular mechanisms implicated.[571,574,575]

Diffuse Axonal Injury

Diffuse traumatic axonal injury (dTAI) refers to a pattern of white matter axonal injury following rapid acceleration-deceleration, characterized pathologically by the accumulation of APP in axonal swellings and bulbs.[576,577] This test is the gold standard for detection of axonal injury in fatal injuries, with injured axons potentially detected within 35 to 45 minutes following head trauma.[576–589]

Although APP is a sensitive marker for axonal injury, it is not specific for mechanical injury, and accumulation occurs in other disease states including hypoxia, infection, and inflammatory disorders, underscoring the necessity for clinicopathologic correlation in all cases.[581,590–592] The inability to reproducibly distinguish mechanical from hypoxic causes of axonal injury using APP staining undermines direct evidence for dTAI since hypoxic-ischemic injury is common in AHT and more specific diagnostic makers are not available. This is further compounded by limited, nonstandardized autopsy data with low case numbers and lack of uniform diagnostic criteria for dTAI.[122,500,517,519,520,542,571,593] Further, older autopsy series predating APP immunohistochemistry lack the requisite sensitivity to detect axonal injury, resulting in inconsistencies when AHT autopsy datasets are reassessed.[122,518,593] Despite the aforementioned limitations of APP staining, the presence of cortical contusions and subcortical white matter lacerations in some cases suggests the etiology of axonal injury might not be adequately explained by hypoxia-ischemia alone in all cases.[519] Several published AHT autopsy series report macroscopic brain descriptions only, and although typical macroscopic features of dTAI such as dorsolateral quadrant brainstem hemorrhages are usually not described, more comprehensive microscopic descriptions of axonal pathology are lacking in several series.[133,269,593]

Localized Axonal Injury

Hyperextension neck injury and cervical spine distraction during shaking or impact are potential mechanisms of spinal cord stretch injury characterized by localized accumulation of APP in axons of white matter brainstem tracts in the cervico-medullary region and pons, a finding described in infants with AHT.[122,133,500,517,519,520,542,571,593] These localized axonal changes are potentially survivable but represent a heightened potential for progression to more severe hypoxic-ischemic injury and cerebral edema, which in turn leads to death.[122] However, apnea complicating cervico-medullary injury does not fully explain the unilateral pattern of cerebral hemispheric injury following AHT seen in some cases, suggesting nonglobal mechanisms of injury are also at play, at least in some instances.[594,595] Localized traumatic axonal injury associated with AHT has been described in brainstem corticospinal tracts and high cervical cord and spinal nerve roots and is associated with cervical epidural hemorrhage in some cases, although complete brainstem data are not reported for all cases.[122,133,286,517,519,596] Isolated epidural or meningeal hemorrhage, reported in some series, is of unclear significance and should be interpreted cautiously without additional supporting evidence of inflicted trauma.[535,597]

Cervical Spinal Cord Injury

Cervical spinal cord injuries are common, although not universal in fatal AHT series, with spinal cord injury reported in up to 80% of cases in some series that document spinal findings.[122,286,519,523] Reported injuries include primary spinal cord trauma, cord edema, spinal nerve root injury, dorsal root ganglion, and extramedullary compartment hemorrhages.[120–123,128,132,133,286,519,598]

Autopsy techniques to assist pathologists in the evaluation of these structures are described.[529,530,535] Localized stretch injury of the spinal cord is postulated to result from hyperextension or distraction movement of the neck, which is thought to predispose to mechanisms of death that include trauma-induced apnea, hypoxic-ischemic injury, and cerebral edema.[120,122,123,599] Suggested diaphragmatic denervation attributable to cervical spinal injury does not fully explain similar changes in AHT cases without cervical cord damage or account for the nonglobal patterns of hypoxic-ischemic injury described in some infants.[122,286,531,594,596,600]

Hypoxic-Ischemic Injury

Hypoxic-ischemic change is a form of secondary brain injury (ie, brain injury that encompasses a reduction in the supply of oxygen [hypoxia] and/or diminished blood supply to the brain) that is frequently reported in AHT series and results in substantial axonal injury burden.[122,517,519] Mechanisms of hypoxic-ischemic change are multifactorial and include concussive-like causes of apnea resulting from cervico-medullary injury, aspiration attributable to muted airway reflexes, perturbation of autoregulation with altered cerebral blood flow, excitotoxicity, altered neurometabolic demands after injury, and seizures in acutely injured brain tissue.[601] Diffuse axonal injury of vascular and ischemic origin is the most frequently reported brain finding across AHT autopsy series.[122,519,528,542,547,583,602]

One small retrospective study found comparable APP staining profiles in cerebral white matter of AHT and hypoxic-ischemic injured cases but brainstem axonal staining only in AHT cases, suggesting cerebral damage in both groups resulted from hypoxia.[519] Another well-annotated neuropathologic series of 37 children found widespread hypoxic-ischemic injury with cerebral edema as the most common finding.[122] A population-based cohort study of perinatal asphyxia in neonatal deaths of preterm and term infants found APP staining patterns could not be reliably distinguished from mechanical axonal injury, although none of these infants had a known history of trauma.[603] The apparent contradictory findings in some series including reports of dTAI in some AHT cases but not controls underscores the lack of standardized diagnostic criteria applied to dTAI across series as well as methodologic issues that can relate to inadequate age-matched controls, confounding, and insufficient brainstem data.[520]

Cortical and Subcortical Contusions

Because of the immaturity of the infant brain, blunt head trauma at younger than 5 months may be associated with subcortical white matter contusional lacerations, with a predilection for the frontal, occipital, and temporal lobes.[604] Occasionally, these extend into overlying cortex as cortical tears or become distended by blood to form intraparenchymal hemorrhages. Data regarding the frequency of subcortical contusional lacerations in fatal AHT are limited.[269,517,518] One larger descriptive series of 16 infants younger than 5 months with contusional lacerations included 9 infants with head trauma history; the remaining infants had autopsy findings either definitive or suspicious for trauma.[604] Evidence to support nontraumatic etiologies of these lesions, such as obstructed superficial venous drainage, is limited.[605]

Sinovenous Thrombosis

Secondary sinovenous thrombosis may occur as a consequence of venous injury following accidental or inflicted head trauma.[543] Further, it is not unusual to find thrombosed venous sinuses at autopsy examination secondary to raised ICP and relative stasis of venous blood flow.

Postmortem Ocular Findings

Postmortem examination of the eye and orbital tissues can reveal abnormalities not appreciated on antemortem clinical examinations. Such findings include hemorrhages of the optic nerve sheath, extraocular muscles, and orbital fat in cases of child fatality and suspected AHT.[606–608] A protocol to assist forensic pathologists in removal of the orbital contents for standardized examination has been described.[533] Optic nerve sheath hemorrhage is not always accompanied by retinal hemorrhage and can also be seen in patients with nAHT. It tends to be most prominent anteriorly and does not necessarily extend the length of the optic nerve.[143,609–611] Optic nerve sheath hemorrhage frequently involves multiple layers around the optic nerve. The location can be subdural (78%), intradural (61%), or subarachnoid (26%) or involve multiple compartments.[607,612] The extent of the optic nerve sheath hemorrhage does not necessarily correlate with the severity of intraocular findings.[610,613,614]

Retinal findings in nonfatal AHT cases are described earlier in detail in the section on ocular findings.

TAKEAWAY POINTS

1. Autopsies are performed as part of the investigation of a child fatality suspected to be attributable to injury to determine the cause and manner of death.
2. SDH, SAH, RH, cerebral edema, hypoxic-ischemic injury, and traumatic injury are the most common autopsy findings in AHT.
3. Pathologists are alerted to the possibility of AHT when the autopsy findings do not comport with the available history.
4. Detailed examination of the central nervous system, orbital contents, and dura are important components of the autopsy in AHT.
5. Optic nerve sheath hemorrhages are less specific for AHT than intraocular hemorrhages, perimacular retinal folds or macular retinoschisis.

OUTCOMES

Research in outcomes in AHT spans many domains. These include series assessing short- and long-term cognitive, behavioral, and motor outcomes with and without comparison to accidental injuries; predictors of outcome based on acute imaging features; predictors of outcome based on acute presentation factors; visual outcomes; post-traumatic epilepsy; and social and legal outcomes.

Cognitive and Behavioral Outcomes and Their Predictors

Mortality in AHT is high compared with head trauma in general in this age group, averaging about 20% among various series.[43,615] Although incidence is higher in infants younger than 1 year, mortality is higher in children between 12 and 23 months of age.[616] Survivors have variable outcomes, with a significant percentage having cognitive and behavioral difficulties, averaging about one-third with "good" outcomes and two-thirds having deficits ranging from mild to severe.

Specific outcomes scales and categories vary among reports, but as a general rule, "good" or "mild" outcomes signify no or mild deficits that do not interfere in a major way with activities of daily living or require major modifications in schooling; "moderately" affected children have needs that require educational adaptations or include physical limitations; and "severe" outcomes include difficulties with activities of daily living. Using these general categories, about one third of children with abusive head trauma are severely disabled, including those who are nonverbal, nonambulatory, and with severe brain atrophy on imaging, even many years after injury.[100,418,599,615,617–619] Of note, of those children who initially seem only mildly or moderately affected, deficits may become more apparent with age, as cognitive and behavioral demands of school and socialization increase.[617,620–625]

Several studies comparing outcomes between children with inflicted and accidental injuries show worse outcomes overall in children in the inflicted category. These include both short-term and longer-term outcomes in the cognitive, verbal, motor, and behavioral domains.[100,384,387,626] Despite significant deficits, however, children with inflicted injuries have been found to have similar health-related quality of life to that of healthy children when assessed by parent questionnaire when children are about 2 years of age.[625]

Imaging predictors of worse outcome include larger areas of loss of grey/white differentiation, hemispheric hypodensity or signal change on CT or MRI, and larger areas of diffusion abnormality on MRI.[91,107,384,600,627,628] Acute predictors of worse cognitive outcomes include early seizures, older age, need for intubation, metabolic perturbations including base deficit, and having a male nonparental perpetrator.[388,481,629–633]

A small number of studies have assessed the results of acute intervention or rehabilitation. Decompressive hemicraniectomy, most often performed for children with a predominantly unilateral subdural hemorrhage and significant mass effect or associated hemispheric brain injury, may help children with inflicted injury as well as children with accidental trauma. But as in other series, the AHT group has worse outcomes, likely reflecting more severe injuries overall.[48,634] Similarly, rehabilitation and early intervention services appear to benefit young children with inflicted and accidental injuries, although those in the former group, especially when injured at younger ages, do worse overall.[626,635]

Visual Outcomes

Visual outcome is good (ie, visual acuity of 20/40 or better) in one-third to one-half of survivors.[145,211] Most intraretinal hemorrhages resolve spontaneously without sequelae. However, serious visual impairment occurs in 25% to 30% of children surviving AHT.[145] The main causes of visual impairment are nonclearing vitreous hemorrhage, which can cause deprivation amblyopia, induced myopia, and refractive amblyopia; retinal scarring or fibrosis, possibly secondary to retinoschisis; optic nerve atrophy; and cortical visual impairment from brain injury.[141,636–638] Direct optic nerve injury from acceleration-deceleration forces within the orbit is the most likely cause of the atrophic damage to the optic nerve. Because papilledema occurs rarely and is commonly transient, it is not a common cause of optic atrophy. Trans-synaptic degeneration and retinal injury are also not likely causes of optic atrophy. In addition to central vision loss, patients may experience peripheral visual field loss, color vision impairment, decreased contrast sensitivity, decreased binocularity, and secondary amblyopia.

RHs are not a major cause of visual loss unless the fovea is directly involved.[145] If the fovea is obscured for a prolonged period of time, vision loss from amblyopia may result. Preretinal dome-shaped hemorrhages can break into the vitreous, usually within 3 to 4 weeks after the injury, causing a dense vitreous hemorrhage that can interfere with vision and may cause amblyopia and induce high axial elongation and myopia in young children. Vitrectomy may be indicated in patients with dense vitreous hemorrhage, although these patients rarely have good visual recovery.[639]

Strabismus develops in up to 30% of children who experience AHT.[640] Sixth nerve palsy, nystagmus, and ophthalmoplegia have been reported. Other ophthalmic sequelae include retinal detachment, dislocation or opacification of the crystalline lens (ectopia lentis and traumatic cataract), and phthisis.[640] Bilateral retinal nonperfusion may also occur in AHT survivors and may lead to optic nerve or retinal neovascularization. Children with positive eye findings require regular follow-up by an ophthalmologist. Visual potential in children with AHT may be limited by retinal, optic nerve, and central nervous system injuries. Children also often have neurologic, cognitive, and psychologic disabilities. With these limitations, the correction of refractive errors and treatment of amblyopia can help maximize the child's visual potential and visual learning ability.[619,640] For children in whom vision cannot be improved, auditory and tactile learning can be promoted through early intervention programs.

Social and Legal Outcomes

Less than one-third of AHT cases are accompanied by a confession by a perpetrator.[30] A 1986 study showed that in fatal cases of child abuse, a minority lead to a conviction in the legal system, and in 78% of cases, no jail time was served.[641] With respect to disposition, of children diagnosed with inflicted head injuries in England, 50% were in foster care or had been adopted. Thirty-two percent lived with their birth mother, and 18% lived with extended family.[418] Physical abuse is associated with a variety of long-term psychological dysfunctions when abused children become adults.[642] However, overall, there is a paucity of data on the true long-term effects of early child abuse from the social, legal, and economic perspectives throughout the lifespan of children with early inflicted head injuries, and these remain target areas for new research.[643]

Economic Outcomes

There is some evidence that children who have experienced AHT or other forms of abuse early in life have a higher risk of detrimental long-term socioeconomic consequences. These consequences include negative socioeconomic effects on the abused children but also on families, caregivers, communities, and societies overall.[644,645] For this reason, some authors have suggested that prevention measures may be considered cost-effective when compared against the high societal and economic consequences for children who sustain AHT early in life.[645]

Motor Outcomes

AHT may cause persistent motor complications including hemiplegia, quadriplegia, and/or fine motor deficits.[646] Several longitudinal studies have measured long-term motor outcomes at 5 or more years following abusive head trauma. Although less common than behavioral or vision problems, fine and gross motor difficulties have been reported in between 25% and 60% of patients.[617,623,624,647,648] Gross motor impairments are primarily spastic hemi- or quadriplegia. These children require ongoing care with pediatric rehabilitation specialists. Factors that predict higher likelihood of long-term disability include the severity of initial presentation (intensive care unit admission, longer hospital stay, lower GCS score, respiratory compromise), extent of injury (cranial fracture, higher brain lesion burden, cerebral edema, seizures) and lower socioeconomic status.[623,648,649] Importantly, multiple studies have found disability incidence or severity was worse at longer follow-up.[647,648] Therefore, long-term longitudinal care of all children after AHT is important, even for patients with initial good recovery.[647]

Post-traumatic Epilepsy

Many children will go on to experience post-traumatic epilepsy (PTE) as a long-term sequela after AHT (10%-40%).[617,623,624,647,650–652] PTE is a long-term seizure disorder defined as having 2 or more unprovoked seizures following traumatic brain injury and is independent of the presence of seizures during the acute period of AHT. For many of these patients, epilepsy is described as intractable, or refractory to multiple antiepileptic medications.[623,651] Although children with PTE following AHT may have multiple seizure types, 1 retrospective study of 10 years of electronic health records at a single center identified hypomotor seizures as the most common seizure type.[651] Severity of injury and having seizures early during the acute presentation and hospitalization for AHT are risk factors for PTE, with the latter increasing the likelihood of PTE by over thirty-fold.[650,651] Although seizure prophylaxis with antiseizure medications can prevent early onset seizures, this practice has not been found to prevent later onset PTE.[653] PTE is notably more frequently found in patients with AHT than accidental or noninflicted head trauma.[623,651]

TAKEAWAY POINTS

1. As a group, children with AHT, in general, have worse outcomes including higher mortality than children in a similar age range with accidental trauma. This likely reflects an increased severity of injury overall in this group.
2. Cognitive and behavioral outcomes range from good to severely impaired. These outcomes may become more apparent as children become older and have more cognitive demands such as school.
3. Although RHs generally clear rapidly, approximately half of children with AHT may have long-term visual impairments attributable to both ocular and cortical injury.
4. Social, legal, and economic outcomes are less well studied but suggest long-term consequences in many children and families after AHT.
5. Fine and gross motor impairments are common after AHT and contribute to significant long-term disability. Similar to cognitive and behavioral deficits, motor deficits may become more apparent over time.
6. Some children may go on to develop PTE.

PREVENTION

Introduction

AHT prevention efforts have targeted various outcomes: improved caregiver or provider knowledge about the dangers of shaking or AHT in general, improved caregiver knowledge about infant crying, reducing infant crying, improved caregiver emotional regulation, and reduction in AHT incidence rates. Current empiric evidence demonstrates efficacy of prevention programs to affect caregiver knowledge and behavior with regards to AHT, infant crying, and emotional-behavioral responses to infant crying. However, replicable effect on AHT incidence rates is lacking.

Improved Knowledge About the Dangers of Shaking or AHT in General

At least 25 studies have examined 12 different initiatives aimed at raising caregiver awareness about AHT and/or the dangers of shaking.[654] The Period of PURPLE Crying program is a multifaceted, hospital-based postpartum program that focuses on parental education about infant sleeping, crying, and soothing behaviors. The program also provides educational materials to caregivers describing AHT and the dangers of shaking. Barr et al found that participants exposed to these educational materials showed a significant increase in knowledge about the risks of shaking an infant.[655] Implementation of the Period of PURPLE Crying program in various countries has confirmed the effect of improved caregiver knowledge about the dangers of shaking.[656–658]

Similarly, the Shaking Your Baby is Just Not the Deal educational program developed in Australia has also demonstrated improved caregiver knowledge about the risks/dangers of shaking.[659] When implemented in other countries, this program has also shown replicable results.[660,661] Several other hospital-based parent education programs, provided in maternity wards, have also demonstrated improvements in caregiver knowledge about the dangers of shaking and AHT.[662,663] These include Love Me...Never Shake Me, The Hand Project: More Hugs, No Shakings, and the Colombia Prevention Program, to name a few. Thus, empiric evidence adequately demonstrates that hospital-based caregiver education programs do improve caregiver knowledge about the dangers of shaking and AHT.

Improved Knowledge About Infant Crying

Another prevention tactic has been to educate caregivers about normal infant crying patterns, given that infant crying is a well-documented triggering event for AHT.[664] Again, there are numerous programs that have studied the effect on caregiver knowledge of infant crying patterns.[657,659,662,665] The most widely implemented and studied has been the Period of PURPLE Crying program discussed earlier. The Period of PURPLE Crying program provides a 12-minute DVD along with a booklet that addresses the normality of crying, suggests strategies to comfort the infant, reinforces the idea that such strategies will not always work, and describes the reasons why inconsolable crying is frustrating. In addition to its demonstrated improvement of caregiver knowledge about the dangers of shaking, the program has showed a significant increase in caregiver knowledge regarding infant crying patterns.[655,657,665]

Reduction of Infant Crying and Modification of Caregiver Behavior or Emotional Regulation

Although knowledge is an important outcome of prevention programs, several initiatives have targeted behavior modifications (either infant or caregiver) as primary outcomes. These initiatives have included efforts to reduce infant crying and efforts to modify caregiver response to the stress/frustration of infant crying.

With regard to reduction in infant crying, at least 7 studies have been published on 5 different initiatives. The REST Routine for Infant Irritability program is a nurse home-visit program aimed at reducing an infant's level of arousal by promoting synchrony in the parent-infant dyad.[666] In a study that included 121 infants between the ages of 2 and 6 weeks, parents of infants were randomly distributed among the experimental group, receiving the REST Routine intervention, and the control group, receiving standard well child care intervention. Keefe et al found that infants in REST Routine group were crying 1.7 hours less per day compared with the control group, and at the end of intervention, 61.8% of infants in the REST Routine group and 28.8% of infants in the control group reduced the crying average to less than 1 hour per day.

Another initiative, The Happiest Baby, involves teaching caregivers a 5-step method to calm infants and stop crying on the basis of the assumption that actions mimicking conditions in the womb will trigger a calming reflex. McRury and Zolotor evaluated the effectiveness of this intervention by randomly assigning 35 parents to 2 conditions: 1) a group that received a video that taught The Happiest Baby method by mail; and 2) a control group that received a video (by mail) with guidelines for standard child care.[667] After 12 weeks of monitoring, McRury and Zolotor found no differences for amount of infant crying and parental stress between the two groups. A similar intervention, the Baby Business intervention, also underwent a randomized controlled trial (RCT) and did not demonstrate reduction in infant crying.[668]

A couple of other methods to reduce infant crying—swaddling and acupuncture—have also been studied. Van Sleuwen et al studied an initiative in which parents were educated about proper swaddling and sleep/play interactions via nursing clinic visits and telephone contact. Parents were randomly assigned to experimental and control groups.[669] Swaddling had no added benefit in the total group, but a small but significant effect was shown in infants aged 1 to 7 weeks. A separate RCT comparing swaddling versus massage in infants with neonatal cerebral insults has shown that swaddling significantly decreases the amount of crying compared with massage.[670]

Landgren et al explored the effects of acupuncture on reducing infant crying by randomly dividing 81 infants with colic into 2 groups.[671] An experimental group underwent 6 sessions of a "minimal, standardised acupuncture" (ie, a sterilized, disposable acupuncture needle inserted at an approximate depth of 2 mm at point LI4 of the hand's first dorsal interossal muscle and left in place for 2 seconds) for 3 weeks. The control group experienced similar pretreatment efforts (ie, nurse soothing and comforting efforts) but without the use of acupuncture. After the intervention, parent surveys reported a significant reduction in the number of hours of crying for both groups, but the reduction was greater in the experimental (acupuncture) group.

With regard to prevention efforts aimed at modifying caregiver behavioral response or emotional regulation, several initiatives have been studied. These include programs that teach caregivers strategies to reduce their daily stress and programs that educate caregivers on behavioral modification approaches to deal with infant crying.[672–674] In addition to other educational materials discussed earlier, the Period of PURPLE Crying suggests 3 steps to deal with the infant crying: (1) increase responses of holding and walking with the infant in the caregiver's arms, comforting and talking to the infant; (2) if the crying becomes very frustrating, place the infant in a safe place, leave for a few minutes to calm down, and return to see how the infant is; and (3) never shake or hurt the infant.

Several studies examining Period of PURPLE Crying materials have demonstrated a higher frequency of caregiver response of walking away when frustrated.[658,665,672]

Additionally, studies have found that learners exposed to Period of PURPLE Crying materials have also shared knowledge with others on normal infant crying patterns and the risks of shaking infants.[655,658] Finally, Barr et al found that implementation of the Period of PURPLE Crying program diminished pediatric emergency department visits for crying.[675] Similar positive results for caregiver response in walking away to frustration events have been reported for the Take Five Safety Plan for Crying initiative and the All Babies Cry initiative.[673,674]

Reduction in AHT Incidence Rates

A few programs have measured the outcome of intervention effect on AHT incidence rates. Although a couple of programs have demonstrated initial reductions of AHT incidence rates in certain regions, no program has yet to demonstrate replicable results in other regions. In 2005, Dias et al reported on a hospital-based program—Prevent Shaken Baby Syndrome!—implemented in the newborn period in which parents were provided written and video content about the dangers of shaking, discussed the risks of shaking with a maternity nurse, and then gave written affirmation that they received and understood the information.[676] This program initially demonstrated a decrease in AHT incidence rates in some regions of New York.[677] However, larger implementation across the state of Pennsylvania by Dias et al failed to demonstrate a reduction in AHT rates.[678]

Similarly, the Period of PURPLE Crying revealed a decrease in AHT incidence rates in British Columbia[679] but failed to demonstrate a reduction in AHT incidence rates in North Carolina when implemented there.[680]

Some additional studies have examined the effect of economic support as a factor in the reduction of AHT incidence rates. In California, Klevens et al reviewed the effect of paid family leave and the earned income tax credit on AHT rates.[681,682] Using difference-in-difference analysis of state level data from 1995–2011, Klevens et al found a significant decrease in AHT admissions in both <1- and <2-year-olds in California after implementation of a 2004 paid family leave policy. In comparison with 7 states with no such paid family leave, Klevens et al found no significant reduction in hospital admissions for AHT in those states. Using a similar analysis on 14 states with an Earned Income Tax Credit (EITC) and 13 states without one, for the time period 1995 to 2013, Klevens et al found that a refundable Earned Income Tax Credit was associated with a decrease of 3.1 AHT admissions per 100 000 population in children aged <2 years.[681] Although these economic policy effect studies demonstrate possible association, further research is needed.

Finally, in-home visitation programs, such as Nurse-Family Partnership,[683] have demonstrated a long-term decrease in child maltreatment in general. Although such programs have not targeted reductions in AHT rates specifically, their holistic approach to bolstering parenting resilience may be a useful approach in addressing AHT.

TAKEAWAY POINTS

1. There is an evidence base among multiple initiatives that demonstrate AHT prevention programs improve caregiver knowledge on infant crying, the consequences of shaking an infant, and AHT in general.
2. There is an evidence base among several initiatives that demonstrate AHT prevention programs improve caregiver response of walking away when frustrated or agitated by a crying infant.
3. There is a small evidence base that indicates initiatives to reduce infant crying are effective.
4. There is a small evidence base that indicates AHT prevention programs reduce AHT incidence rates.

LEAD AUTHORS

Sandeep K. Narang, MD, JD, FAAP
Suzanne Haney, MD, MS, FAAP
Ann-Christine Duhaime, MD, FAAP
Jonathan Martin, MD, FAANS, FACS, FAAP
Gil Binenbaum, MD, MSCE FAAP
Alejandra G. de Alba Campomanes, MD, MPH, FAAP
Rich Barth, MD, FAAP
Gina Bertocci, PhD
Margarite Care, MD
Declan McGuone, MD

AAP COUNCIL ON CHILD ABUSE AND NEGLECT (2018–2024)

Antoinette Laskey, MD, MPH, MBA, FAAP, Chairperson
Andrea Asnes, MD, FAAP
Verena Wyvill Brown, MD, FAAP
Rebecca Girardet, MD, FAAP
Nancy Heavilin, MD, FAAP
Natalie Kissoon, MD, FAAP
Kelly N. McGregory, DO, MS, FAAP
Patricia Morgan, MD, FAAP
Norell Rosado, MD, FAAP
Emalee G. Flaherty, MD, FAAP, Past Chairperson
Andrew Sirotnak, MD, FAAP, Past Chairperson
Suzanne Haney, MD, FAAP, Past Chairperson
Amy R. Gavril, MD MSCI, FAAP
Amanda Bird Hoffert Gilmartin, MD, FAAP
Sheila M. Idzerda, MD, FAAP
Stephen Messner, MD, FAAP
Lori Legano, MD, FAAP
Bethany Mohr, MD, FAAP
Rebecca Moles, MD, FAAP
Vincent Palusci, MD MS, FAAP
Shalon Nienow, MD, FAAP
Ann E. Budzak, MD, FAAP

LIAISONS

Sofia Charania, MD, Section on Pediatric Trainees
Rachael Keefe, MD, MPH, FAAP, Council on Foster Care, Adoption, and Kinship Care
Cara Kelly, PhD, Administration for Children and Families
Anna Kerlak, MD, American Academy of Child and Adolescent Psychiatry
Elizabeth Swedo, MD, FAAP, Centers for Disease Control and Prevention

STAFF

Tammy Piazza Hurley
Jeff Hudson, MA

AAP SECTION ON OPHTHALMOLOGY (2018–2024)

Donny Won Suh, MD, FAAP, Chairperson
Sylvia Yoo, MD, FAAP, Chairperson-Elect
Alina Dumitrescu, MD, FAAP
Douglas Fredrick, MD, FAAP
Ryan Gise, MD, FAAP
Mitchell Strominger, MD, FAAP
Steven E. Rubin, MD, FAAP, Immediate Past Chair
Daniel J. Karr, MD, FAAP
Kanwal Nischal, MD, FAAP
John D. Roarty, MD

LIAISONS

Sylvia R. Kodsi, MD, FAAP, American Academy of Ophthalmology
Geoffrey E. Bradford, MD, FAAP, American Academy of Ophthalmology Council
Christie L. Morse, MD, FAAP, American Association for Pediatric Ophthalmology and Strabismus (AAPOS)
Marguerite C. Weinert, MD, FAAP, AAPOS Committee on Young Ophthalmologists
Jennifer Lambert, CO, American Association of Certified Orthoptists

STAFF

Jennifer Riefe, MEd

AAP SECTION ON RADIOLOGY (2018–2024)

Hansel J. Otero, MD, FAAP, Chairperson)
Sarah Milla, MD, FAAP, Past Chairperson
Maria-Gisela Mercado-Deane, MD, FAAP, Past Chairperson
Adina Alazraki, MD, FAAP
Aparna Annam, DO, FAAP
Ellen Benya, MD, FAAP
Patricia Acharya, MD, FAAP
Brandon Brown, MD, MA, FAAP
Katherine Barton, MD, FAAP
Reza Daugherty, MD, FAAP

STAFF

Laura Laskosz, MPH

AAP SECTION ON NEUROLOGICAL SURGERY (2018–2024)

Greg Albert, MD, MPH, FAAP, Chairperson
David Bauer, MD, MPH, FAAP
Katrina Ducis, MD
Sandi Lam, MD, FAAP
Jonathan Martin, MD, FAAP
Brandon Rocque, MD, MS, FAAP
Philipp R. Aldana, MD, FAAP, Past Chairperson
Douglas Brockmeyer, MD, FAAP
Ann-Christine Duhaime, MD
Andrew Jea, MD, FAAP, Past Chairperson

STAFF

Melissa Marx, MPH

SOCIETY FOR PEDIATRIC RADIOLOGY

AMERICAN ASSOCIATION OF CERTIFIED ORTHOPTISTS

AMERICAN ASSOCIATION FOR PEDIATRIC OPHTHALMOLOGY AND STRABISMUS

AMERICAN ACADEMY OF OPHTHALMOLOGY

APPENDIX A. DEFINITIONS

1. Abusive head trauma: An injury to the skull or intracranial contents of an infant or young child (<5 years of age) attributable to inflicted blunt impact and/or violent shaking (Reference: Centers for Disease Control and Prevention. Pediatric Abusive Head Trauma: Recommended definitions for public health surveillance and research. 2012. Accessed December 18, 2024. https://www.cdc.gov/violenceprevention/pdf/PedHeadTrauma-a.pdf).
2. Acceleration/deceleration: Rate of change of an object's or body's velocity or speed.
3. Accidental head trauma: Injury occurring from mechanisms other than from abusive head trauma or assault.
4. Acute subdural hematoma/hemorrhage: A collection of recent, fresh blood between the arachnoid and the dura, typically (although not always) hyperdense and with a crescent shape on CT. Mixed density may be seen if the collection contains unclotted blood, CSF admixture, and/or active extravasation. On MRI, the acute SDH is iso/hypointense on T1 and very hypointense on T2, GRE, and SW imaging. Although exact timing/dating cannot be determined with absolute certainty, these findings typically characterize hemorrhage that has occurred within hours to a day or so.

5. Animal injury models: Exposing a nonhuman animal to a mechanical phenomenon such as acceleration or force to observe resulting injury so as to understand injury mechanism and threshold.
6. Anthropomorphic test device: A mechanical analogue representing a human that can be used in experiments to simulate potentially injurious events such as falls or motor vehicle crashes to investigate injury risk. ATDs can be equipped with instrumentation to measure acceleration, velocity, force, and other biomechanical outcomes.
7. Autopsy: A medical examination of the body after death that begins with examination of the external surface of the body followed by an examination of the internal organs.
8. Bioengineer: An engineer with expertise in both engineering and life sciences who applies their knowledge of engineering to the human body to better understand injury or disease process.
9. Biofidelity: How well a surrogate or anthropomorphic test device (test dummy) represents its targeted human population in terms of anthropometrics and response to mechanical phenomena (eg, acceleration, force).
10. Biomechanical compatibility: Determines whether the provided history is capable of generating the constellation of injuries and whether the characteristics of injuries are compatible with the provided history.
11. Biomechanical properties: Describes in engineering terms how tissues respond to loading.
12. Biomechanics: Application of mechanical principles to biological systems such as the human body.
13. Bridging veins: Cerebral veins that drain venous blood from the brain surface into the dural venous sinuses
14. Cause and manner of death: The cause of death is the specific disease or injury that initiated the lethal sequence of events. Manner of death is a determination made about the circumstances of death.
15. Center of mass (COM): The location within a body where mass is equally distributed and balanced. The COM of the human body changes as a person moves. The COM of an erect standing person is located at approximately 56% of their height as measured from the soles of their feet within the sagittal plane.
16. Cerebral perfusion pressure: Mean arterial pressure minus mean intracranial pressure.
17. Chronic subdural hematoma/hemorrhage: A collection of nonacute blood between the arachnoid and the dura, typically (although not always) with a crescent shape. On CT, a subacute or chronic SDH will be predominantly iso- or hypodense. On MRI, a subacute SDH will be hyperintense on T1 and will have varying signal intensity on T2. The chronic SDH is slightly hyperintense compared to CSF on both T1- and T2-weighted imaging. FLAIR imaging increases the conspicuity. If rebleeding has occurred in the collection (ie, "chronic recurrent SDH"), the signal may be a variable combination of hypo/iso/hyper-intensity/density on CT and all MR sequences. Internal loculations and septations may be seen on both CT and MRI and these are more conspicuous following intravenous contrast enhancement. Although exact timing/dating cannot be determined with absolute certainty, these findings typically characterize hemorrhage that has occurred in the range of a day or more previously.
18. Computer or computational models: Digitized representations of a human body or regions of a human body and its environment. Models of the human body can be either segmented (rigid body model) or discretized into elements (finite element model); most are 3 dimensional.
19. Computer simulation: Digitized representation of an event such as a fall that includes the includes the fall victim and fall environment.
20. Decompressive craniectomy: A surgical procedure in which portions of the skull are removed (and usually the dura opened widely) to reduce intracranial pressure and/or control dangerous intracranial tissue shifts.
21. Deformation: Change in shape (distortion) of an object under pressure or force.
22. Diffuse traumatic axonal injury: Pattern of white matter injury following rapid acceleration-deceleration characterized by altered consciousness, and the formation of axonal spheroids that contain accumulated amyloid precursor protein.
23. Dura: Tough collagenous connective tissue layer that forms the outer layer of the 3 connective tissue layers covering the brain (dura, arachnoid, and pia mater). The dura is divided into 2 parts: outer periosteal layer adherent to the skull and an inner meningeal layer; the dural venous sinuses are between these layers.
24. Edema: Brain swelling caused by increased fluid accumulation attributable to blood-brain barrier disruption with increased permeability, or intracellular fluid accumulation as a result of cell membrane injury or metabolic derangement, or a combination of both.
25. Epidural hematoma/hemorrhage (EDH): A collection of blood between the skull and dura. On CT, the EDH typically (although not always) has a biconvex shape, an adjacent skull fracture/scalp injury, and classically does not cross sutural margins. (In patients with skull fractures, especially those in children involving the sutures, this rule may not always apply.) The acute EDH appears hyperdense on CT, but may contain hypodense areas representing unclotted blood. As the EDH evolves, it gradually loses its hyperdensity and may appear iso- or hypodense. On MRI, the acute EDH is hypo- or isointense on T1- and very hypointense on

T2-, GRE-, and susceptibility-weighted imaging (SWI). The inwardly displaced dura should be directly visualized on MRI as a thin dark line on all pulse sequences.

26. Fall: An event in which there is a change in the person's center of mass (COM) from a higher elevation to a lower elevation. This includes ground-based falls or falls from an elevated surface. When focusing on head injury, fall height is typically measured from the head COM to the impact surface.
27. Fall dynamics: Describes the motion or movement of the human body or segments of the body during a fall.
28. Force: A push or pull that causes an object to change its velocity (speed), shape or direction of motion. In a free fall, when the body impacts the ground, force is applied to the body.
29. Forensic pathologist: A pathologist with specialized training in the investigation of the cause, mechanism, and manner of death, injury, or disease process.
30. Glasgow coma scale (GCS): A practical means for the assessment of impaired consciousness in response to defined stimuli. The scale allows for a numerical assessment of consciousness ranging from 3 to 15 through the assessment of eye opening, verbal response, and motor response either spontaneously or following either verbal or applied painful stimulus. Although initially developed for adults, several pediatric adaptations of the scale have been developed and adopted for the assessment of children.
31. Head drop testing: Dropping a surrogate or PMHS head from an elevated height to ground or onto an object, often for the purposes of measuring acceleration of the head or determining injury outcomes such as skull fracture.
32. Herniation: Abnormal displacement of brain tissue as a result of raised intracranial pressure. Can be caused by pathologic processes that are diffuse (eg, cerebral edema) or focal (eg, hematoma).
33. Household fall: Falls that occur in the course of domestic activities. As applied to infants and toddlers, they usually involve ground-based falls that occur during crawling, standing or walking or falls from furniture such as beds, couches, or changing tables. Most household falls are low energy events with head to ground fall heights of 3 feet or less.
34. Hypoxic-ischemic injury: Brain injury that encompasses a reduction in the supply of oxygen (hypoxia) and/or diminished blood supply to the brain (hypoperfusion or ischemia).
35. Impact: Occurs when an object comes into forcible contact with another object. In a free fall, impact occurs when the body contacts the ground.
36. Inertial loading: Inertia is a body's resistance to change in speed and direction. When force or acceleration are applied to the body to change its speed or direction of motion, the mass of the body tends to resist the motion. This resistance to motion is the inertial loading.
37. Infarct: An area of tissue necrosis caused by ischemia attributable to arterial or venous occlusion.
38. Injury biomechanics: Field of study focusing on the biomechanical behavior of the human body under potentially injurious conditions (eg, acceleration, force) at both the macroscopic and microscopic levels. Often focused on determining whether forces or accelerations applied to the body will cause injury.
39. Injury mechanism: Macroscopic and microscopic analysis of how injuries occur. Describes how forces or accelerations translated into injuries.
40. Injury threshold or tolerance: The level force or acceleration beyond which there is a risk of a specific injury (eg, skull fracture, SDH).
41. Internal limiting membrane (ILM): One of the layers of the retina that forms the structural interface between the retina and the vitreous.
42. Intracranial hypertension: The elevation of intracranial pressure in response to a disturbance of regulatory intracranial pressure mechanisms. As described by the *Monro-Kellie hypothesis*, intracranial volume is fixed. Any increase in 1 of the 3 fixed intracranial contents (brain parenchyma, intravascular blood, and spinal fluid), or the addition of additional mass, must be balanced by reduction in one of these contents if intracranial pressure is to be maintained within a physiologically normal range. Reduction in intracranial spinal fluid spaces through displacement into the spinal subarachnoid space is the common means of physiologic compensation. Pressure in excess of 20 mm Hg is considered elevated and consistent with intracranial hypertension.
43. Intracranial pressure: Pressure inside the cranial cavity.
44. Intraretinal retinal hemorrhages: Presence of blood in and/or between the different retinal layers.
45. Kinematics: Movement or motion of the body or body region (eg, head) during an event.
46. Kinetic energy: Energy of a body in motion. On impact, this energy has the potential to be converted into an injury.
47. Linear or translational acceleration: Rate of change of linear (straight line) velocity (speed).
48. Macula: The retinal region between the major temporal vascular arcades.
49. Mechanical properties: Properties describe the reaction or response to an applied load. Properties include strength, ductility, elastic modulus, and fracture toughness.
50. Medical examiner/coroner: Responsible for conducting investigations into unnatural, sudden or unexpected deaths to determine the cause and manner of death. Medical examiners are usually appointed

officials and often forensic pathologists. Coroners are usually elected officials and not always physicians.

51. Multilayered retinal hemorrhages: Retinal hemorrhages that are present at multiple locations in relation to the retina (intraretinal, preretinal, and/or subretinal).
52. Neuropathologist: A pathologist with specialized training in the diagnosis of diseases of the central nervous system, peripheral nervous system, and muscle.
53. Optic atrophy: Optic nerve damage caused by the degeneration of retinal ganglion cell axons.
54. Ora serata: The peripheral termination of the retina at its junction with the ciliary body.
55. Papilledema: Optic disc swelling specifically attributable to raised intracranial pressure.
56. Peripapillary: The region around the optic nerve head or optic disc.
57. Posterior pole: Area of the ocular fundus that encompasses the optic nerve and the macula (posterior location should not be confused with "deep," which refers to the layers of the outer retina closer to the choroid).
58. Preretinal retinal hemorrhages: Blood in the space between the vitreous and the retina.
59. Retinal detachment: A separation between the sensory layers of the retina from the underlying retinal pigment epithelium and choroid.
60. Retinal fold: An area of the retina where it is buckled up, projecting up out of the normal plane of the retina.
61. Retinal hemorrhage (RH): Presence of blood under or between the layers of the retina or between the vitreous and the retina.
62. Retinal vascular arcades: The distal branches of the central retinal artery and vein. There are 4 major arcades or branches, each with arterioles and venules: superotemporal, inferotemporal, superonasal, and inferonasal.
63. Retinoschisis: Splitting of the retinal layers.
64. Rotational or angular acceleration: Rate of change of angular (circular or curved) velocity. Rotational and angular may be used interchangeably.
65. Shear: Force applied parallel to a surface.
66. Short distance fall: An event in which there is a change in the person's COM from a higher elevation to a lower elevation. Typically, this fall height is defined as <1 meter (~3 feet).
67. Skull fracture: A break in the normal integrity of the skull, which may be partial or full thickness, caused by presumed mechanical force.
68. Spinal dorsal root ganglion: Collection of sensory nerve cell bodies on the dorsal roots of spinal nerves located near intervertebral foramina.
69. Strain: Deformation or change in shape of an object (attributable to application of stress) normalized to its original shape.
70. Stress: Force per unit area applied to an object. Strength is the stress at which a material fails.
71. Subarachnoid hemorrhage: Macroscopic blood located between the brain surface and the arachnoid membrane. On CT and MR, the blood in this location will follow the contour of the sulci and cisterns. Acute SAH is hyperdense on CT and hyperintense on FLAIR MR imaging. Subacute SAH may be invisible on CT, although the presence of subtle sulcal "effacement" may occasionally be seen. Chronic SAH, or "hemosiderosis" may be seen on MR as hypointense linear areas of cortical "staining" on GRE- and SW-weighted imaging.
72. Subdural hematohygroma: A collection between the arachnoid membrane and dura, typically (although not always) crescentic in shape containing both blood/blood products and fluid-either cerebrospinal fluid or serum. On CT, it is mixed in attenuation depending on the amount and stage of the blood/blood products, but the hemorrhagic collection typically contains areas of low attenuation fluid and higher attenuation blood. On MRI, acute blood components will be T1-hyperintense and T2-hypointense with hypointense signal on GRE and SWI and be mixed with varying amounts of fluid, typically similar to cerebrospinal fluid in signal on T1- and T2-weighted images.
73. Subdural hygroma: A collection of fluid between the arachnoid membrane and dura, typically (although not always) crescentic in shape. The collection may contain proteinaceous or blood-tinged fluid that is simple and without membranes on imaging. It is low-attenuation on CT, although it is often slightly hyper attenuating to cerebrospinal fluid. On MRI, it may be isointense to slightly hyperintense to cerebrospinal fluid on both T1- and T2-weighted sequences, including on FLAIR (fluid attenuated inversion recovery). These may occur in the traumatic setting with a disruption of the arachnoid membrane with cerebrospinal fluid collecting in the subdural space. It may also occur in the setting of low intracranial pressure with fluid or cerebrospinal fluid seeping into the space or formation following disruption of the arachnoid-dural interface. Because they can result from a disruption of the arachnoid membrane, these collections may occur rapidly following trauma. However, they may also collect in a more delayed timeframe, such as in the setting of decreasing brain volume following a brain parenchymal insult.
74. Subgaleal hemorrhage: A collection of blood between the periosteum and aponeurosis of the scalp caused by ruptured emissary veins that connect the intracranial to scalp veins. It is not confined by the sutures and can extend to involve the entire scalp; thus, leading to a potential significant loss of blood and severe hypovolemia.
75. Subretinal RH: Presence of blood between the retina and the choroid.

76. Surrogate: A mechanical analogue representing a human that can be used in experiments simulating potentially injurious events such as falls, shaking or motor vehicle crashes to investigate injury risk. Surrogates can be equipped with instrumentation to measure acceleration, velocity, force, and other biomechanical outcomes.
77. Thrombosis: Formation of blood clot within blood vessels that can cause downstream tissue ischemia.
78. Vitreoretinal traction: A disorder of the vitreoretinal interface with persistently adherent vitreous exerting tractional pull on the retina.
79. Vitreous hemorrhage: Presence of blood in the vitreous cavity of the eye.

FINANCIAL/CONFLICT OF INTEREST DISCLOSURES: The AAP has determined the authors have no conflicts relevant to "Abusive Head Trauma in Infants and Children: Technical Report."

FUNDING: No external funding.

Technical reports from the American Academy of Pediatrics benefit from expertise and resources of liaisons and internal (AAP) and external reviewers. However, technical reports from the American Academy of Pediatrics may not reflect the views of the liaisons or the organizations or government agencies that they represent.

The guidance in this report does not indicate an exclusive course of treatment or serve as a standard of medical care. Variations, taking into account individual circumstances, may be appropriate.

All technical reports from the American Academy of Pediatrics automatically expire 5 years after publication unless reaffirmed, revised, or retired at or before that time.

https://doi.org/10.1542/peds.2024-070457

REFERENCES

1. Reece RM, Christian C. *Child Abuse: Medical Diagnosis and Management*. American Academy of Pediatrics; 2008
2. Laskey A, Sirotnak A. *Child Abuse: Medical Diagnosis and Management*. American Academy of Pediatrics; 2021
3. Duhaime AC, Gean AD, Haacke EM, et al. Common data elements in radiologic imaging of traumatic brain injury. *Arch Phys Med Rehabil*. 2010;91(11):1661–1666. doi: 10.1016/j.apmr.2010.07.238
4. Shouldice M, Ward M. *Joint Statement on Traumatic Head Injury due to Child Maltreatment: An Update to the Joint Statement on Shaken Baby Syndrome*. Government of Canada; 2020. Accessed November 29, 2021. https://www.canada.ca/en/public-health/services/health-promotion/childhood-adolescence/publications/joint-statement-traumatic-head-injury-child-maltreatment.html#a4
5. Parks SE, Annest JL, Hill HA, Karch DL. *Pediatric Abusive Head Trauma: Recommended Definitions for Public Health Surveillance and Research*. Centers for Disease Control and Prevention; April 2012. Accessed September 7, 2020. https://www.cdc.gov/child-abuse-neglect/about/PedHeadTrauma-a.pdf
6. Rebbe R, Mienko JA, Martinson ML. Incidence and risk factors for abusive head trauma: a population-based study. *Child Abuse Rev*. 2020;29(3):195–207. doi: 10.1002/car.2630
7. Nuno M, Shelley CD, Ugiliweneza B, Schmidt AJ, Magana JN. Differences in incidence and case fatality of abusive head trauma. *Child Abuse Negl*. 2020;104:104488. doi: 10.1016/j.chiabu.2020.104488
8. Parrish J, Baldwin-Johnson C, Volz M, Goldsmith Y. Abusive head trauma among children in Alaska: a population-based assessment. *Int J Circumpolar Health*. 2013;72. doi: 10.3402/ijch.v72i0.21216
9. Emrick BB, Smith E, Thompson L, et al. Epidemiology of abusive head trauma in West Virginia children <24 months: 2000–2010. *Child Abuse Negl*. 2019;93:215–221. doi: 10.1016/j.chiabu.2019.05.011
10. Boop S, Axente M, Weatherford B, Klimo P, Jr. Abusive head trauma: an epidemiological and cost analysis. *J Neurosurg Pediatr*. 2016;18(5):542–549. doi: 10.3171/2016.1.PEDS15583
11. Shanahan ME, Zolotor AJ, Parrish JW, Barr RG, Runyan DK. National, regional, and state abusive head trauma: application of the CDC algorithm. *Pediatrics*. 2013;132(6):e1546–e1553. doi: 10.1542/peds.2013-2049
12. Keenan HT, Runyan DK, Marshall SW, Nocera MA, Merten DF, Sinal SH. A population-based study of inflicted traumatic brain injury in young children. *JAMA*. 2003;290(5):621–626. doi: 10.1001/jama.290.5.621
13. Selassie AW, Borg K, Busch C, Russell WS. Abusive head trauma in young children: a population-based study. *Pediatr Emerg Care*. 2013;29(3):283–291. doi: 10.1097/PEC.0b013e31828503ea
14. Barlow KM, Minns RA. Annual incidence of shaken impact syndrome in young children. *Lancet*. 2000;356(9241):1571–1572. doi: 10.1016/S0140-6736(00)03130-5
15. Kelly P, Farrant B. Shaken baby syndrome in New Zealand, 2000–2002. *J Paediatr Child Health*. 2008;44(3):99–107. doi: 10.1111/j.1440-1754.2007.01234.x

16. Joe A, McElwain C, Woodard K, Bell S. A call for culturally-relevant interventions to address child abuse and neglect in American Indian communities. *J Racial Ethn Health Disparities*. 2019;6(3): 447–456. doi: 10.1007/s40615-018-0531-9

17. Wood JN, French B, Fromkin J, et al. Association of pediatric abusive head trauma rates with macroeconomic indicators. *Acad Pediatr*. 2016;16(3):224–232. doi: 10.1016/j.acap.2015.05.008

18. Hymel KP, Laskey AL, Crowell KR, et al. Racial and ethnic disparities and bias in the evaluation and reporting of abusive head trauma. *J Pediatr*. 2018;198:137–143.e1. doi: 10.1016/j.jpeds.2018.01.048

19. Palusci VJ, Botash AS. Race and bias in child maltreatment diagnosis and reporting. *Pediatrics*. 2021;148(1):e2020049625. doi: 10.1542/peds.2020-049625

20. Laskey AL, Stump TE, Perkins SM, Zimet GD, Sherman SJ, Downs SM. Influence of race and socioeconomic status on the diagnosis of child abuse: a randomized study. *J Pediatr*. 2012;160(6): 1003–1008.e1. doi: 10.1016/j.jpeds.2011.11.042

21. Jenny C, Hymel KP, Ritzen A, Reinert SE, Hay TC. Analysis of missed cases of abusive head trauma. *JAMA*. 1999;281(7):621–626. doi: 10.1001/jama.281.7.621

22. Lane WG, Rubin DM, Monteith R, Christian CW. Racial differences in the evaluation of pediatric fractures for physical abuse. *JAMA*. 2002;288(13):1603–1609. doi: 10.1001/jama.288.13.1603

23. Luken A, Nair R, Fix RL. On racial disparities in child abuse reports: exploratory mapping the 2018 NCANDS. *Child Maltreat*. 2021;26(3): 267–281. doi: 10.1177/10775595211001926

24. Leventhal JM. Research strategies and methodologic standards in studies of risk factors for child abuse. *Child Abuse Negl*. 1982;6(2): 113–123. doi: 10.1016/0145-2134(82)90003-5

25. Fingarson AK, Pierce MC, Lorenz DJ, et al. Who's watching the children? Caregiver features associated with physical child abuse versus accidental injury. *J Pediatr*. 2019;212:180–187.e1. doi: 10.1016/j.jpeds.2019.05.040

26. Young A, Pierce MC, Kaczor K, et al. Are negative/unrealistic parent descriptors of infant attributes associated with physical abuse? *Child Abuse Negl*. 2018;80:41–51. doi: 10.1016/j.chiabu.2018.03.020

27. Scribano PV, Makaroff KL, Feldman KW, Berger RP. Association of perpetrator relationship to abusive head trauma clinical outcomes. *Child Abuse Negl*. 2013;37(10):771–777. doi: 10.1016/j.chiabu.2013.04.011

28. Kesler H, Dias MS, Shaffer M, Rottmund C, Cappos K, Thomas NJ. Demographics of abusive head trauma in the Commonwealth of Pennsylvania. *J Neurosurg Pediatr*. 2008;1(5):351–356. doi: 10.3171/PED/2008/1/5/351

29. Kelly P, Thompson JMD, Koh J, et al. Perinatal risk and protective factors for pediatric abusive head trauma: a multicenter case-control study. *J Pediatr*. 2017;187:240–246.e4. doi: 10.1016/j.jpeds.2017.04.058

30. Adamsbaum C, Grabar S, Mejean N, Rey-Salmon C. Abusive head trauma: judicial admissions highlight violent and repetitive shaking. *Pediatrics*. 2010;126(3):546–555. doi: 10.1542/peds.2009-3647

31. Barr RG, Trent RB, Cross J. Age-related incidence curve of hospitalized shaken baby syndrome cases: convergent evidence for crying as a trigger to shaking. *Child Abuse Negl*. 2006;30(1): 7–16. doi: 10.1016/j.chiabu.2005.06.009

32. Kempe CH, Silverman FN, Steele BF, Droegemueller W, Silver HK. The battered-child syndrome. *JAMA*. 1962;181:17–24. doi: 10.1001/jama.1962.03050270019004

33. Christian CW; American Academy of Pediatrics, Committee on Child Abuse and Neglect. The evaluation of suspected child physical abuse. *Pediatrics*. 2015;135(5):e1337–e1354. doi: 10.1542/peds.2015-0356

34. Allasio D, Fischer H. Immersion scald burns and the ability of young children to climb into a bathtub. *Pediatrics*. 2005;115(5): 1419–1421. doi: 10.1542/peds.2004-1550

35. Sirotnak AP, Grigsby T, Krugman RD. Physical abuse of children. *Pediatr Rev*. 2004;25(8):264–277. doi: 10.1542/pir.25-8-264

36. Caffey J. Significance of the history in the diagnosis of traumatic injury to children. Howland Award Address. *J Pediatr*. 1965;67(5 Suppl):1008–1014. doi: 10.1016/s0022-3476(65)82098-4

37. Hettler J, Greenes DS. Can the initial history predict whether a child with a head injury has been abused? *Pediatrics*. 2003; 111(3):602–607. doi: 10.1542/peds.111.3.602

38. Hymel KP, Lee G, Boos S, et al. Estimating the relevance of historical red flags in the diagnosis of abusive head trauma. *J Pediatr*. 2020;218:178–183.e2. doi: 10.1016/j.jpeds.2019.11.010

39. Twentyman CT, Plotkin RC. Unrealistic expectations of parents who maltreat their children: an educational deficit that pertains to child development. *J Clin Psychol*. 1982;38(3):497–503. doi: 10.1002/1097-4679(198207)38:3<497::aid-jclp2270380306>3.0.co;2-x

40. Vinchon M, de Foort-Dhellemmes S, Desurmont M, Delestret I. Confessed abuse versus witnessed accidents in infants: comparison of clinical, radiological, and ophthalmological data in corroborated cases. *Childs Nerv Syst*. 2010;26(5):637–645. doi: 10.1007/s00381-009-1048-7

41. Kennedy JM, Ma J, Lyden ER, Haney SB. Abusive head trauma and a delay in presentation for care. *Pediatr Emerg Care*. 2022;38(1): e170–e172. doi: 10.1097/PEC.0000000000002197

42. Vadivelu S, Esernio-Jenssen D, Rekate HL, Narayan RK, Mittler MA, Schneider SJ. Delay in arrival to care in perpetrator-identified nonaccidental head trauma: observations and outcomes. *World Neurosurg*. 2015;84(5):1340–1346. doi: 10.1016/j.wneu.2015.06.023

43. Sieswerda-Hoogendoorn T, Boos S, Spivack B, Bilo RA, van Rijn RR. Educational paper: abusive head trauma part I. Clinical aspects. *Eur J Pediatr*. 2012;171(3):415–423. doi: 10.1007/s00431-011-1598-z

44. Stiell IG, Bennett C. Implementation of clinical decision rules in the emergency department. *Acad Emerg Med*. 2007;14(11):955–959. doi: 10.1197/j.aem.2007.06.039

45. Berger RP, Fromkin J, Herman B, et al. Validation of the Pittsburgh Infant Brain Injury Score for Abusive Head Trauma. *Pediatrics*. 2016;138(1):e20153756. doi: 10.1542/peds.2015-3756

46. Hymel KP, Fingarson AK, Pierce MC, Kaczor K, Makoroff KL, Wang M. External validation of the PediBIRN Screening Tool for Abusive Head Trauma in pediatric emergency department

settings. *Pediatr Emerg Care.* 2022;38(6):269–272. doi: 10.1097/PEC.0000000000002670

47. Duhaime AC, Christian CW. Abusive head trauma: evidence, obfuscation, and informed management. *J Neurosurg Pediatr.* 2019;24(5):481–488. doi: 10.3171/2019.7.PEDS18394
48. Oluigbo CO, Wilkinson CC, Stence NV, Fenton LZ, McNatt SA, Handler MH. Comparison of outcomes following decompressive craniectomy in children with accidental and nonaccidental blunt cranial trauma. *J Neurosurg Pediatr.* 2012;9(2):125–132. doi: 10.3171/2011.11.PEDS09449
49. Klimo P Jr, Matthews A, Lew SM, Zwienenberg-Lee M, Kaufman BA. Minicraniotomy versus bur holes for evacuation of chronic subdural collections in infants-a preliminary single-institution experience. *J Neurosurg Pediatr.* 2011;8(5):423–429. doi: 10.3171/2011.8.PEDS1131
50. Piteau SJ, Ward MG, Barrowman NJ, Plint AC. Clinical and radiographic characteristics associated with abusive and nonabusive head trauma: a systematic review. *Pediatrics.* 2012;130(2):315–323. doi: 10.1542/peds.2011-1545
51. Maguire SA, Kemp AM, Lumb RC, Farewell DM. Estimating the probability of abusive head trauma: a pooled analysis. *Pediatrics.* 2011;128(3):e550–e64. doi: 10.1542/peds.2010-2949
52. Narang SK, Fingarson A, Lukefahr J; American Academy of Pediatrics, Council on Child Abuse and Neglect. Abusive head trauma in infants and children. *Pediatrics.* 2020;145(4):e20200203. doi: 10.1542/peds.2020-0203
53. Feldman KW, Sugar NF, Browd SR. Initial clinical presentation of children with acute and chronic versus acute subdural hemorrhage resulting from abusive head trauma. *J Neurosurg Pediatr.* 2015;16(2):177–185. doi: 10.3171/2014.12.PEDS14607
54. Bullock MR, Chesnut R, Ghajar J, et al. Surgical management of acute subdural hematomas. *Neurosurgery.* 2006;58(3 Suppl):S16–S24. doi: 10.1227/01.NEU.0000210364.29290.C9
55. De Leeuw M, Beuls E, Parizel P, Jorens P, Jacobs W. Confessed abusive blunt head trauma. *Am J Forensic Med Pathol.* 2013;34(2):130–132. doi: 10.1097/PAF.0b013e31828629ca
56. Arbogast KB, Margulies SS, Christian CW. Initial neurologic presentation in young children sustaining inflicted and unintentional fatal head injuries. *Pediatrics.* 2005;116(1):180–184. doi: 10.1542/peds.2004-2671
57. Graupman P, Winston KR. Nonaccidental head trauma as a cause of childhood death. *J Neurosurg.* 2006;104(4 Suppl):245–250. doi: 10.3171/ped.2006.104.4.245
58. Duhaime AC, Christian CW, Rorke LB, Zimmerman RA. Nonaccidental head injury in infants—the "shaken-baby syndrome." *N Engl J Med.* 1998;338(25):1822–1829. doi: 10.1056/NEJM199806183382507
59. Byard RW, Donald T, Hilton JN, Krous HF. Shaking-impact syndrome and lucidity. *Lancet.* 2000;355(9205):758. doi: 10.1016/S0140-6736(05)72175-9
60. Willman KY, Bank DE, Senac M, Chadwick DL. Restricting the time of injury in fatal inflicted head injuries. *Child Abuse Negl.* 1997;21(10):929–940. doi: 10.1016/s0145-2134(97)00054-9
61. Puls HT, Anderst JD, Bettenhausen JL, et al. Potential opportunities for prevention or earlier diagnosis of child physical abuse in the inpatient setting. *Hosp Pediatr.* 2018;Jan 25:hpeds.2017-0109. doi: 10.1542/hpeds.2017-0109
62. Sheets LK, Leach ME, Koszewski IJ, Lessmeier AM, Nugent M, Simpson P. Sentinel injuries in infants evaluated for child physical abuse. *Pediatrics.* 2013;131(4):701–707. doi: 10.1542/peds.2012-2780
63. Orru E, Calloni SF, Tekes A, Huisman T, Soares BP. The child with macrocephaly: differential diagnosis and neuroimaging findings. *AJR Am J Roentgenol.* 2018;210(4):848–859. doi: 10.2214/AJR.17.18693
64. Choosing Wisely Campaign Toolkit. American Board of Internal Medicine Foundation. Last updated July 18, 2023. Accessed December 18, 2024. https://www.aap.org/en/news-room/campaigns-and-toolkits/choosing-wisely
65. Haws ME, Linscott L, Thomas C, Orscheln E, Radhakrishnan R, Kline-Fath B. A retrospective analysis of the utility of head computed tomography and/or magnetic resonance imaging in the management of benign macrocrania. *J Pediatr.* 2017;182:283–289.e1. doi: 10.1016/j.jpeds.2016.11.033
66. Fisher PG. Does macrocephaly require MRI, CT, ultrasound, or a tape measure? *J Pediatr.* 2017;182:5. doi: 10.1016/j.jpeds.2017.01.011
67. Care M. Macrocephaly and subdural collections. *Pediatr Radiol.* 2021 May;51(6):891–897. doi: 10.1007/s00247-020-04848-1
68. Hobbs C, Childs AM, Wynne J, Livingston J, Seal A. Subdural haematoma and effusion in infancy: an epidemiological study. *Arch Dis Child.* 2005;90(9):952–955. doi: 10.1136/adc.2003.037739
69. Maguire S, Mann M. Systematic reviews of bruising in relation to child abuse-what have we learnt: an overview of review updates. *Evid Based Child Health.* 2013;8(2):255–263. doi: 10.1002/ebch.1909
70. Bennett S, Ward M, Moreau K, et al. Head injury secondary to suspected child maltreatment: results of a prospective Canadian national surveillance program. *Child Abuse Negl.* 2011;35(11):930–966. doi: 10.1016/j.chiabu.2011.05.018
71. Maguire S, Pickerd N, Farewell D, Mann M, Tempest V, Kemp AM. Which clinical features distinguish inflicted from non-inflicted brain injury? A systematic review. *Arch Dis Child.* 2009;94(11):860–867. doi: 10.1136/adc.2008.150110
72. Royal College of Paediatrics and Child Health, Cardiff University. *Child Protection Evidence: Systematic Review on Head and Spinal Injuries.* Cardiff University; August 2019. Accessed December 10, 2021. https://childprotection.rcpch.ac.uk/wp-content/uploads/sites/6/2021/02/Child-Protection-Evidence-Head-and-spinal-injuries.pdf
73. Pierce MC, Kaczor K, Lorenz DJ, et al. Validation of a clinical decision rule to predict abuse in young children based on bruising characteristics. *JAMA Netw Open.* 2021;4(4):e215832. doi: 10.1001/jamanetworkopen.2021.5832
74. Pierce MC, Kaczor K, Aldridge S, O'Flynn J, Lorenz DJ. Bruising characteristics discriminating physical child abuse from

accidental trauma. *Pediatrics.* 2010;125(1):67–74. doi: 10.1542/peds.2008-3632

75. Royal College of Paediatrics and Child Health, Cardiff University. *Child Protection Evidence: Systematic Review on Bruising.* Cardiff University; March 2020. Accessed December 10, 2021. https://childprotection.rcpch.ac.uk/wp-content/uploads/sites/6/2021/02/Child-Protection-Evidence-Chapter-Bruising_Update_final.pdf

76. Carpenter RF. The prevalence and distribution of bruising in babies. *Arch Dis Child.* 1999;80(4):363–366. doi: 10.1136/adc.80.4.363

77. Kemp AM, Dunstan F, Nuttall D, Hamilton M, Collins P, Maguire S. Patterns of bruising in preschool children—a longitudinal study. *Arch Dis Child.* 2015;100(5):426–431. doi: 10.1136/archdischild-2014-307120

78. Kemp AM, Maguire SA, Nuttall D, Collins P, Dunstan F. Bruising in children who are assessed for suspected physical abuse. *Arch Dis Child.* 2014;99(2):108–113. doi: 10.1136/archdischild-2013-304339

79. Sugar NF, Taylor JA, Feldman KW. Bruises in infants and toddlers: those who don't cruise rarely bruise. Puget Sound Pediatric Research Network. *Arch Pediatr Adolesc Med.* 1999;153(4):399–403. doi: 10.1001/archpedi.153.4.399

80. Pierce MC, Magana JN, Kaczor K, et al. The prevalence of bruising among infants in pediatric emergency departments. *Ann Emerg Med.* 2016;67(1):1–8. doi: 10.1016/j.annemergmed.2015.06.021

81. Naidoo S. A profile of the oro-facial injuries in child physical abuse at a children's hospital. *Child Abuse Negl.* 2000;24(4):521–534. doi: 10.1016/s0145-2134(00)00114-9

82. Dunstan FD, Guildea ZE, Kontos K, Kemp AM, Sibert JR. A scoring system for bruise patterns: a tool for identifying abuse. *Arch Dis Child.* 2002;86(5):330–333. doi: 10.1136/adc.86.5.330

83. Lopez MR, Abd-Allah S, Deming DD, et al. Oral, jaw, and neck injury in infants and children: from abusive trauma or intubation? *Pediatr Emerg Care.* 2014;30(5):305–310. doi: 10.1097/PEC.0000000000000124

84. Nazer D, Smyth M.Cutaneous conditions mimicking child abuse. In: Palusci VJ, Fischer H, eds. *Child Abuse and Neglect: A Diagnostic Guide For Physicians, Surgeons, Pathologists, Dentists, Nurses and Social Workers.* Manson Publishing Ltd; 2011:69–90

85. Ward M, Ornstein A, Niec A, Murray C; Canadian Paediatric Society, Child and Youth Maltreatment Section. The medical assessment of bruising in suspected child maltreatment cases: a clinical perspective. *Paediatr Child Health.* 2013;18(8):433–442

86. Vashi NA, Patzelt N, Wirya S, Maymone MB, Kundu RV. Dermatoses caused by cultural practices: cosmetic cultural practices. *J Am Acad Dermatol.* 2018;79(1):19–30. doi: 10.1016/j.jaad.2017.06.160

87. Kemp AM, Maguire SA, Nuttall DE, Collins P, Dunstan FD, Farewell D. Can TEN4 distinguish bruises from abuse, inherited bleeding disorders or accidents? *Arch Dis Child.* 2021;106(8):774–779. doi: 10.1136/archdischild-2020-320491

88. Collins PW, Hamilton M, Dunstan FD, et al. Patterns of bruising in preschool children with inherited bleeding disorders: a longitudinal study. *Arch Dis Child.* 2017;102(12):1110–1117. doi: 10.1136/archdischild-2015-310196

89. Kelly P, John S, Vincent AL, Reed P. Abusive head trauma and accidental head injury: a 20-year comparative study of referrals to a hospital child protection team. *Arch Dis Child.* 2015;100(12):1123–1130. doi: 10.1136/archdischild-2014-306960

90. Bradford R, Choudhary AK, Dias MS. Serial neuroimaging in infants with abusive head trauma: timing abusive injuries. *J Neurosurg Pediatr.* 2013;12(2):110–9. doi: 10.3171/2013.4.PEDS12596

91. Dias MS, Backstrom J, Falk M, Li V. Serial radiography in the infant shaken impact syndrome. *Pediatr Neurosurg.* 1998;29(2):77–85. doi: 10.1159/000028694

92. Matschke J, Voss J, Obi N, et al. Nonaccidental head injury is the most common cause of subdural bleeding in infants <1 year of age. *Pediatrics.* 2009;124(6):1587–1594. doi: 10.1542/peds.2008-3734

93. Bechtel K, Stoessel K, Leventhal JM, et al. Characteristics that distinguish accidental from abusive injury in hospitalized young children with head trauma. *Pediatrics.* 2004;114(1):165–168. doi: 10.1542/peds.114.1.165

94. Feldman KW, Bethel R, Shugerman RP, Grossman DC, Grady MS, Ellenbogen RG. The cause of infant and toddler subdural hemorrhage: a prospective study. *Pediatrics.* 2001;108(3):636–646. doi: 10.1542/peds.108.3.636

95. Kemp AM, Jaspan T, Griffiths J, et al. Neuroimaging: what neuroradiological features distinguish abusive from non-abusive head trauma? A systematic review. *Arch Dis Child.* 2011;96(12):1103–1112. doi: 10.1136/archdischild-2011-300630

96. Duhaime AC, Alario AJ, Lewander WJ, et al. Head injury in very young children: mechanisms, injury types, and ophthalmologic findings in 100 hospitalized patients younger than 2 years of age. *Pediatrics.* 1992;90(2 Pt 1):179–185

97. Hymel KP, Abshire TC, Luckey DW, Jenny C. Coagulopathy in pediatric abusive head trauma. *Pediatrics.* 1997;99(3):371–375. doi: 10.1542/peds.99.3.371

98. Reece RM, Sege R. Childhood head injuries: accidental or inflicted? *Arch Pediatr Adolesc Med.* 2000;154(1):11–15

99. Myhre MC, Grogaard JB, Dyb GA, Sandvik L, Nordhov M. Traumatic head injury in infants and toddlers. *Acta Paediatr.* 2007;96(8):1159–1163. doi: 10.1111/j.1651-2227.2007.00356.x

100. Ewing-Cobbs L, Kramer L, Prasad M, et al. Neuroimaging, physical, and developmental findings after inflicted and noninflicted traumatic brain injury in young children. *Pediatrics.* 1998;102(2 Pt 1):300–307. doi: 10.1542/peds.102.2.300

101. Ewing-Cobbs L, Prasad M, Kramer L, et al. Acute neuroradiologic findings in young children with inflicted or noninflicted traumatic brain injury. *Childs Nerv Syst.* 2000;16(1):25–33. doi: 10.1007/s003810050006

102. Tung GA, Kumar M, Richardson RC, Jenny C, Brown WD. Comparison of accidental and nonaccidental traumatic head injury in children on noncontrast computed tomography. *Pediatrics.* 2006;118(2):626–633. doi: 10.1542/peds.2006-0130

103. Zimmerman RA, Bilaniuk LT, Bruce D, Schut L, Uzzell B, Goldberg HI. Computed tomography of craniocerebral injury in the

abused child. *Radiology.* 1979;130(3):687–690. doi: 10.1148/130.3.687

104. Merten DF, Osborne DR, Radkowski MA, Leonidas JC. Craniocerebral trauma in the child abuse syndrome: radiological observations. *Pediatr Radiol.* 1984;14(5):272–277. doi: 10.1007/BF01601874

105. Hymel KP, Rumack CM, Hay TC, Strain JD, Jenny C. Comparison of intracranial computed tomographic (CT) findings in pediatric abusive and accidental head trauma. *Pediatr Radiol.* 1997;27(9):743–747. doi: 10.1007/s002470050215

106. Wells RG, Vetter C, Laud P. Intracranial hemorrhage in children younger than 3 years: prediction of intent. *Arch Pediatr Adolesc Med.* 2002;156(3):252–257. doi: 10.1001/archpedi.156.3.252

107. Ichord RN, Naim M, Pollock AN, Nance ML, Margulies SS, Christian CW. Hypoxic-ischemic injury complicates inflicted and accidental traumatic brain injury in young children: the role of diffusion-weighted imaging. *J Neurotrauma.* 2007;24(1):106–118. doi: 10.1089/neu.2006.0087

108. Hymel KP, Jenny C, Block RW. Intracranial hemorrhage and rebleeding in suspected victims of abusive head trauma: addressing the forensic controversies. *Child Maltreat.* 2002;7(4):329–348. doi: 10.1177/107755902237263

109. Case ME. Inflicted traumatic brain injury in infants and young children. *Brain Pathol.* 2008;18(4):571–582. doi: 10.1111/j.1750-3639.2008.00204.x

110. Rambaud C. Bridging veins and autopsy findings in abusive head trauma. *Pediatr Radiol.* 2015;45(8):1126–1131. doi: 10.1007/s00247-015-3285-0

111. Ronning MM, Carolan PL, Cutler GJ, Patterson RJ. Parasagittal vertex clots on head CT in infants with subdural hemorrhage as a predictor for abusive head trauma. *Pediatr Radiol.* 2018;48(13):1915–1923. doi: 10.1007/s00247-018-4237-2

112. Choudhary AK, Bradford R, Dias MS, Thamburaj K, Boal DK. Venous injury in abusive head trauma. *Pediatr Radiol.* 2015;45(12):1803–1813. doi: 10.1007/s00247-015-3399-4

113. Hahnemann ML, Kinner S, Schweiger B, et al. Imaging of bridging vein thrombosis in infants with abusive head trauma: the "tadpole sign." *Eur Radiol.* 2015;25(2):299–305. doi: 10.1007/s00330-014-3443-z

114. Zimmerman RA, Bilaniuk LT, Farina L. Non-accidental brain trauma in infants: diffusion imaging, contributions to understanding the injury process. *J Neuroradiol.* 2007;34(2):109–114. doi: 10.1016/j.neurad.2007.01.124

115. Suh DY, Davis PC, Hopkins KL, Fajman NN, Mapstone TB. Nonaccidental pediatric head injury: diffusion-weighted imaging findings. *Neurosurgery.* 2001;49(2):309–318. doi: 10.1097/00006123-200108000-00011

116. Orru E, Huisman T, Izbudak I. Prevalence, patterns, and clinical relevance of hypoxic-ischemic injuries in children exposed to abusive head trauma. *J Neuroimaging.* 2018;28(6):608–614. doi: 10.1111/jon.12555

117. Biousse V, Suh DY, Newman NJ, Davis PC, Mapstone T, Lambert SR. Diffusion-weighted magnetic resonance imaging in shaken baby syndrome. *Am J Ophthalmol.* 2002;133(2):249–255. doi: 10.1016/s0002-9394(01)01366-6

118. Khan NR, Fraser BD, Nguyen V, et al. Pediatric abusive head trauma and stroke. *J Neurosurg Pediatr.* 2017;20(2):183–190. doi: 10.3171/2017.4.PEDS16650

119. McKinney AM, Thompson LR, Truwit CL, Velders S, Karagulle A, Kiragu A. Unilateral hypoxic-ischemic injury in young children from abusive head trauma, lacking craniocervical vascular dissection or cord injury. *Pediatr Radiol.* 2008;38(2):164–174. doi: 10.1007/s00247-007-0673-0

120. Kemp AM, Stoodley N, Cobley C, Coles L, Kemp KW. Apnoea and brain swelling in non-accidental head injury. *Arch Dis Child.* 2003;88(6):472–476. doi: 10.1136/adc.88.6.472

121. Choudhary AK, Ishak R, Zacharia TT, Dias MS. Imaging of spinal injury in abusive head trauma: a retrospective study. *Pediatr Radiol.* 2014;44(9):1130–1140. doi: 10.1007/s00247-014-2959-3

122. Geddes JF, Vowles GH, Hackshaw AK, Nickols CD, Scott IS, Whitwell HL. Neuropathology of inflicted head injury in children. II. Microscopic brain injury in infants. *Brain.* 2001;124(Pt 7):1299–1306. doi: 10.1093/brain/124.7.1299

123. Johnson DL, Boal D, Baule R. Role of apnea in nonaccidental head injury. *Pediatr Neurosurg.* 1995;23(6):305–310. doi: 10.1159/000120976

124. Palifka LA, Frasier LD, Metzger RR, Hedlund GL. Parenchymal brain laceration as a predictor of abusive head trauma. *AJNR Am J Neuroradiol.* 2016;37(1):163–168. doi: 10.3174/ajnr.A4519

125. Jaspan T, Narborough G, Punt JA, Lowe J. Cerebral contusional tears as a marker of child abuse–detection by cranial sonography. *Pediatr Radiol.* 1992;22(4):237–245. doi: 10.1007/BF02019848

126. Au-Yong IT, Wardle SP, McConachie NS, Jaspan T. Isolated cerebral cortical tears in children: aetiology, characterisation and differentiation from non-accidental head injury. *Br J Radiol.* 2009;82(981):735–741. doi: 10.1259/bjr/81603888

127. Barber I, Perez-Rossello JM, Wilson CR, Silvera MV, Kleinman PK. Prevalence and relevance of pediatric spinal fractures in suspected child abuse. *Pediatr Radiol.* 2013;43(11):1507–1515. doi: 10.1007/s00247-013-2726-x

128. Choudhary AK, Bradford RK, Dias MS, Moore GJ, Boal DK. Spinal subdural hemorrhage in abusive head trauma: a retrospective study. *Radiology.* 2012;262(1):216–223. doi: 10.1148/radiol.11102390

129. Kadom N, Khademian Z, Vezina G, Shalaby-Rana E, Rice A, Hinds T. Usefulness of MRI detection of cervical spine and brain injuries in the evaluation of abusive head trauma. *Pediatr Radiol.* 2014;44(7):839–848. doi: 10.1007/s00247-014-2874-7

130. Kleinman PK, Morris NB, Makris J, Moles RL, Kleinman PL. Yield of radiographic skeletal surveys for detection of hand, foot, and spine fractures in suspected child abuse. *AJR Am J Roentgenol.* 2013;200(3):641–644. doi: 10.2214/AJR.12.8878

131. Kemp AM, Joshi AH, Mann M, et al. What are the clinical and radiological characteristics of spinal injuries from physical abuse: a systematic review. *Arch Dis Child.* 2010;95(5):355–360. doi: 10.1136/adc.2009.169110

132. Kemp A, Cowley L, Maguire S. Spinal injuries in abusive head trauma: patterns and recommendations. *Pediatr Radiol.* 2014; 44(Suppl 4):S604–S612. doi: 10.1007/s00247-014-3066-1

133. Hadley MN, Sonntag VK, Rekate HL, Murphy A. The infant whiplash-shake injury syndrome: a clinical and pathological study. *Neurosurgery.* 1989;24(4):536–40. doi: 10.1227/00006123-198904000-00008

134. Karmazyn B, Lewis ME, Jennings SG, Hibbard RA, Hicks RA. The prevalence of uncommon fractures on skeletal surveys performed to evaluate for suspected abuse in 930 children: should practice guidelines change? *AJR Am J Roentgenol.* 2011;197(1): W159–W163. doi: 10.2214/AJR.10.5733

135. Harlan SR, Nixon GW, Campbell KA, Hansen K, Prince JS. Follow-up skeletal surveys for nonaccidental trauma: can a more limited survey be performed? *Pediatr Radiol.* 2009;39(9): 962–968. doi: 10.1007/s00247-009-1313-7

136. Lindberg DM, Harper NS, Laskey AL, Berger RP, Ex SI. Prevalence of abusive fractures of the hands, feet, spine, or pelvis on skeletal survey: perhaps "uncommon" is more common than suggested. *Pediatr Emerg Care.* 2013;29(1):26–29. doi: 10.1097/PEC.0b013e31827b475e

137. Bhardwaj G, Chowdhury V, Jacobs MB, Moran KT, Martin FJ, Coroneo MT. A systematic review of the diagnostic accuracy of ocular signs in pediatric abusive head trauma. *Ophthalmology.* 2010;117(5):983–992.e17. doi: 10.1016/j.ophtha.2009.09.040

138. Song HH, Thoreson WB, Dong P, Shokrollahi Y, Gu L, Suh DW. Exploring the vitreoretinal interface: a key instigator of unique retinal hemorrhage patterns in pediatric head trauma. *Korean J Ophthalmol.* 2022;36(3):253–263. doi: 10.3341/kjo.2021.0133

139. Suh DW, Song HH, Mozafari H, Thoreson WB. Determining the tractional forces on vitreoretinal interface using a computer simulation model in abusive head trauma. *Am J Ophthalmol.* 2021;223: 396–404. doi: 10.1016/j.ajo.2020.06.020

140. Muni RH, Kohly RP, Sohn EH, Lee TC. Hand-held spectral domain optical coherence tomography finding in shaken-baby syndrome. *Retina.* 2010;30(4 Suppl):S45–S50. doi: 10.1097/IAE.0b013e3181dc048c

141. Sturm V, Landau K, Menke MN. Optical coherence tomography findings in shaken baby syndrome. *Am J Ophthalmol.* 2008; 146(3):363–368. doi: 10.1016/j.ajo.2008.04.023

142. Koozekanani DD, Weinberg DV, Dubis AM, Beringer J, Carroll J. Hemorrhagic retinoschisis in shaken baby syndrome imaged with spectral domain optical coherence tomography. *Ophthalmic Surg Lasers Imaging.* 2010 Mar 9:1–3. doi: 10.3928/15428877-20100215-87

143. Kivlin JD, Simons KB, Lazoritz S, Ruttum MS. Shaken baby syndrome. *Ophthalmology.* 2000;107(7):1246–1254. doi: 10.1016/s0161-6420(00)00161-5

144. Mills M. Funduscopic lesions associated with mortality in shaken baby syndrome. *J AAPOS.* 1998;2(2):67–71. doi: 10.1016/s1091-8531(98)90066-0

145. McCabe CF, Donahue SP. Prognostic indicators for vision and mortality in shaken baby syndrome. *Arch Ophthalmol.* 2000;118(3): 373–377. doi: 10.1001/archopht.118.3.373

146. Wilkinson WS, Han DP, Rappley MD, Owings CL. Retinal hemorrhage predicts neurologic injury in the shaken baby syndrome. *Arch Ophthalmol.* 1989;107(10):1472–1474. doi: 10.1001/archopht.1989.01070020546037

147. Breazzano MP, Unkrich KH, Barker-Griffith AE. Clinicopathological findings in abusive head trauma: analysis of 110 infant autopsy eyes. *Am J Ophthalmol.* 2014;158(6):1146–1154.e2. doi: 10.1016/j.ajo.2014.08.011

148. Massicotte SJ, Folberg R, Torczynski E, Gilliland MG, Luckenbach MW. Vitreoretinal traction and perimacular retinal folds in the eyes of deliberately traumatized children. *Ophthalmology.* 1991; 98(7):1124–1127. doi: 10.1016/s0161-6420(91)32167-5

149. Gaynon MW, Koh K, Marmor MF, Frankel LR. Retinal folds in the shaken baby syndrome. *Am J Ophthalmol.* 15 1988;106(4): 423–425. doi: 10.1016/0002-9394(88)90877-x

150. Morad Y, Kim YM, Armstrong DC, Huyer D, Mian M, Levin AV. Correlation between retinal abnormalities and intracranial abnormalities in the shaken baby syndrome. *Am J Ophthalmol.* 2002;134(3):354–359. doi: 10.1016/s0002-9394(02)01628-8

151. Levin AV. Ophthalmology of shaken baby syndrome. *Neurosurg Clin North Am.* 2002;13(2):201–211. doi: 10.1016/s1042-3680(02)00004-9

152. Kivlin JD, Currie ML, Greenbaum VJ, Simons KB, Jentzen J. Retinal hemorrhages in children following fatal motor vehicle crashes: a case series. *Arch Ophthalmol.* 2008;126(6):800–4. doi: 10.1001/archopht.126.6.800

153. Coats B, Binenbaum G, Peiffer RL, Forbes BJ, Margulies SS. Ocular hemorrhages in neonatal porcine eyes from single, rapid rotational events. *Invest Ophthalmol Vis Sci.* 2010;51(9):4792–4797. doi: 10.1167/iovs.10-5211

154. Hughes LA, May K, Talbot JF, Parsons MA. Incidence, distribution, and duration of birth-related retinal hemorrhages: a prospective study. *J AAPOS.* 2006;10(2):102–106. doi: 10.1016/j.jaapos.2005.12.005

155. Callaway NF, Ludwig CA, Blumenkranz MS, Jones JM, Fredrick DR, Moshfeghi DM. Retinal and optic nerve hemorrhages in the newborn infant: one-year results of the newborn eye screen test study. *Ophthalmology.* 2016;123(5):1043–1052. doi: 10.1016/j.ophtha.2016.01.004

156. Watts P, Maguire S, Kwok T, et al. Newborn retinal hemorrhages: a systematic review. *J AAPOS.* 2013;17(1):70–78. doi: 10.1016/j.jaapos.2012.07.012

157. Binenbaum G, Christian CW, Guttmann K, Huang J, Ying GS, Forbes BJ. Evaluation of temporal association between vaccinations and retinal hemorrhage in children. *JAMA Ophthalmol.* 2015;133(11): 1261–1265. doi: 10.1001/jamaophthalmol.2015.2868

158. Togioka BM, Arnold MA, Bathurst MA, et al. Retinal hemorrhages and shaken baby syndrome: an evidence-based review. *J Emerg Med.* 2009;37(1):98–106. doi: 10.1016/j.jemermed.2008.06.022

159. Forbes BJ, Christian CW, Judkins AR, Kryston K. Inflicted childhood neurotrauma (shaken baby syndrome): ophthalmic findings. *J Pediatr Ophthalmol Strabismus.* 2004;41(2):80–88. doi: 10.3928/0191-3913-20040301-07

160. Riffenburgh RS, Sathyavagiswaran L. Ocular findings at autopsy of child abuse victims. *Ophthalmology.* Oct 1991;98(10):1519–24. doi: 10.1016/s0161-6420(91)32095-5

161. Hartley LM, Khwaja OS, Verity CM. Glutaric aciduria type 1 and nonaccidental head injury. *Pediatrics.* Jan 2001;107(1):174–5. doi: 10.1542/peds.107.1.174

162. Ip SS, Zafar S, Liu TYA, et al. Nonaccidental trauma in pediatric patients: evidence-based screening criteria for ophthalmologic examination. *J AAPOS.* 2020;24(4):226.e1–226.e5. doi: 10.1016/j.jaapos.2020.03.012

163. Greiner MV, Berger RP, Thackeray JD, Lindberg DM. Examining Siblings to Recognize Abuse I. Dedicated retinal examination in children evaluated for physical abuse without radiographically identified traumatic brain injury. *J Pediatr.* 2013;163(2):527–531. doi: 10.1016/j.jpeds.2013.01.063

164. Payne BS, Kutz TJ, Di Maio A, Gerard JM. Prevalence of retinal hemorrhages in infants presenting with isolated long bone fractures and evaluation for abuse. *J Emerg Med.* 2016;51(4):365–369. doi: 10.1016/j.jemermed.2016.05.043

165. Vincent AL, Kelly P. Retinal haemorrhages in inflicted traumatic brain injury: the ophthalmologist in court. *Clin Exp Ophthalmol.* 2010;38(5):521–532. doi: 10.1111/j.1442-9071.2010.02324.x

166. DeRidder CA, Berkowitz CD, Hicks RA, Laskey AL. Subconjunctival hemorrhages in infants and children: a sign of nonaccidental trauma. *Pediatr Emerg Care.* 2013;29(2):222–226. doi: 10.1097/PEC.0b013e318280d663

167. Spitzer SG, Luorno J, Noel LP. Isolated subconjunctival hemorrhages in nonaccidental trauma. *J AAPOS.* 2005;9(1):53–56. doi: 10.1016/j.jaapos.2004.10.003

168. Kapoor S, Schiffman J, Tang R, Kiang E, Li H, Woodward J. The significance of white-centered retinal hemorrhages in the shaken baby syndrome. *Pediatr Emerg Care.* 1997;13(3):183–185. doi: 10.1097/00006565-199706000-00002

169. Buys YM, Levin AV, Enzenauer RW, et al. Retinal findings after head trauma in infants and young children. *Ophthalmology.* 1992;99(11):1718–1723. doi: 10.1016/s0161-6420(92)31741-5

170. Elder JE, Taylor RG, Klug GL. Retinal haemorrhage in accidental head trauma in childhood. *J Paediatr Child Health.* 1991;27(5):286–289. doi: 10.1111/j.1440-1754.1991.tb02539.x

171. Johnson DL, Braun D, Friendly D. Accidental head trauma and retinal hemorrhage. *Neurosurgery.* 1993;33(2):231–234.

172. Padron Perez N, Diaz-Cascajosa J, Prat-Bartomeu J, Martin-Begue N, Catala-Mora J. Bilateral retinal detachment in a case of nonaccidental trauma. *Can J Ophthalmol.* 2013;48(3):e44–e45. doi: 10.1016/j.jcjo.2012.11.017

173. Binenbaum G, Christian CW, Ichord RN, et al. Retinal hemorrhage and brain injury patterns on diffusion-weighted magnetic resonance imaging in children with head trauma. *J AAPOS.* 2013;17(6):603–608. doi: 10.1016/j.jaapos.2013.09.002

174. Maguire SA, Watts PO, Shaw AD, et al. Retinal haemorrhages and related findings in abusive and non-abusive head trauma: a systematic review. *Eye (Lond).* 2013;27(1):28–36. doi: 10.1038/eye.2012.213

175. Binenbaum G, Mirza-George N, Christian CW, Forbes BJ. Odds of abuse associated with retinal hemorrhages in children suspected of child abuse. *J AAPOS.* 2009;13(3):268–272. doi: 10.1016/j.jaapos.2009.03.005

176. Minns RA, Jones PA, Tandon A, Fleck BW, Mulvihill AO, Elton RA. Prediction of inflicted brain injury in infants and children using retinal imaging. *Pediatrics.* 2012;130(5):e1227–e1234. doi: 10.1542/peds.2011-3274

177. Aryan HE, Ghosheh FR, Jandial R, Levy ML. Retinal hemorrhage and pediatric brain injury: etiology and review of the literature. *J Clin Neurosci.* 2005;12(6):624–631. doi: 10.1016/j.jocn.2005.05.005

178. Watts P, Obi E. Retinal folds and retinoschisis in accidental and non-accidental head injury. *Eye (Lond).* 2008;22(12):1514–1516. doi: 10.1038/eye.2008.224

179. Lueder GT, Turner JW, Paschall R. Perimacular retinal folds simulating nonaccidental injury in an infant. *Arch Ophthalmol.* 2006;124(12):1782–1783. doi: 10.1001/archopht.124.12.1782

180. Moran K, Reddie I, Jacobs M. Severe haemorrhagic retinopathy and traumatic retinoschisis in a 2 year old infant, after an 11 metre fall onto concrete. *Acta Paediatr.* 2008;97:149–149

181. Lantz PE, Sinal SH, Stanton CA, Weaver RG, Jr. Perimacular retinal folds from childhood head trauma. *BMJ.* 2004;328(7442):754–756. doi: 10.1136/bmj.328.7442.754

182. Shi A, Kulkarni A, Feldman KW, et al. Retinal findings in young children with increased intracranial pressure from nontraumatic causes. *Pediatrics.* 2019;143(2):e20181182. doi: 10.1542/peds.2018-1182

183. Chen WS, Forbes B, Ying G-S, Huang J, Binenbaum G. Natural history of retinal hemorrhage in children with abusive or accidental head trauma. *J AAPOS.* 2013;17(1):e12

184. Binenbaum G, Reid JE, Rogers DL, Jensen AK, Billinghurst LL, Forbes BJ. Patterns of retinal hemorrhage associated with pediatric cerebral sinovenous thrombosis. *J AAPOS.* 2017;21(1):23–27. doi: 10.1016/j.jaapos.2016.10.004

185. Fahmy J. Symptoms and signs of intracranial aneurysms: with particular reference to retinal haemorrhage. *Acta Ophthalmologica.* 1972;50(2):129–136

186. Diaz AG, Carmena JJ, Martin FR, Lopez PD, Casado MJM. Intraocular hemorrhage in sudden increased intracranial pressure (Terson syndrome). *Ophthalmologica.* 1979;179(3):173–176

187. Meyer FB, Sundt TM Jr, Fode NC, Morgan MK, Forbes GS, Mellinger JF. Cerebral aneurysms in childhood and adolescence. *J Neurosurg.* 1989;70(3):420–425. doi: 10.3171/jns.1989.70.3.0420

188. McLellan NJ, Prasad R, Punt J. Spontaneous subhyaloid and retinal haemorrhages in an infant. *Arch Dis Child.* 1986;61(11):1130–1132. doi: 10.1136/adc.61.11.1130

189. Forbes BJ, Cox M, Christian CW. Retinal hemorrhages in patients with epidural hematomas. *J AAPOS.* 2008;12(2):177–180. doi: 10.1016/j.jaapos.2007.07.009

190. Bhardwaj G, Jacobs MB, Moran KT, Tan K. Terson syndrome with ipsilateral severe hemorrhagic retinopathy in a 7-month-old child. *J AAPOS*. 2010;14(5):441–443. doi: 10.1016/j.jaapos.2010.06.009

191. Schloff S, Mullaney PB, Armstrong DC, et al. Retinal findings in children with intracranial hemorrhage. *Ophthalmology*. 2002;109(8): 1472–1476. doi: 10.1016/s0161-6420(02)01086-2

192. Fahmy J. Fundal haemorrhages in ruptured intracranial aneurysms: I. Material, frequency and morphology. *Acta Ophthalmol*. 1973;51(3):289–298

193. Agrawal S, Peters MJ, Adams GG, Pierce CM. Prevalence of retinal hemorrhages in critically ill children. *Pediatrics*. 2012;129(6): e1388–e1396. doi: 10.1542/peds.2011-2772

194. Thau A, Saffren B, Zakrzewski H, Anderst JD, Carpenter SL, Levin A. Retinal hemorrhage and bleeding disorders in children: a review. *Child Abuse Negl*. 2021;112:104901. doi: 10.1016/j.chiabu.2020. 104901

195. Dinakaran S, Chan TK, Rogers NK, Brosnahan DM. Retinal hemorrhages in meningococcal septicemia. *J AAPOS*. 2002;6(4):221–223. doi: 10.1067/mpa.2002.124648

196. Fraser SG, Horgan SE, Bardavio J. Retinal haemorrhage in meningitis. *Eye (Lond)*. 1995;9 (Pt 5):659–660. doi: 10.1038/eye. 1995.165

197. Lopez JP, Roque J, Torres J, Levin AV. Severe retinal hemorrhages in infants with aggressive, fatal Streptococcus pneumoniae meningitis. *J AAPOS*. 2010;14(1):97–98. doi: 10.1016/j.jaapos. 2009.11.013

198. Binenbaum G, Forbes BJ, Topjian AA, Twelves C, Christian CW. Patterns of retinal hemorrhage associated with cardiac arrest and cardiopulmonary resuscitation. *J AAPOS*. 2021;25(6): 324.e1–324.e4. doi: 10.1016/j.jaapos.2021.06.005

199. Odom A, Christ E, Kerr N, et al. Prevalence of retinal hemorrhages in pediatric patients after in-hospital cardiopulmonary resuscitation: a prospective study. *Pediatrics*. 1997;99(6):E3. doi: 10.1542/ peds.99.6.e3

200. Weedn VW, Mansour AM, Nichols MM. Retinal hemorrhage in an infant after cardiopulmonary resuscitation. *Am J Forensic Med Pathol*. 1990;11(1):79–82. doi: 10.1097/00000433-199003000-00012

201. Gilliland MG, Luckenbach MW. Are retinal hemorrhages found after resuscitation attempts? A study of the eyes of 169 children. *Am J Forensic Med Pathol*. 1993;14(3):187–292. doi: 10.1097/ 00000433-199309000-00003

202. Tomasi LG, Rosman NP. Purtscher retinopathy in the battered child syndrome. *Am J Dis Child*. 1975;129(11):1335–1337. doi: 10.1001/archpedi.1975.02120480051012

203. Goldman M, Dagan Z, Yair M, Elbaz U, Lahat E, Yair M. Severe cough and retinal hemorrhage in infants and young children. *J Pediatr*. 2006;148(6):835–836. doi: 10.1016/j.jpeds.2005.12.052

204. Raoof N, Pereira S, Dai S, Neutze J, Grant CC, Kelly P. Retinal haemorrhage in infants with pertussis. *Arch Dis Child*. 2017;102(12): 1158–1160. doi: 10.1136/archdischild-2017-313380

205. Sandramouli S, Robinson R, Tsaloumas M, Willshaw HE. Retinal haemorrhages and convulsions. *Arch Dis Child*. 1997;76(5):449–451. doi: 10.1136/adc.76.5.449

206. Tyagi AK, Scotcher S, Kozeis N, Willshaw HE. Can convulsions alone cause retinal haemorrhages in infants? *Br J Ophthalmol*. 1998;82 (6):659–660. doi: 10.1136/bjo.82.6.659

207. Herr S, Pierce MC, Berger RP, Ford H, Pitetti RD. Does valsalva retinopathy occur in infants? An initial investigation in infants with vomiting caused by pyloric stenosis. *Pediatrics*. 2004;113(6): 1658–1661. doi: 10.1542/peds.113.6.1658

208. Geloneck MM, Forbes BJ, Shaffer J, Ying GS, Binenbaum G. Ocular complications in children with diabetes mellitus. *Ophthalmology*. 2015;122(12):2457–2464. doi: 10.1016/j.ophtha.2015.07.010

209. Chung CW, Levin AV, Forbes BJ, Binenbaum G. Retinal hemorrhage after pediatric neurosurgical procedures. *J AAPOS*. 2022;26(2): 74.e1–74.e5. doi: 10.1016/j.jaapos.2021.11.010

210. Binenbaum G, Chen W, Huang J, Ying G-s, Forbes BJ. The natural history of retinal hemorrhage in pediatric head trauma. *J AAPOS*. 2016;20(2):131–135. doi: 10.1016/j.jaapos.2015.12.008

211. King WJ, MacKay M, Sirnick A; The Canadian Shaken Baby Study Group. Shaken baby syndrome in Canada: clinical characteristics and outcomes of hospital cases. *CMAJ*. 2003;168(2):155–159

212. Barber I, Kleinman PK. Imaging of skeletal injuries associated with abusive head trauma. *Pediatr Radiol*. 2014;44(Suppl 4):S613–S620. doi: 10.1007/s00247-014-3099-5

213. Hoskote A, Richards P, Anslow P, McShane T. Subdural haematoma and non-accidental head injury in children. *Childs Nerv Syst*. 2002; 18(6-7):311–317. doi: 10.1007/s00381-002-0616-x

214. Pontarelli EM, Jensen AR, Komlofske KM, Bliss DW. Infant head injury in falls and nonaccidental trauma: does injury pattern correlate with mechanism? *Pediatr Emerg Care*. 2014;30(10): 677–679. doi: 10.1097/PEC.0000000000000226

215. Roach JP, Acker SN, Bensard DD, Sirotnak AP, Karrer FM, Partrick DA. Head injury pattern in children can help differentiate accidental from non-accidental trauma. *Pediatr Surg Int*. 2014;30(11): 1103–1106. doi: 10.1007/s00383-014-3598-3

216. Adamo MA, Drazin D, Smith C, Waldman JB. Comparison of accidental and nonaccidental traumatic brain injuries in infants and toddlers: demographics, neurosurgical interventions, and outcomes. *J Neurosurg Pediatr*. 2009;4(5):414–419. doi: 10.3171/ 2009.6.PEDS0939

217. Ettaro L, Berger RP, Songer T. Abusive head trauma in young children: characteristics and medical charges in a hospitalized population. *Child Abuse Negl*. 2004;28(10):1099–1111. doi: 10.1016/j. chiabu.2004.06.006

218. Harper NS, Eddleman S, Shukla K, et al. Radiologic assessment of skull fracture healing in young children. *Pediatr Emerg Care*. 2021;37(4):213–217. doi: 10.1097/PEC.0000000000002215

219. Ibrahim NG, Wood J, Margulies SS, Christian CW. Influence of age and fall type on head injuries in infants and toddlers. *Int J Dev Neurosci*. 2012;30(3):201–206. doi: 10.1016/j.ijdevneu.2011.10.007

220. Schutzman SA, Barnes PD, Mantello M, Scott RM. Epidural hematomas in children. *Ann Emerg Med.* 1993;22(3):535–541. doi: 10.1016/s0196-0644(05)81938-9

221. Sieswerda-Hoogendoorn T, Robben SG, Karst WA, et al. Abusive head trauma: differentiation between impact and non-impact cases based on neuroimaging findings and skeletal surveys. *Eur J Radiol.* 2014;83(3):584–588. doi: 10.1016/j.ejrad.2013.11.015

222. Borland ML, Dalziel SR, Phillips N, et al. Delayed Presentations to emergency departments of children with head injury: a PREDICT study. *Ann Emerg Med.* 2019;74(1):1–10. doi: 10.1016/j.annemergmed.2018.11.035

223. Gelernter R, Weiser G, Kozer E. Computed tomography findings in young children with minor head injury presenting to the emergency department greater than 24h post injury. *Injury.* 2018;49(1):82–85. doi: 10.1016/j.injury.2017.09.012

224. Sellin JN, Moreno A, Ryan SL, et al. Children presenting in delayed fashion after minor head trauma with scalp swelling: do they require further workup? *Childs Nerv Syst.* 2017;33(4):647–652. doi: 10.1007/s00381-016-3332-7

225. DiScala C, Sege R, Li G, Reece RM. Child abuse and unintentional injuries: a 10-year retrospective. *Arch Pediatr Adolesc Med.* 2000;154(1):16–22. doi: 10-1001/pubs.Pediatr Adolesc Med.-ISSN-1072-4710-154-1-poa9047

226. Thompson AK, Bertocci G, Rice W, Pierce MC. Pediatric short-distance household falls: biomechanics and associated injury severity. *Accid Anal Prev.* 2011;43(1):143–150. doi: 10.1016/j.aap.2010.07.020

227. Hymel KP, Stoiko MA, Herman BE, et al. Head injury depth as an indicator of causes and mechanisms. *Pediatrics.* 2010;125(4):712–720. doi: 10.1542/peds.2009-2133

228. Meservy CJ, Towbin R, McLaurin RL, Myers PA, Ball W. Radiographic characteristics of skull fractures resulting from child abuse. *AJR Am J Roentgenol.* 1987;149(1):173–175. doi: 10.2214/ajr.149.1.173

229. Ruest S, Kanaan G, Moore JL, Goldberg AP. The prevalence of rib fractures incidentally identified by chest radiograph among infants and toddlers. *J Pediatr.* 2019;204:208–213. doi: 10.1016/j.jpeds.2018.08.067

230. Kemp AM, Dunstan F, Harrison S, et al. Patterns of skeletal fractures in child abuse: systematic review. *BMJ.* 2008;337:a1518. doi: 10.1136/bmj.a1518

231. Paine CW, Fakeye O, Christian CW, Wood JN. Prevalence of abuse among young children with rib fractures: a systematic review. *Pediatr Emerg Care.* 2019;35(2):96–103. doi: 10.1097/PEC.0000000000000911

232. Royal College of Paediatrics and Child Health, Cardiff University. *Child Protection Evidence: Systematic Review on Fractures.* Cardiff University; April 2018. Accessed December 10, 2021. https://childprotection.rcpch.ac.uk/wp-content/uploads/sites/6/2020/05/child_protection_evidence_-_fractures.pdf

233. Love JC, Derrick SM, Wiersema JM, et al. Novel classification system of rib fractures observed in infants. *J Forensic Sci.* 2013;58(2):330–335. doi: 10.1111/1556-4029.12054

234. Kleinman PK. *Diagnostic Imaging of Child Abuse.* Cambridge University Press; 2015

235. Worn MJ, Jones MD. Rib fractures in infancy: establishing the mechanisms of cause from the injuries–a literature review. *Med Sci Law.* 2007;47(3):200–212. doi: 10.1258/rsmmsl.47.3.200

236. Boal DK, Felman AH, Krugman RD. Controversial aspects of child abuse: a roundtable discussion. 43rd Annual Meeting, Society for Pediatric Radiology. *Pediatr Radiol.* 2001;31(11):760–774. doi: 10.1007/s002470100538

237. van Rijn RR, Bilo RA, Robben SG. Birth-related mid-posterior rib fractures in neonates: a report of three cases (and a possible fourth case) and a review of the literature. *Pediatr Radiol.* 2009;39(1):30–34. doi: 10.1007/s00247-008-1035-2

238. Maguire S, Mann M, John N, et al. Does cardiopulmonary resuscitation cause rib fractures in children? A systematic review. *Child Abuse Negl.* 2006;30(7):739–751. doi: 10.1016/j.chiabu.2005.12.007

239. Rehm A, Promod P, Ogilvy-Stuart A. Neonatal birth fractures: a retrospective tertiary maternity hospital review. *J Obstet Gynaecol.* 2020;40(4):485–490. doi: 10.1080/01443615.2019.1631770

240. Franke I, Pingen A, Schiffmann H, et al. Cardiopulmonary resuscitation (CPR)-related posterior rib fractures in neonates and infants following recommended changes in CPR techniques. *Child Abuse Negl.* 2014;38(7):1267–1274. doi: 10.1016/j.chiabu.2014.01.021

241. Pinto DC, Haden-Pinneri K, Love JC. Manual and automated cardiopulmonary resuscitation (CPR): a comparison of associated injury patterns. *J Forensic Sci.* 2013;58(4):904–909. doi: 10.1111/1556-4029.12146

242. Matshes EW, Lew EO. Two-handed cardiopulmonary resuscitation can cause rib fractures in infants. *Am J Forensic Med Pathol.* 2010;31(4):303–307. doi: 10.1097/PAF.0b013e3181e792eb

243. Reyes JA, Somers GR, Taylor GP, Chiasson DA. Increased incidence of CPR-related rib fractures in infants—is it related to changes in CPR technique? *Resuscitation.* 2011;82(5):545–548. doi: 10.1016/j.resuscitation.2010.12.024

244. Chadwick D, Bertocci G, Guenther E. Injuries resulting from falls. *Child Abuse Negl.* 2011:570–578. doi: 10.1016/B978-1-4160-6393-3.00059-2

245. Pierce MC, Bertocci GE, Janosky JE, et al. Femur fractures resulting from stair falls among children: an injury plausibility model. *Pediatrics.* 2005;115(6):1712–1722. doi: 10.1542/peds.2004-0614

246. Dsouza R, Bertocci G. Impact sites representing potential bruising locations associated with bed falls in children. *Forensic Sci Int.* 2018;286:86–95. doi: 10.1016/j.forsciint.2018.02.018

247. Dsouza R, Bertocci G. Impact sites representing potential bruising locations associated with rearward falls in children. *Forensic Sci Int.* 2016;261:129–236. doi: 10.1016/j.forsciint.2016.02.012

248. Hibberd O, Nuttall D, Watson RE, Watkins WJ, Kemp AM, Maguire S. Childhood bruising distribution observed from eight mechanisms of unintentional injury. *Arch Dis Child.* 2017;102(12):1103–1109. doi: 10.1136/archdischild-2017-312847

249. Bertocci G, Pierce MC. Applications of biomechanics aiding in the diagnosis of child abuse. *Clin Pediatr Emerg Med.* 2006;7(3): 194–199. doi: 10.1016/j.cpem.2006.06.006

250. van Zandwijk JP, Vester MEM, Bilo RA, van Rijn RR, Loeve AJ. Modeling of inflicted head injury by shaking trauma in children: what can we learn? Part II: A systematic review of mathematical and physical models. *Forensic Sci Med Pathol.* 2019;15(3): 423–436. doi: 10.1007/s12024-019-00093-7

251. Vester MEM, Bilo RAC, Loeve AJ, van Rijn RR, van Zandwijk JP. Modeling of inflicted head injury by shaking trauma in children: what can we learn? Part I: A systematic review of animal models. *Forensic Sci Med Pathol.* 2019;15(3):408–422. doi: 10.1007/s12024-019-0082-3

252. Mertz HJ.Anthropomorphic test devices. In: Nahum AM, Melvin JW, eds. *Accidental Injury: Biomechanics and Prevention.* Springer New York; 2002:72–88

253. Cory CZ, Jones BM. Can shaking alone cause fatal brain injury? A biomechanical assessment of the Duhaime shaken baby syndrome model. *Med Sci Law.* 2003;43(4):317–333. doi: 10.1258/rsmmsl.43.4.317

254. Jenny CA, Bertocci G, Fukuda T, Rangarajan N, Shams T. Biomechanical response of the infant head to shaking: an experimental investigation. *J Neurotrauma.* 2017;34(8):1579–1588. doi: 10.1089/neu.2016.4687

255. Mertz HJ.Injury risk assessments based on dummy responses. In: Nahum AM, Melvin JW, eds. *Accidental Injury: Biomechanics and Prevention.* Springer New York; 2002:89–102

256. Cory CZ, Jones MD, James DS, Leadbeatter S, Nokes LD. The potential and limitations of utilising head impact injury models to assess the likelihood of significant head injury in infants after a fall. *Forensic Sci Int.* 2001;123(2-3):89–106. doi: 10.1016/s0379-0738(01)00523-0

257. Margulies SS, Coats B.Biomechanics of pediatric TBI. In: Yeates KO, Anderson V, eds. *Pediatric Traumatic Brain Injury: New Frontiers in Clinical and Translational Research.* Cambridge University Press; 2010:7–17

258. Coats B, Margulies SS. Material properties of human infant skull and suture at high rates. *J Neurotrauma.* 2006;23(8):1222–1232. doi: 10.1089/neu.2006.23.1222

259. Prange MT, Margulies SS. Regional, directional, and age-dependent properties of the brain undergoing large deformation. *J Biomech Eng.* 2002;124(2):244–252. doi: 10.1115/1.1449907

260. Maxwell WL. Traumatic brain injury in the neonate, child and adolescent human: an overview of pathology. *Int J Dev Neurosci.* 2012; 30(3):167–183. doi: 10.1016/j.ijdevneu.2011.12.008

261. Thompson AK, Bertocci GE. Paediatric bed fall computer simulation model development and validation. *Comput Methods Biomech Biomed Engin.* 2013;16(6):592–601. doi: 10.1080/10255842.2011.629613

262. Thompson A, Bertocci G. Pediatric bed fall computer simulation model: parametric sensitivity analysis. *Med Eng Phys.* 2014; 36(1):110–118. doi: 10.1016/j.medengphy.2013.10.006

263. Li Z, Hu J, Reed MP, et al. Development, validation, and application of a parametric pediatric head finite element model for impact simulations. *Ann Biomed Eng.* 2011;39(12):2984–2997. doi: 10.1007/s10439-011-0409-z

264. Hajiaghamemar M, Lan IS, Christian CW, Coats B, Margulies SS. Infant skull fracture risk for low height falls. *Int J Legal Med.* 2019;133(3):847–862. doi: 10.1007/s00414-018-1918-1

265. Gennarelli TA, Meaney DF.Mechanisms of primary head injury. In: Wilkins RH, Renachary SS, eds. *Neurosurgery.* Mc-Graw Hill; 1996: 2611–2621

266. Gennarelli TA, Thibault LE. Biomechanics of acute subdural hematoma. *J Trauma.* 1982;22(8):680–686. doi: 10.1097/00005373-198208000-00005

267. Meaney DF. *Biomechanics of Acute Subdural Hematoma in the Subhuman Primate and in Man.* University of Pennsylvania; 1991

268. Raghupathi R, Margulies SS. Traumatic axonal injury after closed head injury in the neonatal pig. *J Neurotrauma.* 2002;19(7): 843–853. doi: 10.1089/08977150260190438

269. Duhaime AC, Gennarelli TA, Thibault LE, Bruce DA, Margulies SS, Wiser R. The shaken baby syndrome. A clinical, pathological, and biomechanical study. *J Neurosurg.* 1987;66(3):409–415. doi: 10.3171/jns.1987.66.3.0409

270. Prange MT, Coats B, Duhaime AC, Margulies SS. Anthropomorphic simulations of falls, shakes, and inflicted impacts in infants. *J Neurosurg.* 2003;99(1):143–150. doi: 10.3171/jns.2003.99.1.0143

271. Miyazaki Y. The mechanism of shaken baby syndrome based on the visualization of intracranial brain motion. *Japan J Neurosurg.* 2015;24(7):468–476. doi: 10.7887/jcns.24.468

272. Coats B, Binenbaum G, Smith C, et al. Cyclic head rotations produce modest brain injury in infant piglets. *J Neurotrauma.* 2017; 34(1):235–247. doi: 10.1089/neu.2015.4352

273. Ibrahim NG, Ralston J, Smith C, Margulies SS. Physiological and pathological responses to head rotations in toddler piglets. *J Neurotrauma.* 2010;27(6):1021–1035. doi: 10.1089/neu.2009.1212

274. Raghupathi R, Mehr MF, Helfaer MA, Margulies SS. Traumatic axonal injury is exacerbated following repetitive closed head injury in the neonatal pig. *J Neurotrauma.* 2004;21(3):307–316. doi: 10.1089/089771504322972095

275. Finnie JW, Blumbergs PC, Manavis J, et al. Neuropathological changes in a lamb model of non-accidental head injury (the shaken baby syndrome). *J Clin Neurosci.* 2012;19(8):1159–1164. doi: 10.1016/j.jocn.2011.12.019

276. Ommaya AK, Hirsch AE. Tolerances for cerebral concussion from head impact and whiplash in primates. *J Biomech.* 1971;4(1): 13–21. doi: 10.1016/0021-9290(71)90011-x

277. Ommaya AK, Faas F, Yarnell P. Whiplash injury and brain damage: an experimental study. *JAMA.* 1968;204(4):285–289

278. Lloyd J, Willey E, Galaznik J, Lee W, Luttner S. Biomechanical evaluation of head kinematics during infant shaking versus pediatric activities of daily living. *J Forens Biomech.* 2011;2(9). doi: 10.4303/jfb/F110601

279. Weber W. [Experimental studies of skull fractures in infants] [Article in German]. *Z Rechtsmed.* 1984;92(2):87–94. doi: 10.1007/BF02116216

280. Weber W. [Biomechanical fragility of the infant skull] [Article in German]. *Z Rechtsmed.* 1985;94(2):93–101. doi: 10.1007/BF00198677

281. Loyd AM, Nightingale RW, Luck JF, Bass C, Cutcliffe HC, Myers BS. The response of the pediatric head to impacts onto a rigid surface. *J Biomech.* 2019;93:167–176. doi: 10.1016/j.jbiomech.2019.06.027

282. Prange MT, Luck JF, Dibb A, Van Ee CA, Nightingale RW, Myers BS. Mechanical properties and anthropometry of the human infant head. *Stapp Car Crash J.* 2004;48:279–299. doi: 10.4271/2004-22-0013

283. Stray-Pedersen A, Strisland F, Rognum TO, Schiks LAH, Loeve AJ. Violent infant surrogate shaking: continuous high-magnitude centripetal force and abrupt shift in tangential acceleration may explain high risk of subdural hemorrhage. *Neurotrauma Rep.* 2021;2(1):224–231. doi: 10.1089/neur.2021.0013

284. Freeman SS, Udomphorn Y, Armstead WM, Fisk DM, Vavilala MS. Young age as a risk factor for impaired cerebral autoregulation after moderate to severe pediatric traumatic brain injury. *Anesthesiology.* 2008;108(4):588–595. doi: 10.1097/ALN.0b013e31816725d7

285. Haviland J, Russell RI. Outcome after severe non-accidental head injury. *Arch Dis Child.* 1997;77(6):504–507. doi: 10.1136/adc.77.6.504

286. Brennan LK, Rubin D, Christian CW, Duhaime AC, Mirchandani HG, Rorke-Adams LB. Neck injuries in young pediatric homicide victims. *J Neurosurg Pediatr.* 2009;3(3):232–239. doi: 10.3171/2008.11.PEDS0835

287. Kochanek PM, Berger RP, Bayir H, Wagner AK, Jenkins LW, Clark RS. Biomarkers of primary and evolving damage in traumatic and ischemic brain injury: diagnosis, prognosis, probing mechanisms, and therapeutic decision making. *Curr Opin Crit Care.* 2008;14(2):135–141. doi: 10.1097/MCC.0b013e3282f57564

288. Smith SL, Andrus PK, Gleason DD, Hall ED. Infant rat model of the shaken baby syndrome: preliminary characterization and evidence for the role of free radicals in cortical hemorrhaging and progressive neuronal degeneration. *J Neurotrauma.* 1998;15(9):693–705. doi: 10.1089/neu.1998.15.693

289. Bonnier C, Mesples B, Carpentier S, Henin D, Gressens P. Delayed white matter injury in a murine model of shaken baby syndrome. *Brain Pathol.* 2002;12(3):320–318. doi: 10.1111/j.1750-3639.2002.tb00446.x

290. Wang G, Zhang YP, Gao Z, et al. Pathophysiological and behavioral deficits in developing mice following rotational acceleration-deceleration traumatic brain injury. *Dis Model Mech.* 2018;11(1):dmm030387. doi: 10.1242/dmm.030387

291. Kawamata Y, Ehara A, Yamaguchi T, Seo Y, Shimoda K, Ueda S. Repeated mild shaking of neonates induces transient cerebral microhemorrhages and anxiety-related behavior in adult rats. *Neurosci Lett.* 2018;684:29–34. doi: 10.1016/j.neulet.2018.06.059

292. Edwards GA, Maguire SA, Gaither JR, Leventhal JM. What do confessions reveal about abusive head trauma? A systematic review. *Child Abuse Rev.* 2020;29(3):253–268. doi: https://doi.org/10.1002/car.2627

293. Gennarelli TA, Thibault LE.Biomechanics of head injury. In: Wilkins RH, Renachary SS, eds. *Neurosurgery.* McGraw Hill; 1985:1531–1536

294. Margulies SS, Thibault LE, Gennarelli TA. Physical model simulations of brain injury in the primate. *J Biomech.* 1990;23(8):823–836. doi: 10.1016/0021-9290(90)90029-3

295. Duhaime AC, Margulies SS, Durham SR, et al. Maturation-dependent response of the piglet brain to scaled cortical impact. *J Neurosurg.* 2000;93(3):455–462. doi: 10.3171/jns.2000.93.3.0455

296. Huang WL, Beazley LD, Quinlivan JA, Evans SF, Newnham JP, Dunlop SA. Effect of corticosteroids on brain growth in fetal sheep. *Obstet Gynecol.* 1999;94(2):213–218. doi: 10.1016/s0029-7844(99)00265-3

297. Anderson RW, Sandoz B, Dutschke JK, et al. Biomechanical studies in an ovine model of non-accidental head injury. *J Biomech.* 2014;47(11):2578–2583. doi: 10.1016/j.jbiomech.2014.06.002

298. Finnie JW, Manavis J, Blumbergs PC. Diffuse neuronal perikaryal amyloid precursor protein immunoreactivity in an ovine model of non-accidental head injury (the shaken baby syndrome). *J Clin Neurosci.* 2010;17(2):237–240. doi: 10.1016/j.jocn.2009.07.001

299. Costine-Bartell BA, McGuone D, Price G, et al. Development of a model of hemispheric hypodensity ("big black brain"). *J Neurotrauma.* 2019;36(5):815–833. doi: 10.1089/neu.2018.5736

300. Durham SR, Duhaime AC. Basic science; maturation-dependent response of the immature brain to experimental subdural hematoma. *J Neurotrauma.* 2007;24(1):5–14. doi: 10.1089/neu.2006.0054

301. Costine-Bartell B, Price G, Shen J, McGuone D, Staley K, Duhaime AC. A perfect storm: the distribution of tissue damage depends on seizure duration, hemorrhage, and developmental stage in a gyrencephalic, multi-factorial, severe traumatic brain injury model. *Neurobiol Dis.* 2021;154:105334. doi: 10.1016/j.nbd.2021.105334

302. Bertocci G, Smalley C, Brown N, Dsouza R, Thompson A. Injuries and biomechancis of falls involving young children in a childcare setting obtained through video recording and wearable biometric devices. Presented at: Shaken Baby Syndrome & Abusive Head Trauma Symposium; September 21-22, 2020 [virtual]

303. Bertocci GE, Pierce MC, Deemer E, Aguel F, Janosky JE, Vogeley E. Using test dummy experiments to investigate pediatric injury risk in simulated short-distance falls. *Arch Pediatr Adolesc Med.* 2003;157(5):480–486. doi: 10.1001/archpedi.157.5.480

304. Bertocci GE, Pierce MC, Deemer E, Aguel F, Janosky JE, Vogeley E. Influence of fall height and impact surface on biomechanics of feet-first free falls in children. *Injury.* 2004;35(4):417–424. doi: 10.1016/S0020-1383(03)00062-7

305. Thompson A, Bertocci G, Pierce MC. Assessment of injury potential in pediatric bed fall experiments using an anthropomorphic

test device. *Accid Anal Prev.* 2013;50:16–24. doi: 10.1016/j.aap.2012.09.011

306. Thompson AK, Bertocci G, Pierce MC. Assessment of head injury risk associated with feet-first free falls in 12-month-old children using an anthropomorphic test device. *J Trauma.* 2009;66(4):1019–1029. doi: 10.1097/TA.0b013e31817dac8b
307. Coats B, Margulies SS. Potential for head injuries in infants from low-height falls. *J Neurosurg Pediatr.* 2008;2(5):321–330. doi: 10.3171/PED.2008.2.11.321
308. Ibrahim NG, Margulies SS. Biomechanics of the toddler head during low-height falls: an anthropomorphic dummy analysis. *J Neurosurg Pediatr.* 2010;6(1):57–68. doi: 10.3171/2010.3.PEDS09357
309. Sullivan S, Coats B, Margulies SS. Biofidelic neck influences head kinematics of parietal and occipital impacts following short falls in infants. *Accid Anal Prev.* 2015;82:143–153. doi: 10.1016/j.aap.2015.05.020
310. Chadwick DL, Bertocci G, Castillo E, et al. Annual risk of death resulting from short falls among young children: less than 1 in 1 million. *Pediatrics.* 2008;121(6):1213–1224. doi: 10.1542/peds.2007-2281
311. Plunkett J. Fatal pediatric head injuries caused by short-distance falls. *Am J Forensic Med Pathol.* 2001;22(1):1–12. doi: 10.1097/00000433-200103000-00001
312. Chaudhary S, Figueroa J, Shaikh S, et al. Pediatric falls ages 0-4: understanding demographics, mechanisms, and injury severities. *Inj Epidemiol.* 2018;5(Suppl 1):7. doi: 10.1186/s40621-018-0147-x
313. Mulligan CS, Adams S, Tzioumi D, Brown J. Injury from falls in infants under one year. *J Paediatr Child Health.* 2017;53(8):754–760. doi: 10.1111/jpc.13568
314. Tarantino CA, Dowd MD, Murdock TC. Short vertical falls in infants. *Pediatr Emerg Care.* 1999;15(1):5–8. doi: 10.1097/00006565-199902000-00002
315. Burrows P, Trefan L, Houston R, et al. Head injury from falls in children younger than 6 years of age. *Arch Dis Child.* 2015;100(11):1032–1037. doi: 10.1136/archdischild-2014-307119
316. Hughes J, Maguire S, Jones M, Theobald P, Kemp A. Biomechanical characteristics of head injuries from falls in children younger than 48 months. *Arch Dis Child.* 2016;101(4):310–315. doi: 10.1136/archdischild-2014-306803
317. Hall JR, Reyes HM, Horvat M, Meller JL, Stein R. The mortality of childhood falls. *J Trauma.* 1989;29(9):1273–1275. doi: 10.1097/00005373-198909000-00015
318. Abder-Rahman H, Jaber MSO, Al-Sabaileh SS. Injuries sustained in falling fatalities in relation to different distances of falls. *J Forensic Leg Med.* 2018;54:69–73. doi: 10.1016/j.jflm.2017.12.001
319. Pomerantz WJ, Gittelman MA, Hornung R, Husseinzadeh H. Falls in children birth to 5 years: different mechanisms lead to different injuries. *J Trauma Acute Care Surg.* 2012;73(4 Suppl 3):S254–S257. doi: 10.1097/TA.0b013e31826b017c
320. Pitone ML, Attia MW. Patterns of injury associated with routine childhood falls. *Pediatr Emerg Care.* 2006;22(7):470–474. doi: 10.1097/01.pec.0000226869.41803.50
321. Love PF, Tepas JJ III, Wludyka PS, Masnita-Iusan C. Fall-related pediatric brain injuries: the role of race, age, and sex. *J Trauma.* 2009;67(1 Suppl):S12–S15. doi: 10.1097/TA.0b013e3181ac7f22
322. Baalmann M, Lu K, Ablah E, Lightwine K, Haan JM. Incidence and circumstances of pediatric fall-related injuries: which fall variables matter? *Am J Surg.* 2020;220(4):1098–1102. doi: 10.1016/j.amjsurg.2020.02.030
323. Johnson K, Fischer T, Chapman S, Wilson B. Accidental head injuries in children under 5 years of age. *Clin Radiol.* 2005;60(4):464–468. doi: 10.1016/j.crad.2004.09.013
324. Williams RA. Injuries in infants and small children resulting from witnessed and corroborated free falls. *J Trauma.* 1991;31(10):1350–1352. doi: 10.1097/00005373-199110000-00005
325. Lyons TJ, Oates RK. Falling out of bed: a relatively benign occurrence. *Pediatrics.* 1993;92(1):125–127
326. Nimityongskul P, Anderson LD. The likelihood of injuries when children fall out of bed. *J Pediatr Orthop.* 1987;7(2):184–186. doi: 10.1097/01241398-198703000-00014
327. Helfer RE, Slovis TL, Black M. Injuries resulting when small children fall out of bed. *Pediatrics.* 1977;60(4):533–535
328. Atkinson N, van Rijn RR, Starling SP. Childhood falls with occipital impacts. *Pediatr Emerg Care.* 2018;34(12):837–841. doi: 10.1097/PEC.0000000000001186
329. Levene S, Bonfield G. Accidents on hospital wards. *Arch Dis Child.* 1991;66(9):1047–1049. doi: 10.1136/adc.66.9.1047
330. Bertocci G, Smalley C, Brown N, et al. Head biomechanics of video recorded falls involving children in a childcare setting. *Sci Rep.* 2022;12(1):8617. doi: 10.1038/s41598-022-12489-7
331. American College of Surgeons. *ATLS Advanced Trauma Life Support: Student Course Manual.* 10th ed. American College of Surgeons; 2018
332. Knight PH, Maheshwari N, Hussain J, et al. Complications during intrahospital transport of critically ill patients: focus on risk identification and prevention. *Int J Crit Illn Inj Sci.* 2015;5(4):256–264. doi: 10.4103/2229-5151.170840
333. Lindberg DM, Shapiro RA, Blood EA, Steiner RD, Berger RP, Ex Si. Utility of hepatic transaminases in children with concern for abuse. *Pediatrics.* 2013;131(2):268–275. doi: 10.1542/peds.2012-1952
334. Anderst JD, Carpenter SL, Abshire TC; American Academy of Pediatrics, Section on Hematology-Oncology, Committee on Child Abuse and Neglect. Evaluation for bleeding disorders in suspected child abuse. *Pediatrics.* 2013;131(4):e1314–e1322. doi: 10.1542/peds.2013-0195
335. Talving P, Lustenberger T, Lam L, et al. Coagulopathy after isolated severe traumatic brain injury in children. *J Trauma.* 2011;71(5):1205–1210. doi: 10.1097/TA.0b013e31820d151d
336. Zhang J, Jiang R, Liu L, Watkins T, Zhang F, Dong JF. Traumatic brain injury-associated coagulopathy. *J Neurotrauma.* 2012;29(17):2597–2605. doi: 10.1089/neu.2012.2348
337. Berger RP, Pak BJ, Kolesnikova MD, et al. Derivation and Validation of a Serum Biomarker Panel to Identify Infants With Acute

Intracranial Hemorrhage. *JAMA Pediatr.* 2017;171(6):e170429. doi: 10.1001/jamapediatrics.2017.0429

338. Expert Panel on Pediatric I, Ryan ME, Pruthi S, et al. ACR Appropriateness Criteria(R) Head Trauma-Child. *J Am Coll Radiol.* 2020;17(5S):S125–S137. doi: 10.1016/j.jacr.2020.01.026

339. Kemp AM, Rajaram S, Mann M, et al. What neuroimaging should be performed in children in whom inflicted brain injury (iBI) is suspected? A systematic review. *Clin Radiol.* 2009;64(5):473–483. doi: 10.1016/j.crad.2008.11.011

340. Expert Panel on Pediatric I, Wootton-Gorges SL, Soares BP, et al. ACR Appropriateness Criteria(R) Suspected Physical Abuse-Child. *J Am Coll Radiol.* 2017;14(5S):S338–S349. doi: 10.1016/j.jacr.2017.01.036

341. Langford S, Panigrahy A, Narayanan S, et al. Multiplanar reconstructed CT images increased depiction of intracranial hemorrhages in pediatric head trauma. *Neuroradiology.* 2015;57(12):1263–1268. doi: 10.1007/s00234-015-1584-7

342. Prabhu SP, Newton AW, Perez-Rossello JM, Kleinman PK. Three-dimensional skull models as a problem-solving tool in suspected child abuse. *Pediatr Radiol.* 2013;43(5):575–581. doi: 10.1007/s00247-012-2546-4

343. Parisi MT, Wiester RT, Done SL, Sugar NF, Feldman KW. Three-dimensional computed tomography skull reconstructions as an aid to child abuse evaluations. *Pediatr Emerg Care.* 2015;31(11):779–786. doi: 10.1097/PEC.0000000000000199

344. Young JY, Duhaime AC, Caruso PA, Rincon SP. Comparison of non-sedated brain MRI and CT for the detection of acute traumatic injury in children 6 years of age or less. *Emerg Radiol.* 2016;23(4):325–331. doi: 10.1007/s10140-016-1392-3

345. Tekes A, Senglaub SS, Ahn ES, Huisman T, Jackson EM. Ultrafast brain MRI can be used for indications beyond shunted hydrocephalus in pediatric patients. *AJNR Am J Neuroradiol.* 2018;39(8):1515–1518. doi: 10.3174/ajnr.A5724

346. Berger RP, Furtado AD, Flom LL, Fromkin JB, Panigrahy A. Implementation of a brain injury screen MRI for infants at risk for abusive head trauma. *Pediatr Radiol.* 2020;50(1):75–82. doi: 10.1007/s00247-019-04506-1

347. Flom L, Fromkin J, Panigrahy A, Tyler-Kabara E, Berger RP. Development of a screening MRI for infants at risk for abusive head trauma. *Pediatr Radiol.* 2016;46(4):519–526. doi: 10.1007/s00247-015-3500-z

348. Barton K, Nickerson JP, Higgins T, Williams RK. Pediatric anesthesia and neurotoxicity: what the radiologist needs to know. *Pediatr Radiol.* 2018;48(1):31–36. doi: 10.1007/s00247-017-3871-4

349. Jevtovic-Todorovic V, Absalom AR, Blomgren K, et al. Anaesthetic neurotoxicity and neuroplasticity: an expert group report and statement based on the BJA Salzburg Seminar. *Br J Anaesth.* 2013;111(2):143–151. doi: 10.1093/bja/aet177

350. Rozovsky K, Ventureyra EC, Miller E. Fast-brain MRI in children is quick, without sedation, and radiation-free, but beware of limitations. *J Clin Neurosci.* 2013;20(3):400–405. doi: 10.1016/j.jocn.2012.02.048

351. Henry M, Riesenburger RI, Kryzanski J, Jea A, Hwang SW. A retrospective comparison of CT and MRI in detecting pediatric cervical spine injury. *Childs Nerv Syst.* 2013;29(8):1333–1338. doi: 10.1007/s00381-013-2092-x

352. Karmazyn B, Reher TA, Supakul N, et al. Whole-spine MRI in children with suspected abusive head trauma. *AJR Am J Roentgenol.* 2022;218(6):1074–1087. doi: 10.2214/AJR.21.26674

353. Zouros A, Bhargava R, Hoskinson M, Aronyk KE. Further characterization of traumatic subdural collections of infancy. Report of five cases. *J Neurosurg.* 2004;100(5 Suppl Pediatrics):512–518. doi: 10.3171/ped.2004.100.5.0512

354. Wittschieber D, Karger B, Pfeiffer H, Hahnemann ML. Understanding subdural collections in pediatric abusive head trauma. *AJNR Am J Neuroradiol.* 2019;40(3):388–395. doi: 10.3174/ajnr.A5855

355. Wittschieber D, Karger B, Niederstadt T, Pfeiffer H, Hahnemann ML. Subdural hygromas in abusive head trauma: pathogenesis, diagnosis, and forensic implications. *AJNR Am J Neuroradiol.* 2015;36(3):432–439. doi: 10.3174/ajnr.A3989

356. Wells RG, Sty JR. Traumatic low attenuation subdural fluid collections in children younger than 3 years. *Arch Pediatr Adolesc Med.* 2003;157(10):1005–1010. doi: 10.1001/archpedi.157.10.1005

357. Postema FA, Sieswerda-Hoogendoorn T, Majoie CB, van Rijn RR. Age determination of subdural hematomas: survey among radiologists. *Emerg Radiol.* 2014;21(4):349–358. doi: 10.1007/s10140-014-1196-2

358. Vezina G. Assessment of the nature and age of subdural collections in nonaccidental head injury with CT and MRI. *Pediatr Radiol.* 2009;39(6):586–590. doi: 10.1007/s00247-009-1212-y

359. Gomori JM, Grossman RI, Goldberg HI, Zimmerman RA, Bilaniuk LT. Intracranial hematomas: imaging by high-field MR. *Radiology.* 1985;157(1):87–93. doi: 10.1148/radiology.157.1.4034983

360. Cramer JA, Rassner UA, Hedlund GL. Limitations of T2*-gradient recalled-echo and susceptibility-weighted imaging in characterizing chronic subdural hemorrhage in infant survivors of abusive head trauma. *AJNR Am J Neuroradiol.* 2016;37(9):1752–1756. doi: 10.3174/ajnr.A4769

361. Lee KS, Bae WK, Bae HG, Doh JW, Yun IG. The computed tomographic attenuation and the age of subdural hematomas. *J Korean Med Sci.* 1997;12(4):353–359. doi: 10.3346/jkms.1997.12.4.353

362. Wright JN, Feyma TJ, Ishak GE, et al. Subdural hemorrhage rebleeding in abused children: frequency, associations and clinical presentation. *Pediatr Radiol.* 2019;49(13):1762–1772. doi: 10.1007/s00247-019-04483-5

363. Duffy SO, Squires J, Fromkin JB, Berger RP. Use of skeletal surveys to evaluate for physical abuse: analysis of 703 consecutive skeletal surveys. *Pediatrics.* 2011;127(1):e47–e52. doi: 10.1542/peds.2010-0298

364. American College of Radiology, Committee on Practice Parameters–Pediatric Radiology, Committee on Practice Parameters–Body Imaging (Musculoskeletal). *ACR–SPR Practice Parameter for the Performance and Interpretation of Skeletal Surveys in Children.* American College of Radiology; Revised

2021. Accessed December 18, 2024. https://www.acr.org/-/media/ACR/Files/Practice-Parameters/Skeletal-Survey.pdf

365. Berger RP, Panigrahy A, Gottschalk S, Sheetz M. Effective radiation dose in a skeletal survey performed for suspected child abuse. *J Pediatr.* 2016;171:310–312. doi: 10.1016/j.jpeds.2016.01.017

366. Maguire S, Cowley L, Mann M, Kemp A. What does the recent literature add to the identification and investigation of fractures in child abuse: an overview of review updates 2005–2013. *Evid-Based Child Health.* 2013;8(5):2044–2057. doi: 10.1002/ebch.1941

367. Zimmerman S, Makoroff K, Care M, Thomas A, Shapiro R. Utility of follow-up skeletal surveys in suspected child physical abuse evaluations. *Child Abuse Negl.* 2005;29(10):1075–1083. doi: 10.1016/j.chiabu.2004.08.012

368. Harper NS, Lewis T, Eddleman S, Lindberg DM, Ex SI. Follow-up skeletal survey use by child abuse pediatricians. *Child Abuse Negl.* 2016;51:336–342. doi: 10.1016/j.chiabu.2015.08.015

369. Halstead S, Scott G, Thust S, Hann G. Review of the new RCR guidelines (2017): the radiological investigation of suspected physical abuse in children. *Arch Dis Child Educ Pract Ed.* 2019;104(6):309–312. doi: 10.1136/archdischild-2017-314591

370. Jain N. The role of diagnostic imaging in the evaluation of child abuse. *BC Med J.* 2015;8:336–340. doi: 10.1016/S2468-2667(24)00166-X

371. McGraw EP, Pless JE, Pennington DJ, White SJ. Postmortem radiography after unexpected death in neonates, infants, and children: should imaging be routine? *AJR Am J Roentgenol.* 2002;178(6):1517–1521. doi: 10.2214/ajr.178.6.1781517

372. Proisy M, Marchand AJ, Loget P, et al. Whole-body post-mortem computed tomography compared with autopsy in the investigation of unexpected death in infants and children. *Eur Radiol.* 2013;23(6):1711–1719. doi: 10.1007/s00330-012-2738-1

373. Christian CW, Levin AV; American Academy of Pediatrics, Council on Child Abuse and Neglect, Section on Ophthalmology; American Association of Certified Orthoptists; American Association for Pediatric Ophthalmology and Strabismus; American Academy of Ophthalmology. The eye examination in the evaluation of child abuse. *Pediatrics.* 2018;142(2):e20181411. doi: 10.1542/peds.2018-1411

374. Binenbaum G, Chen W, Huang J, Ying GS, Forbes BJ. The natural history of retinal hemorrhage in pediatric head trauma. *J AAPOS.* 2016;20(2):131–135. doi: 10.1016/j.jaapos.2015.12.008

375. Levin A. *Abusive Head Trauma/Shaken Baby Syndrome.* American Academy of Ophthalmology; 2015. Accessed September 2, 2022. https://www.aao.org/assets/aa546d05-0d9c-48dc-9569-43ebe56ece47/635616751239170000/shaken-baby-syndrome-2015-final-pdf

376. Morad Y, Kim YM, Mian M, Huyer D, Capra L, Levin AV. Nonophthalmologist accuracy in diagnosing retinal hemorrhages in the shaken baby syndrome. *J Pediatr.* 2003;142(4):431–434. doi: 10.1067/mpd.2003.161

377. Alexander R, Crabbe L, Sato Y, Smith W, Bennett T. Serial abuse in children who are shaken. *Am J Dis Child.* 1990;144(1):58–60. doi: 10.1001/archpedi.1990.02150250068033

378. Sinal SH, Ball MR. Head trauma due to child abuse: serial computerized tomography in diagnosis and management. *South Med J.* 1987;80(12):1505–1512. doi: 10.1097/00007611-198712000-00006

379. Lindberg DM, Shapiro RA, Laskey AL, et al. Prevalence of abusive injuries in siblings and household contacts of physically abused children. *Pediatrics.* 2012;130(2):193–201. doi: 10.1542/peds.2012-0085

380. Groothuis JR, Altemeier WA, Robarge JP, et al. Increased child abuse in families with twins. *Pediatrics.* 1982;70(5):769–73

381. Hansen KK. Twins and child abuse. *Arch Pediatr Adolesc Med.* 1994;148(12):1345–1346. doi: 10.1001/archpedi.1994.02170120107021

382. Mankad K, Sidpra J, Mirsky DM, et al. International consensus statement on the radiological screening of contact children in the context of suspected child physical abuse. *JAMA Pediatr.* 2023;177(5):526–533. doi: 10.1001/jamapediatrics.2022.6184

383. Lindberg DM, Lindsell CJ, Shapiro RA. Variability in expert assessments of child physical abuse likelihood. *Pediatrics.* 2008;121(4):e945–e953. doi: 10.1542/peds.2007-2485

384. Hymel KP, Makoroff KL, Laskey AL, Conaway MR, Blackman JA. Mechanisms, clinical presentations, injuries, and outcomes from inflicted versus noninflicted head trauma during infancy: results of a prospective, multicentered, comparative study. *Pediatrics.* 2007;119(5):922–929. doi: 10.1542/peds.2006-3111

385. National Resource Center for Health and Safety in Child Care and Early Education. Facilities, Supplies, Equipment, and Environmental Health. In: *Caring for Our Children.* Accessed December 13, 2021. https://nrckids.org/CFOC/Database/5

386. Greenes DS, Schutzman SA. Infants with isolated skull fracture: what are their clinical characteristics, and do they require hospitalization? *Ann Emerg Med.* 1997;30(3):253–259. doi: 10.1016/s0196-0644(97)70158-6

387. Keenan HT, Runyan DK, Marshall SW, Nocera MA, Merten DF. A population-based comparison of clinical and outcome characteristics of young children with serious inflicted and noninflicted traumatic brain injury. *Pediatrics.* 2004;114(3):633–639. doi: 10.1542/peds.2003-1020-L

388. Hasbani DM, Topjian AA, Friess SH, et al. Nonconvulsive electrographic seizures are common in children with abusive head trauma. *Pediatr Crit Care Med.* 2013;14(7):709–715. doi: 10.1097/PCC.0b013e3182917b83

389. Duhaime AC, Christian C, Armonda R, Hunter J, Hertle R. Disappearing subdural hematomas in children. *Pediatr Neurosurg.* 1996;25(3):116–122. doi: 10.1159/000121108

390. Hymel KP; American Academy of Pediatrics, Committee on Child Abuse and Neglect. When is lack of supervision neglect? *Pediatrics.* 2006;118(3):1296–1298. doi: 10.1542/peds.2006-1780

391. O'Hara MA. The infant with bilateral skull fractures: diagnostic considerations in consultation with a child abuse pediatrician. *J Inj Violence Res.* 2019;11(1):15–20. doi: 10.5249/jivr.v11i1.938

392. O'Hara MA, Valvano TJ, Kashyap M, et al. Understanding bilateral skull fractures in infancy: a retrospective multicenter case review. *Pediatr Emerg Care.* 2022;39(5):329–334. doi: 10.1097/PEC.0000000000002704

393. Shugerman RP, Paez A, Grossman DC, Feldman KW, Grady MS. Epidural hemorrhage: is it abuse? *Pediatrics.* 1996;97(5):664–668

394. Ciurea AV, Kapsalaki EZ, Coman TC, et al. Supratentorial epidural hematoma of traumatic etiology in infants. *Childs Nerv Syst.* 2007; 23(3):335–341. doi: 10.1007/s00381-006-0230-4

395. Zielinski AE, Rochette LM, Smith GA. Stair-related injuries to young children treated in US emergency departments, 1999-2008. *Pediatrics.* 2012;129(4):721–727. doi: 10.1542/peds.2011-2314

396. Reiber GD. Fatal falls in childhood. How far must children fall to sustain fatal head injury? Report of cases and review of the literature. *Am J Forens Med Pathol.* 1993;14(3):201–207

397. Carpenter SL, Abshire TC, Anderst JD; American Academy of Pediatrics, Section on Hematology-Oncology, Committee on Child Abuse and Neglect. Evaluating for suspected child abuse: conditions that predispose to bleeding. *Pediatrics.* 2013;131(4): e1357–e1373. doi: 10.1542/peds.2013-0196

398. Anderst JD, Carpenter SL, Presley R, et al. Relevance of abusive head trauma to intracranial hemorrhages and bleeding disorders. *Pediatrics.* 2018;141(5):e20173485. doi: 10.1542/peds.2017-3485

399. Rooks V, Eaton J, Ruess L, Petermann G, Keck-Wherley J, Pedersen R. Prevalence and evolution of intracranial hemorrhage in asymptomatic term infants. *Am J Neuroradiol.* 2008;29(6):1082–1089. doi: 10.3174/ajnr.A1004

400. Looney CB, Smith JK, Merck LH, et al. Intracranial hemorrhage in asymptomatic neonates: prevalence on MR images and relationship to obstetric and neonatal risk factors. *Radiology.* 2007; 242(2):535–541. doi: 10.1148/radiol.2422060133

401. Tavani F, Zimmerman RA, Clancy RR, Licht DJ, Mahle WT. Incidental intracranial hemorrhage after uncomplicated birth: MRI before and after neonatal heart surgery. *Neuroradiology.* 2003;45(4): 253–258. doi: 10.1007/s00234-003-0946-8

402. Whitby EH, Griffiths PD, Rutter S, et al. Frequency and natural history of subdural haemorrhages in babies and relation to obstetric factors. *Lancet.* 2004;363(9412):846–851. doi: 10.1016/S0140-6736 (04)15730-9

403. Holden KR, Titus MO, Van Tassel P. Cranial magnetic resonance imaging examination of normal term neonates: a pilot study. *J Child Neurol.* 1999;14(11):708–710. doi: 10.1177/ 088307389901401104

404. Nikam RM, Kandula VV, Yue X, et al. Birth-related subdural hemorrhage: prevalence and imaging morphology. *Pediatr Radiol.* 2021;51(6):939–946. doi: 10.1007/s00247-021-05060-5

405. Kumpulainen V, Lehtola SJ, Tuulari JJ, et al. Prevalence and risk factors of incidental findings in brain MRIs of healthy neonates–The FinnBrain Birth Cohort Study. *Front Neurol.* 2019;10:1347. doi: 10.3389/fneur.2019.01347

406. Hong HS, Lee JY. Intracranial hemorrhage in term neonates. *Child's Nervous System.* 2018;34(6):1135–1143. doi: 10.1007/ s00381-018-3788-8

407. Sirgiovanni I, Avignone S, Groppo M, et al. Intracranial haemorrhage: an incidental finding at magnetic resonance imaging in a cohort of late preterm and term infants. *Pediatr Radiol.* 2014;44(3):289–296. doi: 10.1007/s00247-013-2826-7

408. Brouwer AJ, Groenendaal F, Koopman C, Nievelstein RJ, Han SK, de Vries LS. Intracranial hemorrhage in full-term newborns: a hospital-based cohort study. *Neuroradiology.* 2010;52(6):567–576. doi: 10.1007/s00234-010-0698-1

409. Gupta SN, Kechli AM, Kanamalla US. Intracranial hemorrhage in term newborns: management and outcomes. *Pediatr Neurol.* 2009;40(1):1–12. doi: 10.1016/j.pediatrneurol.2008.09.019

410. Ou-Yang MC, Huang CB, Huang HC, et al. Clinical manifestations of symptomatic intracranial hemorrhage in term neonates: 18 years of experience in a medical center. *Pediatr Neonatol.* 2010;51(4): 208–213. doi: 10.1016/S1875-9572(10)60040-X

411. Zamora C, Sams C, Cornea EA, Yuan Z, Smith JK, Gilmore JH. Subdural hemorrhage in asymptomatic neonates: neurodevelopmental outcomes and MRI findings at 2 years. *Radiology.* 2021;298 (1):173–179. doi: 10.1148/radiol.2020201857

412. Cho IH, Kim MS, Heo NH, Kim SY. Birth-related retinal hemorrhages: The Soonchunhyang University Cheonan Hospital universal newborn eye screening (SUCH-NES) study. *PLoS One.* 2021;16(11): e0259378. doi: 10.1371/journal.pone.0259378

413. Li LH, Li N, Zhao JY, et al. Findings of perinatal ocular examination performed on 3573, healthy full-term newborns. *Br J Ophthalmol.* 2013;97(5):588–591. doi: 10.1136/bjophthalmol-2012-302539

414. Zhao Q, Zhang Y, Yang Y, et al. Birth-related retinal hemorrhages in healthy full-term newborns and their relationship to maternal, obstetric, and neonatal risk factors. *Graefes Arch Clin Exp Ophthalmol.* 2015;253(7):1021–1025. doi: 10.1007/s00417-015-3052-9

415. Emerson MV, Pieramici DJ, Stoessel KM, Berreen JP, Gariano RF. Incidence and rate of disappearance of retinal hemorrhage in newborns. *Ophthalmology.* 2001;108(1):36–39. doi: 10.1016/ s0161-6420(00)00474-7

416. Sezen F. Retinal haemorrhages in newborn infants. *Br J Ophthalmol.* 1971;55(4):248–253. doi: 10.1136/bjo.55.4.248

417. Kaur B, Taylor D. Fundus hemorrhages in infancy. *Surv Ophthalmol.* 1992;37(1):1–17. doi: 10.1016/0039-6257(92)90002-b

418. Wright J, Painter S, Kodagali SS, et al. Disability and visual outcomes following suspected abusive head trauma in children under 2 years. *Arch Dis Child.* 2021;106(6):590–593. doi: 10.1136/ archdischild-2019-318638

419. Sun L, Jiang Z, Li S, et al. What is left after resolution of neonatal retinal hemorrhage: the longitudinal long-term outcome in foveal structure and visual function. *Am J Ophthalmol.* 2021;226: 182–190. doi: 10.1016/j.ajo.2021.01.028

420. Hemalatha BC, Kalpana BN, Shilpa YD, et al. Retinopathy of prematurity screening and retinal hemorrhages - Our experience among Indian babies. *Indian J Ophthalmol.* 2021;69(8):2147–2150. doi: 10.4103/ijo.IJO_3616_20

421. Kim SY, Morgan LA, Baldwin AJ, Suh DW. Comparison of the characteristics of retinal hemorrhages in abusive head trauma versus normal vaginal delivery. *J AAPOS.* 2018;22(2):139–144. doi: 10.1016/j.jaapos.2017.12.006

422. Kleinman PK, Zito JL, Davidson RI, Raptopoulos V. The subarachnoid spaces in children: normal variations in size. *Radiology.* 1983;147(2):455–457. doi: 10.1148/radiology.147.2.6601281

423. Prassopoulos P, Cavouras D, Golfinopoulos S, Nezi M. The size of the intra- and extraventricular cerebrospinal fluid compartments in children with idiopathic benign widening of the frontal subarachnoid space. *Neuroradiology.* 1995;37(5):418–421. doi: 10.1007/BF00588027

424. Ravid S, Maytal J. External hydrocephalus: a probable cause for subdural hematoma in infancy. *Pediatr Neurol.* 2003;28(2): 139–141. doi: 10.1016/s0887-8994(02)00500-3

425. Papasian NC, Frim DM. A theoretical model of benign external hydrocephalus that predicts a predisposition towards extra-axial hemorrhage after minor head trauma. *Pediatr Neurosurg.* 2000; 33(4):188–193. doi: 10.1159/000055951

426. McNeely PD, Atkinson JD, Saigal G, O'Gorman AM, Farmer JP. Subdural hematomas in infants with benign enlargement of the subarachnoid spaces are not pathognomonic for child abuse. *AJNR Am J Neuroradiol.* 2006;27(8):1725–1728

427. Piatt JH Jr. A pitfall in the diagnosis of child abuse: external hydrocephalus, subdural hematoma, and retinal hemorrhages. *Neurosurg Focus.* 1999;7(4):E4. doi: 10.3171/foc.1999.7.4.6

428. Ghosh PS, Ghosh D. Subdural hematoma in infants without accidental or nonaccidental injury: benign external hydrocephalus, a risk factor. *Clin Pediatr (Phila).* 2011;50(10):897–903. doi: 10.1177/0009922811406435

429. Kapila A, Trice J, Spies WG, Siegel BA, Gado MH. Enlarged cerebrospinal fluid spaces in infants with subdural hematomas. *Radiology.* 1982;142(3):669–672. doi: 10.1148/radiology.142.3.6977789

430. Laubscher B, Deonna T, Uske A, van Melle G. Primitive megalencephaly in children: natural history, medium term prognosis with special reference to external hydrocephalus. *Eur J Pediatr.* 1990;149(7):502–507. doi: 10.1007/BF01959405

431. Mori K, Sakamoto T, Nishimura K, Fujiwara K. Subarachnoid fluid collection in infants complicated by subdural hematoma. *Childs Nerv Syst.* 1993;9(5):282–284. doi: 10.1007/BF00306274

432. Greiner MV, Richards TJ, Care MM, Leach JL. Prevalence of subdural collections in children with macrocrania. *AJNR Am J Neuroradiol.* 2013;34(12):2373–2378. doi: 10.3174/ajnr.A3588

433. McKeag H, Christian CW, Rubin D, Daymont C, Pollock AN, Wood J. Subdural hemorrhage in pediatric patients with enlargement of the subarachnoid spaces. *J Neurosurg Pediatr.* 2013;11(4):438–444. doi: 10.3171/2012.12.PEDS12289

434. Tucker J, Choudhary AK, Piatt J. Macrocephaly in infancy: benign enlargement of the subarachnoid spaces and subdural collections. *J Neurosurg Pediatr.* 2016;18(1):16–20. doi: 10.3171/2015.12.PEDS15600

435. Holste KG, Wieland CM, Ibrahim M, et al. Subdural hematoma prevalence and long-term developmental outcomes in patients with benign expansion of the subarachnoid spaces. *J Neurosurg Pediatr.* 2022;29(5):536–542. doi: 10.3171/2021.12.PEDS21436

436. Hansen JB, Frazier T, Moffatt M, Zinkus T, Anderst JD. Evaluations for abuse in young children with subdural hemorrhages: findings based on symptom severity and benign enlargement of the subarachnoid spaces. *J Neurosurg Pediatr.* 2018;21(1):31–37. doi: 10.3171/2017.7.PEDS17317

437. Geddes JF, Talbert DG. Paroxysmal coughing, subdural and retinal bleeding: a computer modelling approach. *Neuropathol Appl Neurobiol.* 2006;32(6):625–634. doi: 10.1111/j.1365-2990.2006.00771.x

438. Cohen MC, Scheimberg I. Evidence of occurrence of intradural and subdural hemorrhage in the perinatal and neonatal period in the context of hypoxic Ischemic encephalopathy: an observational study from two referral institutions in the United Kingdom. *Pediatr Dev Pathol.* 2009;12(3):169–176. doi: 10.2350/08-08-0509.1

439. Geddes JF, Whitwell HL. Neuropathology of fatal infant head injury. *J Neurotrauma.* 2003;20(9):905. doi: 10.1089/089771503322385836

440. Byard RW, Blumbergs P, Rutty G, Sperhake J, Banner J, Krous HF. Lack of evidence for a causal relationship between hypoxic-ischemic encephalopathy and subdural hemorrhage in fetal life, infancy, and early childhood. *Pediatr Dev Pathol.* 2007;10(5): 348–350. doi: 10.2350/06-08-0154.1

441. Hurley M, Dineen R, Padfield CJ, et al. Is there a causal relationship between the hypoxia-ischaemia associated with cardiorespiratory arrest and subdural haematomas? An observational study. *Br J Radiol.* 2010;83(993):736–743. doi: 10.1259/bjr/36871113

442. Punt J, Bonshek R, Jaspan T, McConachie N, Punt N, Ratcliffe J. The 'unified hypothesis' of Geddes et al. is not supported by the data. *Pediatr Rehabil.* 2004;7(3):173–184. doi: 10.1080/13638490410001711515

443. Rao P, Carty H, Pierce A. The acute reversal sign: comparison of medical and non-accidental injury patients. *Clin Radiol.* 1999;54 (8):495–501. doi: 10.1016/s0009-9260(99)90845-0

444. Rafaat KT, Spear RM, Kuelbs C, Parsapour K, Peterson B. Cranial computed tomographic findings in a large group of children with drowning: diagnostic, prognostic, and forensic implications. *Pediatr Crit Care Med.* 2008;9(6):567–572. doi: 10.1097/PCC.0b013e31818c8955

445. Barnes PD, Galaznik J, Gardner H, Shuman M. Infant acute life-threatening event—dysphagic choking versus nonaccidental injury. *Semin Pediatr Neurol.* 2010;17(1):7–11. doi: 10.1016/j.spen.2010.01.005

446. Talbert D. Paroxysmal cough injury, vascular rupture and 'shaken baby syndrome'. *Med Hypotheses.* 2005;64(1):8–13. doi: 10.1016/j.mehy.2004.07.017

447. Altman RL, Forman S, Brand DA. Ophthalmologic findings in infants after an apparent life-threatening event. *Eur J Ophthalmol.* 2007;17(4):648–653. doi: 10.1177/112067210701700426

448. Curcoy AI, Trenchs V, Morales M, Serra A, Pou J. Retinal hemorrhages and apparent life-threatening events. *Pediatr Emerg Care.* 2010;26(2):118–120. doi: 10.1097/PEC.0b013e3181cfdb6b

449. Pitetti RD, Maffei F, Chang K, Hickey R, Berger R, Pierce MC. Prevalence of retinal hemorrhages and child abuse in children who present with an apparent life-threatening event. *Pediatrics.* 2002;110(3):557–562. doi: 10.1542/peds.110.3.557

450. deVeber G, Andrew M, Adams C, et al. Cerebral sinovenous thrombosis in children. *N Engl J Med.* 2001;345(6):417–423. doi: 10.1056/NEJM200108093450604

451. Tuckuviene R, Christensen AL, Helgestad J, Johnsen SP, Kristensen SR. Paediatric arterial ischaemic stroke and cerebral sinovenous thrombosis in Denmark 1994-2006: a nationwide population-based study. *Acta Paediatr.* 2011;100(4):543–549. doi: 10.1111/j.1651-2227.2010.02100.x

452. Carvalho KS, Bodensteiner JB, Connolly PJ, Garg BP. Cerebral venous thrombosis in children. *J Child Neurol.* 2001;16(8): 574–580. doi: 10.1177/088307380101600807

453. Heller C, Heinecke A, Junker R, et al. Cerebral venous thrombosis in children: a multifactorial origin. *Circulation.* 2003;108(11): 1362–1367. doi: 10.1161/01.CIR.0000087598.05977.45

454. Huisman TA, Holzmann D, Martin E, Willi UV. Cerebral venous thrombosis in childhood. *Eur Radiol.* 2001;11(9):1760–1765. doi: 10.1007/s003300100822

455. McLean LA, Frasier LD, Hedlund GL. Does intracranial venous thrombosis cause subdural hemorrhage in the pediatric population? *AJNR Am J Neuroradiol.* 2012;33(7):1281–1284. doi: 10.3174/ajnr.A2967

456. Sebire G, Tabarki B, Saunders DE, et al. Cerebral venous sinus thrombosis in children: risk factors, presentation, diagnosis and outcome. *Brain.* 2005;128(Pt 3):477–489. doi: 10.1093/brain/awh412

457. Barnes PD. Imaging of nonaccidental injury and the mimics: issues and controversies in the era of evidence-based medicine. *Radiol Clin North Am.* 2011;49(1):205–229. doi: 10.1016/j.rcl.2010.08.001

458. Barnes PD, Krasnokutsky M. Imaging of the central nervous system in suspected or alleged nonaccidental injury, including the mimics. *Top Magn Reson Imaging.* 2007;18(1):53–74. doi: 10.1097/RMR.0b013e3180d0a455

459. Uscinski RH. Shaken baby syndrome: an odyssey. *Neurol Med Chir (Tokyo).* 2006;46(2):57–61. doi: 10.2176/nmc.46.57

460. Uscinski RH, McBride DK. The shaken baby syndrome: an odyssey—II origins and further hypotheses. *Neurol Med Chir (Tokyo).* 2008;48(4):151–155. doi: 10.2176/nmc.48.151

461. Datta S, Stoodley N, Jayawant S, Renowden S, Kemp A. Neuroradiological aspects of subdural haemorrhages. *Arch Dis Child.* 2005;90(9):947–951. doi: 10.1136/adc.2002.021154

462. Tien I, Bauchner H, Reece RM. What is the system of care for abused and neglected children in children's institutions? *Pediatrics.* 2002;110(6):1226–1231. doi: 10.1542/peds.110.6.1226

463. Kahneman D. Maps of bounded rationality: a perspective on intuitive judgment and choice. *The American Economic Review.* 2003; 93(5):1449–1475

464. Narang S, Campbell KA, Simonton K. Reporting abuse, managing uncertainty, and other legal issues. In: Laskey A, Sirotnak A, eds. *Child Abuse: Medical Diagnosis and Management.* American Academy of Pediatrics; 2019:875–920

465. McGinn TG, Guyatt GH, Wyer PC, Naylor CD, Stiell IG, Richardson WS. Users' guides to the medical literature: XXII: how to use articles about clinical decision rules. Evidence-Based Medicine Working Group. *JAMA.* 2000;284(1):79–84. doi: 10.1001/jama.284.1.79

466. Pfeiffer H, Cowley LE, Kemp AM, et al. Validation of the PredAHT-2 prediction tool for abusive head trauma. *Emerg Med J.* 2020;37(3): 119–126. doi: 10.1136/emermed-2019-208893

467. Hymel KP, Wang M, Chinchilli VM, et al. Estimating the probability of abusive head trauma after abuse evaluation. *Child Abuse Negl.* 2019;88:266–274. doi: 10.1016/j.chiabu.2018.11.015

468. *Bland v Verizon Wireless (VAW) LLC*, 538 893 (Court of Appeals, 8th Circuit 2008)

469. *Feit v Great-West Life & Annuity Ins. Co*, 271 246 (2008)

470. *Moore v Ashland Chemical Inc*, 151 269 (Court of Appeals, 5th Circuit 1998)

471. Elinder G, Eriksson A, Hallberg B, et al. Traumatic shaking: the role of the triad in medical investigations of suspected traumatic shaking. *Acta Paediatr.* 2018;107(Suppl 472):3–23. doi: 10.1111/apa.14473

472. Leventhal JM, Edwards GA. Flawed theories to explain child physical abuse: what are the medical-legal consequences? *JAMA.* 2017; 318(14):1317–1318. doi: 10.1001/jama.2017.11703

473. Narang SK, Sachdev KK, Bertocci K, et al. Overturned abusive head trauma and shaken baby syndrome convictions in the United States: Prevalence, legal basis, and medical evidence. *Child Abuse Negl.* 2021;122:105380. doi: 10.1016/j.chiabu.2021.105380

474. Paul SR, Narang SK; American Academy of Pediatrics, Committee on Medical Liability and Risk Management. Expert witness participation in civil and criminal proceedings [reaffirmed June 2024]. *Pediatrics.* 2017;139(3):e20163862. doi: 10.1542/peds.2016-3862

475. Bell MJ, Kochanek PM. Pediatric traumatic brain injury in 2012: the year with new guidelines and common data elements. *Crit Care Clin.* 2013;29(2):223–238. doi: 10.1016/j.ccc.2012.11.004

476. Adelson PD, Bratton SL, Carney NA, et al. Guidelines for the acute medical management of severe traumatic brain injury in infants, children, and adolescents. Chapter 1: Introduction. *Pediatr Crit Care Med.* 2003;4(3 Suppl):S2–S4. doi: 10.1097/01.CCM.0000066600.71233.01

477. Kochanek PM, Tasker RC, Carney N, et al. Guidelines for the Management of Pediatric Severe Traumatic Brain Injury, Third Edition: Update of the Brain Trauma Foundation Guidelines, Executive Summary. *Pediatr Crit Care Med.* 2019;20(3):280–289. doi: 10.1097/PCC.0000000000001736

478. Kochanek PM, Tasker RC, Bell MJ, et al. Management of pediatric severe traumatic brain injury: 2019 Consensus and Guidelines-Based Algorithm for First and Second Tier Therapies. *Pediatr Crit Care Med.* 2019;20(3):269–279. doi: 10.1097/PCC.0000000000001737

479. Chung MG, O'Brien NF. Prevalence of early posttraumatic seizures in children with moderate to severe traumatic brain injury despite levetiracetam prophylaxis. *Pediatr Crit Care Med.* 2016; 17(2):150–156. doi: 10.1097/PCC.0000000000000588

480. Liesemer K, Bratton SL, Zebrack CM, Brockmeyer D, Statler KD. Early post-traumatic seizures in moderate to severe pediatric traumatic brain injury: rates, risk factors, and clinical features. *J Neurotrauma.* 2011;28(5):755–762. doi: 10.1089/neu.2010.1518

481. Dingman AL, Stence NV, O'Neill BR, Sillau SH, Chapman KE. Seizure severity is correlated with severity of hypoxic-ischemic injury in abusive head trauma. *Pediatr Neurol.* 2018;82:29–35. doi: 10.1016/j.pediatrneurol.2017.12.003

482. Arndt DH, Lerner JT, Matsumoto JH, et al. Subclinical early post-traumatic seizures detected by continuous EEG monitoring in a consecutive pediatric cohort. *Epilepsia.* 2013;54(10):1780–1788. doi: 10.1111/epi.12369

483. O'Neill BR, Handler MH, Tong S, Chapman KE. Incidence of seizures on continuous EEG monitoring following traumatic brain injury in children. *J Neurosurg Pediatr.* 2015;16(2):167–176. doi: 10.3171/2014.12.PEDS14263

484. Bullock MR, Chesnut R, Ghajar J, et al. Surgical management of depressed cranial fractures. *Neurosurgery.* 2006;58(3 Suppl):S56–S60. doi: 10.1227/01.NEU.0000210367.14043.0E

485. Bullock MR, Chesnut R, Ghajar J, et al. Surgical management of acute epidural hematomas. *Neurosurgery.* 2006;58(3 Suppl):S7–S15

486. Melo JR, Di Rocco F, Bourgeois M, et al. Surgical options for treatment of traumatic subdural hematomas in children younger than 2 years of age. *J Neurosurg Pediatr.* 2014;13(4):456–461. doi: 10.3171/2014.1.PEDS13393

487. Nguyen VN, Wallace D, Ajmera S, et al. Management of Subdural Hematohygromas in Abusive Head Trauma. *Neurosurgery.* 2020;86(2):281–287. doi: 10.1093/neuros/nyz076

488. American College of Surgeons. *TQIP Best Practices Guidelines of Trauma Center Recognition of Child Abuse, Elder Abuse, and Intimate Partner Violence.* American College of Surgeons; 2019. https://www.facs.org/-/media/files/quality-programs/trauma/tqip/abuse_guidelines.ashx

489. Thinnes R, Swanson MB, Wetjen K, Harland KK, Mohr NM. Preferences for emergency medical service transport after childhood injury: an emergency department-based multi-methods study. *Injury.* 2020;51(9):1961–1969. doi: 10.1016/j.injury.2020.04.036

490. Palusci VJ, Kay AJ, Batra E, et al. Identifying child abuse fatalities during infancy. *Pediatrics.* 2019;144(3):e20192076. doi: 10.1542/peds.2019-2076

491. Hanzlick R. Medical examiners, coroners, and public health: a review and update. *Arch Pathol Lab Med.* 2006;130(9):1274–1282. doi: 10.1043/1543-2165(2006)130[1274:Mecaph]2.0.Co;2

492. American Academy of Pediatrics, Committee on Child Abuse and Neglect, Committee on Injury, Violence, and Poison Prevention, Council on Community Pediatrics. Policy statement: Child fatality review. *Pediatrics.* 2010;126(3):592–596. doi: 10.1542/peds.2010-2006

493. Fleming P, Byard RW. Subdural haemorrhage in infants: abuse or natural causes? The importance of thorough child death review. Editorial. *Acta Paediatr.* 2018;107(3):382–383. doi: 10.1111/apa.14185

494. Kairys SW, Alexander RC, Block RW, et al; American Academy of Pediatrics, Committee on Child Abuse and Neglect, Committee on Community Health Services. Investigation and review of unexpected infant and child deaths. *Pediatrics.* 1999;104(5 Pt 1):1158–1160

495. Hanzlick R, Hunsaker JC, Davis GJ. *A Guide for Manner of Death Classification.* National Association of Medical Examiners; 2002:46–59

496. National Center for Health Statistics. *Physicians' Handbook on Medical Certification of Death.* Centers for Disease Control and Prevention; 2004

497. Collins KA. *American College of American Pathologists Autopsy Performance & Reporting.* 3rd ed. CAP Press; 2017

498. Hanzlick R. Principles for including or excluding 'mechanisms' of death when writing cause-of-death statements. *Arch Pathol Lab Med.* 1997;121(4):377

499. Pinneri K, Matshes EW. Recommendations for the autopsy of an infant who has died suddenly and unexpectedly. *Acad Forensic Pathol.* 2017;7(2):171–181. doi: 10.23907/2017.019

500. Gill JR, Andrew T, Gilliland MGF, Love J, Matshes E, Reichard RR. National Association of Medical Examiners position paper: recommendations for the postmortem assessment of suspect head trauma in infants and young children. *Acad Forensic Pathol.* 2014;4(2):206–213

501. Case ME, Graham MA, Handy TC, Jentzen JM, Monteleone JA. Position paper on fatal abusive head injuries in infants and young children. *Am J Forensic Med Pathol.* 2001;22(2):112–122

502. Bundock E, Corey T. *Unexplained Pediatric Deaths: Investigation, Certification, and Family Needs.* Academic Forensic *Pathology International*; 2019

503. Sadler DW. The value of a thorough protocol in the investigation of sudden infant deaths. *J Clin Pathol.* 1998;51(9):689–694. doi: 10.1136/jcp.51.9.689

504. Rinaldo P, Yoon HR, Yu C, Raymond K, Tiozzo C, Giordano G. Sudden and unexpected neonatal death: a protocol for the post-mortem diagnosis of fatty acid oxidation disorders. *Semin Perinatol.* 1999;23(2):204–210. doi: 10.1016/s0146-0005(99)80052-4

505. Bove KE. Practice guidelines for autopsy pathology: the perinatal and pediatric autopsy. Autopsy Committee of the College of American Pathologists. *Arch Pathol Lab Med.* 1997;121(4):368–376

506. Royal College of Pathologists. *Sudden Unexpected Death in Infancy and Childhood: Multi-agency Guidelines for Care and Investigation.* 2nd ed. Royal College of Pathologists; 2016

507. National Association of Medical Examiners. *National Association of Medical Examiners - Public Position Papers.* Accessed December 8, 2021. https://www.thename.org/name-public-position-papers

508. Peterson GF, Clark SC. Forensic autopsy performance standards. *Am J Forensic Med Pathol.* 2006;27(3):200–225. doi: 10.1097/01.paf.0000243580.43150.3c

509. Byard RW. "Shaken baby syndrome" and forensic pathology: an uneasy interface. *Forensic Sci Med Pathol.* 2014;10(2):239–241. doi: 10.1007/s12024-013-9514-7

510. Case M. "Shaken baby syndrome" and forensic pathology. *Forensic Sci Med Pathol.* 2014;10(2):246–247. doi: 10.1007/s12024-014-9532-0

511. Cohen MC, Ramsay DA. "Shaken baby syndrome" and forensic pathology. *Forensic Sci Med Pathol.* 2014;10(2):244–245. doi: 10.1007/s12024-013-9525-4

512. Greeley CS. "Shaken baby syndrome" and forensic pathology. *Forensic Sci Med Pathol.* 2014;10(2):253–255. doi: 10.1007/s12024-014-9540-0

513. Scheimberg I, Mack J. "Shaken baby syndrome" and forensic pathology. *Forensic Sci Med Pathol.* Jun 2014;10(2):242–243. doi: 10.1007/s12024-013-9527-2

514. Smith C. "Shaken baby syndrome" and forensic pathology. *Forensic Sci Med Pathol.* 2014;10(2):256–258. doi: 10.1007/s12024-014-9557-4

515. Sperhake JP, Matschke J. "Shaken baby syndrome" and forensic pathology. *Forensic Sci Med Pathol.* 2014;10(2):251–252. doi: 10.1007/s12024-014-9546-7

516. Squier W. "Shaken baby syndrome" and forensic pathology. *Forensic Sci Med Pathol.* 2014;10(2):248–250. doi: 10.1007/s12024-014-9533-z

517. Geddes JF, Hackshaw AK, Vowles GH, Nickols CD, Whitwell HL. Neuropathology of inflicted head injury in children. I. Patterns of brain damage. *Brain.* 2001;124(Pt 7):1290–1298. doi: 10.1093/brain/124.7.1290

518. Vowles GH, Scholtz CL, Cameron JM. Diffuse axonal injury in early infancy. *J Clin Pathol.* 1987;40(2):185–189

519. Shannon P, Smith CR, Deck J, Ang LC, Ho M, Becker L. Axonal injury and the neuropathology of shaken baby syndrome. *Acta Neuropathol.* 1998;95(6):625–631

520. Gleckman AM, Bell MD, Evans RJ, Smith TW. Diffuse axonal injury in infants with nonaccidental craniocerebral trauma: enhanced detection by beta-amyloid precursor protein immunohistochemical staining. *Arch Pathol Lab Med.* 1999;123(2):146–151. doi: 10.1043/0003-9985(1999)123<0146:Daiiiw>2.0.Co;2

521. Gill JR, Goldfeder LB, Armbrustmacher V, Coleman A, Mena H, Hirsch CS. Fatal head injury in children younger than 2 years in New York City and an overview of the shaken baby syndrome. *Arch Pathol Lab Med.* 2009;133(4):619–627

522. Gilliland MG, Folberg R. Shaken babies–some have no impact injuries. *J Forensic Sci.* 1996;41(1):114–116

523. Serinelli S, Arunkumar P, Filkins JA, Gitto L. Deaths Due to Child Abuse: A 6-Year Review of Cases in The Cook County Medical Examiner's Office. *J Forensic Sci.* 2017;62(1):107–118. doi: 10.1111/1556-4029.13219

524. Munger CE, Peiffer RL, Bouldin TW, Kylstra JA, Thompson RL. Ocular and associated neuropathologic observations in suspected whiplash shaken infant syndrome. A retrospective study of 12 cases. *Am J Forensic Med Pathol.* 1993;14(3):193–200. doi: 10.1097/00000433-199309000-00004

525. Hart BL, Dudley MH, Zumwalt RE. Postmortem cranial MRI and autopsy correlation in suspected child abuse. *Am J Forensic Med Pathol.* 1996;17(3):217–224. doi: 10.1097/00000433-199609000-00008

526. Matschke J, Büttner A, Bergmann M, Hagel C, Püschel K, Glatzel M. Encephalopathy and death in infants with abusive head trauma is due to hypoxic-ischemic injury following local brain trauma to vital brainstem centers. *Int J Legal Med.* 2015;129(1):105–114. doi: 10.1007/s00414-014-1060-7

527. Johnson MW, Stoll L, Rubio A, et al. Axonal injury in young pediatric head trauma: a comparison study of β-amyloid precursor protein (β-APP) immunohistochemical staining in traumatic and nontraumatic deaths. *J Forensic Sci.* 2011;56(5):1198–1205. doi: 10.1111/j.1556-4029.2011.01814.x

528. Oehmichen M, Schleiss D, Pedal I, Saternus KS, Gerling I, Meissner C. Shaken baby syndrome: re-examination of diffuse axonal injury as cause of death. *Acta Neuropathol.* 2008;116(3):317–29. doi: 10.1007/s00401-008-0356-4

529. Judkins AR, Hood IG, Mirchandani HG, Rorke LB. Technical communication: rationale and technique for examination of nervous system in suspected infant victims of abuse. *Am J Forensic Med Pathol.* 2004;25(1):29–32

530. Peterson JE, Love JC, Pinto DC, Wolf DA, Sandberg G. A novel method for removing a spinal cord with attached cervical ganglia from a pediatric decedent. *J Forensic Sci.* 2016;61(1):241–244. doi: 10.1111/1556-4029.12925

531. Matshes EW, Evans RM, Pinckard JK, Joseph JT, Lew EO. Shaken infants die of neck trauma, not of brain trauma. *Acad Forens Pathol.* 2011;1(1):82–91. doi: 10.23907/2011.009

532. Cheshire EC, Malcomson RD, Joseph S, Biggs MJ, Adlam D, Rutty GN. Optical clearing of the dura mater using glycerol: a reversible process to aid the post-mortem investigation of infant head injury. *Forensic Sci Med Pathol.* 2015;11(3):395–404. doi: 10.1007/s12024-015-9691-7

533. Gilliland MG, Levin AV, Enzenauer RW, et al. Guidelines for postmortem protocol for ocular investigation of sudden unexplained infant death and suspected physical child abuse. *Am J Forensic Med Pathol.* 2007;28(4):323–329. doi: 10.1097/PAF.0b013e31815b4c00

534. Collins KA. *Special Autopsy Dissections.* College of American Pathologists; 2010

535. Ali Z, Fowler DR. En bloc examination of the neck in pediatric homicide cases: a proper way for complete assessment of neck trauma. *Acad Forensic Pathol.* 2016;6(4):622–637. doi: 10.23907/2016.059

536. Brooks C.Medical Examiner and Coroner Offices, 2018. US Department of Justice, Office of Justice Programs, Bureau of Justice Statistics. Bulletin NCJ 302051. November 2021. Accessed December 18, 2024. https://bjs.ojp.gov/content/pub/pdf/meco18.pdf

537. Weedn VW, Menendez MJ. Reclaiming the autopsy as the practice of medicine: a pathway to remediation of the forensic pathology workforce shortage? *Am J Forensic Med Pathol.* 2020;41(4):242–248. doi: 10.1097/paf.0000000000000589

538. Case ME. Forensic pathology of child brain trauma. *Brain Pathol.* 2008;18(4):562–564. doi: 10.1111/j.1750-3639.2008.00202.x

539. Case ME. Abusive head injuries in infants and young children. *Leg Med (Tokyo).* 2007;9(2):83–87. doi: 10.1016/j.legalmed.2006.11.017

540. Gill JR, Goldfeder LB, Armbrustmacher V, Coleman A, Mena H, Hirsch CS. Fatal head injury in children younger than 2 years in New York City and an overview of the shaken baby syndrome. *Arch Pathol Lab Med.* 2009;133(4):619–627. doi: 10.1043/1543-2165-133.4.619

541. Oehmichen M, Meissner C, Schmidt V, Pedal I, Konig HG, Saternus KS. Axonal injury–a diagnostic tool in forensic neuropathology? A review. *Forensic Sci Int.* 1998;95(1):67–83

542. Matschke J, Buttner A, Bergmann M, Hagel C, Puschel K, Glatzel M. Encephalopathy and death in infants with abusive head trauma is due to hypoxic-ischemic injury following local brain trauma to vital brainstem centers. *Int J Legal Med.* 2015;129(1):105–114. doi: 10.1007/s00414-014-1060-7

543. Choudhary AK, Servaes S, Slovis TL, et al. Consensus statement on abusive head trauma in infants and young children. *Pediatr Radiol.* 2018;48(8):1048–1065. doi: 10.1007/s00247-018-4149-1

544. Bauer R, Fritz H. Pathophysiology of traumatic injury in the developing brain: an introduction and short update. *Exp Toxicol Pathol.* 2004;56(1-2):65–73. doi: 10.1016/j.etp.2004.04.002

545. Bittigau P, Sifringer M, Felderhoff-Mueser U, Hansen HH, Ikonomidou C. Neuropathological and biochemical features of traumatic injury in the developing brain. *Neurotox Res.* 2003;5(7):475–490. doi: 10.1007/bf03033158

546. Pinto PS, Meoded A, Poretti A, Tekes A, Huisman TA. The unique features of traumatic brain injury in children. review of the characteristics of the pediatric skull and brain, mechanisms of trauma, patterns of injury, complications, and their imaging findings–part 2. *J Neuroimaging.* 2012;22(2):e18–e41. doi: 10.1111/j.1552-6569.2011.00690.x

547. Johnson MW, Stoll L, Rubio A, et al. Axonal injury in young pediatric head trauma: a comparison study of beta-amyloid precursor protein (beta-APP) immunohistochemical staining in traumatic and nontraumatic deaths. *J Forensic Sci.* 2011;56(5):1198–1205. doi: 10.1111/j.1556-4029.2011.01814.x

548. Atwal GS, Rutty GN, Carter N, Green MA. Bruising in non-accidental head injured children; a retrospective study of the prevalence, distribution and pathological associations in 24 cases. *Forensic Sci Int.* 1998;96(2-3):215–230

549. Wood JN, Christian CW, Adams CM, Rubin DM. Skeletal surveys in infants with isolated skull fractures. *Pediatrics.* 2009;123(2):e247–e252. doi: 10.1542/peds.2008-2467

550. Fajardo GC, Hanzlick RL. A 10-year epidemiologic review of homicide cases in children younger than 5 years in Fulton County, GA: 1996-2005. *Am J Forensic Med Pathol.* 2010;31(4):355–358. doi: 10.1097/PAF.0b013e3181fc3593

551. Reece RM, Christian CW. *Child Abuse: Medical Diagnosis and Management.* American Academy of Pediatrics; 2009

552. Adamsbaum C, Rambaud C. Abusive head trauma: don't overlook bridging vein thrombosis. *Pediatr Radiol.* 2012;42(11):1298–1300. doi: 10.1007/s00247-012-2434-y

553. Stein KM, Ruf K, Ganten MK, Mattern R. Representation of cerebral bridging veins in infants by postmortem computed tomography. *Forensic Sci Int.* 2006;163(1-2):93–101. doi: 10.1016/j.forsciint.2005.11.015

554. Maxeiner H. Demonstration and interpretation of bridging vein ruptures in cases of infantile subdural bleedings. *J Forensic Sci.* 2001;46(1):85–93

555. Busuttil A, Keeling J. *Paediatric Forensic Medicine and Pathology.* 2nd ed. Routledge; 2008

556. Squier W, Mack J. The neuropathology of infant subdural haemorrhage. *Forensic Sci Int.* 2009;187(1-3):6–13. doi: 10.1016/j.forsciint.2009.02.005

557. Edlmann E, Giorgi-Coll S, Whitfield PC, Carpenter KLH, Hutchinson PJ. Pathophysiology of chronic subdural haematoma: inflammation, angiogenesis and implications for pharmacotherapy. *J Neuroinflammation.* 2017;14(1):108. doi: 10.1186/s12974-017-0881-y

558. Nomura S, Kashiwagi S, Fujisawa H, Ito H, Nakamura K. Characterization of local hyperfibrinolysis in chronic subdural hematomas by SDS-PAGE and immunoblot. *J Neurosurg.* 1994;81(6):910–913. doi: 10.3171/jns.1994.81.6.0910

559. Castellani RJ, Mojica-Sanchez G, Schwartzbauer G, Hersh DS. Symptomatic acute-on-chronic subdural hematoma: a clinicopathological study. *Am J Forensic Med Pathol.* 2017;38(2):126–130. doi: 10.1097/paf.0000000000000300

560. Gerlach R, Dittrich S, Schneider W, Ackermann H, Seifert V, Kieslich M. Traumatic epidural hematomas in children and adolescents: outcome analysis in 39 consecutive unselected cases. *Pediatr Emerg Care.* 2009;25(3):164–169. doi: 10.1097/PEC.0b013e31819a8966

561. Case ME. Accidental traumatic head injury in infants and young children. *Brain Pathol.* 2008;18(4):583–589. doi: 10.1111/j.1750-3639.2008.00203.x

562. Jamieson KG, Yelland JD. Extradural hematoma. Report of 167 cases. *J Neurosurg.* 1968;29(1):13–23. doi: 10.3171/jns.1968.29.1.0013

563. Rivas JJ, Lobato RD, Sarabia R, Cordobés F, Cabrera A, Gomez P. Extradural hematoma: analysis of factors influencing the courses of 161 patients. *Neurosurgery.* 1988;23(1):44–51. doi: 10.1227/00006123-198807000-00010

564. Case ME. Distinguishing accidental from inflicted head trauma at autopsy. Review. *Pediatric Radiology.* 2014;44(4):632–640. doi: 10.1007/s00247-014-3061-6

565. Berney J, Favier J, Froidevaux AC. Paediatric head trauma: influence of age and sex. I. Epidemiology. *Childs Nerv Syst.* 1994;10(8):509–516. doi: 10.1007/bf00335073

566. Case ME. Distinguishing accidental from inflicted head trauma at autopsy. *Pediatr Radiol.* 2014;44(Suppl 4):S632–S640. doi: 10.1007/s00247-014-3061-6

567. Graham DI, Ford I, Adams JH, et al. Fatal head injury in children. *J Clin Pathol.* 1989;42(1):18–22. doi: 10.1136/jcp.42.1.18

568. Quinn TJ, Smith C, Murray L, Stewart J, Nicoll JA, Graham DI. There is no evidence of an association in children and teenagers

between the apolipoprotein E epsilon4 allele and post-traumatic brain swelling. *Neuropathol Appl Neurobiol.* 2004;30(6):569–575. doi: 10.1111/j.1365-2990.2004.00581.x

569. Adelson PD, Kochanek PM. Head injury in children. *J Child Neurol.* 1998;13(1):2–15. doi: 10.1177/088307389801300102

570. Bruce DA, Alavi A, Bilaniuk L, Dolinskas C, Obrist W, Uzzell B. Diffuse cerebral swelling following head injuries in children: the syndrome of "malignant brain edema." *J Neurosurg.* 1981;54(2):170–178. doi: 10.3171/jns.1981.54.2.0170

571. Smith C, Lo M. The neuropathological features of fatal pediatric brain trauma. Review. *Acad Forens Pathol.* 2012;2(1):36–41. doi: 10.23907/2012.005

572. Aldrich EF, Eisenberg HM, Saydjari C, et al. Diffuse brain swelling in severely head-injured children. A report from the NIH Traumatic Coma Data Bank. *J Neurosurg.* 1992;76(3):450–454. doi: 10.3171/jns.1992.76.3.0450

573. Adelson PD, Clyde B, Kochanek PM, Wisniewski SR, Marion DW, Yonas H. Cerebrovascular response in infants and young children following severe traumatic brain injury: a preliminary report. *Pediatr Neurosurg.* 1997;26(4):200–207. doi: 10.1159/000121192

574. Bauer R, Walter B, Fritz H, Zwiener U. Ontogenetic aspects of traumatic brain edema–facts and suggestions. *Exp Toxicol Pathol.* 1999;51(2):143–150. doi: 10.1016/s0940-2993(99)80088-8

575. Unterberg AW, Stover J, Kress B, Kiening KL. Edema and brain trauma. *Neuroscience.* 2004;129(4):1021–1029. doi: 10.1016/j.neuroscience.2004.06.046

576. Johnson VE, Stewart W, Smith DH. Axonal pathology in traumatic brain injury. *Exp Neurol.* 2013;246:35–43. doi: 10.1016/j.expneurol.2012.01.013

577. Johnson VE, Stewart W, Weber MT, Cullen DK, Siman R, Smith DH. SNTF immunostaining reveals previously undetected axonal pathology in traumatic brain injury. *Acta Neuropathol.* 2016;131(1):115–135. doi: 10.1007/s00401-015-1506-0

578. Gentleman SM, Nash MJ, Sweeting CJ, Graham DI, Roberts GW. Beta-amyloid precursor protein (beta APP) as a marker for axonal injury after head injury. *Neurosci Lett.* 1993;160(2):139–144

579. Sherriff FE, Bridges LR, Gentleman SM, Sivaloganathan S, Wilson S. Markers of axonal injury in post mortem human brain. *Acta Neuropathol.* 1994;88(5):433–439. doi: 10.1007/bf00389495

580. Grady MS, McLaughlin MR, Christman CW, Valadka AB, Fligner CL, Povlishock JT. The use of antibodies targeted against the neurofilament subunits for the detection of diffuse axonal injury in humans. *J Neuropathol Exp Neurol.* 1993;52(2):143–152. doi: 10.1097/00005072-199303000-00007

581. Reichard RR, Smith C, Graham DI. The significance of beta-APP immunoreactivity in forensic practice. *Neuropathol Appl Neurobiol.* 2005;31(3):304–313. doi: 10.1111/j.1365-2990.2005.00645.x

582. Dolinak D, Reichard R. An overview of inflicted head injury in infants and young children, with a review of beta-amyloid precursor protein immunohistochemistry. *Arch Pathol Lab Med.* 2006;130(5):712–717. doi: 10.1043/1543-2165(2006)130[712:Aooihi]2.0.Co;2

583. Reichard RR, White CL III, Hladik CL, Dolinak D. Beta-amyloid precursor protein staining of nonaccidental central nervous system injury in pediatric autopsies. *J Neurotrauma.* 2003;20(4):347–355. doi: 10.1089/089771503765172309

584. Reichard RR, White CL III, Hladik CL, Dolinak D. Beta-amyloid precursor protein staining in nonhomicidal pediatric medicolegal autopsies. *J Neuropathol Exp Neurol.* 2003;62(3):237–247. doi: 10.1093/jnen/62.3.237

585. McKenzie KJ, McLellan DR, Gentleman SM, Maxwell WL, Gennarelli TA, Graham DI. Is beta-APP a marker of axonal damage in short-surviving head injury? *Acta Neuropathol.* 1996;92(6):608–613

586. Geddes JF, Vowles GH, Beer TW, Ellison DW. The diagnosis of diffuse axonal injury: implications for forensic practice. *Neuropathol Appl Neurobiol.* 1997;23(4):339–347

587. Morrison C, MacKenzie JM. Axonal injury in head injuries with very short survival times. *Neuropathol Appl Neurobiol.* 2008;34(1):124–125. doi: 10.1111/j.1365-2990.2007.00876.x

588. Hortobágyi T, Wise S, Hunt N, et al. Traumatic axonal damage in the brain can be detected using beta-APP immunohistochemistry within 35 min after head injury to human adults. *Neuropathol Appl Neurobiol.* 2007;33(2):226–237. doi: 10.1111/j.1365-2990.2006.00794.x

589. Gorrie C, Oakes S, Duflou J, Blumbergs P, Waite PM. Axonal injury in children after motor vehicle crashes: extent, distribution, and size of axonal swellings using beta-APP immunohistochemistry. *J Neurotrauma.* 2002;19(10):1171–1182. doi: 10.1089/08977150260337976

590. Ferguson B, Matyszak MK, Esiri MM, Perry VH. Axonal damage in acute multiple sclerosis lesions. *Brain.* 1997;120(Pt 3):393–399. doi: 10.1093/brain/120.3.393

591. Bitsch A, Schuchardt J, Bunkowski S, Kuhlmann T, Brück W. Acute axonal injury in multiple sclerosis. Correlation with demyelination and inflammation. *Brain.* 2000;123(Pt 6):1174–1183. doi: 10.1093/brain/123.6.1174

592. Medana IM, Day NP, Hien TT, et al. Axonal injury in cerebral malaria. *Am J Pathol.* 2002;160(2):655–666. doi: 10.1016/s0002-9440(10)64885-7

593. Calder IM, Hill I, Scholtz CL. Primary brain trauma in non-accidental injury. *J Clin Pathol.* 1984;37(10):1095–1100

594. Duhaime AC, Durham S. Traumatic brain injury in infants: the phenomenon of subdural hemorrhage with hemispheric hypodensity ("big black brain"). *Progr Brain Res.* 2007;161:293–302. doi: 10.1016/s0079-6123(06)61020-0

595. Luyet FM, Feldman KW, Knox BL. The big black brain: subdural hemorrhage with hemispheric swelling and low attenuation. *J Child Adolesc Trauma.* 2018;11(2):241–247. doi: 10.1007/s40653-017-0132-5

596. Feldman KW, Weinberger E, Milstein JM, Fligner CL. Cervical spine MRI in abused infants. *Child Abuse Negl.* 1997;21(2):199–205. doi: 10.1016/s0145-2134(96)00145-7

597. Rutty GN, Squier WM, Padfield CJ. Epidural haemorrhage of the cervical spinal cord: a post-mortem artefact? *Neuropathol Appl*

Neurobiol. 2005;31(3):247–257. doi: 10.1111/j.1365-2990.2004.00633.x

598. Feldman KW, Avellino AM, Sugar NF, Ellenbogen RG. Cervical spinal cord injury in abused children. *Pediatr Emerg Care.* 2008;24(4):222–227. doi: 10.1097/PEC.0b013e31816b7aa4

599. Ewing-Cobbs L, Prasad M, Kramer L, Landry S. Inflicted traumatic brain injury: relationship of developmental outcome to severity of injury. *Pediatr Neurosurg.* 1999;31(5):251–258. doi: 10.1159/000028872

600. Foster KA, Recker MJ, Lee PS, Bell MJ, Tyler-Kabara EC. Factors associated with hemispheric hypodensity after subdural hematoma following abusive head trauma in children. *J Neurotrauma.* 2014;31(19):1625–1631. doi: 10.1089/neu.2014.3372

601. Ruppel RA, Clark RS, Bayir H, Satchell MA, Kochanek PM. Critical mechanisms of secondary damage after inflicted head injury in infants and children. *Neurosurg Clin North Am.* 2002;13(2):169–182. doi: 10.1016/s1042-3680(01)00005-5

602. Blumenthal I. Shaken baby syndrome. *Postgrad Med J.* 2002;78(926):732–735

603. Bell JE, Becher JC, Wyatt B, Keeling JW, McIntosh N. Brain damage and axonal injury in a Scottish cohort of neonatal deaths. *Brain.* 2005;128(Pt 5):1070–1081. doi: 10.1093/brain/awh436

604. Lindenberg R, Freytag E. Morphology of brain lesions from blunt trauma in early infancy. *Arch Pathol.* 1969;87(3):298–305

605. Larsen KB, Barber Z, Squier W. The pathology and aetiology of subcortical clefts in infants. *Forens Sci Int.* 2019;296:115–122. doi: 10.1016/j.forsciint.2019.01.011

606. Puanglumyai S, Lekawanvijit S. The importance of optic nerve sheath hemorrhage as a postmortem finding in cases of fatal abusive head trauma: a 13-year study in a tertiary hospital. *Forensic Sci Int.* 2017;276:5–11. doi: 10.1016/j.forsciint.2017.04.008

607. Wygnanski-Jaffe T, Levin AV, Shafiq A, et al. Postmortem orbital findings in shaken baby syndrome. *Am J Ophthalmol.* 2006;142(2):233–240. doi: 10.1016/j.ajo.2006.03.038

608. Gilliland MG, Luckenbach MW, Chenier TC. Systemic and ocular findings in 169 prospectively studied child deaths: retinal hemorrhages usually mean child abuse. *Forensic Sci Int.* 1994;68(2):117–132. doi: 10.1016/0379-0738(94)90309-3

609. Lambert SR, Johnson TE, Hoyt CS. Optic nerve sheath and retinal hemorrhages associated with the shaken baby syndrome. *Arch Ophthalmol.* 1986;104(10):1509–1512. doi: 10.1001/archopht.1986.01050220103037

610. Budenz DL, Farber MG, Mirchandani HG, Park H, Rorke LB. Ocular and optic nerve hemorrhages in abused infants with intracranial injuries. *Ophthalmology.* 1994;101(3):559–565. doi: 10.1016/s0161-6420(94)31300-5

611. Marshall DH, Brownstein S, Dorey MW, Addison DJ, Carpenter B. The spectrum of postmortem ocular findings in victims of shaken baby syndrome. *Can J Ophthalmol.* 2001;36(7):377–383. doi: 10.1016/s0008-4182(01)80081-8

612. Wygnanski-Jaffe T, Morad Y, Levin AV. Pathology of retinal hemorrhage in abusive head trauma. *Forensic Sci Med Pathol.* 2009;5(4):291–297. doi: 10.1007/s12024-009-9134-4

613. Gnanaraj L, Gilliland MG, Yahya RR, et al. Ocular manifestations of crush head injury in children. *Eye (Lond).* 2007;21(1):5–10. doi: 10.1038/sj.eye.6702174

614. Gleckman AM, Evans RJ, Bell MD, Smith TW. Optic nerve damage in shaken baby syndrome. *Am J Ophthalmol.* 2000;129(6):831. doi: 10.1016/s0002-9394(00)00508-0

615. Fanconi M, Lips U. Shaken baby syndrome in Switzerland: results of a prospective follow-up study, 2002-2007. *Eur J Pediatr.* 2010;169(8):1023–1028. doi: 10.1007/s00431-010-1175-x

616. Nuno M, Pelissier L, Varshneya K, Adamo MA, Drazin D. Outcomes and factors associated with infant abusive head trauma in the US. *J Neurosurg Pediatr.* 2015;16(5):515–522. doi: 10.3171/2015.3.PEDS14544

617. Barlow KM, Thomson E, Johnson D, Minns RA. Late neurologic and cognitive sequelae of inflicted traumatic brain injury in infancy. *Pediatrics.* 2005;116(2):e174–e185. doi: 10.1542/peds.2004-2739

618. Duhaime AC, Christian C, Moss E, Seidl T. Long-term outcome in infants with the shaking-impact syndrome. *Pediatr Neurosurg.* 1996;24(6):292–298. doi: 10.1159/000121058

619. Bonnier C, Nassogne MC, Evrard P. Outcome and prognosis of whiplash shaken infant syndrome; late consequences after a symptom-free interval. *Dev Med Child Neurol.* 1995;37(11):943–956. doi: 10.1111/j.1469-8749.1995.tb11949.x

620. Narang S, Clarke J. Abusive head trauma: past, present, and future. *J Child Neurol.* Dec 2014;29(12):1747–56. doi: 10.1177/0883073814549995

621. Stipanicic A, Nolin P, Fortin G, Gobeil MF. Comparative study of the cognitive sequelae of school-aged victims of Shaken Baby Syndrome. *Child Abuse Negl.* Mar 2008;32(3):415–28. doi: 10.1016/j.chiabu.2007.07.008

622. Laurent-Vannier A, Toure H, Vieux E, Brugel DG, Chevignard M. Long-term outcome of the shaken baby syndrome and medicolegal consequences: a case report. *Ann Phys Rehabil Med.* 2009;52(5):436–447. doi: 10.1016/j.rehab.2009.03.001

623. Chevignard MP, Lind K. Long-term outcome of abusive head trauma. *Pediatr Radiol.* 2014;44(Suppl 4):S548–S558. doi: 10.1007/s00247-014-3169-8

624. Lind K, Toure H, Brugel D, Meyer P, Laurent-Vannier A, Chevignard M. Extended follow-up of neurological, cognitive, behavioral and academic outcomes after severe abusive head trauma. *Child Abuse Negl.* 2016;51:358–367. doi: 10.1016/j.chiabu.2015.08.001

625. Eismann EA, Theuerling J, Cassedy A, Curry PA, Colliers T, Makoroff KL. Early developmental, behavioral, and quality of life outcomes following abusive head trauma in infants. *Child Abuse Negl.* 2020;108:104643. doi: 10.1016/j.chiabu.2020.104643

626. Merritt DH, Klein S. Do early care and education services improve language development for maltreated children? Evidence from a national child welfare sample. *Child Abuse Negl.* 2015;39:185–196. doi: 10.1016/j.chiabu.2014.10.011

627. Gilles EE, Nelson MD, Jr. Cerebral complications of nonaccidental head injury in childhood. *Pediatr Neurol.* 1998;19(2):119–128. doi: 10.1016/s0887-8994(98)00038-1

628. Tanoue K, Aida N, Matsui K. Apparent diffusion coefficient values predict outcomes of abusive head trauma. *Acta Paediatr.* 2013; 102(8):805–808. doi: 10.1111/apa.12281

629. Scribano PV, Makoroff KL, Feldman KW, Berger RP. Association of perpetrator relationship to abusive head trauma clinical outcomes. *Child Abuse Negl.* 2013;37(10):771–777. doi: 10.1016/j.chiabu.2013.04.011

630. Barlow KM, Spowart JJ, Minns RA. Early posttraumatic seizures in non-accidental head injury: relation to outcome. *Dev Med Child Neurol.* 2000;42(9):591–594. doi: 10.1017/s0012162200001110

631. Greiner MV, Lawrence AP, Horn P, Newmeyer AJ, Makoroff KL. Early clinical indicators of developmental outcome in abusive head trauma. *Childs Nerv Syst.* 2012;28(6):889–896. doi: 10.1007/s00381-012-1714-z

632. Chen CC, Hsieh PC, Chen CPC, et al. Clinical characteristics and predictors of poor hospital discharge outcome for young children with abusive head trauma. *J Clin Med.* 2019;8(3):390. doi: 10.3390/jcm8030390

633. Stewart CL, Holscher CM, Moore EE, et al. Base deficit correlates with mortality in pediatric abusive head trauma. *J Pediatr Surg.* 2013;48(10):2106–2111. doi: 10.1016/j.jpedsurg.2013.05.009

634. Adamo MA, Drazin D, Waldman JB. Decompressive craniectomy and postoperative complication management in infants and toddlers with severe traumatic brain injuries. *J Neurosurg Pediatr.* 2009;3(4):334–339. doi: 10.3171/2008.12.PEDS08310

635. Risen SR, Suskauer SJ, Dematt EJ, Slomine BS, Salorio CF. Functional outcomes in children with abusive head trauma receiving inpatient rehabilitation compared with children with nonabusive head trauma. *J Pediatr.* 2014;164(3):613–9.e1-2. doi: 10.1016/j.jpeds.2013.10.075

636. Weldy E, Shimoda A, Patnaik J, Jung J, Singh J. Long-term visual outcomes following abusive head trauma with retinal hemorrhage. *J AAPOS.* 2019;23(6):329.e1–329.e4. doi: 10.1016/j.jaapos.2019.08.276

637. Kelly JP, Feldman KW, Weiss A. Optical coherence tomography and visual outcomes in pediatric abusive head trauma. *Retin Cases Brief Rep.* 2024;18(2):225–229. doi: 10.1097/ICB.0000000000001353

638. Kelly JP, Feldman KW, Wright JN, Metz JB, Weiss A. Pediatric abusive head trauma: visual outcomes, evoked potentials, diffusion tensor imaging, and relationships to retinal hemorrhages. *Doc Ophthalmol.* 2023;147(1):1–14. doi: 10.1007/s10633-023-09927-w

639. Matthews GP, Das A. Dense vitreous hemorrhages predict poor visual and neurological prognosis in infants with shaken baby syndrome. *J Pediatr Ophthalmol Strabismus.* 1996;33(4):260–265. doi: 10.3928/0191-3913-19960701-13

640. Levin A. Ocular manifestations of child abuse. *Ophthalmol Clin North Am.* 1990;3:249–264

641. Showers J, Apolo J. Criminal disposition of persons involved in 72 cases of fatal child abuse. *Medicine, Science, and the Law.* 1986; 26(3):243–247

642. Strathearn L, Giannotti M, Mills R, Kisely S, Najman J, Abajobir A. Long-term cognitive, psychological, and health outcomes associated with child abuse and neglect. *Pediatrics.* 2020;146(4):e20200438. doi: 10.1542/peds.2020-0438

643. Dubowitz H, Christian CW, Hymel K, Kellogg ND. Forensic medical evaluations of child maltreatment: a proposed research agenda. *Child Abuse Negl.* 2014;38(11):1734–1746. doi: 10.1016/j.chiabu.2014.07.012

644. Currie J, Widom CS. Long-term consequences of child abuse and neglect on adult economic well-being. *Child Maltreat.* 2010;15(2):111–120. doi: 10.1177/1077559509355316

645. Beaulieu E, Rajabali F, Zheng A, Pike I. The lifetime costs of pediatric abusive head trauma and a cost-effectiveness analysis of the Period of Purple crying program in British Columbia, Canada. *Child Abuse Negl.* 2019;97:104133. doi: 10.1016/j.chiabu.2019.104133

646. Joyce T, Gossman W, Huecker MR.Pediatric abusive head trauma. In: *StatPearls* [internet]. StatPearls Publishing; 2024 Jan. 2023 May 22

647. Manfield J, Oakley K, Macey JA, Waugh MC. Understanding the Five-Year Outcomes of Abusive Head Trauma in Children: A Retrospective Cohort Study. *Dev Neurorehabil.* 2021;24(6):361–367. doi: 10.1080/17518423.2020.1869340

648. Jackson JE, Beres AL, Theodorou CM, Ugiliweneza B, Boakye M, Nuno M. Long-term impact of abusive head trauma in young children: outcomes at 5 and 11 years old. *J Pediatr Surg.* 2021;56(12):2318–2325. doi: 10.1016/j.jpedsurg.2021.02.019

649. Badger S, Waugh MC, Hancock J, Marks S, Oakley K. Short term outcomes of children with abusive head trauma two years post injury: a retrospective study. *J Pediatr Rehabil Med.* 2020;13(3):241–253. doi: 10.3233/PRM-190624

650. DeGrauw X, Thurman D, Xu L, Kancherla V, DeGrauw T. Epidemiology of traumatic brain injury-associated epilepsy and early use of anti-epilepsy drugs: an analysis of insurance claims data, 2004-2014. *Epilepsy Res.* 2018;146:41–49. doi: 10.1016/j.eplepsyres.2018.07.012

651. Park JT, Chugani HT. Post-traumatic epilepsy in children-experience from a tertiary referral center. *Pediatr Neurol.* 2015;52(2):174–181. doi: 10.1016/j.pediatrneurol.2014.09.013

652. Chevignard M, Câmara-Costa H, Dellatolas G.Pediatric traumatic brain injury and abusive head trauma. In: *Handbook of Clinical Neurology.* Elsevier; 2020:451–484

653. Lucke-Wold BP, Nguyen L, Turner RC, et al. Traumatic brain injury and epilepsy: Underlying mechanisms leading to seizure. *Seizure.* 2015;33:13–23. doi: 10.1016/j.seizure.2015.10.002

654. Lopes NRL, Williams LCA. Pediatric Abusive Head Trauma Prevention Initiatives: A Literature Review. *Trauma Violence Abuse.* 2018;19(5):555–566. doi: 10.1177/1524838016675479

655. Barr RG, Rivara FP, Barr M, et al. Effectiveness of educational materials designed to change knowledge and behaviors regarding crying and shaken-baby syndrome in mothers of newborns: a randomized, controlled trial. *Pediatrics.* 2009;123(3):972–980. doi: 10.1542/peds.2008-0908

656. Stewart TC, Polgar D, Gilliland J, et al. Shaken baby syndrome and a triple-dose strategy for its prevention. *J Trauma.* 2011;71(6):1801–1807. doi: 10.1097/TA.0b013e31823c484a

657. Fujiwara T, Yamada F, Okuyama M, Kamimaki I, Shikoro N, Barr RG. Effectiveness of educational materials designed to change knowledge and behavior about crying and shaken baby syndrome: a replication of a randomized controlled trial in Japan. *Child Abuse Negl.* 2012;36(9):613–620. doi: 10.1016/j.chiabu.2012.07.003

658. Reese LS, Heiden EO, Kim KQ, Yang J. Evaluation of Period of PURPLE Crying, an abusive head trauma prevention program. *J Obstet Gynecol Neonatal Nurs.* 2014;43(6):752–761. doi: 10.1111/1552-6909.12495

659. Tolliday F, Simons M, Foley S, Benson S, Stephens A, Rose D. From inspiration to action: The Shaken Baby prevention project in Western Sydney. *Communities, Children and Families Australia.* 2010;5(2):31–47

660. Foley S, Kovacs Z, Rose J, et al. International collaboration on prevention of shaken baby syndrome - an ongoing project/intervention. *Paediatr Int Child Health.* 2013;33(4):233–238. doi: 10.1179/2046905513Y.0000000093

661. Taşar MA, Dallar Bilge Ylz, Şahin F, et al. Shaken Baby Syndrome prevention programme: a pilot study in Turkey. *Child Abuse Review.* 2015;24(2):120–128

662. Deyo G, Skybo T, Carroll A. Secondary analysis of the "Love Me… Never Shake Me" SBS education program. *Child Abuse Negl.* 2008;32(11):1017–1025. doi: 10.1016/j.chiabu.2008.02.006

663. Ríos J. The hand project: more hugs, no shakings. *Boletin de la Asociacion Medica de Puerto Rico.* 2011;103(1):9–13

664. Barr RG. Crying as a trigger for abusive head trauma: a key to prevention. *Pediatr Radiol.* 2014;44(Suppl 4):S559–S564. doi: 10.1007/s00247-014-3100-3

665. Barr RG, Barr M, Fujiwara T, Conway J, Catherine N, Brant R. Do educational materials change knowledge and behaviour about crying and shaken baby syndrome? A randomized controlled trial. *CMAJ.* 2009;180(7):727–733. doi: 10.1503/cmaj.081419

666. Keefe MR, Lobo ML, Froese-Fretz A, Kotzer AM, Barbosa GA, Dudley WN. Effectiveness of an intervention for colic. *Clin Pediatr (Phila).* 2006;45(2):123–133. doi: 10.1177/000992280604500203

667. McRury JM, Zolotor AJ. A randomized, controlled trial of a behavioral intervention to reduce crying among infants. *J Am Board Fam Med.* 2010;23(3):315–322. doi: 10.3122/jabfm.2010.03.090142

668. Hiscock H, Cook F, Bayer J, et al. Preventing early infant sleep and crying problems and postnatal depression: a randomized trial. *Pediatrics.* 2014;133(2):e346–e354. doi: 10.1542/peds.2013-1886

669. van Sleuwen BE, L'Hoir M P, Engelberts AC, et al. Comparison of behavior modification with and without swaddling as interventions for excessive crying. *J Pediatr.* 2006;149(4):512–517. doi: 10.1016/j.jpeds.2006.06.068

670. Ohgi S, Akiyama T, Arisawa K, Shigemori K. Randomised controlled trial of swaddling versus massage in the management of excessive crying in infants with cerebral injuries. *Arch Dis Child.* 2004;89(3):212–216. doi: 10.1136/adc.2002.025064

671. Landgren K, Kvorning N, Hallstrom I. Acupuncture reduces crying in infants with infantile colic: a randomised, controlled, blind clinical study. *Acupunct Med.* 2010;28(4):174–19. doi: 10.1136/aim.2010.002394

672. Fujiwara T. Effectiveness of public health practices against shaken baby syndrome/abusive head trauma in Japan. *Public Health.* 2015;129(5):475–482. doi: 10.1016/j.puhe.2015.01.018

673. Bechtel K, Le K, Martin KD, Shah N, Leventhal JM, Colson E. Impact of an educational intervention on caregivers' beliefs about infant crying and knowledge of shaken baby syndrome. *Acad Pediatr.* 2011;11(6):481–486. doi: 10.1016/j.acap.2011.08.001

674. Morrill AC, McElaney L, Peixotto B, VanVleet M, Sege R. Evaluation of All Babies Cry, a second generation universal abusive head trauma prevention program. *J Community Psychol.* 2015;43(3):296–314. doi: 10.1002/jcop.21679

675. Barr RG, Rajabali F, Aragon M, Colbourne M, Brant R. Education about crying in normal infants is associated with a reduction in pediatric emergency room visits for crying complaints. *J Dev Behav Pediatr.* 2015;36(4):252–257. doi: 10.1097/DBP.0000000000000156

676. Dias MS, Smith K, DeGuehery K, Mazur P, Li V, Shaffer ML. Preventing abusive head trauma among infants and young children: a hospital-based, parent education program. *Pediatrics.* 2005;115(4):e470–e487. doi: 10.1542/peds.2004-1896

677. Altman RL, Canter J, Patrick PA, Daley N, Butt NK, Brand DA. Parent education by maternity nurses and prevention of abusive head trauma. *Pediatrics.* 2011;128(5):e1164–e1172. doi: 10.1542/peds.2010-3260

678. Dias MS, Rottmund CM, Cappos KM, et al. Association of a postnatal parent education program for abusive head trauma with subsequent pediatric abusive head trauma hospitalization rates. *JAMA Pediatr.* 2017;171(3):223–229. doi: 10.1001/jamapediatrics.2016.4218

679. Barr RG, Barr M, Rajabali F, et al. Eight-year outcome of implementation of abusive head trauma prevention. *Child Abuse Negl.* 2018;84:106–114. doi: 10.1016/j.chiabu.2018.07.004

680. Zolotor AJ, Runyan DK, Shanahan M, et al. Effectiveness of a statewide abusive head trauma prevention program in North Carolina. *JAMA Pediatr.* 2015;169(12):1126–1131. doi: 10.1001/jamapediatrics.2015.2690

681. Klevens J, Schmidt B, Luo F, Xu L, Ports KA, Lee RD. Effect of the Earned Income Tax Credit on hospital admissions for pediatric abusive head trauma, 1995-2013. *Public Health Rep.* 2017;132(4):505–511. doi: 10.1177/0033354917710905

682. Klevens J, Luo F, Xu L, Peterson C, Latzman NE. Paid family leave's effect on hospital admissions for pediatric abusive head trauma. *Inj Prev.* 2016;22(6):442–445. doi: 10.1136/injuryprev-2015-041702

683. Eckenrode J, Campa MI, Morris PA, et al. The prevention of child maltreatment through the nurse family partnership program: mediating effects in a long-term follow-up study. *Child Maltreat.* 2017;22(2):92–99. doi: 10.1177/1077559516685185

Advanced Practice Nursing in Neonatology

- *Clinical Report*

CLINICAL REPORT Organizational Principles to Guide and Define the Child Health Care System and/or Improve the Health of All Children

American Academy of Pediatrics
DEDICATED TO THE HEALTH OF ALL CHILDREN™

Advanced Practice Nursing in Neonatology: Clinical Report

Lisa M. Grisham, PhD, DNP, NNP-BC,[1,2,3] Jay P. Goldsmith, MD, FAAP,[4] Ashley M. Lucke, MD FAAP,[5] Sheila M. Gephart, PhD, RN, FAAN,[6] the AAP Committee on Fetus and Newborn

Under Review: The American Academy of Pediatrics has identified sections of this report that require clarification regarding the description of APRN scope of practice for different neonatal care settings and patients. A revision will be published and linked to this page accordingly. In addition, shared attribution to the National Association of Neonatal Nurses (NANN) has been removed by request.

abstract

The participation of advanced practice registered nurses (APRNs) in neonatal care continues to be supported by the American Academy of Pediatrics. Traditionally, neonatal nurse practitioners and neonatal clinical nurse specialists were the two roles well established within the Neonatal Intensive Care Unit (NICU). With ongoing shortages of these roles, some institutions have turned toward pediatric nurse practitioners (acute and primary care) and family nurse practitioners to meet patient care needs. This clinical report aims to review the roles, scope of practice, collaboration, and credentialling of these categories of APRNs with recommendations for the safe and effective utilization of these providers in neonatal care. This clinical report will not address other roles in the NICU, including hospitalists or physician assistants in the NICU, nor speak to the potential shortages and solutions these professions are experiencing, as those topics are well covered in the Standards for Levels of Neonatal Care: II, III, IV and Neonatal Provider Workforce Technical Report.

INTRODUCTION

Advanced Practice Registered Nurses (APRNs) have served in the Neonatal Intensive Care Unit (NICU) for nearly 50 years. The Neonatal Clinical Nurse Specialist (NCNS) was one of the two APRN roles that filled a much-needed position of a neonatal nursing expert who facilitates education, patient advocacy, practice improvements, and quality initiatives.[1] The Board-Certified Neonatal Nurse Practitioner (NNP-BC) was the second APRN role, which started as a certificate program and has evolved over the last 40 years into a master's or doctoral-prepared, with a defined scope of practice, functioning provider caring for the full range of infants in all levels of newborn care. These two roles met many of the patient and family care needs in the nation's NICUs for decades, but recent changes have suggested

[1]*National Association of Neonatal Nurses, Chicago, Illinois;* [2]*Department of Pediatrics, University of Arizona, Tucson, Arizona;* [3]*Edson College of Nursing and Health Innovation, Arizona State University, Tempe, Arizona;* [4]*Department of Pediatrics, Division of Newborn Medicine, Tulane University School of Medicine, New Orleans, Louisiana;* [5]*Dell Medical School, University of Texas at Austin, Austin, Texas; and* [6]*College of Nursing, University of Arizona, Tucson, Arizona*

CONFLICT OF INTEREST DISCLOSURES: The authors have indicated they have no potential conflicts of interest to disclose. The authors have indicated they do not have a financial relationship relevant to this article to disclose.

FUNDING: No external funding.

To cite: Grisham LM, Goldsmith JP, Lucke AM, et al; American Academy of Pediatrics, the AAP Committee on Fetus and Newborn. Advanced Practice Nursing in Neonatology: Clinical Report. *Pediatrics.* 2025;156(3):e2025073170

the need for additional APRN roles in the NICU. Although neonatal physician assistants and pediatric hospitalists supplement the neonatal workforce, this report will focus on advanced practice nursing roles in the NICU.

According to the American Academy of Nurse Practitioners (AANP) Certification Board, there are more than 385 000 nurse practitioners (NPs) licensed in the US, and more than 39 000 new NPs completed their academic programs in 2021–2022. Neonatal and pediatric acute care comprise 1.1% of the total number of NPs by primary certification area.[2] These numbers support a relative shortage of APRNs in the NICU. There are several factors contributing to this shortage and the need for more APRN roles in the NICU. The first started in 2003, when the Accreditation Council for Graduate Medical Education (ACGME) reviewed and modified hospital resident physician hours, including significant limitations on how much time pediatric residents could spend in NICU rotations. This limitation of resident hours in the NICU shifted the workload onto neonatal APRNs, Neonatal Fellows, Neonatologists, and other providers such as pediatric hospitalists and physician assistants. This increased workload has persisted, with a report from 2021 showing that NNP-BCs work almost 250 extra hours a year beyond what they are contracted.[3] The extra time and extra shifts have led to burnout and fewer NNP-BC preceptors, creating a relative shortage of clinical placements for students, limiting enrollment.[3] Additionally, between 2016 and 2021, NICU admissions increased by 2%, even though there was a 7% decrease in births.[4] The increased workload, increased APRN positions to account for decreased resident hours, natural attrition patterns, and increased NICU admissions have resulted in a prolonged shortage of APRNs in the NICU.[5]

The American Academy of Pediatrics (AAP) endorses the role of the APRN.[6] Current training and educational objectives for the NNP-BC were developed by the National Association of Neonatal Nurses (NANN).[7] These guidelines are specifically designed to educate neonatal APRNs at the graduate level to manage well newborns, critically ill neonates, and convalescing infants to two years of age. With the recent shortage of neonatal APRNs in the NICU, many institutions have included the certified primary care pediatric nurse practitioner (CPNP-PC), certified acute care pediatric nurse practitioner (CPNP-AC), and certified or board-certified family nurse practitioner (FNP-C and FNP-BC) to augment the role of neonatal APRNs in providing care and medical management of premature and sick infants while hospitalized. However, training and certification for CPNP-PC, CPNP-AC, FNP-C, and FNP-BC are different from an NNP-BC (see Table 1: Education, Certification, and Training for ARPNs), and this education alone does not ensure competency for CPNP-PCs, CPNP-ACs, FNP-Cs, and FNP-BCs to care for all neonatal patients. The purpose of this clinical report is to outline recommendations for the scope of practice for APRNs in neonatal nursing and advanced care practices in the NICU.

Licensure, Accreditation, Certification, & Education (LACE)

In 2008, the APRN Consensus Work Group and the National Council of State Boards of Nursing APRN Advisory Committee published the LACE Consensus Model for APRN Regulation.[8] LACE stands for licensure, accreditation, certification, and education and outlines the necessity of having these four elements in alignment to define and support the APRN scope of practice. For an APRN to practice safely, the patient population they care for 1) must have been covered in their formal academic education (by an accredited institution), 2) the APRN must pass a national board certification that includes testing of the knowledge on that patient population, and 3) the APRN be granted state licensure, which verifies that the individual has completed the necessary education, clinical training, and certification giving them the authority to practice in their specialty as outlined in the LACE guidelines. Furthermore, there are individual state nursing laws and rules that define the scope of practice for APRNs. The CNS (clinical nurse specialist) and CNP (certified nurse practitioner) are two types of APRNs that practice in the NICU and were identified in the LACE Consensus Model for APRN Regulation.[8] All APRNs are required to complete a graduate-level education program of study and supervised practice beyond the level of the Registered Nurse (RN). However, there are different course requirements, clinical hours, and patient experiences to ensure the provider has trained appropriately in the corresponding neonatal or pediatric patient population. Although there are five APRN roles that can provide care to neonatal patients (see Table 2: APRN Roles in the NICU), the types and acuity of patients for whom each specific APRN can provide care is dependent upon the education, training, certification, and licensure required for each role, as described below.

DESCRIPTION OF ROLES AND SCOPE OF PRACTICE

Neonatal Clinical Nurse Specialist (NCNS)

An NCNS is a registered nurse with a Master's or Doctor of Nursing Practice (DNP) degree who, through study and supervised practice at the graduate level, has become an expert in the theory and practice of neonatal nursing. Completion of 500 (for masters) or 1000 (for doctorate) supervised clinical hours is required as part of the training, as well as certification by the American Association of Critical-Care Nurses (AACN).[9,10] If the program is a post-baccalaureate practice doctorate program, there is an additional 500 clinical hours required for a total of 1000 clinical hours.[10] An NCNS is poised to influence care by linking the individual domains of the patient, the nurse, and the

TABLE 1. Education, Training, and Certification for APRNs

Role	Education and Description	Training	Certification
Neonatal Clinical Nurse Specialist (NCNS)	Master's or doctorate in theory and practice of neonatal nursing.	Master's program: 500 supervised clinical hours Doctorate program: 1000 clinical hours required	American Association of Critical-Care Nurses (AACN)
Board-Certified Neonatal Nurse Practitioner (NNP-BC)	Master's prepared or Doctor of Nursing Practice (DNP): minimum of 200 neonatal-specific didactic hours including neonatal pathophysiology, pharmacology, and neonatal assessment.[7,38,a]	Minimum 750 h of supervised clinical experience. Clinical experience in delivery rooms, level II-IV NICUs, follow-up and well-infant programs, (majority of the time in level III or IV NICUs)	National Certification Corporation (NCC)
Acute Care – Pediatric Nurse Practitioner (CPNP-AC)	Master's prepared or Doctor of Nursing Practice (DNP). Focus on children with or without unstable physiology. Training includes content on sepsis, chronic lung disease, and congenital heart lesions.	Pediatric-specific didactic hours plus a minimum of 750 supervised clinical hours.	Pediatric Nursing Certification Board® Certification does not contain content on fetal or preterm neonatal pathologies and physiology.
Primary Care - Pediatric Nurse Practitioner (CPNP-PC)	Master's prepared or Doctor of Nursing Practice (DNP). Focus on prevention, wellness, and continuous care of chronic conditions. Training in stabilization of acute and episodic conditions. Neonatal training includes newborn history and physical exam, breastfeeding, immunizations, and management of common newborn conditions.	Pediatric-specific didactic hours plus minimum of 750 supervised clinical hours.	Pediatric Nursing Certification Board® Certification does not contain content on fetal or preterm neonatal pathologies and physiology.
Certified Family Nurse Practitioner (FNP-C) Board-Certified Family Nurse Practitioner (FNP-BC)	Master's prepared or Doctor of Nursing Practice (DNP). Education is focused on health promotion, harm reduction, and disease prevention across the lifespan. Clinical experiences emphasize primary care concerns. The FNP-BC contains content on healthcare policy.	Pediatric-specific didactic hours (90) can count towards the minimum of 750 supervised clinical hours. *Note - pediatric clinical hours are not specific to neonates and all hours could be completed with adolescent patient population.	FNP-C – American Academy of Nurse Practitioners Certification Board® (AANP) FNP-BC – American Nurses Credentialing Center® (ANCC)

[a] Credentialed NNP-BCs who hold certificates or other non-master's degrees can continue to practice but should be encouraged to complete formal graduate education.

system, and is responsible for fostering continuous quality improvement in neonatal nursing care and developing and educating staff.[8,9] Training for the NCNS includes core content in theory, clinical inquiry, leadership, systems thinking, quality improvement and safety, and evidence-based practice (EBP).[10] The NCNS models expert nursing practice and applies and promotes EBP within a neonatal setting. The primary role of the NCNS is to influence direct patient care through education of competent nurses and influence for sound nursing practice in health care systems and organizations, although the role can also function to diagnose and treat states of illness, including direct patient care.[8,10,11] In the NICU or Special Care Nursery (SCN) setting, collaborative practice between clinical nurse managers and the NCNS is essential in maintaining current practice guidelines and policies, which can be instrumental in obtaining certifications such as The Joint Commission (JC), Magnet recognition, or Det Norske Veritas (DNV) programs.[12]

Board-Certified Neonatal Nurse Practitioner (NNP-BC)

A board-certified neonatal nurse practitioner (NNP-BC) is an experienced neonatal nurse with clinical expertise in neonatal nursing who has obtained a master's or DNP degree with supervised clinical experience in the management of newborn infants and their families. Some accelerated programs are designed to have the student complete the curriculum for the RN license and certification in the first year and then practice gaining experience while completing APRN coursework in the following years of the program. Education and clinical experiences address the care of infants with any pathology that may present at birth or during the neonatal period. NNP-BCs are nationally

TABLE 2. APRN Roles in the NICU

Role	Patient Population	Neonatal Setting	Procedural Competencies
Neonatal Clinical Nurse Specialist (NCNS)	Birth to age two years old	Newborn Nursery Special Care Nursery NICU - levels I-IV	No required procedural competencies No direct patient care
Board-Certified Neonatal Nurse Practitioner (NNP-BC)	Birth to age two years old	Newborn Nursery Special Care Nursery NICU - levels I-IV Developmental Follow-up Clinic	• Resuscitation and stabilization • Endotracheal intubation • Laryngeal airway (LMA) placement • Umbilical vessel catheterization • Percutaneous arterial and venous catheterization • Arterial puncture • Lumbar puncture • Chest tube thoracentesis and needle aspiration • Exchange transfusion • Assisted ventilation • Other procedures with demonstrated education and competency (e.g., circumcision).
Acute Care – Pediatric Nurse Practitioner (CPNP-AC)	Care for children from birth to young adult May include infants who are ≥ 32 weeks, and conditions such as[a]: - respiratory distress - clinical sepsis - feeding discoordination due to prematurity - bronchopulmonary dysplasia (BPD) - congenital heart lesions	Newborn Nursery Special Care Nursery NICU - levels I-IV Developmental Follow-up Clinic	• Resuscitation and stabilization of term infants • Endotracheal intubation • LMA placement • Percutaneous arterial and venous catheters • Arterial puncture • Lumbar puncture • Intraosseous placement • Needle aspiration of pneumothorax • Chest-tube insertion and removal • Assisted ventilation • Other procedures with demonstrated education and competency (e.g., circumcision).
Primary Care - Pediatric Nurse Practitioner (CPNP-PC)	Care for children from birth to young adult May include infants who are ≥35 weeks with minor pathologies	Newborn Nursery Special Care Nursery NICU - levels I-IV Developmental Follow-up Clinic	Neonatal procedural competencies are outside the scope of practice as CPNP-PCs do not receive education and training for them.
Certified Family Nurse Practitioner (FNP-C) Board-Certified Family Nurse Practitioner (FNP-BC)	Can provide care for children from birth through adulthood May include infants who are ≥35 weeks with minor pathologies	Newborn Nursery Special Care Nursery NICU - levels I-IV Developmental Follow-up Clinic	Neonatal procedural competencies are outside the scope of practice as FNP-C/FNP-BCs do not receive education and training for them.

[a] This list is not inclusive.

board-certified to care for children from birth to age two.[7,13] Some examples of disorders addressed in their education include prematurity, respiratory distress, necrotizing enterocolitis, congenital heart disease, chronic lung disease, and genetic abnormalities. The NNP-BC curriculum must include a minimum of 200 neonatal-specific didactic hours plus a minimum of 750 directly supervised clinical hours with critically ill neonates/infants, with a majority of the clinical hours in level III or IV NICUs.[14] Clinical simulation may be used to augment the educational experience but does not count toward the 750 minimum clinical hour requirement. Training on neonatal procedures includes didactic content and simulation on resuscitation and stabilization, endotracheal intubation, administration of surfactant, laryngeal airway (LMA) placement, umbilical vessel catheterization, percutaneous arterial and venous catheterization, arterial puncture, lumbar puncture, chest tube thoracentesis and needle aspiration, exchange transfusion, and assisted ventilation. Procedural confidence is developed through supervised clinical and simulation experiences, whereas competency is achieved beyond degree completion through the supervision of procedures by experienced colleagues and neonatologists as part of the credentialing process with the employer. Currently, credentialed NNP-BCs who have graduated from non-master's degree programs or certificate programs are preauthorized or "grandfathered in," meaning they can continue to practice in most states but should be encouraged to complete formal graduate education.[15] The AAP supports the documented competency of the master's degree-prepared APRN for entry into practice as an NNP-BC.[6] The AAP also supports APRNs who wish to pursue the highest level of educational preparation in nursing, either the Doctor of Philosophy (PhD) or the Doctor of Nursing Practice (DNP), but recognizes that such degrees are not required for clinical practice. The PhD maintains a focus on advanced training in research, whereas the DNP maintains a focus on leadership and quality improvement; both are considered terminal degrees in nursing. In addition to patient care, the NNP-BC may also be responsible for educating staff, engaging in research, participating in quality improvement initiatives, and developing standards of nursing care.[16]

Acute Care Pediatric Nurse Practitioner (CPNP-AC)

An acute care pediatric nurse practitioner (CPNP-AC) is an experienced pediatric nurse with training in the management of acute, critical, and chronic pediatric health care illnesses, including emergent and life-threatening conditions.[17,18] The CPNP-AC works closely with an interprofessional team to provide the highest level of evidence-based care for infants, children, adolescents, and young adults with life-threatening illnesses and organ dysfunction or failure. Young adult patients with chronic medical needs outside the traditionally defined pediatric age parameters may benefit from management by the CPNP-AC. In addition to preventative and health care maintenance, education and clinical experiences include preparation for congenital birth defects (eg, congenital heart disease), common acute childhood illnesses (eg, respiratory syncytial virus, strep throat), post-surgical care, trauma, and more. The CPNP-AC curriculum includes pediatric-specific didactic content plus a minimum of 750 directly supervised clinical hours.[14,19,20] Clinical hours can be completed in acute care settings such as hospitals (including intensive care units), subspecialty clinics, and emergency departments. There is no requirement for a rotation in the NICU or newborn nursery as part of the clinical hours. Simulation or alternative clinical experiences (eg, community settings) cannot count in the required 750 hours, but may be counted above the 750 direct clinical hours.[20] Certification is achieved through the Pediatric Nursing Certification Board® and covers content on assessment, diagnosis, management, and the professional practice role; additionally, multiple clinical pathologies (respiratory, oncologic, endocrine, immunologic, metabolic, toxicology, etc.) are included as test content.[18] The CPNP-AC also receives education and training on ventilator management and procedures, including airway management, central line placement, procedural sedation, chest tubes, and lumbar puncture. Employers wishing to deploy these providers in a neonatal setting are responsible for assessing initial and ongoing neonatal cognitive and procedural competency as part of the credentialing process.

Primary Care Pediatric Nurse Practitioner (CPNP-PC)

A primary care pediatric nurse practitioner (CPNP-PC) is an experienced pediatric nurse with advanced training in pediatric conditions. Some CPNP-PCs have nursing experience prior to beginning an NP program, but given that it is not an application requirement, not all students enter the program with experience. Additionally, accelerated programs are designed to have the student complete the curriculum for the RN license and certification in the first year and then complete APRN coursework in the following two years, meaning they graduate without bedside nursing experience. CPNP-PCs receive didactic and clinical training focused on physiologic and psychological needs in children from birth to young adulthood. CPNP-PCs assess, screen, evaluate, and diagnose children from birth through young adults to provide the full spectrum of primary care health services. They prescribe a comprehensive therapeutic treatment plan, including pharmacological and non-pharmacological strategies, provide patient and family education, and refer patients to collaborative members of the health care team when indicated.[21] The CPNP-PC curriculum includes pediatric-specific didactic hours plus a minimum of 750 directly supervised clinical hours.[19] Clinical hours are outpatient and can include private practice, ambulatory, school-based clinics, home care, and subspecialty clinics. Clinical training in the NICU and newborn nursery can be included for interested students, but it is not part of the required curriculum. CPNP-PCs provide pediatric primary care in a variety of health care settings including, but not limited to, private practice, ambulatory and school-based clinics, the home, hospital, and subspecialty clinics. Patient management often focuses on prevention and medical continuity.[21] Education on neonatal populations includes low-risk late preterm and term infants as well as long-term complications from prematurity that extend beyond the stay in the NICU. Training on neonatal procedures is not part of the standard CPNP-PC academic curriculum, but employers may wish to provide training and clinical experiences of neonatal procedures that fall within the scope of practice for a CPNP-PC. Employers are responsible for assessing ongoing cognitive and procedural competency in neonatal care as part of the credentialing process. Some examples of neonatal procedures performed by a CPNP-PC with additional training and credentialing could include resuscitation and stabilization (Neonatal Resuscitation Program), laryngeal mask airway (LMA) placement, and chest needle aspiration. The Pediatric Nursing Certification Board® administers the certifying exam for CPNP-PC, which covers content on health maintenance and promotion, assessment and diagnosis, management, and professional roles and responsibilities.[22]

Certified Family Nurse Practitioner (FNP-C) and Board-Certified Family Nurse Practitioner (FNP-BC)

A certified family nurse practitioner (FNP-C) and a board-certified family nurse practitioner (FNP-BC) both have foundational nursing education and advanced training in the management of individuals and families across the lifespan.[19] The difference between the two designations is that the FNP-C emphasizes a focus on clinical practice, whereas the FNP-BC includes clinical practice, policy, and education. The FNP-C/FNP-BC can provide primary care for all patients, including prenatal, pediatric, adolescent, adult, and elderly primary care.[19,23] Education for the FNP-C/FNP-BC is focused on health promotion, harm reduction, and disease prevention, and clinical experiences aim to include preparation for primary care concerns (eg, common childhood illnesses, hypertension, type II diabetes, etc.). An FNP-C/FNP-BC may or may not have nursing experience prior to being accepted into their graduate program. The FNP-C and FNP-BC curricula require a minimum of 750 directly supervised clinical hours but recognize that proper training to care for multiple age groups will far exceed this minimum. Of the 750 hours, only 90 are required in a pediatric setting, which is generally an outpatient setting. There is no requirement for clinical hours in the NICU or newborn nursery. Simulation or alternative clinical experiences (eg, community settings) can count for clinical experience beyond the required 750 hours.[19] Certification for the FNP-C is achieved through the American Academy of Nurse Practitioners Certification Board® and covers content on assessment, diagnosis, management, and evaluation across multiple age groups as outlined above.[23] Certification for the FNP-BC is achieved through the American Nurses Credentialing Center (ANCC) and covers content on diagnosis, management, evaluation, and nursing policy. Both FNP-C and FNP-BC receive training on the following procedures: minor skin lesion removal, microscopy, Papanicolaou tests, joint aspirations and injections, skin biopsy, arterial puncture, therapeutic injections, wound closure, splinting, casting, and wound management. Training on neonatal procedures is not included in the curriculum. Additional procedures may be performed with proper training, evaluation, and credentialing by the employer. Employers wishing to utilize FNP-C/FNP-BCs in a neonatal setting are responsible for assessing initial and ongoing neonatal cognitive and procedural competency as part of the credentialing process.

Competency and Scope of Practice

Initial and ongoing competency for all types of nurse practitioners is defined by the National Organization of Nurse Practitioner Faculties (NONPF) and includes nine domains: Knowledge of Practice, Person-Centered Care, Population Health, Practice Scholarship and Translational Science, Quality and Safety, Interprofessional Collaboration in Practice, Health Systems, Technology and Information Literacy, Professionalism, and Personal, Professional and Leadership Development.[24,25] Competency and scope of practice for NCNSs are defined by the National Association of Clinical Nurse Specialists (NACNS).[10] Academic centers develop their curricula around the competencies; national certification boards incorporate the competencies into their respective exams; and professional organizations use the competencies to develop policy statements. Therefore, all APRN roles that practice within the NICU follow either the NONPF or NACNS competency guidelines. Some roles have expanded the competency checklist to provide additional guidance to organizations assessing competency. The National Association of Neonatal Nurses (NANN), the professional organization for neonatal nurses and APRNs, applies the NONPF competency framework to the neonatal population for management by NNP-BCs.[7] The NACNS has defined a separate competency framework for the management of neonates by NCNSs.[10] Both include specific requirements such as maternal and fetal physiology for initial and ongoing practice.[7,26] For CPNP-PC and CPNP-AC roles, the competencies are specific to the education, training, and certification of a pediatric nurse practitioner.[16] For the FNC-C/FNP-BC roles, the competencies are broad and less specific (eg, pulmonary diseases). Competencies are aimed at creating a framework to ensure congruence with the APRN LACE Consensus Model, which aligns with the scope of practice for each role.[8] However, each state has the ultimate responsibility of defining the legal scope of practice for APRN roles.

In the NICU, APRNs manage a variety of diseases as allowed by applicable scope of practice laws as governed by the state. To demonstrate the differences in scope of practice for the different APRN roles in the NICU, respiratory distress will be used as an example. NNP-BCs could manage respiratory distress syndrome (RDS), bronchopulmonary dysplasia (BPD), transient tachypnea of the newborn (TTN), persistent pulmonary hypertension (PPHN), and a pneumothorax in an infant of any gestational age because the education for an NNP-BC aligns with the clinical experiences and certification received. A CPNP-AC could manage RDS in the late preterm infant, convalescing BPD, TTN, and a pneumothorax in a late preterm or term infant (but not in a preterm infant <34 weeks). A CPNP-PC could manage term and late preterm infants with TTN, or a preterm infant now corrected to term with convalescing BPD but would not manage other respiratory pathologies in the NICU. An FNP-C/FNP-BC could similarly manage TTN in term and late preterm infants and convalescing BPD, as these would fall within their scope of practice.

SUPERVISION AND COLLABORATION

At the time of this publication, 29 states and territories grant NPs full practice authority,[27] meaning that an NP can legally provide inpatient and/or outpatient management and care within their scope of practice without a supervising or collaborating physician (see Table 3: Practice Authority by State). Reduced practice authority is present in 12 states/territories and allows the NP to perform parts of their role without a supervising or

TABLE 3. Practice Authority by State

Full Practice Authority[a] (29 states)	Reduced Practice Authority[b] (12 states)	Restricted Practice Authority[c] (10 states)
Alaska	Alabama	California
Arizona	Arkansas	Georgia
Colorado	Illinois	Michigan
Connecticut	Indiana	Missouri
Delaware	Kentucky	North Carolina
District of Columbia	Louisiana	Oklahoma
	Mississippi	South Carolina
Florida	New Jersey	Tennessee
Hawaii	Ohio	Texas
Idaho	Pennsylvania	Virginia
Iowa	West Virginia	
Kansas	Wisconsin	
Maine		
Maryland		
Massachusetts		
Minnesota		
Montana		
Nebraska		
Nevada		
New Hampshire		
New Mexico		
New York		
North Dakota		
Oregon		
Rhode Island		
South Dakota		
Utah		
Vermont		
Washington		
Wyoming		

[a] Full practice authority is defined as the ability to practice without restriction to evaluation, diagnosis, management, and prescribing medications, including controlled substances.[39]
[b] Reduced practice authority includes a restriction on one or more of these elements and mandates a collaborative agreement with another health provider for the NP to practice.
[c] Restricted practice includes a restriction on one or more elements and requires supervision by another health provider for the NP to practice.

collaborating physician. Restricted practice authority constrains the NP to work with a supervising or a collaborating physician for all patient care management and is a requirement in 10 states. In usual practice, the NNP-BC and NCNS roles includes patient management and education in collaboration with a physician, usually a pediatrician or neonatologist depending on the level of care provided in the NICU although the NCNS often practiced independently.[10]

Using the acquired knowledge from pathophysiology, pharmacology, and physiology, the NNP-BC may exercise independent judgment in the assessment, diagnosis, and management of infants and in the performance of credentialed procedures, under direct or indirect supervision of a neonatologist. In 2023, the AAP published Standards for Levels of NICU Care: II, III, IV which delineated national standards for training and supervision privileged care providers, including NNPs, in NICUs. Under these standards, Level III and IV NICUs must have a neonatologist as Medical Director, and if a neonatologist is not available on-site 24/7, there should be a policy in place which defines criteria and timeframe for on-site physician presence and supervision. In addition, privileged care providers in the NICU must complete annual continuing education specific to neonatology, with credentials reviewed by the medical director at least every two years. These standards are currently being adopted in many states.

WORKFORCE DIVERSITY

Enhancing representation among neonatal providers under-represented in the workforce can help address inequities and reduce outcome disparities.[28,29] Differential neonatal care delivery can occur along a continuum of structural and process inequities such as, care in lower quality NICUs, lower likelihood to receive human milk, and less access to the benefits of innovation. Such inequities can lead to clinical complications and other outcome disparities.[30–32] When gaps in care emerge, families have reported that bias and cultural incongruence often interfere with the ability to advocate for their infants. This is commonly experienced by families of color.[33] A more diverse neonatal provider workforce could potentially help address differential patient-family experiences rooted in bias, implicit or otherwise, and mitigate real, or perceived, outcome disparities.[28]

Because APRNs need a minimum of a Master's degree to practice, successful completion of initial RN preparation at a BSN level and matriculation into graduate school is necessary. Yet, NP education has been shifting to eliminate the master's degree and prepare new NPs at the doctoral level, which could be a barrier to some applicants.[34] Barriers such as lack of financial resources, absence of access to role models, and inflexibility of program delivery can be influenced by targeted interventions to support nurses under-represented in the workforce to advance their education and practice. Policies and programs to support the success of NP students under-represented in the workforce and incentivize completion of graduate education, such as loan forgiveness or increased scholarships in underserved areas, could alter this imbalance to support broader workforce diversity.

CONCLUSION

The relative shortage of NNP-BCs and NCNSs in addition to the limitations of other providers (residents, fellows and attending staff) has created staffing challenges for many NICUs. Increased incentives for potential students (ie, loan forgiveness) and for training programs (ie, financial incentives for clinical training sites) are necessary to address this shortage. In the interim, institutions that have added CPNP-AC, CPNP-PC, and FNP-C/FNP-BC positions in the NICU need to ensure that education, training, and certification align with the population receiving care by the certification the APRN holds. The spectrum of duties performed by the neonatal APRN will vary among institutions, but a nationally defined scope of practice must remain a priority when APRNs provide care for neonatal patients. CPNP-ACs, CPNP-PCs, and FNP-C/FNP-BCs may complement the care provided by NNP-BCs and NCNSs. Their scope of practice includes late preterm, low acuity, and chronic care populations. This, in turn, allows the NNP-BC to care for higher acuity and extremely premature infants. Each of these Neonatal APRN roles requires advanced education and a master's degree (except for those who practiced prior to these requirements). Nationally recognized certification examinations and requirements for the maintenance of education also exist within each role.[35] Credentialing for practice is currently governed by individual states, and inpatient care privileges are granted by the individual institution. Each institution should develop a procedure for the initial granting and subsequent maintenance of privileges, ensuring that the proper professional credentials are in place and that nationally defined scope of practice and competencies are maintained. These procedures are best developed by the collaborative efforts of the nursing administration, APRNs, and the medical and APRN provider staff.

RECOMMENDATIONS

1. APRNs must practice within their scope of practice, which is defined by their state to ensure that education, training, and certification by a nationally recognized organization are in alignment with the provision of safe and effective care in a given patient population.[8]
2. CPNP-ACs, CPNP-PCs, and FNP-C/FNP-BCs may complement the care provided by NNP-BCs and NCNSs in the neonatal population. Their scope of practice includes late preterm, low acuity, and chronic care populations.
3. Medical care for patients in level III or IV newborn intensive care units may be provided by appropriately trained and credentialed APRNs, in collaboration with a neonatologist.
4. Medical care provided by the APRN for patients receiving level I and II care may be provided independently in collaboration with a physician with a special interest and experience in neonatal medicine, usually a pediatrician, family medicine provider, or neonatologist.
5. Determination of whether the APRN practices in collaboration with or under the direct supervision of a physician outside of the NICU setting (eg, independent billing in the newborn nusery) will be in accordance with the board of nursing regulations in the state in which the APRN is practicing.[26,35]
6. Once certified, APRNs will need to maintain their certification through continuing education and periodic demonstration of competency skills checklists and practices.[8,36]
7. The APRN should comply with hospital policy regarding credentialing and re-credentialing.[37]
8. Employers and institutions providing APRN education may consider incentives and flexible program schedules to accommodate a more diverse student and provider population to decrease the disparities present in the current neonatal medicine workforce.

LEAD AUTHORS

Lisa M. Grisham, PhD, DNP, NNP-BC
Jay P. Goldsmith, MD, FAAP
Ashley M. Lucke, MD, FAAP
Sheila M. Gephart, PhD, RN, FAAN

COMMITTEE ON FETUS AND NEWBORN, 2024–2025

Eric Eichenwald, MD, Chairperson
Namasivayam Ambalavanan, MD
Charleta Guillory, MD
Mark Hudak, MD
David Kaufman, MD
Camilia Martin, MD
Ashley Lucke, MD
Margaret Parker, MD
Arun Pramanik, MD
Kelly Wade, MD

LIAISONS

Timothy Jancelewicz, MD - AAP Section on Surgery
Michael Narvey, MD - Canadian Paediatric Society
Stacy Beck, MD - American College of Obstetricians and Gynecologists
Lisa M. Grisham, PhD, DNP, NNP-BC - National Association of Neonatal Nurses

STAFF

Jim Couto, MA

ABBREVIATIONS

AACN: American Association of Critical-Care Nurses
AAP: American Academy of Pediatrics
AANP: American Academy of Nurse Practitioners

ANCC: American Nurses Credentialing Center
ACGME: Accreditation Council for Graduate Medical Education
APRN: Advanced Practice Registered Nurse
BPD: Bronchopulmonary Dysplasia
CNS: Clinical Nurse Specialist
CNP: Certified Nurse Practitioner
CPNP-AC: Certified Pediatric Nurse Practitioner - Acute Care
CPNP-PC: Certified Pediatric Nurse Practitioner - Primary Care
DNP: Doctorate in Nursing Practice
DNV: Det Norske Veritas
EBP: evidence-based practice
FNP-BC: Family Nurse Practitioner - Board Certified
FNP-C: Family Nurse Practitioner - Certified
JC: Joint Commission
LACE: Licensure, Accreditation, Certification, & Education
LMA: laryngeal airway
NACNS: National Association of Clinical Nurse Specialists
NANN: National Association of Neonatal Nurses
NCNS: Neonatal Clinical Nurse Specialist
NICU: Neonatal Intensive Care Unit
NNP-BC: Neonatal Nurse Practitioner - Board Certified
NONPF: National Organization of Nurse Practitioner Faculties
NP: Nurse Practitioner
PhD: Doctor of Philosophy
PPHN: Persistent Pulmonary Hypertension of the Newborn
RDS: Respiratory Distress Syndrome
RN: Registered Nurse
SCN: Special Care Nursery
TTN: Transient Tachypnea of the Newborn

All policy statements from the American Academy of Pediatrics automatically expire 5 years after publication unless reaffirmed, revised, or retired at or before that time.

https://doi.org/10.1542/peds.2025-073170

REFERENCES

1. Storr G. The clinical nurse specialist: from the outside looking in. *J Adv Nurs*. 1988;13(2):265–272. PubMed doi: 10.1111/j.1365-2648.1988.tb01416.x
2. American Association of Nurse Practitioners. *NP Facts*. 2024. https://storage.aanp.org/www/documents/NPFacts.pdf?_gl=1*1kp2ht1*_gcl_au*MTg1OTQ4MzA3MC4xNzA5MzI1ODg2
3. Snapp B, Moore TA, Wallman C, Staebler S. 2020 Neonatal Nurse Practitioner Workforce Survey: An Executive Summary. *Adv Neonatal Care*. 2021;21(3):242–246. PubMed doi: 10.1097/ANC.0000000000000903
4. Gamber RA, Blonsky H, McDowell M, Lakshminrusimha S. Declining birth rates, increasing maternal age and neonatal intensive care unit admissions. *J Perinatol*. 2024;44(2):203–208. PubMed doi: 10.1038/s41372-023-01834-x
5. Pressler JL, Kenner CA. The NNP/DNP shortage: transforming neonatal nurse practitioners into DNPs. *J Perinat Neonatal Nurs*. 2009;23(3):272–278. PubMed doi: 10.1097/JPN.0b013e3181b0bd79
6. American Academy of Pediatrics. Advanced practice registered nurse: role, preparation, and scope of practice. *Pediatrics*. 2014;134(2):e619–e619. doi: 10.1542/peds.2014-1390
7. National Association of Neonatal Nurses. *Education standards and curriculum guidelines for neonatal nurse practitioner programs*. 2017. http://nann.org/uploads/2017_NNP_Education_Standards_completed_FINAL.pdf
8. APRN Consensus Work Group & the National Council of State Boards of Nursing APRN Advisory Committee. *Consensus model for APRN regulation: Licensure, accreditation, certification & education*. 2008. https://www.ncsbn.org/Consensus_Model_Report.pdf
9. National Task Force on the Guidelines for Clinical Nurse Specialist Education. *Criteria for the Evaluation of Clinical Nurse Specialist Master's, Practice Doctorate, and Post-Graduate Certificate Educational Programs*. 2011. https://nacns.org/wp-content/uploads/2016/11/CNSEducationCriteria.pdf
10. National Association of Clinical Nurse Specialists. *Statement on Clinical Nurse Specialist Practice and Education*. 2019. https://nacns.org/resources/practice-and-cns-role/cns-competencies/
11. Staebler S, Meier SR, Bagwell G, Conway-Orgel M. The Future of Neonatal Advanced Practice Registered Nurse Practice: White Paper. *Adv Neonatal Care*. 2016;16(1):8–14. PubMed doi: 10.1097/ANC.0000000000000243
12. Edwardson T, Irvin K. Key players in collaboration: clinical nurse manager and clinical nurse specialist. *Nurs Manage*. 2013;44(6):40–46. PubMed doi: 10.1097/01.NUMA.0000428201.37260.c9
13. National Association of Neonatal Nurse Practitioners. *Curriculum guidelines and education competencies for neonatal*

nurse practitioner programs. 2023. https://nann.org/uploads/About/PositionPDFS/NNP_Curriculum_Guidelines_and_Education_Competencies_042523_Final.pdf

14. National Task Force. *Standards for quality nurse practitioner education, A report of the national task force on quality nurse practitioner education, 6th Edition.* 2022. https://cdn.ymaws.com/www.nonpf.org/resource/resmgr/2022/ntfs_/ntfs_final.pdf
15. National Council of State Boards of Nursing (NCSBN). Guidelines for grandfathering APRNs by endorsement. Accessed May 14th, 2022, https://www.ncsbn.org/Grandfathering_Guidelines_(3).pdf
16. National Organization of Nurse Practitioner Faculties. *Nurse practitioner core competencies content.* 2017.
17. National Association of Pediatric Nurse Practitioners. NAPNAP position statement on the acute care pediatric nurse practitioner. *J Pediatr Health Care.* 2011;25(3):e11–e12. PubMed doi: 10.1016/j.pedhc.2010.12.004
18. Pediatric Nursing Certification Board. Certified Pediatric Nurse Practitioner – Acute Care (CPNP-AC®) Detailed Exam Content Outline. https://www.pncb.org/sites/default/files/resources/CPNP-AC_Exam_Content_Outline_June_2019.pdf
19. National Task Force on Quality Nurse Practitioner Education. *2016 Criteria for Evaluation of Nurse Practitioner Programs.* 2016. https://cdn.ymaws.com/www.nonpf.org/resource/resmgr/Docs/EvalCriteria2016Final.pdf
20. Pediatric Nursing Certification Board. *Statement regarding nurse practitioner students and direct care clinical hours.* 2020:1–2.
21. National Association of Pediatric Nurse Practitioners. NAPNAP Position Statement on Age Parameters for Pediatric Nurse Practitioner Practice. *J Pediatr Health Care.* 2014;28(4):A15–A16. doi: 10.1016/j.pedhc.2014.03.001
22. Pediatric Nursing Certification Board. *Certified Pediatric Nurse Practitioner – Primary Care (CPNP-PC®).* Exam Detailed Content Outline; 2018.
23. American Academy of Nurse Practitioners Certification Board. Family Nurse Practitioner (FNP). https://www.aanpcert.org/certs/fnp
24. American Association of Colleges of Nursing. *The Essentials: Core Competencies for Professional Nursing Education.* 2021. https://www.aacnnursing.org/portals/42/academicnursing/pdf/essentials-2021.pdf
25. National Organization of Nurse Practitioner Faculties. NONPF NP Role Core Competencies Table. Accessed October 23, 2022, https://cdn.ymaws.com/www.nonpf.org/resource/resmgr/competencies/20220825_nonpf_np_role_core_.pdf
26. Keels EL, Goldsmith JP, Cummings JJ, et al; COMMITTEE ON FETUS AND NEWBORN. Neonatal Provider Workforce. *Pediatrics.* 2019;144(6):e20193147. PubMed doi: 10.1542/peds.2019-3147
27. NurseJournal.org. Nurse practitioner practice authority: A stat-by-state guide. Updated April 21, 2022. Accessed June 3, 2022, https://nursejournal.org/nurse-practitioner/np-practice-authority-by-state/
28. Poghosyan L, Carthon JMB. The Untapped Potential of the Nurse Practitioner Workforce in Reducing Health Disparities. *Policy Polit Nurs Pract.* 2017;18(2):84–94. PubMed doi: 10.1177/1527154417721189
29. Greenwood BN, Hardeman RR, Huang L, Sojourner A. Physician-patient racial concordance and disparities in birthing mortality for newborns. *Proc Natl Acad Sci U S A.* 2020;117(35):21194–21200. PubMed doi: 10.1073/pnas.1913405117
30. Goldstein GP, Pai VV, Liu J, et al. Racial/ethnic disparities and human milk use in necrotizing enterocolitis. *Pediatr Res.* 2020;88(S1)(suppl 1):3–9. PubMed doi: 10.1038/s41390-020-1073-5
31. Horbar JD, Edwards EM, Greenberg LT, et al. Racial Segregation and Inequality in the Neonatal Intensive Care Unit for Very Low-Birth-Weight and Very Preterm Infants. *JAMA Pediatr.* 2019;173(5):455–461. PubMed doi: 10.1001/jamapediatrics.2019.0241
32. Sigurdson K, Mitchell B, Liu J, et al. Racial/Ethnic Disparities in Neonatal Intensive Care: A Systematic Review. *Pediatrics.* 2019;144(2):e20183114. PubMed doi: 10.1542/peds.2018-3114
33. Sigurdson K, Profit J, Dhurjati R, et al. Former NICU Families Describe Gaps in Family-Centered Care. *Qual Health Res.* 2020;30(12):1861–1875. PubMed doi: 10.1177/1049732320932897
34. Phillips J, Julion WA, Dallas C, et al. Pursuing a doctorate in nursing: Implications for underrepresented minority nurses. *J Prof Nurs.* 2022;39:117–121. PubMed doi: 10.1016/j.profnurs.2022.01.008
35. Shugerman RP, Rimsza ME, Basco WT, Hotaling AJ, Sigrest TD, Simon FA; Committee on Pediatric Workforce. Scope of practice issues in the delivery of pediatric health care. *Pediatrics.* 2013;131(6):1211–1216. PubMed doi: 10.1542/peds.2013-0943
36. National Certification Corporation. 2022 Candidate Guide Neonatal Nurse Practitioner NNP-BC®. https://www.nccwebsite.org/content/documents/cms/nnp-candidate_guide.pdf
37. Bellini S. State of the state: NNP program update 2013. *Adv Neonatal Care.* 2013;13(5):346–348. PubMed doi: 10.1097/ANC.0b013e3182a35a7e
38. National Organization of Nurse Practitioner Faculties. *Population-Focused nurse practitioner competencies: Family/across the lifespan, neonatal, acute care pediatric, primary care pediatric, psychiatric-mental health, & women's health/gender-related.* 2013. https://www.aacnnursing.org/Portals/42/AcademicNursing/pdf/Population-Focused-NP-Competencies-2013.pdf
39. American Association of Nurse Practitioners. State practice environment. https://www.aanp.org/advocacy/state/state-practice-environment

Atopic Dermatitis: Update on Skin-Directed Management

- *Clinical Report*

CLINICAL REPORT Guidance for the Clinician in Rendering Pediatric Care

American Academy of Pediatrics

DEDICATED TO THE HEALTH OF ALL CHILDREN™

Atopic Dermatitis: Update on Skin-Directed Management: Clinical Report

Jennifer J. Schoch, MD, FAAD, FAAP,[1] Katelyn R. Anderson, MD, FAAP, FAAD,[2,3] Amie E. Jones, MD, FAAP,[3] Megha M. Tollefson, MD, FAAP, FAAD,[2,3] and the Section on Dermatology

abstract

Atopic dermatitis affects 20% to 25% of children and has significant impact on quality of life of patients and families. Recent studies of the pathogenesis of AD highlight the interplay between a defective skin barrier, immune dysfunction, and the cutaneous microbiome. Standard of care for AD treatment includes topical corticosteroids for active disease and moisturization to repair the barrier defect. Emerging treatments include dupilumab and Janus kinase (JAK) inhibitors. Reduction of triggers and proactive treatment with topical corticosteroids and/or topical calcineurin inhibitors can reduce flares. Treatment plans should be clear and as simple as possible to maximize adherence.

[1]Department of Dermatology, University of Florida, Gainesville, Florida; [2]Department of Dermatology, Mayo Clinic, Rochester, Minnesota; and [3]Department of Pediatric and Adolescent Medicine, Mayo Clinic, Rochester, Minnesota

Corresponding Author: Megha M. Tollefson, MD, FAAP, FAAD. Email: tollefson.megha@mayo.edu

Dr Schoch drafted the initial manuscript, critically reviewed the manuscript for important intellectual content, and reviewed and revised the manuscript. Dr Anderson drafted the initial manuscript and reviewed and revised the manuscript. Dr Jones reviewed and revised the manuscript. Dr Tollefson conceptualized and designed the study, drafted the initial manuscript, and reviewed and revised the manuscript. All authors approved the final manuscript as submitted and agree to be accountable for all aspects of the work.

FINANCIAL/CONFLICT OF INTEREST DISCLOSURE: Dr Jennifer Schoch has disclosed a financial relationship with Janssen Biotech as an advisory board member and has a family member with a financial relationship with Exactech as a consultant. Any other disclosures were reviewed and determined not relevant to the work related to "Atopic Dermatitis: Update on Skin-Directed Management." Disclosures are reviewed and mitigated through a Conflict-of-Interest process that consists of reviewing pertinent information which is then used to decide what action is required to maintain content integrity. There may be instances where no action is necessary. This process has been approved by the AAP Board of Directors.

To cite: Schoch JJ, Anderson KR, Jones AE, et al; American Academy of Pediatrics, Section on Dermatology. Atopic Dermatitis: Update on Skin-Directed Management: Clinical Report. *Pediatrics.* 2025;155(6):e2025071812

INTRODUCTION

Atopic dermatitis (AD) is a common chronic skin condition often seen in children and adolescents. Its prevalence has been increasing in industrialized countries, including the United States and may reach as high as 25% in some populations.[1,2] The number of health care visits for AD in the United States is also increasing; however, the burden of those visits is disproportionately on general pediatricians and other pediatric primary care providers, in part because of lack of access to subspecialists.[3,4] Outpatient primary care visits for AD have nearly doubled over the last 20 years, while during that same period of time, outpatient dermatology visits for AD have decreased. Children account for most of these visits, with approximately one-third of visits being for children younger than 5 years.

Many pediatricians may not feel comfortable treating AD or other dermatologic conditions. Studies show that most pediatricians believe that their residency training in the management of AD was "enough to get by or inadequate."[5] In addition, variability in practice recommendations, especially regarding bathing, moisturizing, topical medications, and the role of food allergies in AD, can lead to frustration for both pediatricians and families. Because the professional competence of the physician treating AD has been shown to be an important determinant of treatment satisfaction, improving primary care provider comfort with treating pediatric AD is of paramount importance.

STATEMENT OF THE PROBLEM

Since the American Academy of Pediatrics published its initial clinical report on AD in 2014,[6] the landscape of pediatric AD has been rapidly changing, particularly as it relates to comorbidities and treatment options. This clinical report reviews pediatric AD and provides an up-to-date approach to skin-directed management that incorporates recent advances, including mental health and quality of life in children with AD, implications of the Learning Early About Peanut allergy (LEAP) trial for children with AD, and emerging topical therapies. This information will allow pediatricians and other pediatric primary care clinicians to provide effective and up-to-date care for most children with AD.

CLINICAL FEATURES AND DIAGNOSIS

The diagnosis of AD remains primarily clinical, based on the presence of characteristic features (Table 1).[6] Major clinical features include relapsing and remitting dermatitis that is pruritic, with onset of the disease usually occurring before 1 year of age. A family history of atopic dermatitis and/or a personal or family history of other atopic conditions may be supportive. Erythema, scaling, excoriations, and lichenification are often present in typical plaques of AD (Figure 1). In patients with darkly-pigmented skin, erythema may be more subtle (Figure 2), while dyspigmentation and follicular eczema may be more prominent. The distribution of the eczematous plaques varies with age, with cheeks, trunk, and extremities being the most characteristic areas of involvement in infancy (Figure 3), flexures being most characteristic in childhood, and hands and feet being most characteristic in teenagers and young adults.[7] It is important to consider other skin conditions that may mimic AD, including scabies, contact dermatitis, psoriasis, and seborrheic dermatitis. In young infants, there may be an overlap of concurrent seborrheic dermatitis and AD, consisting of characteristic features of both conditions.[8] Generally, tests such as laboratory testing and skin biopsies are not needed nor helpful in confirming the diagnosis of AD but may be useful when alternate diagnoses are being considered.

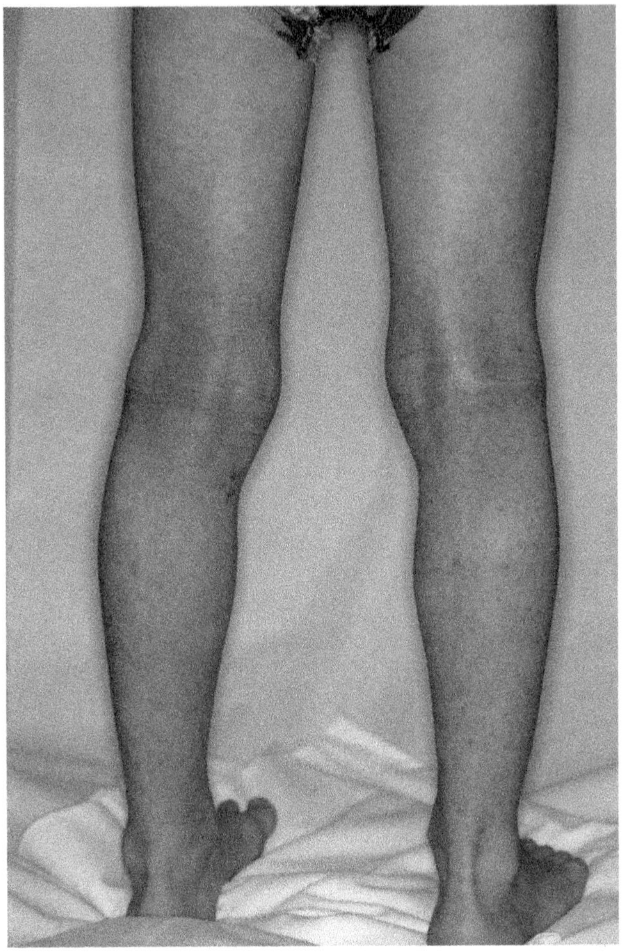

FIGURE 1.
Poorly-defined erythema in the popliteal fossae, a typical distribution for pediatric atopic dermatitis.

TABLE 1. Clinical Features in Atopic Dermatitis

Major Clinical Features	Minor Clinical Features
Itching/pruritus	Early age of onset
Typical dermatitis with a chronic/relapsing history	Dry skin/xerosis
Patient or family member(s) with atopy	Keratosis pilaris
Typical distribution and age-specific patterns	Ichthyosis vulgaris
	Lip dermatitis
	Hand eczema
	Lichenification
	Elevated IgE level
	Itching with sweating
	Recurrent infections
	Pityriasis alba
	Dermatographism
	Eye symptoms: cataracts, keratoconus, inflammation

Black and Hispanic children are disproportionally affected by AD. Black infants are more likely to develop AD.[2] Compared with white children, eczema severity is increased in both Black and Hispanic children,[9] and both groups are more likely to miss school because of AD.[10] Black and Hispanic children are also more likely to receive medical care for AD in the primary care and emergency

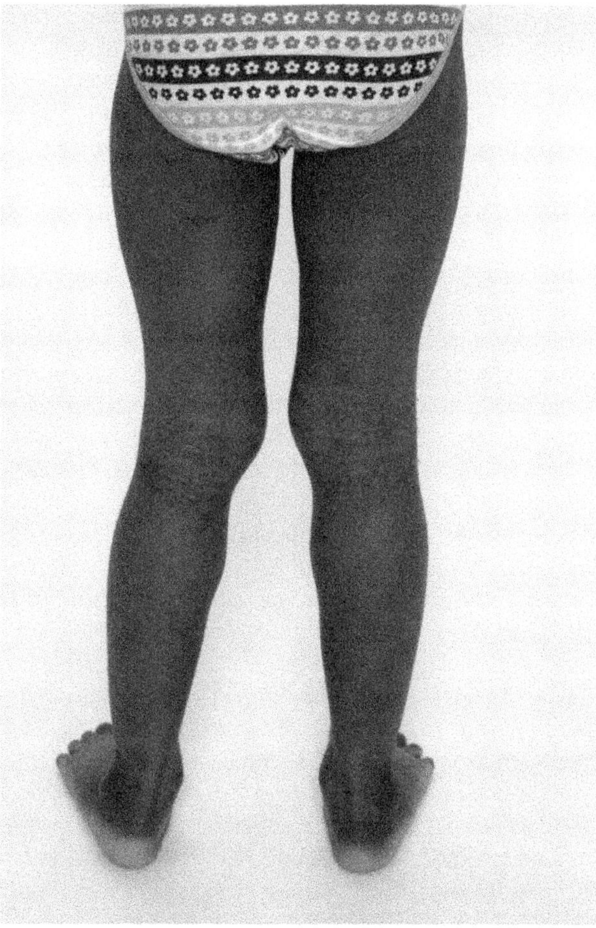

FIGURE 2.
Erythema in the popliteal fossae and posterior legs is deeper red and less prominent in darker skin compared to lighter skin; lichenification and dyspigmentation are apparent.

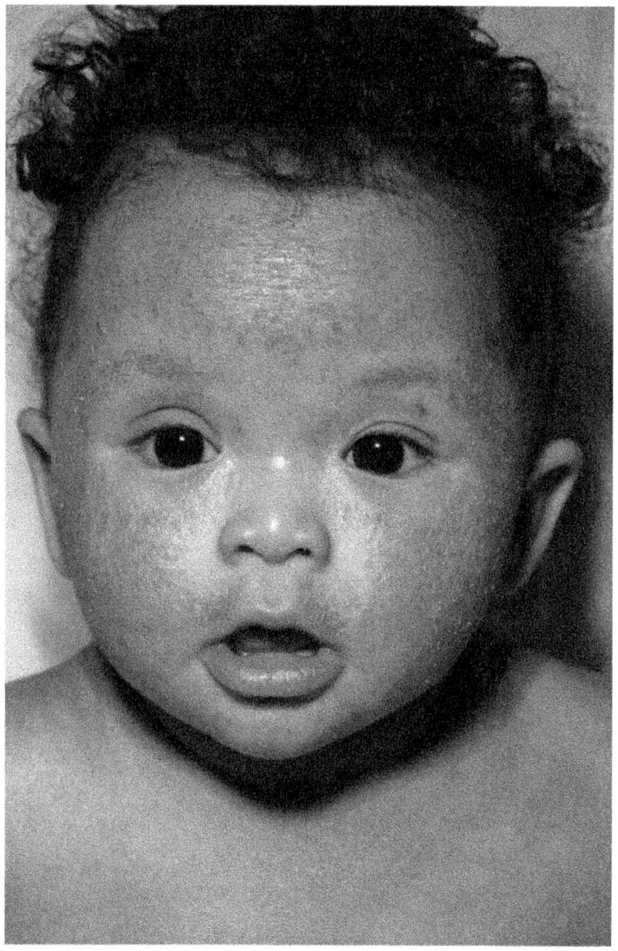

FIGURE 3.
Prominent cheek involvement is typical of infantile atopic dermatitis.

settings, although Black children are significantly less likely than white children to be referred to a dermatologist for poorly controlled AD.[11]

PATHOGENESIS AND NATURAL HISTORY

The pathogenesis of AD is complex and multifactorial, involving an interplay of genetic predisposition, skin barrier disruption, environmental triggers, and immune dysfunction. Skin barrier dysfunction is central to the pathophysiology of AD.[12,13] While early studies identified increased stratum corneum lipids in Black patients compared with patients of other races, more recent and larger studies have shown lower ceramide levels in Black patients compared with white and Asian patients.[14–16] Studies examining racial differences in transepidermal water loss and stratum corneum hydration are conflicting.[15,17–20] Differences in skin barrier physiology may explain morphologic variations in the appearance of AD between patients of different races. However, it is unclear whether the disparity in AD severity between racial groups is explained by differences in the skin barrier or attributable to contextual differences including socioeconomic, health care, and/or environmental factors.[14,21] Loss-of-function mutations in the gene that encodes filaggrin (*FLG*) have also been found in those with AD and other atopic disorders, likely attributable to impact on the function of the skin barrier. Inheritance of this loss-of-function mutation increases the risk of developing AD and allergic disorders, potentially by allowing the entry of external antigens, which then trigger a systemic immune response.[13] Children of parents with a history of atopic disease have an increased risk of developing AD.[22]

The most recent advances in understanding the pathogenesis of AD have been regarding the accompanying complex immune dysfunction, particularly the Th2 immune response and its impact on AD. The initial immune dysfunction triggered in AD has been identified in the Th2 immune response, which includes the cytokines IL-4 and IL-13, both of which are involved in the development of AD.[23] This Th2-mediated inflammation continues in chronic lesions of AD, along with upregulation of Th1 cytokines such as interferon gamma.[24] In addition, the Th2 immune response is involved in driving the synthesis of immunoglobulin E (IgE); however, IgE is not consistently elevated in patients with AD.[25] Recent therapeutic advances have focused on targets along the Th2 immune response.

In the majority of children, AD starts before 1 year of age and before 5 years of age in nearly all children.[1] Many will outgrow the disease, but the specific predictors of prognosis are not yet understood. A prospective study in a cohort of children followed longitudinally indicated that approximately 60% of children who developed AD by the age of 2 years had resolution of their symptoms by 4 years of age.[26] Those who have mutations in the filaggrin gene are more likely to have persistent disease.[27]

COMORBITIES

The effects of AD extend beyond the skin, influencing quality of life and mental health. AD impacts quality of life in multiple domains in affected children and their families.[28] Itching, treatment burden, sleep, embarrassment related to appearance of the skin, and ability to participate in sports have the most bearing on quality of life.[29] Not surprisingly, impact on quality of life correlates with severity of disease. AD also affects mental health and has been linked to depression and anxiety in both patients and parents.[30–32] Cognitive behavioral therapy may be effective in reducing self-reported symptoms of eczema and anxiety.[33]

Sleep disturbance affects approximately two-thirds of pediatric patients with AD, and disturbed sleep is associated with increased depression, anxiety, and inattention.[34] Lower nocturnal melatonin secretion was also associated with sleep disturbance in children with AD.[35] A randomized, double-blinded, placebo-controlled trial of melatonin in children 6 to 12 years old demonstrated subjective improvement in AD severity and sleep quality.[36] Behavioral therapy, including progressive muscle relaxation and optimization of sleep hygiene, can serve as an effective adjunct in the care of patients with AD.[37]

Although sedating antihistamines have historically been used as adjunctive treatment of eczema, there is limited evidence to support their efficacy in the treatment of AD.[38] Children with AD have increased attention-deficit symptoms compared with healthy controls, which have been linked to sedating antihistamine use. It is unclear whether there is a causal relationship between early antihistamine exposure and increased attention deficit, or whether antihistamine use is a surrogate for more severe AD or poor sleep quality.[39] Infantile exposure to H1-antihistamines has been linked to development of attention-deficit/hyperactivity disorder (ADHD).[40] Nonsedating second-generation antihistamines are not associated with the same side effect profile as first-generation antihistamines and have been shown to be safe to use long-term, particularly in patients who also have comorbid environmental allergies.[41]

AD has been viewed as the first step in the "atopic march," whereby the defective skin barrier leads to immune sensitization to antigens, resulting in food allergy, asthma, and allergic rhinitis.[42] Although parents may suspect food allergies as a cause of AD, food-induced AD is rare. Instead, the conditions tend to co-occur in patients with atopic disease, and up to 40% of children with AD develop food allergy.[42] Food allergy typically manifests with IgE-mediated hypersensitivity, with symptoms including urticaria and angioedema. In the rare patient in whom food allergy drives eczematous dermatitis (delayed-type hypersensitivity), an immediate-type hypersensitivity reaction has preceded it.[43] Food allergy testing should only be pursued in children with a history consistent with immediate-type allergy, because more than half of children with AD will have high food-specific IgE concentrations (even without true food allergy).[44] Overemphasis on food allergy as a cause of AD leads to unnecessary, and potentially dangerous, elimination diets[45] and may result in intolerance of previously tolerated foods.[43] Avoidance diets should only be recommended in patients who have failed a diagnostic food challenge. Treatment should instead focus on skin-directed therapies.

Increasing rates of food allergy prompted the hypothesis that decreased exposure to antigens leads to decreased immune tolerance and, thus, increased sensitization (the "hygiene hypothesis"). The Learning Early About Peanut allergy (LEAP) trial demonstrated that early exposure to peanut in a cohort of at-risk infants reduced the risk of peanut allergy compared with a control group.[46] The effect was persistent after 12 months of peanut avoidance, strengthening the argument for induction of immune tolerance via early exposure to the antigen.[47] This landmark study led to changes in clinical practice, emphasizing early antigen exposure to the gastrointestinal tract (rather than through the skin) to induce tolerance. New guidelines from the National Institute of Allergy and Infectious Disease (NIAID) for early peanut introduction[48] relied heavily on the results of the LEAP trial. In these guidelines, infants are stratified based on their risk for peanut allergy, which is determined by the presence and severity of AD as well as the presence of egg allergy. In the highest-risk group—infants with severe eczema and/or egg allergy—a peanut-specific IgE and/or skin prick test is recommended before introduction of peanut; if infants do not show evidence of sensitization, then peanut introduction is recommended at 4 to 6 months of age. Infants with mild to moderate eczema comprise the moderate-risk group, and introduction of peanut-containing foods is recommended around 6 months of age to reduce the risk of peanut allergy. In low-risk infants (infants without eczema or any food allergy), peanut-containing foods may be introduced according to family preference.

TREATMENT PRINCIPLES

Successful treatment of AD revolves around the triad of maintenance skin care, topical anti-inflammatory medications, and avoidance of triggers. For most patients with mild to moderate AD, following these treatment principles results in good disease control. However, for a subset of patients with severe or treatment-refractory AD, systemic therapies such as phototherapy, immunosuppressants, or biologic medications are warranted, necessitating referral to a pediatric subspecialist. It is worth noting that many cases of perceived treatment failure are attributable to misunderstanding of the recommended treatment plan or difficulty in adhering to the treatment regimen. Barriers to adherence include fear of adverse medication effects, misunderstanding of the chronic nature of the disease, and lack of time and/or resources needed to follow treatment recommendations. Educating families about the expected disease course and safety of treatments can build a therapeutic foundation of trust and understanding. Individual patient circumstances, including socioeconomic status, work/time constraints, language preference, cultural practices, and beliefs, may all contribute to treatment adherence and should be considered when designing a treatment regimen. Online resources may help increase patient and family engagement.[49] The use of a written action plan has been shown to increase parent understanding of AD treatment and may positively impact patient outcomes.[50] Older children and adolescents can also participate in action plan development as a way to support chronic disease understanding, self-management, and treatment adherence.[51] Additionally, physicians have found action plans to be useful in their own understanding and management of AD.[52] Therefore, consideration should be given to the use of a written AD action plan, such as the sample shown in Figure 4.

SAMPLE DERMATITIS ACTION PLAN

1. Bath daily in lukewarm water for up to 10-15 minutes. Use a gentle, fragrance-free soap or non-soap cleanser to soiled areas only. Your doctor may recommend bleach baths.

   Bleach baths:
   ☐ In some cases, dilute bleach baths may be helpful. You may add ¼ cup of household bleach for every half bathtub full of water. Please do bleach baths ___ times per week.

2. After patting skin dry with a clean towel, apply prescription medications to any active areas of dermatitis (rough, red, or itchy), followed by a cream or ointment-based moisturizer over the entire body.

   Prescription medications:
   ☐ Apply ______________ to affected areas of the face, neck, armpits, and groin.
   Apply ______________ to affected areas of the body.

3. For severe flares, apply wet wraps after medications and moisturizer.

   Wet wrap instructions:
   ☐ After applying prescription medications and moisturizer, soak a pair of cotton pajamas (as close to 100% cotton as possible) in warm tap water, then wring out until damp. Put on pajamas. Cover with robe or extra clothing to keep warm during treatment. Take off wet pajamas after recommended amount of time (_______ minutes/hours), and rub in any residual topical medications or moisturizer.

   ☐ Your doctor may recommend adding a small amount of distilled white vinegar to the tap water (1/8 cup vinegar to every 2 cups tap water) used to dampen the pajamas to help treat and prevent infection.

4. Repeat application of medications and moisturizer, with or without wet wraps, a second time during the day.

5. For maintenance and prevention, continue daily baths and moisturization even when dermatitis is not active. Your doctor may recommend proactive treatment.

   Proactive treatment:
   ☐ Apply ________________ on typical problem areas 2-3x per week before bed/after bathing even when skin is clear.

6. Restart prescription medications when eczema flares.

FIGURE 4.
Sample Atopic Dermatitis Action Plan

Maintenance Skin Care

The mainstay of preventive care in AD is moisturization. Moisturizers work by enhancing the skin barrier to protect from allergens, pathogens, and injury while simultaneously reducing transepidermal water loss. Regular use of moisturizers has been shown to reduce the frequency of flares in AD and the amount of topical corticosteroid needed to control disease.[53] Ideally, moisturizers should be applied liberally to the entire body skin surface at least daily in patients with AD, especially after a bath, shower, or hand washing. Younger children should be encouraged to assist in the application process, empowering them to help manage their skin disease. To increase adherence to the treatment plan and include adolescents in decision making, adolescents should be encouraged to trial various emollients and choose one that they feel most comfortable applying to their skin.

Moisturizers are emulsions of oil and water and can be categorized based on water content as lotions (higher water content) or creams (lower water content). Moisturizer selection should consider cost, accessibility, and tolerability. Evidence has not strongly supported any specific brand or formulation over another. In general, moisturizers should be fragrance free and thick in texture with low water content (creams). If a stinging sensation is encountered, ointments such as petrolatum may be substituted to allow for greater patient comfort. Although emollients have also historically been used as bath additives, evidence does not support their efficacy in reducing severity of skin disease in patients with AD.[54]

Although moisturizers are beneficial in patients with AD, recent data suggest that they may not have a role in *preventing* the disease. This finding is in contrast to previously published studies that suggested a preventive benefit.[55,56] In the BEEP (Barrier Enhancement for Eczema Protection) and PreventADALL (Preventing Atopic Dermatitis and Allergy in Children) studies, two large randomized controlled trials of prophylactic emollients, there was no statistically significant change in incidence of AD in those who were treated with daily emollient vs those that used only routine infant skin care.[57,58] In the preterm infant population, application of petrolatum-based ointments in the neonatal intensive care unit has been associated with increased rates of candidemia and coagulase-negative *Staphylococcus* infection.[59–61] Together, these data suggest that there is currently no role for recommendation of daily emollient application to all infants, because doing so does not appear to prevent AD.[62]

Historically, bleach (sodium hypochlorite) baths have been considered part of maintenance skin care for patients with AD. However, the research regarding the efficacy of dilute bleach baths has been conflicting. Patients with AD have higher rates of skin surface colonization with *Staphylococcus aureus* than their non-AD counterparts, with increased density of *S aureus* associated with greater severity of AD.[63–65] Bleach theoretically may help reduce the skin surface colonization of *S aureus* without inducing bacterial resistance. One systematic review and meta-analysis concluded that, although dilute bleach baths were helpful in decreasing AD severity, they showed no statistical advantage over water baths alone,[66] whereas another review found slight improvement in AD with bleach baths.[67] Dilute bleach baths appear to be safe and relatively well-tolerated, although some patients may experience transient burning, stinging, or xerosis. Thus, dilute unscented bleach baths may be recommended as an adjunct in the care of AD, because they are unlikely to cause harm; however, further well-designed studies are needed to determine their efficacy.

Frequency of bathing has been a controversial topic in AD, and parents often receive conflicting advice from different providers. Although good quality studies are generally lacking, studies favor more frequent bathing,[68,69] with daily baths being the most common recommendation made by pediatric dermatologists.[70] In general, it is reasonable to recommend frequent, short baths with lukewarm water and gentle cleansers. Emphasis should be given to the importance of moisturizer application immediately after the bath.

Environmental triggers may precipitate or worsen an AD flare and should, therefore, be avoided if possible. These include low humidity, skin irritants such as harsh soaps or detergents, and contact allergens. Although the data are conflicting,[71] some studies find contact allergies to be more common in people with AD than in those without atopic disease.[72,73] Patients with AD may become sensitized to various allergens via application of topical products to non-intact skin. Although not necessary for all patients with atopic disease, it is reasonable to consider patch testing in patients with dermatitis that is unresponsive to usual treatment measures, extends beyond the typical skin locations, or is temporally flared after application of a specific product. As a preventative measure, patients with AD should be counseled to avoid products with added fragrance, dyes, or essential oils, as these do little to treat AD and are known potential contact allergens.

Topical Anti-inflammatory Medications

For decades, topical corticosteroids have been the standard of care for treatment of AD.[74] Despite concerns about potential side effects, topical corticosteroids have long been an effective and safe treatment for eczema when used with appropriate supervision.[75] A common misconception about topical steroids in the treatment of eczema is that steroids discolor or bleach the skin. Although rare cases of hypopigmentation secondary to intralesional corticosteroid use have been reported,[76] typical use of topical steroids does not alter skin pigmentation. Instead, the skin affected by the AD can be lightened either because of the inflammation associated with the eczema and/or tanning of the skin around the actively inflamed eczema patch. Hypopigmentation is, thus, a secondary feature of the eczema itself rather than an adverse effect of the topical medications.

Topical steroids are available in a variety of vehicles, including cream, ointment, solution, foam, oil, and spray. Potency of topical corticosteroids is ranked from class I (superpotent) to class VII (least potent). In some instances, the vehicle affects the potency of the corticosteroid. For example, mometasone 0.1% cream is a "mid-strength" topical steroid, and mometasone 0.1% ointment is classified as "potent."[77] In addition to potency, body site should be considered when selecting topical corticosteroids in the treatment of AD. For example, a solution, foam, or scalp oil may be preferable for treatment of scalp dermatitis rather than a cream.

Wet wrap therapy, with or without topical corticosteroids, is a useful adjunctive therapy in patients with moderate-severe or focally recalcitrant AD. Wet wraps are performed by applying topical corticosteroid or emollient to affected areas and then covering the area with damp wet wraps (typically cotton pajamas, tight-fitting clothing, or gauze wraps). Distilled white vinegar is sometimes added to the wet wrap as an antimicrobial. If desired for comfort, an additional dry layer of clothing or a blanket may be applied on top of the wet wraps. Wet wraps may be left on for a minimum of 20 to 30 minutes or as long as overnight. The proposed mechanism of wet wrap therapy is that the occlusion and moisture of the wrap enhances penetration of the topical steroid.[78]

Topical calcineurin inhibitors (TCIs), tacrolimus 0.03% and 0.1% ointments, and pimecrolimus 1% cream, are steroid-sparing topical immunosuppressive agents that are approved as second-line therapy in the treatment of atopic dermatitis (for children 2 years and older). Both tacrolimus and pimecrolimus are effective in the treatment of mild to moderate AD, although tacrolimus is more effective than pimecrolimus.[79] However, TCIs are rarely effective in cases of AD that are recalcitrant to topical steroids. TCIs have a favorable side effect profile in that there is no concern for striae, atrophy, or adrenal suppression. They are particularly useful in patients with AD in locations where concern for long-term topical steroid side effects is highest, such as the face and eyelids. However, TCI use is associated with burning and pruritus, primarily in the first few days of use. This, combined with the cost of these medications and US Food and Drug Administration (FDA) approval down to only 2 years of age, may limit use of TCIs for some patients.

Concern has been raised regarding the safety of TCIs because of their immunosuppressive properties. The FDA issued a "black box" warning for TCIs because of the observation that laboratory animals exposed to high systemic doses of calcineurin inhibitors developed malignancies and because of isolated reports of melanoma and lymphoma in adults who were using TCIs.[80] Further studies did not identify an association between TCIs and malignancy risk, although there may be a baseline increased lymphoma risk in those with more severe AD.[81,82] A recent study found no increased long-term cancer risk in children who used topical tacrolimus for AD.[83] Similarly reassuring findings have been reported regarding the use of pimecrolimus in children with AD.[84] Thus, TCIs are believed to be extremely safe in the management of pediatric AD, with little evidence to support increased risk of malignancy.

There is increasing interest in and demand for nonsteroidal topical therapies in the treatment of AD because of concerns and perceptions regarding potential side effects. The first nonsteroidal/non-TCI topical medication to be approved to treat AD was topical crisaborole 2%. Crisaborole is a phosphodiesterase (PDE) 4 inhibitor that has been shown to be safe and have some efficacy in the treatment of mild to moderate AD in patients 3 months or older.[85] The effect, however, was modest when compared with vehicle; only 32.8% with improvement of AD in the crisaborole group vs 25.4% improvement rate in the vehicle group.[86] Because crisaborole has not been compared head-to-head against topical steroids or TCIs, the relative efficacy is difficult to determine, although it appears to be considerably lower than either of those medications. Thus, because of lower relative efficacy, cost, and a higher prevalence of side effects of application site burning and stinging, use of crisaborole in the treatment of AD is somewhat limited.

There are multiple emerging topical therapies that have the potential for safe and efficacious use in the treatment of AD. Topical ruxolitinib, a topical Janus kinase (JAK) inhibitor, was approved for use in people 12 years and older in 2022, although cost currently limits access for many patients. In addition, alternative PDE4 inhibitors and medications with other mechanisms, such as aryl hydrocarbon receptor agonists, are currently being developed and studied. It is likely that the number of topical medications available to treat AD will increase in the coming years.

Proactive Treatment

Standard dogma in the treatment of AD has been to use topical prescription medications to areas of active, eczema-involved skin only. However, recent evidence indicates a role for so-called "proactive" treatment, especially in children who experience recurrent flares at the same body site. This strategy has been both efficacious and cost-effective in patients with moderate to severe AD. Twice weekly treatment with topical tacrolimus to areas of previously recurrent AD was found to reduce the number of AD flares and to increase the time between flares, with potential cost-savings.[87,88] In addition, topical steroids used in proactive fashion in children with moderate to severe AD led to improved disease severity and quality of life scores when compared with similar children not using topical steroids proactively.[89] This strategy should be considered in children with recurrent flares in similar locations of involvement. Specific medication and dosing may depend on individual characteristics, such as patient's age, location of disease, and cost.

Probiotics

Spurred in part by the Human Microbiome Project initiative sponsored by the National Institutes of Health,[90] there has been an increased emphasis on the interplay between the human microbiome and disease. The microbiome includes the bacteria, viruses, fungi, and other sources of external genetic material present on the host. Researchers hypothesize that inflammatory diseases, such as AD, are caused or sustained by dysbiosis, resulting in a proinflammatory state.[91] A randomized controlled trial of children with AD treated with 12 weeks of oral probiotics demonstrated reduced severity of AD and reduction in topical corticosteroid use compared with children who received a placebo.[92] However the evidence for oral probiotics in *prevention* of AD is conflicting, and administration of probiotics to a group of preterm infants did not result in reduction of AD incidence.[93] Larger prospective placebo-controlled trials are needed to better understand the complex relationship between manipulation of the gut microbiome via probiotics and AD.

Systemic Treatment

When skin-directed therapies fail to adequately control AD, systemic therapies are considered. Pediatricians should consider referral to subspecialists when a patient's AD is not controlled with the use of topical corticosteroids for flares, plus proactive treatment to reduce flares. Until recently, oral immunosuppressants were the only options but were suboptimal in the treatment of AD, with modest efficacy and considerable risk of side effects. Dupilumab, a human monoclonal interleukin-4 and interleukin-13 blocker, has recently been approved in the treatment of moderate to severe AD in patients 6 months or older, with demonstration of good efficacy and a favorable side effect profile, thus changing the AD treatment landscape.[94,95] Tralokinumab, which targets IL-13, was approved in 2023 for moderate to severe AD in patients 12 years and older. JAK inhibitors have also recently gained FDA approval for refractory moderate to severe AD in people 12 years and older, including upadacitinib in 2022 and abrocitinib in 2023. There are multiple other systemic agents showing promise in the treatment of AD in various stages of development and testing, including several other biologic agents (eg, lebrikizumab and nemolizumab).

Itch Control

Pruritus is significantly disruptive for affected patients and their families and is one of the most difficult components of AD. The associated pruritus may contribute to ongoing damage to the skin barrier, superinfection, sleep disturbance, and decreased quality of life. The factors contributing to itch are multiple, and there is a complex interplay of both physical and immunologic factors.[96] It can be difficult to eliminate itch; however, some supportive measures include avoiding contact with irritants such as wool and aeroallergens, minimizing other triggers, and continuing skin-directed treatments aimed at reducing inflammation and restoring the skin barrier. Treatment of active AD has the greatest impact on improvement of itch. The role of histamine in AD-related itch is not completely clear, and although oral antihistamines do not have a direct effect on dermatitis, some patients may find benefit from antihistamines. Nonsedating second-generation antihistamines are not associated with the same side effect profile as first-generation antihistamines and have been shown to be safe to use long-term, particularly in patients who also have comorbid environmental allergies or dermatographism.[97] Emerging treatments for AD have shown promise in having a directly beneficial effect on the associated pruritus.[96]

Managing Infectious Triggers

Advances in skin microbiome research have led to an increased understanding of the pathophysiology of AD.[98] AD flares are associated with a reduction of skin microbial diversity and increased prevalence of *Staphylococcus* species.[99] Patients with intermittent treatment between AD flares, including either maintenance application of topical corticosteroids or dilute bleach baths, had higher microbial diversity and decreased *S aureus* prevalence. For this reason, intermittent/maintenance treatment ("proactive" treatment) with topical corticosteroids and/or topical calcineurin inhibitors can lead to a reduction in AD flares. Commensal *Staphylococcal* species protect from pathogenic *Staphylococcal* strains,[100] supporting the notion that widespread eradication of cutaneous *Staphylococcus* does not lead to long-term improvement in AD. Treatment of *S aureus* in AD has, thus, moved toward treatment of underlying eczema and utilization of maintenance therapies rather than focusing on eradication of *Staphylococcus*. However, in patients with clear impetiginization, short-term anti-staphylococcal oral or topical antibiotics may be appropriate in treatment of severe AD flares. Other bacteria, particularly group A *Streptococcus* species, have also been implicated in severe flares of AD. In one retrospective, culture-based study, children with AD and streptococcal infection were more likely to have herpetiform lesions and invasive disease compared with children infected by staphylococcal species.[101] However, prospective, microbiome-based

TABLE 2. General Recommendations for the Treatment of Pediatric Atopic Dermatitis
• Bathing should be frequent (daily to every other day) and short, with lukewarm water and gentle cleanser.
• Avoid products with added fragrance, dyes, or essential oils, as these are potential irritants and/or contact allergens.
• Topical anti-inflammatories (corticosteroids, calcineurin inhibitors, etc) should be applied once to twice daily to active eczema patches. Topical medications should not be mixed with topical emollients unless specifically instructed, as this dilutes the potency of the medication.
• Moisturizers should be applied liberally to the entire body skin surface at least daily in patients with atopic dermatitis, especially after a bath or shower.
• "Proactive" treatment with topical anti-inflammatories can reduce flares of recurrent AD.

studies are needed to corroborate this finding, which may have been biased by culture-based and retrospective methodology.

Children with AD also have increased risk of viral skin infections. Molluscum contagiosum (MC) is a common viral infection in children and is 5 times more prevalent in patients with AD vs those without eczema.[102] MC can trigger or flare eczema in patients with AD, often leading to dermatitis concentrated around MC lesions.[103] Children with AD are at increased risk for MC because of their compromised skin barrier and tend to have more widespread disease, in part resulting from autoinoculation via scratching. MC may persist from weeks to years, and there are currently no consistently effective treatments, which can be a source of significant frustration for parents.

Eczema herpeticum, which occurs nearly exclusively in patients with AD, can rarely lead to life-threatening disseminated herpes simplex virus infection. Eczema herpeticum presents as monomorphic, grouped vesicles and shallow erosions, concentrated in areas of underlying AD. In patients who require hospitalization, early recognition and treatment with systemic antivirals shortens hospitalization.[104] Treatment of underlying AD with topical corticosteroids does not prolong hospitalization and, therefore, should not be withheld during eczema herpeticum.

Children with AD may have flares of eczema with enteroviral infection, described as "eczema coxsackium."[105] Eczema coxsackium is characterized by polymorphous vesicles and bullae, distributed in areas previously or currently involved with AD, as well as an acral distribution (cheeks, buttocks, hands, and feet). The irregular and larger vesicles, as well as the presence of lesions on the palms and soles, may be helpful clues in distinguishing eczema coxsackium from eczema herpeticum. There may be an eczematous background surrounding the vesicular or bullous lesions. A similar presentation may occur in patients without a history of AD, but without flaring of background eczema, and is termed "atypical hand, foot, and mouth disease." Patients often have concurrent oral lesions and/or exposure to hand, foot, and mouth disease, which helps to distinguish the disease from eczema herpeticum. Supportive care and treatment of the underlying AD often leads to resolution in 1 to 2 weeks without sequelae.

CONCLUSIONS

AD is one of the most common skin complaints presenting to the pediatric primary care provider. The information reviewed here will equip pediatricians with the tools required to diagnose and treat the majority of patients with AD. Treatment recommendations are summarized in Table 2. Patients with severe, recalcitrant, and/or complicated AD should be referred to subspecialists, such as pediatric dermatologists. In some regions, wait times to see subspecialists exceed many months; thus, pediatric primary care providers should feel comfortable prescribing standard of care treatments, including topical corticosteroids. Ongoing collaboration between pediatric primary care providers and AD specialists can optimize care for patients with complex AD.

LEAD AUTHORS

Jennifer J. Schoch, MD, FAAD, FAAP
Katelyn R. Anderson, MD, FAAP, FAAD
Amie E. Jones, MD, FAAP
Megha M. Tollefson, MD, FAAP, FAAD

SECTION ON DERMATOLOGY EXECUTIVE COMMITTEE, 2023-2024

Teresa Wright, MD, FAAP, Chairperson
Raegan Hunt, MD, PhD, FAAP
Christine Lauren, MD, FAAP
Christina Boull, MD, FAAP
Deepti Gupta, MD, FAAP
Brandi Kenner-Bell, MD, FAAP

FORMER EXECUTIVE COMMITTEE MEMBERS

Sheilagh Maguiness, MD, FAAP
Megha M. Tollefson, MD, FAAP
Miriam Weinstein, MD, FRCPC, FAAP
Albert Yan, MD, FAAP

EX OFFICIO

Kim Horii, MD, FAAP

STAFF

Melissa Marx

ABBREVIATIONS

AD: atopic dermatitis
IgE: immunoglobulin E
JAK: Janus kinase
LEAP: Learning Early About Peanut (allergy)
MC: molluscum contagiosum
PDE: phosphodiesterase
TCI: topical calcineurin inhibitor

Clinical reports from the American Academy of Pediatrics benefit from expertise and resources of liaisons and internal (AAP) and external reviewers. However, clinical reports from the American Academy of Pediatrics may not reflect the views of the liaisons or the organizations or government agencies that they represent.

The guidance in this report does not indicate an exclusive course of treatment or serve as a standard of medical care. Variations, taking into account individual circumstances, may be appropriate.

All clinical reports from the American Academy of Pediatrics automatically expire 5 years after publication unless reaffirmed, revised, or retired at or before that time.

FUNDING: No external funding.

Accepted for Publication Date: March 28, 2025

https://doi.org/10.1542/peds.2025-071812

REFERENCES

1. Shaw TE, Currie GP, Koudelka CW, Simpson EL. Eczema prevalence in the United States: data from the 2003 National Survey of Children's Health. *J Invest Dermatol.* 2011;131(1):67–73. PubMed doi: 10.1038/jid.2010.251
2. Monir RL, Schoch JJ, Garvan CW, Neu J, Lemas DJ. Association between atopic dermatitis and race from infancy to early childhood: a retrospective cohort study. *Int J Dermatol.* 2022;61(6): 727–732. PubMed doi: 10.1111/ijd.15805
3. Horii KA, Simon SD, Liu DY, Sharma V. Atopic dermatitis in children in the United States, 1997–2004: visit trends, patient and provider characteristics, and prescribing patterns. *Pediatrics.* 2007;120(3): e527–e534. PubMed doi: 10.1542/peds.2007-0289
4. Pletcher BA, Rimsza ME, Cull WL, Shipman SA, Shugerman RP, O'Connor KG. Primary care pediatricians' satisfaction with subspecialty care, perceived supply, and barriers to care. *J Pediatr.* 2010;156(6):1011–1015.e1. PubMed doi: 10.1016/j.jpeds.2009.12.032
5. Resnick SD, Hornung R, Konrad TR. A comparison of dermatologists and generalists. Management of childhood atopic dermatitis. *Arch Dermatol.* 1996;132(9):1047–1052. PubMed doi: 10.1001/archderm.1996.03890330061011
6. Tollefson MM, Bruckner AL; Section On Dermatology. Atopic dermatitis: skin-directed management. *Pediatrics.* 2014;134(6): e1735–e1744. PubMed doi: 10.1542/peds.2014-2812
7. Eichenfield LF, Tom WL, Chamlin SL, et al. Guidelines of care for the management of atopic dermatitis: section 1. Diagnosis and assessment of atopic dermatitis. *J Am Acad Dermatol.* 2014;70 (2):338–351. PubMed doi: 10.1016/j.jaad.2013.10.010
8. Schoch JJ, Monir RL, Satcher KG, Harris J, Triplett E, Neu J. The infantile cutaneous microbiome: A review. *Pediatr Dermatol.* 2019;36(5):574–580. PubMed doi: 10.1111/pde.13870
9. Silverberg JI, Simpson EL. Associations of childhood eczema severity: a US population-based study. *Dermatitis.* 2014;25(3): 107–114. PubMed doi: 10.1097/DER.0000000000000034
10. Wan J, Margolis DJ, Mitra N, Hoffstad OJ, Takeshita J. Racial and ethnic differences in atopic dermatitis-related school absences among US children. *JAMA Dermatol.* 2019;155(8):973–975. PubMed doi: 10.1001/jamadermatol.2019.0597
11. Wan J, Oganisian A, Spieker AJ, et al. Racial/ethnic variation in use of ambulatory and emergency care for atopic dermatitis among US children. *J Invest Dermatol.* 2019;139(9):1906–1913.e1901. doi: https://doi.org/10.1016/j.jid.2019.02.024
12. Egawa G, Kabashima K. Multifactorial skin barrier deficiency and atopic dermatitis: Essential topics to prevent the atopic march. *J Allergy Clin Immunol.* 2016;138(2):350–358.e1. PubMed doi: 10.1016/j.jaci.2016.06.002
13. Kelleher M, Dunn-Galvin A, Hourihane JO, et al. Skin barrier dysfunction measured by transepidermal water loss at 2 days and 2 months predates and predicts atopic dermatitis at 1 year. *J Allergy Clin Immunol.* 2015;135(4):930–935.e1. PubMed doi: 10.1016/j.jaci.2014.12.013
14. Vachiramon V, Tey HL, Thompson AE, Yosipovitch G. Atopic dermatitis in African American children: addressing unmet needs of a common disease. *Pediatr Dermatol.* 2012;29(4):395–402. PubMed doi: 10.1111/j.1525-1470.2012.01740.x
15. Muizzuddin N, Hellemans L, Van Overloop L, Corstjens H, Declercq L, Maes D. Structural and functional differences in barrier properties of African American, Caucasian and East Asian skin. *J*

Dermatol Sci. 2010;59(2):123–128. PubMed doi: 10.1016/j.jdermsci.2010.06.003

16. Reinertson RP, Wheatley VR. Studies on the chemical composition of human epidermal lipids. *J Invest Dermatol.* 1959;32(1):49–59. PubMed doi: 10.1038/jid.1959.11
17. Wesley NO, Maibach HI. Racial (ethnic) differences in skin properties: the objective data. *Am J Clin Dermatol.* 2003;4(12):843–860. PubMed doi: 10.2165/00128071-200304120-00004
18. Alexis AF, Woolery-Lloyd H, Williams K, et al. Racial/ethnic variations in skin barrier: implications for skin care recommendations in skin of color. *J Drugs Dermatol.* 2021;20(9):932–938. PubMed doi: 10.36849/JDD.6312
19. Young MM, Franken A, du Plessis JL. Transepidermal water loss, stratum corneum hydration, and skin surface pH of female African and Caucasian nursing students. *Skin Res Technol.* 2019;25(1):88–95. PubMed doi: 10.1111/srt.12614
20. McColl M, Boozalis E, Aguh C, Eseonu AC, Okoye GA, Kwatra SG. Pruritus in black skin: unique molecular characteristics and clinical features. *J Natl Med Assoc.* 2021;113(1):30–38. PubMed doi: 10.1016/j.jnma.2020.07.002
21. Croce EA, Levy ML, Adamson AS, Matsui EC. Reframing racial and ethnic disparities in atopic dermatitis in Black and Latinx populations. *J Allergy Clin Immunol.* 2021;148(5):1104–1111. PubMed doi: 10.1016/j.jaci.2021.09.015
22. Ravn NH, Halling AS, Berkowitz AG, et al. How does parental history of atopic disease predict the risk of atopic dermatitis in a child? A systematic review and meta-analysis. *J Allergy Clin Immunol.* 2020;145(4):1182–1193. PubMed doi: 10.1016/j.jaci.2019.12.899
23. Esaki H, Brunner PM, Renert-Yuval Y, et al. Early-onset pediatric atopic dermatitis is T_H2 but also T_H17 polarized in skin. *J Allergy Clin Immunol.* 2016;138(6):1639–1651. PubMed doi: 10.1016/j.jaci.2016.07.013
24. Gittler JK, Shemer A, Suárez-Fariñas M, et al. Progressive activation of T(H)2/T(H)22 cytokines and selective epidermal proteins characterizes acute and chronic atopic dermatitis. *J Allergy Clin Immunol.* 2012;130(6):1344–1354. PubMed doi: 10.1016/j.jaci.2012.07.012
25. Werfel T. The role of leukocytes, keratinocytes, and allergen-specific IgE in the development of atopic dermatitis. *J Invest Dermatol.* 2009;129(8):1878–1891. PubMed doi: 10.1038/jid.2009.71
26. Roduit C, Frei R, Depner M, et al; the PASTURE study group. Phenotypes of atopic dermatitis depending on the timing of onset and progression in childhood. *JAMA Pediatr.* 2017;171(7):655–662. PubMed doi: 10.1001/jamapediatrics.2017.0556
27. Paternoster L, Savenije OEM, Heron J, et al. Identification of atopic dermatitis subgroups in children from 2 longitudinal birth cohorts. *J Allergy Clin Immunol.* 2018;141(3):964–971. PubMed doi: 10.1016/j.jaci.2017.09.044
28. Yang EJ, Beck KM, Sekhon S, Bhutani T, Koo J. The impact of pediatric atopic dermatitis on families: A review. *Pediatr Dermatol.* 2019;36(1):66–71. PubMed doi: 10.1111/pde.13727
29. Drucker AM, Wang AR, Li W-Q, Sevetson E, Block JK, Qureshi AA. The burden of atopic dermatitis: summary of a report for the National Eczema Association. *J Invest Dermatol.* 2017;137(1):26–30. PubMed doi: 10.1016/j.jid.2016.07.012
30. Teichgräber F, Jacob L, Koyanagi A, Shin JI, Seiringer P, Kostev K. Association between skin disorders and depression in children and adolescents: A retrospective case-control study. *J Affect Disord.* 2021;282:939–944. PubMed doi: 10.1016/j.jad.2021.01.002
31. Kyung Y, Lee JS, Lee JH, Jo SH, Kim SH. Health-related behaviors and mental health states of South Korean adolescents with atopic dermatitis. *J Dermatol.* 2020;47(7):699–706. PubMed doi: 10.1111/1346-8138.15386
32. Durovic MR, Jankovic J, Cirkovic A, et al. Impact of atopic dermatitis on the quality of life of children and their families. *Ital J Dermatol Venereol.* 2021;156(1). doi: 10.23736/s2784-8671.19.06447-2.
33. Hedman-Lagerlöf E, Bergman A, Lindefors N, Bradley M. Exposure-based cognitive behavior therapy for atopic dermatitis: an open trial. *Cogn Behav Ther.* 2019;48(4):300–310. PubMed doi: 10.1080/16506073.2018.1504320
34. Fishbein AB, Cheng BT, Tilley CC, et al. Sleep disturbance in school-aged children with atopic dermatitis: prevalence and severity in a cross-sectional sample. *J Allergy Clin Immunol Pract.* 2021;9(8):3120–3129.e3. PubMed doi: 10.1016/j.jaip.2021.04.064
35. Schwarz W, Birau N, Hornstein OP, et al. Alterations of melatonin secretion in atopic eczema. *Acta Derm Venereol.* 1988;68(3):224–229. PubMed
36. Taghavi Ardakani A, Farrehi M, Sharif MR, et al. The effects of melatonin administration on disease severity and sleep quality in children with atopic dermatitis: A randomized, double-blinded, placebo-controlled trial. *Pediatr Allergy Immunol.* 2018;29(8):834–840. PubMed doi: 10.1111/pai.12978
37. Patel D, Levoska M, Shwayder T. Managing sleep disturbances in children with atopic dermatitis. *Pediatr Dermatol.* 2018;35(4):428–433. PubMed doi: 10.1111/pde.13444
38. He A, Feldman SR, Fleischer AB Jr. An assessment of the use of antihistamines in the management of atopic dermatitis. *J Am Acad Dermatol.* 2018;79(1):92–96. PubMed doi: 10.1016/j.jaad.2017.12.077
39. Schmitt J, Buske-Kirschbaum A, Tesch F, et al. Increased attention-deficit/hyperactivity symptoms in atopic dermatitis are associated with history of antihistamine use. *Allergy.* 2018;73(3):615–626. PubMed doi: 10.1111/all.13326
40. Fuhrmann S, Tesch F, Romanos M, Abraham S, Schmitt J. ADHD in school-age children is related to infant exposure to systemic H1-antihistamines. *Allergy.* 2020;75(11):2956–2957. PubMed doi: 10.1111/all.14411
41. Warner JO; ETAC Study Group. Early Treatment of the Atopic Child. A double-blinded, randomized, placebo-controlled trial of cetirizine in preventing the onset of asthma in children with atopic dermatitis: 18 months' treatment and 18 months' posttreatment follow-up. *J Allergy Clin Immunol.* 2001;108(6):929–937. PubMed doi: 10.1067/mai.2001.120015

42. Tham EH, Leung DYM. Mechanisms by which atopic dermatitis predisposes to food allergy and the atopic march. *Allergy Asthma Immunol Res.* 2019;11(1):4–15. PubMed doi: 10.4168/aair.2019.11.1.4

43. Singh AM, Anvari S, Hauk P, et al. Atopic dermatitis and food allergy: best practices and knowledge gaps-a work group report from the AAAAI Allergic Skin Diseases Committee and Leadership Institute Project. *J Allergy Clin Immunol Pract.* 2022;10(3):697–706. PubMed doi: 10.1016/j.jaip.2021.12.037

44. Wahn U, Warner J, Simons FER, et al; EPAAC Study Group. IgE antibody responses in young children with atopic dermatitis. *Pediatr Allergy Immunol.* 2008;19(4):332–336. PubMed doi: 10.1111/j.1399-3038.2007.00643.x

45. Eigenmann PA, Beyer K, Lack G, et al. Are avoidance diets still warranted in children with atopic dermatitis? *Pediatr Allergy Immunol.* 2020;31(1):19–26. PubMed doi: 10.1111/pai.13104

46. Du Toit G, Roberts G, Sayre PH, et al; LEAP Study Team. Randomized trial of peanut consumption in infants at risk for peanut allergy. *N Engl J Med.* 2015;372(9):803–813. PubMed doi: 10.1056/NEJMoa1414850

47. Du Toit G, Sayre PH, Roberts G, et al; Immune Tolerance Network LEAP-On Study Team. Effect of avoidance on peanut allergy after early peanut consumption. *N Engl J Med.* 2016;374(15):1435–1443. PubMed doi: 10.1056/NEJMoa1514209

48. Togias A, Cooper SF, Acebal ML, et al. Addendum guidelines for the prevention of peanut allergy in the United States: Report of the National Institute of Allergy and Infectious Diseases-sponsored expert panel. *J Allergy Clin Immunol.* 2017;139(1):29–44. PubMed doi: 10.1016/j.jaci.2016.10.010

49. National Eczema Association website. Accessed February 23, 2024. www.nationaleczema.org

50. Sauder MB, McEvoy A, Sampson M, et al. The effectiveness of written action plans in atopic dermatitis. *Pediatr Dermatol.* 2016;33(2):e151–e153. PubMed doi: 10.1111/pde.12774

51. Bodenheimer T, Wagner EH, Grumbach K. Improving primary care for patients with chronic illness. *JAMA.* 2002;288(14):1775–1779. PubMed doi: 10.1001/jama.288.14.1775

52. Brown J, Weitz NW, Liang A, Stockwell MS, Friedman S. Does an eczema action plan improve atopic dermatitis? A single-site randomized controlled trial. *Clin Pediatr (Phila).* 2018;57(14):1624–1629. PubMed doi: 10.1177/0009922818795906

53. van Zuuren EJ, Fedorowicz Z, Christensen R, Lavrijsen A, Arents BWM. Emollients and moisturisers for eczema. *Cochrane Database Syst Rev.* 2017;2(2):CD012119. PubMed doi: 10.1002/14651858.cd012119.pub2

54. Santer M, Ridd MJ, Francis NA, et al. Emollient bath additives for the treatment of childhood eczema (BATHE): multicentre pragmatic parallel group randomised controlled trial of clinical and cost effectiveness. *BMJ.* 2018;361:k1332. PubMed doi: 10.1136/bmj.k1332

55. Simpson EL, Chalmers JR, Hanifin JM, et al. Emollient enhancement of the skin barrier from birth offers effective atopic dermatitis prevention. *J Allergy Clin Immunol.* 2014;134(4):818–823. PubMed doi: 10.1016/j.jaci.2014.08.005

56. Horimukai K, Morita K, Narita M, et al. Application of moisturizer to neonates prevents development of atopic dermatitis. *J Allergy Clin Immunol.* 2014;134(4):824–830.e6. PubMed doi: 10.1016/j.jaci.2014.07.060

57. Chalmers JR, Haines RH, Bradshaw LE, et al; BEEP study team. Daily emollient during infancy for prevention of eczema: the BEEP randomised controlled trial. *Lancet.* 2020;395(10228):962–972. PubMed doi: 10.1016/S0140-6736(19)32984-8

58. Skjerven HO, Rehbinder EM, Vettukattil R, et al. Skin emollient and early complementary feeding to prevent infant atopic dermatitis (PreventADALL): a factorial, multicentre, cluster-randomised trial. *Lancet.* 2020;395(10228):951–961. PubMed doi: 10.1016/S0140-6736(19)32983-6

59. Campbell JR, Zaccaria E, Baker CJ. Systemic candidiasis in extremely low birth weight infants receiving topical petrolatum ointment for skin care: a case-control study. *Pediatrics.* 2000;105(5):1041–1045. PubMed doi: 10.1542/peds.105.5.1041

60. AlKharfy T, Ba-Abbad R, Hadi A, AlFaleh K. Use of topical petroleum jelly for prevention of sepsis in very low-birthweight infants: a prospective, randomised controlled trial. *Paediatr Int Child Health.* 2014;34(3):194–197. PubMed doi: 10.1179/2046905514Y.0000000117

61. Edwards WH, Conner JM, Soll RF; Vermont Oxford Network Neonatal Skin Care Study Group. The effect of prophylactic ointment therapy on nosocomial sepsis rates and skin integrity in infants with birth weights of 501 to 1000 g. *Pediatrics.* 2004;113(5):1195–1203. PubMed doi: 10.1542/peds.113.5.1195

62. Kelleher MM, Phillips R, Brown SJ, et al. Skin care interventions in infants for preventing eczema and food allergy. *Cochrane Database Syst Rev.* 2022;11(11):CD013534. PubMed doi: 10.1002/14651858.cd013534.pub3

63. Clausen ML, Edslev SM, Andersen PS, Clemmensen K, Krogfelt KA, Agner T. *Staphylococcus aureus* colonization in atopic eczema and its association with filaggrin gene mutations. *Br J Dermatol.* 2017; 177(5):1394–1400. PubMed doi: 10.1111/bjd.15470

64. Totté JE, van der Feltz WT, Hennekam M, van Belkum A, van Zuuren EJ, Pasmans SG. Prevalence and odds of *Staphylococcus aureus* carriage in atopic dermatitis: a systematic review and meta-analysis. *Br J Dermatol.* 2016;175(4):687–695. PubMed doi: 10.1111/bjd.14566

65. Guzik TJ, Bzowska M, Kasprowicz A, et al. Persistent skin colonization with *Staphylococcus aureus* in atopic dermatitis: relationship to clinical and immunological parameters. *Clin Exp Allergy.* 2005;35(4):448–455. PubMed doi: 10.1111/j.1365-2222.2005.02210.x

66. Chopra R, Vakharia PP, Sacotte R, Silverberg JI. Efficacy of bleach baths in reducing severity of atopic dermatitis: A systematic review and meta-analysis. *Ann Allergy Asthma Immunol.* 2017; 119(5):435–440. PubMed doi: 10.1016/j.anai.2017.08.289

67. Bakaa L, Pernica JM, Couban RJ, et al. Bleach baths for atopic dermatitis: a systematic review and meta-analysis including unpublished data, Bayesian interpretation, and GRADE. *Ann Allergy Asthma Immunol.* 2022;128(6):660–668.e669. doi: https://doi.org/10.1016/j.anai.2022.03.024

68. Cardona ID, Stillman L, Jain N. Does bathing frequency matter in pediatric atopic dermatitis? *Ann Allergy Asthma Immunol.* 2016; 117(1):9–13. PubMed doi: 10.1016/j.anai.2016.05.014

69. Cardona ID, Kempe EE, Lary C, Ginder JH, Jain N. Frequent versus infrequent bathing in pediatric atopic dermatitis: a randomized clinical trial. *J Allergy Clin Immunol Pract.* 2020;8(3):1014–1021. PubMed doi: 10.1016/j.jaip.2019.10.042

70. Cardona ID, Kempe E, Hatzenbeuhler JR, Antaya RJ, Cohen B, Jain N. Bathing frequency recommendations for children with atopic dermatitis: results of three observational pilot surveys. *Pediatr Dermatol.* 2015;32(4):e194–e196. PubMed doi: 10.1111/pde.12618

71. Hamann CR, Hamann D, Egeberg A, Johansen JD, Silverberg J, Thyssen JP. Association between atopic dermatitis and contact sensitization: A systematic review and meta-analysis. *J Am Acad Dermatol.* 2017;77(1):70–78. PubMed doi: 10.1016/j.jaad.2017.02.001

72. Shaughnessy CN, Malajian D, Belsito DV. Cutaneous delayed-type hypersensitivity in patients with atopic dermatitis: reactivity to topical preservatives. *J Am Acad Dermatol.* 2014;70(1):102–107. PubMed doi: 10.1016/j.jaad.2013.08.046

73. Malajian D, Belsito DV. Cutaneous delayed-type hypersensitivity in patients with atopic dermatitis. *J Am Acad Dermatol.* 2013;69(2): 232–237. PubMed doi: 10.1016/j.jaad.2013.03.012

74. Weidinger S, Novak N. Atopic dermatitis. *Lancet.* 2016;387(10023): 1109–1122. PubMed doi: 10.1016/S0140-6736(15)00149-X

75. Mooney E, Rademaker M, Dailey R, et al. Adverse effects of topical corticosteroids in paediatric eczema: Australasian consensus statement. *Australas J Dermatol.* 2015;56(4):241–251. PubMed doi: 10.1111/ajd.12313

76. Bjorklund KA, Fernandez Faith E. Branching hypopigmentation following intralesional corticosteroid injection: Case report and review of the literature. *Pediatr Dermatol.* 2020;37(1):235–236. PubMed doi: 10.1111/pde.14050

77. Topical SPC. National Psoriasis Foundation. Last updated October 25, 2022. Accessed September 7, 2021, 2021. https://www.psoriasis.org/potency-chart/

78. Schoch J, Davis DM. Practical guide to outpatient wet dressings for pediatric atopic dermatitis. *Curr Dermatol Rep.* 2013;2(4): 212–215. doi: 10.1007/s13671-013-0057-7

79. Chen SL, Yan J, Wang FS. Two topical calcineurin inhibitors for the treatment of atopic dermatitis in pediatric patients: a meta-analysis of randomized clinical trials. *J Dermatolog Treat.* 2010;21(3): 144–156. PubMed doi: 10.3109/09546630903401470

80. Legendre L, Barnetche T, Mazereeuw-Hautier J, Meyer N, Murrell D, Paul C. Risk of lymphoma in patients with atopic dermatitis and the role of topical treatment: A systematic review and meta-analysis. *J Am Acad Dermatol.* 2015;72(6):992–1002. PubMed doi: 10.1016/j.jaad.2015.02.1116

81. Tennis P, Gelfand JM, Rothman KJ. Evaluation of cancer risk related to atopic dermatitis and use of topical calcineurin inhibitors. *Br J Dermatol.* 2011;165(3):465–473. PubMed doi: 10.1111/j.1365-2133.2011.10363.x

82. Arellano FM, Wentworth CE, Arana A, Fernández C, Paul CF. Risk of lymphoma following exposure to calcineurin inhibitors and topical steroids in patients with atopic dermatitis. *J Invest Dermatol.* 2007;127(4):808–816. PubMed doi: 10.1038/sj.jid.5700622

83. Paller AS, Fölster-Holst R, Chen SC, et al. No evidence of increased cancer incidence in children using topical tacrolimus for atopic dermatitis. *J Am Acad Dermatol.* 2020;83(2):375–381. PubMed doi: 10.1016/j.jaad.2020.03.075

84. Wahn U, Bos JD, Goodfield M, et al; Flare Reduction in Eczema with Elidel (Children) Multicenter Investigator Study Group. Efficacy and safety of pimecrolimus cream in the long-term management of atopic dermatitis in children. *Pediatrics.* 2002;110(1 Pt 1):e2. PubMed doi: 10.1542/peds.110.1.e2

85. Eichenfield LF, Call RS, Forsha DW, et al. Long-term safety of crisaborole ointment 2% in children and adults with mild to moderate atopic dermatitis. *J Am Acad Dermatol.* 2017;77(4):641–649.e5. PubMed doi: 10.1016/j.jaad.2017.06.010

86. Paller AS, Tom WL, Lebwohl MG, et al. Efficacy and safety of crisaborole ointment, a novel, nonsteroidal phosphodiesterase 4 (PDE4) inhibitor for the topical treatment of atopic dermatitis (AD) in children and adults. *J Am Acad Dermatol.* 2016;75(3): 494–503.e6. PubMed doi: 10.1016/j.jaad.2016.05.046

87. Thaci D, Chambers C, Sidhu M, Dorsch B, Ehlken B, Fuchs S. Twice-weekly treatment with tacrolimus 0.03% ointment in children with atopic dermatitis: clinical efficacy and economic impact over 12 months. *J Eur Acad Dermatol Venereol.* 2010;24(9): 1040–1046. PubMed doi: 10.1111/j.1468-3083.2010.03577.x

88. Healy E, Bentley A, Fidler C, Chambers C. Cost-effectiveness of tacrolimus ointment in adults and children with moderate and severe atopic dermatitis: twice-weekly maintenance treatment vs. standard twice-daily reactive treatment of exacerbations from a third party payer (U.K. National Health Service) perspective. *Br J Dermatol.* 2011;164(2):387–395. PubMed doi: 10.1111/j.1365-2133.2010.10141.x

89. Fukuie T, Hirakawa S, Narita M, et al. Potential preventive effects of proactive therapy on sensitization in moderate to severe childhood atopic dermatitis: A randomized, investigator-blinded, controlled study. *J Dermatol.* 2016;43(11):1283–1292. PubMed doi: 10.1111/1346-8138.13408

90. Integrative HMP; Integrative HMP (iHMP) Research Network Consortium. The Integrative Human Microbiome Project. *Nature.* 2019;569(7758):641–648. PubMed doi: 10.1038/s41586-019-1238-8

91. Hammond AM, Monir RL, Schoch JJ. The role of the pediatric cutaneous and gut microbiomes in childhood disease: A review. *Semin Perinatol.* 2021;45(6):151452. PubMed doi: 10.1016/j.semperi.2021.151452

92. Navarro-López V, Ramírez-Boscá A, Ramón-Vidal D, et al. Effect of oral administration of a mixture of probiotic strains on SCORAD Index and use of topical steroids in young patients with moderate atopic dermatitis. *JAMA Dermatol.* 2018;154(1):37–43. PubMed doi: 10.1001/jamadermatol.2017.3647

93. Damm JA, Smith B, Greisen G, Krogfelt KA, Clausen M-L, Agner T. The influence of probiotics for preterm neonates on the incidence

of atopic dermatitis-results from a historically controlled cohort study. *Arch Dermatol Res.* 2017;309(4):259–264. PubMed doi: 10.1007/s00403-017-1725-4

94. Paller AS, Siegfried EC, Thaçi D, et al. Efficacy and safety of dupilumab with concomitant topical corticosteroids in children 6 to 11 years old with severe atopic dermatitis: A randomized, double-blinded, placebo-controlled phase 3 trial. *J Am Acad Dermatol.* 2020;83(5):1282–1293. PubMed doi: 10.1016/j.jaad.2020.06.054
95. Simpson EL, Paller AS, Siegfried EC, et al. Efficacy and safety of dupilumab in adolescents with uncontrolled moderate to severe atopic dermatitis: a phase 3 randomized clinical trial. *JAMA Dermatol.* 2020;156(1):44–56. PubMed doi: 10.1001/jamadermatol.2019.3336
96. El Hachem M, Di Mauro G, Rotunno R, et al. Pruritus in pediatric patients with atopic dermatitis: a multidisciplinary approach - summary document from an Italian expert group. *Ital J Pediatr.* 2020;46(1):11. PubMed doi: 10.1186/s13052-020-0777-9
97. Diepgen TL; Early Treatment of the Atopic Child Study Group. Long-term treatment with cetirizine of infants with atopic dermatitis: a multi-country, double-blind, randomized, placebo-controlled trial (the ETAC trial) over 18 months. *Pediatr Allergy Immunol.* 2002;13(4):278–286. PubMed doi: 10.1034/j.1399-3038.2002.01047.x
98. Monir RL, Schoch JJ. Clinical relevance of the microbiome in pediatric skin disease: a review. *Dermatol Clin.* 2022;40(2):117–126. PubMed doi: 10.1016/j.det.2021.12.001
99. Kong HH, Oh J, Deming C, et al; NISC Comparative Sequence Program. Temporal shifts in the skin microbiome associated with disease flares and treatment in children with atopic dermatitis. *Genome Res.* 2012;22(5):850–859. PubMed doi: 10.1101/gr.131029.111
100. Nakatsuji T, Chen TH, Narala S, et al. Antimicrobials from human skin commensal bacteria protect against *Staphylococcus aureus* and are deficient in atopic dermatitis. *Sci Transl Med.* 2017;9(378):eaah4680. PubMed doi: 10.1126/scitranslmed.aah4680
101. Sugarman JL, Hersh AL, Okamura T, Howard R, Frieden IJ. A retrospective review of streptococcal infections in pediatric atopic dermatitis. *Pediatr Dermatol.* 2011;28(3):230–234. PubMed doi: 10.1111/j.1525-1470.2010.01377.x
102. Ren Z, Silverberg JI. Association of atopic dermatitis with bacterial, fungal, viral, and sexually transmitted skin infections. *Dermatitis.* 2020;31(2):157–164. PubMed doi: 10.1097/DER.0000000000000526
103. Silverberg NB. Molluscum contagiosum virus infection can trigger atopic dermatitis disease onset or flare. *Cutis.* 2018;102(3):191–194. PubMed
104. Aronson PL, Yan AC, Mittal MK, Mohamad Z, Shah SS. Delayed acyclovir and outcomes of children hospitalized with eczema herpeticum. *Pediatrics.* 2011;128(6):1161–1167. PubMed doi: 10.1542/peds.2011-0948
105. Mathes EF, Oza V, Frieden IJ, et al. "Eczema coxsackium" and unusual cutaneous findings in an enterovirus outbreak. *Pediatrics.* 2013;132(1):e149–e157. PubMed doi: 10.1542/peds.2012-3175

Contraception for Adolescents

• *Policy Statement*

POLICY STATEMENT Organizational Principles to Guide and Define the Child Health Care System and/or Improve the Health of All Children

American Academy of Pediatrics

DEDICATED TO THE HEALTH OF ALL CHILDREN™

Contraception for Adolescents: Policy Statement

Mary A. Ott, MD, MA, FAAP,[1] Andrea J. Hoopes, MD, MPH, FAAP,[2,3] Gina S. Sucato, MD, MPH, FSAHM, FAAP,[2,3] Maayan Leroy-Melamed, MD, MPH, FAAP,[4] and the Committee on Adolescence

abstract

The American Academy of Pediatrics recommends that pediatricians provide contraceptive care for adolescents. Contraceptive prescribing and counseling skills ensure the safety and well-being of adolescents, enabling pediatricians to help adolescents achieve optimal reproductive health. This policy statement updates the 2014 policy statement on contraception for adolescents and is designed to be used in tandem with the accompanying clinical report, "Contraceptive Counseling and Methods for Adolescents" and the series of method-specific policy statements and clinical reports from the Academy. This policy statement provides the pediatrician with evidence-informed and equity-informed practices in contraceptive care for adolescents.

INTRODUCTION

Contraception counseling, prescribing, and management are important skills that enable pediatricians to advance adolescent safety and well-being. The proportion of US high school students who have ever had sexual intercourse range from 16% of 9th graders to 48% of 12th graders.[1] With 52% of sexually active high school students reporting condom use and 33% any hormonal contraceptive use at last sex, many adolescents are at risk for pregnancy and sexually transmitted infections (STIs).[1] Unfortunately, adolescents face barriers to accessing effective, equitable contraceptive care.[2] This policy statement is an update of the 2014 policy statement, applying a sexual and reproductive health equity framework to contraceptive care. It is designed to be used with the companion clinical report.[3]

Adolescents consider pediatricians to be a trustworthy source of medically accurate sexual health care information.[4–6] Thus, pediatricians are well-positioned to address adolescents' unmet contraceptive needs with developmentally tailored approaches. Pediatricians' long-term relationships with adolescents and families can provide the trust and accessibility needed for private conversations about sensitive topics such as sexuality and contraception and timely care when contraceptive needs arise.

[1]*Departments of Global Health and Health Systems Design and Pediatrics, Icahn School of Medicine at Mount Sinai, New York, New York;* [2]*Adolescent Medicine Program, Washington Permanente Medical Group, Kaiser Permanente Washington Health Research Institute, Seattle, Washington;* [3]*Department of Pediatrics, University of Washington, Seattle, Washington; and* [4]*The Warren Alpert Medical School of Brown University, Division of Adolescent Medicine, Hasbro Children's Hospital, Rhode Island Hospital, Providence, Rhode Island*

Address correspondence to: Mary A. Ott, MD, MA. Email: maryaott8@gmail.com

Drs Ott and Hoopes conceptualized and organized the policy statement, reviewed the literature, drafted the document, and provided critical review. Drs Sucato and Leroy-Melamed contributed to the conceptualization and organization and provided critical review.

CONFLICT OF INTEREST DISCLOSURE: The authors have indicated they have no potential conflicts of interest to disclose.

To cite: Ott MA, Hoopes AJ, Sucato GS, et al; American Academy of Pediatrics, Committee on Adolescence. Contraception for Adolescents: Policy Statement. *Pediatrics.* 2025;156(1):e2025072217

SEXUAL AND REPRODUCTIVE HEALTH EQUITY

Sexual and reproductive health equity occurs when "systems ensure that all people, across the range of age, gender, race, and other intersectional identities, have what they need to attain their highest level of sexual and reproductive health, and includes self-determining and achieving their reproductive goals."[7] Achieving sexual and reproductive health equity requires that policies, programs, and services account for historical and current forces that lead to inequities based on race, location, income, and other factors and center the needs of those who have been most harmed. Table 1 highlights threats to adolescent sexual and reproductive health equity.

A foundational framework of sexual and reproductive health equity is reproductive justice. Conceptualized by Black women activists and subsequent activism of Indigenous and other women of color, the reproductive justice framework sheds light on the impacts of racism on adolescent contraceptive care.[8–10] This includes recognizing coercive and nonconsensual contraception provision experienced by minoritized and marginalized populations and acknowledging the existence of inequitable structures that afford differential educational and economic opportunities based on race, income status, ability, or other social determinants, all of which can impact an adolescent's motivations and ability to prevent pregnancy.[11–14] See Table 2 to learn more about reproductive justice.

For adolescents, sexual and reproductive health equity-informed care avoids stigmatizing healthy and developmentally appropriate sexually intimate relationships, supports young people's autonomy regarding contraception, and considers the social and structural drivers which impact their ability to access and use effective contraception.[8,14] Acknowledging that adolescents with disabilities experience additional barriers to accessing comprehensive reproductive health care,[15–17] pediatricians can ensure that counseling and services are inclusive of and accessible to adolescents of all abilities. The AAP policy statement "Promoting Healthy Sexuality for Children and Adolescents with Disabilities" provides additional guidance and resources specific to this population.[17]

TABLE 1. Threats to Sexual and Reproductive Health Equity

Threat	Examples in Contraception Care
Implicit bias among healthcare providers	Young people report experiencing biased counseling from providers to use or continue high efficacy long-acting methods even if the method does not align with their needs and preferences.[11,73,74]
A restrictive legal landscape of reproductive healthcare access	State laws that limit access to confidential contraceptive services for minors create barriers to adolescent use of contraception.[2,28,30,75]
Inequitable societal systems	Communities that afford differential educational and economic opportunities based on race, income status, or other social and structural drivers may impact a young person's motivations and ability to use contraception.[76–78]

TABLE 2. Reproductive Justice Learning Resources

Equitable Access to Sexual and Reproductive Health Care for all Youth Resources and Acknowledgements (website)	https://www.aap.org/en/patient-care/adolescent-sexual-health/equitable-access-to-sexual-and-reproductive-health-care-for-all-youth/equitable-access-to-sexual-and-reproductive-health-care-for-all-youth-resources/
Youth Reproductive Justice: Beyond Choice, Toward Health Equity (journal article)	Gilliam M. Health Educ Behav 2020 Vol. 47 Issue 4 Pages 640–641. Avaliable at: https://journals.sagepub.com/doi/full/10.1177/1090198119876309
What is Reproductive Justice? (video)	McLemore MR, Scott K (2019). USC Annenberg. Available at: https://www.youtube.com/watch?v=I4mwQhKLBiM

CONSENT AND CONFIDENTIALITY

Adolescence is a time when youth expand their social networks from families into peer groups, have their first intimate relationships, and gain clarity about their gender and sexual identities.[18] A positive youth development approach allows professionals working with adolescents to acknowledge and support sexuality as a part of normal, healthy development.[19,20] It also honors the capacity of adolescents to make thoughtful, informed decisions about contraception.

The American Academy of Pediatrics (AAP) considers policies supporting adolescent self-consent for contraception and protecting adolescent confidentiality to be in the best interest of adolescent safety and well-being.[21–23] Data show that limitations on confidentiality and consent are associated with decreased access to sexual and reproductive health care, lower use of contraceptives, and higher adolescent pregnancy rates.[24–30]

Globally, human rights frameworks emphasize the importance of adolescent access to confidential sexual and reproductive health services.[31,32] Human rights are dependent not on citizenship or local laws, but on our shared humanity and recognition of adolescents' emerging capacity. Human rights frameworks emphasize the evolving role of the parents/caregivers from decision making for the child to providing a safe and supportive environment for the adolescent to make autonomous decisions, and the role of the state to provide systems of care that respect confidentiality and provide access.[31] In the United States, legal support for minors to consent to contraception or to receive confidential care is complex, with a changing landscape of state laws. Currently, 27 states have laws explicitly allowing minors' consent to contraception, and another 19 states allow certain classes of minors to consent to contraception.[33] The AAP encourages pediatricians to become familiar with relevant minor consent laws in their jurisdiction. With the rapid changes in state laws after the US Supreme Court *Dobbs* decision, the AAP State Advocacy team can provide pediatricians with an update on their state's legal landscape and opportunities for advocacy by pediatricians at the state level (stgov@aap.org). For states without specific state laws, federal statutes (eg, Title X and Medicaid) and federal case law may provide some support for minor confidentiality and consent for contraception.[22,34,35] For example, Title X of the federal Public Health Services Act (42 USC §300–300a-6 [1970]) requires family planning clinics funded by Title X to provide confidential services for minors. (For a detailed discussion, see *State Minor Consent Laws*, 3rd Edition.[35])

The Health Insurance Portability and Accountability Act (HIPAA [Pub L No. 104–191, 1996]) also addresses minor confidentiality. Under HIPAA, a pediatrician may protect minor confidentiality when the minor can legally consent for contraceptive care in their jurisdiction or when the parent/caregiver agrees to confidentiality.[36] HIPAA additionally states that even when there is no applicable law, providers may exercise professional judgment to maintain confidentiality (with the reasoning documented in the health record).[36] An office policy that explicitly describes confidential services and a practice habit to discuss confidentiality policies with both parents/caregivers and adolescents can assist pediatricians with HIPAA compliance.

Insurance billing and explanations of benefits (EOBs), electronic health records (EHRs), and patient online portals create system-level threats to the confidentiality of visits, visit content, laboratory test results, and payment for contraceptive care.[37] The 21st Century Cures Act has amplified these threats to confidentiality. A common response to provisions prohibiting information blocking is to make EHR notes accessible through the patient portal, yet parent/caregiver access to patient portals is common, with adolescent portals frequently registered with parent/caregiver emails.[37–39] The AAP policy statement on health information technology provides additional discussion of EHRs and confidentiality.[40–42]

On a more pragmatic level, although some parents/caregivers may not want to honor teen confidentiality, data show that many parents/caregivers are supportive of both confidentiality and adolescent time alone with providers to address sexual and reproductive health care.[43–45] As a best practice, pediatricians can offer contraception as a confidential service when legally able to do so, allowing the adolescent the choice to involve parents, caregivers, or another trusted adult. To decrease parent/caregiver and adolescent reluctance about time alone with a provider, pediatricians can introduce confidentiality and time alone during early adolescence.[46] When adolescents present for contraception care together with a parent/caregiver, the parent/caregiver may benefit from anticipatory guidance and educational materials from pediatricians regarding confidentiality, adolescent development, emerging autonomy for decision making, and general contraceptive care approaches.

ADOLESCENT-CENTERED COUNSELING

The AAP recommends the use of a sexual and reproductive health equity-informed and adolescent-centered approach to counseling about contraception (see companion clinical report[3]). This approach applies shared decision making and person-centered care principles to center adolescents' priorities and helps them choose a method that best fits their goals, preferences, and life circumstances.[7,8,47–49] Equity-informed, adolescent-centered counseling involves reflection upon one's own biases, assessing the adolescent's stated goals and preferences, assessing the adolescent's developmental needs and contextual barriers and facilitators, presenting method options based on the adolescent's stated preferences and developmental needs, and addressing any barriers to method choice and continuation (Table 3). This is a departure from counseling approaches based entirely on efficacy. The pediatrician starts with the adolescent's goals, preferences, and needs then provides method-specific information and counseling to enable the adolescent to meet those goals. For adolescents for whom pregnancy prevention is their most important goal, a highly effective LARC could be recommended. For adolescents for whom it is very important to have no hormones and no devices, a barrier method supported by pediatrician education and counseling could be how they meet their goals. On a practical note, adolescents' buy-in is critical to contraceptive use, and a less-effective method that is consistently and correctly used may provide better pregnancy protection than a more effective method that is discontinued.

CONTRACEPTIVE METHODS

Within a sexual and reproductive health equity framework, almost all forms of reversible contraception are available to adolescents. Therefore, it is important that pediatricians are familiar with the range of contraceptive methods, including LARC methods, progestin-only and combined hormonal methods, barrier methods, and emergency contraception. These options are described in detail in the method-specific policy statements from the AAP on LARCs,[50] barrier methods,[51] and emergency contraception,[52] as well as in the companion clinical report to this policy statement.[3] The update provides clinical information about additional progestin-only methods, combined hormonal contraceptive methods (pills, patches, rings), and barrier methods. Methods are listed by effectiveness in Table 4. When an adolescent expresses a preference for a LARC method, but a provider is unable to provide the same-day LARC method

TABLE 3. Contraceptive Counseling for Adolescents Within a Sexual and Reproductive Health Equity Framework

Step	Actions
(1) Reflect upon your own biases and assumptions about an adolescent's contraceptive need prior to counseling	• Assume a position of curiosity and empathy • Ask yourself: - *What personal values and beliefs about adolescent sexuality and contraception may influence how I counsel this adolescent?* - *What structural factors may impact this adolescent's reproductive health goals and behaviors and comfort/trust discussing these with a healthcare provider?*
(2) Assess the adolescent's stated preferences	• Mirror the adolescent's language regarding gender and body parts and normalize adolescent sexuality[54] • Ask the adolescent: - *Have you had or are you thinking about having sex with someone who makes sperm?* - *How do you feel about becoming pregnant?* - *Why or why isn't it important for you to avoid pregnancy right now?* - *What things are important to you in a birth control method? (Prompts: Effectiveness, how often used, start and stop it when you'd like, confidential from partner and/or parents, non-contraceptive benefits like helping acne or cramps?)* - *What concerns or questions do you have about birth control risks or side effects? What experiences have you had using birth control (positive or negative)?*
(3) Assess the adolescent's developmental needs and contextual factors	• What is this adolescent's maturity level and prior experience with pregnancy and/or contraception? • What challenges might this adolescent face if they experience pregnancy? • Who in their life supports their health decisions and can help them follow through on reproductive health goals? (eg, friend, partner, parent/caregiver or other family member) • Are there individuals who are trying to control this adolescent's sexual behaviors, ability to become pregnant or access birth control?
(4) Present method options based on the adolescent's stated preferences and developmental needs	• Consider using a visual tool like the CDC's "Birth Control Methods" webpage,[79] Bedsider's "Explore Birth Control Options,"[80] Reproductive Health Access Project's "Your Birth Control Choices Fact Sheet,"[81] or Pharmacy Access Forms Provider Toolkit.[62] • Highlight the role of condoms for STI prevention throughout your discussion of contraceptive methods. • Motivational interviewing approaches can be useful.[82,83]
(5) Assess for and address any barriers to method choice and continuation	• Are they able to maintain confidentiality when obtaining method? • Do they need financial support to start or continue the method? • Follow up visits can reassess: - Contraceptive needs, method choice, satisfaction, and adherence. - Relationship safety and sexual behaviors. - STI surveillance and prevention counseling, and other sexual health prevention measures (eg, HPV immunization).

in their office, the provider can offer adolescents a bridging method until the adolescent can access a LARC.

GENDER-DIVERSE ADOLESCENTS

Contraception in adolescents who are transgender and gender diverse (TGD) and capable of pregnancy involves inclusive language, adolescents' preferences around pregnancy prevention and menstrual regulation, and knowledge about the effects of gender-affirming treatments on fertility and sexual health.[53–57] Pediatricians can sensitively inquire about and mirror patients' language when referring to patient and/or partner reproductive organs,[56] and when relevant, discuss the lack of evidence and poor efficacy of exogenous testosterone (or exogenous estrogen in a sperm-producing partner) as a contraceptive method. In some patients who are TGD, gender-affirming care, such as menstrual suppression using hormonal methods, significantly improves dysphoria.[54,58] The Society for Family Planning published clinical recommendations for contraceptive counseling with individuals who are TGD.[56]

ACCESS AND HEALTH SYSTEMS APPROACHES

Expanded Access

Many adolescents face barriers to accessing contraception, such as transportation, costs, and privacy.[2] Expanded contraceptive access addresses these barriers and includes innovations such as telehealth (within and outside the medical home), online and mobile application-based prescribing, pharmacist prescribing, and OTC access.[59,60] The SARS-CoV-2 global pandemic highlighted the need for

TABLE 4. Contraception Effectiveness[79]

Effectiveness for Pregnancy Prevention	
Method	Typical use[a] failure rate %
Contraceptive implant	0.1
Hormonal IUD	0.1–0.4
Copper IUD	0.8
Progestin-only injection	4
Pill,[b] patch, ring	7
External condom	13
Sponge	14 (nulliparous) 27 (parous)
Diaphragm	17
Internal condom	21
Cervical cap	17–23[c]
Fertility awareness methods[d]	Up to 23
No method	85

[a] The number of pregnancies expected per 100 women (population as described by study authors) who use a method for one year.
[b] Combined estrogen-progestin and progestin-only pills are not distinguished in the data.
[c] https://www.fda.gov/consumers/free-publications-women/birth-control#BarrierMethods
[d] A description of fertility awareness methods (also called natural family planning) is discussed in detail in the accompanying clinical report.

low-touch and no-touch approaches, accelerating the availability of many of these expanded-access approaches.[59]

Of relevance to expanding contraceptive access, the pandemic saw a marked increase in the number of pediatricians integrating telehealth into the medical home.[61] For both medical home and other providers, low-touch (detailed medical history with limited physical examination, such as a blood pressure) and no-touch (clinician can be remote and prescribe based on detailed medical history alone) innovations to expand contraceptive access are ideal for adolescents as most adolescents are healthy and few have medical contraindications.[60] In the US Selected Practice Recommendations, the Centers for Disease Control and Prevention (CDC) has a series of basic clinical questions to be reasonably certain that an individual is not pregnant.[57] Multiple self-screening tools exist to identify potential contraindications (eg, pharmacyaccessforms.org provider toolkit[62]), and a recent blood pressure is the only component of a physical examination needed for low-touch and no-touch CHCs.[59] Research demonstrates that minors are interested in expanded access[63,64] and are as capable as young adults in reporting potential contraindications.[65] Telehealth algorithms have been developed for prescribing of combined hormonal contraceptives and subcutaneous depo medroxyprogesterone acetate to adolescents without an in-person visit.[59] The authors note that mobile application-based contraceptive access is generally based on principles of telehealth, with a provider reviewing information entered by the young person and prescribing the contraception.

A patient-centered pediatric medical home offers the continuity, trust, and accessibility for adolescents in need of contraceptive services. However, expanded-access avenues are critical to adolescents who face barriers to medical home-based care or have concerns about confidentiality of care within their medical home.[4] More than 19 million pregnancy-capable people live in contraceptive deserts, or counties without a single health center providing the full range of contraceptive options.[66] For adolescents who cannot access contraceptive care through their medical home and live in a contraceptive desert, expanded-access options such as pharmacist prescribing, online or mobile application-based approaches, and OTC access can promote reproductive equity. Developmentally appropriate counseling and efforts to communicate and coordinate care with the patient's medical home are important aspects of these expanded-access initiatives.

Pharmacist prescribing allows a single interaction with a pharmacist, and almost every community has at least 1 pharmacy. As of March 1, 2023, 17 states and the District of Columbia have specific legislation allowing pharmacists to prescribe contraception,[67] and pharmacists in other states may potentially prescribe through collaborative drug therapy management agreements with physician groups.[68] For pharmacist prescribing, most states identify specific protocols for screening for contraindications, counseling about contraceptive options, and referrals. Adolescent expanded access varies state-to-state because of variation in states' minor consent statutes, pharmacy regulations, and telehealth laws.

Health System Considerations

To provide high-quality, evidence-informed contraceptive services to adolescents, pediatricians require the support of the health systems in which they provide care, including payers, regulators, EHR vendors, and health care corporations. Optimized systems allow extended time for adolescent visits, have clear processes for documentation, and billing/payment practices that both protect confidential care and account for time spent counseling.[69,70] Health system practices to reduce barriers to contraceptive use can improve adolescent sexual and reproductive health. Examples include (but are not limited to) the onsite advanced provision of barrier methods and emergency contraception, the use of standing telephone orders for emergency contraception, provision of contraception in school-based clinics, same-day access for contraception initiation, training adolescents and/or families in the administration of subcutaneous depo medroxyprogesterone acetate, on-site same-day LARC placement and removal services, and not allowing EOBs to be sent for sexual health services.[2,71,72] When LARC services are not available on-site, health systems can support pediatricians to provide bridging contraceptive options, adolescent-friendly referral pathways to LARC services, and follow-up support after referrals. To support access, payers and policy makers need to cover provider contraceptive counseling and all contraceptive services, including low- and no-touch pathways (eg, telehealth, pharmacist provision, online and mobile application-based prescribing) and OTC access for young people. With the recent changes at the state level in laws addressing abortion care, advocacy by pediatricians to ensure minor consent for, and continued access to, contraception is paramount.

RECOMMENDATIONS

1. As a best practice, pediatricians provide access to contraceptive information and counseling to all adolescents within a sexual and reproductive health equity framework. A developmentally appropriate approach informed by principles of shared decision-making and person-centered care enables adolescents to choose the best method for their goals, preferences, and needs, regardless of gender, age, race, ethnicity, sexual orientation, illness, or ability status. A working knowledge of the risks and benefits of the full range of contraceptive methods allows the pediatrician to best meet adolescent contraceptive preferences and medical needs.
2. Adolescent contraception counseling accounts for, and educates about, diminished access to abortion services based on state law, including the limited options an individual might have if they become pregnant.
3. As a best practice, pediatricians provide adolescents with their contraceptive of choice, when there are no medical contraindications, on the same day as contraceptive counseling. When this is not possible, best practice is to offer a bridging contraceptive method and/or prescription for emergency contraception when indicated, and offer an appointment at earliest convenience or referral to a provider that can provide the requested contraceptive.
4. Governments, insurers, EHR vendors, and health care systems should design policies and products that support pediatricians in providing confidential and timely contraceptive care to adolescents, including adequate appointment time, adequate payment, attention to confidentiality in the EHR and billing practices, support staff with skills and training in confidentiality and reproductive health, and access to the full range of methods.
5. Pediatric training programs and continuing medical education should prepare pediatricians to provide the full spectrum of contraceptive care to adolescents, including LARC methods. Counseling and prescribing skills include a working knowledge about appropriate referrals for contraceptive methods practicing pediatricians do not offer themselves.
6. It is safe to prescribe many contraceptive methods based on medical history, without a physical examination other than a recent blood pressure for combined hormonal contraceptives. Pediatricians may offer telehealth contraceptive counseling and prescription.
7. Contraceptive counseling includes addressing adolescents' broader sexual health needs, including healthy relationships and interpersonal violence, HPV vaccination, and STI prevention and screening.
8. When an adolescent is not able to access contraception through their medical home, expanded access should be available. Expanded access includes telehealth approaches (within and outside of the medical home), confidential and low-cost reproductive health care services in the community, school or college health services, state and federally subsidized programs, pharmacist contraceptive prescribing, and online and mobile applications.
9. Counseling adolescents on access to all over-the-counter contraceptive methods, including OTC progestin-only contraceptive pills, is a necessary part of contraceptive counseling for adolescents. Health care systems, including health care insurers and pharmacies, should design processes to make OTC contraceptive methods accessible to adolescents.

LEAD AUTHORS

Mary A. Ott, MD, MA, FAAP
Andrea J. Hoopes, MD, MPH, FAAP
Gina S. Sucato, MD, MPH, FSAHM, FAAP
Maayan Leroy-Melamed MD, MPH, FAAP

COMMITTEE ON ADOLESCENCE, 2020–2022

Elizabeth M. Alderman, MD, FSAHM, FAAP, Chairperson
Elise Berlan, MD, MPH, FAAP
Richard J. Chung, MD, FAAP
Michael Colburn, MD, MEd, FAAP
Laura K. Grubb, MD, MPH, FAAP
Janet Lee, MD, FAAP
Stephenie B. Wallace, MD, MSPH, FAAP

LIAISONS

Anne-Marie Amies, MD – American College of Obstetricians and Gynecologists
Liwei L. Hua, MD, PhD – American Academy of Child and Adolescent Psychiatry
Seema Menon, MD – North American Society of Pediatric and Adolescent Gynecology
Maria H. Rahmandar, MD, FAAP – AAP Section on Adolescent Health
Ellie Vyver, MD – Canadian Pediatric Society

STAFF

Karen Smith
James Baumberger, MPP

ABBREVIATIONS

AAP: American Academy of Pediatrics
EHR: electronic health record
EOB: explanation of benefits
HIPAA: Health Insurance Portability and Accountability Act
HPV: Human Papillomavirus
IUD: intrauterine device
LARC: long-acting reversible contraceptives
OTC: over-the-counter
STI: sexually transmitted infection

All policy statements from the American Academy of Pediatrics automatically expire 5 years after publication unless reaffirmed, revised, or retired at or before that time.

FUNDING: No external funding.

https://doi.org/10.1542/peds.2025-072217

COMPANION PAPER: A companion to this article can be found online at www.pediatrics.org/cgi/doi/10.1542/peds.2025-072218.

REFERENCES

1. Centers for Disease Control and Prevention. High School YRBS - United States 2021 Results. Published 2023. Accessed August 5, 2023. https://nccd.cdc.gov/Youthonline/App/Results.aspx
2. Brittain AW, Loyola Briceno AC, Pazol K, et al. Youth-friendly family planning services for young people: a systematic review update. *Am J Prev Med.* 2018;55(5):725–735. PubMed doi: 10.1016/j.amepre.2018.06.010
3. Ott MA, Sucato GS, Leroy-Melamed M, Hoopes AJ; American Academy of Pediatrics, Committee on Adolescence. Contraceptive counseling and methods for adolescents: Clinical report. *Pediatrics.* 2025;156(1):e2025072218. doi: 10.1542/peds.2025-072218
4. Sieving RE, McRee AL, Mehus C, et al. Sexual and reproductive health discussions during preventive visits. *Pediatrics.* 2021;148(2):e2020049411. PubMed doi: 10.1542/peds.2021-054751
5. Mahony H, Spinner C, Vamos CA, Daley EM. Social network influences on young women's choice to use long-acting reversible contraception: a systematic review. *J Midwifery Womens Health.* 2021;66(6):758–771. PubMed doi: 10.1111/jmwh.13280
6. Ott MA, Rosenberger JG, McBride KR, Woodcox SG. How do adolescents view health? Implications for state health policy. *J Adolesc Health.* 2011;48(4):398–403. PubMed doi: 10.1016/j.jadohealth.2010.07.019
7. Hart J, Crear-Perry J, Stern L. US sexual and reproductive health policy: which frameworks are needed now, and next steps forward. *Am J Public Health.* 2022;112(S5):S518–S522. PubMed doi: 10.2105/ajph.2022.306929
8. Cohen RE, Wilkinson TA, Staples-Horne M. The need for reproductive justice in pediatrics. *JAMA Pediatr.* 2021;175(12):1207–1208. PubMed doi: 10.1001/jamapediatrics.2021.2978
9. Trent M, Dooley DG, Dougé J; SECTION ON ADOLESCENT HEALTH; COUNCIL ON COMMUNITY PEDIATRICS; COMMITTEE ON ADOLESCENCE. The impact of racism on child and adolescent health. *Pediatrics.* 2019;144(2):e20191765. PubMed doi: 10.1542/peds.2019-1765
10. Ross L, Solinger R. *Reproductive Justice: An Introduction.* University of California Press; 2017.
11. Allison BA, Angelino A, Joshua KH, Strayhorn L, Rogers P, Mann ES. "It means being safe, having power over one's body": black female adolescent experiences with reproductive health counseling in primary care. *J Pediatr Adolesc Gynecol.* 2024;37(4):389–395. PubMed doi: 10.1016/j.jpag.2024.01.165
12. Bryson A, Koyama A, Hassan A. Addressing long-acting reversible contraception access, bias, and coercion: supporting adolescent and young adult reproductive autonomy. *Curr Opin Pediatr.* 2021;33(4):345–353. PubMed doi: 10.1097/mop.0000000000001008
13. Rowley S, Broomfield C, Min J, Quinn S, Campbell K, Wood S. Racial inequities in adolescent contraceptive care delivery: a reproductive justice issue. *J Pediatr Adolesc Gynecol.* 2023;36(3):298–303. PubMed doi: 10.1016/j.jpag.2022.11.004
14. Gilliam M. Youth reproductive justice: beyond choice, toward health equity. *Health Educ Behav.* 2020;47(4):640–641. PubMed doi: 10.1177/1090198119876309
15. Singh Shrestha P, Ishak A, Maskey U, et al. Challenges in providing reproductive and gynecologic care to women with intellectual disabilities: a review of existing literature. *J Family Reprod Health.* 2022;16(1):9–15. PubMed doi: 10.18502/jfrh.v16i1.8589
16. Horner-Johnson W, Klein KA, Campbell J, Guise JM. "It would have been nice to have a choice": barriers to contraceptive decision-making among women with disabilities. *Womens Health Issues.* 2022;32(3):261–267. PubMed doi: 10.1016/j.whi.2022.01.001
17. Houtrow A, Elias ER, Davis BE; COUNCIL ON CHILDREN WITH DISABILITIES. Promoting healthy sexuality for children and adolescents with disabilities. *Pediatrics.* 2021;148(1):e2021052043. PubMed doi: 10.1542/peds.2021-052043

18. National Academies of Sciences, Engineering, and Medicine. *The Promise of Adolescence: Realizing Opportunity for All Youth.* National Academies Press; 2019.

19. Gavin LE, Catalano RF, Markham CM. Positive youth development as a strategy to promote adolescent sexual and reproductive health. *J Adolesc Health.* 2010;46(3)(suppl):S1–S6. PubMed doi: 10.1016/j.jadohealth.2009.12.017

20. National Academies of Sciences, Engineering, and Medicine. *Promoting Positive Adolescent Health Behaviors and Outcomes: Thriving in the 21st Century.* National Academies Press; 2020.

21. Chung RJ, Lee JB, Hackell JM, Alderman EM; COMMITTEE ON ADOLESCENCE; COMMITTEE ON PRACTICE & AMBULATORY MEDICINE. Confidentiality in the care of adolescents: Policy statement. *Pediatrics.* 2024;153(5):e2020007252. PubMed doi: 10.1542/peds.2024-066326

22. AMERICAN ACADEMY OF PEDIATRICS; COMMITTEE ON ADOLESCENCE. The adolescent's right to confidential care when considering abortion. *Pediatrics.* 2022;150(3):e2022058780. PubMed doi: 10.1542/peds.2022-058780

23. COMMITTEE ON ADOLESCENCE. Achieving quality health services for adolescents. *Pediatrics.* 2016;138(2):e20161347. PubMed doi: 10.1542/peds.2016-1347

24. Pampati S, Liddon N, Dittus PJ, Adkins SH, Steiner RJ. Confidentiality matters but how do we improve implementation in adolescent sexual and reproductive health care? *J Adolesc Health.* 2019;65(3):315–322. PubMed doi: 10.1016/j.jadohealth.2019.03.021

25. Fuentes L, Ingerick M, Jones R, Lindberg L. Adolescents' and young adults' reports of barriers to confidential health care and receipt of contraceptive services. *J Adolesc Health.* 2018;62(1):36–43. PubMed doi: 10.1016/j.jadohealth.2017.10.011

26. Copen CE, Dittus PJ, Leichliter JS. Confidentiality concerns and sexual and reproductive health care among adolescents and young adults aged 15-25. *NCHS Data Brief.* 2016;(266):1–8. PubMed

27. Guldi M. Fertility effects of abortion and birth control pill access for minors. *Demography.* 2008;45(4):817–827. PubMed doi: 10.1353/dem.0.0026

28. Lehrer JA, Pantell R, Tebb K, Shafer MA. Forgone health care among U.S. adolescents: associations between risk characteristics and confidentiality concern. *J Adolesc Health.* 2007;40(3):218–226. PubMed doi: 10.1016/j.jadohealth.2006.09.015

29. Zavodny M. Fertility and parental consent for minors to receive contraceptives. *Am J Public Health.* 2004;94(8):1347–1351. PubMed doi: 10.2105/ajph.94.8.1347

30. Reddy DM, Fleming R, Swain C. Effect of mandatory parental notification on adolescent girls' use of sexual health care services. *JAMA.* 2002;288(6):710–714. PubMed doi: 10.1001/jama.288.6.710

31. Office of the United Nations High Commissioner for Human Rights. *Committee on the Rights of the Child: General Comment on the implementation of the rights of the child during adolescence, CRC/GC/2003/4.* United Nations; 2016.

32. World Health Organization. *Ensuring Human Rights in the Provision of Contraceptive Information and Services: Guidance and Recommendations.* World Health Organization; 2014.

33. Guttmacher Institute. An Overview of Consent to Reproductive Health Services by Young People. Published 2023. Accessed July 25, 2024. https://www.guttmacher.org/state-policy/explore/overview-minors-consent-law

34. Ford C, English A, Sigman G. Confidential Health Care for Adolescents: position paper for the society for adolescent medicine. *J Adolesc Health.* 2004;35(2):160–167. PubMed doi: 10.1016/j.jadohealth.2004.03.002

35. *State Minor Consent Laws: A Summary.* 3rd ed. Center for Adolescent Health and the Law; 2010.

36. English A, Ford CA. The HIPAA privacy rule and adolescents: legal questions and clinical challenges. *Perspect Sex Reprod Health.* 2004;36(2):80–86. PubMed doi: 10.1363/psrh.36.80.04

37. Carlson J, Goldstein R, Hoover K, Tyson N. NASPAG/SAHM Statement: The 21st Century Cures Act and Adolescent Confidentiality. *J Adolesc Health.* 2021;68(2):426–428. PubMed doi: 10.1016/j.jpag.2020.12.015

38. Pasternak RH, Alderman EM, English A. 21st Century Cures Act ONC Rule: implications for adolescent care and confidentiality protections. *Pediatrics.* 2023;151(suppl 1):e2022057267K. PubMed doi: 10.1542/peds.2022-057267k

39. Xie J, McPherson T, Powell A, et al. Ensuring adolescent patient portal confidentiality in the age of the Cures Act Final Rule. *J Adolesc Health.* 2021;69(6):933–939. PubMed doi: 10.1016/j.jadohealth.2021.09.009

40. Council on Clinical Information Technology. Health information technology and the medical home. *Pediatrics.* 2011;127(5):978–982. PubMed doi: 10.1542/peds.2011-0454

41. American Academy of Pediatrics. Guiding principles for information sharing and blocking in pediatric care. Published 2021. Accessed January 27, 2022. https://www.aap.org/en/practice-management/health-information-technology/guiding-principles-for-information-sharing-and-blocking-in-pediatric-care/

42. Pageler NM, Webber EC, Lund DP. Implications of the 21st Century Cures Act in Pediatrics. *Pediatrics.* 2021;147(3):e2020034199. PubMed doi: 10.1542/peds.2020-034199

43. Dempsey AF, Singer DD, Clark SJ, Davis MM. Adolescent preventive health care: what do parents want? *J Pediatr.* 2009;155(5):689–94.e1. PubMed doi: 10.1016/j.jpeds.2009.05.029

44. Gilbert AL, Rickert VI, Aalsma MC. Clinical conversations about health: the impact of confidentiality in preventive adolescent care. *J Adolesc Health.* 2014;55(5):672–677. PubMed doi: 10.1016/j.jadohealth.2014.05.016

45. Eisenberg ME, Oliphant JA, Plowman S, Forstie M, Sieving RE. Increased parent support for comprehensive sexuality education over 15 years. *J Adolesc Health.* 2022;71(6):744–750. PubMed doi: 10.1016/j.jadohealth.2022.08.005

46. Hagan JF, Shaw JS, Duncan PM, eds. *Bright Futures: Guidelines for Health Supervision of Infants, Children, and Adolescents.* 4th ed. American Academy of Pediatrics; 2017.

47. Nguyen AT, Curtis KM, Tepper NK, et al; Contributors. U.S. medical eligibility criteria for contraceptive use, 2024. *MMWR Recomm Rep.* 2024;73(4):1–126. PubMed doi: 10.15585/mmwr.rr7304a1

48. Dehlendorf C, Grumbach K, Schmittdiel JA, Steinauer J. Shared decision making in contraceptive counseling. *Contraception.* 2017;95(5):452–455. PubMed doi: 10.1016/j.contraception.2016.12.010

49. Holt K, Reed R, Crear-Perry J, Scott C, Wulf S, Dehlendorf C. Beyond same-day long-acting reversible contraceptive access: a person-centered framework for advancing high-quality, equitable contraceptive care. *Am J Obstet Gynecol.* 2020;222(4S):S878.e871–S878.e876. PubMed doi: 10.1016/j.ajog.2019.11.1279

50. Menon S; COMMITTEE ON ADOLESCENCE. Long-acting reversible contraception: specific issues for adolescents. *Pediatrics.* 2020;146(2):e2020007252. PubMed doi: 10.1542/peds.2020-007252

51. Grubb LK; COMMITTEE ON ADOLESCENCE. Barrier protection use by adolescents during sexual activity. *Pediatrics.* 2020;146(2):e2020007237. PubMed doi: 10.1542/peds.2020-007237

52. Upadhya KK; COMMITTEE ON ADOLESCENCE. Emergency Contraception. *Pediatrics.* 2019;144(6):e20193149. PubMed doi: https://doi.org/10.1542/peds.2019-3149

53. Rafferty J; COMMITTEE ON PSYCHOSOCIAL ASPECTS OF CHILD AND FAMILY HEALTH; COMMITTEE ON ADOLESCENCE; SECTION ON LESBIAN, GAY, BISEXUAL, AND TRANSGENDER HEALTH AND WELLNESS. Ensuring comprehensive care and support for transgender and gender-diverse children and adolescents. *Pediatrics.* 2018;142(4):e20182162. PubMed doi: 10.1542/peds.2023-063756

54. Hembree WC, Cohen-Kettenis PT, Gooren L, et al. Endocrine treatment of gender-dysphoric/gender-incongruent persons: an Endocrine Society Clinical Practice Guideline. *J Clin Endocrinol Metab.* 2017;102(11):3869–3903. PubMed doi: 10.1210/jc.2017-01658

55. American College of Obstetricians and Gynecologists. Committee Opinion No. 685: Care for transgender adolescents. *Obstet Gynecol.* 2017;129(1):e11–e16. PubMed doi: 10.1097/aog.0000000000001861

56. Bonnington A, Dianat S, Kerns J, et al. Society of Family Planning clinical recommendations: Contraceptive counseling for transgender and gender diverse people who were female sex assigned at birth. *Contraception.* 2020;102(2):70–82. PubMed doi: 10.1016/j.contraception.2020.04.001

57. Curtis KM, Nguyen AT, Tepper NK, et al; Contributors. US selected practice recommendations for contraceptive use, 2024. *MMWR Recomm Rep.* 2024;73(3):1–77. PubMed doi: 10.15585/mmwr.rr7303a1

58. American College of Obstetricians and Gynecologists' Committee on Clinical Consensus–Gynecology. General approaches to medical management of menstrual suppression: ACOG Clinical Consensus No. 3. *Obstet Gynecol.* 2022;140(3):528–541. PubMed doi: 10.1097/aog.0000000000004899

59. Wilkinson TA, Kottke MJ, Berlan ED. Contraception for adolescents during the coronavirus disease 2019 pandemic. *JAMA Pediatr.* 2021;175(3):322. PubMed doi: 10.1001/jamapediatrics.2020.5091

60. Williams RL, Meredith AH, Ott MA. Expanding adolescent access to hormonal contraception: an update on over-the-counter, pharmacist prescribing, and web-based telehealth approaches. *Curr Opin Obstet Gynecol.* 2018;30(6):458–464. PubMed doi: 10.1097/gco.0000000000000497

61. Heinrich L, Hernandez AK, Laurie AR. Telehealth considerations for the adolescent patient. *Prim Care.* 2022;49(4):597–607. PubMed doi: 10.1016/j.pop.2022.04.006

62. Pharmacy Access Forms. Provider Toolkit. Published 2021. Accessed July 22, 2024. https://www.pharmacyaccessforms.org/toolkit-materials

63. Manski R, Kottke M. A Survey of teenagers' attitudes toward moving oral contraceptives over the counter. *Perspect Sex Reprod Health.* 2015;47(3):123–129. PubMed doi: 10.1363/47e3215

64. Meredith AH, Vahary EB, Wilkinson TA, Meagher CG, Vielott T, Ott MA. Adolescents' perceptions of contraception access through pharmacies. *Pharmacy (Basel).* 2020;8(2):53. PubMed doi: 10.3390/pharmacy8020053

65. Wilkinson TA, Meredith AH, Rafie S, et al. Adolescents' and young adults' ability to self-screen for contraindications to hormonal contraception and the role of chronic illness. *J Adolesc Health.* 2021;69(4):566–573. PubMed doi: 10.1016/j.jadohealth.2021.04.032

66. Access to Birth Control and Contraceptive Deserts. Published 2019. Accessed August 11, 2024. https://powertodecide.org/what-we-do/information/resource-library/access-birth-control-and-contraceptive-deserts

67. Guttmacher Institute. Pharmacist-Prescribed Contraceptives. Published 2023. Accessed April 15, 2023. https://www.guttmacher.org/state-policy/explore/pharmacist-prescribed-contraceptives

68. Ahmad ZM, Noel NL, Rudd TM, et al. Implementation of a pharmacist-led hormonal contraceptive prescribing service in a campus community pharmacy in Indiana, United States. *Contraception.* 2022;113:113–118. PubMed doi: 10.1016/j.contraception.2022.05.004

69. Marcell AV, Breuner CC, Hammer L, Hudak ML; COMMITTEE ON ADOLESCENCE; COMMITTEE ON CHILD HEALTH FINANCING. Targeted reforms in health care financing to improve the care of adolescents and young adults. *Pediatrics.* 2018;142(6):e20182998. PubMed doi: 10.1542/peds.2018-2998

70. Society for Adolescent Health and Medicine; American Academy of Pediatrics. Confidentiality protections for adolescents and young adults in the health care billing and insurance claims process. *J Adolesc Health.* 2016;58(3):374–377. PubMed doi: 10.1016/j.jadohealth.2015.12.009

71. Berlan E, Valenti O, Long W, et al. Practice facilitation improves adolescent reproductive health preventive services in primary care. *Pediatrics.* 2022;149(1):e2020035774. PubMed doi: 10.1542/peds.2020-035774

72. Kohn JE, Berlan ED, Tang JH, Beasley A. Society of Family Planning committee consensus on self-administration of subcutaneous depot medroxyprogesterone acetate (DMPA-SC). *Contraception.* 2022;112:11–13. PubMed doi: 10.1016/j.contraception.2022.03.023

73. Gomez AM, Wapman M. Under (implicit) pressure: young Black and Latina women's perceptions of contraceptive care.

Contraception. 2017;96(4):221–226. PubMed doi: 10.1016/j.contraception.2017.07.007

74. Rocca CH, Harper CC. Do racial and ethnic differences in contraceptive attitudes and knowledge explain disparities in method use? *Perspect Sex Reprod Health.* 2012;44(3):150–158. PubMed doi: 10.1363/4415012
75. Sharko M, Jameson R, Ancker JS, Krams L, Webber EC, Rosenbloom ST. State-by-state variability in adolescent privacy laws. *Pediatrics.* 2022;149(6):e2021053458. PubMed doi: 10.1542/peds.2021-053458
76. Shneyderman Y, Schwartz SJ. Contextual and intrapersonal predictors of adolescent risky sexual behavior and outcomes. *Health Educ Behav.* 2013;40(4):400–414. PubMed doi: 10.1177/1090198112447800
77. White CN, Warner LA. Influence of family and school-level factors on age of sexual initiation. *J Adolesc Health.* 2015;56(2):231–237. PubMed doi: 10.1016/j.jadohealth.2014.09.017
78. Ti A, Soin K, Rahman T, Dam A, Yeh PT. Contraceptive values and preferences of adolescents and young adults: A systematic review. *Contraception.* 2022;111:22–31. PubMed doi: 10.1016/j.contraception.2021.05.018
79. Centers for Disease Control and Prevention. Contraception: Birth Control Methods. Published 2024. Accessed July 22, 2024. https://www.cdc.gov/reproductive-health/contraception/index.html
80. Bedsider. Explore Birth Control Options. Published 2024. Accessed July 22, 2024. https://www.bedsider.org/birth-control
81. Reproductive Health Access Project. Your Birth Control Choices Fact Sheet. Published 2022. Accessed July 22, 2024. https://www.reproductiveaccess.org/resource/birth-control-fact-sheet/
82. Centers for Disease Control and Prevention. A Guide to Taking a Sexual History. Published 2022. Accessed January 28, 2022. https://www.cdc.gov/sti/hcp/clinical-guidance/taking-a-sexual-history.html
83. Lopez LM, Grey TW, Chen M, Tolley EE, Stockton LL. Theory-based interventions for contraception. *Cochrane Database Syst Rev.* 2016;11(11):CD007249. PubMed doi: 10.1002/14651858.cd007249.pub5

Contraceptive Counseling and Methods for Adolescents

- *Clinical Report*

CLINICAL REPORT Guidance for the Clinician in Rendering Pediatric Care

American Academy of Pediatrics

DEDICATED TO THE HEALTH OF ALL CHILDREN™

Contraceptive Counseling and Methods for Adolescents: Clinical Report

Mary A. Ott, MD, MA, FAAP,[1] Gina S. Sucato, MD, MPH, FSAHM, FAAP,[2,3] Maayan Leroy-Melamed, MD, MPH, FAAP,[4] Andrea J. Hoopes, MD, MPH, FAAP,[2,3] and the Committee on Adolescence

abstract

To provide contraceptive care to adolescents, pediatricians need a working knowledge about counseling basics as well as a full range of contraceptive methods. Pediatricians may provide contraception for pregnancy prevention or for menstrual suppression and other medical indications. This clinical report is a companion to the revised policy statement "Contraception for Adolescents," and it provides updates for pediatricians on adolescent-centered counseling approaches and contraceptive methods, including long-acting reversible contraceptives, hormonal contraceptives, barrier methods, and emergency contraceptives. Together, these documents provide the pediatrician with evidence-informed and equity-informed practices in counseling and prescribing contraception for adolescents.

INTRODUCTION

It is important for pediatricians to be knowledgeable about basic contraceptive counseling and the range of contraceptive methods. Adolescents have an unmet need for contraception. In 2021, 30% of all high school students reported ever having sex.[1] Among sexually active students in 2021, 52% reported using a condom at last sexual intercourse and 33% reported that they or a partner used an effective form of contraception (either long acting reversible method [LARC] or hormonal method) at last sexual intercourse; of those, 10% reported dual use of condom and a more effective hormonal or LARC method together.[1] Almost 14% of sexually active youth used no method of contraception at last sexual intercourse.[2]

Contraception is an important tool in optimizing adolescent reproductive health, and the majority of the declines in adolescent pregnancy since the 1990s are attributable to increased use of contraception.[3] However, many adolescents continue to face barriers to accessing effective, equitable contraceptive care.[4] As trusted health care professionals, many with

[1]Departments of Global Health and Health Systems Design and Pediatrics, Icahn School of Medicine at Mount Sinai, New York, New York; [2]Adolescent Medicine, Washington Permanente Medical Group, Seattle, Washington; [3]Department of Pediatrics, University of Washington, Seattle, Washington; and [4]The Warren Alpert Medical School of Brown University, Division of Adolescent Medicine, Hasbro Children's Hospital, Rhode Island Hospital, Providence, Rhode Island

Address correspondence to: Mary A. Ott, MD, MA. maryaott8@gmail.com

Drs Ott, Sucato, Leroy-Melamed and Hoopes conceptualized the manuscript, reviewed the literature, drafted sections of the manuscript, and provided critical review.

FINANCIAL/CONFLICT OF INTEREST DISCLOSURE: The authors have indicated they have no potential conflicts of interest to disclose.

To cite: Ott MA, Sucato GS, Leroy-Melamed M, et al; American Academy of Pediatrics, Committee on Adolescence. Contraceptive Counseling and Methods for Adolescents: Clinical Report. *Pediatrics.* 2025;156(1):e2025072218

long-term relationships with adolescents, pediatricians are often the first health care provider that adolescents speak to about sexual and reproductive health concerns[5,6] and pediatricians are well-positioned to meet adolescents' contraceptive needs with patient-centered, evidence-informed, developmentally tailored, equity-focused counseling. In addition to using contraception for pregnancy prevention, many adolescents, particularly adolescents with medical complexity, use hormonal contraception for menstrual regulation and other medical indications.

This clinical report is a companion to the revised policy statement "Contraception for Adolescents,"[7] provides an overview of contraceptive methods available to adolescents in the United States, and expands on counseling guidance in the policy statement. This report builds on the series of method-specific statements and clinical reports from the American Academy of Pediatrics (AAP) on LARCs,[8] barrier methods,[9] and emergency contraception (EC).[10] It also includes new information on progestin-only pills (POPs) as well as combined hormonal, barrier, and other methods not included in the method-specific statements. Together, this family of documents supports the pediatrician in providing evidence-informed and equity-informed practices in counseling and prescribing contraception for adolescents. Table 1 lists contraceptive methods and the effectiveness of each. Other sources of information on contraception that may be useful to the pediatrician are listed in Table 2, including the contraceptive guidance documents from the Centers for Disease Control and Prevention (CDC), the US Medical Eligibility Criteria (US MEC)[11] and its companion document, the US Selected Practice Recommendations (US SPR).[12] Both are available online and as free applications for mobile devices. The US-MEC reviews data on medical conditions and contraceptives and categorizes methods as 1 - no restrictions; 2 - advantages generally outweigh theoretical or proven risks; 3 - theoretical or proven risks usually outweigh advantages, but may be used with a specific patient using a shared decision making approach; and 4 - unacceptable health risk.[11] The most recent version of the US-MEC, released in August 2024, includes many important updates. Even experienced clinicians are advised to consult this reference when prescribing for adolescents with ongoing medical conditions, using it in conjunction with shared decision making and consideration of an adolescent's preferences and circumstances to make an individualized treatment plan.

TABLE 1. Contraception Effectiveness and Continuation

Effectiveness for Pregnancy Prevention		
Method	Typical Use Failure Rate,[a] %	Continuation Rate,[b] %
Contraceptive implant	0.1	81
Hormonal IUD	0.1–0.4	82
Copper IUD	0.8	76
Progestin-only injection	4	47
Pill,[c] patch, ring	7	47 (pills), 41 (patch), and 31 (ring)
External condom	13	—
Sponge	17 (overall), 14 (nulliparous), 27 (parous)	—
Diaphragm	17	—
Cervical cap	17–23[b]	—
Fertility awareness	17 (range 2–23)	—
Internal condom	21	—
No method	85	—

—, not applicable.
Hormonal contraception effectiveness from the CDC,[133] and continuation rates from Rosenstock.[49]
[a] The number of pregnancies expected per 100 pregnancy-capable individuals who use a method for 1 year.
[b] The proportion of individuals who continue a method for 1 year.
[c] Combined estrogen-progestin and progestin-only pills not distinguished in the data.

TABLE 2. Online Contraception Resources for Pediatricians

Resource (Sponsor)	Where to Find It
US Medical Eligibility Criteria, 2024 (CDC)	U.S. Medical Eligibility Criteria for Contraceptive Use, 2024 (U.S. MEC) | Contraception | CDC
US Selected Practice Recommendations, 2024 (CDC)	U.S. Selected Practice Recommendations for Contraceptive Use, 2024 (U.S. SPR) | Contraception | CDC
CDC Contraception Information	Contraception and Birth Control Methods | Contraception | CDC
FDA Birth Control Information	https://www.fda.gov/consumers/free-publications-women/birth-control
Bedsider Providers (Power Through Choices)	https://providers.bedsider.org/
Reproductive Health Access Project	https://www.reproductiveaccess.org/contraception/

ADOLESCENT-CENTERED COUNSELING

Effective contraceptive counseling with adolescents applies principles of shared decision making and person-centered care within a sexual and reproductive health equity framework.[13–15] The pediatrician provides medical knowledge about contraception, while the adolescent offers perspective on their goals, preferences and life circumstances, and together they make a collaborative decision about contraception initiation, continuation, or discontinuation.[14] Shared decision-making may involve a parent/caregiver or trusted adult as preferred by the adolescent, as adolescents frequently identify family as sources of sexual health values, information, and support for method choice.[16] Additionally, peers and partners can be sources of influence or support for contraceptive choice and continuation.[6,17–20] If the adolescent chooses, a partner can be included in contraceptive visits and decision making.[21]

Bright Futures: Guidelines for Health Supervision of Infants, Children, and Adolescents, 4th edition, recommends that pediatricians obtain a developmentally tailored sexual history from the adolescent alone, assess STI and pregnancy risk, and provide appropriate screening, counseling, and, when needed, contraception.[22] Taking a sexual history is facilitated by an honest, caring, nonjudgmental attitude and a comfortable, matter-of-fact approach to asking questions. Tools for sexual history taking include the "5 Ps" of sexual history: partners, practices, protection from STIs, past history of STIs, and pregnancy intention[23] and motivational interviewing focused on future goals, validating adolescents' capacity to reach those goals, and engaging adolescents in adoption of health-promoting behaviors.[23–25]

Gender-inclusive language ensures that adolescents maintain trust and confidence with their care team.[26] Providers may introduce themselves with their personal pronouns and inquire about the adolescent's gender identity, pronouns, and sexual identity as part of the confidential interview. Pediatricians may consider using terms like "a person who can become pregnant" or "someone with a uterus" rather than "women" to include those individuals who identify as transmasculine or nonbinary and have contraceptive needs. Beyond pregnancy-capable individuals, pediatricians can ensure that contraceptive information and counseling is available to all individuals who can contribute to a pregnancy, including those who make sperm, such as birth-assigned males (ie, cisgender males, transgender females, and gender diverse youth with testicles).[21]

If adolescents have experienced prior sexual abuse, sexual assault, human trafficking, and other forms of trauma, a healing-centered approach may be necessary.[27] Of particular importance, adolescents involved in the child welfare and juvenile justice systems have high rates of sexual trauma and high rates adverse sexual health outcomes; many have also experienced biases from providers.[28–30] A healing-centered approach includes using language and skills to promote trust building, as well as screening for trauma, and referring to trauma-specific health care services as indicated.[31,32]

For adolescents and young adults with diminished decision-making capacity due to cognitive impairment or intellectual disability, the pediatrician can involve a parent/caregiver to partner in decision-making that centers the best interests of the adolescent. An alternative framework is *supported* decision-making, in which the adolescent or young adult with cognitive impairment identifies a trusted adult (frequently a parent) to help communicate their preferences to the clinician.[33,34]

Research suggests that adolescents make decisions differently than adults—for example, adolescents may be less risk averse, have more challenges considering multiple perspectives, and make different decisions in "hot" (high emotion and distraction) decision-making scenarios.[35–37] Nonetheless, studies of overall capacity for health decisions demonstrate that adolescents have adult-type capacity to understand health information, weigh risks and benefits, and make rational, voluntary choices.[35,38–41] In a study of contraceptive decision making, by 14 years of age, participants demonstrated the capacity to self-screen for medical contraindications, understand contraceptive information, appreciate how it affects them personally, balance risks and benefits, and make voluntary decisions.[41,42]

An adolescent-centered counseling approach within a sexual and reproductive health equity framework starts with a pediatrician reflecting on their own biases and assumptions about an adolescent's contraceptive needs. Pediatricians who choose not to provide contraceptive care because of claims of conscience are directed to the AAP policy statement, "Physician Refusal to Provide Information or Treatment on the Basis of Claims of Conscience."[43] Referrals need to be time-sensitive, respectful, nonjudgmental and done with an awareness of the power differential between adolescents and providers.

Self-reflection is followed by assessing the adolescent's stated goals and preferences, (independent of the preferences of interested family members, partners, or friends), developmental needs and contextual factors. Stated preferences might include how a method is used (and whether it requires a prescription or procedure) or method efficacy at preventing pregnancy. Developmental needs and contextual factors might include an adolescent's prior (or lack of) contraceptive experiences, need for more interactive counseling, school and family characteristics, social norms, and relevant cultural perspectives.[44–46]

After this assessment, the pediatrician can then present method options based on the adolescent's stated preferences, developmental needs, and context. Ideally, a pediatrician will be able to provide a range of methods based on access, from over-the-counter (OTC) options like emergency contraception, condoms, and progestin-only contraceptive pills, which do not require a prescription and are not disclosed to guardians through the EHR or EOB, to prescription-based options such as combined hormonal contraceptive methods, the contraceptive injection, and long-acting reversible contraceptive (LARC) devices such as implants and intrauterine devices (IUDs). Important guidance on counseling about LARC methods using sexual and reproductive equity principles can be found in the Patient-Centered LARC Counseling Section of the AAP Clinical Report on Long-Acting Reversible Contraception.[8] Pediatricians additionally need to take into account and educate adolescents about access to contraception and abortion services based on state law, which may limit options an adolescent might have if they become pregnant.[47]

TABLE 3. Contraceptive Counseling for Adolescents Within a Sexual and Reproductive Health Equity Framework

Step	Actions
(1) Reflect upon your own biases and assumptions about an adolescent's contraceptive need prior to counseling	• Assume a position of curiosity and empathy • Ask yourself: - *What personal values and beliefs about adolescent sexuality and contraception may influence how I counsel this adolescent?* - *What structural factors may impact this adolescent's reproductive health goals, behaviors, and comfort discussing these with a healthcare provider?*
(2) Assess the adolescent's stated goals and preferences	• Mirror the adolescent's language regarding gender and body parts and normalize adolescent sexuality[57] • Ask the adolescent: - *Have you had or are you thinking about having sex with someone who makes sperm?* - *How do you feel about becoming pregnant?* - *Why or why isn't it important for you to avoid pregnancy right now?* - *What things are important to you in a birth control method? (Prompts: Effectiveness, how often used, start and stop it when you'd like, confidential from partner and/or parents, non-contraceptive benefits like helping acne or cramps?)* - *What concerns or questions do you have about birth control risks or side effects? What experiences have you had using birth control (positive or negative)?*
(3) Assess the adolescent's developmental needs and contextual factors	• What is this adolescent's maturity level and prior experience with pregnancy and/or contraception? • What circumstances might this adolescent face if they experience pregnancy? • Who in their life supports their health decisions and can help them follow through on reproductive health goals? (eg, friend, partner, parent/caregiver or other family member) • Are there individuals who are trying to control this adolescent's sexual behaviors, ability to become pregnant or access birth control?
(4) Present method options based on the adolescent's stated goals, preferences, and needs	• Consider using a visual tool like the CDC's "Birth Control Methods" webpage,[133] Bedsider's "Explore Birth Control Options,"[134] Reproductive Health Access Project's "Your Birth Control Choices Fact Sheet,"[135] or Pharmacy Access Forms Provider Toolkit.[136] • Highlight the role of condoms for STI prevention throughout your discussion of contraceptive methods. • Motivational interviewing approaches can be useful.[23,25]
(5) Assess for and address any barriers to method choice and continuation	• Are they able to maintain confidentiality when obtaining method? • Do they need financial support to start, continue, or change the method? • Follow up visits can reassess: - Contraceptive needs, method choice, satisfaction, and adherence. - Relationship safety and sexual behaviors. - STI surveillance and prevention counseling, and other sexual health prevention measures (eg, HPV immunization).

Pediatricians may use contraceptive decision aids to improve knowledge and provide additional support to adolescents making contraception decisions.[48] (See Table 3 for examples of decision aids.) For many adolescents seeking contraception, pregnancy prevention is a key priority, and counseling should proceed from most effective to least effective methods.[46] Other adolescents may prioritize menstrual control, not taking a daily pill, or privacy; for these adolescents, method preferences will be different.

Table 3 provides a step-by-step summary of this sexual and reproductive equity-informed counseling framework. Shared contraception decision-making with adolescents is often an iterative process. Adolescents may need to try more than one method, working together with their pediatrician to address barriers and facilitators to effective use, including access, payment, transportation for continuity of care, burden of use, and side effects. It may be helpful to schedule a follow-up visit 1 to 3 months after starting a contraceptive method to check in on this process.

For the pediatrician, comprehensive contraceptive counseling relies on familiarity with the full range of contraceptive methods. The purpose of this clinical report is to provide pediatricians with an updated review of effectiveness and method characteristics to help inform shared decision making with their patients.

METHOD OVERVIEW

LARCs (ie, intrauterine devices [IUDs] and contraceptive implants) are safe and provide the most effective pregnancy prevention for adolescents. Although only one aspect of an adolescent-centered approach to contraceptive decision making, effectiveness has become particularly salient given recent restrictions on access to safe abortion care.[47] Compared with other methods, LARCs have both higher effectiveness and higher continuation. In the CHOICE study, the 14- to 19-year-old participants (who had parental permission to participate and a higher rate of prior pregnancy than teens in the general population) had a 12-month continuation rate of LARCs of 81%, compared with 44% for non-LARC methods.[49] Also from the CHOICE study, the contraceptive failure rate was 20 times higher in women 14 to 45 years of age who used combined hormonal pills, patches, or rings than in those using LARC methods.[50] This was an especially notable finding in those women younger than 21 years in whom the pill, patch, and ring contraceptive failure rates were twice as high as in women 21 years or older.[50] Permanent contraception (eg, tubal ligation, hysterectomy, vasectomy), although listed in many adult-oriented resources, raises legal, ethical, and medical concerns for adolescents and is addressed in a separate AAP policy statement.[51]

Shorter-acting contraceptives include combined hormonal contraceptive (CHC) methods and progestin-only methods. CHC methods contain a combination of progestin and estrogen and include pills, vaginal rings, and transdermal patches. All progestin-only methods, including levonorgestrel IUDs, implants, injections, and pills, are safer for health conditions in which estrogen use is contraindicated. Shorter-acting hormonal contraceptives (pills, patches, rings) are highly effective but are often discontinued after less than 6 months of use, most commonly because of reported side effects.[52] Emergency contraception (EC [eg, designated oral products, IUDs, pills]) are important tools and account for a significant part of the decrease in adolescent pregnancy rates. Pediatricians should be aware of any restrictions on contraceptive methods for minors in their states. With states considering legislation restricting EC, IUDs, and other methods, the AAP State Advocacy team can provide pediatricians with an update on their state's legal landscape and opportunities for advocacy by pediatricians at the state level (stgov@aap.org).

STARTING CONTRACEPTION

Contraception should always be started on the day of visit ("quick start") if the health care provider is reasonably certain the adolescent is not pregnant, remembering that menstrual periods can be irregular in adolescents and the urine pregnancy tests may not detect a very early pregnancy, especially prior to missed menses. (See the CDC algorithm in the US selected Practice Recommendations for Contraceptive Use, 2024[12]). However, even when the health care provider is not reasonably certain the adolescent is not pregnant, the benefit of starting almost all contraceptive methods may outweigh the risks of delaying contraceptive initiation, and shared decision making with the adolescent is recommended. To prevent pregnancy as soon as possible after unprotected intercourse, EC is indicated and can be provided with oral levonorgestrel, oral ulipristal acetate or an IUD (see EC and IUD method sections below).[10]

If a pediatrician is unable to provide a specific method, the pediatrician should be knowledgeable about adolescent-friendly locations where patients can access the full range of methods.[43] A "bridge method" that is easily accessed can be useful for any patients experiencing a delay in obtaining their preferred method of ongoing contraception—for example, prescribing oral contraceptive pills that can be procured at a local pharmacy and used until a patient can obtain a clinician-placed LARC method. Online resources exist to help identify the nearest health center offering LARCs—for example, https://www.bedsider.org/find-health-care/clinics.

Providers should counsel adolescents to use a backup method (ie, condom or other barrier method) for 7 days after initiation of a hormonal contraceptive method and encourage adolescents to use a condom and/or latex sheet for all sexual encounters to protect against sexually transmitted infections (STIs).[9] Contraception should be provided within the context of routine sexual health care, and pediatricians should address topics such as human papillomavirus (HPV) vaccination and routine screening for STIs.[22] Except for IUD placement, a pelvic examination is not necessary to start contraception. Following contraception initiation, patients should be provided with clear instructions on how to contact the office with problems or questions and with additional sources of information about their method, including how to manage missed doses, in the format (eg, online links, QR codes, or taking a photo of the instructions) preferred by the patient. Some adolescents do not want to receive paper copies of instructions that may be discovered by others. Contraception counseling can be an iterative process, and some patients may need to try multiple contraceptive methods to find the one that best fits their needs. Scheduling a routine follow-up visit can help address the management of side effects or minimize a gap prior to changing to a different method if necessary or desired. Virtual visits (telehealth or telephonic) are well-suited to these types of visits.

CONTRACEPTIVE METHODS

Progestin Implants

Nexplanon (Organon, Whitehouse Station, New Jersey) is a single-rod implant that contains 68 mg of etonogestrel, the active metabolite of the progestin desogestrel, that provides highly effective pregnancy prevention for up to 2 years beyond the US Food and Drug Administration (FDA)-approved 3 years (5 years total).[53–55] Nexplanon is currently the only available subdermal contraceptive implant in the United States. Implants are suitable for adolescents who prefer a method that does not require regularly scheduled adherence and who desire an extended length of protection.[8,56] Training is widely available at no cost through the manufacturer, and increasing numbers of general pediatricians are learning to place and remove implants.[57] Additional information can be found in the AAP clinical report on LARC methods.[8]

TABLE 4. IUDs Available in the United States, 2025

Device	Hormone	Length of Use[56,137,138]	Manufacturer
Liletta	52 mg levonorgestrel	6 y	AbbVie and Medicines360
Mirena	52 mg levonorgestrel	8 y	Bayer HealthCare Pharmaceuticals Inc
Kyleena	19.5 mg levonorgestrel	5 y	Bayer HealthCare Pharmaceuticals Inc
Skyla	13.5 mg levonorgestrel	3 y	Bayer HealthCare Pharmaceuticals Inc
Copper T380-A, ParaGard	None	10 y	Cooper
Miudella (175 mm^2 copper in nitinol frame)[a]	None	3 y	Sebela Women's Health Inc

[a] US Food and Drug Administration. Miudella Full Prescribing Information. Updated February 2025. Accessed May 14, 2025. https://sebelapharma.com/assets/media/miudella-PI.pdf

Intrauterine Devices

The IUD is a LARC medical device inserted into the uterus. There are 6 FDA-approved IUDs (Table 4). IUDs are safe for nulliparous individuals, do not cause infertility, and provide rapid return to fertility after removal.[58,59] The copper T380-A IUD has been shown to be effective emergency contraception within 5 days of unprotected intercourse,[10] and a study of adult patients showed similar effectiveness of the 52-mg levonorgestrel IUD as emergency contraception.[60] Patients desiring an IUD after the EC window but before pregnancy can be reliably ruled out may choose to quick start another contraceptive method that can be more easily discontinued as a bridge method until pregnancy can be reliably excluded and an IUD can be safely placed. If an IUD is placed, providers may recommend another pregnancy test 2 weeks after the last episode of unprotected intercourse. If an IUD user is found to be pregnant, the increased risks of spontaneous abortion and preterm delivery can be decreased by IUD removal.[12] Menstrual cups have been shown to increase the risk of IUD expulsion, whereas tampons have not been shown to do so.[61–63] The AAP clinical report on LARC methods and the ACOG provide additional information on risks, benefits, and counseling for implants and IUDs.[8,64] Because IUD insertion can cause severe cramping, pain management options, including insertion under sedation for select patients, should be included in counseling. There is no consensus on a single, evidence-informed, best practice. However, options for pain management are presented in the SPR.[12]

Progestin-Only Injectable Contraception

Depo medroxyprogesterone acetate (DMPA, Depo-Provera [Pfizer, New York, New York]) is a long-acting progestin that is injected every 3 months, using a dose of either 150 mg intramuscularly or 104 mg subcutaneously.[12] As an off-label use, patients can self-inject the subcutaneous formulation after instruction, which has demonstrated improved contraceptive continuation rates.[12,65] Both regimens have similar side effects and are highly effective in preventing pregnancy.[65,66] DMPA may be administered up to 2 weeks late (15 weeks after last injection) without requiring backup contraception, and there is no time limit for early injections.[12]

DMPA advantages include easy use, reduction of uterine bleeding, and improvement in dysmenorrhea. Disadvantages include the need for regular injections and menstrual cycle irregularities that occur in nearly all patients initially but typically improve over time.[66] Other potential side effects include headache, mastalgia, hair loss, change in libido, and weight gain. Studies in both adolescents and adults suggest that DMPA-related weight gain occurs in a minority of users and that weight gain status at 6 months after initiation is a strong predictor of future excessive weight gain with ongoing DMPA use.[67,68]

In 2004, the FDA issued a "boxed warning" (the highest safety-related warning that medications can have) regarding the risk of decreased bone mineral density (BMD) among DMPA users. The ACOG, citing substantial recovery of BMD after discontinuing DMPA, does not advise limiting the duration of DMPA use nor routinely monitoring bone density but does recommend a shared decision-making approach.[69] With the emergence of limited data linking bone fracture to more than 2 years of DMPA use, the risk-benefit discussion for hormonal contraception may be more challenging when prescribing DMPA for teens for medical uses rather for contraception.[70,71] It is good practice to include counseling to promote skeletal health, including meeting recommended daily intake of 1300 mg of calcium and 600 IU of vitamin D, and regular weight-bearing exercise.[72]

Progestin-Only Pills

There are 3 progestin-only oral contraceptives (sometimes called "mini-pill") currently available in the United States. Norethindrone 0.35 mg has been available since the late 1960s. In July 2023, norgestrel 0.75 mg (brand name Opill, Perrigo, Dublin, Ireland) became the first oral birth control pill approved by the FDA to be available in the US without a prescription and without age restrictions.[73] Both of these POPs have no placebo interval. They prevent pregnancy by thickening cervical mucus and do not reliably inhibit ovulation.[74] It is recommended they are taken within the same 3-hour window each day to maintain efficacy. Adolescents' access to over-the-counter contraceptive options will be affected by retail pricing and insurance coverage which warrant ongoing attention, particularly as more options become available.[75]

A newer POP containing the progestin drospirenone (brand name Slynd, Exeltis USA Inc, Florham Park, New Jersey) provides another POP alternative for individuals with estrogen contraindications (eg, migraine headaches with aura, severe and uncontrolled hypertension) who struggle with traditional POPs because of breakthrough bleeding or adherence issues. Similar to the mechanism of action of CHC, Slynd suppresses ovulation, including even when a pill is delayed by 24 hours, and has a built in 4-day placebo interval intended to create more predictable monthly bleeding.[76] Slynd contains an analog of spironolactone and, thus, has the potential to cause hyperkalemia in those at risk, for example patients with renal disorders or using medications with elevated potassium as a potential side effect.[77]

Combined Hormonal Contraception

CHC methods (pills, transdermal patches, and vaginal rings) are the most used methods of hormonal contraception for adolescents. Although more data are available from studies of combined oral contraceptive (COC) pills than the other modalities, all have the same mechanism of action and similar contraindications to use, which are minimal in healthy adolescents. CHCs are identified as an unacceptable health risk (MEC category 4) for adolescents with severe and uncontrolled hypertension (systolic pressure ≥160 mm Hg or diastolic pressure ≥100 mm Hg), <21 days postpartum, peripartum cardiomyopathy (with normal or mildly impaired cardiac function <6 months postpartum or with moderately or severely impaired cardiac function) liver tumors (hepatocellular adenoma or malignant hepatoma), severe (decompensated) cirrhosis, acute viral hepatitis, nephrotic syndrome, dialysis, major surgery with prolonged immobilization, current history of thromboembolism or thrombophilia, sickle cell disease, lupus (with positive or unknown antiphospholipid antibodies), history of and current ischemic heart disease, history of cerebrovascular accident (stroke), complications of diabetes (eg, nephropathy, retinopathy, neuropathy, or other vascular disease), migraines with aura or focal neurologic symptoms, and continuation in a patient with multiple risk factors for atherosclerotic cardiovascular disease.[11,78,79] Given the frequency of headache symptoms, careful attention to headache classification[80] will prevent unnecessarily limiting access to CHC. Complicated valvular heart disease (pulmonary hypertension, risk for atrial fibrillation or history of subacute bacterial endocarditis), and complicated solid organ transplant are additionally identified as an unacceptable health risk (MEC category 4),[11] and collaboration with the patient's specialty team is prudent. Smoking, although discouraged, is not a contraindication for adolescents or adults younger than 35 years of age (MEC category 2).[11]

Venous thromboembolism (VTE) is the most serious adverse event associated with CHC, which increases from a baseline risk of 1 per 10 000 to 3 to 4 per 10 000 person-years during CHC use.[81–83] In comparison, the incidence of venous thromboembolism during pregnancy and postpartum is 10 to 20 per 10 000 person-years, of which 1% to 2% are fatal.[84] Although there are some conflicting data suggesting higher VTE risk using the patch[85] and other data showing small differences in VTE risk with different progestins, the absolute VTE risk for CHC is low and similar across CHC methods.[86]

Numerous studies have investigated the risk of breast cancer associated with use of hormonal contraception with inconsistent findings, but overall, the additional risk of premenopausal breast cancer conferred by hormonal contraception is generally thought to be low and a family history of breast cancer is not considered a contraindication to any hormonal contraceptive method.[11,87] In contrast, there is a demonstrated decrease in the risk of ovarian and endometrial and possibly colon cancer with the use of COC pills.[88]

CHCs have similar common side effects including transient irregular bleeding, headache, and nausea. Recommendations for managing adverse effects are available elsewhere and online.[12,89–91] Pediatricians are advised to use caution to avoid drug interactions with CHCs, particularly with medications that decrease contraceptive effectiveness (eg, some anticonvulsants and rare antiretroviral drugs).[12,92,93] Antibiotics, except for rifamycin antibiotics such as rifampin, are unlikely to affect the contraceptive effectiveness.[94]

All CHC methods can be started on the day of visit (quick start as described above) in healthy, nonpregnant adolescents with advice to use a back-up method (eg, condoms) for at least the first 7 days if sexually active. The US SPR has clear and comprehensive guidance on managing late or missed doses of pills, patches, and rings.[12]

Providers may authorize sufficient refills for a full year (13 four-week cycles). Method continuation is higher when patients receive a full-year prescription at one time, a practice recommended by the CDC[12] and legally required in some states when requested by patients (see, for example, the state of Washington[95]). A routine follow-up visit at 1 to 3 months may be useful for addressing adverse effects or adherence issues but is not necessary.

Combined Oral Contraceptive Pills

In most COC pills, the estrogen component is ethinyl estradiol in amounts varying from 10 to 50 μg. A common approach is to begin with a COC containing 30 to 35 μg of ethinyl estradiol (EE). Lower doses of EE are available and not contraindicated but may have an adverse impact on bone mineral density acquisition[72] and be associated with more irregular bleeding compared with higher doses of estrogen.[96] Higher doses (ie, 50 µg EE) increase thrombotic risk.[86] In addition, one pill (Nextstellis, Mayne Pharma LLC, Raleigh, North Carolina) combines a plant-synthesized version of the naturally occurring estrogen, estetrol, with drospirenone. Although theoretically it has the potential for an improved safety profile, based on the currently available data, prescribing considerations are the same as for all other COC pills.[97,98]

Pill packs typically include a combination of hormone-containing pills and hormone-free or "reminder" pills. While taking reminder pills, uterine bleeding occurs because of the absence of hormones. Pills are packaged to support a variety of regimens, from monthly cycling (4–7 hormone-free days per month) to extended cycling to continuous active pills with zero hormone-free pills per year.[99] For example, a commonly used extended cycling regimen includes 12 weeks of hormone pills and 7 hormone-free pills. Any commonly prescribed brands of monophasic COC pills can be used in any of the aforementioned regimens. Comprehensive counseling includes strategies to promote daily adherence, such as mobile device alarms, tracker mobile applications, and support from a family member or partner.

Contraceptive Vaginal Ring

There are 2 vaginal rings. NuvaRing (Merck, Whitehouse Station, NJ) requires insertion of a new ring each month. Patients insert the contraceptive ring into the vagina and leave it in place for 3 weeks, with removal for 1 week to induce withdrawal bleeding. A new ring is inserted after 7 days even if bleeding continues. Annovera, a ring that can be used for up to a year, is a similar diameter (2.25" vs 2.13") to the Nuvaring but twice as thick (0.33" vs 0.16"). It is removed after 21 days of use and stored unrefrigerated for 7 days to allow a withdrawal bleed, and then reinserted each month. In addition to other CHC side effects, ring users may experience vaginal discharge or discomfort and problems related to the device (eg, expulsion or inability to locate).[100] The NuvaRing contains sufficient medication for use up to 35 days[101] and, thus, can be used continuously and replaced without a period of removal to skip menses.[99] There are no data on continuous use of Annovera. Patients do not need to remove rings for tampon use, menstrual cup use, or intercourse, but if the adolescent chooses, they can remove them for up to 2 hours for Annovera and 3 hours for NuvaRing without diminished efficacy for pregnancy prevention.[102]

Transdermal Contraceptive Patches

There are 2 types of transdermal patches available in the United States; beige/peach is the only color available. The square patch (Xulane, Viatris Pharmaceuticals, Inc, Canonsburg, Pennsylvania, and Zafemy, Amneal, Bridgewater, New Jersey) delivers 150 µg/d norelgestromin and 35 µg/d ethinyl estradiol, but its labeling notes that overall estrogen exposure is about 60% higher than with an oral birth control pill containing 35 µg of ethinyl estradiol. The larger (28 cm^2 vs 14 cm^2) circular patch (Twirla, Agile Therapeutics, Princeton, New Jersey) delivers 120 µg/d levonorgestrel and 30 µg/d ethinyl estradiol. Both patches are labeled for use only by individuals with a body mass index (BMI) <30 kg/m^2. Patches are placed on the abdomen, upper torso, or buttocks (and also upper outer arm for Xulane), using 1 patch per week for 3 weeks in a row, followed by 1 week off the patch, during which time a withdrawal bleed usually occurs. Similarly to the pill and ring, the patch-off week can be eliminated for continuous use to reduce bleeding.[99,103] In addition to other CHC side effects, users may also experience dislodged patches and skin effects (hyperpigmentation, contact dermatitis, and other irritation).[104,105]

Barrier Methods

Barrier methods include the external (formerly called "male") condom, internal (formerly "female") condom, latex sheets (dental dams), diaphragms, cervical caps, sponges, spermicides, and vaginal pH modulators. A recent AAP policy statement and technical report on barrier methods provides detailed information for the pediatrician on external and internal condoms and dental dams.[9]

Diaphragms are shallow, dome-shaped silicone cups used with spermicide and placed inside the vagina prior to intercourse. The Milex diaphragm (Cooper Surgical, Trumbull, Connecticut) requires fitting by a provider. A newer contoured diaphragm (Caya, HPSRx Enterprises, Salem, Virginia) is one-size-fits-most and does not require fitting. Both can remain in the vagina for up to 24 hours. Cervical caps are 1.5 × 1 inch silicone cups that fit over the cervix with spermicide inside. Contraceptive sponges are 2-inch pieces of plastic foam impregnated with spermicide. The single-use sponge is wetted to activate the spermicide, can be placed up to 24 hours prior to sex, and remains in for up to 30 hours. All 3 methods (diaphragm, cervical cap, sponge) require remaining in for at least 6 hours after intercourse. The typical use failure rates for diaphragms and sponges are high (see Table 1), and they do not protect from STIs. Younger adolescents use these methods less frequently, but older adolescents may desire these event-specific and hormone-free methods.[106]

Two contraceptive vaginal gels are available. Nonoxynol-9 spermicide is available OTC as gel, cream, foam, film, or suppository. Nonoxynol-9 gels are used with diaphragms and cervical caps, and nonoxynol-9 is impregnated in sponges. The typical use failure rate of nonoxynol-9 alone is 21%.[90] Nonoxynol-9 does not protect against STIs. Because repeated and high-dose use may cause vaginal or anal lesions that may increase HIV transmission, the CDC considers its use an unacceptable health risk (MEC category 4) for individuals at risk for HIV.[11] For individuals living with HIV, use of nonoxynol-9 is usually not recommended unless other more appropriate methods are not available or acceptable (MEC category 3).[11] A newer vaginal pH modulator (Phexxi, Evofem Biosciences, San Diego, California) is a prescription contraceptive acidifying gel with active ingredients lactic acid 1.8%, citric acid 1%, and sodium bitartrate 0.4%. It prevents pregnancy by modulating vaginal pH and impairing sperm motility. It is applied immediately before or up to an hour before sexual intercourse and reapplied every hour thereafter. Population-based effectiveness data are not available; clinical trials from the manufacturer reported a typical use failure rate of 14%.[76,107] A new applicator should be used for each vaginal sexual act,[76] and the vaginal pH modulator may be used with other methods except the vaginal ring.

Emergency Contraception

When used within 120 hours after unprotected intercourse, EC reduces the risk of pregnancy, and the sooner EC is initiated, the more effective it is. ECs include FDA-indicated oral EC products, levonorgestrel and ulipristal acetate (a progesterone receptor modulator), and IUDs. Oral levonorgestrel and ulipristal acetate are more effective the sooner they are taken after unprotected intercourse and may be less effective in individuals with higher BMI.[108] While individuals may start another hormonal contraceptive method immediately after taking oral levonorgestrel EC, starting another hormonal method within 5 days of using ulipristal acetate may decrease the effectiveness of ulipristal.[12] Shared decision-making is recommended to weigh this risk against potentially delaying care for patients who choose an ongoing contraceptive method that requires an office visit (LARC or DMPA) to start. A recent study demonstrated that the levonorgestrel IUD was noninferior to the copper IUD for use as EC,[60] an off-label use for both. Body weight and timing (≤5 days) do not affect the effectiveness of the IUD as EC. The AAP policy statements on LARC methods[8] and emergency contraception[10] provide additional detailed information.

Withdrawal, Abstinence, and Fertility Awareness-Based Methods

Withdrawal, abstinence, and fertility awareness-based methods are less effective methods but are practiced by many adolescents.[2] Withdrawal, or coitus interruptus, is a method in which the penis is pulled out of the vagina before ejaculation. Withdrawal has limited effectiveness, with a 20% overall failure rate (adolescent data not available).[109] Although less than 4% of individuals report currently using withdrawal,[110] lifetime use is common, and 65% of sexually active 15- to 19-year-old adolescents reported ever using withdrawal.[111] In fertility awareness-based methods, individuals abstain during fertile days of their menstrual cycle, identified via menstrual calendar, basal body temperature, observations of cervical mucus, or a combination of these three. Fertility awareness places a high responsibility on users, and it may be less effective for adolescents, as ovulation is often not predictable in the first few years after menarche. Fertility awareness-based mobile applications are available but have not been tested in people younger than 18 years and are not indicated for persons with irregular periods.[112]

As a contraceptive method, abstinence has a perfect use efficacy of 100%; however, in nationally representative surveys, many adolescents who plan to be abstinent become sexually active,[113,114] making the typical use effectiveness much lower. These data suggest that pediatricians should not rely on abstinence counseling alone and need to provide comprehensive sexual health information including when and how to access to EC.

YOUTH WITH MEDICAL COMPLEXITY AND MEDICAL INDICATIONS

Youth With Medical Complexity

An estimated 16% to 25% of adolescents have special health care needs, including physical disability, intellectual disability, and medically complex conditions.[115] Sexuality and sexual health care needs in this population are often overlooked, yet compared with healthy adolescents, adolescents with chronic medical conditions have similar levels of sexual behaviors and STIs.[116] In addition to pregnancy prevention, medically complex adolescents may have medical indications for contraceptives. For example, patients with intellectual disability or mobility limitations may benefit from menstrual suppression.[117] Collaboration with a patient's managing subspecialist about contraception can enhance a pediatrician's knowledge of the underlying condition, how that may impact contraceptive effectiveness, and side effects (such as hypertension with renal disease, low bone density with celiac disease, or seizure management).[79,81,118] When applicable, adolescents with medical complexity should be made aware of the additional risks that an unplanned pregnancy could pose to their health.

Medications that are teratogenic are commonly prescribed for adolescents, and many teenagers are not counseled about contraceptives.[119,120] Pediatricians prescribing teratogens or caring for adolescents who are prescribed teratogenic medications, such as isotretinoin, spironolactone, or mycophenolate, should discuss pregnancy prevention with patients[120–122] For example, anticonvulsants are widely prescribed for both seizure disorder and behavioral indications and interact with many contraceptives.[79,120] The CDC addresses contraception considerations for certain medical conditions and medication interactions in the US MEC (see Table 2),[11] and the ACOG provides guidance on the hormonal contraception use for adolescents and adults with coexisting medical conditions as well as medical management of menstrual suppression.[81,99,120,123]

Contraceptive care in adolescents with a uterus who are transgender and gender diverse (TGD) includes pregnancy prevention and menstrual regulation as desired by the patient. For both these indications, all hormonal methods, including those including estrogen, can be used by patients also taking testosterone. Testosterone may or may not provide amenorrhea and is not to be used as a contraceptive method. Ideally, communication around amenorrhea, anatomy, and physical examinations will be healing centered and consider individual dysphoria.[124] The Society for Family Planning published clinical recommendations for contraceptive counseling with individuals who are TGD.[26]

Medical Indications for Contraception

Many adolescents need or desire menstrual regulation or suppression, and contraceptives can treat medical conditions such as anemia, acne, severe dysmenorrhea, endometriosis, bleeding disorders, abnormal or heavy menstrual bleeding, and thrombocytopenia related to chemotherapy.[81,118,125–127] Given the relative safety of hormonal contraceptives, adolescents may use them to reduce bleeding or move toward amenorrhea. Contraceptives may be useful for ovarian suppression for conditions with catamenial exacerbation, such as migraines, epilepsy, irritable bowel syndrome, inflammatory bowel disease, and some psychiatric and behavioral symptoms.[79,118,120,123]

Extended Cycling

Menstrual management involves a variety of methods, and providers can use shared decision-making approaches in counseling. CHC methods offer patients some control over when withdrawal bleeding occurs. When using continuously or with extended cycling, there is the "tailored approach" of taking active pills until bleeding reoccurs, and the "scheduled approach" of a break every 3 to 4 months to reduce unscheduled breakthrough bleeding.[103,128,129] In the tailored approach, patients stop pills for 3 to 5 days when they begin spotting and then reinitiate active pills. Some pills are packaged and marketed for 3-month cycles or continuously. The most common adverse effect of extended/continuous cycles is unscheduled bleeding.[130] A common approach to continuous and extended cycling with COC pills is to use monophasic, 30-μg or 35-μg ethinyl estradiol pills and a second- (levonorgestrel or norgestrel) or third-generation (desogestrel or norgestimate) progestin.[103] Prescribers can indicate extended cycling to help the pharmacy and insurance dispense refills earlier. See Table 5 for rates of amenorrhea and anovulation for contraceptive methods.

TABLE 5. Rates of No Bleeding for 90 Days and Anovulation for Medical Uses Contraception

Method	Amenorrhea Rate at 1 Year	Anovulation Rate
Continuous combined oral contraceptive pills	49–88%[139]	95–99%[140]
Depot medroxyprogesterone acetate (DMPA)	50–70%[141]	Over 99%[142]
Oral progestins	Up to 76%[143]	98.75% (desogestrel), 67% (norethindrone 0.35 and norgestrel 0.75)[140,144]
Levonorgestrel IUD (52 mg)	0.2–30%[145]	50%[131]
Contraceptive implant	21.4%[146]	99%[132]

For those with contraindications to estrogens or who wish to avoid estrogen, progestin-only options can be used for menstrual suppression and extended cycling. Users can start and stop POPs more quickly than progestin-only shots, implants, or IUDs; however, adolescents using POPs may experience more breakthrough bleeding. DMPA effectively suppresses ovulation and menstruation, is safe for most patients with chronic illness,[11] and is used for medical conditions such as anemia[126] and seizure disorders,[79,120] as described above. The 19.5-mg and 52-mg levonorgestrel IUDs can reduce uterine bleeding with minimal hormonal exposure but do not reliably suppress ovulation; in contrast, the implant suppresses ovulation but has higher rates of breakthrough bleeding.[8,131,132]

CONCLUSION

Access to a full range of contraceptive methods is an important component of safe, equitable, and adolescent-centered health care, and pediatricians are well-placed to address contraceptive needs. Together with the companion policy statement, "Contraception for Adolescents," and the family of policy statements and clinical reports on contraception and sexual health, the AAP provides guidance for a comprehensive, equity-informed approach to contraception for adolescents.

LEAD AUTHORS

Mary A. Ott, MD, MA, FAAP
Gina S. Sucato, MD, MPH, FSAHM, FAAP
Maayan Leroy-Melamed, MD, MPH, FAAP
Andrea J. Hoopes MD, MPH, FAAP

COMMITTEE ON ADOLESCENCE, 2020–2022

Elizabeth M. Alderman, MD, FSAHM, FAAP, Chairperson
Elise Berlan, MD, MPH, FAAP
Richard J. Chung, MD, FAAP
Michael Colburn, MD, MEd, FAAP
Laura K. Grubb, MD, MPH, FAAP

Janet Lee, MD, FAAP
Stephenie B. Wallace, MD, MSPH, FAAP

LIAISONS

Anne-Marie Amies, MD – American College of Obstetricians and Gynecologists
Liwei L. Hua, MD, PhD – American Academy of Child and Adolescent Psychiatry
Seema Menon, MD – North American Society of Pediatric and Adolescent Gynecology
Maria H. Rahmandar, MD, FAAP – AAP Section on Adolescent Health
Ellie Vyver, MD – Canadian Pediatric Society

STAFF

Karen Smith
James Baumberger, MPP

ABBREVIATIONS

AAP: American Academy of Pediatrics
ACOG: American College of Obstetricians and Gynecologists
BMD: bone mineral density
BMI: body mass index
CDC: Centers for Disease Control and Prevention
CHC: combined hormonal contraceptive
COC: combined oral contraceptive
IUD: intrauterine device
DMPA: depot medroxyprogesterone acetate
EC: emergency contraception
LARC: long-acting reversible contraceptive
MEC: Medical Eligibility Criteria
POP: progestin-only pill
SPR: Selected Practice Recommendations
STI: sexually transmitted infection
VTE: venous thromboembolism

All clinical reports from the American Academy of Pediatrics automatically expire 5 years after publication unless reaffirmed, revised, or retired at or before that time.

FUNDING: No external funding.

https://doi.org/10.1542/peds.2025-072218

COMPANION PAPER: A companion to this article can be found online at www.pediatrics.org/cgi/doi/10.1542/peds.2025-072217.

REFERENCES

1. Centers for Disease Control and Prevention. Youth Risk Behavior Survey Data Summary and Trends Report 2011–2021. Published 2023. Accessed July 24, 2024. https://www.cdc.gov/yrbs/dstr/pdf/YRBS_Data-Summary-Trends_Report2023_508.pdf
2. Centers for Disease Control and Prevention. High School YRBS - United States 2021 Results. Published 2023. Accessed August 5, 2023. https://nccd.cdc.gov/Youthonline/App/Results.aspx
3. Lindberg L, Santelli J, Desai S. Understanding the decline in adolescent fertility in the United States, 2007–2012. *J Adolesc Health.* 2016;59(5):577–583. PubMed doi: 10.1016/j.jadohealth.2016.06.024
4. Brittain AW, Loyola Briceno AC, Pazol K, et al. Youth-friendly family planning services for young people: a systematic review update. *Am J Prev Med.* 2018;55(5):725–735. PubMed doi: 10.1016/j.amepre.2018.06.010
5. Sieving RE, McRee AL, Mehus C, et al. Sexual and reproductive health discussions during preventive visits. *Pediatrics.* 2021;148(2):e2020049411. PubMed doi: 10.1542/peds.2020-049411
6. Mahony H, Spinner C, Vamos CA, Daley EM. Social network influences on young women's choice to use long-acting reversible contraception: a systematic review. *J Midwifery Womens Health.* 2021;66(6):758–771. PubMed doi: 10.1111/jmwh.13280
7. Ott MA, Hoopes AJ, Sucato GS, Leroy-Melamed M; American Academy of Pediatrics, Committee on Adolescence. Contraception for adolescents: policy statement. *Pediatrics.* 2025;156(1):e2025072217. doi: 10.1542/peds.2025-072217
8. Menon S, Alderman EM, Chung RJ, et al; COMMITTEE ON ADOLESCENCE. Long-acting reversible contraception: specific issues for adolescents. *Pediatrics.* 2020;146(2):e2020007252. PubMed doi: 10.1542/peds.2020-007252
9. Grubb LK, Alderman EM, Chung RJ, et al; COMMITTEE ON ADOLESCENCE. Barrier protection use by adolescents during sexual activity. *Pediatrics.* 2020;146(2):e2020007237. PubMed doi: 10.1542/peds.2020-007237
10. Upadhya KK, Breuner CC, Alderman EM, et al; COMMITTEE ON ADOLESCENCE. Emergency Contraception. *Pediatrics.* 2019;144(6):e20193149. PubMed doi: 10.1542/peds.2019-3149
11. Nguyen AT, Curtis KM, Tepper NK, et al; Contributors. U.S. medical eligibility criteria for contraceptive use, 2024. *MMWR Recomm Rep.* 2024;73(4):1–126. PubMed doi: 10.15585/mmwr.rr7304a1

12. Curtis KM, Nguyen AT, Tepper NK, et al; Contributors. U.S. selected practice recommendations for contraceptive use, 2024. *MMWR Recomm Rep.* 2024;73(3):1–77. PubMed doi: 10.15585/mmwr.rr7303a1

13. Holt K, Reed R, Crear-Perry J, Scott C, Wulf S, Dehlendorf C. Beyond same-day long-acting reversible contraceptive access: a person-centered framework for advancing high-quality, equitable contraceptive care. *Am J Obstet Gynecol.* 2020;222(4S):S878.e871–S878.e876. doi: 10.1016/j.ajog.2019.11.1279

14. Dehlendorf C, Grumbach K, Schmittdiel JA, Steinauer J. Shared decision making in contraceptive counseling. *Contraception.* 2017;95(5):452–455. PubMed doi: 10.1016/j.contraception.2016.12.010

15. Hart J, Crear-Perry J, Stern L. US sexual and reproductive health policy: which frameworks are needed now, and next steps forward. *Am J Public Health.* 2022;112(S5):S518–S522. PubMed doi: 10.2105/AJPH.2022.306929

16. Ghobadzadeh M, Sieving RE, Gloppen K. Positive youth development and contraceptive use consistency. *J Pediatr Health Care.* 2016;30(4):308–316. PubMed doi: 10.1016/j.pedhc.2015.08.006

17. Cohen R, Sheeder J, Kane M, Teal SB. Factors associated with contraceptive method choice and initiation in adolescents and young women. *J Adolesc Health.* 2017;61(4):454–460. PubMed doi: 10.1016/j.jadohealth.2017.04.008

18. Hoopes AJ, Teal SB, Akers AY, Sheeder J. Low acceptability of certain contraceptive methods among young women. *J Pediatr Adolesc Gynecol.* 2018;31(3):274–280. PubMed doi: 10.1016/j.jpag.2017.11.008

19. Yee L, Simon M. The role of the social network in contraceptive decision-making among young, African American and Latina women. *J Adolesc Health.* 2010;47(4):374–380. PubMed doi: 10.1016/j.jadohealth.2010.03.014

20. Sucato GS, Bhatt SK, Murray PJ, Ott MA. Transdermal contraception as a model for adolescent use of new methods. *J Adolesc Health.* 2011;49(4):357–362. PubMed doi: 10.1016/j.jadohealth.2011.01.008

21. Grubb LK, Powers M; COMMITTEE ON ADOLESCENCE. Emerging issues in male adolescent sexual and reproductive health care. *Pediatrics.* 2020;145(5):e20200627. PubMed doi: 10.1542/peds.2020-0627

22. Hagan JF, Shaw JS, Duncan PM, eds. *Bright Futures: Guidelines for Health Supervision of Infants, Children, and Adolescents.* 4th ed. American Academy of Pediatrics; 2017.

23. Centers for Disease Control and Prevention. A Guide to Taking a Sexual History. Published 2022. Accessed January 28, 2022. https://www.cdc.gov/sti/hcp/clinical-guidance/taking-a-sexual-history.html

24. Barnes AJ, Gold MA. Promoting healthy behaviors in pediatrics: motivational interviewing. *Pediatr Rev.* 2012;33(9):e57–e68. PubMed doi: 10.1542/pir.33.9.e57

25. Lopez LM, Grey TW, Chen M, Tolley EE, Stockton LL. Theory-based interventions for contraception. *Cochrane Database Syst Rev.* 2016;11(11):CD007249. PubMed doi: 10.1002/14651858.cd007249.pub5

26. Bonnington A, Dianat S, Kerns J, et al. Society of Family Planning clinical recommendations: Contraceptive counseling for transgender and gender diverse people who were female sex assigned at birth. *Contraception.* 2020;102(2):70–82. PubMed doi: 10.1016/j.contraception.2020.04.001

27. Blaustein ME, Kinniburgh KM. *Treating Traumatic Stress in Children and Adolescents: How to Foster Resilience Through Attachment, Self-Regulation, and Competency.* 2nd ed. The Guilford Press; 2018.

28. Wilson E, Casanueva C, Smith KR, Koo H, Tueller SJ, Webb MB. Risk of early sexual initiation and pregnancy among youth reported to the child welfare system. *Child Welfare.* 2014;93(1):127–147. PubMed

29. Barnert E, Sun A, Abrams L, Chung PJ. Reproductive health needs of recently incarcerated youth during community reentry: a systematic review. *BMJ Sex Reprod Health.* 2020;46(3):161–171. PubMed doi: 10.1136/bmjsrh-2019-200386

30. Romero EG, Teplin LA, McClelland GM, Abram KM, Welty LJ, Washburn JJ. A longitudinal study of the prevalence, development, and persistence of HIV/sexually transmitted infection risk behaviors in delinquent youth: implications for health care in the community. *Pediatrics.* 2007;119(5):e1126–e1141. PubMed doi: 10.1542/peds.2006-0128

31. Racine N, Killam T, Madigan S. Trauma-informed care as a universal precaution: beyond the adverse childhood experiences questionnaire. *JAMA Pediatr.* 2020;174(1):5–6. PubMed doi: 10.1001/jamapediatrics.2019.3866

32. American Academy of Family Practice. The National Child Traumatic Stress Network: Screening and Assessment. Published 2017. Accessed July 17, 2022. https://www.nctsn.org/treatments-and-practices/screening-and-assessment

33. Kripke C. Adults with developmental disabilities: a comprehensive approach to medical care. *Am Fam Physician.* 2018;97(10):649–656. PubMed

34. Turchi RM, Kuo DZ, Rusher JW, et al; COUNCIL ON CHILDREN WITH DISABILITIES; COMMITTEE ON MEDICAL LIABILITY AND RISK MANAGEMENT. Considerations for alternative decision-making when transitioning to adulthood for youth with intellectual and developmental disabilities: policy statement. *Pediatrics.* 2024;153(6):e2024066841. PubMed doi: 10.1542/peds.2024-066841

35. Andrews JL, Ahmed SP, Blakemore SJ. Navigating the social environment in adolescence: the role of social brain development. *Biol Psychiatry.* 2021;89(2):109–118. PubMed doi: 10.1016/j.biopsych.2020.09.012

36. Prencipe A, Kesek A, Cohen J, Lamm C, Lewis MD, Zelazo PD. Development of hot and cool executive function during the transition to adolescence. *J Exp Child Psychol.* 2011;108(3):621–637. PubMed doi: 10.1016/j.jecp.2010.09.008

37. Strang NM, Chein JM, Steinberg L. The value of the dual systems model of adolescent risk-taking. *Front Hum Neurosci.* 2013;7:223. PubMed doi: 10.3389/fnhum.2013.00223

38. Maslowsky J, Owotomo O, Huntley ED, Keating D. Adolescent risk behavior: differentiating reasoned and reactive risk-taking.

J Youth Adolesc. 2019;48(2):243–255. PubMed doi: 10.1007/s10964-018-0978-3

39. Steinberg L. Does recent research on adolescent brain development inform the mature minor doctrine? *J Med Philos.* 2013;38(3):256–267. PubMed doi: 10.1093/jmp/jht017
40. Grootens-Wiegers P, Hein IM, van den Broek JM, de Vries MC. Medical decision-making in children and adolescents: developmental and neuroscientific aspects. *BMC Pediatr.* 2017;17(1):120. PubMed doi: 10.1186/s12887-017-0869-x
41. Wilkinson TA, Meredith AH, Katz AJ, Meagher CG, Ott MA. Assessment of adolescent decision-making capacity for pharmacy access to hormonal contraception. *Contraception.* 2023;123:110002. PubMed doi: 10.1016/j.contraception.2023.110002
42. Wilkinson TA, Meredith AH, Rafie S, et al. Adolescents' and young adults' ability to self-screen for contraindications to hormonal contraception and the role of chronic illness. *J Adolesc Health.* 2021;69(4):566–573. PubMed doi: 10.1016/j.jadohealth.2021.04.032
43. Committee on Bioethics. Policy statement–Physician refusal to provide information or treatment on the basis of claims of conscience. *Pediatrics.* 2009;124(6):1689–1693. PubMed doi: 10.1542/peds.2009-2222
44. Shneyderman Y, Schwartz SJ. Contextual and intrapersonal predictors of adolescent risky sexual behavior and outcomes. *Health Educ Behav.* 2013;40(4):400–414. PubMed doi: 10.1177/1090198112447800
45. White CN, Warner LA. Influence of family and school-level factors on age of sexual initiation. *J Adolesc Health.* 2015;56(2):231–237. PubMed doi: 10.1016/j.jadohealth.2014.09.017
46. Ti A, Soin K, Rahman T, Dam A, Yeh PT. Contraceptive values and preferences of adolescents and young adults: A systematic review. *Contraception.* 2022;111:22–31. PubMed doi: 10.1016/j.contraception.2021.05.018
47. Guttmacher Institute. An Overview of Consent to Reproductive Health Services by Young People. Published 2023. Accessed July 25, 2024. https://www.guttmacher.org/state-policy/explore/overview-minors-consent-law
48. Jones A, Allison BA, Perry M. Effectiveness of contraceptive decision aids in adolescents and young adults: a systematic review. *J Pediatr Adolesc Gynecol.* 2022;35(1):7–17. PubMed doi: 10.1016/j.jpag.2021.08.005
49. Rosenstock JR, Peipert JF, Madden T, Zhao Q, Secura GM. Continuation of reversible contraception in teenagers and young women. *Obstet Gynecol.* 2012;120(6):1298–1305. PubMed doi: 10.1097/AOG.0b013e31827499bd
50. Winner B, Peipert JF, Zhao Q, et al. Effectiveness of long-acting reversible contraception. *N Engl J Med.* 2012;366(21):1998–2007. PubMed doi: 10.1056/NEJMoa1110855
51. Geis GM, Saunders BS, Hillard P, et al; COMMITTEE ON BIOETHICS; COUNCIL ON CHILDREN WITH DISABILITIES. Examining permanent contraception for children, adolescents, and young adults with intellectual developmental disorder: ethical, legal, and medical considerations: Clinical report. *Pediatrics.* 2024;154(5):e2024068955. PubMed doi: 10.1542/peds.2024-068955
52. Raine TR, Foster-Rosales A, Upadhyay UD, et al. One-year contraceptive continuation and pregnancy in adolescent girls and women initiating hormonal contraceptives. *Obstet Gynecol.* 2011;117(2 Pt 1):363–371. PubMed doi: 10.1097/AOG.0b013e31820563d3
53. American College of Obstetricians and Gynecologists. Practice Bulletin No. 186 Summary: Long-acting reversible contraception: implants and intrauterine devices. *Obstet Gynecol.* 2017;130(5):1173–1175. PubMed doi: 10.1097/AOG.0000000000002394
54. Ali M, Akin A, Bahamondes L, et al; WHO study group on subdermal contraceptive implants for women. Extended use up to 5 years of the etonogestrel-releasing subdermal contraceptive implant: comparison to levonorgestrel-releasing subdermal implant. *Hum Reprod.* 2016;31(11):2491–2498. PubMed doi: 10.1093/humrep/dew222
55. McNicholas C, Swor E, Wan L, Peipert JF. Prolonged use of the etonogestrel implant and levonorgestrel intrauterine device: 2 years beyond Food and Drug Administration-approved duration. *Am J Obstet Gynecol.* 2017;216(6):586 e581–586 e586. doi: 10.1016/j.ajog.2017.01.036
56. American College of Obstetricians and Gynecologists. Committee Opinion No. 735: Adolescents and long-acting reversible contraception: implants and intrauterine devices. *Obstet Gynecol.* 2018;131(5):e130–e139. PubMed doi: 10.1097/AOG.0000000000002632
57. Berlan E, Valenti O, Long W, et al. Practice facilitation improves adolescent reproductive health preventive services in primary care. *Pediatrics.* 2022;149(1):e2020035774. PubMed doi: 10.1542/peds.2020-035774
58. Hubacher D, Lara-Ricalde R, Taylor DJ, Guerra-Infante F, Guzmán-Rodríguez R. Use of copper intrauterine devices and the risk of tubal infertility among nulligravid women. *N Engl J Med.* 2001;345(8):561–567. PubMed doi: 10.1056/NEJMoa010438
59. Girum T, Wasie A. Return of fertility after discontinuation of contraception: a systematic review and meta-analysis. *Contracept Reprod Med.* 2018;3(1):9. PubMed doi: 10.1186/s40834-018-0064-y
60. Turok DK, Gero A, Simmons RG, et al. Levonorgestrel vs. copper intrauterine devices for emergency contraception. *N Engl J Med.* 2021;384(4):335–344. PubMed doi: 10.1056/NEJMoa2022141
61. Bowman N, Thwaites A. Correction: Menstrual cup and risk of IUD expulsion - a systematic review. *Contracept Reprod Med.* 2023;8(1):23. PubMed doi: 10.1186/s40834-023-00219-x
62. Bowman N, Thwaites A. Menstrual cup and risk of IUD expulsion - a systematic review. *Contracept Reprod Med.* 2023;8(1):15. PubMed doi: 10.1186/s40834-022-00203-x
63. van Eijk AM, Zulaika G, Lenchner M, et al. Menstrual cup use, leakage, acceptability, safety, and availability: a systematic review and meta-analysis. *Lancet Public Health.* 2019;4(8):e376–e393. PubMed doi: 10.1016/S2468-2667(19)30111-2
64. American College of Obstetricians and Gynecologists' Committee on Gynecologic PracticeLong-Acting Reversible Contraceptive Expert Work Group. Committee Opinion No 672: Clinical challenges of long-acting reversible contraceptive methods. *Obstet Gynecol.* 2016;128(3):e69–e77. PubMed doi: 10.1097/AOG.0000000000001644

65. Kennedy CE, Yeh PT, Gaffield ML, Brady M, Narasimhan M. Self-administration of injectable contraception: a systematic review and meta-analysis. *BMJ Glob Health.* 2019;4(2):e001350. PubMed doi: 10.1136/bmjgh-2018-001350

66. Kaunitz AM, Darney PD, Ross D, Wolter KD, Speroff L. Subcutaneous DMPA vs. intramuscular DMPA: a 2-year randomized study of contraceptive efficacy and bone mineral density. *Contraception.* 2009; 80(1):7–17. PubMed doi: 10.1016/j.contraception.2009.02.005

67. Lopez LM, Ramesh S, Chen M, et al. Progestin-only contraceptives: effects on weight. *Cochrane Database Syst Rev.* 2016;2016(8): CD008815. PubMed doi: 10.1002/14651858.CD008815.pub4

68. Dianat S, Fox E, Ahrens KA, et al. Side effects and health benefits of depot medroxyprogesterone acetate: a systematic review. *Obstet Gynecol.* 2019;133(2):332–341. PubMed doi: 10.1097/AOG.0000000000003089

69. American College of Obstetricians and Gynecologists. Committee Opinion No. 602: Depot medroxyprogesterone acetate and bone effects. *Obstet Gynecol.* 2014;123(6):1398–1402. PubMed doi: 10.1097/01.AOG.0000450758.95422.c8

70. Raine-Bennett T, Chandra M, Armstrong MA, Alexeeff S, Lo JC. Depot Medroxyprogesterone acetate, oral contraceptive, intrauterine device use, and fracture risk. *Obstet Gynecol.* 2019; 134(3):581–589. PubMed doi: 10.1097/AOG.0000000000003414

71. Lopez LM, Chen M, Mullins Long S, Curtis KM, Helmerhorst FM. Steroidal contraceptives and bone fractures in women: evidence from observational studies. *Cochrane Database Syst Rev.* 2015; 2015(7):CD009849. PubMed doi: 10.1002/14651858.CD009849.pub3

72. Weaver CM, Gordon CM, Janz KF, et al. The National Osteoporosis Foundation's position statement on peak bone mass development and lifestyle factors: a systematic review and implementation recommendations. *Osteoporos Int.* 2016;27(4):1281–1386. PubMed doi: 10.1007/s00198-015-3440-3

73. US Food and Drug Administration. FDA Approves First Nonprescription Daily Oral Contraceptive. Published 2023. Accessed July 30, 2023. https://www.fda.gov/news-events/press-announcements/fda-approves-first-nonprescription-daily-oral-contraceptive

74. Han L, Creinin MD, Hemon A, Glasier A, Chen MJ, Edelman A. Mechanism of action of a 0.075 mg norgestrel progestogen-only pill 2. Effect on cervical mucus and theoretical risk of conception. *Contraception.* 2022;112:43–47. PubMed doi: 10.1016/j.contraception.2022.03.016

75. Otto AK, Klein DA, Lau M, et al. It's time for over-the-counter oral contraceptive pills. *J Adolesc Health.* 2023;72(6):829–830. PubMed doi: 10.1016/j.jadohealth.2023.02.035

76. Baker CC, Chen MJ. New Contraception Update - Annovera, Phexxi, Slynd, and Twirla. *Curr Obstet Gynecol Rep.* 2022;11(1):21–27. PubMed doi: 10.1007/s13669-021-00321-4

77. US Food and Drug Administration. Multi-disciplinary Review and Evaluation NDA 211367 Slynd (drospirenone). Published 2019. Accessed April 15, 2023. www.fda.gov/media/129539/download

78. Ardura MI, Coscia LA, Meyers MR. Promoting safe sexual practices and sexual health maintenance in pediatric and young adult solid organ transplant recipients. *Pediatr Transplant.* 2021;25(1): e13949. PubMed doi: 10.1111/petr.13949

79. Kirkpatrick L, Van Cott AC, Kazmerski TM, Bravender T. Contraception and reproductive health care for adolescent and young adult women with epilepsy. *J Pediatr.* 2022;241:229–236. PubMed doi: 10.1016/j.jpeds.2021.10.056

80. Headache Classification Committee of the International Headache Society (IHS) The International Classification of Headache Disorders. 3rd edition. *Cephalalgia.* 2018;38(1):1–211. doi: 10.1177/0333102417738202

81. American College of Obstetricians and Gynecologists. Practice Bulletin No. 206: Use of hormonal contraception in women with coexisting medical conditions. *Obstet Gynecol.* 2019;133(2): e128–e150. PubMed doi: 10.1097/AOG.0000000000003072

82. Trenor CC III, Chung RJ, Michelson AD, et al. Hormonal contraception and thrombotic risk: a multidisciplinary approach. *Pediatrics.* 2011;127(2):347–357. PubMed doi: 10.1542/peds.2010-2221

83. Vandenbroucke JP, Rosing J, Bloemenkamp KW, et al. Oral contraceptives and the risk of venous thrombosis. *N Engl J Med.* 2001; 344(20):1527–1535. PubMed doi: 10.1056/NEJM200105173442007

84. Walker ID. Venous and arterial thrombosis during pregnancy: epidemiology. *Semin Vasc Med.* 2003;3(1):25–32. PubMed doi: 10.1055/s-2003-38330

85. Tepper NK, Dragoman MV, Gaffield ME, Curtis KM. Nonoral combined hormonal contraceptives and thromboembolism: a systematic review. *Contraception.* 2017;95(2):130–139. PubMed doi: 10.1016/j.contraception.2016.10.005

86. Dragoman MV, Tepper NK, Fu R, Curtis KM, Chou R, Gaffield ME. A systematic review and meta-analysis of venous thrombosis risk among users of combined oral contraception. *Int J Gynaecol Obstet.* 2018;141(3):287–294. PubMed doi: 10.1002/ijgo.12455

87. Mørch LS, Skovlund CW, Hannaford PC, Iversen L, Fielding S, Lidegaard Ø. Contemporary hormonal contraception and the risk of breast cancer. *N Engl J Med.* 2017;377(23):2228–2239. PubMed doi: 10.1056/NEJMoa1700732

88. Iversen L, Sivasubramaniam S, Lee AJ, Fielding S, Hannaford PC. Lifetime cancer risk and combined oral contraceptives: the Royal College of General Practitioners' Oral Contraception Study. *Am J Obstet Gynecol.* 2017;216(6):580 e581–580 e589. doi: 10.1016/j.ajog.2017.02.002

89. Dickey RP, Seymour ML. *Managing Contraceptive Pill Patients.* 17th ed. EMIS, Inc, Medical Publishers; 2021.

90. Hatcher RA, Nelson AL, Trussell J, et al. *Contraceptive Technology.* 21st ed. Ayer Co Publishers, Inc; 2018.

91. Zieman M, Hatcher RA, Allen AZ, Haddad L. *Managing Contraception.* 16th ed. Bridging the Gap Publications; 2021.

92. Sun H, Sivasubramanian R, Vaidya S, Barve A, Jarugula V. Drug-drug interaction studies with oral contraceptives: pharmacokinetic/pharmacodynamic and study design considerations. *J Clin Pharmacol.* 2020;60(S2)(suppl 2):S49–S62. PubMed doi: 10.1002/jcph.1765

93. Nanda K, Stuart GS, Robinson J, Gray AL, Tepper NK, Gaffield ME. Drug interactions between hormonal contraceptives and antiretrovirals. *AIDS.* 2017;31(7):917–952. PubMed doi: 10.1097/QAD.0000000000001392

94. Simmons KB, Haddad LB, Nanda K, Curtis KM. Drug interactions between non-rifamycin antibiotics and hormonal contraception: a systematic review. *Am J Obstet Gynecol.* 2018;218(1):88–97.e14. PubMed doi: 10.1016/j.ajog.2017.07.003

95. Washington State Legistlature. RCW 48.43.195. Contraceptive drugs—Twelve-month refill coverage. Published 2017. Accessed January 28, 2022. https://app.leg.wa.gov/RCW/default.aspx?cite=48.43.195

96. Bitzer J, Simon JA. Current issues and available options in combined hormonal contraception. *Contraception.* 2011;84(4):342–356. PubMed doi: 10.1016/j.contraception.2011.02.013

97. Chen MJ, Jensen JT, Kaunitz AM, et al. Tolerability and safety of the estetrol/drospirenone combined oral contraceptive: Pooled analysis of two multicenter, open-label phase 3 trials. *Contraception.* 2022;116:44–50. PubMed doi: 10.1016/j.contraception.2022.10.004

98. US Food and Drug Administration. Nextellis Prescribing Information. Published 2021. Accessed April 21, 2023. https://www.accessdata.fda.gov/drugsatfda_docs/label/2021/214154s000lbl.pdf

99. American College of Obstetricians and Gynecologists' Committee on Clinical Consensus–Gynecology. General approaches to medical management of menstrual suppression: ACOG Clinical Consensus No. 3. *Obstet Gynecol.* 2022;140(3):528–541. PubMed doi: 10.1097/AOG.0000000000004899

100. Edwardson J, Jamshidi R. The contraceptive vaginal ring. *Semin Reprod Med.* 2010;28(2):133–139. PubMed doi: 10.1055/s-0030-1248138

101. Timmer CJ, Mulders TM. Pharmacokinetics of etonogestrel and ethinylestradiol released from a combined contraceptive vaginal ring. *Clin Pharmacokinet.* 2000;39(3):233–242. PubMed doi: 10.2165/00003088-200039030-00005

102. US Food and Drug Administration. Annovera Prescribing Information. Published 2022. Accessed April 21, 2023. https://www.annovera.com/pi.pdf

103. Edelman A, Micks E, Gallo MF, Jensen JT, Grimes DA. Continuous or extended cycle vs. cyclic use of combined hormonal contraceptives for contraception. *Cochrane Database Syst Rev.* 2014;2014(7):CD004695. PubMed doi: 10.1002/14651858.cd004695.pub3

104. Stricker T, Sennhauser FH. Allergic contact dermatitis due to transdermal contraception patch. *J Pediatr.* 2006;148(6):845. PubMed doi: 10.1016/j.jpeds.2005.12.010

105. Harel Z, Riggs S, Vaz R, Flanagan P, Dunn K, Harel D. Adolescents' experience with the combined estrogen and progestin transdermal contraceptive method Ortho Evra. *J Pediatr Adolesc Gynecol.* 2005;18(2):85–90. PubMed doi: 10.1016/j.jpag.2004.11.016

106. Berglas NF, Kimport K, Mays A, Kaller S, Biggs MA. "It's worked well for me": young women's reasons for choosing lower-efficacy contraceptive methods. *J Pediatr Adolesc Gynecol.* 2021;34(3):341–347. PubMed doi: 10.1016/j.jpag.2020.12.012

107. Evofem Inc. Phexxi Full Prescribing Information. Revised June 2023. Accessed May 14, 2025. https://22077562.fs1.hubspotusercontent-na1.net/hubfs/22077562/PhexxiUSPI.pdf

108. Shen J, Che Y, Showell E, Chen K, Cheng L. Interventions for emergency contraception. *Cochrane Database Syst Rev.* 2019;1(1):CD001324. PubMed doi: 10.1002/14651858.cd001324.pub6

109. Sundaram A, Vaughan B, Kost K, et al. Contraceptive Failure in the United States: Estimates from the 2006–2010 National Survey of Family Growth. *Perspect Sex Reprod Health.* 2017;49(1):7–16. PubMed doi: 10.1363/psrh.12017

110. Centers for Disease Control and Prevention. Key Statistics from the National Survey of Family Growth - Contraception. Published 2020. Accessed July 25, 2024. https://www.cdc.gov/nchs/nsfg/key_statistics/c-keystat.htm#contraception

111. Martinez G, Abma JC. *Sexual activity and contraceptive use among teenagers aged 15–19 in the United States, 2015–2019.* National Center for Health Statistics; 2023.

112. Berglund Scherwitzl E, Lundberg O, Kopp Kallner H, Gemzell Danielsson K, Trussell J, Scherwitzl R. Perfect-use and typical-use Pearl Index of a contraceptive mobile app. *Contraception.* 2017;96(6):420–425. PubMed doi: 10.1016/j.contraception.2017.08.014

113. Brückner H, Bearman P. After the promise: the STD consequences of adolescent virginity pledges. *J Adolesc Health.* 2005;36(4):271–278. PubMed doi: 10.1016/j.jadohealth.2005.01.005

114. Pinkerton SD. A relative risk-based, disease-specific definition of sexual abstinence failure rates. *Health Educ Behav.* 2001;28(1):10–20. PubMed doi: 10.1177/109019810102800102

115. Bethell CD, Read D, Blumberg SJ, Newacheck PW. What is the prevalence of children with special health care needs? Toward an understanding of variations in findings and methods across three national surveys. *Matern Child Health J.* 2008;12(1):1–14. PubMed doi: 10.1007/s10995-007-0220-5

116. McRee AL, Haydon AA, Halpern CT. Reproductive health of young adults with physical disabilities in the U.S. *Prev Med.* 2010;51(6):502–504. PubMed doi: 10.1016/j.ypmed.2010.09.006

117. Quint EH, O'Brien RF, Braverman PK, et al; COMMITTEE ON ADOLESCENCE; North American Society for Pediatric and Adolescent Gynecology. Menstrual management for adolescents with disabilities. *Pediatrics.* 2016;138(1):e20160295. PubMed doi: 10.1542/peds.2016-0295

118. Scott N, Maslyanskaya S. Contraceptive needs of adolescents with chronic illness. *Pediatr Ann.* 2019;48(2):e78–e85. PubMed doi: 10.3928/19382359-20190121-01

119. Stancil SL, Miller M, Briggs H, Lynch D, Goggin K, Kearns G. Contraceptive provision to adolescent females prescribed teratogenic medications. *Pediatrics.* 2016;137(1):e20151454. PubMed doi: 10.1542/peds.2015-1454

120. American College of Obstetricians and Gynecologists. Committee Opinion No. 806, Summary: Gynecologic management of adolescents and young women with seizure disorders. *Obstet Gynecol.* 2020;135(5):1242–1243. PubMed doi: 10.1097/AOG.0000000000003828

121. Carandang K, Mruk V, Ardoin SP, et al. Reproductive health needs of adolescent and young adult women with pediatric rheumatic diseases. *Pediatr Rheumatol Online J.* 2020;18(1):66. PubMed doi: 10.1186/s12969-020-00460-7

122. Zaenglein AL, Pathy AL, Schlosser BJ, et al. Guidelines of care for the management of acne vulgaris. *J Am Acad Dermatol.* 2016; 74(5):945–73.e33. PubMed doi: 10.1016/j.jaad.2015.12.037

123. American College of Obstetricians and Gynecologists' Committee on Adolescent Health Care. Committee Opinion No. 668: Menstrual manipulation for adolescents with physical and developmental disabilities. *Obstet Gynecol.* 2016;128(2):e20–e25. PubMed doi: 10.1097/AOG.0000000000001585

124. Rafferty J, Yogman M, Baum R, et al; COMMITTEE ON PSYCHOSOCIAL ASPECTS OF CHILD AND FAMILY HEALTH; COMMITTEE ON ADOLESCENCE; SECTION ON LESBIAN, GAY, BISEXUAL, AND TRANSGENDER HEALTH AND WELLNESS. Ensuring comprehensive care and support for transgender and gender-diverse children and adolescents. *Pediatrics.* 2018;142(4):e20182162. PubMed doi: 10.1542/peds.2018-2162

125. Williams NM, Randolph M, Rajabi-Estarabadi A, Keri J, Tosti A. Hormonal contraceptives and dermatology. *Am J Clin Dermatol.* 2021;22(1):69–80. PubMed doi: 10.1007/s40257-020-00557-5

126. Bellizzi S, Ali MM. Effect of oral contraception on anemia in 12 low- and middle-income countries. *Contraception.* 2018;97(3):236–242. PubMed doi: 10.1016/j.contraception.2017.11.001

127. American College of Obstetricians and Gynecologists. Committee Opinion No. 747: Gynecologic issues in children and adolescent cancer patients and survivors. *Obstet Gynecol.* 2018;132(2):e67–e77. PubMed doi: 10.1097/AOG.0000000000002763

128. MacGregor EA, Guillebaud J. The 7-day contraceptive hormone-free interval should be consigned to history. *BMJ Sex Reprod Health.* 2018;Jun 26:bmjsrh–2017–200036. doi: 10.1136/bmjsrh-2017-200036

129. Stephenson J, Shawe J, Panicker S, et al. Randomized trial of the effect of tailored versus standard use of the combined oral contraceptive pill on continuation rates at 1 year. *Contraception.* 2013;88(4):523–531. PubMed doi: 10.1016/j.contraception.2013.03.014

130. Sulak PJ, Smith V, Coffee A, Witt I, Kuehl AL, Kuehl TJ. Frequency and management of breakthrough bleeding with continuous use of the transvaginal contraceptive ring: a randomized controlled trial. *Obstet Gynecol.* 2008;112(3):563–571. PubMed doi: 10.1097/AOG.0b013e3181842071

131. Alvarez F, Brache V, Fernandez E, et al. New insights on the mode of action of intrauterine contraceptive devices in women. *Fertil Steril.* 1988;49(5):768–773. PubMed doi: 10.1016/S0015-0282(16)59881-1

132. Croxatto HB. Mechanisms that explain the contraceptive action of progestin implants for women. *Contraception.* 2002;65(1):21–27. PubMed doi: 10.1016/S0010-7824(01)00294-3

133. Centers for Disease Control and Prevention. Contraception: Birth Control Methods. Published 2024. Updated Aug 6, 2024. Accessed August 30, 2024. https://www.cdc.gov/contraception/about/index.html

134. Bedsider. Explore Birth Control Options. Published 2024. Accessed July 22, 2024. https://www.bedsider.org/birth-control

135. Reproductive Health Access Project. Your Birth Control Choices Fact Sheet. Published 2022. Accessed July 22, 2024. https://www.reproductiveaccess.org/resource/birth-control-fact-sheet/

136. Pharmacy Access Forms. Provider Toolkit. Published 2021. Accessed July 22, 2024. https://www.pharmacyaccessforms.org/toolkit-materials

137. McNicholas C, Maddipati R, Zhao Q, Swor E, Peipert JF. Use of the etonogestrel implant and levonorgestrel intrauterine device beyond the U.S. Food and Drug Administration-approved duration. *Obstet Gynecol.* 2015;125(3):599–604. PubMed doi: 10.1097/AOG.0000000000000690

138. Heinemann K, Reed S, Moehner S, Minh TD. Comparative contraceptive effectiveness of levonorgestrel-releasing and copper intrauterine devices: the European Active Surveillance Study for Intrauterine Devices. *Contraception.* 2015;91(4):280–283. PubMed doi: 10.1016/j.contraception.2015.01.011

139. Miller L, Hughes JP. Continuous combination oral contraceptive pills to eliminate withdrawal bleeding: a randomized trial. *Obstet Gynecol.* 2003;101(4):653–661. PubMed 10.1016/s0029-7844(03)00014-0

140. Milsom I, Korver T. Ovulation incidence with oral contraceptives: a literature review. *J Fam Plann Reprod Health Care.* 2008;34(4):237–246. PubMed doi: 10.1783/147118908786000451

141. Schwallie PC, Assenzo JR. Contraceptive use–efficacy study utilizing medroxyprogesterone acetate administered as an intramuscular injection once every 90 days. *Fertil Steril.* 1973;24(5):331–339. PubMed doi: 10.1016/S0015-0282(16)39669-8

142. Jain J, Dutton C, Nicosia A, Wajszczuk C, Bode FR, Mishell DR Jr. Pharmacokinetics, ovulation suppression and return to ovulation following a lower dose subcutaneous formulation of Depo-Provera. *Contraception.* 2004;70(1):11–18. PubMed doi: 10.1016/j.contraception.2004.01.011

143. Mölsä PK. Inducement of therapeutic amenorrhea in mentally retarded women: two-year follow-up study. *Am J Ment Defic.* 1986;90(5):591–593. PubMed

144. US Food and Drug Administration. OPill Label and Patient Information. Revised August 2017. Accessed May 14, 2025. https://www.accessdata.fda.gov/drugsatfda_docs/label/2017/017031s035s036lbl.pdf

145. Sergison JE, Maldonado LY, Gao X, Hubacher D. Levonorgestrel intrauterine system associated amenorrhea: a systematic review and metaanalysis. *Am J Obstet Gynecol.* 2019;220(5):440–448.e8. PubMed doi: 10.1016/j.ajog.2018.12.008

146. Hohmann H. Examining the efficacy, safety, and patient acceptability of the etonogestrel implantable contraceptive. *Patient Prefer Adherence.* 2009;3:205–211. PubMed doi: 10.2147/PPA.S4299

Disclosure of Adverse Events in Pediatrics

- *Policy Statement*

POLICY STATEMENT Organizational Principles to Guide and Define the Child Health Care System and/or Improve the Health of All Children

American Academy of Pediatrics

DEDICATED TO THE HEALTH OF ALL CHILDREN™

Disclosure of Adverse Events in Pediatrics: Policy Statement

Laura Sigman, MD, JD, FAAP,[1] Robert Turbow, MD, JD, FAAP,[2] Daniel Neuspiel, MD, MPH, FAAP,[3] Julia M. Kim, MD, MPH, FAAP,[4] and the Committee on Medical Liability and Risk Management, and Council on Quality Improvement and Patient Safety

abstract

Disclosure of adverse events has become the expectation in medicine and is widely regarded as the appropriate path when medical errors occur. Although data are limited on adverse events in pediatrics, that they occur frequently is uncontested. Types and rates of errors vary depending on the care setting and patient population. Patients with complex medical conditions or from historically marginalized groups or minoritized communities likely suffer disparate health and safety outcomes. Systemic factors, including nonpunitive safety cultures and supportive environments within institutions, are essential to promoting disclosure. State laws protecting apologies from use in legal proceedings can also help to encourage open communication. Some states have adopted laws to advance disclosure, and governmental agencies provide materials encouraging open communication and early resolution after adverse events occur. Many programs emphasize the importance of supporting health care workers involved in adverse events. Shame, fear of professional and legal repercussions, and lack of training remain barriers to disclosure. Education for health care clinicians, support in health care settings, additional research on programs and disparities, and governmental and regulatory initiatives can support disclosure of adverse events.

INTRODUCTION

Over the last 2 decades, there has been increased recognition of the frequency and impact of adverse events in health care, accompanied by a transformation in how disclosure of such events takes place. Patients and their families expect such disclosure in a timely fashion. Additionally, data suggest that prompt and accurate disclosure of adverse events may be associated with decreased legal liability for the health care clinician. This policy statement updates a previous version[1]; discusses the current

[1]Armstrong Institute for Patient Safety and Quality, Department of Pediatrics, Johns Hopkins University School of Medicine, Baltimore, Maryland; [2]Dignity Health- Central Coast California and Adjunct Professor Biomedical Engineering California Polytechnic State University, San Luis Obispo, California; [3]Department of Pediatrics, Atrium Health; and [4]Department of Pediatrics, Johns Hopkins University School of Medicine, Armstrong Institute for Patient Safety and Quality, Baltimore, Maryland

All authors contributed substantially to the conception and design; review and interpretation of relevant literature; drafting and revisions; and final approval of the version to the published.

CONFLICT OF INTEREST DISCLOSURE: The authors have indicated they have no potential conflicts of interest to disclose.

FUNDING: No external funding.

https://doi.org/10.1542/peds.2025-070880

To cite: Sigman L, Turbow R, Neuspiel D, et al; American Academy of Pediatrics, Committee on Medical Liability and Risk Management, and Council on Quality Improvement and Patient Safety. Disclosure of Adverse Events in Pediatrics: Policy Statement. *Pediatrics.* 2025;155(4):e2025070880

Table 1. Definitions

Term	Definition
Patient safety	Prevention of patient harm and freedom from accidental injury in health care setting
Adverse event	Patient harm caused by medical care
Medical error	Act of commission or omission that unreasonably increases risk of an undesirable patient outcome
Preventable adverse event	Patient harm related to a medical error
Nonpreventable adverse event	Patient harm in absence of medical error
Potential adverse event (near miss)	Medical error with potential to cause patient harm that does not do so
Disclosure	Communication from health care personnel to affected patient and/or family about an adverse event
Reporting	Exchange of information about adverse events among clinicians and regulators
Just culture/safety culture	An organization's shared perceptions, beliefs, values, and attitudes that promote safety and minimize harm

state of disclosure in pediatrics and issues surrounding it, including legal and ethical implications; and provides recommendations for pediatricians.

Patient safety is the prevention of patient harm and freedom from accidental injury in the health care setting.[2] An adverse event (AE) occurs when patient harm is caused by medical care.[3] A medical error (ME) is an act of commission or omission that increases risk of an unintended patient outcome. AEs may be preventable (when patient harm is related to an ME) or nonpreventable (when patient harm occurs in the absence of an ME). An ME that causes patient harm becomes a preventable AE. An ME that has the potential to cause patient harm but does not do so is referred to as a potential AE or "near miss."[4] These concepts and their relationships are explained in Table 1 and illustrated in Figure 1.

Estimates of total annual mortality in the United States attributable to preventable AEs vary widely, from 22 000[5] to as high as 250 000 deaths.[6] It is estimated that 6% of patients have experienced preventable harm.[7] The American Academy of Pediatrics (AAP) has called attention to the importance of pediatric patient safety since 2001[8] and has recommended improved identification and reporting of MEs and AEs to improve the culture of safety in pediatric care.[9]

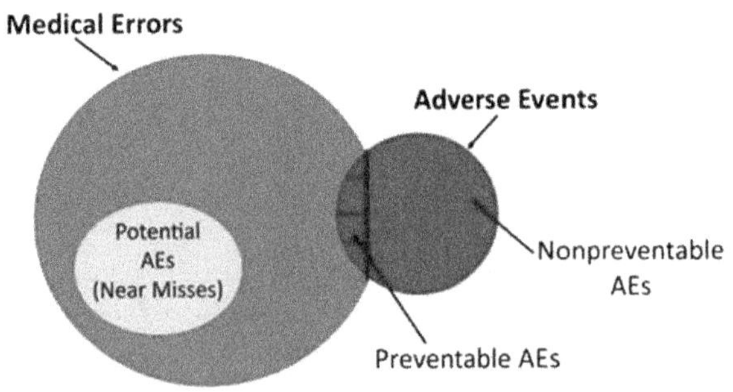

Figure 1.
Graphical Depiction of Adverse Events and Medical Errors

The economic cost of AEs in the United States is substantial, although estimates have varied. In 2006, costs of AEs were estimated between $393 and $958 billion, equal to 18% to 45% of total US health care spending.[10] In 2008, an estimate of the cost of MEs in the United States based on claims data was $17.1 billion.[11] Another study estimated that MEs in the United States cost $985 million in 2008 and over $1 billion in 2009, with median costs per error of $892 in 2008 and $939 in 2009.[12] Specific costs for AEs involving children and adolescents have not been quantified.

ADVERSE EVENTS AND MEDICAL ERRORS IN PEDIATRIC POPULATIONS

While the exact magnitude of harm to pediatric patients from AEs is not well established, pediatric AEs occur frequently, with significant morbidity and mortality. Among Canadian inpatient pediatric AEs, the overall rate was 9.2%, and those related to surgery were most frequent[13]; almost half of these AEs were determined to be preventable. There are wide variations in estimates of the incidence of AEs among pediatric inpatients.[9,14,15] Error rates related to medications in pediatrics have been noted to be 3 times higher than in adult patients.[16]

Types and rates of MEs vary depending on the health care setting and patient population. The majority of research to date has focused on errors in inpatient or emergency department settings. Emergency care settings involve high risks for errors, given the often busy, high-volume environment with frequent interruptions and transitions in care; complex patients who may not be well-known to staff; boarding; and commonly, a lack of standardized dosing, formulary, or information technology systems with pediatric safety features.[17–19] Most pediatric care occurs in ambulatory settings, and studies have reported significant numbers of errors related to medications, vaccines, diagnoses, and coordination and transition of care.[20,21] Medication administration errors account for the majority of preventable adverse drug events in the outpatient pediatric setting.[21–24] Although diagnostic errors occur frequently in pediatrics, relatively little research has been performed on their incidence and epidemiology.[25,26]

Children with special health care needs and/or medical complexity likely have higher rates of AEs than the general population because of frequent interactions with the health care system, clinicians in multiple settings, and medical needs. They are particularly vulnerable to medical errors during care transitions.[24,27–32] Families are an underused resource for detecting and reporting safety events in these populations and can provide valuable perspectives, including in ambulatory settings.[33–36]

Although research is limited on rates of AEs in historically marginalized or minoritized populations, evidence shows that these communities are more likely to suffer disparate health and safety outcomes.[37,38] Recent data have shown higher rates of AEs in hospitalized Latino children and publicly insured children, including serious AEs.[39,40] Hospitalized children of parents with limited comfort with English were twice as likely to experience AEs from medical care.[41] Language barriers have been associated with increased rates of AEs[42,43]; underreporting of AEs in hospitals relying on voluntary event reports[44]; and less willingness to question health care clinicians, which may contribute to increased safety events.[45]

THE SYSTEMS APPROACH AND SAFETY CULTURE

The Institute of Medicine (IOM) noted that most MEs are attributable to flaws in systems rather than individuals and called for a "dramatic improvement in the reliability and safety" of the health care process.[3] For this improvement to occur, AEs must first be identified and analyzed to understand their preventable causes and to allow for systematic safety improvements. Disclosure and open communication with patients and their families after an AE may benefit the patient and health care clinicians, reduce consequential harms, allow for better follow-up, and promote a safety culture.

Safety culture refers to an environment that facilitates open and honest communication to promote safety and minimize harm[46] and is particularly important when potentially uncomfortable topics such as MEs or preventable harm are being addressed. A growing body of literature, including subspecialty publications in pediatrics, demonstrate that safer culture is associated with safer care. Increasingly, the culture of pediatrics, and health care in general, is to promptly disclose to patients and families after an AE has taken place. Multiple factors are considered when disclosing MEs, including safety culture, clinician and patient level factors, and the type of error itself (see Figure 2).

REPORTING VS DISCLOSURE

The concepts of *reporting* and *disclosure* of AEs should be distinguished. *Reporting* refers to the exchange of information among clinicians and regulators. Reporting systems may be internal to health care organizations or may be

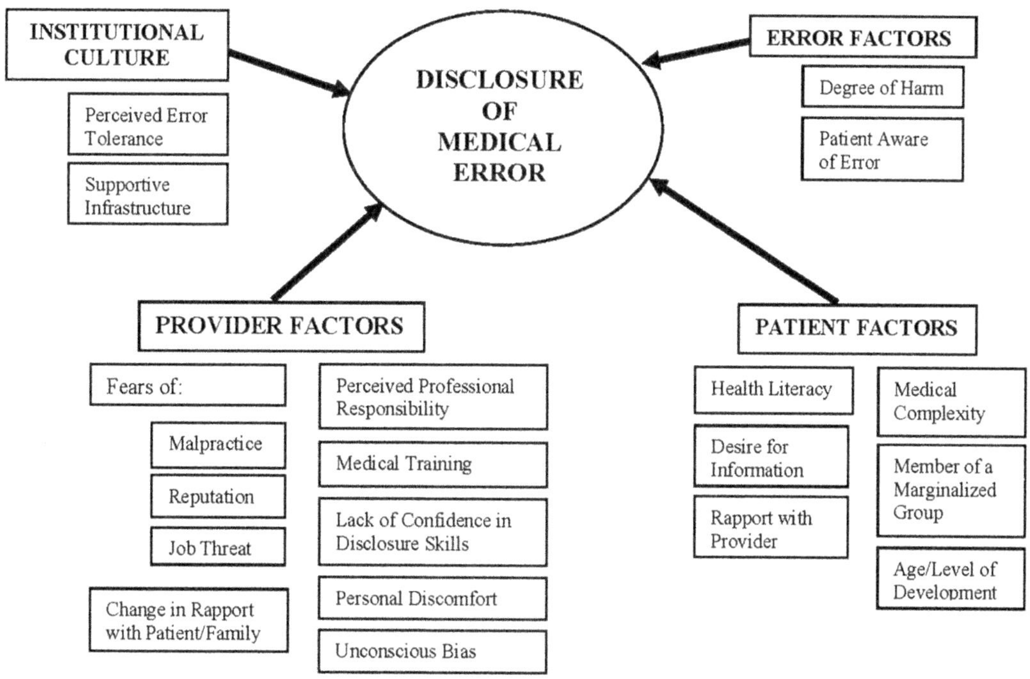

Figure 2.
Influences on the Decision to Disclose a Medical Error (adapted from Fein et al[91] [https://www.ahrq.gov/downloads/pub/advances/vol2/Fein.pdf])

required by licensing boards and governmental regulations. These systems may be voluntary or mandatory, depending on state and institutional policies, and some organizations may use automated AE reporting. Prior reporting systems often focused on punitive consequences, which was found to deter further reporting. More recent trends emphasize the adoption of "just culture," promote reporting of AEs by all clinicians and staff, and utilize reports to develop systematic improvements and a safer patient care environment.[47,48] Additionally, there is emerging evidence that including family reports in safety surveillance systems, which is not typical in many health care institutions, may help to identify more AEs.[34]

DISCLOSURE TO PATIENTS AND FAMILIES

Historically, physicians were not often advised to disclose MEs to patients and their families, but early disclosure and resolution is now routinely encouraged. A variety of programs have been initiated around the United States, including the CANDOR (communication and optimal resolution) approach (https://www.ahrq.gov/patient-safety/settings/hospital/candor/index.html).[49] The CANDOR program consists of 2 main components:

1. Prompt and accurate disclosure to families
2. Care for the caregiver (see "Effects on Health Care Clinicians" section)

Clinicians involved are expected to notify their malpractice attorney(s) or institutional legal and risk management contacts as soon as possible. It is important for trainees to immediately notify appropriate supervisors and involve them, whenever possible, in conversations with families. Additional personnel, such as office managers, unit directors, and social workers, can aid in responding and provide support and guidance. Prompt and accurate discussion is encouraged, and whenever possible, a care team should have an organized plan, including predisclosure huddles and checklists, such as those available through the AHRQ, prior to meeting with families. In the immediate aftermath of a serious event, and when there may not be time to involve additional resources, conversations with families are usually limited to statements that something went wrong and that a formal investigation—usually in the form of a "root cause analysis" or "apparent cause analysis"—is forthcoming. At the initial discussion, clinicians can advise families that not all the facts are known and can assure them that additional meetings will be scheduled as more information is available. Apologies, including statements of sympathy with or without expressions of fault, may be included in initial conversations depending on the institutions and clinicians involved as well as the legal landscape around disclosures and protections for apologies and statements of fault in the local jurisdiction.[50,51] A more formal disclosure is usually done after an investigation has been conducted, and at times in conjunction with an early offer for resolution. Attorneys or risk management staff usually direct such discussions. Veracity, meaning that communication should be honest, is one of the guiding principles of bioethics and a moral foundation of disclosure. The principle of truth is deeply rooted in the practice of medicine and is essential for building trust between clinicians and patients or families. Although in the past, patients and their families were often "shielded" from the truth by paternalistic physicians, they should be viewed as partners in shared decision making. Families cannot make informed decisions for their loved ones if they have not been given relevant facts.

ENGAGEMENT OF CHILDREN AND ADOLESCENTS

Children and adolescents, including those with chronic illnesses, have expressed their desire to be involved in disclosures of errors affecting their care,[52] and consideration should be given to involving them in such discussions when appropriate. Disclosure to children should be individualized and should not be determined simply by age and developmental parameters. Koller et al[53] have suggested that the development of policies on disclosure "must begin by examining children's understanding of medical errors and what they expect from their health care clinicians when errors occur."

ADOLESCENT CONFIDENTIALITY

There may be circumstances when AEs occur during the confidential treatment of adolescents, including conditions involving behavioral health, substance use, or sexual activity. Although state laws vary depending on exact age and condition, adolescents are usually legally entitled to seek treatment without needing consent from a parent or guardian for these conditions.[54] In such cases, disclosures are limited to the adolescent alone. Clinicians need to remain cognizant that subsequent care for medical consequences of the AE may fall outside adolescent confidentiality protections, and state laws protecting parental rights may impose further complications. Consultation with legal and/or risk management advisors in the relevant jurisdiction is recommended because of the complexity and variety of these protections.

BEST PRACTICES FOR DISCLOSURE

Disclosure practices may vary depending on setting, type of error, and patient population. Important aspects of disclosure include an explanation of what happened, acknowledgment that something has gone wrong and of responsibility, expression of sincere regret and apology, and commitment to preventing recurrences.[55] These should be conducted with the involvement of appropriate parties in each practice setting. Participants may include leaders, risk managers, and possibly attorneys. Immediately after an AE occurs, clinicians can follow recommended steps such as involving team members, practice or unit leaders, risk managers, or attorneys; apologizing when appropriate; and communicating with the involved patient and/or family. Resources for responding to AEs are provided in the Toolkit Appendix.

EFFECTS ON HEALTH CARE CLINICIANS

AEs and MEs not only affect patients and their families but also may have devastating effects on health care clinicians, who may suffer emotional consequences both from preventable AEs and from subsequent malpractice litigation.[56–58] Affected clinicians may feel guilt, shame, and isolation, and these feelings may be exacerbated by negative reactions from their colleagues. They may experience depression, anxiety, and/or posttraumatic stress disorder.[59] Anticipated or actual punitive consequences can add further emotional and financial burdens on clinicians. Although the terminology is evolving, the concepts of "second victims" or more recently "care for the caregiver" acknowledge that clinicians often experience significant personal turmoil if an AE occurs and focus on the important need to support health care clinicians involved in these events. Support systems for affected clinicians may reduce distress among health care clinicians.[60–62] The tragedy in 2011 of a pediatric intensive care unit nurse's suicide following a medication error highlights the devastating effects that MEs can have on the health care workers as well.[59]

BARRIERS TO AND PROMOTERS OF DISCLOSURE

Numerous barriers to disclosure have been identified, including shame, fear of litigation and punishment, concern about the impact on professional reputation, decreased patient trust, situational complexity, lack of training or confidence in how to disclose, inconsistent guidelines on disclosure, and the lack of a nonpunitive patient safety culture.[63] Language and cultural barriers may hinder communication about AEs. Even with institutional policies advocating for disclosure, errors may not always be disclosed. In some cases, failure to disclose may impact patients at other institutions. For example, an outbreak of carbapenem-resistant *Enterobacter* infections related to duodenoscope contamination at one institution was associated with later deaths in other hospitals and states.[64]

Factors that promote disclosure include a safe setting for reporting AEs and availability of guidelines and education on how to disclose errors.[65,66] Peer support for disclosure, just-in-time disclosure coaching, refresher trainings, medical school and residency disclosure training and modeling, and organizational and national policies supporting disclosure also influence the likelihood and implementation of disclosure.[55]

LEGAL RISKS AND OUTCOMES

Patients and caregivers most often desire complete disclosure of AEs.[67,68] Yet historically, lawyers advised their physician-clients not to disclose MEs and did so with sound legal justification, because of the risk of statements of apology being used against physicians if an AE should result in a lawsuit.[51,69,70] Physicians were trained that admitting fault would increase the risk of being sued.

However, studies suggest that affected patients and families may be less likely to pursue litigation against their health care clinicians if such disclosure is provided.[71–76] Lack of such communication may make patients feel worse and may erode the sense of trust in their caregivers that is key to healing and to optimal health care. Although there is some disagreement in the legal literature on the impact of apologies and admissions of fault,[77–79] the preponderance of the data, as well as the guiding ethical principles, support prompt and accurate disclosure.[80] Patients and families expect information about the error, sincere remorse, and a pledge of improvement.[66]

Numerous states have passed so-called "apology laws," which protect statements of apologies from being used in court against health care clinicians. As of 2022, 39 states and the District of Columbia have such statutes.[81] Most of these states protect only sympathetic statements, such as saying "I'm sorry for your suffering" or "I regret that this happened," while 9 states also protect statements of fault.[50] These apology laws, along with institutional, state, and federal efforts to implement disclosure programs, may help to encourage candid discussions after AEs.[74] More recently, several states have developed "candor laws" that provide a process for investigating and communicating openly about AEs. Under the Colorado Candor Act, for example, discussions and offers of compensation held in the process are privileged and confidential, meaning they cannot be used against clinicians if the injured party later decides to file a lawsuit.[82]

A case in which a nurse was convicted of negligent homicide after a medication error highlights the need for broader legal protections for statements about AEs. In this case in Tennessee, which was decided in 2022, the nurse's words to state investigators were used against her in court. Widespread concern has been expressed that health care workers will be hesitant to disclose errors if their cooperation will be used as part of criminal prosecutions.[83,84] Although this type of legal case is extremely rare, the potential deterring effect on self-reporting could not only undermine the disclosure of AEs but also reverse gains in establishing a culture of safety and other patient safety initiatives.[85]

EDUCATION ON DISCLOSURE OF PREVENTABLE ADVERSE EVENTS

In 2019, disclosure of AEs was included as a common program requirement for resident education and experience, highlighting the importance of disclosure as a patient safety skill by the Accreditation Council for Graduate Medical Education (ACGME) (https://www.acgme.org/What-We-Do/Accreditation/Common-Program-Requirements). With increased focus on experiential learning, trainees have been involved in real or simulation scenarios, including disclosure of AEs.[86,87] Disclosure practices are also included as one of 13 core professional activities for medical school graduates by the Association of American Medical Colleges, as part of identifying system failures and contributing to a culture of safety and improvement.[88,89] Continued education in patient safety and developing communication skills for effective disclosure is needed at all training and career levels.[55,90]

CONCLUSION

Progress has been made toward routine disclosure of adverse events over the past decades. Further efforts to better understand adverse events in pediatrics, focusing on risks, different health care settings, and inequitable practices that disproportionately impact historically marginalized or minoritized populations, may help to improve trends in disclosure. Support from institutions and legal protections can facilitate a culture of safety, reduce fear of disclosure, and provide enhanced education and support for health care clinicians involved in adverse events.

RECOMMENDATIONS

For Pediatric Health Care Clinicians, Practices, and Institutions

1. Develop and implement policies and procedures for identifying and disclosing AEs to patients and families in an honest and empathetic manner as part of a nonpunitive safety culture.
2. Develop policies and procedures and provide resources to support clinicians and other staff involved in AEs.
3. Encourage a culture of safety, just culture, and reporting by all staff as well as by patients and families.
4. Identify populations and situations with higher risk for AEs, such as patients with chronic illnesses and those from historically marginalized or minoritized communities, and partner with families and care teams to help prevent them.

For Medical Educators

5. Develop and implement educational programs regarding identification and prevention of MEs and communication about AEs with patients and their families as part of a comprehensive patient safety curriculum.

For Researchers

6. Investigate the consequences of various approaches to disclosure as well as of the effectiveness of disclosure education.
7. Further explore and address disparities in AEs and disclosure. More data are needed on trends in AEs and disclosure by race, ethnicity, chronic conditions, and preferred language; impact of AEs and disclosure on historically marginalized or minoritized communities; structural factors related to disclosure; and impact on clinicians underrepresented in medicine.

For Pediatric Advocates

8. Encourage states and the federal government to adopt laws protecting apologies, programs supporting disclosure, and other mechanisms to reduce liability risks associated with disclosure in order to avoid detrimental effects on health care clinicians' reactions to AEs.

For more information about advocating for these issues, contact the AAP state advocacy team at stgov@aap.org.

Policy statements from the American Academy of Pediatrics benefit from expertise and resources of liaisons and internal (AAP) and external reviewers. However, policy statements from the American Academy of Pediatrics may not reflect the views of the liaisons or the organizations or government agencies that they represent.

The guidance in this statement does not indicate an exclusive course of treatment or serve as a standard of medical care. Variations, taking into account individual circumstances, may be appropriate.

All policy statements from the American Academy of Pediatrics automatically expire 5 years after publication unless reaffirmed, revised, or retired at or before that time.

LEAD AUTHORS

Laura Sigman, MD, JD, FAAP
Robert Turbow, MD, JD, FAAP
Daniel Neuspiel, MD, MPH, FAAP
Julia M. Kim, MD, MPH, FAAP

COMMITTEE ON MEDICAL LIABILITY AND RISK MANAGEMENT, 2023-2024

Steven A. Bondi, JD, MD, FAAP, Chairperson
Craig Howard Gosdin, MD, FAAP

David A. Horowitz, MD, FAAP
Kajal Khanna, MD, JD, FAAP
Jonathan Muraskas, MD, FAAP
Alan L. Nager, MD, MHA, FAAP
Sarah W. Northrop, MD, FAAP
Preethi Srinivasakumar, MD, FAAP
Michelle Terry, MD, FAAP
Ryan Earl Alanzalon, MD, FAAP

COMMITTEE ON MEDICAL LIABILITY AND RISK MANAGEMENT, PAST CONTRIBUTING MEMBERS

James Peter Scibilia, MD, FAAP, Immediate Past Chairperson
Laura Sigman, MD, JD, FAAP
Robert Turbow, MD, JD, FAAP

STAFF

Julie Kersten Ake
Sunnah Kim

COUNCIL ON QUALITY IMPROVEMENT AND PATIENT SAFETY, 2023-2024

Ulfat Shaikh, MD, FAAP Chairperson
Francisco Javier Alvarez, MD, FAAP
John Chuo, MD, FAAP
Meghan Drayton Jackson, DO, FAAP
Julia M. Kim, MD, FAAP
Mary Beth Miotto, MD, FAAP
Raina Paul, MD, FAAP
Corinna Rea, MD, FAAP
Sandra Spencer, MD, FAAP
Amy Tyler, MD, FAAP
Joyee Vachani, MD, FAAP

STAFF

Cathleen Guch

ABBREVIATIONS

AAP: American Academy of Pediatrics
AEs: adverse events
AHRQ: Agency for Healthcare Research and Quality
IOM: Institute of Medicine
MEs: medical errors.

REFERENCES

1. McDonnell WM, Altman RL, Bondi SA, et al; COMMITTEE ON MEDICAL LIABILITY AND RISK MANAGEMENT; COUNCIL ON QUALITY IMPROVEMENT AND PATIENT SAFETY. Disclosure of adverse events in pediatrics. *Pediatrics*. 2016;138(6):e20163215. PubMed doi: 10.1542/peds.2016-3215
2. Institute of Medicine, Committee on Quality of Health Care in America. *Crossing the Quality Chasm: A New Health System for the 21st Century*. National Academy Press; 2001.
3. Institute of Medicine, Committee on Quality of Health Care in America. *To Err Is Human: Building a Safer Health System*. Kohn LT, Corrigan JM, Donaldson MS, eds. National Academies Press; 2000.
4. Rodziewicz TL, Houseman B, Hipskin J. *Medical Error Reduction and Prevention*. StatPearls Publishing; 2022.
5. Rodwin BA, Bilan VP, Merchant NB, et al. Rate of preventable mortality in hospitalized patients: a systematic review and meta-analysis. *J Gen Intern Med*. 2020;35(7):2099–2106. PubMed doi: 10.1007/s11606-019-05592-5
6. Makary MA, Daniel M. Medical error-the third leading cause of death in the US. *BMJ*. 2016;353:i2139. PubMed doi: 10.1136/bmj.i2139
7. Panagioti M, Khan K, Keers RN, et al. Prevalence, severity, and nature of preventable patient harm across medical care settings: systematic review and meta-analysis. *BMJ*. 2019;366:l4185. PubMed doi: 10.1136/bmj.l4185
8. Lannon CM, Coven BJ, Lane France F, et al; National Initiative for Children's Health Care Quality Project Advisory Committee. Principles of patient safety in pediatrics. *Pediatrics*. 2001;107(6):1473–1475. PubMed doi: 10.1542/peds.107.6.1473
9. Mueller BU, Neuspiel DR, Fisher ERS, et al; COUNCIL ON QUALITY IMPROVEMENT AND PATIENT SAFETY, COMMITTEE ON HOSPITAL CARE. Policy Statement. Principles of pediatric patient safety: reducing harm due to medical care. *Pediatrics*. 2019;143(2):e20183649. PubMed doi: 10.1542/peds.2018-3649
10. Goodman JC, Villarreal P, Jones B. The social cost of adverse medical events, and what we can do about it. *Health Aff (Millwood)*. 2011;30(4):590–595. PubMed doi: 10.1377/hlthaff.2010.1256
11. Van Den Bos J, Rustagi K, Gray T, Halford M, Ziemkiewicz E, Shreve J. The $17.1 billion problem: the annual cost of measurable medical errors. *Health Aff (Millwood)*. 2011;30(4):596–603. PubMed doi: 10.1377/hlthaff.2011.0084
12. David G, Gunnarsson CL, Waters HC, Horblyuk R, Kaplan HS. Economic measurement of medical errors using a hospital claims database. *Value Health*. 2013;16(2):305–310. PubMed doi: 10.1016/j.jval.2012.11.010
13. Matlow AG, Baker GR, Flintoft V, et al. Adverse events among children in Canadian hospitals: the Canadian Paediatric Adverse Events Study. *CMAJ*. 2012;184(13):E709–E718. PubMed doi: 10.1503/cmaj.112153
14. Gates PJ, Meyerson SA, Baysari MT, Lehmann CU, Westbrook JI. Preventable adverse drug events among inpatients: a systematic review. *Pediatrics*. 2018;142(3):e20180805. PubMed doi: 10.1542/peds.2018-0805
15. Schroeder L, Stockwell DC. The persistent challenge of understanding preventable adverse drug events. *Pediatrics*. 2018;142(3):e20181841. PubMed doi: 10.1542/peds.2018-1841

16. Kaushal R, Bates DW, Landrigan C, et al. Medication errors and adverse drug events in pediatric inpatients. *JAMA.* 2001;285(16): 2114–2120. PubMed doi: 10.1001/jama.285.16.2114

17. Benjamin L, Frush K, Shaw K, et al; AMERICAN ACADEMY OF PEDIATRICS Committee on Pediatric Emergency Medicine; AMERICAN COLLEGE OF EMERGENCY PHYSICIANS Pediatric Emergency Medicine Committee; EMERGENCY NURSES ASSOCIATION Pediatric Emergency Medicine Committee. Pediatric medication safety in the emergency department. *Pediatrics.* 2018;141(3): e20174066. PubMed doi: 10.1542/peds.2017-4066

18. Gross TK, Lane NE, Timm NL, et al; COMMITTEE ON PEDIATRIC EMERGENCY MEDICINE. Crowding in the emergency department: challenges and best practices for the care of children. *Pediatrics.* 2023;151(3):e2022060972. PubMed doi: 10.1542/peds.2022-060972

19. Joseph MM, Mahajan P, Snow SK, Ku BC, Saidinejad M; AMERICAN ACADEMY OF PEDIATRICS COMMITTEE ON PEDIATRIC EMERGENCY MEDICINE, AMERICAN COLLEGE OF EMERGENCY PHYSICIANS PEDIATRIC EMERGENCY MEDICINE COMMITTEE, and EMERGENCY NURSES ASSOCIATION PEDIATRIC COMMITTEE. Optimizing pediatric patient safety in the emergency care setting. *Pediatrics.* 2022; 150(5):e2022059673. PubMed doi: 10.1542/peds.2022-059673

20. Neuspiel DR, Stubbs EH. Patient safety in ambulatory care. *Pediatr Clin North Am.* 2012;59(6):1341–1354. PubMed doi: 10.1016/j.pcl.2012.08.006

21. Huth K, Hotz A, Starmer AJ. Patient safety in ambulatory pediatrics. *Curr Treat Options Pediatr.* 2020;6(4):350–365. PubMed doi: 10.1007/s40746-020-00213-4

22. Kaushal R, Goldmann DA, Keohane CA, et al. Adverse drug events in pediatric outpatients. *Ambul Pediatr.* 2007;7(5):383–389. PubMed doi: 10.1016/j.ambp.2007.05.005

23. Yin HS, Parker RM, Sanders LM, et al. Liquid medication errors and dosing tools: a randomized controlled experiment. *Pediatrics.* 2016;138(4):e20160357. PubMed doi: 10.1542/peds.2016-0357

24. Yin HS, Neuspiel DR, Paul IM, et al; American Academy of Pediatrics, Council on Quality Improvement and Patient Safety, Committee on Drugs. Policy statement. Preventing home medication administration errors. *Pediatrics.* 2021;148(6):e2021054666. PubMed doi: 10.1542/peds.2021-054666

25. Rinke ML, Singh H, Heo M, et al. Diagnostic errors in primary care pediatrics: Project RedDE. *Acad Pediatr.* 2018;18(2):220–227. PubMed doi: 10.1016/j.acap.2017.08.005

26. Marshall TL, Rinke ML, Olson APJ, Brady PW. Diagnostic error in pediatrics: a narrative review. *Pediatrics.* 2022;149(suppl 3): e2020045948D. PubMed doi: 10.1542/peds.2020-045948D

27. Rinke ML, Bundy DG, Shore AD, Colantuoni E, Morlock LL, Miller MR. Pediatric antidepressant medication errors in a national error reporting database. *J Dev Behav Pediatr.* 2010;31(2):129–136. PubMed doi: 10.1097/DBP.0b013e3181ce6509

28. Taylor JA, Winter L, Geyer LJ, Hawkins DS. Oral outpatient chemotherapy medication errors in children with acute lymphoblastic leukemia. *Cancer.* 2006;107(6):1400–1406. PubMed doi: 10.1002/cncr.22131

29. Walsh KE, Mazor KM, Stille CJ, et al. Medication errors in the homes of children with chronic conditions. *Arch Dis Child.* 2011;96(6):581–586. PubMed doi: 10.1136/adc.2010.204479

30. Stone BL, Boehme S, Mundorff MB, Maloney CG, Srivastava R. Hospital admission medication reconciliation in medically complex children: an observational study. *Arch Dis Child.* 2010;95(4): 250–255. PubMed doi: 10.1136/adc.2009.167528

31. Feinstein JA, Feudtner C, Kempe A. Adverse drug event-related emergency department visits associated with complex chronic conditions. *Pediatrics.* 2014;133(6):e1575–e1585. PubMed doi: 10.1542/peds.2013-3060

32. Huth K, Vandecruys P, Orkin J, Patel H. Medication Safety for children with medical complexity. Canadian Pediatric Society. *Paediatr Child Health.* 2020;25(7):473–474. doi: 10.1093/pch/pxaa105

33. Khan A, Baird J, Kelly MM, et al. Family safety reporting in medically complex children: parent, staff, and leader perspectives. *Pediatrics.* 2022;149(6):e2021053913. PubMed doi: 10.1542/peds.2021-053913

34. Khan A, Furtak SL, Melvin P, Rogers JE, Schuster MA, Landrigan CP. Parent-reported errors and adverse events in hospitalized children. *JAMA Pediatr.* 2016;170(4):e154608. PubMed doi: 10.1001/jamapediatrics.2015.4608

35. Daniels JP, Hunc K, Cochrane DD, et al. Identification by families of pediatric adverse events and near misses overlooked by health care providers. *CMAJ.* 2012;184(1):29–34. PubMed doi: 10.1503/cmaj.110393

36. Lang S, Garrido MV, Heintze C. Patients' views of adverse events in primary and ambulatory care: a systematic review to assess methods and the content of what patients consider to be adverse events. *BMC Fam Pract.* 2016;17:6. PubMed doi: 10.1186/s12875-016-0408-0

37. Jean-Pierre P. Medical error and vulnerable communities. *Boston Univ Law Rev.* 2022;102:327–392.

38. Raman J, Johnson TJ, Hayes K, Balamuth F. Racial differences in sepsis recognition in the emergency department. *Pediatrics.* 2019;144(4):e20190348. PubMed doi: 10.1542/peds.2019-0348

39. Stockwell DC, Landrigan CP, Toomey SL, et al; GAPPS Study Group. Racial, ethnic, and socioeconomic disparities in patient safety events for hospitalized children. *Hosp Pediatr.* 2019;9(1):1–5. PubMed doi: 10.1542/hpeds.2018-0131

40. Lion KC, Rafton SA, Shafii J, et al. Association between language, serious adverse events, and length of stay among hospitalized children. *Hosp Pediatr.* 2013;3(3):219–225. PubMed doi: 10.1542/hpeds.2012-0091

41. Khan A, Yin HS, Brach C, et al; Patient and Family Centered I-PASS Health Literacy Subcommittee. Patient and Family Centered I-PASS Health Literacy Subcommittee. Association between parent comfort with English and adverse events among hospitalized children. *JAMA Pediatr.* 2020;174(12):e203215. PubMed doi: 10.1001/jamapediatrics.2020.3215

42. Cohen AL, Rivara F, Marcuse EK, McPhillips H, Davis R. Are language barriers associated with serious medical events in hospitalized pediatric patients? *Pediatrics.* 2005;116(3):575–579. PubMed doi: 10.1542/peds.2005-0521

43. Divi C, Koss RG, Schmaltz SP, Loeb JM. Language proficiency and adverse events in US hospitals: a pilot study. *Int J Qual Health Care*. 2007;19(2):60–67. PubMed doi: 10.1093/intqhc/mzl069

44. Halvorson EE, Thurtle DP, Easter A, Lovato J, Stockwell D. Disparities in adverse event reporting for hospitalized children. *J Patient Saf*. 2022;18(6):e928–e933. PubMed doi: 10.1097/PTS.0000000000001049

45. Khan A, Parente V, Baird JD, et al; Patient and Family Centered I-PASS SCORE Scientific Oversight Committee. Association of patient and family reports of hospital safety climate with language proficiency in the US. *JAMA Pediatr*. 2022;176(8):776–786. PubMed doi: 10.1001/jamapediatrics.2022.1831

46. Weaver SJ, Lubomksi LH, et al. Promoting a culture of safety as a patient safety strategy: a systematic review. *Ann Int Med*. 2013;158(5.2):369–374. PubMed doi: 10.7326/0003-4819-158-5-201303051-00002

47. Boysen PG II. Just culture: a foundation for balanced accountability and patient safety. *Ochsner J*. 2013;13(3):400–406. PubMed

48. Marx D. Patient safety and the just culture. *Obstet Gynecol Clin North Am*. 2019;46(2):239–245. PubMed doi: 10.1016/j.ogc.2019.01.003

49. Agency for Healthcare Research and Quality. Communication and Optimal Resolution (CANDOR). Accessed July 19, 2024. https://www.ahrq.gov/patient-safety/settings/hospital/candor/index.html

50. Ross NE, Newman WJ. The role of apology laws in medical malpractice. *J Am Acad Psychiatry Law*. 2021;49(3):406–414. PubMed

51. Mastroianni AC, Mello MM, Sommer S, Hardy M, Gallagher TH. The flaws in state 'apology' and 'disclosure' laws dilute their intended impact on malpractice suits. *Health Aff (Millwood)*. 2010;29(9):1611–1619. PubMed doi: 10.1377/hlthaff.2009.0134

52. Koller D, Binder MJ, Alexander S, Darch J. "Everybody makes mistakes": children's views on medical errors and disclosure. *J Pediatr Nurs*. 2019;49:1–9. PubMed doi: 10.1016/j.pedn.2019.07.014

53. Koller D, Rummens A, Le Pouesard M, et al. Patient disclosure of medical errors in paediatrics: A systematic literature review. *Paediatr Child Health*. 2016;21(4):e32–e38. PubMed doi: 10.1093/pch/21.4.e32

54. Chung RJ, Lee JB, Hackell JM, et al; COMMITTEE ON ADOLESCENCE; COMMITTEE ON PRACTICE & AMBULATORY MEDICINE. Confidentiality in the care of adolescents: policy statement. *Pediatrics*. 2024;153(5):e2024066326. PubMed doi: 10.1542/peds.2024-066326

55. Wu AW, Boyle DJ, Wallace G, Mazor KM. Disclosure of adverse events in the United States and Canada: an update, and a proposed framework for improvement. *J Public Health Res*. 2013;2(3):e32. PubMed doi: 10.4081/jphr.2013.e32

56. Wu AW. Medical error: the second victim. The doctor who makes the mistake needs help too. *BMJ*. 2000;320(7237):726–727. PubMed doi: 10.1136/bmj.320.7237.726

57. Seys D, Wu AW, Van Gerven E, et al. Health care professionals as second victims after adverse events: a systematic review. *Eval Health Prof*. 2013;36(2):135–162. PubMed doi: 10.1177/0163278712458918

58. Coughlan B, Powell D, Higgins MF. The second victim: a review. *Eur J Obstet Gynecol Reprod Biol*. 2017;213:11–16. PubMed doi: 10.1016/j.ejogrb.2017.04.002

59. Grissinger M. Too many abandon the "second victims" of medical errors. *P&T*. 2014;39(9):591–592. PubMed

60. Edrees H, Connors C, Paine L, Norvell M, Taylor H, Wu AW. Implementing the RISE second victim support programme at the Johns Hopkins Hospital: a case study. *BMJ Open*. 2016;6(9):e011708. PubMed doi: 10.1136/bmjopen-2016-011708

61. Busch IM, Moretti F, Campagna I, et al. Promoting the psychological well-being of healthcare providers facing the burden of adverse events: a systematic review of second victim support resources. *Int J Environ Res Public Health*. 2021;18(10):5080. PubMed doi: 10.3390/ijerph18105080

62. Shapiro J, Galowitz P. Peer support for clinicians: a programmatic approach. *Acad Med*. 2016;91(9):1200–1204. PubMed doi: 10.1097/ACM.0000000000001297

63. Edwards MT. An assessment of the impact of just culture on quality and safety in US hospitals. *Am J Med Qual*. 2018;33(5):502–508. PubMed doi: 10.1177/1062860618768057

64. Centers for Disease Control and Prevention. Los Angeles County/UCLA investigation of CRE transmission and duodenoscopes. July 10, 2015. Accessed July 19, 2024. https://archive.cdc.gov/www_cdc_gov/hai/outbreaks/cdcstatement-la-cre.html#:~:text=In%20this%20investigation%2C%20exposure%20to,associated%20with%20transmission%20of%20CRE

65. Ock M, Lim SY, Jo MW, Lee SI. Frequency, expected effects, obstacles, and facilitators of disclosure of patient safety incidents: a systematic review. *J Prev Med Public Health*. 2017;50(2):68–82. PubMed doi: 10.3961/jpmph.16.105

66. Sattar R, Johnson J, Lawton R. The views and experiences of patients and health-care professionals on the disclosure of adverse events: A systematic review and qualitative meta-ethnographic synthesis. *Health Expect*. 2020;23(3):571–583. PubMed doi: 10.1111/hex.13029

67. Coffey M, Espin S, Hahmann T, et al. Parent preference for medical error disclosure: a qualitative study. *Hosp Pediatr*. 2017;7(1):24–30. PubMed doi: 10.1542/hpeds.2016-0048

68. Hobgood C, Tamayo-Sarver JH, Elms A, Weiner B. Parental preferences for error disclosure, reporting, and legal action after medical error in the care of their children. *Pediatrics*. 2005;116(6):1276–1286. PubMed doi: 10.1542/peds.2005-0946

69. Hyman DA. When and why lawyers are the problem. *Depaul L Rev*. 2008;57(2):267–280.

70. Tabler N. Should physicians apologize for medical errors? *Health Lawyer*. 2007;19:23–30.

71. Helmchen LA, Richards MR, McDonald TB. How does routine disclosure of medical error affect patients' propensity to sue and their assessment of provider quality? Evidence from survey data. *Med Care*. 2010;48(11):955–961. PubMed doi: 10.1097/MLR.0b013e3181eaf84d

72. Kachalia A, Kaufman SR, Boothman R, et al. Liability claims and costs before and after implementation of a medical error

disclosure program. *Ann Intern Med.* 2010;153(4):213–221. PubMed doi: 10.7326/0003-4819-153-4-201008170-00002

73. Adams MA, Elmunzer BJ, Scheiman JM. Effect of a health system's medical error disclosure program on gastroenterology-related claims rates and costs. *Am J Gastroenterol.* 2014;109(4): 460–464. PubMed doi: 10.1038/ajg.2013.375
74. Mello MM, Kachalia A, Roche S, et al. Outcomes in two Massachusetts hospital systems give reason for optimism about communication-and-resolution programs. *Health Aff (Millwood).* 2017;36(10):1795–1803. PubMed doi: 10.1377/hlthaff.2017.0320
75. Kachalia A, Sands K, Niel MV, et al. Effects of a communication-and-resolution program on hospitals' malpractice claims and costs. *Health Aff (Millwood).* 2018;37(11):1836–1844. PubMed doi: 10.1377/hlthaff.2018.0720
76. Gallagher TH, Mello MM, Sage WM, Bell SK, McDonald TB, Thomas EJ. Can communication-and-resolution programs achieve their potential? Five key questions. *Health Aff (Millwood).* 2018;37(11): 1845–1852. PubMed doi: 10.1377/hlthaff.2018.0727
77. McMichael BJ, Van Horn RL, Viscusi WK. "Sorry" is never enough: how state apology laws fail to reduce medical malpractice liability risk. *Stanford Law Rev.* 2019;71(2):341–409. PubMed
78. Berlin L. Will "sorry" make things worse? *Radiology.* 2020;294(1): 239–240. PubMed doi: 10.1148/radiol.2019192231
79. Painter LM, Kidwell KM, Kidwell RP, et al. Do written disclosures of serious events increase risk of malpractice claims? One health care system's experience. *J Patient Saf.* 2018;14(2):87–94. PubMed doi: 10.1097/PTS.0000000000000178
80. Phillips-Bute B. Transparency and disclosure of medical errors: it's the right thing to do, so why the reluctance? *Campbell Law Rev.* 2013;35(3):332–354.
81. National Conference of State Legislatures. Medical Professional Apologies Statutes. Accessed July 19, 2024. https://www.ncsl.org/research/financial-services-and-commerce/medical-professional-apologies-statutes.aspx
82. Martin J. An Overview of the Colorado Candor Act. *Colorado Med.* 2019;116(4):53–54.
83. Dolansky MA, Barg-Walkow L, Barnsteiner J, et al. A call to action following the Radonda Vaught case. *J Nurses Prof Dev.* 2022;38(6): 329–332. PubMed doi: 10.1097/NND.0000000000000945
84. Harrington L. The RaDonda Vaught case: a critical conversation on nursing practice and technology. *AACN Adv Crit Care.* 2023;34(1): 11–15. PubMed doi: 10.4037/aacnacc2023873
85. Institute for Safe Medication Practices. Criminalization of Human Error and a Guilty Verdict: A Travesty of Justice that Threatens Patient Safety. April 7, 2022. Accessed July 19, 2024. https://psnet.ahrq.gov/issue/criminalization-human-error-and-guilty-verdict-travesty-justice-threatens-patient-safety
86. Aubin J, Rivolet O, Taunay AL, Ragot S, Ghazali DA, Oriot D. Benefit of simulation-based training in medical adverse events disclosure in pediatrics. *Pediatr Emerg Care.* 2022;38(2):e622–e627. PubMed doi: 10.1097/PEC.0000000000002454
87. Stroud L, Wong BM, Hollenberg E, Levinson W. Teaching medical error disclosure to physicians-in-training: a scoping review. *Acad Med.* 2013;88(6):884–892. PubMed doi: 10.1097/ACM.0b013e31828f898f
88. Amiel JM, Andriole DA, Biskobing DM, et al; Association of American Medical Colleges Core EPAs for Entering Residency Pilot Team. Revisiting the core entrustable professional activities for entering residency. *Acad Med.* 2021;96(7S):S14–S21. PubMed doi: 10.1097/ACM.0000000000004088
89. AAMC. Core Entrustable Professional Activities for Entering Residency Curriculum Developers' Guide. AAMC; 2014. Accessed April 5, 2024. https://store.aamc.org/downloadable/download/sample/sample_id/63/%20
90. Lin M, Famiglietti H. Closing the disclosure gap: medical errors in pediatrics. *Pediatrics.* 2019;143(4):e20190221. PubMed doi: 10.1542/peds.2019-0221
91. Fein S, Hilborne L, Kagawa-Singer M, et al. A conceptual model for disclosure of medical errors. In: Henriksen K, Battles JB, Marks ES, et al, eds. *Advances in Patient Safety: From Research to Implementation (Volume 2: Concepts and Methodology).* Agency for Healthcare Research and Quality; 2005.

Environmental Issues in Global Pediatric Health

- *Policy Statement*

POLICY STATEMENT Organizational Principles to Guide and Define the Child Health Care System and/or Improve the Health of all Children

American Academy of Pediatrics

DEDICATED TO THE HEALTH OF ALL CHILDREN™

Environmental Issues in Global Pediatric Health: Policy Statement

Lauren Zajac, MD, MPH, FAAP,[1] Philip J. Landrigan, MD, MSc, FAAP,[2] and the Council on Environmental Health and Climate Change

abstract

Pediatricians and pediatric trainees in North America are increasingly involved in caring for children and adolescents in or from low- and middle-income countries (LMICs). In many LMICs, hazardous environmental exposures—notably outdoor and household air pollution, water pollution, lead, pesticides, and other manufactured chemicals—are highly prevalent and account for twice the proportion of disease and deaths among young children as in North America. Climate change will likely worsen these exposures.

It is important that pediatricians and other pediatric health professionals from high-income countries who work in LMICs be aware of the disproportionately severe impacts of toxic environmental hazards, become knowledgeable about the major local/regional environmental threats, and consider environmental factors in their differential diagnoses. Likewise, pediatricians in high-income countries who care for patients who have emigrated from LMICs need to be aware that these children may be at elevated risk of toxic environmental diseases from past exposures to toxic environmental hazards in their countries of origin as well as ongoing exposures in products imported from their home countries, including traditional foods, medications, and cosmetics.

Because diseases of toxic environmental origin seldom have unique physical signatures, pediatricians can utilize the environmental screening history, supplemented by laboratory testing, as a diagnostic tool. To prepare pediatricians to care for children in and from LMICs, pediatric organizations could increase the amount of environmental health and climate change content offered in continuing medical education (CME) credits, maintenance of certification (MOC) credits, and certification and recertification examinations. Broadly, it is important that governments and international agencies increase resources directed to pollution prevention, strengthen the environmental health workforce, and expand public health infrastructure in all countries.

[1]Department of Environmental Medicine and Public Health and Department of Pediatrics, Icahn School of Medicine at Mount Sinai, New York, New York; and [2]Program for Global Public Health and the Common Good, Boston College, Chestnut Hill, Massachusetts; Centre Scientifique de Monaco, Monaco, MC

Dr Zajac was the lead author and Drs Zajac and Landrigan were both responsible for conceptualizing, writing, and revising the manuscript and considering input from all reviewers and the board of directors, and all authors approved the final manuscript as submitted.

CONFLICT OF INTEREST DISCLOSURES: The authors have indicated they have no potential conflicts of interest to disclose.

FUNDING: No external funding.

Policy statements from the American Academy of Pediatrics benefit from expertise and resources of liaisons and internal (AAP) and external reviewers. However, policy statements from the American Academy of Pediatrics may not reflect the views of the liaisons or the organizations or government agencies that they represent.

The guidance in this statement does not indicate an exclusive course of treatment or serve as a standard of medical care. Variations, taking into account individual circumstances, may be appropriate.

All policy statements from the American Academy of Pediatrics automatically expire 5 years after publication unless reaffirmed, revised, or retired at or before that time.

To cite: Zajac L and Landrigan PJ; American Academy of Pediatrics, Council on Environmental Health and Climate Change. Environmental Issues in Global Pediatric Health: Policy Statement. *Pediatrics*. 2025;155(2):e2024070075

INTRODUCTION

Pediatricians and pediatric trainees in North America are increasingly involved in providing care to children and adolescents in low- and middle-income countries (LMICs). Pediatricians in North America also care for children who have emigrated from across the globe[1]; their may increase in future years in consequence of climate change,[2] armed conflicts, complex sociopolitical circumstances, and changing immigration policies.[3]

Toxic environmental hazards are major causes of disease and death among children in all countries, especially LMICs, but the great magnitude of the environment's impact on children's health is not generally appreciated.[4–6] Globally, environmental pollution is responsible for an estimated 9 million deaths each year—3 times as many as are caused by AIDS, tuberculosis, and malaria combined.[7] Nearly 92% of all pollution-related deaths occur in LMICs, where environmental hazards account for twice as great a proportion of deaths in children younger than 5 years as in high-income countries.[8] Environmental threats to children's health in LMICs are worsening: two-thirds of global chemical and pesticide manufacturing is now located there, and ambient air pollution as well as contamination by pesticides and other toxic chemicals is growing rapidly. The impacts of environmental factors on children's health in all countries, and especially in LMICs, will likely be magnified by climate change.

STATEMENT OF THE PROBLEM

It is important that pediatricians, pediatric trainees, and other pediatric health professionals from high-income countries who plan to work in LMICs be aware that hazardous environmental exposures account for a much higher proportion of disease, disability, and death among children there than among children in high-income countries. Thus, it is important that they become knowledgeable about the major environmental threats to children's health in the countries where they will be working and incorporate this information into their clinical practice. Similarly, it is important that pediatricians in high-income countries who care for children and adolescents who have emigrated from LMICs be aware that these children may be at elevated risk of diseases caused by hazardous environmental exposures in their countries of origin. The intent of this policy statement and the accompanying technical report[9] is to provide pediatricians and pediatric trainees an overview of the following:

1. Key environmental issues in global pediatric health, with a particular focus on the major environmental hazards contributing to pediatric morbidity and mortality in LMICs.
2. Strategies and resources to recognize, diagnose, manage, and prevent disease in children caused by hazardous environmental exposures in LMICs.
3. Opportunities for increased education and training on environmental health issues for pediatricians and other pediatric health professionals.
4. Roles of the pediatricians and other clinicians practicing in the United States and LMICs in the prevention of environmental exposures and the diseases that they cause, with a particular focus on prevention of disease caused by toxic chemical hazards.
5. Role of governmental and nongovernmental organizations to increase resources and capacity to address children's environmental health.

Environmental Justice

Significant social, ethnic, racial, and economic inequities are evident in the global distribution of environmental hazards. Nearly 92% of all disease and death attributable globally to environmental risk factors occur in LMICs.[10] In countries at every economic level, disease caused by hazardous environmental exposures is most prevalent among poor people and historically marginalized groups, an inequitable pattern of exposure and disease termed "environmental injustice."[11]

Environmental injustice is also seen in high-income countries, including the United States. Examples include the disproportionate siting of polluting industries, hazardous waste sites, and major roadways in low-income communities where the majority of the residents are people of color. Another example is the disproportionally high levels of lead found in drinking water in communities that are predominantly people of color, such as Flint, Michigan. The disproportionate exposures of Native American and Alaska Native children to high levels of household air pollution and unsafe drinking water are further examples of environmental injustice in the United States.[12–27]

Diseases Caused by Hazardous Environmental Exposures Can Be Prevented

Toxic environmental exposures and the diseases that they cause are the result of human activity and can, therefore, be prevented. This is a key point, and it is the basis for all pollution control policy.

The strongest evidence that diseases of environmental origin can be prevented is seen in the experience of the United States and other high-income countries in controlling pollution and preventing pollution-related disease.[10] In the United States, for example, air pollutant emissions have fallen by 77% since passage of the Clean Air Act in 1970[28]; air and drinking water are now cleaner, polluted rivers no longer catch fire, and the worst hazardous waste sites have been remediated. Disease and premature death of environmental origin have been prevented.

The two factors that made possible these gains were (1) research to discover the environmental causes of disease in children; and (2) evidence-based advocacy that translated research findings into laws, policies, and prevention programs. Pediatricians are trusted advisors, uniquely well qualified to address environmental threats to children's health. For this reason, pediatricians have repeatedly been leaders in environmental health research, and individual pediatricians and pediatric organizations have been key players in successful intervention efforts. Examples of environmental health efforts led by pediatricians include the removal of lead from gasoline, which resulted in a more than 95% reduction in blood lead levels of American children and an approximate 5-point gain in population mean IQ[29]; reduction in children's exposure to urban air pollution, which resulted in improvements in lung function and reduction in childhood asthma[30]; bans on the use of neurotoxic insecticides such as chlorpyrifos; and reduction of arsenic levels in drinking water.

The High Costs of Disease Caused by Hazardous Environmental Exposures

A powerful ancillary argument for the prevention of pediatric disease of environmental origin is that these diseases result in large economic costs and their prevention is highly cost-effective.[31] This argument is valid in all countries and especially in LMICs, where the costs of diseases caused by hazardous environmental exposures are so great that they can undermine national economies and undercut prospects for human development.[32,33]

The economic costs of pediatric diseases caused by toxic environmental exposures include health care costs as well as increased costs for special education, accommodation for disabilities, and other developmental services. In addition, environmentally related disease and disability have negative economic impacts on children's futures, because they diminish children's educational attainment, their lifelong earning potential, and their ability to contribute to society by reducing cognitive function, decreasing IQ, and impairing physical function.[10] Globally, the economic losses attributable to pollution-related disease are estimated to amount to $4.6 trillion per year, approximately 6% of global economic output.[10]

Prevention of Disease Caused by Hazardous Environmental Exposures is Highly Cost-Effective

Prevention of diseases caused by toxic environmental exposures has not only improved children's health and well-being but also benefited the economy.[28] Improvements in air quality in the United States have been associated with benefits of nearly $30 for every dollar invested in pollution control since passage of the Clean Air Act in 1970.[34] Removal of lead from gasoline has not only reduced childhood lead poisoning by over 95% but also returned an estimated $200 billion to the US economy each year since 1980 through the increased creativity and economic productivity of generations of more intelligent and creative children not impaired by lead.[29]

Information on the cost-effectiveness of disease prevention programs provides pediatricians with another powerful argument for persuading policy makers to take preventive action to safeguard children's health.[29,34]

Key Environmental Exposures in LMICs

The key toxic environmental exposures for children in LMICs include: water pollution, ambient air pollution, household air pollution from indoor fuel-burning stoves, toxic chemical pollution including heavy metals (lead, mercury, arsenic), industrial chemicals, pesticides, and hazardous waste (Table 1). A review of the evidence on the health hazards of these exposures is presented in the accompanying technical report.[9] In addition, the impacts of global climate change fall most severely on children in LMICs and will magnify the effects of pollution on children's health. The health impacts of climate change have been extensively reviewed[35,36] and are addressed in a statement from the American Academy of Pediatrics (AAP) Council on Environmental Health and Climate Change focused on climate change and children's health.[37,38]

Role of the Pediatrician and Other Health Care Professionals

It is important for pediatric clinicians to be alert to the possibility that any illness or exacerbation of illness in a child or adolescent may have an environmental etiology. Given the disproportionately heavy burden of environmental exposures in LMICs, environmental causation is an especially likely diagnostic possibility among children evaluated clinically in LMICs. Because diseases of environmental origin in children seldom have unique physical signatures, an exposure history, supplemented as appropriate by laboratory testing, is the principal diagnostic tool. A targeted environmental history is also an important part of pediatric care during well visits and management of an environmentally related illness (eg, asthma). The environmental screening history includes questions about hazardous exposures in the home, neighborhood, and other places the child spends time; questions can be tailored to reflect the most prominent environmental exposures in a particular country and community.[39] Positive responses on the screening history can trigger deeper inquiry and/or referral to a Pediatric Environmental Health Specialty Unit (PEHSU).

Pediatricians and other pediatric health professionals in high-income countries are increasingly likely to care for foreign-born children and to have an important role in promoting these children's health and wellness. It is important for these providers to be aware of the possibility that children who have come to high-income countries from LMICs may have been exposed to toxic environmental hazards in their countries of origin. Such exposures might include heavy metals (lead, mercury, arsenic), pesticides, and air pollution. In addition, once they arrive in the United States, immigrant

TABLE 1. Select Key Environmental Exposures of Concern in Low- and Middle-Income Countries (LMICs)

Environmental Concern	Sources of Exposure	Health Impacts and Disease Burden
Water, sanitation, and hygiene (WASH)	• Water contaminated by biological waste (human and animal) and chemical waste. • 2.4 billion people use unimproved sanitation facilities; 946 million people practice open defecation.[10]	• Acute and chronic gastrointestinal tract diseases such as diarrheal diseases, paratyphoid fever, and parasitic infections; affecting more than 1 billion people (most in LMICs).[61,62] • Unknown impact of chemical pollution because of sparse data.[63]
Ambient air pollution	• Increasing coal combustion and growing car ownership,[10] along with wildfires,[64] leads to higher concentrations of fine particulate matter ($PM_{2.5}$). • 88% of urban residents globally live in cities that fail to meet WHO air quality guidelines.[65]	• $PM_{2.5}$ exposure is linked to asthma, impaired lung function, cardiovascular disease, preterm births, low birth weight, impaired cognitive function, lung cancer. • $PM_{2.5}$-related deaths expected to rise sharply over next 3 decades, especially in South and East Asia.[66] • May increase morbidity and mortality from SARS-CoV-2 infection (COVID-19).[67–70]
Household air pollution (HAP)	• Burning of biomass and solid fuels in unvented indoor stoves for cooking and heating, leading to exceedingly high levels of $PM_{2.5}$.	• Women and young children are disproportionately exposed to HAP because of traditional gender roles in many LMICs.[17,71]
Lead	• Lead "hot spots"—battery recycling operations, smelters, mines, hazardous waste sites. • Lead paint. • Medicinal products (eg, Ayurveda). • Cosmetics (eg, Sindoor). • Ceramic glazes. • Spices, solder in food cans. • Contaminated soil.	• Lead exposure is linked to neurocognitive impairment, anemia, kidney impairment, gastrointestinal tract effects. • 40% of the world's children have blood lead levels exceeding 5 µg/dL, and 90% of these live in LMICs.[72] • Episodes of pediatric lead poisoning in LMICs have been extremely severe or fatal.[73]
Mercury	• Artisanal and small-scale gold mining. • Consumption of large predator fish contaminated with methylmercury is the major route of exposure.[74,75]	• Mercury is a neurotoxicant. • Methylmercury crosses the placenta, passes easily into the tissues of fetuses and young children, and causes permanent injury to the developing brain.[74]
Arsenic	• Contaminated drinking water is the principal source of arsenic exposure, especially in areas with high levels of naturally occurring arsenic in bedrock. • Rice-based food products	• Chronic exposure to inorganic arsenic is linked to several cancers (lung, bladder, skin).[76] • Prenatal exposures are linked to late fetal/neonatal/postneonatal mortality, neurodevelopmental abnormalities, adult cancers, and bronchiectasis.[77–79]
Pesticides	• Highly toxic pesticides banned in the United States are shipped or sold to LMICs and widely used.[80]	• 99% of all acute pesticide poisonings occur in LMICs.[81]
Hazardous wastes	• Asbestos exported into LMICs (more than 2 million tons/year) to be used in construction of homes and schools.[82] • Electronic waste (e-waste) shipped into LMICs (45 million tons per year).[18] Women and young children are employed in e-waste recycling and are exposed to mixture of heavy metals and other chemicals during the process.	• Asbestos exposure can cause lung cancer and malignant mesothelioma.[82] • Children at e-waste sites can have elevated levels of multiple toxic chemicals, including lead and nickel.[83] These exposures are associated with injury to children's immune, cardiovascular, gastrointestinal, renal, endocrine, and hematological systems as well as adverse birth outcomes.[18,84]
Unintentional injuries	• Road traffic accidents, drowning, falls. • Poisonings: household chemicals/pesticides, medications, fuels and solvents, methanol (informally produced alcoholic drinks).	• Approximately 2000 children globally die from unintentional injuries each day.[85]

$PM_{2.5}$= particulate matter with aerodynamic diameter of 2.5 microns or less; also known as "fine particulate matter."

children may face ongoing environmental exposures if they move into substandard housing, have parents who bring home work-related exposures (eg, pesticides with agricultural workers), or have family members who use toxic products imported from the home country (eg, Ayurvedic medicines) (Table 2). It is also important to assess the mental health of children who have come from LMICs, because these children may have been exposed to environmental stressors (eg, violence, famine) and can be referred to appropriate social services and mental health support.

Comprehensive resources on the identification, management, and prevention of environmental exposures are available to guide clinicians caring for children and adolescents in LMICs and children in the United States who have come from LMICs (for full details, see Table 2). For example, the World Health Organization (WHO) provides clinicians with a

TABLE 2. Sources of Environmental Exposures Among Immigrant, Refugee, and Internationally Adopted Children and Adolescents in the United States

	Possible Sources of Exposure	Clinical Resources
General Environmental Health Considerations		
	• For new patients, include key questions about possible environmental and para-occupational exposures • In patients with suspected environmental etiology of disease, consider a consultation with specialists in the PEHSU network for assistance with the diagnosis, management, or treatment of complex environmental health issues.	Use environmental health history forms from WHO (https://www.who.int/publications/m/item/children-s-environmental-record–green-page) or NEEF (https://www.neefusa.org/resource/asthma-environmental-history-form). In the United States, access expert guidance from the Pediatric Environmental Health Specialty Units (PEHSU): www.pehsu.net The WHO has a collaborating network of expert centers in pediatric environmental health: www.niehs.nih.gov/research/programs/geh/partnerships/network/index.cfm
Toxic Stress		
	Violence, extreme poverty, racism, nativism, trauma in unaccompanied minors, effects of climate change	AAP Immigrant Child Health Toolkit provides guidance on screening for trauma, assessing risk and protective factors for mental health and developmental outcomes.[43] AAP policy statement on preventing childhood toxic stress[86] provides recommendations on how to integrate relational health into pediatric care to buffer adversity and build resilience. The CDC provides guidance on health care for immigrants and refugees: www.cdc.gov/immigrantrefugeehealth
Specific Toxicants		
Lead	Upon arrival in the United States, consider: • Lead paint (homes built before 1978) • Imported consumer products, cosmetics, spices, medications, candies wrapped in lead foil • Glazed ceramic cookware, dishes	Obtain a blood lead level on all foreign-born children. CDC has additional guidance on testing immigrant and refugee children for lead.[87]
Mercury	• Large ocean fish • Religious rituals (eg, Santeria, Espiritismo) • Skin-lightening creams/soaps • Exposure to small-scale gold mining	EPA and FDA provide fish consumption guidance.[88] EPA has information on mercury in consumer products.[89]
Arsenic	• Groundwater contamination (children from Bangladesh and other Southeast Asian countries) • Ayurvedic medications • Rice-centered diet	FDA has guidance to reduce arsenic in rice-based diet.[90]
Pesticides	Para-occupational exposure from caregivers working in agriculture	Migrant Clinicians Network provides clinical tools on reducing environmental exposures among migrant farmworker families.[91]
Tobacco or nicotine products	Secondhand exposure to cigarette smoke, electronic cigarettes, hookahs	AAP Richmond Center has extensive clinical resources on tobacco.[92]
Alcohol	Prenatal exposure – risk of fetal alcohol syndrome disorder (FASD)	AAP provides clinical guidelines[93] for diagnosis of FASD and a management toolkit.[94]
Exposure Categories		
Substandard housing and asthma triggers	• Peeling lead-based paint (pre-1978 home) • Mold, pests, and other asthma triggers • Secondhand smoke • Housing instability	CDC recommends screening foreign-born children for lead exposure. Tools are available to screen for environmental triggers in the homes of children with asthma.[95]
Contaminated consumer products	• Imported cosmetics (Kohl, Kajal, Surma, Sindoor, skin-lightening creams) • Herbal supplements, Ayurvedic medications • Amulets	New York City Department of Health (NYCDOH) has compiled an extensive list of consumer products that may be contaminated with heavy metals.[96]
Diet	• Large ocean fish (mercury) • Rice-based diet (arsenic) • Spices purchased abroad (lead)	EPA and FDA provide fish consumption guidance.[88] FDA has guidance to reduce arsenic in a rice-based diet.[90] NYCDOH has guidance on lead-contaminated spices.[97]

CDC, Centers for Disease Control and Prevention; EPA, US Environmental Protection Agency; FDA, US Food and Drug Administration.

pediatric environmental health history tool called the "Green Page" to assist in the identification of critical environmental exposures, including key issues in LMICs.[40] The national network of PEHSUs in the United States provides consultation, guidance, and education for health care providers, public health agencies, and communities on key pediatric environmental health issues.[39,41,42] The WHO has launched an international network of Children's Environmental Health Units, including the Unidades de Pediátrica Ambiental (UPAs) in Latin America, and has created a comprehensive training program in pediatric environmental health that can serve as a resource for clinicians. The AAP has published resources to assist providers in the clinical care of immigrant children[43] and internationally-adopted children.[44]

Role of Pediatric and Public Health Organizations

Pediatric organizations can make important contributions to protecting children against environmental threats to health by complementing and magnifying the voices of individual pediatricians. The informed and trusted voices of district, state, and national pediatric organizations can powerfully influence environmental policy decisions by reminding policy makers that almost any environmental decision has implications for children's health and that these implications must be explicitly considered before decisions are made.

Need for Expanded Education in Children's Environmental Health

Recent decades have seen a dramatic rise in interest in environmental health among medical and public health professionals in the United States and across the globe. Gains have been made in adding topics on environmental health and climate change into medical education. These educational programs are, however, not yet comprehensive, and many of them do not fully prepare physicians to address environmental concerns among their patients, especially patients in LMICs.[45–48] Environmental health training for medical personnel, public health professionals, environmental public health technicians, and community health workers could be expanded to raise knowledge of and capacity to address environmental health concerns in the clinical setting. The curricula of such training can also be structured to provide pediatricians with the knowledge and tools they will need to be effective, science-based advocates for children's environmental health.

To fill the gap in medical education, organizations such as the AAP, the Academic Pediatric Association, and the WHO have launched initiatives to build capacity in pediatric environmental health. The Academic Pediatric Association has launched an environmental health fellowship that has trained more than 50 clinicians and scientists who have become leaders in the field[49,50] and has formed an environmental health special interest group. The AAP has convened pediatric environmental health champions (including trainees), raised the national profile of the field, and published the *Pediatric Environmental Health* clinical handbook (known as the "Green Book"), now in its 4th edition.[39] A *Textbook on Children's Environmental Health* has also been published.[51] However, greater integration of environmental health and climate change topics into existing educational structures (eg, medical school curricula, pediatric residency competencies, continuing education for providers) is needed to reach more providers and increase their ability to address key environmental exposures in their patients.[52] A growing network of health professional schools and programs around the world have begun integrating climate change into their educational curricula,[48,52,53] providing a model for replication in additional settings and covering a broader range of topics in environmental health.

Need for Increased Resources in Children's Environmental Health

Given the immense burden of disease attributable to modifiable environmental factors, increased financial support and capacity building in environmental public health and research is urgently needed in all countries, and especially LMICs. Programs such as the WHO-National Institute of Environmental Health Sciences (NIEHS) Collaborating Centers and the Fogarty International Center (of the National Institutes of Health) offer international training programs, research, capacity building, and information sharing across countries, which have reduced disease burden around the world.[54,55] However, substantially more funding and investment in these types of programs is needed to fully address the complex and changing scope of environmentally related disease.

Role of Governmental and Nongovernmental Agencies

Despite the great magnitude of their effects on human health, environmental hazards in LMICs have been neglected in the international development and global health agendas as well as in the planning strategies of many countries. The foreign aid budgets of the European Commission, the US Agency for International Development, and bilateral development agencies allocate only minimal resources to the prevention and control of ambient air pollution and chemical pollution.[56,57] No major foundation has made pollution control a priority. Despite the great impact of pollution on global morbidity and mortality, the average investment by international development agencies in preventing an environmentally related death (caused by ambient air pollution and chemical pollution) is \$14/death compared with \$1250/death for malaria, \$190/death for tuberculosis, and \$165/death for HIV/AIDS.[58]

It is critical that governmental and nongovernmental agencies prioritize the funding of primary environmental interventions such as implementing safely managed drinking water systems, ending open defecation through installation of safe toilet facilities, increasing access to cleaner fuels and more efficient indoor cook stoves, and improving surveillance of chemical products.[59] These preventive interventions produce crosscutting health, social, and economic co-benefits and support the ambitious vision of United Nation's Sustainable Development Goals. The 17 Sustainable Development Goals aim to eradicate global poverty by 2030 by focusing on sustainable strategies to ensure healthy environments for all, especially women and children.[60]

As climate change accelerates and LMICs continue their passage through the epidemiological and environmental transitions with increasing urbanization and industrialization, increased investment in research and infrastructure is needed to ensure a resilient future for all children and future generations.

SUMMARY AND RECOMMENDATIONS

The AAP provides additional details on the topics discussed in this policy statement in the accompanying technical report.[9] Combined, these 2 documents provide guidance to pediatricians and trainees on recognizing, diagnosing, managing, and preventing environmentally related diseases in children and adolescents living in LMICs and those who have relocated to high-income countries from LMICs. Given the importance of environmental exposures to the health and well-being of children around the world, the AAP offers recommendations for pediatricians, trainees, and other health professionals.

Recommendations for Pediatricians and Other Health Care Professionals

1. Understand the importance of environmental hazards, including climate change, and their impacts on children's health, especially on children in LMICs and children who have come to high-income countries from LMICs.
2. Recognize the importance of environmental hazards and their impacts on the health of children in communities experiencing environmental injustice in areas that you serve in clinical practice and engage in appropriate needs-based collaboration with these communities to identify and reduce environmental threats to children's health.
3. Include environmental health in histories for new patients via standardized questions about possible environmental and para-occupational (exposures to toxic materials brought into the home by parents on clothing, shoes, or vehicles) exposures. Refer to general environmental history guides, such as the World Health Organization's "Green Page," the AAP's textbook *Pediatric Environmental Health* (known as the "Green Book"), or tailored guidance from local health agencies if available.
4. Include environmental health questions during appropriate medical encounters with existing patients who have environmentally related disease (eg, asthma).
5. Refer patients with suspected environmental exposures to PEHSUs, public health or environmental health agencies, or community organizations for further help with exposure assessment and management.
6. In patients with suspected environmental etiology of disease, consider a consultation with specialists in the PEHSU network for assistance with the diagnosis, management, or treatment of complex environmental health issues.
7. Contact local public health and environmental health authorities about previously unknown or unrecognized community environmental exposures to allow for further community-based assessment of potential impacts on children's health and management of the problem.

Recommendations for Pediatric Organizations

1. Increase the amount of environmental health and climate change content offered as continuing medical education (CME) credits and in maintenance of certification (MOC) credits as well as in certification and recertification examinations.
2. Collaborate with other pediatric and environmental organizations (national and international), as well as with the WHO, to advocate for prevention strategies and policies that protect children against environmental hazards in all countries.
3. Collaborate with health departments and research institutions to develop standardized data sets to enhance surveillance, analysis, and reporting of environmental exposures and environmentally related diseases.
4. Collaborate with other national or international pediatric and health organizations to prevent and ameliorate the impact of environmental factors on the health of children, and address child poverty as a determinant of health. These goals can be further achieved by supporting progress on the Sustainable Development Goals.

Recommendations for Governmental and Nongovernmental Agencies

1. Nations, states, territories, and cities must take action to end the exposure of all children to known toxic chemicals and to prevent the entry of untested new chemicals into markets.
2. Nations, states, and cities must put the protection of children's health at the center of all environmental legislation and rule making and deliberately consider potential impacts on children's health in all environmental decision making.
3. When setting environmental regulations, use the best available scientific evidence that adequately considers the unique vulnerabilities of children as well as the impacts on children's health and development of cumulative exposures to chemical mixtures.
4. When setting environmental regulations, seek whenever possible to regulate entire classes of chemicals such as the organophosphate insecticides rather than individual chemicals within such classes.
5. Increase the resources directed to global public health and pollution prevention to better protect children against environmental threats to health.
6. Increase resources for the surveillance, analysis, and reporting of environmental exposures and environmentally related diseases.

7. Create channels of communication for dissemination of information among governmental and nongovernmental organizations regarding pediatric environmental exposures, effects, and management strategies.
8. Increase opportunities and resources for training pediatric health workers in environmental and occupational health to provide the global health workforce needed to address these health problems.
9. Create more opportunities and resources for research on global pediatric environmental health issues to include characterizations of environmental exposures and study of efficacy of interventions to evaluate, decrease, and/or prevent exposures.
10. Create opportunities for increased collaboration between high-income and low- and middle-income countries in achieving the above recommendations.

LEAD AUTHORS

Lauren Zajac, MD, MPH, FAAP
Philip J. Landrigan, MD, MSc, FAAP

COUNCIL ON ENVIRONMENTAL HEALTH AND CLIMATE CHANGE EXECUTIVE COMMITTEE, 2022–2023

Lauren Zajac, MD, MHP, FAAP; Chairperson
Sophie J. Balk, MD, FAAP
Lori G. Byron, MD, FAAP
Gredia Maria Huerta-Montañez MD, FAAP
Philip J. Landrigan, MD, FAAP
Steven M. Marcus, MD, FAAP
Abby L. Nerlinger, MD, FAAP
Lisa H. Patel, MD, FAAP
Rebecca Philipsborn, MD, FAAP
Alan D. Woolf, MD, MPH, FAAP

LIAISONS

Kimberly A. Gray, PhD – National Institute of Environmental Health Sciences
Grace Robiou – US Environmental Protection Agency
Nathaniel G. DeNicola, MD, MSc – American College of Obstetricians and Gynecologists
CDR Matt Karwowski, MD, MPH, FAAP – Centers for Disease Control and Prevention National Center for Environmental Health and Agency for Toxic Substances and Disease Registry
Mary H. Ward, PhD – National Cancer Institute

STAFF

Paul Spire

ABBREVIATIONS

AAP: American Academy of Pediatrics
LMICs: low- and middle-income countries
PEHSU: Pediatric Environmental Health Specialty Unit
WHO: World Health Organization

Accepted for Publication Date: November 22, 2024

https://doi.org/10.1542/peds.2024-070075

COMPANION PAPER: A companion to this article can be found online at www.pediatrics.org/cgi/doi/10.1542/peds.2024-070076.

REFERENCES

1. Suchdev PS, Howard CR. The role of pediatricians in global health. *Pediatrics.* 2018;142(6):e20182997. doi:10.1542/peds.2018-2997
2. Philipsborn RP, Chan K. Climate change and global child health. *Pediatrics.* 2018;141(6):e20173774. doi: 10.1542/peds.2017-3774
3. Linton JM, Green A, Chilton LA, et al. Providing care for children in immigrant families. *Pediatrics.* 2019;144(3):e20192077. doi: 10.1542/peds.2019-2077
4. Miller MD, Marty MA, Landrigan PJ. Children's environmental health: beyond national boundaries. *Pediatr Clin North Am.* 2016;63(1):149–165. doi: 10.1016/j.pcl.2015.08.008
5. Landrigan PJ, Fuller R, Fisher S, et al. Pollution and children's health. *Sci Total Environ.* 2019;650(Pt 2):2389–2394. doi: 10.1016/j.scitotenv.2018.09.375
6. Suk WA, Ahanchian H, Asante KA, et al. Environmental pollution: an underrecognized threat to children's health, especially in low- and middle-income countries. *Environ Health Perspect.* 2016;124(3):A43–A45. doi: 10.1289/ehp.1510517
7. Landrigan PJ, Fuller R. The impact of pollution on planetary health: emergence of an underappreciated risk factor. *UN Environment Perspective.* 2017;29:1–12
8. World Health Organization. *Inheriting a Sustainable World: Atlas on Children's Health and the Environment.* World Health Organization; 2017. Available at: https://www.who.int/publications/i/item/9789241511773. Accessed May 19, 2020
9. Zajac L, Landrigan PJ; American Academy of Pediatrics, Council on Environmental Health and Climate Change. Technical report. Environmental issues in global pediatric health. *Pediatrics.* 2023; in press

10. Landrigan PJ, Fuller R, Acosta NJR, et al. The Lancet Commission on pollution and health. *Lancet.* 2018;391(10119):462–512. doi: 10.1016/S0140-6736(17)32345-0

11. Bullard RD, Robert D. *Dumping in Dixie : Race, Class, and Environmental Quality.* Westview Press; 1990

12. Foote EM, Singleton RJ, Holman RC, et al. Lower respiratory tract infection hospitalizations among American Indian/Alaska Native children and the general United States child population. *Int J Circumpolar Health.* 2015;74:29256. doi: 10.3402/IJCH.V74.29256

13. Singleton R, Salkoski AJ, Bulkow L, et al. Impact of home remediation and household education on indoor air quality, respiratory visits and symptoms in Alaska Native children. *Int J Circumpolar Health.* 2018;77(1):1422669. doi: 10.1080/22423982.2017.1422669

14. Hennessy TW, Ritter T, Holman RC, et al. The relationship between in-home water service and the risk of respiratory tract, skin, and gastrointestinal tract infections among rural Alaska Natives. *Am J Public Health.* 2008;98(11):2072. doi: 10.2105/AJPH.2007.115618

15. Smith KR, Ezzati M. How environmental health risks change with development: the epidemiologic and environmental risk transitions revisited. *Annu Rev Environ Resour.* 2005;30:291–333. doi: 10.1146/annurev.energy.30.050504.144424

16. Omran AR. The epidemiologic transition: a theory of the epidemiology of population change. *Milbank Q.* 2005;83(4):731–757. doi: 10.1111/j.1468-0009.2005.00398.x

17. Yadama GN. *Fires, Fuel, and the Fate of Three Billion: Portraits of the Energy Impoverished.* Oxford University Press; 2013

18. Grant K, Goldizen FC, Sly PD, et al. Health consequences of exposure to e-waste: a systematic review. *Lancet Glob Heal.* 2013;1(6):e350–e361. doi: 10.1016/S2214-109X(13)70101-3

19. Spitz PH. *The Chemical Industry at the Millennium : Maturity, Restructuring, and Globalization.* Chemical Heritage Press; 2003

20. Pronczuk J, Bruné MN GF. Children's environmental health in developing countries. In: Nriagu JO, Kacew S, Kawamoto T, Patz JA RD, ed. *Encyclopedia of Environmental Health.* Amsterdam, Netherlands: Elsevier; 2011:601–610. https://www.sciencedirect.com/referencework/9780444522726/encyclopedia-of-environmental-health. Accessed May 19, 2020

21. Stanaway JD, Afshin A, Gakidou E, et al. Global, regional, and national comparative risk assessment of 84 behavioural, environmental and occupational, and metabolic risks or clusters of risks for 195 countries and territories, 1990-2017: a systematic analysis for the Global Burden of Disease Study 2017. *Lancet.* 2018;392(10159):1923–1994. doi: 10.1016/S0140-6736(18)32225-6

22. Yen C, Tate JE, Hyde TB, et al. Rotavirus vaccines: current status and future considerations. *Hum Vaccines Immunother.* 2014;10(6):1436–1448. doi: 10.4161/hv.28857

23. Florez ID, Al-Khalifah R, Sierra JM, et al. The effectiveness and safety of treatments used for acute diarrhea and acute gastroenteritis in children: protocol for a systematic review and network meta-analysis. *Syst Rev.* 2016;5(1). doi: 10.1186/s13643-016-0186-8

24. Branca F, Piwoz E, Schultink W, Sullivan LM. Nutrition and health in women, children, and adolescent girls. *BMJ.* 2015;351:h4173. doi: 10.1136/bmj.h4173

25. Landrigan PJ, Sly JL, Ruchirawat M, et al. Health consequences of environmental exposures: changing global patterns of exposure and disease. *Ann Glob Health.* 2016;82(1):10–19. doi: 10.1016/j.aogh.2016.01.005

26. Remais JV, Zeng G, Li G, Tian L, Engelgau MM. Convergence of non-communicable and infectious diseases in low-and middle-income countries. *Int J Epidemiol.* 2013;42:221–227. doi: 10.1093/ije/dys135

27. Fuller R, Rahona E, Fisher S, et al. Pollution and non-communicable disease: time to end the neglect. *Lancet Planet Health.* 2018;2(3):e96–e98. doi: 10.1016/S2542-5196(18)30020-2

28. Samet JM, Burke TA, Goldstein BD. The Trump administration and the environment—heed the science. *N Engl J Med.* 2017;376(12):1182–1188. doi: 10.1056/NEJMms1615242

29. Grosse SD, Matte TD, Schwartz J, Jackson RJ. Economic gains resulting from the reduction in children's exposure to lead in the United States. *Environ Health Perspect.* 2002;110(6):563–569. doi: 10.1289/ehp.02110563

30. Gauderman WJ, Urman R, Avol E, et al. Association of improved air quality with lung development in children. *N Engl J Med.* 2015;372(10):905–913. doi: 10.1056/NEJMoa1414123

31. Galvez M, Collins G, Amler RW, et al. Building New York state centers of excellence in children's environmental health: a replicable model in a time of uncertainty. *Am J Public Health.* 2019;109(1):108–112. doi: 10.2105/AJPH.2018.304742

32. Barreto M. The globalization of epidemiology: critical thoughts from Latin America. *Int J Epidemiol.* 2004;33(5):1132–1137. Available at: https://www.researchgate.net/publication/8490293_The_globalization_of_epidemiology_Critical_thoughts_from_Latin_America. Accessed May 19, 2020

33. De Maio FG. Understanding chronic non-communicable diseases in Latin America: towards an equity-based research agenda. *Global Health.* 2011;7(1):36. doi: 10.1186/1744-8603-7-36

34. US Environmental Protection Agency, Office of Air and Radiation. Overview of the Clean Air Act and Air Pollution. 2020. Available at: https://www.epa.gov/clean-air-act-overview. Accessed May 19, 2020

35. Watts N, Amann M, Arnell N, et al. The 2019 report of The Lancet Countdown on Health and Climate Change: ensuring that the health of a child born today is not defined by a changing climate. *Lancet.* 2019;394(10211):1836–1878. doi: 10.1016/S0140-6736(19)32596-6

36. Anderko L, Chalupka S, Du M, Hauptman M. Climate changes reproductive and children's health: a review of risks, exposures, and impacts. *Pediatr Res.* 2020;87(2):414–419. doi: 10.1038/s41390-019-0654-7

37. Ahdoot S, Baum CR, Cataletto M, Hogan P, Wu CB, Bernstein A; American Academy of Pediatrics, Council on Enviornmental Health and Climate Change, Council on Children and Disasters, Section on Pediatric Pulmonology and Sleep Medicine, Section on Minority Health, Equity, and Inclusion. Policy statement. Climate change and children's health: building a healthy future for every child. *Pediatrics* 2024;153(3):e2023065504

38. Ahdoot S, Baum CR, Cataletto M, Hogan P, Wu CB, Bernstein A, Council on Enviornmental Health and Climate Change, Council

on Children and Disasters, Section on Pediatric Pulmonology and Sleep Medicine, Section on Minority Health, Equity, and Inclusion. Technical report. Climate Change and Children's Health: Building a Healthy Future for Every Child. *Pediatrics* March 2024; 153(3): e2023065505. 10.1542/peds.2023-065505

39. American Academy of Pediatrics, Council on Environmental Health. *Pediatric Environmental Health*. Etzel RA, Balk SJ, eds. Itasca, IL: American Academy of Pediatrics; 2018
40. World Health Organization. The Paediatric Environmental History Recording Children's Exposure to Environmental Health Threats: A "Green Page" in the Medical Record. World Health Organization; 2018. Available at: https://www.who.int/news-room/questions-and-answers/item/q-a-the-paediatric-environmental-history. Accessed May 16, 2023
41. Paulson JA, Karr CJ, Seltzer JM, et al. Development of the pediatric environmental health specialty unit network in North America. *Am J Public Health*. 2009;99(Suppl 3)S511–S516. doi: 10.2105/ajph.2008.154641
42. Wilborne-Davis P, Kirkland KH, Mulloy KB. A model for physician education and consultation in pediatric environmental health —the Pediatric Environmental Health Specialty Units (PEHSU) Program. *Pediatr Clin North Am*. 2007;54(1):1–13. doi: 10.1016/j.pcl.2006.11.001
43. American Academy of Pediatrics, Council on Community Pediatrics. Immigrant Child Health Toolkit. 2020. Available at: https://www.aap.org/en-us/advocacy-and-policy/aap-health-initiatives/Immigrant-Child-Health-Toolkit/Pages/Immigrant-Child-Health-Toolkit.aspx. Accessed December 1, 2022
44. Jones VF, Schulte EE, Springer S, et al. Comprehensive health evaluation of the newly adopted child. *Pediatrics*. 2019;143(5): e20190657. doi: 10.1542/peds.2019-0657
45. Trasande L, Schapiro ML, Falk R, et al. Pediatrician attitudes, clinical activities, and knowledge of environmental health in Wisconsin. *Wis Med J*. 2006;105(2):45–49
46. Trasande L, Boscarino J, Graber N, et al. The environment in pediatric practice: a study of New York pediatricians' attitudes, beliefs, and practices towards children's environmental health. *J Urban Heal*. 2006;83(4):760–772. doi: 10.1007/s11524-006-9071-4
47. Trasande L, Newman N, Long L, et al. Translating knowledge about environmental health to practitioners: are we doing enough? *Mt Sinai J Med*. 2010;77(1):114–123. doi: 10.1002/msj.20158
48. Philipsborn RP, Sheffield P, White A, Osta A, Anderson MS, Bernstein A. Climate change and the practice of medicine: essentials for resident education. *Acad Med*. 2021;96(3):355–367. doi: 10.1097/ACM.0000000000003719
49. Landrigan PJ, Woolf AD, Gitterman B, et al. The ambulatory pediatric association fellowship in pediatric environmental health: a 5-year assessment. *Environ Health Perspect*. 2007;115(10):1383–1387. doi: 10.1289/ehp.10015
50. Landrigan PJ, Braun JM, Crain EF, et al. Building capacity in pediatric environmental health: the Academic Pediatric Association's professional development program. *Acad Pediatr*. 2019;19(4): 421–427. doi: 10.1016/j.acap.2019.01.001
51. Etzel RA, Landrigan PJ, eds. *Textbook of Children's Environmental Health*. Oxford University Press; 2024. ISBN 978 019 766 2533
52. Goldman RH, Zajac L, Geller RJ, Miller MD. Developing and implementing core competencies in children's environmental health for students, trainees and healthcare providers: a narrative review. *BMC Med Educ*. 2021;21(1). doi: 10.1186/S12909-021-02921-3
53. Columbia University Mailman School of Public Health. Global Consortium on Climate and Health Education. 2020. Available at: https://www.publichealth.columbia.edu/research/global-consortium-climate-and-health-education. Accessed December 1, 2022
54. Drain PK HK. The Fogarty International Center at 50: Accomplishments and Priorities for the Next 50 Years. *Clin Infect Dis*. 2018;66(9):1323–1325. doi: 10.1093/cid/ciy078
55. World Health Organization. *Collaboration between the World Health Organization and the National Institute of Environmental Health Sciences: Highlights from 30 Years of Partnership*. Geneva: World Health Organization; 2011. Available at: https://www.who.int/publications/i/item/978924502078. Accessed June 26, 2020
56. Greenberg H, Leeder SR, Raymond SU. And why so great a "no?" The donor and academic communities' failure to confront global chronic disease. *Glob Heart*. 2016;11(4):381–385. doi: 10.1016/j.gheart.2016.10.018
57. Nugent R. A chronology of global assistance funding for NCD. *Glob Heart*. 2016;11(4):371–374. doi: 10.1016/j.gheart.2016.10.027
58. Swinehart S, Fuller R, Kupka R, Conte MN. Rethinking aid allocation: analysis of official development spending on modern pollution reduction. *Ann Glob Heal*. 2019;85(1). doi: 10.5334/aogh.2633
59. World Health Organization. *Healthy Environments for Healthier Populations: Why Do They Matter, and What Can We Do?* Geneva: World Health Organization; 2019
60. United Nations. Sustainable Development Goals. 2015. Available at: https://sustainabledevelopment.un.org. Accessed June 23, 2020
61. Forouzanfar MH, Afshin A, Alexander LT, et al. Global, regional, and national comparative risk assessment of 79 behavioural, environmental and occupational, and metabolic risks or clusters of risks, 1990–2015: a systematic analysis for the Global Burden of Disease Study 2015. *Lancet*. 2016;388(10053):1659–1724. doi: 10.1016/S0140-6736(16)31679-8
62. Wang H, Naghavi M, Allen C, et al. Global, regional, and national life expectancy, all-cause mortality, and cause-specific mortality for 249 causes of death, 1980–2015: a systematic analysis for the Global Burden of Disease Study 2015. *Lancet*. 2016;388(10053): 1459–1544. doi: 10.1016/S0140-6736(16)31012-1
63. Landrigan PJ, Goldman LR. Children's vulnerability to toxic chemicals: a challenge and opportunity to strengthen health and environmental policy. *Health Aff*. 2011;30(5):842–850. doi: 10.1377/hlthaff.2011.0151
64. Kelly FJ, Fussell JC. Global nature of airborne particle toxicity and health effects: a focus on megacities, wildfires, dust storms and residential biomass burning. *Toxicol Res (Camb)*. 2020;9(4):331–345. doi: 10.1093/toxres/tfaa044

65. World Health Organization. Air Pollution. Available at: https://www.who.int/health-topics/air-pollution#tab=tab_1. Accessed May 25, 2020

66. Lelieveld J, Evans JS, Fnais M, Giannadaki D, Pozzer A. The contribution of outdoor air pollution sources to premature mortality on a global scale. *Nature.* 2015;525(7569):367–371. doi: 10.1038/nature15371

67. Dettori M, Deiana G, Balletto G, et al. Air pollutants and risk of death due to COVID-19 in Italy. *Environ Res.* 2021;192:110459. doi: 10.1016/j.envres.2020.110459

68. Copat C, Cristaldi A, Fiore M, et al. The role of air pollution (PM and NO2) in COVID-19 spread and lethality: a systematic review. *Environ Res.* 2020;191:110129. doi: 10.1016/j.envres.2020.110129

69. Paital B, Agrawal PK. Air pollution by NO2 and PM2.5 explains COVID-19 infection severity by overexpression of angiotensin-converting enzyme 2 in respiratory cells: a review. *Environ Chem Lett.* 2021;19(1):25–42. doi: 10.1007/s10311-020-01091-w

70. Zoran MA, Savastru RS, Savastru DM, Tautan MN. Assessing the relationship between surface levels of PM2.5 and PM10 particulate matter impact on COVID-19 in Milan, Italy. *Sci Total Environ.* 2020;738:139825. doi: 10.1016/j.scitotenv.2020.139825

71. Balakrishnan K, Cohen A, Smith KR. Addressing the burden of disease attributable to air pollution in India: the need to integrate across household and ambient air pollution exposures. *Environ Health Perspect.* 2014;122(1):A6–A7. doi: 10.1289/ehp.1307822

72. Fewtrell LJ, Prüss-Üstün A, Landrigan P, Ayuso-Mateos JL. Estimating the global burden of disease of mild mental retardation and cardiovascular diseases from environmental lead exposure. *Environ Res.* 2004;94(2):120–133. doi: 10.1016/S0013-9351(03)00132-4

73. Haefliger P, Mathieu-Nolf M, Lociciro S, et al. Mass lead intoxication from informal used lead-acid battery recycling in Dakar, Senegal. *Environ Health Perspect.* 2009;117(10):1535–1540. doi: 10.1289/ehp.0900696

74. United Nations Environment Programme. *Global Mercury Assessment 2018. UNEP-UN Environment Programme.* Geneva: United Nations; 2019. doi:ISBN: 978-92-807-3744-8

75. World Health Organization. Mercury and health. 2017. Available at: https://www.who.int/news-room/fact-sheets/detail/mercury-and-health. Accessed May 25, 2020

76. Hopenhayn-Rich C, Browning SR, Hertz-Picciotto I, Ferreccio C, Peralta C, Gibb H. Chronic arsenic exposure and risk of infant mortality in two areas of Chile. *Environ Health Perspect.* 2000;108(7):667–673. doi: 10.1289/ehp.00108667

77. Smith AH, Marshall G, Liaw J, Yuan Y, Ferreccio C, Steinmaus C. Mortality in young adults following in utero and childhood exposure to arsenic in drinking water. *Environ Health Perspect.* 2012;120(11):1527–1531. doi: 10.1289/ehp.1104867

78. Von Ehrenstein OS, Poddar S, Yuan Y, et al. Children's intellectual function in relation to arsenic exposure. *Epidemiology.* 2007;18(1):44–51. doi: 10.1097/01.ede.0000248900.65613.a9

79. Wasserman GA, Liu X, Parvez F, et al. Water arsenic exposure and children's intellectual function in Araihazar, Bangladesh. *Environ Health Perspect.* 2004;112(13):1329–1333. doi: 10.1289/ehp.6964

80. Food and Agriculture Organization of the United Nations. Prevention and Disposal of Obsolete Pesticides: Pesticide Bans. Available at: http://www.fao.org/agriculture/crops/obsolete-pesticides/why-problem/pesticide-bans/en. Accessed May 20, 2020

81. United Nations Environment Programme. *Childhood Pesticide Poisoning: Information for Advocacy and Action.* Chatelaine, Switzerland: United Nations Environment Programme; 2004

82. Frank AL, Joshi TK. The global spread of asbestos. *Ann Glob Heal.* 2014;80(4):257–262. doi: 10.1016/j.aogh.2014.09.016

83. Xu X, Yang H, Chen A, et al. Birth outcomes related to informal e-waste recycling in Guiyu, China. *Reprod Toxicol.* 2012;33(1):94–98. doi: 10.1016/j.reprotox.2011.12.006

84. Heacock M, Kelly CB, Asante KA, et al. E-waste and harm to vulnerable populations: a growing global problem. *Environ Health Perspect.* 2016;124(5):550–555. doi: 10.1289/ehp.1509699

85. Peden M, Oyegbite K, Ozanne-Smith J, et al. *World Report on Child Injury Prevention.* Geneva, Switzerland; 2008. Available at: https://www.who.int/publications/i/item/9789241563574. Accessed June 4, 2020

86. Garner A, Yogman M; Committee on Psychosocial Aspects of Child and Family Health, Section on Developmental and Behavioral Pediatrics, Council on Early Childhood. Preventing childhood toxic stress: partnering with families and communities to promote relational health. *Pediatrics.* 2021;148(2):e2021052582

87. Centers for Disease Control and Prevention. Refugees and Other Newcomer Persons Resettled to the United States. Available at: https://www.cdc.gov/nceh/lead/prevention/refugees.htm. Accessed May 16, 2023

88. US Environmental Protection Agency, US Food and Drug Administration. Fish and Shellfish Advisories and Safe Eating Guidelines. Choose Fish and Shellfish Wisely. 2020. Available at: https://www.epa.gov/choose-fish-and-shellfish-wisely/fish-and-shellfish-advisories-and-safe-eating-guidelines. Accessed June 16, 2020

89. US Environmental Protection Agency. Mercury in Consumer Products. 2019. Available at: https://www.epa.gov/mercury/mercury-consumer-products. Accessed June 19, 2020.

90. US Food and Drug Administration. What You Can Do to Limit Exposure to Arsenic. 2019. Available at: https://www.fda.gov/food/metals-and-your-food/what-you-can-do-limit-exposure-arsenic. Accessed June 16, 2020

91. Migrant Clinicians Network. Environmental and Occupational Health Screening Questions for Primary Care. 2020. Available at: https://www.migrantclinician.org/toolsource/288/environmental-and-occupational-health/index.html. Accessed June 16, 2020

92. American Academy of Pediatrics, Julius B. Richmond Center of Excellence. Tobacco Control and Prevention. 2020. Available at: https://www.aap.org/en-us/advocacy-and-policy/aap-health-initiatives/Richmond-Center/Pages/default.aspx. Accessed June 19, 2020.

93. Hoyme HE, Kalberg WO, Elliott AJ, et al. Updated clinical guidelines for diagnosing fetal alcohol spectrum disorders. *Pediatrics.* 2016;138(2):e20154256. doi: 10.1542/peds.2015-4256

94. American Academy of Pediatrics. The Fetal Alcohol Spectrum Disorders (FASD) Toolkit. Available at: https://www.aap.org/en/patient-care/fetal-alcohol-spectrum-disorders/. Accessed May 20, 2020

95. National Environmental Education Foundation. Asthma Environmental History Form. 2020. Available at: https://www.neefusa.org/resource/asthma-environmental-history-form. Accessed June 19, 2020

96. New York City Department of Health. Hazardous Consumer Products. 2020. Available at: https://www1.nyc.gov/site/doh/health/health-topics/lead-poisoning-hazardous-consumer-products.page. Accessed June 16, 2020

97. New York City Department of Health. Hazardous Foods and Spices. 2020. Available at: https://www1.nyc.gov/site/doh/health/health-topics/hazardous-foods-spices.page. Published 2020. Accessed June 16, 2020

Environmental Issues in Global Pediatric Health (Technical Report)

- *Technical Report*

TECHNICAL REPORT

American Academy of Pediatrics
DEDICATED TO THE HEALTH OF ALL CHILDREN™

Environmental Issues in Global Pediatric Health: Technical Report

Lauren Zajac, MD, MPH, FAAP,[1] Philip J. Landrigan, MD, MSc, FAAP,[2] and the COUNCIL ON ENVIRONMENTAL HEALTH AND CLIMATE CHANGE

Pediatricians and pediatric trainees in North America are increasingly involved in caring for children and adolescents in or from low- and middle-income countries (LMICs). In many LMICs, toxic environmental exposures—notably outdoor and household air pollution, water pollution, lead, hazardous waste disposal, pesticides, and other manufactured chemicals—are highly prevalent and account for twice as great a proportion of disease and deaths among young children as in North America. Climate change will likely worsen these exposures.

It is important that pediatricians and other pediatric health professionals from high-income countries who plan to work in LMICs be aware of the disproportionately severe impacts of environmental hazards, become knowledgeable about the major toxic threats to children's health in the countries and communities where they will be working, and consider environmental factors in their differential diagnoses. Likewise, pediatricians in high-income countries who care for children and adolescents who have emigrated from LMICs need to be aware that these children may be at elevated risk of diseases caused by past exposures to toxic environmental hazards in their countries of origin as well as ongoing exposures in products such as traditional foods, medications, and cosmetics imported from their original home countries.

Because diseases of toxic environmental origin seldom have unique physical signatures, the environmental screening history, supplemented by laboratory testing, is the principal diagnostic tool. The goal of this technical report is to enhance pediatricians' ability to recognize, diagnose, and manage disease caused by hazardous environmental exposures, especially toxic chemical exposures, in all countries and especially in LMICs.

abstract

[1]*Department of Environmental Medicine and Public Health and Department of Pediatrics, Icahn School of Medicine at Mount Sinai, New York, New York; and* [2]*Program for Global Public Health and the Common Good, Boston College, Chestnut Hill, Massachusetts; Centre Scientifique de Monaco, Monaco, MC*

Dr Zajac was the lead author and Drs Zajac and Landrigan were both responsible for conceptualizing, writing, and revising the manuscript and considering input from all reviewers and the board of directors, and all authors approved the final manuscript as submitted.

CONFLICT OF INTEREST DISCLOSURE: The authors have indicated they have no potential conflicts of interest to disclose.

FUNDING: No external funding.

Accepted for Publication Date: November 22, 2024

https://doi.org/10.1542/peds.2024-070076

COMPANION PAPER: A companion to this article can be found online at www.pediatrics.org/cgi/doi/10.1542/peds.2024-070075.

To cite: Zajac L and Landrigan PJ; American Academy of Pediatrics, Council on Environmental Health and Climate

BACKGROUND INFORMATION

Pediatricians and pediatric trainees in North America are increasingly involved in directly providing clinical care to children and adolescents in low- and middle-income countries (LMICs). North American pediatricians also care for children who have emigrated from across the globe,[1]; their number may increase in future years in consequence of climate change,[2] armed conflicts, complex sociopolitical circumstances, and changing immigration policies.[3]

Pediatric educators have come to recognize the great value of global health experiences.[4,5] Clinical and educational experiences in LMICs increase trainees' appreciation of the importance of social and economic factors in shaping patterns of health and disease in children. They enhance trainees' ability to operate across cultural and linguistic divides and provide competent, compassionate care in low-resource settings. To support global health training programs and enrich their curricula, the American Academy of Pediatrics (AAP) and the American Board of Pediatrics have jointly developed a comprehensive guide for education in pediatric global health.[6] The AAP Section on International Child Health (currently named the Section on Global Health) released a policy statement titled "The Role of Pediatricians in Global Health."[1]

Environmental hazards are major causes of disease and death among children in LMICs, but the great magnitude of environmental impacts on children's health in these countries is not generally appreciated.[7–9] In LMICs, environmental hazards account for twice as great a proportion of deaths in children younger than 5 years as in high-income countries—26% versus 17%.[10] Pollution is a major risk factor and is responsible for an estimated 9 million deaths annually in persons of all ages—3 times as many deaths as AIDS, tuberculosis, and malaria combined. Nearly 92% of pollution-related deaths occur in LMICs.[11] Environmental threats to children's health in LMICs are worsening, and ambient air pollution and contamination by pesticides and other toxic chemicals are growing especially rapidly.

STATEMENT OF THE PROBLEM

It is important that pediatricians, pediatric trainees, and other pediatric health professionals from high-income countries who plan to work in LMICs be aware that toxic environmental exposures account for a much higher proportion of disease, disability, and death among children and adolescents in these countries than among youth in high-income countries. It is important also that they become knowledgeable about the major environmental threats to children's health in the countries and communities where they will be working and incorporate this information into their clinical practice. Similarly, it is important that pediatricians in high-income countries who care for children and adolescents who have emigrated from LMICs be aware that these patients may be at elevated risk of diseases caused by past exposures to toxic environmental hazards in their countries of origin as well as ongoing exposures in products such as traditional foods, medications, and cosmetics imported from their home countries.

This technical report provides an overview of key environmental issues in global pediatric health with a particular focus on toxic chemical hazards. The goals are to increase awareness of the great impacts these hazards on children's health both among pediatricians who may be directly providing care to children in LMICs as well as among pediatricians in North America who may be caring for children who have emigrated from LMICs. The report provides summary reviews of the major environmental hazards in LMICs and a listing of resources for further information.

The goal of this technical report, along with the accompanying policy statement,[12] is to enhance pediatricians' ability to recognize, diagnose, and manage disease caused by hazardous environmental exposures, especially toxic chemical exposures, in all countries and especially in LMICs.

REVIEW OF EVIDENCE

The Environmental Risk Transition and the Epidemiological Transition

The twin concepts of the "environmental risk transition"[13] and the "epidemiological transition"[14] provide a useful framework for understanding how environmental threats to children's health vary across countries and how these threats change as countries develop. In the world's poorest, least developed countries, the prevalent environmental hazards are the ancient scourges of household air pollution and water pollution. Household air pollution arises mainly from the combustion of biomass fuels—wood, straw, dung, and charcoal—in poorly ventilated home cook stoves.[15] Household air pollution is responsible for nearly 570 000 deaths each year in children younger than 5 years, mainly from lower respiratory tract infections.[10] Water pollution accounts for 360 000 deaths annually in children younger than 5 years, mainly from diarrheal diseases.[10] Malnutrition magnifies the impacts of these exposures.

As countries develop, urbanize, industrialize, and become integrated into global supply chains, patterns of environmental exposure change. This is termed the "environmental risk transition."[13] In this transition, countries move from biomass to cleaner fuels, and the traditional hazards of household air pollution and contaminated drinking water are replaced by ambient air pollution, toxic chemical pollution, and hazardous waste exposures.[16] An important driver of this transition has been the relocation in recent decades of nearly two-thirds of the global chemical manufacturing industry to LMICs.[17]

As countries develop, patterns of disease in children change.[18] This is the "epidemiological transition"[14] and it parallels the environmental risk transition. In the epidemiological transition, deaths from pneumonia and diarrheal disease decline, infant mortality plummets, and life expectancy increases. In Africa, for example, infant mortality has decreased by almost 75%—from 187 deaths per 1000 live births in 1950 to 51 per 1000 today, and in the same time, life expectancy has nearly doubled—from 36.5 years to 64.1 years.[19] Drivers of the epidemiological transition include the introduction of cleaner fuels,[15] increased access to safe drinking water, the dissemination of pneumococcal vaccine and rotavirus vaccine,[20] the introduction of new treatment protocols such as oral rehydration therapy,[21] improved infant nutrition,[22] and enhanced access to medical care.

In the aftermath of the environmental risk and epidemiological transitions, noncommunicable diseases (NCDs)—asthma, birth defects, cancer, neurodevelopmental disorders, diabetes, obesity, and disorders of reproduction—replace infectious diseases as the major causes of disease and death in children.[19,23] Even in LMICs where they were previously rare, pediatric NCDs have now become common.[19,24] The once very separate patterns of disease and death in low-, middle-, and high-income countries are converging.[25] Children in many LMICs today suffer a double burden of environmentally attributable disease that reflects their simultaneous exposures to both traditional and more modern environmental hazards.[18,26]

The environmental risk and epidemiological transitions have taken place at different times in different countries. High-income countries such as the United States and Canada went through their transitions in the late 19th and early 20th centuries. Many LMICs are in transition now, and different countries and even different regions within countries are at various stages of transition. Accordingly, patterns of disease vary greatly from country to country and from region to region. Some of the sharpest contrasts are seen between rural and urban areas within LMICs.

Environmental Justice

Significant social, ethnic, racial, and economic inequities are evident in the global distribution of environmental hazards. Nearly 92% of all disease and death attributable globally to environmental risk factors occurs in LMICs.[11] In countries at every economic level, disease caused by hazardous environmental exposures is most prevalent among poor people and historically marginalized groups, an inequitable pattern of exposure and disease termed "environmental injustice."[27]

Environmental injustice is seen also in high-income countries, including the United States. Examples include the disproportionate siting of polluting industries, hazardous waste sites and major roadways in low-income communities where the majority of the residents are people of color. Another example is the disproportionally high levels of lead found in drinking water in communities comprising predominantly people of color, such as Flint, Michigan. The disproportionate exposures of Native American and Alaska Native children to high levels of household air pollution and unsafe drinking water are further examples of environmental injustice in the United States.[28–30]

In LMICs, disparities based on social class, economics, race, and ethnicity can shape the environmental risk and epidemiological transitions.[11,18,24] Some countries, notably middle-income countries with effective central governments and fairly equitable distributions of resources, have largely completed their epidemiological transitions and have increased the well-being of families across the economic spectrum. Some countries are passing through the transition now. In still other countries, typically the world's lowest-income and most economically unjust and politically corrupt nations, the transition has not yet begun, and infectious diseases remain the predominant causes of disease and death in children.

The "off-shoring" of hazardous industries from high-income countries to LMICs where wages are low and environmental protections and the health infrastructure are often weak—so-called "pollution havens"—contributes to the disproportionate concentration in these countries of toxic pollution and diseases caused by hazardous environmental exposures. The disproportionate distribution of these hazards may be expected to become still greater in future years with increasing globalization of supply chains.[31,32]

The High Costs of Disease Caused by Hazardous Environmental Exposures

Disease, disability, and death caused by toxic environmental exposures result in large economic and social costs in all countries, and especially in heavily polluted LMICs (Table 1). These include health care costs as well as increased costs for special education, accommodation for disabilities, and other developmental services. In addition, environmentally related disease and disability have negative economic impacts on children's futures because they diminish children's educational attainment, their lifelong learning potential, and their ability to contribute to society by reducing cognitive function, decreasing IQ, and

TABLE 1. Economic Costs of Hazardous Environmental Exposures
Direct Medical Costs: These include physician costs, hospital costs, and costs of medications
Indirect Health-Related Costs: These include time lost from school and work, costs of rehabilitation, and costs of special education.
Costs to Health Systems: These include the heavy and unnecessary load imposed by environmental diseases on health care delivery systems, particularly in LMICs, that already are overextended, understaffed, and underfunded
Opportunity Costs: These include the lifelong decreases in educational attainment, earnings potential, and economic productivity resulting from diminished cognitive capacity and other impairments in children caused by early life exposures to environmental hazards.

impairing physical function.[11] The economic losses caused by disease of environmental origin are so massive in heavily polluted LMICs that they can undercut these countries' ability to develop and to invest in children's health, education, and social welfare,[33,34] thus perpetuating the cycle of poverty.

Diseases Caused by Hazardous Environmental Exposures Can Be Prevented

Hazardous environmental exposures and the diseases they cause are the result of human activity and can, therefore, be prevented. This is a key point, and it is the basis for all pollution control policy. The strongest evidence that diseases of environmental origin can be prevented is seen in the experience of the United States and other high-income countries in controlling pollution and preventing pollution-related disease.[11] In the United States, for example, air pollutant emissions have been driven down by 77% since passage of the Clean Air Act in 1970,[35] drinking water is now cleaner, polluted rivers no longer catch fire, and the worst hazardous waste sites have been remediated. Disease and premature death of environmental origin have been prevented and tens of thousands of lives have been saved.[35]

Prevention of environmental hazards requires a combination of research to discover the environmental causes of disease coupled with evidence-based advocacy that translates research findings into policies and prevention programs. Pediatricians are trusted advisors, uniquely well qualified to address environmental threats to children's health and to advocate for prevention of children's exposures to environmental hazards. Successful prevention efforts in environmental health, many of them led by pediatricians, have included:

- Removal of lead from automotive gasoline, which resulted in a more than 95% reduction in blood lead levels of American children and an approximate 5-point gain in population mean IQ.[36] Every country around the world has now removed lead from automotive gasoline.
- A ban on production of polychlorinated biphenyls (PCBs) that was incorporated into the Toxic Substances Control Act.[37] This has resulted in reductions of PCB levels in children's blood and reduction in the number of children suffering from PCB-induced loss of intelligence.
- Elimination of residential uses of organophosphate pesticides, such as chlorpyrifos, with subsequent reductions in the numbers of infants born with lower birth weight and small head circumference caused by prenatal exposure to chlorpyrifos.[38]
- Reduction in children's exposure to arsenic in drinking water with subsequent reduction in risk of skin and liver cancer.[39,40]
- Reduction in rates of childhood asthma and improvement in lung function following reduction in children's exposure to urban air pollution and widespread education about the hazards of second-hand tobacco smoke, cooking fumes, cockroach droppings, and other indoor air pollutants.[41]

Prevention of Disease Caused by Hazardous Environmental Exposures is Highly Cost-Effective

Prevention of diseases caused by hazardous environmental exposures has not only improved children's health and well-being, but also created economic benefits.[35] Examples include the great economic gains that have resulted from reductions in air pollution[42] and from removal of lead from gasoline.[36] Information on the cost-effectiveness of disease prevention programs provides pediatricians with another powerful argument for persuading policy makers to take preventive action to safeguard children's health.[36,42]

Key Environmental Exposures in LMICs

Lack of Clean Water, Sanitation, and Hygiene (WASH)

Contaminated water is a major source of disease and death among children in LMICs.[11] It is responsible for an estimated 360 000 deaths annually in children younger than 5 years. Water supplies in LMICs can be contaminated by biological waste (human and animal) and also by chemical waste. In rural areas and in the least developed countries, biological contamination predominates, but as countries develop and industrialize, chemical pollution becomes increasingly important. Some of the worst pollution of drinking water is seen in and around the megacities of rapidly industrializing LMICs, where local waterways and groundwater are heavily polluted by both biological waste and chemical discharges, and there are no alternative water sources.[43] Treatments that control infectious agents are generally not effective in removing toxic chemicals from drinking water.

Substantial progress has been made in reducing water pollution globally. Between 1990 and 2015, 2.6 billion people worldwide gained access to improved drinking water sources, and 2.1 billion people gained access to improved sanitation. In this time, the number of children dying from diarrheal diseases decreased by almost 60%. However, despite this progress, 2.4 billion people are still using unimproved sanitation facilities, including 946 million people who still practice open defecation.[11]

Burden of Disease Attributable to Water Pollution

The principal diseases linked to water pollution are acute and chronic gastrointestinal tract diseases—diarrheal diseases, typhoid fever, and paratyphoid fever.[44] Polluted water and inadequate sanitation are linked additionally to a range of parasitic infections. These diseases affect more than 1 billion people worldwide, predominantly in LMICs.[44,45] Large numbers of deaths are seen also in some

Southeast Asian countries. In the past 2 decades, China has greatly reduced mortality from waterborne infectious disease.[44] These burden-of-disease data do not adequately reflect disease and death caused by chemical pollution of water, because data on levels of chemical contamination of drinking water are not available for most LMICs, patterns of exposure have not been mapped, and the potential toxicity of many chemical pollutants has never been assessed.[46]

Air Pollution

Household air pollution (HAP) and ambient air pollution are major sources of disease and death in children worldwide, and especially in LMICs.[11] HAP and ambient air pollution are both products of combustion and thus originate from the same sources—coal, oil, natural gas, and biomass fuels—as the carbon dioxide that drives global climate change. HAP and ambient air pollution contain many of the same chemical constituents, and they often coexist and exert synergistic effects. Fine particulate pollution comprised of airborne particles of median diameter of 2.5 microns and below ($PM_{2.5}$ pollution) is the most extensively studied form of air pollution.

Household Air Pollution

Burning of biomass and solid fuels in unvented indoor stoves for cooking and heating is the major source of HAP. HAP concentrations inside poorly ventilated homes in LMICs can reach exceedingly high levels. Women and young children are disproportionately exposed to HAP because of traditional gender roles involving cooking and food preparation in many LMICs placing women and their children in close and prolonged proximity to polluting stoves.[15,47]

Ambient Air Pollution

Many LMICs are experiencing large increases in ambient air pollution today as they develop economically and industrialize.[11] These increases are driven by increased combustion of coal and other fossil fuels for the generation of electricity and other industrial activities as well as by growing car ownership. Wildfires contribute additionally to particulate matter pollution, and air pollution from this source will likely increase as climate change increases the frequency and scale of wildfires.[48] The World Health Organization (WHO) compiles information on $PM_{2.5}$ concentrations from more than 1000 cities around the globe. This information indicates that LMICs generally have higher concentrations of $PM_{2.5}$ pollution than high-income countries, and shows that 88% of urban residents globally live in cities that fail to meet WHO air quality guidelines.[49] Children in LMICs are at greatly increased risk of adverse health effects from air pollution. Emerging evidence suggests that exposure to air pollution, including airborne particulate matter, can increase morbidity and mortality from SARS-CoV-2 infection (COVID-19).[50–53]

A projection of future trends in mortality associated with ambient $PM_{2.5}$ air pollution predicts that, in the absence of aggressive intervention, the numbers of air pollution-related deaths will rise sharply over the next 3 decades. Greatest increases will be seen in South and East Asia.[54] In the worst case scenario, these trends are anticipated to produce a more than 50% increase in the number of deaths attributable to air pollution by 2050.[54] Not included in this projection are likely increases in numbers of deaths attributable to pollution-related low birth weight and preterm birth.[55,56]

Burden of Disease Attributable to Air Pollution

$PM_{2.5}$ air pollution from both household and outdoor sources is linked to a number of adverse health outcomes in children. In infancy, these include preterm birth, low birth weight, and intrauterine growth restriction.[57] The impacts of air pollution in children include increased incidence of lower respiratory infection, increased prevalence of asthma, increased frequency of acute asthmatic attacks, and impaired lung growth.[41] Chronic exposure to $PM_{2.5}$ pollution in childhood may increase disk of cardiovascular disease, chronic obstructive pulmonary disease, and other NCDs in adult life.[58] Recent studies suggest associations between $PM_{2.5}$ pollution exposure during pregnancy and increased risk of impaired cognitive function,[59,60] attention deficit/hyperactivity disorder (ADHD), and autism spectrum disorder (ASD).[61] All of the health impacts of air pollution fall very heavily on children in LMICs, especially on children in countries where concentrations of $PM_{2.5}$ and other air pollutants are orders of magnitude higher than those typically encountered in high-income countries.[49]

Toxic Chemical Exposures

Lead

Acute and chronic lead poisoning are problems of enormous importance for child health worldwide. Global consumption of lead is increasing because of rising demand for batteries and energy-efficient vehicles. An estimated 40% of the world's children have blood lead levels exceeding 5 μg/dL, and 90% of these children live in LMICs.[62] Patterns and sources of exposure to lead (Table 2), prevalence rates of lead poisoning, and the severity of outcomes vary greatly from country to country. Countries with strong prevention programs have imposed bans on certain uses of lead, have set environmental standards, and have deployed screening programs. Lead "hot spots" are common in LMICs; these include battery recycling operations, smelters, mines, hazardous waste sites, and sites where hazardous waste is burned.[63]

TABLE 2. Sources of Child and Adolescent Exposure to Lead
Industry, such as mining, smelting, and informal battery recycling
Lead-based paints and pigments
Lead solder in food cans
Ceramic glazes (eg, traditional glazed ceramic cookware, dishes)
Drinking water systems with lead solder and lead pipes
Medicinal products, such as herbal, Ayurvedic, and traditional medicines, folk remedies
Consumer products such as cosmetics (eg, Kohl, Surma, Sindoor) and toys
Incineration of lead-containing waste
Electronic waste (e-waste)
Food chain (eg, spices) and contaminated soil
Contamination (eg, soil and water) as a legacy of historical contamination from former industrial sites
Aviation and marine fuel

Mercury

Mercury is a highly toxic metal. It occurs in the environment in several forms, of which methylmercury is the most hazardous. Methylmercury, an organic form of mercury, is a potent developmental neurotoxicant. Human exposure to methylmercury is of great concern, especially exposures occurring in utero during pregnancy. Methylmercury crosses the placenta, passes easily into the tissues of fetuses and young children, and causes permanent injury to the developing brain.[64]

Polluting industries are the main source of mercury emission to the environment.[65] Four industries are especially problematic:

- Coal-burning electricity generation plants are the major global source of mercury emission, as all coal contains mercury. When coal is burned, microscopic droplets of metallic mercury are released into the air and eventually reach rivers, lakes, and oceans. Metallic mercury is converted to methylmercury in the aquatic environment and enters the marine food chain.
- Waste incinerators, including hospital incinerators, which, like coal-fired power plants, release metallic mercury to the atmosphere.
- Chloralkali facilities that use metallic mercury as a catalyst to produce chlorine gas.
- Artisanal and small-scale gold mining (ASGM) operations that use metallic mercury to form an amalgam to separate gold from ore. ASGM operations release mercury to the environment through vaporization and also through runoff of spilled mercury into waterways.[64] Most ASGM operations are located in LMICs.

Consumption of fish contaminated by methylmercury is the major route of human exposure.[64,66] Methylmercury concentrates as it moves up the food chain to reach very high levels in the predatory fish at the top of the chain, such as tuna, mackerel, and striped bass, as well as marine mammals consumed by humans in the circumpolar regions.[65] Children and adolescents in fishing communities in LMICs and in Indigenous communities whose traditional diets are rich in fish and marine mammals are at especially high risk of exposure to methylmercury in seafood.[67] A 2019 AAP technical report details the benefits and risks associated with fish and shellfish consumption.[68] In addition, individuals can be exposed to elemental or inorganic mercury from its use in rituals and folk remedies including Santeria (Cuba), Voodoo (Haiti), Espiritismo (Puerto Rico), and Ayurvedic medicine (India).[69]

Arsenic

Arsenic is a metalloid element that occurs naturally in the earth's crust. It is also released into the environment by polluting industries such as mines and ore smelters. Near such industries, inhalation is an important exposure route. Worldwide, drinking water is the principal source of arsenic exposure, especially in areas with high levels of naturally occurring arsenic in bedrock that leaches into ground water accessed by small wells (eg, in areas of Bangladesh, Chile, Argentina, the southwestern United States, and northern New England). Children born to mothers who reside in such areas during pregnancy are at risk of exposure in utero. Children can also be exposed to arsenic through ingestion of contaminated soil—eg, soil contaminated by industrial activity or agricultural land contaminated by current or past use of arsenic-containing pesticides. Further, given that rice plants can uptake and accumulate arsenic from the soil, food can be a significant source or arsenic exposure, especially in children who eat rice-centered diets.[70,71]

Chronic exposure to inorganic arsenic is associated with several human cancers, including lung, bladder, and skin cancer.[72] Prenatal exposures to arsenic in drinking water have been linked to increases in late fetal, neonatal, and postneonatal mortality as well as to neurodevelopmental abnormalities, pediatric and adult cancers, and bronchiectasis.[40,73,74] Lifetime risks of lung and bladder cancer are 2 to 4 times greater among children whose exposure to arsenic begins in early life than among children whose exposures that begin later in childhood or in adult life.[75]

Industrial Chemicals

Global production of industrial chemicals and plastics has grown dramatically in the past half-century, and children's exposures to synthetic chemicals have become a focus of great concern in environmental pediatrics. More than 350 000 new synthetic chemicals and pesticides have been invented since 1950.[76] Most did not previously exist in nature. These manufactured chemicals are now used in millions of consumer products and have become extensively disseminated in the global environment. Only a minority have ever been tested for safety or potential toxicity.[46] As is documented by the Centers for Disease Control and

Prevention (CDC)'s National Biomonitoring Program, children's exposure to these largely untested chemicals is almost universal.[77]

With globalization of trade, toxic chemicals that previously were used only in high-income countries are entering LMICs in ever-increasing volumes.[17] Nearly 70% of global chemical and pesticide production now takes place in LMICs.[78] Most new growth in global chemical production is occurring in LMICs, much of it concentrated in so-called "pollution havens" where labor costs are low and environmental and public health protections are often few.[79]

Catastrophes involving chemical exposures have resulted and have caused disease and death in children in LMICs, including the following:

- **Bhopal catastrophe:** In 1984, a massive explosion occurred in a poorly maintained chemical plant in Bhopal, India. Large quantities of highly toxic, methyl isocyanate gas were released and spread across the city. Hundreds of persons died, including many children, and tens of thousands suffered permanent injury.[80] The plant had been transported to India from the United States.
- **Asbestos:** More than 2 million tons of newly mined asbestos are exported each year to LMICs. Russia is the major producer. The material is widely used in the construction of homes and schools. The resulting exposures to persons of all ages will result in epidemics of lung cancer and malignant mesothelioma that extend over much of the century.[81]
- **Lead:** Recycling of used lead-acid batteries takes place in virtually all LMICs. Battery recycling often takes place in "backyard" establishments in close proximity to homes and schools. Multiple episodes of pediatric lead poisoning have been documented to result, some of them extremely severe and even fatal.[82]
- **Mercury:** Mercury poisoning from artisanal and small-scale gold mining is a major global hazard.[83]
- **Electronic waste (e-waste):** An estimated 45 million tons per year of e-waste are shipped each year into LMICs.[16] Thousands of women and young children are employed in e-waste recycling and are exposed to mixtures of heavy metals, flame retardants, toxic products of combustion, and other chemicals during the recycling process.
- **Polybrominated diphenyl ethers (PBDEs):** PBDEs are chemical flame retardants that were extensively added to electronics, building materials, and other consumer products. Despite a global phase-out for use in new products, the environmental persistence and lipid bioaccumulation of PBDEs contributes to an ongoing exposure risk through contaminated soil, dust, and fatty foods (eg, fish, meat, dairy). Individuals involved in e-waste recycling, especially through village-based recycling processes, can be exposed to large amounts of PBDEs.[84,85] Exposure to PBDEs has been linked to cognitive deficits in children[86] and disruption of the endocrine system, including thyroid hormones.[87]
- **Per- and poly-fluoroalkyl substances (PFAS):** PFAS (the "forever chemicals") are a class of synthetic chemicals that have been widely utilized by industry because of properties such as heat-resistance, stain-resistance, and friction reduction. They are found in products such as food packing, nonstick cookware, and firefighting foam. PFAS are extremely persistent in the environment and have been found across the globe in water, soil, and dust, and nearly universal human exposure has been documented.[88,89] Emerging evidence has linked PFAS exposure to a range of health effects such as high cholesterol, alterations in thyroid and liver function tests, lower birth weight, immunotoxicity, and cancer (kidney, testicular).[90,91]
- **Phthalates**: Phthalates are plasticizers added to plastic products, polyvinyl chloride (PVC), and cosmetics in the amount of millions of tons annually. They migrate easily out of products and lead to human exposure through inhalation, ingestion, and skin absorption. Phthalates exposure is associated with obesity, type 2 diabetes mellitus/insulin resistance, alterations in thyroid function, and adverse reproductive system impacts. These compounds have also been linked to increased risk of allergy and asthma as well as neurodevelopmental delays.[92]

Pesticides

Pesticides are potent molecules specifically designed to kill living organisms. They include insecticides, rodenticides, fungicides, and herbicides. More than 700 unique pesticide chemicals and thousands of commercial formulations are currently on world markets. Several billion pounds are used annually. Approximately 75% of current global pesticide use is in LMICs. The sale and widespread use in LMICs of highly toxic pesticides that are banned in the United States and Western Europe poses a growing threat to children's health.[93,94]

Pesticide use has evolved over time. Some highly toxic and environmentally persistent older pesticides such as lead arsenate, dichloro-diphenyl-trichloroethane (DDT), and lindane have been largely phased out. However, use of newer pesticides such as the pyrethroid insecticides and the neurotoxic neonicotinoid insecticides have increased sharply.

The herbicide glyphosate (marketed as Roundup), the world's most widely used herbicide, has become a chemical of particular concern. Global use of glyphosate has increased more than 10-fold in recent decades. Use is increasing very rapidly in LMICs as these countries adopt industrialized farming technologies to produce commodity crops such as genetically modified organism (GMO) corn and soybeans for world markets.[95] Glyphosate was long considered a relatively innocuous chemical. In 2015, however, the International Agency for Research on Cancer, the cancer agency of the WHO, determined on the basis of extensive review by international experts that glyphosate is "probably carcinogenic to humans."[95] Glyphosate exposure is associated with non-Hodgkin lymphoma.[97]

Pesticides can cause both acute poisoning and chronic toxicity in children. An estimated 99% of all acute pesticide poisonings occur in LMICs. Children in LMICs are at very high risk of acute pesticide poisoning because of their potential exposure to highly toxic pesticides no longer used in high-income countries, labels that are not printed in local languages, low literacy, inadequate training of pesticide applicators,[98] and storage of pesticides in unsafe containers such as soda bottles.[99] It is important that pediatricians and pediatric trainees working in LMICS be able to recognize and treat pesticide poisoning and be able to provide guidance on how to reduce pesticide exposures.

Hazardous Waste Sites

Electronic waste (e-waste) disposal sites containing discarded electronic devices and their components represent a relatively new and rapidly growing type of hazardous waste site in countries around the world.[16] More than 45 million tons of e-waste is generated globally each year,[16] and this volume is expected to increase in coming years. Significant amounts of e-waste are exported from high-income countries to LMICs where recycling of valuable compounds from e-waste, such as copper and gold, has evolved into an important business, predominantly in home-based and village-based industry.[100]

E-waste contains a vast number of hazardous chemicals, including lead, cadmium, mercury, nickel, barium, and lithium as well as persistent organic pollutants, such as PCBs and brominated flame retardants. Unsafe recycling activities, such as open burning and acid leaching of e-waste, produce toxic combustion products including dioxin-like PCBs and polychlorinated dibenzo-dioxins and dibenzofurans.[101]

Young children and pregnant women are often employed at e-waste disposal sites, and e-waste poses significant health risks to child workers.[85] Children may also encounter hazardous substances through take-home exposures and home-based e-recycling workshops. Children at e-waste sites have been reported to display elevated levels of multiple toxic chemicals, including lead and nickel.[102] These exposures are associated with a range of adverse health effects, including injury to children's immune, cardiovascular, gastrointestinal, renal, endocrine, and hematological systems; and adverse birth outcomes.[16,103]

Global Climate Change and Children's Health

The main driver of global climate change is increasing release into the atmosphere of carbon dioxide (CO_2), methane, and other long-lived greenhouse gases that trap heat energy.[104] Human activity is the main source of greenhouse gas emissions. The consequences of rising CO_2 levels include rising temperatures at the surface of the earth, sea surface warming, glacial melting, rising sea levels, increased frequency of violent storms, increased frequency of floods and droughts, increased frequency of heat waves, increased frequency of wildfires, and expanded geographic ranges of vectorborne diseases, such as malaria and dengue, and waterborne diseases, including cholera.[104]

Each of the consequences of global climate change has myriad impacts on children's health. These health effects of climate change have been extensively reviewed[105,106] and are addressed in a statement from the AAP focused on climate change and children's health.[107,108] Therefore, these are considered only briefly here.

A key consideration in the context of this report is that the health impacts of climate change fall most severely on children in LMICs. Children in LMICs who have underlying health conditions and have limited access to essentials necessary for life will be least resilient and most severely affected. Climate change has potential to magnify the impacts on children's health of other hazardous environmental exposures.[109]

The impacts of climate change on child and adolescent health can be divided into direct and indirect effects (Table 3).[7] Sustained high temperatures, air pollution, infectious diseases, and extreme weather and natural disasters will directly affect health. Climate change will also reduce agricultural yields and thus create food shortages; decrease access to clean water, increase social unrest, and trigger migration and war, all of which, in turn, may endanger child health and welfare. The pediatric community can play a critical role in addressing climate change, explaining the connections between climate and child health to policy makers and the public and advocating for the protection of children's health against climate-related hazards.

Other Selected Topics in Pediatric Global Health

Child Labor

Child labor is defined as "work that deprives children of their childhood, their potential and their dignity, and that is harmful to physical and mental development."[110] Child labor can lead to dangerous environmental exposures such as pesticides and organic dusts in agriculture[111]; lead and other toxic metals from smelting, battery recovery, and mining[112]; and solvents from cleaning or leather tanning activities.[113] It is linked to multiple adverse physical, developmental, emotional and behavioral outcomes.[114] Hazardous child labor conditions have also been documented in the United States (eg, agriculture work among young migrant Latinx children).[115] Although a critical global health issue, child labor goes beyond the scope of this

TABLE 3. Direct and Indirect Effects of Climate Change on Child and Adolescent Health

Direct Impacts	Indirect Impacts
Heat Stress • Preterm delivery • Dehydration, hyperthermia	**Water Insecurity** • Need for increasing agriculture production despite current overuse • Increased water stress in some areas
Increase in Air Pollution (Including Wildfires) and Airborne Allergens • Asthma • Exacerbation other lung disease • Impaired lung development	**Malnutrition** • Shortage in food supply (eg, failed harvests and diminished fish stocks in coastal communities) • Decreases in food quality or protein content of staple grains and legumes
Infectious Diseases • Expanded ranges of vectorborne disease (eg, malaria, West Nile virus infection, viral encephalitis, and dengue) and the appearance of previously unrecognized vectorborne diseases (eg, Zika and Chikungunya virus infections). • Diarrheal illnesses attributable to waterborne pathogens	**Population Displacement and Community Stress, Including Climate-Related Displacement and Stress** • Malnutrition • Psychosocial stress, traumatic stress • Anxiety about climate change and its effects • Mental health issues • Armed conflict, societal breakdown • Increases in child abuse/neglect
Extreme Weather Events • Heavy precipitation and flood, drought, hurricanes, monsoons, heat waves	**Unexpected Impacts** • Emerging impacts of climate change related issues such as seawater intrusion into groundwater (eg, preeclampsia and water salinity)

Adapted from Miller M, Marty M, Landrigan P. Children's environmental health: beyond national boundaries. *Pediatr Clin North Am.* 2016;63(1):149–165.

report, and interested providers are encouraged to review available resources.[110,113,114,116]

Injuries

Each day, approximately 2000 children globally die from unintentional injuries such as road traffic injuries, drowning, fire-related burns, falls, and poisonings. More than 95% of these deaths occur in LMICs.[117] Within LMICs, children facing chronic poverty, conflict, or displacement are at greatest risk.[117] Of particular concern are road traffic injuries, which are the leading cause of death for persons 5 to 29 years of age in LMICs.[118] Many childhood and adolescent injuries do not lead to death but can have serious sequelae. Head injuries are the most common nonfatal child injury and the most severe type of injury sustained by children around the world. Many children who suffer head injuries and other types of trauma are left with disabilities.[117] In LMICs, there is limited public health funding and infrastructure dedicated to injury prevention or to rehabilitation.[117]

Transboundary Exposures

Many types of environmental pollution affect the health of communities living far from their points of origin. A prime example of such "transboundary" exposure is ambient air pollution (see section "Ambient Air Pollution"). Air pollutants such as fine particulate matter ($PM_{2.5}$) can be transported long distances in the atmosphere across regions and continents. A study found that 12% of the 3.45 million deaths attributable to $PM_{2.5}$ in 2007 were attributable to pollutants emitted in another region of the world.[119] Similarly, chemical and biological water pollutants can travel downstream, crossing jurisdictional boundaries within rivers, aquifers, lake basins, and marine ecosystems. Depletion of aquifers, construction of large dams, and climate change further impact the availability and quality of water in LMICs.[120]

The international trade in toxic products, both through official and illegal mechanisms, poses disproportionate risk to communities in LMICs. Although multinational agreements regulate some international trade of chemicals, illegal trafficking of hazardous products remains widespread. Pesticides are a common entity in this illegal market, and agricultural workers and their children are at particular risk from dangerous exposures to banned pesticides such as aldicarb, paraquat, and parathion. Mercury is informally imported into LMICs that engage in ASGM.[121] Families in high-income countries such as the United States can be exposed to toxic chemicals in products imported from LMICs, including cosmetics, amulets, ceramics, religious powders, and pesticides.[122,123]

Clinical Care for Children and Adolescents in LMICs

Informed suspicion is key to the correct diagnosis of disease in children and adolescents caused by hazardous exposures in the environment.[124] The alert clinician needs to be open to the possibility that any child or adolescent may have an illness caused or exacerbated by an environmental exposure. Because diseases of environmental origin in children seldom have unique physical signatures, an exposure history, supplemented by laboratory testing, is the principal diagnostic tool. A targeted environmental history is an important part of pediatric care during well visits, management of an environmentally related illness (eg, asthma), and the diagnostic assessment of a new illness.[125] It is important that the environmental history include questions about the home, neighborhood, and other places the child spends time; these questions can be tailored to reflect the most prominent environmental exposures in a particular community and country.[69] It is important to use a qualified interpreter in every patient encounter in which English is not the family's first language.

The WHO provides clinicians with a pediatric environmental health history tool, the "Green Page," to assist in the identification of critical environmental exposures.[126] This tool is especially important for providers who are practicing outside the United States, as it includes key issues facing children in LMICs (eg, sanitation, potable water, household air pollution, and highly toxic pesticides). The Green Page contains 4 sections:

1. Demographics: Includes type of residential setting, school, work, and activities.
2. Exposure history: Includes parent occupations, overcrowding in home, pets, vectors of disease transmission, history of injuries (traffic, fire, chemical), venomous/poisonous animals, extreme temperatures.
3. Environmental exposure ratings (A/B/C): for various environmental conditions (air, water, soil/floor, sewage, waste, noise, chemicals, traffic) among the child's environments including home, school, recreation, workplace, community.
4. Public services: Availability of basic services across the home, school, community; services include electricity, communication, waste collection/disposal, transportation, public lighting, health care centers, excreta treatment plant, sewage system, water supply.

Further, the WHO's Pediatric Environmental Health Training Package provides specific guidance on the diagnosis and management of environmental health issues commonly encountered in LMICs.[127]

To further assist pediatricians and pediatric trainees in making a diagnosis of environmental disease in children, a two-stage systematic approach to obtaining a history of environmental exposure is suggested.[128,129] In the first stage, pediatricians may wish to routinely ask a series of screening questions of every new patient, of every patient with a new disease, and of every patient with an exacerbation of disease. If positive responses are elicited to any of these screening questions, more detailed follow-up or referral to a Pediatric Environmental Health Specialty Unit (PEHSU), toxicologist, or another resource may be indicated (Table 4).

1. ***In the History of the Present Illness,*** consider any temporal relationship between onset of illness and exposures in the child's environment. For example, did symptoms begin shortly after the child moved to a new school or day care center? Did they abate during vacation and then recrudesce after the child resumed school? Were symptoms temporally related to an event such as pesticide application, chemical spill, or air pollution episode? Were there similar symptoms or illness among other children in the same school or community?
2. ***In the Social and Family History,*** ask where the child attends school and what industrial facilities are near by the child's home and school. Ask about the caregiver/parents' employment, with particular attention to the possibility that a parent may inadvertently be bringing toxic materials home from work on their shoes or clothing (eg, pesticides, heavy metals, asbestos).
3. ***In the Review of Systems,*** routinely include this question: "Does the child now or previously have exposures to lead, fumes, chemicals, pesticides, dust, asbestos, loud noise, radiation, or other environmental hazards?"

Clinical Care for Foreign-born Children and Adolescents in the United States

Pediatricians in high-income countries are increasingly likely to care for foreign-born children and adolescents and have an important role in promoting these children's health and wellness. The AAP has published resources to assist providers in the clinical care of immigrant children[130] and internationally adopted children.[131]

It is important for pediatric providers in the United States to be aware of the possibility that children and adolescents who have come to high-income countries from LMICs may have been exposed to toxic chemicals and other environmental hazards in their countries of origin. Such exposures might include lead from mining and smelting, arsenic from contaminated groundwater, mercury from artisanal gold mining, and pesticides from agriculture or extreme psychosocial stress. In addition, once arriving in the United States, immigrant children may face ongoing environmental exposures if they move into substandard housing, have parents who bring home work-related exposures (eg, pesticides in agricultural workers), or have family members who use toxic products imported from the home country (eg, Ayurvedic medicines, lead-containing cosmetics, or candies wrapped in lead foil). Appropriate histories might be difficult to obtain if the patient was adopted, and/or if there are language barriers. Using a qualified interpreter with every such encounter is key.

It is also important to assess the mental health of children who have emigrated from LMICs, because these children may have been exposed to poverty, complex sociopolitical circumstances, war, other forms of violence and famine, and may require referral for appropriate social services or mental health support.[3] Mental health issues may be of particular concern in children who are refugees, and

TABLE 4. Educational Resources and Clinical Tools in Pediatric Environmental Health

Pediatric Environmental Health Specialty Centers

- Pediatric Environmental Health Specialty Unit (PEHSU). One PEHSU is located in each of the 10 federal regions in the United States. The PEHSUs provide online classroom materials, resources, and access to network of experts in pediatric and reproductive environmental health: www.pehsu.net
- New York State network of Centers of Excellence in Children's Environmental Health (NYSCHECK) https://nyscheck.org/. A statewide network of 7 centers modeled on the PEHSUs spanning New York from Long Island to Buffalo
- International Pediatric Environmental Health Specialty Units:
  - Buenos Aires, Argentina:
    Hospital Elizalde: https://www.youtube.com/watch?v=D3qCpBzy59g
    Hospital Gutiérrez: http://www.scielo.org.ar/scielo.php?script=sci_arttext&pid=S0325-00752014000600022
    Hospital Garraham: www.garrahan.gov.ar/salud-ambiental/contenidos/salud-ambiental
  - Edmonton, Alberta, Canada: Children's Environmental Health Clinic: www.ChEHC.ca
  - Cuernavaca, Mexico: Unidad Pediátrica Ambiental Hospital del Nino Morelense
  - Murcia, Spain: www.pehsu.org/wp/
  - Montevideo, Uruguay: www.ciat.hc.edu.uy/
- World Health Organization (WHO) Network of Collaborating Centres for Children's Environmental Health: www.niehs.nih.gov/research/programs/geh/partnerships/network/index.cfm

Pediatric Environmental Health Clinical Tools

- WHO Paediatric Environmental Health History (Green Page) provides a series of concise questions to assess potential exposures: https://www.who.int/publications/m/item/children-s-environmental-record–green-page
- National Environmental Education Foundation (NEEF) provides Pediatric Environmental Health history forms – both a general form and an asthma-specific form: www.neefusa.org/resource/pediatric-environmental-history
- The Pediatric Environmental Health Toolkit is an online clinical tool that providers can use to access information on common exposures, including identification of sources of exposure and provision of targeted anticipatory guidance: https://peht.ucsf.edu
- Prescriptions for Prevention are tools that link patients to evidence-based simple steps to reduce or prevent common environmental exposures: https://nyscheck.org/rx

Pediatric Environmental Health Educational Tools

- WHO training series in Children's Environmental Health: www.who.int/ceh/capacity/training_modules/en/
- The "Green Book": American Academy of Pediatrics, Committee on Environmental Health. *Pediatric Environmental Health.* 4th ed. Etzel RA, Balk SJ, eds. Itasca, IL: American Academy of Pediatrics; 2018
- *Textbook on Children's Environmental Health.* Etzel RA, Landrigan PJ, eds. London: Oxford University Press, 2024
- *Environmental Health Perspectives*, the peer-reviewed, open-access journal of the National Institute of Environmental Health Sciences, regularly publishes articles on topics in children's environmental health: http://ehp.niehs.nih.gov
- A Story of Health. Multimedia e-book explores how environments interact with genes to influence health across the lifespan (free continuing medical education credits): wspehsu.ucsf.edu/main-resources/for-clinical-professionals/training/a-story-of-health-a-multi-media-ebook/
- The Power of Prevention Video Series (including "Little Things Matter") illustrates key concepts in children's environmental health in multiple languages: http://littlethingsmatter.ca/

Professional Societies, Networking, and Career Resources

- American Academy of Pediatrics (AAP), Council on Environmental Health: https://services.aap.org/en/community/aap-councils/council-on-environmental-health/
- Academic Pediatric Association (APA), Special Interest Group on Environmental Health: www.academicpeds.org/sig/environmental-health/
- Children's Environmental Health Network (CEHN): http://cehn.org/
- International Network on Children's Health, Environment and Safety (INCHES): http://inchesnetwork.net/
- International Society for Children's Health and the Environment (ISCHE): www.ische.ca/

the CDC has developed guidance for mental health screening of refugee children.[132]

Environmental Health in Medical Training

Recent decades have seen a dramatic rise in interest in environmental health among medical and public health professionals in the United States and across the globe. There have been small gains made in adding topics in environmental health, including climate change, into routine medical education. These educational programs are, however, not yet comprehensive, and they do not fully prepare physicians to address environmental concerns among their patients, especially patients in LMICs.[133–135] It is very important to include training in cultural humility and cultural competency in such education. Training in advocacy that provides pediatricians with the knowledge and tools they will need to be effective, science-based advocates for children's environmental health is another important component of such training.

To fill this gap in medical education, organizations such as the AAP, the Academic Pediatric Association, and the WHO have launched initiatives to build capacity in pediatric environmental health. The Academic Pediatric Association has launched an environmental health fellowship that has trained more than 50 clinicians and scientists who have become leaders in the field[136,137] and has formed an Environmental Health Special Interest Group. The AAP Council on Environmental Health and Climate Change has convened pediatric environmental health champions (including trainees), raised the national profile of the

TABLE 5. Resources on Common Environmental Exposures in Global Pediatric Health

Water, Sanitation, and Hygiene (WASH) • Centers for Disease Control and Prevention (CDC) information on WASH, including safe water and sewage systems, health promotion materials, and training materials: www.cdc.gov/healthywater/global • World Health Organization (WHO) resources on WASH: www.who.int/water_sanitation_health/en/
Outdoor Air Pollution • US Environmental Protection Agency (EPA) air pollution website: www.epa.gov/environmental-topics/air-topics • California Air Resource Board information on how the state has been a leader in managing air pollution: www.arb.ca.gov, and information on how regulatory efforts have reduced exposures and ways individuals can reduce pollution, primarily applicable to the developed world: www.arb.ca.gov/html/cando.htm • WHO information on the impacts of air pollution: www.who.int/health-topics/air-pollution • Air Quality Index (AQI)—a color-coded numerical scale that indicates how healthy or unhealthy the outdoor air is for certain key air pollutants (eg, particulate matter and ozone) around the world: https://aqicn.org/map/world/
Indoor Air Pollution • WHO information on the impact of indoor air quality, including from cookstoves, and strategies to reduce exposures: www.who.int/news-room/fact-sheets/detail/household-air-pollution-and-health • The Global Alliance for Clean Cookstoves information on overcoming market barriers that currently impede the production, deployment, and use of clean cookstoves in LMICs: http://cleancookstoves.org • WHO Tobacco Free Initiative:https://www.who.int/westernpacific/about/how-we-work/programmes/tobacco-free-initiative
Pesticides • EPA Clinical manual: Recognition and Management of Pesticide Poisonings, 6th ed: https://www.epa.gov/pesticide-worker-safety/recognition-and-management-pesticide-poisonings • Migrant Clinicians Network has developed resources to educate clinicians on the recognition and management of pesticide exposure, and also has patient education materials: www.migrantclinician.org/issues/occupational-health/pesticides.html • The WHO pesticide program: www.who.int/topics/pesticides/en/ • United Nations Children's Fund report: "Understanding the Impact of Pesticides on Children": www.unicef.org/csr/files/Understanding_the_impact_of_pesticides_on_children-_Jan_2018.pdf
Heavy Metals: Lead, Mercury, and Arsenic • PEHSU Factsheet: Recommendations on Medical Management of Childhood Lead Exposure and Poisoning, including low level exposure: https://www.pehsu.net/_Library/facts/medical-mgmnt-childhood-lead-exposure-June-2013.pdf • CDC Guidelines for Screening and Management of Lead Poisoning: www.cdc.gov/nceh/lead/publications/default.htm#screening • WHO Guideline for clinical management of exposure to lead: www.who.int/publications/i/item/9789240037045 • WHO: Mercury and Health: www.who.int/news-room/fact-sheets/detail/mercury-and-health • WHO Exposure to Arsenic: A Major Public Health Concern: www.who.int/publications/i/item/WHO-CED-PHE-EPE-19.4.1
Climate Change • WHO climate change resources: www.who.int/health-topics/climate-change • UN Children's Fund information on a child's physical and social environment playing a key role in their health and development: www.unicef.org/environment-and-climate-change • Global Change Research Program's Climate and Health Assessment: health2016.globalchange.gov • Harvard Center for Climate, Health, and the Global Environment (engages physicians to become climate leaders, including the Climate MD program): www.hsph.harvard.edu/c-change/ • The Medical Consortium on Climate & Health (brings together multiple medical societies to collectively work on the issue of climate change): https://medsocietiesforclimatehealth.org/
Care of Immigrant, Refugee, and Adopted Children in the United States • CDC Lead Poisoning Prevention in Newly Arrived Refugee Children: www.cdc.gov/nceh/lead/publications/refugeetoolkit/refugee-tool-kit.htm • AAP Immigrant Child Health Toolkit: www.aap.org/en-us/advocacy-and-policy/aap-health-initiatives/Immigrant-Child-Health-Toolkit/Pages/Immigrant-Child-Health-Toolkit.aspx • CDC guidance on screening and treatment of immigrants, refugees, and migrant groups: www.cdc.gov/immigrantrefugeehealth/

field, and published the clinical handbook Pediatric Environmental Health (also known as the "Green Book"), now in its 4th edition.[69]

A national network of PEHSUs was established in 1998 by the US EPA and the Agency for Toxic Substances and Disease Registry (ATSDR). PEHSUs span the United States, and they provide consultation, guidance, and education for healthcare providers, public health agencies, and communities on key pediatric environmental health issues.[69,138,139] The WHO has launched an international network of Children's Environmental Health Units, including the Unidades de Pediátrica Ambiental (UPAs) in Latin America, and created a comprehensive training program in pediatric environmental health. In addition to these valuable resources, additional online training materials, research journals, and clinical tools have been developed (Table 5).

Funding of Global Environmental Health

Despite the great magnitude of their effects on human health, environmental hazards in LMICs have been neglected in the international development and global health agendas, as well as in the planning strategies of many countries. The foreign aid budgets of the European

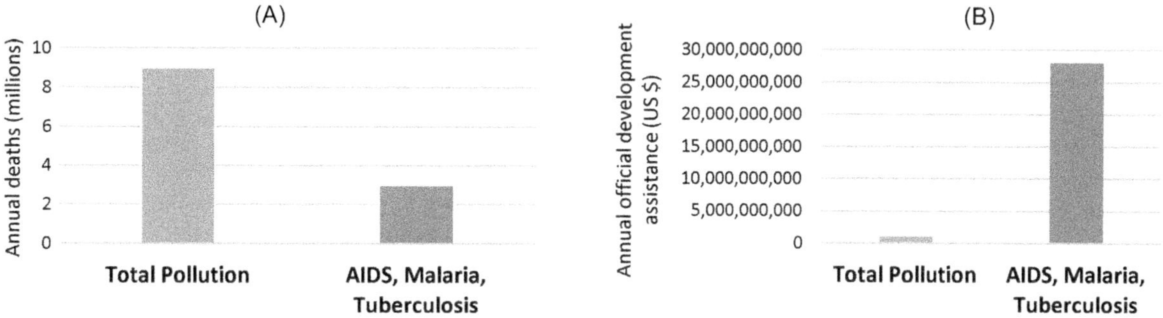

FIGURE 1.
The annual impact of environmental pollution on global mortality versus global mortality from AIDS, malaria, and tuberculosis combined (A) in comparison to the annual official development assistance directed to pollution control versus official development assistance directed to AIDS, malaria, and tuberculosis combined (B).
Adapted from Landrigan PJ, Fuller R. The impact of pollution on planetary health: emergence of an underappreciated risk factor. *UN Environment Perspective.* 2017;29:1–12.

Commission, the US Agency for International Development, and bilateral development agencies allocate only minimal resources to the prevention control of ambient air pollution and chemical pollution.[140,141] No major foundation has made pollution control a priority. The data presented in Figure 1 illustrate the striking imbalance between pollution's impacts on human health and the meager resources devoted towards its prevention and control (Figure 1).[142] The investment by international development agencies in preventing a death caused by pollution is $14 versus $1250/death for malaria, $190/death for tuberculosis, and $165/death for HIV/AIDS.[143]

Increasing Capacity in the Field of Environmental Health

Given the immense burden of disease attributable to modifiable environmental factors, increased financial support and capacity building in environmental health are urgently needed in all countries, and especially LMICs. Programs such as the WHO-National Institute of Environmental Health Sciences (NIEHS) Collaborating Centers and the Fogarty International Center (of the National Institutes of Health) offer international training programs, research, capacity building, and information sharing across countries, which have reduced disease burden around the world.[144,145] However, substantially more funding and investment in these type of programs are needed to fully address the complex and changing scope of environmentally related disease.

Environmental health training for medical personnel, public health professionals, and environmental technicians is critical for the development of locally tailored and sustainable environmental interventions. Primary prevention interventions in environmental health include strategies such as: implementing safely managed drinking water system, ending open defecation through installation of safe toilet facilities, increasing access to cleaner fuels and more efficient indoor cook stoves, and improving surveillance and control of chemical products.[146]

These environmental interventions produce crosscutting health, social, and economic co-benefits, and support the vision of United Nation's Sustainable Development Goals (SDGs). The 17 ambitious SDGs aim to eradicate global poverty by 2030 by focusing on sustainable strategies to ensure healthy environments for all, especially women and children.[147] As climate change accelerates and LMICs continue their trajectories on the epidemiological and environmental transitions, increased investment in research and infrastructure are needed to ensure a resilient future for all children and future generations.

SUMMARY/CONCLUSION

Hazardous environmental exposures including air pollution, water pollution, and toxic chemical exposures have disproportionately great impacts on the health and development of children and adolescents in LMICs. Although advances have been made in improving environmental conditions for children in LMICs, their risk of environmentally related morbidity and mortality remains much higher than for children in high-income countries. To equip pediatricians to address these persistent problems, an increased emphasis on environmental health needs to be incorporated into medical education and into the clinical care of children and youth worldwide.

It is important that pediatric health care providers have knowledge of the environmental health exposures affecting the communities they serve in North America and in LMICs and that they are aware of the many resources available at the local national and international levels to address these hazards. Pediatricians and other child health experts can play key roles in protecting children's health against environmental threats by routinely considering the possibility of environmental causation in the assessment of each child and through remaining ever alert to "sentinel events" that may signal the presence of a previously unrecognized environmental danger. Pediatricians can contribute additionally to protecting children against environmental hazards by participating in relevant policy and decision-making processes in their communities and by incorporating measures to protect children against environmental threats into primary care pediatrics and public health systems.

The already great need for pediatricians to be involved in protecting children against environmental threats to health will become still greater in the years ahead as climate change continues to cause direct and indirect impacts on the health and well-being of children around the world and to magnify the impacts on children's health of other harmful exposures in the environment.

LEAD AUTHORS

Lauren Zajac, MD, MPH, FAAP
Philip J. Landrigan, MD, MSc, FAAP

COUNCIL ON ENVIRONMENTAL HEALTH AND CLIMATE CHANGE EXECUTIVE COMMITTEE, 2022–2023

Lauren Zajac, MD, MHP, FAAP; Chairperson
Sophie J. Balk, MD, FAAP
Lori G. Byron, MD, FAAP
Gredia Maria Huerta-Montañez, MD, FAAP
Philip J. Landrigan, MD, FAAP
Steven M. Marcus, MD, FAAP
Abby L. Nerlinger, MD, FAAP
Lisa H. Patel, MD, FAAP
Rebecca Philipsborn, MD, FAAP
Alan D. Woolf, MD, MPH, FAAP

LIAISONS

Kimberly A. Gray, PhD – National Institute of Environmental Health Sciences
Grace Robiou – US Environmental Protection Agency
Nathaniel G. DeNicola, MD, MSc – American College of Obstetricians and Gynecologists
CDR Matt Karwowski, MD, MPH, FAAP – Centers for Disease Control and Prevention National Center for Environmental Health and Agency for Toxic Substances and Disease Registry
Mary H. Ward, PhD – National Cancer Institute

STAFF

Paul Spire

ABBREVIATIONS

AAP: American Academy of Pediatrics
ASGM: artisanal and small-scale gold mining
CDC: Centers for Disease Control and Prevention
CO_2: carbon dioxide
LMICs: low- and middle-income countries
NCD: noncommunicable disease
PBDE: polybrominated diphenyl ether
PCBs: polychlorinated biphenyls
PEHSU: Pediatric Environmental Health Specialty Unit
PFAS: per- and polyfluoroalkyl substances
SDG: Sustainable Development Goals
WHO: World Health Organization

REFERENCES

1. Suchdev PS, Howard CR. The role of pediatricians in global health. *Pediatrics*. 2018;142(6):e20182997. doi: 10.1542/peds.2018-2997
2. Philipsborn RP, Chan K. Climate change and global child health. *Pediatrics*. 2018;141(6):e20173774. doi: 10.1542/peds.2017-3774
3. Linton JM, Green A, Chilton LA, et al. Providing care for children in immigrant families. *Pediatrics*. 2019;144(3):e20192077. doi: 10.1542/peds.2019-2077
4. Chan K, Sisk B, Yun K, St Clair NE. Global health experience and interest: results from the AAP Periodic Survey. *Pediatrics*. 2020;145(1):e20191655. doi: https://doi.org/10.1542/peds.2019-1655
5. Crouse HL, Watts J, St Clair NE, et al. Global health opportunities in pediatric fellowships. *Pediatrics*. 2020;145(2):e20191589. doi: 10.1542/peds.2019-1589
6. St Clair NE, Abdul-Mumin A, Banker SL, et al. Global guide: a comprehensive global health education resource for pediatric program directors. *Pediatrics*. 2020;145(2):e20192138. doi: 10.1542/peds.2019-2138
7. Miller MD, Marty MA, Landrigan PJ. Children's environmental health: beyond national boundaries. *Pediatr Clin North Am*. 2016;63(1):149–165. doi: 10.1016/j.pcl.2015.08.008
8. Landrigan PJ, Fuller R, Fisher S, et al. Pollution and children's health. *Sci Total Environ*. 2019;650(Pt 2):2389–2394. doi: 10.1016/j.scitotenv.2018.09.375
9. Suk WA, Ahanchian H, Asante KA, et al. Environmental pollution: An underrecognized threat to children's health, especially in low- and middle-income countries. *Environ Health Perspect*. 2016;124(3):A43–A45. doi: 10.1289/ehp.1510517
10. World Health Organization. *Inheriting a Sustainable World: Atlas on Children's Health and the Environment*. Geneva, Switzerland: World Health Organization; 2018. Available at: https://www.who.int/publications/i/item/9789241511773. Accessed May 19, 2020
11. Landrigan PJ, Fuller R, Acosta NJR, et al. The Lancet Commission on pollution and health. *Lancet*. 2018;391(10119):462–512. doi: 10.1016/S0140-6736(17)32345-0
12. Zajac L, Landrigan PJ; American Academy of Pediatrics, Council on Environmental Health and Climate Change. Policy statement. Environmental issues in global pediatric health. *Pediatrics*. 2023; in press
13. Smith KR, Ezzati M. How Environmental health risks change with development: the epidemiologic and environmental risk transitions revisited. *Ann Rev Environ Res*. 2005;30:291–333. doi: 10.1146/annurev.energy.30.050504.144424

14. Omran AR. The epidemiologic transition: a theory of the epidemiology of population change. *Milbank Q.* 2005;83(4):731–757. doi: 10.1111/j.1468-0009.2005.00398.x

15. Yadama GN. *Fires, Fuel, and the Fate of Three Billion: Portraits of the Energy Impoverished.* Oxford, England: Oxford University Press; 2013

16. Grant K, Goldizen FC, Sly PD, et al. Health consequences of exposure to e-waste: a systematic review. *Lancet Glob Health.* 2013; 1(6):e350–e361. doi: 10.1016/S2214-109X(13)70101-3

17. Spitz PH. *The Chemical Industry at the Millennium: Maturity, Restructuring, and Globalization.* Philadelphia, PA: Chemical Heritage Press; 2003

18. Pronczuk J, Bruné M-N, Gore F.Children's environmental health in developing countries. In: Nriagu JO, Kacew S, Kawamoto T, et al, eds. *Encyclopedia of Environmental Health.* Amsterdam, Netherlands: Elsevier; 2011:601–610. Available at: https://www.sciencedirect.com/referencework/9780444522726/encyclopedia-of-environmental-health. Accessed May 19, 2020

19. Stanaway JD, Afshin A, Gakidou E, et al. Global, regional, and national comparative risk assessment of 84 behavioural, environmental and occupational, and metabolic risks or clusters of risks for 195 countries and territories, 1990–2017: a systematic analysis for the Global Burden of Disease Study 2017. *Lancet.* 2018; 392(10159):1923–1994. doi: 10.1016/S0140-6736(18)32225-6

20. Yen C, Tate JE, Hyde TB, et al. Rotavirus vaccines: current status and future considerations. *Hum Vaccines Immunother.* 2014;10(6): 1436–1448. doi: 10.4161/hv.28857

21. Florez ID, Al-Khalifah R, Sierra JM, et al. The effectiveness and safety of treatments used for acute diarrhea and acute gastroenteritis in children: protocol for a systematic review and network meta-analysis. *Syst Rev.* 2016;5(1):14. doi: 10.1186/s13643-016-0186-8

22. Branca F, Piwoz E, Schultink W, Sullivan LM. Nutrition and health in women, children, and adolescent girls. *BMJ.* 2015;351:h4173. doi: 10.1136/bmj.h4173

23. Shaffer RM, Sellers SP, Baker MG, et al. Improving and expanding estimates of the global burden of disease due to environmental health risk factors. *Environ Health Perspect.* 2019;127(10):105001-1-105001-105016. doi: 10.1289/EHP5496

24. Landrigan PJ, Sly JL, Ruchirawat M, et al. Health consequences of environmental exposures: changing global patterns of exposure and disease. *Ann Glob Health.* 2016;82(1):10–19. doi: 10.1016/j.aogh.2016.01.005

25. Remais JV, Zeng G, Li G, Tian L, Engelgau MM. Convergence of non-communicable and infectious diseases in low-and middle-income countries. *Int J Epidemiol.* 2013;42:221–227. doi: 10.1093/ije/dys135

26. Fuller R, Rahona E, Fisher S, et al. Pollution and non-communicable disease: time to end the neglect. *Lancet Planet Health.* 2018;2(3):e96–e98. doi: 10.1016/S2542-5196(18)30020-2

27. Bullard RD, Robert D. *Dumping in Dixie: Race, Class, and Environmental Quality.* Boulder, CO: Westview Press; 1990

28. Foote EM, Singleton RJ, Holman RC, et al. Lower respiratory tract infection hospitalizations among American Indian/Alaska Native children and the general United States child population. *Int J Circumpolar Health.* 2015;74(1). doi: 10.3402/IJCH.V74.29256

29. Singleton R, Salkoski AJ, Bulkow L, et al. Impact of home remediation and household education on indoor air quality, respiratory visits and symptoms in Alaska Native children. *Int J Circumpolar Health.* 2018;77(1). doi: 10.1080/22423982.2017.1422669

30. Hennessy TW, Ritter T, Holman RC, et al. The relationship between in-home water service and the risk of respiratory tract, skin, and gastrointestinal tract infections among rural Alaska Natives. *Am J Public Health.* 2008;98(11):2072. doi: 10.2105/AJPH.2007.115618

31. Berry H, Kaul A, Lee N. Follow the smoke: the pollution haven effect on global sourcing. *Strateg Manag J.* 2021;42(13):2420–2450. doi: 10.1002/SMJ.3288

32. Duan Y, Ji T, Yu T. Reassessing pollution haven effect in global value chains. *J Clean Prod.* 2021;284:124705. doi: 10.1016/J.JCLEPRO.2020.124705

33. Barreto M. The globalization of epidemiology: critical thoughts from Latin America. *Int J Epidemiol.* 2004;33(5):1132–1137

34. De Maio FG. Understanding chronic non-communicable diseases in Latin America: towards an equity-based research agenda. *Glob Health.* 2011;7(1):36. doi: 10.1186/1744-8603-7-36

35. Samet JM, Burke TA, Goldstein BD. The trump administration and the environment—heed the science. *N Engl J Med.* 2017;376(12): 1182–1188. doi: 10.1056/NEJMms1615242

36. Grosse SD, Matte TD, Schwartz J, Jackson RJ. Economic gains resulting from the reduction in children's exposure to lead in the United States. *Environ Health Perspect.* 2002;110(6):563–569. doi: 10.1289/ehp.02110563

37. US Environmental Protection Agency. Summary of the Toxic Substances Control Act. Available at: https://www.epa.gov/laws-regulations/summary-toxic-substances-control-act. Published 2019. Accessed May 25, 2020

38. Whyatt RM, Rauh V, Barr DB, et al. Prenatal insecticide exposures and birth weight and length among an urban minority cohort. *Environ Health Perspect.* 2004;112(10):1125–1132. doi: 10.1289/ehp.6641

39. Graziano JH, van Geen A. Reducing arsenic exposure from drinking water: different settings call for different approaches. *Environ Health Perspect.* 2005;113(6): A360–A361. doi: 10.1289/ehp.113-a360

40. Smith AH, Marshall G, Liaw J, Yuan Y, Ferreccio C, Steinmaus C. Mortality in young adults following in utero and childhood exposure to arsenic in drinking water. *Environ Health Perspect.* 2012; 120(11):1527–1531. doi: 10.1289/ehp.1104867

41. Gauderman WJ, Urman R, Avol E, et al. Association of improved air quality with lung development in children. *N Engl J Med.* 2015; 372(10):905–913. doi: 10.1056/NEJMoa1414123

42. US Environmental Protection Agency, Office of Air and Radiation. Overview of the Clean Air Act and Air Pollution. Available at: https://www.epa.gov/clean-air-act-overview. Published 2020. Accessed May 19, 2020

43. Schwarzenbach RP, Egli T, Hofstetter TB, von Gunten U, Wehrli B. Global water pollution and human health. *Ann Rev Environ Res.* 2010;35(1):109–136. doi: 10.1146/annurev-environ-100809-125342

44. Forouzanfar MH, Afshin A, Alexander LT, et al. Global, regional, and national comparative risk assessment of 79 behavioural, environmental and occupational, and metabolic risks or clusters of risks, 1990–2015: a systematic analysis for the Global Burden of Disease Study 2015. *Lancet.* 2016;388(10053):1659–1724. doi: 10.1016/S0140-6736(16)31679-8

45. Wang H, Naghavi M, Allen C, et al. Global, regional, and national life expectancy, all-cause mortality, and cause-specific mortality for 249 causes of death, 1980–2015: a systematic analysis for the Global Burden of Disease Study 2015. *Lancet.* 2016;388(10053):1459–1544. doi: 10.1016/S0140-6736(16)31012-1

46. Landrigan PJ, Goldman LR. Children's vulnerability to toxic chemicals: a challenge and opportunity to strengthen health and environmental policy. *Health Aff (Millwood).* 2011;30(5):842–850. doi: 10.1377/hlthaff.2011.0151

47. Balakrishnan K, Cohen A, Smith KR. Addressing the burden of disease attributable to air pollution in India: the need to integrate across household and ambient air pollution exposures. *Environ Health Perspect.* 2014;122(1):A6–A7. doi: 10.1289/ehp.1307822

48. Kelly FJ, Fussell JC. Global nature of airborne particle toxicity and health effects: a focus on megacities, wildfires, dust storms and residential biomass burning. *Toxicol Res (Camb).* 2020;9(4):331–345. doi: 10.1093/toxres/tfaa044

49. World Health Organization. Air pollution. Available at: https://www.who.int/health-topics/air-pollution#tab=tab_1. Accessed May 25, 2020

50. Dettori M, Deiana G, Balletto G, et al. Air pollutants and risk of death due to COVID-19 in Italy. *Environ Res.* 2021;192:110459. doi: 10.1016/j.envres.2020.110459

51. Copat C, Cristaldi A, Fiore M, et al. The role of air pollution (PM and NO2) in COVID-19 spread and lethality: a systematic review. *Environ Res.* 2020;191:110129. doi: 10.1016/j.envres.2020.110129

52. Paital B, Agrawal PK. Air pollution by NO2 and PM2.5 explains COVID-19 infection severity by overexpression of angiotensin-converting enzyme 2 in respiratory cells: a review. *Environ Chem Lett.* 2020;191:110129. doi: 10.1007/s10311-020-01091-w

53. Zoran MA, Savastru RS, Savastru DM, Tautan MN. Assessing the relationship between surface levels of PM2.5 and PM10 particulate matter impact on COVID-19 in Milan, Italy. *Sci Total Environ.* 2020;738:139825. doi: 10.1016/j.scitotenv.2020.139825

54. Lelieveld J, Evans JS, Fnais M, Giannadaki D, Pozzer A. The contribution of outdoor air pollution sources to premature mortality on a global scale. *Nature.* 2015;525(7569):367–371. doi: 10.1038/nature15371

55. Porpora MG, Piacenti I, Scaramuzzino S, Masciullo L, Rech F, Panici PB. Environmental contaminants exposure and preterm birth: a systematic review. *Toxics.* 2019;7(1):11. doi: 10.3390/toxics7010011

56. Chen J, Fang J, Zhang Y, et al. Associations of adverse pregnancy outcomes with high ambient air pollution exposure: results from the Project ELEFANT. *Sci Total Environ.* 2021;761:143218. doi: 10.1016/j.scitotenv.2020.143218

57. Klepac P, Locatelli I, Korošec S, Künzli N, Kukec A. Ambient air pollution and pregnancy outcomes: a comprehensive review and identification of environmental public health challenges. *Environ Res.* 2018;167:144–159. doi: 10.1016/j.envres.2018.07.008

58. Heindel JJ, Balbus J, Birnbaum L, et al. Developmental origins of health and disease: integrating environmental influences. *Endocrinology.* 2015;156(10):3416–3421. doi: 10.1210/EN.2015-1394

59. Wang P, Tuvblad C, Younan D, et al. Socioeconomic disparities and sexual dimorphism in neurotoxic effects of ambient fine particles on youth IQ: a longitudinal analysis. *PLoS One.* 2017;12(12):e0188731. doi: 10.1371/journal.pone.0188731

60. Perera FP. Multiple threats to child health from fossil fuel combustion: impacts of air pollution and climate change. *Environ Health Perspect.* 2017;125(2):141–148. doi: 10.1289/EHP299

61. Raz R, Roberts AL, Lyall K, et al. Autism spectrum disorder and particulate matter air pollution before, during, and after pregnancy: a nested case–control analysis within the nurses' health study II cohort. *Environ Health Perspect.* 2015;123(3):264–270. doi: 10.1289/ehp.1408133

62. Fewtrell LJ, Prüss-Üstün A, Landrigan P, Ayuso-Mateos JL. Estimating the global burden of disease of mild mental retardation and cardiovascular diseases from environmental lead exposure. *Environ Res.* 2004;94(2):120–133. doi: 10.1016/S0013-9351(03)00132-4

63. World Health Organization. *Childhood Lead Poisoning.* Geneva, Switzerland: World Health Organization; 2010. Available at: https://apps.who.int/iris/handle/10665/136571. Accessed May 25, 2020

64. United Nations Environment Programme. *Global Mercury Assessment 2018. UNEP-UN Environment Programme.* Geneva, Switzerland: United Nations Environment Programme; 2019. Available at: https://www.unep.org/resources/publication/global-mercury-assessment-2018. Accessed December 7, 2022

65. National Research Council, *Committee on the Toxicological Effects of Methylmercury. Toxicological Effects of Methylmercury.* Washington, DC: National Academies Press; 2000. doi: 10.17226/9899

66. World Health Organization. Mercury and health. 2017. Available at: https://www.who.int/news-room/fact-sheets/detail/mercury-and-health. Accessed May 25, 2020

67. Debes F, Weihe P, Grandjean P. Cognitive deficits at age 22 years associated with prenatal exposure to methylmercury. *Cortex.* 2016;74:358–369. doi: 10.1016/j.cortex.2015.05.017

68. Bernstein AS, Oken E, De Ferranti S, et al. Fish, shellfish, and children's health: an assessment of benefits, risks, and sustainability. *Pediatrics.* 2019;143(6):e20190999. doi: https://doi.org/10.1542/peds.2019-0999

69. American Academy of Pediatrics, Council on Environmental Health. Pediatric Environmental Health.Etzel RA, Balk SJ, eds. Itasca, IL: American Academy of Pediatrics; 2018

70. Munera-Picazo S, Cano-Lamadrid M, Castaño-Iglesias MC, Burló F, Carbonell-Barrachina AA. Arsenic in your food: potential health hazards from arsenic found in rice. *Nutr Diet Suppl.* 2015;7:1–10

71. Mawia AM, Hui S, Zhou L, et al. Inorganic arsenic toxicity and alleviation strategies in rice. *J Haz Mat.* 2021;408:124751

72. Hopenhayn-Rich C, Browning SR, Hertz-Picciotto I, Ferreccio C, Peralta C, Gibb H. Chronic arsenic exposure and risk of infant mortality in two areas of Chile. *Environ Health Perspect.* 2000;108(7):667–673. doi: 10.1289/ehp.00108667

73. Von Ehrenstein OS, Poddar S, Yuan Y, et al. Children's intellectual function in relation to arsenic exposure. *Epidemiology.* 2007;18(1):44–51. doi: 10.1097/01.ede.0000248900.65613.a9

74. Wasserman GA, Liu X, Parvez F, et al. Water arsenic exposure and children's intellectual function in Araihazar, Bangladesh. *Environ Health Perspect.* 2004;112(13):1329–1333. doi: 10.1289/ehp.6964

75. Steinmaus C, Ferreccio C, Acevedo J, et al. Increased lung and bladder cancer incidence in adults after in utero and early-life arsenic exposure. *Cancer Epidemiol Biomarkers Prev.* 2014;23(8):1529–1538. doi: 10.1158/1055-9965.EPI-14-0059

76. Wang Z, Walker GW, Muir DCG, Nagatani-Yoshida K. Toward a global understanding of chemical pollution: a first comprehensive analysis of national and regional chemical inventories. *Environ Sci Technol.* 2020;54(5):2575–2584. doi: 10.1021/ACS.EST.9B06379/ASSET/IMAGES/LARGE/ES9B06379_0002.JPEG

77. Centers for Disease Control and Prevention. National Report on Human Exposure to Environmental Chemicals. March 2022. Available at: https://www.cdc.gov/exposurereport/index.html. Accessed December 7, 2022

78. World Health Organization. *Children and Chemicals: WHO Training Package for the Health Sector: Children's Health and the Environment: Improving the Capacity to Diagnose, Prevent and Manage Paediatric Diseases Linked to the Environment.* Geneva, Switzerland: World Health Organization; 2019. Available at: https://apps.who.int/iris/handle/10665/330296. Accessed December 7, 2022

79. Cole MA, Elliott RJR, Okubo T. Trade, environmental regulations and industrial mobility: an industry-level study of Japan. *Ecol Econ.* 2010;69(10):1995–2002. doi: 10.1016/j.ecolecon.2010.05.015

80. Dhara VR, Dhara R, Acquilla SD, Cullinan P. Personal exposure and long-term health effects in survivors of the Union Carbide disaster at Bhopal. *Environ Health Perspect.* 2002;110(5):487–500. doi: 10.1289/ehp.02110487

81. Frank AL, Joshi TK. The global spread of asbestos. *Ann Glob Heal.* 2014;80(4):257–262. doi: 10.1016/j.aogh.2014.09.016

82. Haefliger P, Mathieu-Nolf M, Lociciro S, et al. Mass lead intoxication from informal used lead-acid battery recycling in Dakar, Senegal. *Environ Health Perspect.* 2009;117(10):1535–1540. doi: 10.1289/ehp.0900696

83. Wade L. Gold's dark side. *Science.* 2013;341(6153):1448–1449. doi: 10.1126/science.341.6153.1448

84. Cai K, Song Q, Yuan W, et al. Human exposure to PBDEs in e-waste areas: a review. *Environ Pollut.* 2020;267:115634. doi: 10.1016/J.ENVPOL.2020.115634

85. Wu K, Xu X, Liu J, Guo Y, Li Y, Huo X. Polybrominated diphenyl ethers in umbilical cord blood and relevant factors in neonates from Guiyu, China. *Environ Sci Technol.* 2010;44(2):813–819. doi: 10.1021/es9024518

86. Lam J, Lanphear BP, Bellinger D, et al. Developmental PBDE exposure and IQ/ADHD in childhood: a systematic review and meta-analysis. *Environ Health Perspect.* 2017;125(8). doi: 10.1289/EHP1632

87. Sheikh IA, Beg MA. Structural studies on the endocrine-disrupting role of polybrominated diphenyl ethers (PBDEs) in thyroid diseases. *Environ Sci Pollut Res Int.* 2020;27(30):37866–37876. doi: 10.1007/S11356-020-09913-8

88. Fan X, Tang S, Wang Y, et al. Global exposure to per- and polyfluoroalkyl substances and associated burden of low birthweight. *Environ Sci Technol.* 2022;56(7):4282–4294. doi: 10.1021/ACS.EST.1C08669/SUPPL_FILE/ES1C08669_SI_002.XLSX

89. Podder A, Sadmani AHMA, Reinhart D, Chang N Bin, Goel R. Per and poly-fluoroalkyl substances (PFAS) as a contaminant of emerging concern in surface water: a transboundary review of their occurrences and toxicity effects. *J Hazard Mater.* 2021;419:126361. doi: 10.1016/J.JHAZMAT.2021.126361

90. Agency for Toxic Substances and Disease Registry. PFAS Clinician Fact Sheet. 2019. Available at: https://www.atsdr.cdc.gov/pfas/resources/clinical-guidance.html. Accessed May 19, 2022

91. Fenton SE, Ducatman A, Boobis A, et al. Per- and polyfluoroalkyl substance toxicity and human health review: current state of knowledge and strategies for informing future research. *Environ Toxicol Chem.* 2021;40(3):606–630. doi: 10.1002/ETC.4890

92. Wang Y, Qian H. Phthalates and their impacts on human health. *Healthcare (Basel).* 2021;9(5):603. doi: 10.3390/HEALTHCARE9050603

93. Food and Agriculture Organization of the United Nations. Prevention and Disposal of Obsolete Pesticides: Pesticide Bans. Available at: http://www.fao.org/agriculture/crops/obsolete-pesticides/why-problem/pesticide-bans/en. Accessed May 20, 2020

94. Food and Agriculture Organization of the United Nations. *International Code of Conduct on the Distribution and Use of Pesticides (Revised Version): Adopted by the Hundred and Twenty-Third Session of the FAO Council in November 2002.* Rome, Italy: Food and Agriculture Organization of the United Nations; 2003

95. Abrams SA, Lewis Albin J, Landrigan PJ; American Academy of Pediatrics, Committee on Nutrition and Council on Environmental Health and Climate Change. Use of genetically modified organism (GMO)-containing food products in children. *Pediatrics.* 2024;153(1):e2023064774

96. Guyton KZ, Loomis D, Grosse Y, et al. Carcinogenicity of tetrachlorvinphos, parathion, malathion, diazinon, and glyphosate. *Lancet Oncol.* 2015;16(5):490–491. doi: 10.1016/S1470-2045(15)70134-8

97. Zhang L, Rana I, Shaffer RM, Taioli E, Sheppard L. Exposure to glyphosate-based herbicides and risk for non-Hodgkin lymphoma: a meta-analysis and supporting evidence. *Mutat Res Rev Mutat Res.* 2019;781:186–206. doi: 10.1016/j.mrrev.2019.02.001

98. United Nations Environment Programme. *Childhood Pesticide Poisoning: Information for Advocacy and Action.* Chatelaine, Switzerland: United Nations Environment Programme; 2004

99. Naidoo S, London L, Rother HA, Burdorf A, Naidoo RN, Kromhout H. Pesticide safety training and practices in women working in small-scale agriculture in South Africa. *Occup Environ Med.* 2010;67(12):823–828. doi: 10.1136/oem.2010.055863

100. United Nations Department of Economic and Social Affairs. Sustainable Development. The Partnership Platform. Available at: https://sdgs.un.org/partnerships. Accessed May 25, 2020

101. Frazzoli C, Orisakwe OE, Dragone R, Mantovani A. Diagnostic health risk assessment of electronic waste on the general population in developing countries' scenarios. *Environ Impact Assess Rev.* 2010; 30(6):388–399. doi: 10.1016/j.eiar.2009.12.004

102. Xu X, Yang H, Chen A, et al. Birth outcomes related to informal e-waste recycling in Guiyu, China. *Reprod Toxicol.* 2012;33(1):94–98. doi: 10.1016/j.reprotox.2011.12.006

103. Heacock M, Kelly CB, Asante KA, et al. E-waste and harm to vulnerable populations: a growing global problem. *Environ Health Perspect.* 2016;124(5):550–555. doi: 10.1289/ehp.1509699

104. Intergovernmental Panel on Climate Change. *AR5 Synthesis Report: Climate Change 2014.* Geneva, Switzerland: Intergovernmental Panel on Climate Change; 2014. Available at: https://www.ipcc.ch/report/ar5/syr/. Accessed May 25, 2020

105. Watts N, Amann M, Arnell N, et al. The 2019 report of The Lancet Countdown on health and climate change: ensuring that the health of a child born today is not defined by a changing climate. *Lancet.* 2019;394(10211):1836–1878. doi: 10.1016/S0140-6736(19)32596-6

106. Anderko L, Chalupka S, Du M, Hauptman M. Climate changes reproductive and children's health: a review of risks, exposures, and impacts. *Pediatr Res.* 2020;87(2):414–419. doi: 10.1038/s41390-019-0654-7

107. Ahdoot S, Baum CR, Cataletto M, Hogan P, Wu CB, Bernstein A; American Academy of Pediatrics, Council on Enviornmental Health and Climate Change, Council on Children and Disasters, Section on Pediatric Pulmonology and Sleep Medicine, Section on Minority Health, Equity, and Inclusion. Policy statement. Climate change and children's health: building a healthy future for every child. *Pediatrics.* 2024;153(3):e2023065504

108. Ahdoot S, Baum CR, Cataletto M, Hogan P, Wu CB, Bernstein A; Council on Enviornmental Health and Climate Change, Council on Children and Disasters, Section on Pediatric Pulmonology and Sleep Medicine, Section on Minority Health, Equity, and Inclusion. Technical report. Climate change and children's health: building a healthy future for every child. *Pediatrics.* 2024;153(3):e2023065505

109. Balbus JM, Boxall ABA, Fenske RA, McKone TE, Zeise L. Implications of global climate change for the assessment and management of human health risks of chemicals in the natural environment. *Environ Toxicol Chem.* 2013;32(1):62–78. doi: 10.1002/etc.2046

110. International Labour Organization. Child Labour. Decent Work for Sustainable Development (DW4SD) Resource Platform. Available at: https://www.ilo.org/global/topics/dw4sd/themes/child-labour/lang--en/index.htm. Published 2018. Accessed June 10, 2020

111. Hurst P. Health and child labor in agriculture. *Food Nutr Bull.* 2007; 28(2 Suppl). doi: 10.1177/15648265070282s216

112. Ide LSR, Parker DL. Hazardous child labor: lead and neurocognitive development. *Public Health Rep.* 2005;120(6):607–613. doi: 10.1177/003335490512000608

113. Shendell DG, Noomnual S, Chishti S, Allacci MS, Madrigano J. Exposures resulting in safety and health concerns for child laborers in less developed countries. *J Environ Public Health.* 2016;2016. doi: 10.1155/2016/3985498

114. Ibrahim A, Abdalla S, Jafer M, Abdelgadir J, de Vries N. Child labor and health: a systematic literature review of the impacts of child labor on child's health in low- and middle-income countries. *J Public Health (Bangkok).* 2019;41(1):18–26. Available at: https://academic.oup.com/jpubhealth/article/41/1/18/4835667. Accessed June 4, 2020

115. Iannacci-Manasia L. Unprotected youth workers in US agriculture. *Front Public Health.* 2023;11:1064143

116. Habib RR, El Khayat M, Ghanawi J, Katrib RS, Hneiny L, Halwani DA. Child labor and associated risk factors in the wake of the COVID-19 pandemic: a scoping review. *Front Public Health.* 2024;11:1240988

117. Peden M, Oyegbite K, Ozanne-Smith J, et al. *World Report on Child Injury Prevention.* Geneva, Switzerland: World Health Organization; 2008. Available at: https://pubmed.ncbi.nlm.nih.gov/26269872/. Accessed June 4, 2020

118. World Health Organization. *Global Status Report On Road Safety 2018 Summary.* Geneva, Switzerland: World Health Organization; 2018. Available at: https://www.who.int/publications/i/item/9789241565684. Accessed June 4, 2020

119. Zhang Q, Jiang X, Tong D, et al. Transboundary health impacts of transported global air pollution and international trade. *Nature.* 2017;543(7647):705–709. doi: 10.1038/nature21712

120. United Nations Environment Programme. *Transboundary Waters Systems – Status and Trends: Crosscutting Analysis.* Nairobi, Kenya: United Nations Environment Programme; 2016. Available at: https://uneplive.unep.org/media/docs/assessments/transboundary_waters_systems_status_and_trends_crosscutting_analysis.pdf. Accessed June 19, 2020

121. United Nations Environment Programme. The Illegal Trade in Chemicals. 2020. Available at: https://wedocs.unep.org/bitstream/handle/20.500.11822/32021/Chemicals.pdf. Accessed June 19, 2020

122. New York City Department of Health. Hazardous Consumer Products. 2020. Available at: https://www1.nyc.gov/site/doh/health/health-topics/lead-poisoning-hazardous-consumer-products.page. Accessed June 16, 2020

123. Centers for Disease Control and Prevention. Poisoning by an illegally imported chinese rodenticide containing tetramethylenedisulfotetramine—New York City, 2002. *MMWR Morb Mortal Wkly Rep.* 2003;52(10):199–201

124. Miller RW. How environmental hazards in childhood have been discovered: carcinogens, teratogens, neurotoxicants, and others. *Pediatrics.* 2004;113(Suppl 3):945–951

125. Zajac L, Johnson SA, Hauptman M. Doc, can you test me for "toxic metals"? Challenges of testing for toxicants in patients with environmental concerns. *Curr Probl Pediatr Adolesc Health Care.* 2020;50(2). doi: 10.1016/j.cppeds.2020.100762

126. World Health Organization. *The Paediatric Environmental History: Green Page*. Geneva, Switzerland: World Health Organization; 2018. Available at: https://www.who.int/publications/m/item/children-s-environmental-record–green-page. Accessed December 7, 2022

127. World Health Organization. *Training Modules and Instructions for Health Care Providers*. Geneva, Switzerland: World Health Organization; 2020

128. Goldman R, Peters J. The Occupational and Environmental Health History. *JAMA*. 1981;246(24):2831–2836

129. Landrigan P, Baker P. The recognition and control of occupational disease. *JAMA*. 1991;266(5):676–680

130. American Academy of Pediatrics, Council on Community Pediatrics. Immigrant Child Health Toolkit. 2020. Available at: https://www.aap.org/en-us/advocacy-and-policy/aap-health-initiatives/Immigrant-Child-Health-Toolkit/Pages/Immigrant-Child-Health-Toolkit.aspx. Accessed December 7, 2022

131. Jones VF, Schulte EE, Springer S, et al. Comprehensive health evaluation of the newly adopted child. *Pediatrics*. 2019;143(5): e20190657. doi: 10.1542/peds.2019-0657

132. Centers for Disease Control and Prevention. Guidance for Mental Health Screening during the Domestic Medical Examination for Newly Arrived Refugees. 2022. Available at: https://www.cdc.gov/immigrantrefugeehealth/guidelines/domestic/mental-health-screening-guidelines.html. Accessed May 19, 2022

133. Trasande L, Schapiro ML, Falk R, et al. Pediatrician attitudes, clinical activities, and knowledge of environmental health in Wisconsin. *Wis Med J*. 2006;105(2):45–49

134. Trasande L, Boscarino J, Graber N, et al. The environment in pediatric practice: a study of New York pediatricians' attitudes, beliefs, and practices towards children's environmental health. *J Urban Heal*. 2006;83(4):760–772. doi: 10.1007/s11524-006-9071-4

135. Trasande L, Newman N, Long L, et al. Translating knowledge about environmental health to practitioners: are we doing enough? *Mt Sinai J Med*. 2010;77(1):114–123. doi: 10.1002/msj.20158

136. Landrigan PJ, Woolf AD, Gitterman B, et al. The ambulatory pediatric association fellowship in pediatric environmental health: a 5-year assessment. *Environ Health Perspect*. 2007;115(10): 1383–1387. doi: 10.1289/ehp.10015

137. Landrigan PJ, Braun JM, Crain EF, et al. Building capacity in pediatric environmental health: the Academic Pediatric Association's Professional Development Program. *Acad Pediatr*. 2019;19(4): 421–427. doi: 10.1016/j.acap.2019.01.001

138. Paulson JA, Karr CJ, Seltzer JM, et al. Development of the pediatric environmental health specialty unit network in North America. *Am J Public Health*. 2009;99(Suppl 3). doi: 10.2105/ajph.2008.154641

139. Wilborne-Davis P, Kirkland KH, Mulloy KB. A model for physician education and consultation in pediatric environmental health—The Pediatric Environmental Health Specialty Units (PEHSU) Program. *Pediatr Clin North Am*. 2007;54(1):1–13. doi: 10.1016/j.pcl.2006.11.001

140. Greenberg H, Leeder SR, Raymond SU. And why so great a "no?": the donor and academic communities' failure to confront global chronic disease. *Glob Heart*. 2016;11(4):381–385. doi: 10.1016/j.gheart.2016.10.018

141. Nugent R. A chronology of global assistance funding for NCD. *Glob Heart*. 2016;11(4):371–374. doi: 10.1016/j.gheart.2016.10.027

142. Landrigan PJ, Fuller R. The Impact of Pollution on Planetary Health: Emergence of an Underappreciated Risk Factor. *UN Environment Perspectives*. 2017;29:1–12. Available at: https://wedocs.unep.org/bitstream/handle/20.500.11822/22416/Perspective_No_29_web.pdf?isAllowed=y&sequence=1. Accessed December 7, 2022

143. Swinehart S, Fuller R, Kupka R, Conte MN. Rethinking aid allocation: analysis of official development spending on modern pollution reduction. *Ann Glob Heal*. 2019;85(1). doi: 10.5334/aogh.2633

144. Drain PK, Holmes KK. The Fogarty International Center at 50: accomplishments and priorities for the next 50 years. *Clin Infect Dis*. 2018;66(9):1323–1325. doi: 10.1093/cid/ciy078

145. World Health Organization. *Collaboration between the World Health Organization and the National Institute of Environmental Health Sciences: Highlights from 30 Years of Partnership*. Geneva, Switzerland: World Health Organization; 2011. Available at: https://www.who.int/publications/i/item/978924502078. Accessed June 26, 2020

146. World Health Organization. *Healthy Environments for Healthier Populations: Why Do They Matter, and What Can We Do?* Geneva, Switzerland: 2019. Available at: https://www.who.int/publications/i/item/WHO-CED-PHE-DO-19.01. Accessed December 7, 2022

147. United Nations Department of Economic and Social Affairs. Make the SDGs a Reality. Available at: https://sustainabledevelopment.un.org. Published 2015. Accessed June 23, 2020

Evaluating Young Children With Fractures for Child Abuse

- *Clinical Report*

CLINICAL REPORT Guidance for the Clinician in Rendering Pediatric Care

American Academy of Pediatrics

DEDICATED TO THE HEALTH OF ALL CHILDREN™

Evaluating Young Children With Fractures for Child Abuse: Clinical Report

Suzanne Haney, MD, FAAP,[1] Susan Scherl, MD, FAAP,[2] Linda DiMeglio, MD, FAAP,[3] Jeannette Perez-Rossello, MD, FAAP,[4] Sabah Servaes, MD, FAAP,[5] Nadia Merchant, MD, FAAP[6]; and the COUNCIL ON CHILD ABUSE AND NEGLECT; SECTION ON ORTHOPAEDICS; SECTION ON RADIOLOGY; and SECTION ON ENDOCRINOLOGY; and the SOCIETY FOR PEDIATRIC RADIOLOGY

abstract

Fractures are common injuries in childhood and can be caused by unintentional injury, medical conditions, and child abuse. Although the consequences of failing to diagnose an abusive injury in a child can be grave, the consequences of incorrectly diagnosing child abuse in a child whose fractures have another etiology are also significant. This report aims to review recent advances in the understanding of fracture specificity, fracture mechanisms, and other medical conditions that predispose infants and children to fracture. This clinical report will aid pediatricians and pediatric care providers in developing an evidence-based differential diagnosis and performing appropriate evaluations when assessing a child with fractures.

[1]Department of Pediatrics, University of Nebraska Medical Center, Children's Nebraska, Omaha, Nebraska; [2]Department of Orthopedics, University of Nebraska Medical Center, Children's Nebraska, Omaha, Nebraska; [3]Division of Pediatric Endocrinology and Diabetology, Riley Hospital for Children, Indiana University School of Medicine, Indianapolis, IN; [4]Department of Radiology Boston Children's Hospital, Harvard Medical School, Boston Massachusetts; [5]Department of Radiology, West Virginia University Children's Hospital, Morgantown, WV; and [6]Division of Endocrinology, Department of Pediatrics, University of Texas Southwestern, Dallas, Texas

Dr. Suzanne Haney wrote new content and edited content from the previous AAP statement and responded to reviews. Dr. Susan Scherl wrote new content and edited content from the previous AAP statement and responded to reviews. Dr. Nadia Merchant wrote new content and edited content from the previous AAP statement and responded to reviews

CONFLICT OF INTEREST DISCLOSURE: Dr Nadia Merchant has disclosed a financial relationship as an advisory board member with BioMarin, a financial relationship as an advisory board member with Pfizer, a financial relationship as an advisory board member with Catalyst and a financial relationship as an advisory board member with Alexion. Any other disclosures were reviewed and determined not relevant to the work related to "Evaluating Young Children With Fractures for Child Abuse." Disclosures are reviewed and mitigated through a Conflict of Interest process that consists of reviewing pertinent information which is then used to decide what action is required to maintain content integrity. (Continued)

To cite: Haney S, Scherl S, DiMeglio L, et al; American Academy of Pediatrics, Council on Child Abuse and Neglect; Section on Orthopaedics; Section on Radiology; Section on Endocrinology; Society for Pediatric Radiology. Evaluating Young Children With Fractures for Child Abuse: Clinical Report. *Pediatrics.* 2025;155(2):e2024070074

INTRODUCTION

Fractures are one of the most common injuries from child physical abuse, second only to bruising.[1–3] However, it can be difficult to determine whether a child's injury is the result of abuse or attributable to another cause, such as an unintentional injury or a medical condition, and whether or not neglect played a role in the child's presentation. Failure to identify an abusive injury and to intervene appropriately may place a child at risk of further abuse, with potentially permanent consequences for the child.[4–6] On the other hand, incorrectly diagnosing physical abuse in a child with a nonabusive injury has serious consequences for the child and family.

An appropriate diagnosis of abuse involves a thorough history and physical examination, including the age and developmental ability of the child; the reported mechanism, location, and type(s) of fracture; and the presence of other injuries.[7] Children whose fractures are the result of abuse commonly present with histories of either no trauma or minor trauma.[6,7] In children younger than 3 years, as many as 20% of fractures caused by abuse may be misdiagnosed initially as unintentional or attributed to other causes.[6] In addition, fractures may not be visible on initial radiography if studies are performed early, before bony radiographic changes become obvious.[8] Finally, there is significant concern for racial and ethnic bias in the diagnosis of child abuse.[4,9] Standardized pathways, decision support processes, and even applications for smartphones can help pediatricians and pediatric care providers reduce bias, and it is important for providers to recognize and acknowledge these concerns.[9]

TABLE 1. Features of Fractures That Might Raise Suspicion for Abuse

- No history of injury
- History of injury not plausible—mechanism described not consistent with the type of fracture, the energy load needed to cause the fracture, or the severity of the injury
- Inconsistent histories or changing histories provided by caregiver
- Fracture in a nonambulatory child
- Fracture of high specificity for child abuse (eg, rib fractures)
- Multiple fractures
- Fractures of different ages
- Other injuries suspicious for child abuse
- Delay in seeking care for an injury

MEDICAL EVALUATION

History of Present Illness

It is essential to obtain a detailed history to determine how an injury occurred. When injuries in a child are witnessed or there are witnesses after the fact, details about the child's activity and position prior to an injury and the child's final position and location after the injury occurred are helpful in addressing plausibility.[10] Lack of a history of trauma is also concerning, and caregivers may be able to help narrow the time frame of injury if they are asked when the child was last observed to be well, such as using the affected extremity. In a study of abusive fractures, caregivers commonly provided either no history of an injury or related a low-energy event. By contrast, 29% of caregivers of children with unintentional injuries provided some high-energy explanation, such as a motor vehicle collision or that the child fell from a height.[11] Most low-energy mechanisms provided for injuries involved falls and siblings landing on the injured child during play.[10,11]

The child's response to the event may also provide important clues for the evaluation. Most children with long bone fractures will manifest external signs of injury such as pain, swelling, or decreased use of the extremity.[12,13] However, some children, especially those with nondisplaced fractures, may have less severe responses and/or minimal external signs of injury.[14] The absence of any history of injury; a vague description of the event; delay in seeking care; the absence of an explanation for an injury, particularly in a nonambulatory child; or an inconsistent explanation should increase the medical care provider's concern that an injury was caused by child abuse (see Table 1).[11,15]

Medical History

The medical history of the patient is important and should include details about the child's birth history, including the pregnancy of the delivering parent.[7] Preterm infants, especially those requiring prolonged hospitalization, parenteral nutrition, or diuretic or corticosteroid therapy may have reduced bone mineral content, and therefore, may be more vulnerable to fracture with relatively minor trauma. In addition, bone strength can be affected by chronic diseases, such as renal insufficiency, metabolic acidosis, malabsorption, cerebral palsy or other neuromuscular disorders, other illnesses that limit mobility, and genetic diseases that affect skeletal development. Of note, fractures in children with overt rickets are rare.[16] The child's developmental history is important in differentiating unintentional fractures from abusive fractures. A thorough dietary history and history of medications that can predispose to fractures are important. The pediatrician or pediatric care provider should inquire about previous injuries including bruises.

Family History

A family history of multiple fractures (especially with minor trauma), early-onset hearing loss, abnormally developed dentition, blue sclerae, hypermobility, and short stature may suggest the possibility of osteogenesis imperfecta (OI) or other inherited bone diseases. However, a reported history of a familial bone disease does not preclude the diagnosis of abuse and can be appropriately verified during the evaluation.

Social History

It is important to obtain a complete psychosocial history, including asking who lives in the home and who has provided care for the child.[7] This history includes inquiries about social risk factors such as intimate partner violence, substance use/misuse including drugs and alcohol, mental illness, and previous involvement with child protective services and/ or law enforcement. Social risk factors can aid in safety planning and provision of family support; however, it is important to remember that these risk factors cannot be used to determine whether a fracture is the result of abuse.

Physical Examination

It is important to perform a comprehensive physical examination, including careful review of the growth parameters.[7] Growth parameters outside of expected may indicate neglect or may suggest genetic (eg, OI), endocrine, or metabolic disorders. It is important to document any signs or symptoms of fractures, such as swelling, limitation of motion, and point tenderness. A complete skin examination is important to look for bruises or other injures as well as an inspection of the oral cavity to look for signs of trauma and abnormal dentition.[17,18] The majority of children with fractures do not have bruising associated with the fracture; the presence or absence of bruising does not help to determine which fractures are caused by child abuse.[19,20] Bruising in a child who is not yet cruising or bruising in unusual locations, such as the ears, neck, or trunk, raises concern for child abuse and may prompt further evaluation.[17,21] In addition to looking for other injuries, a physical examination can help elucidate signs of other medical conditions such as those associated with bone fragility. For example, blue sclerae can be a marker in certain types of OI; dentinogenesis imperfecta is occasionally identified in older children with OI; and sparse, kinky hair is associated with Menkes disease.

IMAGING APPROACH

Radiological imaging can be guided with the assistance of a pediatric radiologist and/or a child abuse pediatrician. In cases of suspected abuse, it may be most prudent to consult local specialists or even transfer a child to a higher level of care.

It is recommended that children younger than 24 months who present with fracture(s) with increased concern for child abuse have a radiographic skeletal survey to look for other bone injuries or osseous abnormalities.[22,23] Additional fractures are identified in approximately 10% of skeletal surveys, with infants having the highest yields of additional fractures, up to 13% to 26%.[24–26] Skeletal surveys may be appropriate in some children 24 to 60 months of age, depending on the clinical suspicion of abuse. If specific clinical findings indicate an injury at a particular site, imaging of that area can be obtained regardless of the child's age.

The American College of Radiology has developed specific practice guidelines for skeletal surveys in children including the need for an appropriately skilled facility and radiology team.[27] A total of 21 images are obtained: frontal images of the appendicular skeleton, frontal and lateral views of the axial skeleton, and oblique views of the chest. Oblique views of the chest have been shown to increase the sensitivity, specificity, and accuracy of the identification of rib fractures.[28] Some institutions add lateral views of the long bones to improve detection of metaphyseal fractures.[29,30] A full 4 skull series is also obtained if there are concerns of head injury. Computed tomography (CT) 3-dimensional models may replace the skull series if performed with thin cuts and bone algorithm.[31–34] Fractures may be missed if the guidelines are not followed or if the images are of poor quality.[35] It is also recommended that a follow-up skeletal survey be performed approximately 2 weeks after the initial skeletal when the initial study is positive or has equivocal findings or when the initial study is negative and there is still strong clinical suspicion of abuse.[22,36] The follow-up examination may identify fractures not seen on the initial skeletal survey, clarify uncertain findings identified by the initial skeletal survey, and improve both sensitivity and specificity of the skeletal survey.[36,37] A large multicenter study found the follow-up study added new information in 21.5% of the patients with concern for nonaccidental trauma.[38] The number of images on the follow-up examination may be limited to 15 views by omitting the views of the skull, pelvis, and lateral spine.[39,40]

Radiography may assist in assessing the approximate time when an injury occurred, because, in an otherwise healthy child, long bone fractures heal following a particular sequence.[41–43] If the healing pattern of the injury is not consistent with the history provided, the concern for child abuse is increased.

Head imaging (CT and/or magnetic resonance imaging [MRI]) is indicated in children younger than 6 months and can be considered for any child younger than 1 year with a fracture suspicious for abuse.[44]

Bone scintigraphy may be used to complement the skeletal survey but cannot be the sole method of identifying fractures in infants. Although it has high overall sensitivity, it lacks specificity for fracture detection and may fail to identify classic metaphyseal lesions (CMLs) and skull fractures.[22,41,45] In addition, the radiation exposure is high, and in young children, sedation may be required. Scintigraphy does have high sensitivity for identifying rib fractures, which can be difficult to detect prior to healing. In toddlers and older children, bone scintigraphy or skeletal survey is only useful in cases where there are concerns for developmental delay as older children are able to express pain and/or loss of function.[22]

Chest CT can identify rib fractures that are not visualized on chest radiographs.[46–48] CT is particularly useful in detecting anterior rib fractures and rib fractures at all stages of healing. Although CT may be more sensitive in identifying these injuries, a routine chest CT exposes the child to significantly more radiation than chest radiography; modified CT parameters can help identify rib fractures at lower radiation doses.[49] It is important to minimize children's exposure to radiation while at the same time considering the risk to the child if abuse is not identified.[50] Therefore, selective application of this technique in certain clinical settings is appropriate.

Other modalities may become available in the future that provide more accurate identification of skeletal injuries. Whole-body short Tau inverse recovery (STIR) imaging, an MRI technique, may identify rib fractures not recognized on the radiographic skeletal survey.[51] In a study of 21 infants with suspected abuse, whole-body MRI at 1.5 Tesla was insensitive in the detection of CMLs and rib fractures.[52] Whole-body MRI can identify soft tissue injuries, such as muscle and subcutaneous edema, ligamentous injuries, and joint effusions, that can lead to the identification of skeletal injuries with additional radiographs.[52,53]

Bone scintigraphy with 18F-sodium fluoride positron emission tomography (18F-NaF PET) bone scan, although not widely available, may be useful in cases of equivocal or negative skeletal surveys when there is high clinical suspicion of abuse. If available, 18F-NaF PET bone scan has better contrast and spatial resolution than technetium 99m-labeled methylene diphosphonate.[45] The radiation dose is similar to bone scintigraphy with technetium 99m-labeled methylene diphosphonate but much higher than a skeletal survey; therefore, the use of bone scintigraphy is recommended only for cases when the findings of the study would significantly change the outcome of the case, for example when the findings are urgently needed to determine child safety or placement.

Although bone densitometry by dual energy x-ray absorptiometry (DXA) is useful to predict bone fragility and fracture risk in older adults, interpretation of bone densitometry in children and adolescents is often more problematic.[54] Peak bone mass is not achieved until early adulthood. In children, Z-scores are used to interpret bone density. The Z-score express the child's bone mineral density as a function of SDs above or below the average for an age- and sex-matched norm control population. [55] In addition, because bone size influences DXA, Z-scores can be adjusted for height Z-scores,[56] and for children with early or late puberty, interpreted in the context of pubertal status and/or bone age assessment. The International Society for Clinical Densitometry recommends that the diagnosis of osteoporosis in childhood not be made on the basis of low bone mass alone but, in the absence of vertebral fractures, also include a clinically significant history of low impact fracture.[57] A clinically significant fracture history is defined as two or more long bone fractures prior to the age of 10 or three or more long bone fractures before age 19. The recommendations currently apply to children 5 years and older, although reference data are available for children as young as 3 years.[58,59] Unfortunately, there are very limited reference data for infants and toddlers who are most at risk of suffering fractures caused by child abuse. Proper positioning for interpretable measurements in very young children is also often difficult.

LABORATORY EVALUATION

The clinical evaluation guides the laboratory evaluation. In children with fractures suspicious for abuse, serum calcium, phosphorus, and alkaline phosphatase are important, noting that alkaline phosphatase may be elevated because of bone remodeling associated with healing fractures. Other helpful laboratory tests include serum concentrations of parathyroid hormone (with a serum creatinine) and 25-hydroxyvitamin D, especially if there is clinical evidence of rickets or radiographic evidence of osteopenia or metabolic bone disease. Screening for abdominal trauma with liver enzymes as well as amylase and lipase concentration is important when severe or multiple injuries are identified. A urinalysis will screen for occult blood and any injuries to the renal system. Serum copper, ceruloplasmin concentrations, and vitamin C levels may be considered if the child has a dietary history that suggests copper deficiency or scurvy and has radiographic findings that include metaphyseal abnormalities.

If OI is suspected clinically or radiographically, *COL1A1* and *COL1A2* genes are sequenced first, because autosomal dominant mutations in these genes are associated with 80% to 85% of cases of OI.[60,61] If there is suspicion of OI and *COL1A1/COL1A2* sequencing is unremarkable, then testing of other genes associated with less common autosomal recessive or x-linked inherited forms of OI can be performed, because this testing is more sensitive than biochemical tests of type I collagen and may identify variants to guide testing of other family members.[62] Molecular testing is preferred over skin biopsy if there is clinical suspicion for OI. It is important to consult with a pediatric geneticist or genetic counselor in deciding which children to test and the preferred testing to order.[63] A child with OI can still be at risk for child abuse; hence, it is important to perform a comprehensive evaluation if there is a suspicion for child abuse.

DIAGNOSIS

When evaluating a child with a fracture, it is important that providers take a careful history of any injury event and then determine whether the mechanism described and the severity and timing are likely consistent with the injury identified (see Table 1).[64] The child's specific gross motor developmental abilities are important to assess if an offered injury mechanism is plausible. In addition, it is important to consider other nonabusive explanations for the injuries, including medical conditions or unintentional injury. A careful evaluation for other injuries is important, because the presence of additional injuries that are associated with child abuse increases the likelihood that a particular fracture was the result of abuse.[11,65] It is important to remember that even if a child has an underlying disorder or disability that could increase the likelihood of a fracture, the child may also have been abused, as children with disabilities and other special health care needs are at increased risk of child abuse.[66,67] If a provider is uncertain about how to evaluate an injury or if there is suspicion for abuse, a child abuse pediatrician or multidisciplinary child abuse team can assist in the evaluation.[68] In certain circumstances, the provider may need to consult an orthopedic surgeon, endocrinologist, radiologist, geneticist, or other subspecialist(s). In circumstances in which these specialists are not available in a timely fashion, a discussion with investigators on options to ensure child safety may be necessary.

All US states, commonwealths, and territories have mandatory reporting requirements for physicians and other health care providers. These requirements vary by state and it is important that providers are aware of and comply with the reporting requirements of their state. Typically, the standard for making a report is when the reporter "has reason to believe" that a child has been abused or neglected. This belief typically is a higher level of concern than that needed for a workup for suspected abuse. Sometimes, determining whether that "reasonable belief" or "reasonable suspicion" standard has been met can be nuanced and complex. Incontrovertible proof of abuse or neglect is not required for a child abuse report by state statutes, and on the other hand, one can initiate a workup for possible abuse but then not have enough concern to warrant a report. The assistance of a hospital child protection team and/or child abuse pediatrician can help with decision making.

It is important that providers recognize the existing bias that occurs in child abuse evaluations related to historically marginalized racial and ethnic populations.[9] Some processes that can assist in mitigating bias include education for medical and child welfare professionals, electronic medical record screening tools, and standardized pathways.[9,69]

Child's Age and Development

Approximately 80% of all fractures caused by child abuse occur in children younger than 18 months,[70] and approximately one quarter of fractures in children younger than 1 year are caused by child abuse.[3,15,71–73] Physical abuse is more likely to be the cause of femoral and humeral fractures in children who are not yet walking, compared with children who are ambulatory,[11,73–75] and the percentage of fractures caused by abuse declines sharply after the child begins to walk.[3,76,77]

Fracture Specificity for Abuse

There are no specific fractures that are pathognomonic for child abuse. However, fractures have differing levels of specificity for child abuse (see Table 2).[78] Knowing whether a specific fracture corresponds to high-, mid-, or low-specificity for child abuse can be helpful in work-up and diagnosis.

TABLE 2. Specificity of Radiologic Findings in Infants and Toddlers[78]

High specificity[a]	• Classic metaphyseal lesions (CMLs) • Rib fractures, especially posteromedial • Scapular fractures • Spinous process fractures • Sternal fractures
Moderate specificity	• Multiple fractures, especially bilateral • Fractures of different ages • Epiphyseal separations • Vertebral body fractures and subluxations • Digital fractures • Complex skull fractures
Common, but low specificity	• Subperiosteal new bone formation • Clavicular fractures • Long-bone shaft fractures • Linear skull fractures

[a] Highest specificity applies in infants.

Fractures With High Specificity for Abuse

Rib fractures have a high probability of being caused by abuse.[73,74,79] The positive predictive value of rib fractures for child abuse in children younger than 3 years was 95% in 1 retrospective study.[80] A systematic review of 10 studies that included infant data found a prevalence of abuse in 91% of children with rib fractures if motor vehicle collisions and metabolic bone diseases were excluded.[81] Rib fractures encountered in abuse may be the result of anterior to posterior compression of the chest, as when the perpetrator squeezes the chest, or a direct impact.[82] Historically, posterior rib fractures were thought to be most indicative of abuse, with a classic pattern described as fractures of 3 or 4 consecutive ribs, corresponding to the placement of the hand of the perpetrator while he or she squeezed or shook the child. In contrast, Kemp's meta-analysis from 2008 included 2 studies in which anterior rib fractures were found to be more common in abuse, and overall, rib fracture location did not correlate to the likelihood of abuse.[83] However, more recent studies with better imaging techniques confirm that posterior rib fractures are more commonly found in abuse.[49,84–86] Other less common causes of rib fractures in infants include motor vehicle collisions, minor trauma in infants who have increased bone fragility and, very rarely, trauma sustained during childbirth.[87–90]

Cardiopulmonary resuscitation (CPR) has been proposed as a cause of rib fractures, but conventional CPR with 2 fingers of 1 hand rarely causes fractures in children.[91–93] Since 2005, it has been recommended that in infants CPR be performed with both thumbs using 2 hands encircling the rib cage. There is evidence that this technique might cause increased incidence of rib fractures compared with the former technique. An analysis of infants who were discovered during autopsy to have rib fractures and had received 2-handed chest compressions antemortem suggested that 2-handed CPR is associated with anterior-lateral rib fractures of the third to sixth ribs.[94] In this small study, no posterior rib fractures were observed. The fractures in these infants were always multiple, uniformly involved the fourth rib, and were sometimes bilateral. An autopsy study that compared a cohort from 1997–2005 with one from 2006–2008 found a statistically significant increase in rib fractures in the later cohort in whom CPR was performed with the 2-hand technique, however there were no identified posterior rib fractures.[95] Although rib fractures have been reported with the 2-thumb technique, there have been no reports of posterior rib fractures.[96]

Classic metaphyseal lesions (CMLs) have high specificity for child abuse in infants.[79,97] CMLs are the most common long bone fracture found in infants who die with evidence of abusive injury.[98] CMLs are planar fractures through the primary spongiosa of the metaphysis. These fractures are thought to be caused when torsional and tractional shearing strains are applied across the metaphysis, as may occur with vigorous pulling or twisting of the infant's extremity, or from varus and valgus bending, as when there is an inversion or eversion strain to the joint.[99–102] Fractures resembling CMLs radiographically have been reported following difficult deliveries[103] and as a result of treatment for clubfoot.[104]

Depending on the projection of the radiograph, CMLs can have a corner, partial bucket handle, or bucket handle appearance.[101] CMLs frequently heal without subperiosteal new bone formation, because the tightly adherent periosteum in the metaphysis does not generate subperiosteal hemorrhage.[29] These fractures can heal quickly and be undetectable on plain radiographs 4 to 8 weeks after the injury.[99]

Fractures of the sternum, scapula, and pelvis are typically the result of high-energy trauma, such as a motor vehicle collision, pedestrian-struck, or a fall from a height. They are rare in children and should trigger concern for abuse in the absence of a plausible, verifiable incident.[85,105–108]

Long bone fractures in nonambulatory children are highly suspicious for abuse. The femur, humerus, and tibia are the most common long bones to be injured in child abuse.[71,109] A fracture of the humeral shaft in a child younger than 18 months has a high likelihood of having been caused by abuse.[83,110,111] Up to 54% of humerus fractures in children younger than 3 years are attributable to abuse, with a statistically significantly higher prevalence in those younger than 15 months.[83,111,112] Hymel and Jenny described a plausible unintentional mechanism resulting in a spiral-oblique fracture of the humerus in an infant.[113] When a young infant is rolled from the prone position to the supine while the child's arm is extended, the torsion and stress placed on the extended arm appeared to cause a spiral-oblique fracture of the midshaft of the humerus. Similarly, a cohort study of lower extremity injuries in children younger than 18 months found that nearly 75% were the result of abuse.[114] Although there are reports of isolated transverse femur fractures resulting from unintentional injury, these fractures still need a complete evaluation.[115,116] An isolated long-bone fracture in an ambulatory child without a plausible history presents a diagnostic challenge to clinicians. Although not as suspicious as the case of a long-bone fracture in a nonambulatory child, this situation should prompt a consideration for abuse. One multicenter study proposed initiating a child-abuse workup for a child younger than 12 months with any fracture, younger than 18 months with a femur fracture, and younger than 2 years with a humerus fracture.[117] However, in the absence of other corroborative injuries or skeletal survey findings, a definitive determination may not be possible in these cases.

Fractures With Moderate Specificity for Abuse

The presence of multiple fractures, fractures of different ages and/or stages of healing, and complex skull fractures have moderate specificity for physical abuse.[83,118] The likelihood of abuse for infants with 3 or more fractures is four- to sixfold when compared with infants with only 1 fracture.[3] In this study, 85.4% of cases (n = 298 infants) involving more than 3 fractures were determined to be child abuse versus 18.5% of cases (n = 5076 infants) involving a single fracture. In children in whom abuse is diagnosed, 50% overall and 80% of those younger than 1 year will have more than 1 fracture diagnosed.[106,119,120] Children in whom abusive head trauma is diagnosed can have bilateral acute symmetrical fractures from being shaken.[121–123]

Displaced physeal fractures or "epiphyseal separations" can be the result of abuse, particularly in the distal humerus. This fracture, also known as a transphyseal humerus fracture, is 13 times more likely to be abusive compared with displaced supracondylar humerus fractures in children.[124] The typical pattern is a displaced Salter-Harris 1 fracture in a child younger than 1 year. In these very young children, the distal humerus is still nonossified, which makes visualization on plain radiography challenging. Ultrasonography, MRI, or arthrography can aid in visualization, but these fractures are often diagnosed late, after healing has begun to occur and periosteal new bone formation is visible. One study found the diagnosis was missed on 56% of plain radiography but confirmed by ultrasonography in 100% of cases, with 38% of cases (all in children younger than 1 month old) secondary to birth trauma and 40% the result of abuse.[125] Skeletal survey is necessary not only in infants with distal humerus fracture with epiphyseal separation but also in children 12 through 23 months of age when the mechanism of injury provided is a short fall.[25]

Spine fractures are rare in children and account for 1% to 3% of both unintentional and abusive pediatric fractures.[126] Similarly to pelvic, scapular, and sternal fractures, spine fractures are typically the result of a high-energy injury and are, therefore, concerning in the absence of a verifiable incident, although not as specifically as those listed above. Spine fractures are frequently asymptomatic and can be the only finding on skeletal survey.[127] Flexion-extension injuries can cause a variety of fracture patterns in the posterior vertebral elements and are more likely to be symptomatic and associated with neurologic deficit.[128,129]

Fractures of the hands and feet, although common unintentional injuries in older children, are rare in nonambulatory children, with a prevalence ranging from 1% to 5%.[130,131] In skeletal surveys for suspected abuse, the prevalence of digital fractures increases to 20% in children with more than one fracture.[130]

Common Fractures With Low Specificity for Child Abuse

Clavicle fractures have been reported in 3% to 10% of cases of child abuse.[109,132] Clavicle fractures are a common birth-related injury. These fractures will demonstrate callus within the first 7 to 10 days of life; therefore, an acute clavicle (or humeral) fracture with no signs of healing in an infant older than 10 days is unlikely to be a birth injury. Although mid-shaft clavicular fractures can occur from short falls, distal and proximal clavicle fractures are uncommon in children younger than 3 years and likewise would prompt an evaluation for abuse.

Supracondylar humerus fractures are usually unintentional, and a history of a fall from playground equipment or a trampoline is typical.[111,112,133] One study of 388 supracondylar humerus fractures found that only 0.5% were the result of abuse.[133] However, younger children are more at risk for abuse, as another study reported 30% of supracondylar humerus fractures in children younger than 3 years to be the result of abuse.[111]

Distal radius and ulna buckle fractures are common compressive injuries caused by a fall on an outstretched arm or by running into a barrier with an outstretched arm. They are almost always unintentional in ambulatory children.

Femoral fractures in the nonambulatory child are more likely caused by child abuse, whereas these fractures in ambulatory children are most commonly unintentional.[11,65,134–136] In fact, ambulatory status is the single most important predictive factor for abuse in children with a femur fracture.[83,134,137] Several studies have demonstrated that a short fall to the knee may produce a torus or impacted transverse fracture of the distal femoral metadiaphysis.[10,138] Oblique distal femur metaphyseal fractures have been reported in children playing in a stationary activity center.[139] Although transverse distal femur fractures in nonambulatory children can result from abuse, this pattern can also result from an adult falling onto the child's femur while holding a child on their hip.[115,116] In both ambulatory and nonambulatory children, under some circumstances, falls on a stairway can cause a spiral femoral fracture. For example, a fall down several steps and landing with one leg folded or twisted underneath a child can lead to excessive torsional loading of the femur and a spiral fracture.[10] In ambulatory children, unintentional femoral fractures have been described in children who fell while running or who fell and landed in a split-leg position.[65]

"Toddler's fracture" refers to an isolated, nondisplaced, spiral fracture of the distal tibial metaphysis or diaphysis often most clearly visualized on an internal oblique radiograph. These fractures occur in children who have recently become ambulatory, often during seemingly trivial incidents such as a misstep off a stair or a trip over a toy or a playground fall.[140] A well-documented etiology is getting a foot caught on the edge of a slide while riding down on the lap of an adult or older child.[140] Similarly, a nondisplaced transverse or torus fracture of the proximal tibia is a common trampoline injury, caused by compression from "double-bounce"—the recoil of the mat as one child jumps and the other lands.[141]

Skull fractures are also common in both the unintentional and abusive settings. A simple, linear parietal fracture is the most common pattern in both unintentional and abusive trauma and in lower risk skull fractures, some researchers have recommended eliminating a skeletal survey.[15,142–144] Complex fractures such as stellate, depressed, diastatic, multiple, bilateral, or fractures crossing suture lines are more specific for abuse than simple fractures.[15,145,146] Therefore, corroborative history is especially important in evaluating skull fractures, and an implausible or inconsistent history is cause for concern. Household falls of fewer than 3 feet are associated with a low incidence of complex skull fracture.[147,148]

DIFFERENTIAL DIAGNOSIS OF FRACTURES

Trauma: Child Abuse Versus Unintentional Injuries

Fractures are a common childhood injury and account for between 8% and 12% of all pediatric injuries.[149–151] In infants and toddlers, physical abuse is the cause of 12% to 20% of fractures.[3] Although unintentional fractures are much more common than fractures caused by child abuse, the clinician should remain aware of the possibility of abusive injury. Although some fracture types are highly suggestive of physical abuse, no pattern can exclude child abuse.[134,152] Specifically, it is important to recognize that any fracture, even fractures that are commonly unintentional injuries, can be caused by child abuse. Certain details that can help the clinician determine whether a fracture was caused by abuse rather than unintentional injury include the history, the child's age and developmental stage, the type and location of the fracture, the age of the fracture, and an understanding of the mechanism that causes the fracture type. The presence of multiple fractures, fractures of different ages or stages of healing, delay in obtaining medical treatment, and the presence of other injuries suspicious for abuse (eg, coexisting injuries to the skin, internal organs, or central nervous system) raises the likelihood of abuse.

An understanding of the extent and type of load that is necessary to cause a particular long bone fracture can help to determine whether a specific fracture is consistent with the injury described by the caregiver.[153,154] Transverse fractures of the long bones are caused by the application of a bending load in a direction that is perpendicular to the bone, while spiral fractures are caused by torsion or twisting of a long bone along its long axis. Oblique fractures are caused by a combination of bending and torsion loads.[155] Torus or buckle fractures are the result of compression from axial loading along the length of the bone. Although earlier studies had suggested that spiral fractures should always raise suspicion for child abuse,[70] more recent studies do not show that any particular fracture pattern can distinguish between abuse and nonabuse with certainty.[11,156]

Falls are common in childhood.[157] Short falls can cause fractures, but they rarely result in additional significant injury (eg, neurologic injury).[152,158–160] In a retrospective study of short falls, parents reported that 40% of the children before 2 years of age had suffered at least one fall from a height of between 6 inches and 4 feet. Approximately one quarter of these children suffered an injury; bruises were the most common injury observed.[65]

Syndromes, Metabolic Disorders, Systemic Disease

Preexisting medical conditions and bone disease may increase the bone vulnerability to fracture. Some of these conditions may manifest with skeletal changes, such as metaphyseal irregularity and subperiosteal new bone formation. These entities are considered in the differential diagnosis of childhood fractures.

Osteogenesis Imperfecta

OI is a group of inherited connective tissue disorders with remarkable clinical and genetic heterogeneity. The hallmark feature is bone fragility with susceptibility to fractures from minimal trauma and low bone mineral density or osteopenia.[161] Other secondary features include growth failure, macrocephaly, Wormian bones of the skull, blue sclera, dentinogenesis imperfecta (weak, discolored, or translucent teeth), hearing loss, scoliosis, limb deformities, hyperextensible joints, bruising, and cardiopulmonary complications. Sometimes OI symptoms resolve or lessen after puberty.[60,162] When OI is suspected, multidisciplinary clinical management and genetic analysis are needed.

Approximately 80% to 85% of cases are autosomal dominantly inherited and present with a full spectrum of OI severity because of heterozygous mutations of the *COL1A1* and *COL1A2* genes, which encode type I collagen that forms the structural framework of bone.[60,162] This includes perinatal lethal OI (previously OI type II), classic nondeforming OI with blue sclera (previously OI type I), progressively deforming OI (previously OI type III), and common variable OI with normal sclera (previously OI type IV). Rare autosomal recessive forms of OI are caused by variants in genes whose protein products interact with collagen for post-translational modification or folding.[60]

TABLE 3. Characteristics of Osteogenesis Imperfecta

Fragile, bones with few, some, or many of the following findings:	• Poor linear growth • Macrocephaly • Triangular-shaped face • Blue sclerae • Hearing impairment as a result of otosclerosis (usually manifests in adulthood) • Hypoplastic, translucent, carious, late-erupting, or discolored teeth • Easy bruisability • Inguinal and/or umbilical hernias • Limb deformities • Hyperextensible joints • Scoliosis and/or kyphosis • Wormian bones of the skull • Undermineralized bones

Although OI is a genetic disorder, many children have de novo mutations or autosomal recessive disease and, therefore, have no family history of bone fragility. In addition, the disease presentation within affected members of the same family can be quite variable. Phenotypic disease expression depends on the nature of the variant and its expression in target tissues.[163]

The diagnosis of OI is often suggested by features outlined in Table 3. The types of fractures can help determine whether the diagnosis is likely. For example, transverse and diaphyseal humerus and olecranon fractures are most likely to indicate OI compared with physeal and supracondylar humerus fractures that were least likely to indicate OI.[164,165] It is unusual to have multiple long bone fractures or rib fractures, particularly in infancy, without other clinical and radiographic evidence of OI.[166,167]

OI can be misdiagnosed as child abuse.[168] On the other hand, OI is sometimes also suggested as the cause of fractures in children who have been abused. When fractures continue to occur when a child is placed in a protective environment, a more thorough evaluation for an underlying bone disease is needed. Child abuse is more common than OI, and children with OI and other metabolic or genetic conditions may also be abused.[169–171]

Preterm Birth

Preterm infants have decreased bone mineralization at birth, but after the first year of life, bone density normalizes. Metabolic bone disease of prematurity (MBDP), defined as preterm infant skeletal undermineralization arising from inadequate prenatal and postnatal calcium and phosphate accretion, has been well described as a complication in low birth weight infants.[172,173] Infants born at less than 28 weeks' gestation or who weigh less than 1500 g at birth are particularly vulnerable. This condition is defined as reduced bone mineral content with characteristic biochemical and/or radiographic changes.[174,175] MBDP is estimated to occur in 16% to 40% of infants with very low birth weight (<1500 g) and extremely low birth weight (<1000 g). MBDP is multifactorial. Infants are at higher risk if they receive prolonged (for 4 or more weeks) total parenteral nutrition, have bronchopulmonary dysplasia, and/or received a prolonged course of diuretics, antacids, or steroids.[176] MBDP can be ameliorated and even avoided if infants are monitored closely and adequate nutritional and mineral supplementation is initiated in the neonatal intensive care unit.

Osteopenia commonly manifests biochemically between 6 and 12 weeks of life. Fractures associated with MBDP usually occur in the first year of life.[17,177] Rib fractures are typically encountered incidentally, whereas long bone fractures commonly present with extremity swelling. MBDP can be associated with rickets, and in such cases, metaphyseal irregularities, like fraying and cupping of the metaphyses, may be present.[178]

Vitamin D Deficiency Rickets

Vitamin D insufficiency in otherwise healthy infants and toddlers is common. Approximately 40% of infants and toddlers ages 8 to 24 months in an urban clinic had laboratory evidence of suboptimal vitamin D (serum 25-hydroxyvitamin D concentrations of ≤30 ng/mL).[179] Fewer had vitamin D insufficiency or deficiency, generally defined as ≤20 ng/mL for insufficiency and <12 ng/mL for deficiency.[180] Maternal vitamin D deficiency and prolonged breastfeeding without vitamin D supplementation is a common feature placing infants at risk of low circulating vitamin D, although increased skin pigmentation and/or lack of sunlight exposure can contribute. Prolonged vitamin D deficiency may leads to rickets, characterized by bone changes including demineralization, loss of the zone of provisional calcification, widening and irregularity of the physis, and fraying and cupping of the metaphysis.[181] Of note, despite the high prevalence of suboptimal serum vitamin D levels in infants and toddlers, rickets is uncommon.[182]

Low vitamin D concentrations and rickets have been proposed as causes of infant fracture.[183] However, no evidence supports that vitamin D deficiency or insufficiency predisposes a child to fracture. Radiographs of children with rickets and osteomalacia will sometimes demonstrate "looser zones;" these areas likely represent insufficiency/stress fractures and are not associated with bony angulation, discontinuity, or displacement.[16] A systematic clinical, laboratory, and radiologic assessment along with history will exclude that vitamin D insufficiency or deficiency is the cause of fracture(s).[184–186] Schilling et al found no difference in serum concentrations of 25-hydroxyvitamin D in young children with fractures suspicious for abuse and noninflicted fractures.[187] Vitamin D insufficiency was not associated with multiple fractures, in particular rib fractures or CMLs.

In a study of 45 young children with radiographic evidence of rickets, investigators found that fractures occurred only in those infants and toddlers who were mobile.[174] Fractures were seen in 17.5% of the children, and these children were 8 to 19 months of age. The fractures involved long bones, anterior and anterior-lateral ribs, and metatarsal and metaphyseal regions. The metaphyseal fractures occurred closer to the diaphysis in the background of florid metaphyseal rachitic changes and did not resemble the juxtaphyseal corner or bucket handle appearance of the CML.[174] In a series of infant fatalities with head trauma, CMLs, and other skeletal injuries, radiographic or histologic rachitic changes were not present.[188]

Fractures Secondary to Demineralization From Disuse

Any child with a severe disability that limits or prevents ambulation can be at risk of fractures secondary to disuse demineralization, even with normal handling, physical therapy and range of motion exercises.[189,190] They may also be less able to report symptoms (because of cognitive or communication impairments) or less likely to display signs.[191] These fractures, however, are usually diaphyseal rather than CMLs. Often, these fractures occur during physical therapy and range-of-motion exercises. It can be difficult to distinguish between abusive and unintentional fractures occurring in these children. At the same time, children with disabilities are at an increased risk of maltreatment.[192–194]

Scurvy

Scurvy is caused by insufficient intake of vitamin C, which is important for the synthesis of collagen. Although extremely rare today because formula, human milk, fruits, and vegetables contain vitamin C, scurvy may develop in older infants and children exclusively given cow milk without vitamin supplementation and in children who eat foods containing no vitamin C.[195,196] Although scurvy can result in metaphyseal irregularity, other osseous changes, including osteopenia, increased sclerosis of the zones of provisional calcification, dense epiphyseal rings, and extensive calcification of subperiosteal and soft tissue hemorrhages, will point to the diagnosis of scurvy.

Copper Deficiency

Copper plays a role in cartilage formation. Preterm infants are born with lower stores of copper than term infants, because copper is accumulated at a faster rate during the last trimester.[197] Copper insufficiency may be observed in children with severe nutritional disorders, for example, liver failure or short gut syndrome.[198] This deficiency is not likely to be observed in full-term children younger than 6 months or preterm infants younger than 2.5 months of age, because fetal copper stores are sufficient for this length of time. In addition, human milk and formula contain sufficient copper to prevent deficiency. Psychomotor retardation, hypotonia, hypopigmentation, pallor, and a sideroblastic anemia are some of the characteristic findings of copper deficiency in infants. Radiologic changes that may increase suspicion for possible deficiency include cupping and fraying of the metaphyses, sickle-shaped metaphyseal spurs, significant demineralization, and subperiosteal new bone formation.[197] Copper deficiency is a rare condition that may result in metaphyseal fragmentation; however, these will be accompanied by other clinical and biochemical findings of copper deficiency.

Menkes Disease

Menkes disease, formerly known as Menkes kinky hair syndrome, is a very rare congenital defect of copper metabolism.[199] Menkes disease is an X-linked recessive condition that occurs only in the male sex; it is attributable to pathogenic variants in the *ATP7A* gene, that encodes a copper-transporting ATPase. Although it has many of the features of dietary copper deficiency, anemia is not associated with Menkes disease. Classic Menkes disease typically presents after 6 to 12 weeks of normal health and pregnancy, usually initially presenting with feeding difficulties and/or seizure. Metaphyseal fragmentation and subperiosteal new bone formation may be observed on radiographs, and the findings may be difficult to distinguish from fractures caused by abuse.[200] Other signs of Menkes disease include sparse, kinky hair, Wormian bones, anterior rib flaring, failure to thrive, and developmental delay. A characteristic finding is tortuous cerebral vessels. Intracranial hemorrhage can occur in Menkes disease but has not been reported in infants with nutritional copper deficiency.[199]

Systemic Disease

Chronic renal disease affects bone metabolism, because it interferes with vitamin D metabolism. Chronic renal disease can cause renal osteodystrophy, resulting in the same radiographic changes as nutritional rickets.[201] Chronic liver disease (eg, biliary atresia) can interfere with vitamin D metabolism; children with chronic liver disease are at an increased risk of rickets, low bone mineral density, and fractures.[202] Fanconi syndrome, hypophosphatasia, hypophosphatemic (vitamin D-resistant) rickets, hyperparathyroidism, and renal tubular acidosis also cause clinical variants of rickets with bone changes associated with alterations in calcium, phosphate, alkaline phosphatase, parathyroid hormone, and/or vitamin D metabolites.

EVALUATION OF SIBLINGS

Siblings, especially twins, and other young household contacts of children who have been physically abused are at high risk of also being abused, and it is recommended that they also be evaluated for possible abuse.[203] In a study of 795 siblings in 400 households of a child who had been abused or neglected, all siblings in 37% of households and some siblings in 20% of households had suffered some form of maltreatment.[204] In this study, which included all manifestations of maltreatment, siblings were found to be more at risk of maltreatment if the index child suffered moderate or severe maltreatment. In addition to a careful evaluation, imaging should be considered for any siblings younger than 2 years, especially if there are signs of abuse.

LEGAL CHALLENGES

Alternative, nonevidence-based explanations for child abuse have been proffered by a few vocal physicians both in the medical literature and in legal civil and criminal proceedings. These explanations have been used in court to assert that the evidence supporting the diagnosis of abuse is suspect. A false, fabricated condition is "temporary brittle bone disease" (TBBD).[205] TBBD has been invoked for cases in which infants younger than 6 months are said to experience multiple initial (often painless) fractures in a home environment that cease when the child is removed from the home. TBBD is described as a self-limited bone demineralization attributable to antacid use by the mother during pregnancy, transient copper deficiency, or limited prenatal movement. Experts from many subspecialties have exposed TBBD as an unproven, dishonest sham.[206] Another flawed explanation for fractures during infancy is an undiagnosed genetic disease like hypermobile Ehlers-Danlos syndrome (EDS).[207] Again, this represents a false explanation for multiple infant fractures without evidence, particularly for syndromes such as hypermobile EDS in which long bone and rib fractures are not components of the clinical disease presentation or diagnostic criteria for the hypermobile EDS.[208,209] Other "experts" maintain that CMLs and posterior rib fractures nearly pathognomonic of child abuse are often instead rachitic changes.[210] Yet, data suggest that these findings are distinct and distinguishable radiographically.[188,211,212] These false explanations and irresponsible legal testimony put forth by these denialists undoubtedly have resulted, at times, in children being returned to life-threatening home environments.

CONCLUSION

Optimal assessment of the child with fractures and suspected child abuse requires careful review of the clinical history, a thorough physical examination, rigorous imaging evaluation, and correlation with bone health laboratory studies. A multidisciplinary evaluation with consultation as indicated to a child abuse pediatrician, orthopaedic surgeon, radiologist, endocrinologist, and/or geneticist can help ensure a correct diagnosis of unintentional injury, abuse, or disease process.

KEY POINTS AND RECOMMENDATIONS

1. Fractures that are more concerning for abuse include fractures in a nonambulatory child, fractures that are not consistent with the history provided or for which no history of injury is given, and fractures that have a high or moderate specificity for abuse.
2. In children in whom abuse is suspected, the following is recommended:
   a. On physical examination, a close evaluation of all areas of the skin to look for other injuries is important, as well as closely looking for indications of a medical condition, such as OI.
   b. Medical history and family history are important to evaluate for prior injuries, fractures, or medical conditions that would predispose a child to fracture more easily.
   c. A head CT is recommended in children up to 6 months of age to rule out a head injury; a skeletal survey is recommended up to 2 years of age to evaluate for occult fractures, although the survey may be performed up to 5 years of age in certain situations. All children with significant concern for abuse will also need a follow up skeletal survey 2 weeks after the initial evaluation to assess for occult fractures.
   d. The laboratory evaluation is important, to include serum calcium, phosphorus, and alkaline phosphatase. Also helpful are serum parathyroid hormone and 25-hydroxyvitamin D. In severe trauma, liver enzymes, lipase, amylase, and a urinalysis are helpful to evaluate for abdominal trauma. Finally, more detailed evaluation for metabolic bone disease, such as OI, can be conducted on the basis of clinical suspicion.
3. Reporting suspected abusive fractures to authorities is based on reasonable concern/suspicion for abuse and subject to individual state statutes.
4. Bias is known to exist in child abuse diagnosis and reporting. It is important to be aware of that bias and attempt to limit its effects.

LEAD AUTHORS

Suzanne Haney, MD, FAAP
Susan Scherl, MD, FAAP
Linda DiMeglio, MD, FAAP
Jeanette Perez-Rossello, MD, FAAP
Sabah Servaes, MD, FAAP
Nadia Merchant, MD, FAAP

COUNCIL ON CHILD ABUSE AND NEGLECT EXECUTIVE COMMITTEE, 2023–2024

Antoinette Laskey, MD, MPH, MBA, FAAP, Chairperson
Suzanne Breen Haney, MD, MS, FAAP, Immediate Past Chairperson
Andrea Gottsegen Asnes, MD, FAAP
Verena Wyvill Brown, MD, FAAP
Amanda Bird Hoffert Gilmartin, MD, FAAP
Rebecca Girardet, MD, FAAP
Nancy Dayzie Heavilin, MD, FAAP
Natalie Kissoon, MD, FAAP
Bethany Anne Mohr, MD, FAAP
Patricia Dinalynn Morgan, MD, FAAP
Shalon Marie Nienow, MD, FAAP
Norell Rosado, MD, FAAP

LIAISONS

Sofia Charania, MD – Section on Pediatric Trainees
Rachael Keefe, MD, MPH, FAAP – Council on Foster Care, Adoption, and Kinship Care
Cara Kelly – Administration for Children, Youth, and Families
Anna Kerlek – American Academy of Child and Adolescent Psychiatry
Elizabeth Anne Swedo – Centers for Disease Control and Prevention

STAFF

Tammy Piaza Hurley
Jeff Hudson, MA

SECTION ON ORTHOPAEDICS EXECUTIVE COMMITTEE, 2023–2024

Joshua Abzug, MD, FAAP, Chairperson
Yi-Meng Yen, MD, FAAP, Vice chairperson
Martin J. Herman, MD, FAAP, Immediate Past Chairperson
Lindsay Andras, MD, FAAP
Aristides Cruz, Jr, MD, FAAP
Christine Ho, MD, FAAP
Alexa Karkenny, MD, FAAP
J. Todd Lawrence, MD, PhD, FAAP
Susan Scherl, MD, FAAP

LIAISONS

Blaise Nemeth, MD, FAAP, Non-operative Subcommittee Chairperson
Natalie Stork, MD, FAAP, Non-operative Subcommittee Vice Chairperson

STAFF

Niccole Alexander, MPP

SECTION ON RADIOLOGY EXECUTIVE COMMITTEE, 2023–2024

Hansel J. Otero, MD, FAAP, Chairperson
Patricia Trinidad Acharya, MD, FAAP
Katherine Barton, MD, FAAP
Ellen Benya, MD, FAAP
Brandon Patrick Brown, MD MA, FAAP
Reza James Daugherty, MD, FAAP

STAFF

Laura Laskosz, MPH

SECTION ON ENDOCRINOLOGY EXECUTIVE COMMITTEE, 2023–2024

Kupper Anthony Wintergerst, MD, FAAP, Chairperson
Jane Lockwood Lynch, MD, Immediate Past Chairperson
Lucy Diane Mastrandrea, MD, PhD, FAAP
Jennifer Marie Barker, MD, FAAP
Kathleen Elizabeth Bethin, MD, FAAP
Chineze Ebo, MD, FAAP
David H. Jelley, MD, FAAP
Bess Adkins Marshall, MD, FAAP

STAFF

Laura Laskosz, MPH

ABBREVIATIONS

CML: classic metaphyseal lesion
CT: computed tomography
CPR: cardiopulmonary resuscitation
DXA: dual energy x-ray absorptiometry
EDS: Ehlers Danlos syndrome
MRI: magnetic resonance imaging
MBDP: metabolic bone disease of prematurity
OI: osteogenesis imperfecta
TBBD: temporary brittle bone disease

There may be instances where no action is necessary. This process has been approved by the AAP Board of Directors.

FUNDING: No external funding.

Clinical reports from the American Academy of Pediatrics benefit from expertise and resources of liaisons and internal (AAP) and external reviewers. However, clinical reports from the American Academy of Pediatrics may not reflect the views of the liaisons or the organizations or government agencies that they represent.

The guidance in this report does not indicate an exclusive course of treatment or serve as a standard of medical care. Variations, taking into account individual circumstances, may be appropriate. All clinical reports from the American Academy of Pediatrics automatically expire 5 years after publication unless reaffirmed, revised, or retired at or before that time.

Accepted for Publication Date: November 22, 2024

https://doi.org/10.1542/peds.2024-070074

REFERENCES

1. Pierce MC, Magana JN, Kaczor K, et al. The Prevalence of Bruising Among Infants in Pediatric Emergency Departments. *Ann Emerg Med.* Jan 2016;67(1):1–8. doi: 10.1016/j.annemergmed.2015.06.021
2. Loder RT, Feinberg JR. Orthopaedic injuries in children with non-accidental trauma: demographics and incidence from the 2000 kids' inpatient database. *J Pediatr Orthop.* Jun 2007;27(4):421–6. doi: 10.1097/01.bpb.0000271328.79481.07
3. Leventhal JM, Martin KD, Asnes AG. Incidence of fractures attributable to abuse in young hospitalized children: results from analysis of a United States database. *Pediatrics.* 2008;122(3):599–604. doi: 10.1542/peds.2007-1959
4. Jenny C, Hymel KP, Ritzen A, Reinert SE, Hay TC. Analysis of missed cases of abusive head trauma. *JAMA.* Feb 17 1999;281(7):621–6. doi: 10.1001/jama.281.7.621
5. Sheets LK, Leach ME, Koszewski IJ, Lessmeier AM, Nugent M, Simpson P. Sentinel injuries in infants evaluated for child physical abuse. *Pediatrics.* Apr 2013;131(4):701–7. doi: 10.1542/peds.2012-2780
6. Ravichandiran N, Schuh S, Bejuk M, et al. Delayed identification of pediatric abuse-related fractures. *Pediatrics.* Jan 2010;125(1):60–6. doi: 10.1542/peds.2008-3794
7. Christian CW, Committee on Child A, Neglect AAoP. The evaluation of suspected child physical abuse. *Pediatrics.* May 2015;135(5):e1337–54. doi: 10.1542/peds.2015-0356
8. Harper NS, Lewis T, Eddleman S, Lindberg DM, Ex SI. Follow-up skeletal survey use by child abuse pediatricians. *Child Abuse Negl.* Jan 2016;51:336–42. doi: 10.1016/j.chiabu.2015.08.015
9. Palusci VJ, Botash AS. Race and Bias in Child Maltreatment Diagnosis and Reporting. *Pediatrics.* Jul 2021;148(1). doi: 10.1542/peds.2020-049625
10. Pierce MC, Bertocci GE, Janosky JE, et al. Femur fractures resulting from stair falls among children: an injury plausibility model. *Pediatrics.* Jun 2005;115(6):1712–22. doi: 10.1542/peds.2004-0614
11. Hui C, Joughin E, Goldstein S, et al. Femoral fractures in children younger than three years: the role of nonaccidental injury. *Journal of Pediatric Orthopedics.* 2008;28(3):297–302.

12. Rivara FP, Parish RA, Mueller BA. Extremity injuries in children: predictive value of clinical findings. *Pediatrics.* 1986;78(5):803–807.

13. Taitz J, Moran K, O'Meara M. Long bone fractures in children under 3 years of age: is abuse being missed in Emergency Department presentations? *J Paediatr Child Health.* 2004;40(4):170–4.

14. Farrell C, Rubin DM, Downes K, Dormans J, Christian CW. Symptoms and time to medical care in children With accidental extremity fractures. *Pediatrics.* 2011;doi: 10.1542/peds.2010-0691

15. Leventhal JM, Thomas SA, Rosenfield NS, Markowitz RI. Fractures in young children. Distinguishing child abuse from unintentional injuries. *Am J Dis Child.* 1993;147(1):87–92.

16. Aldana Sierra MC, Christian CW. Vitamin D, rickets and child abuse: controversies and evidence. *Pediatr Radiol.* May 2021; 51(6):1014–1022. doi: 10.1007/s00247-020-04893-w

17. Pierce MC, Kaczor K, Aldridge S, O'Flynn J, Lorenz DJ. Bruising characteristics discriminating physical child abuse from accidental trauma. *Pediatrics.* Jan 2010;125(1):67–74. doi: 10.1542/peds.2008-3632

18. Pierce MC, Kaczor K, Lorenz DJ, et al. Validation of a Clinical Decision Rule to Predict Abuse in Young Children Based on Bruising Characteristics. *JAMA Netw Open.* Apr 1 2021;4(4): e215832. doi: 10.1001/jamanetworkopen.2021.5832

19. Peters ML, Starling SP, Barnes-Eley ML, Heisler KW. The presence of bruising associated with fractures. *Arch Pediatr Adolesc Med.* 2008;162(9):877–881. doi: 10.1001/archpedi.162.9.877

20. Valvano TJ, Binns HJ, Flaherty EG, Leonhardt DE. Does bruising help determine which fractures are caused by abuse? *Child Maltreat.* 2009;14:376–381. doi: 10.1177/1077559508326356

21. Sugar NF, Taylor JA, Feldman KW. Bruises in infants and toddlers: those who don't cruise rarely bruise. Puget Sound Pediatric Research Network. *Archives of Pediatrics & Adolescent Medicine.* 1999;153(4):399–403.

22. Section on R, American Academy of P. Diagnostic imaging of child abuse. *Pediatrics.* May 2009;123(5):1430–5. doi: 10.1542/peds.2009-0558

23. Kellogg ND, American Academy of Pediatrics Committee on Child A, Neglect. Evaluation of suspected child physical abuse. *Pediatrics.* Jun 2007;119(6):1232–41. doi: 10.1542/peds.2007-0883

24. Duffy SO, Squires J, Fromkin JB, Berger RP. Use of skeletal surveys to evaluate for physical abuse: analysis of 703 consecutive skeletal surveys. *Pediatrics.* Jan 2011;127(1):e47–52. doi: 10.1542/peds.2010-0298

25. Wood JN, Fakeye O, Feudtner C, Mondestin V, Localio R, Rubin DM. Development of guidelines for skeletal survey in young children with fractures. *Pediatrics.* Jul 2014;134(1):45–53. doi: 10.1542/peds.2013-3242

26. Paine CW, Wood JN. Skeletal surveys in young, injured children: A systematic review. *Child Abuse Negl.* Feb 2018;76:237–249. doi: 10.1016/j.chiabu.2017.11.004

27. Expert Panel on Pediatric I. ACR–SPR PRACTICE PARAMETER FOR THE PERFORMANCE AND INTERPRETATION OF SKELETAL SURVEYS *IN CHILDREN.* American College of Radiology. https://www.acr.org/-/media/ACR/Files/Practice-Parameters/Skeletal-Survey.pdf

28. Ingram J, Connell J, Hay T, Strain J, Mackenzie T. Oblique radiographs of the chest in nonaccidental trauma. *Emergency Radiology.* 2000;7(1):42–46.

29. Tsai A, Connolly SA, Ecklund K, Johnston PR, Kleinman PK. Subperiosteal new bone formation with the distal tibial classic metaphyseal lesion: prevalence on radiographic skeletal surveys. *Pediatr Radiol.* Apr 2019;49(4):551–558. doi: 10.1007/s00247-018-4329-z

30. Karmazyn B, Duhn RD, Jennings SG, et al. Long bone fracture detection in suspected child abuse: contribution of lateral views. *Pediatr Radiol.* Apr 2012;42(4):463–9. doi: 10.1007/s00247-011-2248-3

31. Prabhu SP, Newton AW, Perez-Rossello JM, Kleinman PK. Three-dimensional skull models as a problem-solving tool in suspected child abuse. *Pediatr Radiol.* Mar 2013;43(5):575–81. doi: 10.1007/s00247-012-2546-4

32. Culotta PA, Crowe JE, Tran QA, et al. Performance of computed tomography of the head to evaluate for skull fractures in infants with suspected non-accidental trauma. *Pediatr Radiol.* Jan 2017; 47(1):74–81. doi: 10.1007/s00247-016-3707-7

33. Sharp SR, Patel SM, Brown RE, Landes C. Head imaging in suspected non accidental injury in the paediatric population. In the advent of volumetric CT imaging, has the skull X-ray become redundant? *Clin Radiol.* May 2018;73(5):449–453. doi: 10.1016/j.crad.2017.11.027

34. Martin A, Paddock M, Johns CS, et al. Avoiding skull radiographs in infants with suspected inflicted injury who also undergo head CT: "a no-brainer?". *Eur Radiol.* Mar 2020;30(3):1480–1487. doi: 10.1007/s00330-019-06579-w

35. van Rijn RR. How should we image skeletal injuries in child abuse? *Pediatric radiology.* 2009;39:226.

36. Kleinman PK, Nimkin K, Spevak MR, et al. Follow-up skeletal surveys in suspected child abuse. *AJR Am J Roentgenol.* Oct 1996;167(4):893–6. doi: 10.2214/ajr.167.4.8819377

37. Bennett BL, Chua MS, Care M, Kachelmeyer A, Mahabee-Gittens M. Retrospective review to determine the utility of follow-up skeletal surveys in child abuse evaluations when the initial skeletal survey is normal. *BMC Res Notes.* Sep 12 2011;4:354. doi: 10.1186/1756-0500-4-354

38. Harper NS, Eddleman S, Lindberg DM, Ex SI. The utility of follow-up skeletal surveys in child abuse. *Pediatrics.* Mar 2013;131(3):e672–8. doi: 10.1542/peds.2012-2608

39. Hansen KK, Keeshin BR, Flaherty E, et al. Sensitivity of the limited view follow-up skeletal survey. *Pediatrics.* Aug 2014;134(2):242–8. doi: 10.1542/peds.2013-4024

40. Harlan SR, Nixon GW, Campbell KA, Hansen K, Prince JS. Follow-up skeletal surveys for nonaccidental trauma: can a more limited survey be performed? *Pediatr Radiol.* Sep 2009;39(9):962–8. doi: 10.1007/s00247-009-1313-7

41. Mandelstam SA, Cook D, Fitzgerald M, Ditchfield MR. Complementary use of radiological skeletal survey and bone

scintigraphy in detection of bony injuries in suspected child abuse. *Arch Dis Child.* May 2003;88(5):387–90; discussion 387–90. doi: 10.1136/adc.88.5.387

42. Messer DL, Adler BH, Brink FW, Xiang H, Agnew AM. Radiographic timelines for pediatric healing fractures: a systematic review. *Pediatr Radiol.* Jul 2020;50(8):1041–1048. doi: 10.1007/s00247-020-04648-7

43. Walters MM, Forbes PW, Buonomo C, Kleinman PK. Healing patterns of clavicular birth injuries as a guide to fracture dating in cases of possible infant abuse. *Pediatr Radiol.* Oct 2014; 44(10):1224–9. doi: 10.1007/s00247-014-2995-z

44. Rubin DM, Christian CW, Bilaniuk LT, Zazyczny KA, Durbin DR. Occult head injury in high-risk abused children. *Pediatrics.* Jun 2003;111 (6 Pt 1):1382–6. doi: 10.1542/peds.111.6.1382

45. Drubach LA, Johnston PR, Newton AW, Perez-Rossello JM, Grant FD, Kleinman PK. Skeletal trauma in child abuse: detection with 18F-NaF PET. *Radiology.* Apr 2010;255(1):173–81. doi: 10.1148/radiol.09091368

46. Wootton-Gorges SL, Stein-Wexler R, Walton JW, Rosas AJ, Coulter KP, Rogers KK. Comparison of computed tomography and chest radiography in the detection of rib fractures in abused infants. *Child abuse & neglect.* 2008;32(6):659–663.

47. Sanchez TR, Lee JS, Coulter KP, Seibert JA, Stein-Wexler R. CT of the chest in suspected child abuse using submillisievert radiation dose. *Pediatr Radiol.* Jul 2015;45(7):1072–6. doi: 10.1007/s00247-014-3245-0

48. Pomeranz CB, Barrera CA, Servaes SE. Value of chest CT over skeletal surveys in detection of rib fractures in pediatric patients. *Clin Imaging.* Feb 2022;82:103–109. doi: 10.1016/j.clinimag.2021.11.008

49. Sanchez TR, Grasparil AD, Chaudhari R, Coulter KP, Wootton-Gorges SL. Characteristics of Rib Fractures in Child Abuse-The Role of Low-Dose Chest Computed Tomography. *Pediatr Emerg Care.* Feb 2018;34(2):81–83. doi: 10.1097/PEC.0000000000000608

50. Brody AS, Frush DP, Huda W, Brent RL, American Academy of Pediatrics Section on R. Radiation risk to children from computed tomography. *Pediatrics.* Sep 2007;120(3):677–82. doi: 10.1542/peds.2007-1910

51. Stranzinger E, Kellenberger CJ, Braunschweig S, Hopper R, Huisman TAGM. Whole-body STIR MR imaging in suspected child abuse: an alternative to skeletal survey radiography? *European Journal of Radiology Extra.* 2007;63(1):43–47.

52. Perez-Rossello JM, Connolly SA, Newton AW, Zou KH, Kleinman PK. Whole-body MRI in suspected infant abuse. *AJR Am J Roentgenol.* Sep 2010;195(3):744–50. doi: 10.2214/AJR.09.3364

53. Proisy M, Vivier PH, Morel B, et al. Whole-body MR imaging in suspected physical child abuse: comparison with skeletal survey and bone scintigraphy findings from the PEDIMA prospective multicentre study. *Eur Radiol.* Nov 2021;31(11):8069–8080. doi: 10.1007/s00330-021-07896-9

54. Bachrach LK, Sills IN, Endocrinology So. Bone densitometry in children and adolescents. *Pediatrics.* 2011;127(1):189–194.

55. Khoury DJ, Szalay EA. Bone mineral density correlation with fractures in nonambulatory pediatric patients. *J Pediatr Orthop.* Jul-Aug 2007;27(5):562–6. doi: 10.1097/01.bpb.0000279021.04000.d3

56. Zemel BS, Kalkwarf HJ, Gilsanz V, et al. Revised reference curves for bone mineral content and areal bone mineral density according to age and sex for black and non-black children: results of the bone mineral density in childhood study. *The Journal of Clinical Endocrinology & Metabolism.* 2011;96(10):3160–3169.

57. Bishop N, Arundel P, Clark E, et al. Fracture prediction and the definition of osteoporosis in children and adolescents: the ISCD 2013 Pediatric Official Positions. *J Clin Densitom.* Apr-Jun 2014;17(2): 275–80. doi: 10.1016/j.jocd.2014.01.004

58. Gordon CM, Baim S, Bianchi ML, et al. Special report on the 2007 Pediatric Position Development Conference of the International Society for Clinical Densitometry. *South Med J.* Jul 2008;101(7): 740–3. doi: 10.1097/SMJ.0b013e31817a8b55

59. Henderson RC, Lark RK, Newman JE, et al. Pediatric reference data for dual X-ray absorptiometric measures of normal bone density in the distal femur. *AJR Am J Roentgenol.* Feb 2002;178(2):439–43. doi: 10.2214/ajr.178.2.1780439

60. Marini JC, Dang Do AN.Osteogenesis Imperfecta. In: Feingold KR, Anawalt B, Boyce A, et al, eds. *Endotext.* 2000.

61. Zarate YA, Clingenpeel R, Sellars EA, et al. COL1A1 and COL1A2 sequencing results in cohort of patients undergoing evaluation for potential child abuse. *Am J Med Genet A.* Jul 2016;170(7): 1858–62. doi: 10.1002/ajmg.a.37664

62. Shapiro JR, Sponsellor PD. Osteogenesis imperfecta: questions and answers. *Curr Opin Pediatr.* Dec 2009;21(6):709–16. doi: 10.1097/MOP.0b013e328332c68f

63. Marlowe A, Pepin MG, Byers PH. Testing for osteogenesis imperfecta in cases of suspected non-accidental injury. *Journal of Medical Genetics.* 2002;39(6):382–386. doi: 10.1136/jmg.39.6.382

64. Asnes AG, Leventhal JM. Managing child abuse. *Pediatrics in Review.* 2010;31(2):47–55. doi: 10.1542/pir.31-2-47

65. Thomas SA, Rosenfield NS, Leventhal JM, Markowitz RI. Long-bone fractures in young children: distinguishing accidental injuries from child abuse. *Pediatrics.* 1991;88(3):471–6.

66. Sullivan PM, Knutson JF. Maltreatment and disabilities: a population-based epidemiological study. *Child Abuse & Neglect.* 2000; 24(10):1257–73.

67. Sullivan PM, Knutson JF. The association between child maltreatment and disabilities in a hospital-based epidemiological study. *Child Abuse & Neglect.* 1998;22(4):271–88.

68. Banaszkiewicz PA, Scotland TR, Myerscough EJ. Fractures in children younger than age 1 year: importance of collaboration with child protection services. *Journal of Pediatric Orthopaedics.* 2002;22(6):740–744.

69. Rumball-Smith J, Fromkin J, Rosenthal B, et al. Implementation of routine electronic health record-based child abuse screening in General Emergency Departments. *Child abuse & neglect.* 2018;85: 58–67.

70. Worlock P, Stower M, Barbor P. Patterns of fractures in accidental and non-accidental injury in children: a comparative study. *British Medical Journal.* 1986;293(6539):100–2.

71. Loder RT, Feinberg JR. Orthopaedic injuries in children with non-accidental trauma: demographics and incidence from the 2000 kids' inpatient database.[Erratum appears in J Pediatr Orthop. 2008 Sep;28(6):699]. *Journal of Pediatric Orthopedics.* 2007;27 (4):421–6.

72. Leventhal JM, Larson IA, Abdoo D, et al. Are abusive fractures in young children becoming less common? Changes over 24 years. *Child Abuse & Neglect.* 2007;31(3):311–322. doi: 10.1016/j.chiabu.2006.07.004

73. Kemp AM, Dunstan F, Harrison S, et al. Patterns of skeletal fractures in child abuse: systematic review. [Review] [24 refs]. *BMJ.* 2008;337:a1518.

74. Pandya NK, Baldwin K, Wolfgruber H, Christian CW, Drummond DS, Hosalkar HS. Child Abuse and Orthopaedic Injury Patterns: Analysis at a Level I Pediatric Trauma Center. *Journal of Pediatric Orthopaedics.* 2009;29(6):618–625.

75. Coffey C, Haley K, Hayes J, Groner JI. The risk of child abuse in infants and toddlers with lower extremity injuries. *Journal of Pediatric Surgery.* 2005;40(1):120–123. doi: 10.1016/j.jpedsurg.2004.09.003

76. Kleinman PK.The Spectrum of Non-accidental Injuries (Child Abuse) and Its Imitators. In: Hodler J, Zollikofer CL, Schulthess GK, eds. *Musculoskeletal Diseases 2009–2012.* Springer Milan; 2009:227–233.

77. Clarke NMP, Shelton FRM, Taylor CC, Khan T, Needhirajan S. The incidence of fractures in children under the age of 24 months – In relation to non-accidental injury. *Injury.* 2011;(0). doi: 10.1016/j.injury.2011.08.024

78. Kleinman PK. *Diagnostic imaging of child abuse.* Cambridge University Press; 2015.

79. Kleinman PK. *Diagnostic imaging of child abuse.* 2nd ed. Mosby; 1998:xxiii, 439 p.

80. Barsness KA, Cha E-S, Bensard DD, et al. The positive predictive value of rib fractures as an indicator of nonaccidental trauma in children.[see comment]. *J Trauma.* 2003;54(6):1107–10.

81. Paine CW, Fakeye O, Christian CW, Wood JN. Prevalence of Abuse Among Young Children With Rib Fractures: A Systematic Review. *Pediatr Emerg Care.* Feb 2019;35(2):96–103. doi: 10.1097/PEC.0000000000000911

82. Tsai A, Coats B, Kleinman PK. Stress profile of infant rib in the setting of child abuse: A finite element parametric study. *J Biomech.* Jul 26 2012;45(11):1861–8. doi: 10.1016/j.jbiomech.2012.05.049

83. Kemp AM, Dunstan F, Harrison S, et al. Patterns of skeletal fractures in child abuse: systematic review. *BMJ.* Oct 2 2008;337:a1518. doi: 10.1136/bmj.a1518

84. Kriss S, Thompson A, Bertocci G, Currie M, Martich V. Characteristics of rib fractures in young abused children. *Pediatr Radiol.* May 2020;50(5):726–733. doi: 10.1007/s00247-019-04599-8

85. Barber I, Perez-Rossello JM, Wilson CR, Kleinman PK. The yield of high-detail radiographic skeletal surveys in suspected infant abuse. *Pediatr Radiol.* Jan 2015;45(1):69–80. doi: 10.1007/s00247-014-3064-3

86. Brennan B, Henry MK, Altaffer A, Wood JN. Prevalence of Abuse and Additional Injury in Young Children With Rib Fractures as Their Presenting Injury. *Pediatr Emerg Care.* Dec 1 2021;37(12): e1451–e1456. doi: 10.1097/PEC.0000000000002071

87. Bulloch B, Schubert CJ, Brophy PD, Johnson N, Reed MH, Shapiro RA. Cause and Clinical Characteristics of Rib Fractures in Infants. *Pediatrics.* 2000;105(4):e48.

88. Kleinman PK, Schlesinger AE. Mechanical factors associated with posterior rib fractures: laboratory and case studies. *Pediatric Radiology.* 1997;27(1):87–91.

89. Bixby SD, Abo A, Kleinman PK. High-impact trauma causing multiple posteromedial rib fractures in a child. *Pediatric Emergency Care.* 2011;27(3):218–219.

90. Ruest S, Kanaan G, Moore JL, Goldberg AP. The Prevalence of Rib Fractures Incidentally Identified by Chest Radiograph among Infants and Toddlers. *J Pediatr.* Jan 2019;204:208–213. doi: 10.1016/j.jpeds.2018.08.067

91. Feldman KW,Brewer DK.Child Abuse, Cardiopulmonary Resuscitation, and Rib Fractures. *Pediatrics.* 1984;73(3):339–342.

92. Spevak MR, Kleinman PK, Belanger PL, Primack C, Richmond JM. Cardiopulmonary Resuscitation and Rib Fractures in Infants. *JAMA.* 1994;272(8):617–618. doi: 10.1001/jama.1994.03520080059044

93. Maguire S, Mann M, John N, et al. Does cardiopulmonary resuscitation cause rib fractures in children? A systematic review. *Child Abuse Negl.* Jul 2006;30(7):739–51. doi: 10.1016/j.chiabu.2005.12.007

94. Matshes EW, Lew EO. Two-Handed Cardiopulmonary Resuscitation Can Cause Rib Fractures in Infants. *American Journal of Forensic Medicine and Pathology.* 2010;31(4):303–307.

95. Reyes JA, Somers GR, Taylor GP, Chiasson DA. Increased incidence of CPR-related rib fractures in infants–is it related to changes in CPR technique? *Resuscitation.* May 2011;82(5):545–8. doi: 10.1016/j.resuscitation.2010.12.024

96. Franke I, Pingen A, Schiffmann H, et al. Cardiopulmonary resuscitation (CPR)-related posterior rib fractures in neonates and infants following recommended changes in CPR techniques. *Child Abuse Negl.* Jul 2014;38(7):1267–74. doi: 10.1016/j.chiabu.2014.01.021

97. Kleinman PK, Perez-Rossello JM, Newton AW, Feldman HA, Kleinman PL. Prevalence of the classic metaphyseal lesion in infants at low versus high risk for abuse. *American Journal of Roentgenology.* 2011;197(4):1005–1008. doi: 10.2214/ajr.11.6540

98. Kleinman PK, Marks SC, Jr, Richmond JM, Blackbourne BD. Inflicted skeletal injury: a postmortem radiologic-histopathologic study in 31 infants. *American Journal of Roentgenology.* 1995; 165(3):647–50.

99. Kleinman PK. Problems in the diagnosis of metaphyseal fractures. *Review. Pediatric Radiology.* 2008;38 Suppl 3:S388–94.

100. Adamsbaum C, De Boissieu P, Teglas JP, Rey-Salmon C. Classic Metaphyseal Lesions among Victims of Abuse. *J Pediatr.* Jun 2019;209:154–159 e2. doi: 10.1016/j.jpeds.2019.02.013

101. Tsai A, Coats B, Kleinman PK. Biomechanics of the classic metaphyseal lesion: finite element analysis. *Pediatr Radiol.* Nov 2017;47(12):1622–1630. doi: 10.1007/s00247-017-3921-y

102. Bertocci G, Smalley C, Brown N, Dsouza R, Thompson A. Injuries and biomechancis of falls involving young children in a childcare setting obtained through video recording and wearable biometric devices. presented at: Shaken Baby Syndrome & Abusive Head Trauma Symposium; 2020; Virtual.

103. O'Connell A, Donoghue VB. Can classic metaphyseal lesions follow uncomplicated caesarean section? Case Reports. *Pediatric Radiology.* 37(5):488–91.

104. Grayev AM, Boal DK, Wallach DM, Segal LS. Metaphyseal fractures mimicking abuse during treatment for clubfoot.[see comment]. *Pediatric Radiology.* 2001;31(8):559–63.

105. Starling SP, Heller RM, Jenny C. Pelvic fractures in infants as a sign of physical abuse. *Child Abuse Negl.* May 2002;26(5):475–80. doi: 10.1016/s0145-2134(02)00323-x

106. Kocher MS, Kasser JR. Orthopaedic aspects of child abuse. *J Am Acad Orthop Surg.* Jan-Feb 2000;8(1):10–20. doi: 10.5435/00124635-200001000-00002

107. Perez-Rossello JM, Connolly SA, Newton AW, et al. Pubic ramus radiolucencies in infants: the good, the bad, and the indeterminate. *AJR Am J Roentgenol.* Jun 2008;190(6):1481–6. doi: 10.2214/AJR.07.3251

108. Bixby SD, Wilson CR, Barber I, Kleinman PK. Ischial apophyseal fracture in an abused infant. *Pediatr Radiol.* Sep 2014;44(9):1175–8. doi: 10.1007/s00247-014-2960-x

109. King J, Diefendorf D, Apthorp J, Negrete VF, Carlson M. Analysis of 429 fractures in 189 battered children. *Journal of Pediatric Orthopedics.* 1988;8(5):585–9.

110. Pandya NK, Baldwin KD, Wolfgruber H, Drummond DS, Hosalkar HS. Humerus fractures in the pediatric population: an algorithm to identify abuse. *J Pediatr Orthop B.* 2010;19(6):535–41.

111. Strait RT, Siegel RM, Shapiro RA. Humeral fractures without obvious etiologies in children less than 3 years of age: when is it abuse? *Pediatrics.* Oct 1995;96(4 Pt 1):667–71.

112. Shaw BA, Murphy KM, Shaw A, Oppenheim WL, Myracle MR. Humerus shaft fractures in young children: accident or abuse? *J Pediatr Orthop.* May-Jun 1997;17(3):293–7.

113. Hymel KP, Jenny C. Abusive spiral fractures of the humerus: a videotaped exception. *Archives of Pediatrics & Adolescent Medicine.* 1996;150(2):226–7.

114. Coffey C, Haley K, Hayes J, Groner JI. The risk of child abuse in infants and toddlers with lower extremity injuries. *J Pediatr Surg.* Jan 2005;40(1):120–3. doi: 10.1016/j.jpedsurg.2004.09.003

115. Haney SB, Boos SC, Kutz TJ, Starling SP. Transverse fracture of the distal femoral metadiaphysis: a plausible accidental mechanism. *Pediatr Emerg Care.* Dec 2009;25(12):841–4. doi: 10.1097/PEC.0b013e3181c330f0

116. Arkader A, Friedman JE, Warner WC, Jr, Wells L. Complete distal femoral metaphyseal fractures: a harbinger of child abuse before walking age. *J Pediatr Orthop.* Oct-Nov 2007;27(7):751–3. doi: 10.1097/BPO.0b013e3181558b13

117. Mitchell PD, Brown R, Wang T, et al. Multicentre study of physical abuse and limb fractures in young children in the East Anglia Region, UK. *Arch Dis Child.* Oct 2019;104(10):956–961. doi: 10.1136/archdischild-2018-315035

118. McGraw EP, Pless JE, Pennington DJ, White SJ. Postmortem radiography after unexpected death in neonates, infants, and children: should imaging be routine? *AJR Am J Roentgenol.* Jun 2002;178(6):1517–21. doi: 10.2214/ajr.178.6.1781517

119. Stewart GM, Rosenberg NM. Conditions mistaken for child abuse: Part I. *Pediatr Emerg Care.* Apr 1996;12(2):116–21. doi: 10.1097/00006565-199604000-00014

120. Krishnan J, Barbour PJ, Foster BK. Patterns of osseous injuries and psychosocial factors affecting victims of child abuse. *Aust N Z J Surg.* Jun 1990;60(6):447–50. doi: 10.1111/j.1445-2197.1990.tb07400.x

121. Caffey J. On the theory and practice of shaking infants. Its potential residual effects of permanent brain damage and mental retardation. *Am J Dis Child.* Aug 1972;124(2):161–9. doi: 10.1001/archpedi.1972.02110140011001

122. Caffey J. The parent-infant traumatic stress syndrome; (Caffey-Kempe syndrome), (battered babe syndrome). *Am J Roentgenol Radium Ther Nucl Med.* Feb 1972;114(2):218–29.

123. Kleinman PK. Diagnostic imaging in infant abuse. *AJR Am J Roentgenol.* Oct 1990;155(4):703–12. doi: 10.2214/ajr.155.4.2119097

124. Crowe M, Byerly L, Mehlman CT. Transphyseal Distal Humeral Fractures: A 13-Times-Greater Risk of Non-Accidental Trauma Compared with Supracondylar Humeral Fractures in Children Less Than 3 Years of Age. *J Bone Joint Surg Am.* Jul 6 2022;104(13):1204–1211. doi: 10.2106/JBJS.21.01534

125. Supakul N, Hicks RA, Caltoum CB, Karmazyn B. Distal humeral epiphyseal separation in young children: an often-missed fracture-radiographic signs and ultrasound confirmatory diagnosis. *AJR Am J Roentgenol.* Feb 2015;204(2):W192–8. doi: 10.2214/AJR.14.12788

126. Akbarnia BA. Pediatric spine fractures. *Orthop Clin North Am.* Jul 1999;30(3):521–36, x. doi: 10.1016/s0030-5898(05)70103-6

127. Lindberg DM, Harper NS, Laskey AL, Berger RP, Ex SI. Prevalence of abusive fractures of the hands, feet, spine, or pelvis on skeletal survey: perhaps "uncommon" is more common than suggested. *Pediatr Emerg Care.* Jan 2013;29(1):26–9. doi: 10.1097/PEC.0b013e31827b475e

128. Diamond P, Hansen CM, Christofersen MR. Child abuse presenting as a thoracolumbar spinal fracture dislocation: a case report. *Pediatr Emerg Care.* Apr 1994;10(2):83–6. doi: 10.1097/00006565-199404000-00005

129. Rooks VJ, Sisler C, Burton B. Cervical spine injury in child abuse: report of two cases. *Pediatr Radiol.* Mar 1998;28(3):193–5. doi: 10.1007/s002470050330

130. Kleinman PK, Morris NB, Makris J, Moles RL, Kleinman PL. Yield of radiographic skeletal surveys for detection of hand, foot, and spine fractures in suspected child abuse. *AJR Am J Roentgenol.* Mar 2013;200(3):641–4. doi: 10.2214/AJR.12.8878

131. Karmazyn B, Lewis ME, Jennings SG, Hibbard RA, Hicks RA. The prevalence of uncommon fractures on skeletal surveys performed to evaluate for suspected abuse in 930 children: should practice guidelines change? *AJR Am J Roentgenol.* Jul 2011;197 (1):W159–63. doi: 10.2214/AJR.10.5733

132. Merten DF, Radkowski MA, Leonidas JC. The abused child: a radiological reappraisal. *Radiology.* Feb 1983;146(2):377–81. doi: 10.1148/radiology.146.2.6849085

133. Farnsworth CL, Silva PD, Mubarak SJ. Etiology of supracondylar humerus fractures. *J Pediatr Orthop.* Jan-Feb 1998;18(1):38–42.

134. Schwend RM, Werth C, Johnston A. Femur shaft fractures in toddlers and young children: rarely from child abuse. *Journal of Pediatric Orthopedics.* 2000;20(4):475–81.

135. Loder RT, O"Donnell PW, Feinberg JR. Epidemiology and mechanisms of femur fractures in children. *Journal of Pediatric Orthopaedics.* 2006;26(5):561–566.

136. Baldwin K, Pandya N, Wolfgruber H, Drummond D, Hosalkar H. Femur fractures in the pediatric population: abuse or accidental trauma? *Clinical Orthopaedics and Related Research®.* 2011;469 (3):798–804. doi: 10.1007/s11999-010-1339-z

137. Son-Hing JP, Deniz Olgun Z. The frequency of nonaccidental trauma in children under the age of 3 years with femur fractures: is there a better cutoff point for universal workups? *J Pediatr Orthop B.* Jul 2018;27(4):366–368. doi: 10.1097/BPB.0000000000000495

138. Haney SB, Boos SC, Kutz TJ, Starling SP. Transverse fracture of the distal femoral metadiaphysis: a plausible accidental mechanism. *Pediatr Emerg Care.* 2009;25(12):841–844.

139. Grant P, Mata MB, Tidwell M. Femur fracture in infants: a possible accidental etiology. *Case Reports. Pediatrics.* 2001;108(4):1009–11.

140. Gaffney JT. Tibia fractures in children sustained on a playground slide. *J Pediatr Orthop.* Sep 2009;29(6):606–8. doi: 10.1097/BPO.0b013e3181b2ba2f

141. Kakel R. Trampoline fracture of the proximal tibial metaphysis in children may not progress into valgus: a report of seven cases and a brief review. *Orthop Traumatol Surg Res.* Jun 2012;98(4): 446–9. doi: 10.1016/j.otsr.2012.02.007

142. Harwood-Nash DC, Hendrick EB, Hudson AR. The significance of skull fractures in children. A study of 1,187 patients. *Radiology.* Oct 1971;101(1):151–6. doi: 10.1148/101.1.151

143. Meservy CJ, Towbin R, McLaurin RL, Myers PA, Ball W. Radiographic characteristics of skull fractures resulting from child abuse. *AJR Am J Roentgenol.* Jul 1987;149(1):173–5. doi: 10.2214/ajr.149.1.173

144. Isaac R, Greeley C, Marinello M, et al. Skeletal survey yields in low vs. high risk pediatric patients with skull fractures. *Child Abuse Negl.* May 2023;139:106130. doi: 10.1016/j.chiabu.2023.106130

145. Arnholz D, Hymel KP, Hay TC, Jenny C. Bilateral pediatric skull fractures: accident or abuse? *J Trauma.* Jul 1998;45(1):172–4. doi: 10.1097/00005373-199807000-00039

146. Hobbs CJ. Skull fracture and the diagnosis of abuse. *Arch Dis Child.* Mar 1984;59(3):246–52. doi: 10.1136/adc.59.3.246

147. Helfer RE, Slovis TL, Black M. Injuries resulting when small children fall out of bed. *Pediatrics.* Oct 1977;60(4):533–5.

148. Tarantino CA, Dowd MD, Murdock TC. Short vertical falls in infants. *Pediatr Emerg Care.* Feb 1999;15(1):5–8. doi: 10.1097/00006565-199902000-00002

149. Gallagher SS, Finison K, Guyer B, Goodenough S. The incidence of injuries among 87,000 Massachusetts children and adolescents: results of the 1980–81 Statewide Childhood Injury Prevention Program Surveillance System. *Am J Public Health.* 1984;74(12): 1340–7.

150. Spady DW, Saunders DL, Schopflocher DP, Svenson LW. Patterns of injury in children: a population-based approach. *Pediatrics.* 2004; 113(3 Pt 1):522–9.

151. Rennie L, Court-Brown CM, Mok JYQ, Beattie TF. The epidemiology of fractures in children. *Injury.* 2007;38(8):913–922. doi: 10.1016/j.injury.2007.01.036

152. Hennrikus WL, Shaw BA, Gerardi JA. Injuries when children reportedly fall from a bed or couch. *Clin Orthop.* 2003;407:148–51.

153. Pierce MC, Bertocci G. Injury biomechanics and child abuse. *Review. Annu Rev Biomed Eng.* 2008;10:85–106.

154. Pierce MC, Bertocci GE, Vogeley E, Moreland MS. Evaluating long bone fractures in children: a biomechanical approach with illustrative cases. *Child Abuse & Neglect.* 2004;28(5):505–24.

155. Pierce MC, Bertocci G. Fractures resulting from inflicted trauma: assessing injury and history compatibility. *Clin Ped Emerg Med.* 2006;7:143–148.

156. Rex C, Kay PR. Features of femoral fractures in nonaccidental injury. *Journal of Pediatric Orthopedics.* 2000;20(3):411–3.

157. Haney SB, Starling SP, Heisler KW, Okwara L. Characteristics of falls and risk of injury in children younger than 2 years. *Pediatric Emergency Care.* 2010;26(12):914–918.

158. Nimityongskul P, Anderson LD. The likelihood of injuries when children fall out of bed. *Journal of Pediatric Orthopaedics.* 1987;7(2): 184–186.

159. Lyons TJ, Oates RK. Falling out of bed: a relatively benign occurrence. *Pediatrics.* 1993;92(1):125–127.

160. Hansoti B, Beattie T. Can the height of fall predict long bone fracture in children under 24 months? *Eur J Emerg Med.* 2005;12(6): 285–6.

161. Barsh GS, Byers PH. Reduced secretion of structurally abnormal type I procollagen in a form of osteogenesis imperfecta. *Proc Natl Acad Sci U S A.* Aug 1981;78(8):5142–6. doi: 10.1073/pnas.78.8.5142

162. Byers PH, Steiner RD. Osteogenesis imperfecta. *Annu Rev Med.* 1992;43:269–82. doi: 10.1146/annurev.me.43.020192.001413

163. Wallis GA, Starman BJ, Zinn AB, Byers PH. Variable expression of osteogenesis imperfecta in a nuclear family is explained by somatic mosaicism for a lethal point mutation in the alpha 1(I) gene (COL1A1) of type I collagen in a parent. *Am J Hum Genet.* Jun 1990;46(6):1034–40.

164. Peddada KV, Sullivan BT, Margalit A, Sponseller PD. Fracture Patterns Differ Between Osteogenesis Imperfecta and Routine Pediatric Fractures. *J Pediatr Orthop.* Apr 2018;38(4):e207–e212. doi: 10.1097/BPO.0000000000001137

165. Fortin K, Bertocci G, Nicholas JL, Lorenz DJ, Pierce MC. Long bone fracture characteristics in children with medical conditions linked to bone health. *Child Abuse Negl.* May 2020;103:104396. doi: 10.1016/j.chiabu.2020.104396

166. Greeley CS, Donaruma-Kwoh M, Vettimattam M, Lobo C, Williard C, Mazur L. Fractures at diagnosis in infants and children with osteogenesis imperfecta. *J Pediatr Orthop.* Jan 2013;33(1):32–6. doi: 10.1097/BPO.0b013e318279c55d

167. Sprigg A. Temporary brittle bone disease versus suspected non-accidental skeletal injury. *Arch Dis Child.* May 2011;96(5):411–3. doi: 10.1136/adc.2009.180463

168. Singh Kocher M, Dichtel L. Osteogenesis imperfecta misdiagnosed as child abuse. *J Pediatr Orthop B.* Nov 2011;20(6):440–3. doi: 10.1097/BPB.0b013e328347a2e1

169. Ablin DS, Sane SM. Non-accidental injury: confusion with temporary brittle bone disease and mild osteogenesis imperfecta. *Pediatr Radiol.* Feb 1997;27(2):111–3. doi: 10.1007/s002470050079

170. Gahagan S, Rimsza ME. Child abuse or osteogenesis imperfecta: how can we tell? *Pediatrics.* Nov 1991;88(5):987–92.

171. Knight DJ, Bennet GC. Nonaccidental injury in osteogenesis imperfecta: a case report. *J Pediatr Orthop.* Jul-Aug 1990;10(4):542–4.

172. Backstrom MC, Kuusela AL, Maki R. Metabolic bone disease of prematurity. *Ann Med.* Aug 1996;28(4):275–82. doi: 10.3109/07853899608999080

173. Jenny C, Committee on Child A, Neglect. Evaluating infants and young children with multiple fractures. *Pediatrics.* Sep 2006; 118(3):1299–303. doi: 10.1542/peds.2006-1795

174. Chapman T, Sugar N, Done S, Marasigan J, Wambold N, Feldman K. Fractures in infants and toddlers with rickets. *Pediatr Radiol.* Jul 2010;40(7):1184–9. doi: 10.1007/s00247-009-1470-8

175. Naylor KE, Eastell R, Shattuck KE, Alfrey AC, Klein GL. Bone turnover in preterm infants. *Pediatr Res.* Mar 1999;45(3):363–6. doi: 10.1203/00006450-199903000-00012

176. Harrison CM, Johnson K, McKechnie E. Osteopenia of prematurity: a national survey and review of practice. Article. *Acta Paediatrica.* 2008;97(4):407–413. doi: 10.1111/j.1651-2227.2007.00721.x

177. Amir J, Katz K, Grunebaum M, Yosipovich Z, Wielunsky E, Reisner SH. Fractures in premature infants. *J Pediatr Orthop.* Jan-Feb 1988;8(1):41–4. doi: 10.1097/01241398-198801000-00010

178. Harrison CM, Johnson K, McKechnie E. Osteopenia of prematurity: a national survey and review of practice. *Acta Paediatr.* Apr 2008; 97(4):407–13. doi: 10.1111/j.1651-2227.2007.00721.x

179. Gordon CM, Feldman HA, Sinclair L, et al. Prevalence of Vitamin D deficiency among healthy infants and toddlers. *Archives of Pediatrics and Adolescent Medicine.* 2008;162(6):505–512. doi: 10.1001/archpedi.162.6.505

180. Munns CF, Shaw N, Kiely M, et al. Global Consensus Recommendations on Prevention and Management of Nutritional Rickets. *J Clin Endocrinol Metab.* Feb 2016;101(2):394–415. doi: 10.1210/jc.2015-2175

181. A G. *Orthopedic imaging: a practical approach.* Lippincott Williams & Wilkins. 2004.

182. Perez-Rossello JM, Feldman HA, Kleinman PK, et al. Rachitic changes, demineralization, and fracture risk in healthy infants and toddlers with vitamin D deficiency. *Radiology.* Jan 2012;262 (1):234–41. doi: 10.1148/radiol.11110358

183. Keller KA, Barnes PD. Rickets vs. abuse: a national and international epidemic. *Pediatr Radiol.* Nov 2008;38(11):1210–6. doi: 10.1007/s00247-008-1001-z

184. Jenny C. Rickets or abuse? *Pediatr Radiol.* Nov 2008;38(11):1219–20. doi: 10.1007/s00247-008-0995-6

185. Slovis TL, Chapman S. Vitamin D insufficiency/deficiency - a conundrum. *Pediatr Radiol.* Nov 2008;38(11):1153. doi: 10.1007/s00247-008-0997-4

186. Slovis TL, Chapman S. Evaluating the data concerning vitamin D insufficiency/deficiency and child abuse. *Pediatr Radiol.* Nov 2008;38(11):1221–4. doi: 10.1007/s00247-008-0994-7

187. Schilling S, Wood JN, Levine MA, Langdon D, Christian CW. Vitamin D status in abused and nonabused children younger than 2 years old with fractures. *Pediatrics.* May 2011;127(5):835–41. doi: 10.1542/peds.2010-0533

188. Perez-Rossello JM, McDonald AG, Rosenberg AE, Tsai A, Kleinman PK. Absence of rickets in infants with fatal abusive head trauma and classic metaphyseal lesions. *Radiology.* Jun 2015;275(3):810–21. doi: 10.1148/radiol.15141784

189. Presedo A, Dabney KW, Miller F. Fractures in patients with cerebral palsy. *J Pediatr Orthop.* Mar 2007;27(2):147–53. doi: 10.1097/BPO.0b013e3180317403

190. Whedon GD. Disuse osteoporosis: physiological aspects. *Calcif Tissue Int.* 1984;36 Suppl 1:S146–50. doi: 10.1007/BF02406148

191. Legano LA, Desch LW, Messner SA, et al. Maltreatment of Children With Disabilities. *Pediatrics.* May 2021;147(5)doi: 10.1542/peds.2021-050920

192. Sullivan PM, Knutson JF. The association between child maltreatment and disabilities in a hospital-based epidemiological study. *Child Abuse Negl.* Apr 1998;22(4):271–88. doi: 10.1016/s0145-2134(97)00175-0

193. Sullivan PM, Knutson JF. Maltreatment and disabilities: a population-based epidemiological study. *Child Abuse Negl.* Oct 2000;24 (10):1257–73. doi: 10.1016/s0145-2134(00)00190-3

194. Westcott H. The abuse of disabled children: a review of the literature. *Child Care Health Dev.* Jul-Aug 1991;17(4):243–58. doi: 10.1111/j.1365-2214.1991.tb00695.x

195. Larralde M, Santos Munoz A, Boggio P, Di Gruccio V, Weis I, Schygiel A. Scurvy in a 10-month-old boy. *Int J Dermatol.* Feb 2007;46(2):194–8. doi: 10.1111/j.1365-4632.2007.02856.x

196. Olmedo JM, Yiannias JA, Windgassen EB, Gornet MK. Scurvy: a disease almost forgotten. *Int J Dermatol.* Aug 2006;45(8):909–13. doi: 10.1111/j.1365-4632.2006.02844.x

197. Shaw JC. Copper deficiency and non-accidental injury. *Arch Dis Child.* Apr 1988;63(4):448–55. doi: 10.1136/adc.63.4.448

198. Marquardt ML, Done SL, Sandrock M, Berdon WE, Feldman KW. Copper deficiency presenting as metabolic bone disease in extremely low birth weight, short-gut infants. *Pediatrics.* Sep 2012;130(3):e695–8. doi: 10.1542/peds.2011-1295

199. Tumer Z, Moller LB. Menkes disease. *Eur J Hum Genet.* May 2010;18(5):511–8. doi: 10.1038/ejhg.2009.187

200. Bacopoulou F, Henderson L, Philip SG. Menkes disease mimicking non-accidental injury. *Arch Dis Child.* Nov 2006;91(11):919. doi: 10.1136/adc.2006.081836

201. Bakkaloglu SA, Bacchetta J, Lalayiannis AD, et al. Bone evaluation in paediatric chronic kidney disease: clinical practice points from the European Society for Paediatric Nephrology CKD-MBD and Dialysis working groups and CKD-MBD working group of the ERA-EDTA. *Nephrol Dial Transplant.* Feb 20 2021;36(3):413–425. doi: 10.1093/ndt/gfaa210

202. Ruuska S, Laakso S, Leskinen O, et al. Impaired Bone Health in Children With Biliary Atresia. *J Pediatr Gastroenterol Nutr.* Dec 2020;71(6):707–712. doi: 10.1097/MPG.0000000000002896

203. Lindberg DM, Shapiro RA, Laskey AL, et al. Prevalence of Abusive Injuries in Siblings and Household Contacts of Physically Abused Children. *Pediatrics.* 2012;130(2):193–201. doi: 10.1542/peds.2012-0085

204. Hamilton-Giachritsis CE, Browne KD. A retrospective study of risk to siblings in abusing families. *Journal of Family Psychology.* 2006;19(4):619–24.

205. Egge MK, Berkowitz CD. Controversies in the evaluation of young children with fractures. *Adv Pediatr.* 2010;57(1):63–83. doi: 10.1016/j.yapd.2010.08.002

206. Hicks R. Relating to methodological shortcomings and the concept of temporary brittle bone disease. *Calcif Tissue Int.* May 2001;68(5):316–9. doi: 10.1007/BF02390839

207. George MP, Shur NE, Perez-Rossello JM. Ehlers-Danlos syndrome: what the radiologist needs to know. *Pediatr Radiol.* May 2021;51(6):1023–1028. doi: 10.1007/s00247-020-04856-1

208. Leventhal JM, Edwards GA. Flawed Theories to Explain Child Physical Abuse: What Are the Medical-Legal Consequences? *JAMA.* Oct 10 2017;318(14):1317–1318. doi: 10.1001/jama.2017.11703

209. Malfait F, Francomano C, Byers P, et al. The 2017 international classification of the Ehlers-Danlos syndromes. *Am J Med Genet C Semin Med Genet.* Mar 2017;175(1):8–26. doi: 10.1002/ajmg.c.31552

210. Pfeifer CM, Henry MK, Care MM, et al. Debunking Fringe Beliefs in Child Abuse Imaging: AJR Expert Panel Narrative Review. *AJR Am J Roentgenol.* Sep 2021;217(3):529–540. doi: 10.2214/AJR.21.25655

211. Tadepalli V, Schultz JD, Rees AB, et al. Nonaccidental Trauma in Pediatric Elbow Fractures: When You Should Be Worried. *J Pediatr Orthop.* Jul 1 2022;42(6):e601–e606. doi: 10.1097/BPO.0000000000002145

212. Karmazyn B, Marine MB, Jones RH, et al. Radiologists' Diagnostic Performance in Differentiation of Rickets and Classic Metaphyseal Lesions on Radiographs: A Multicenter Study. *AJR Am J Roentgenol.* Dec 2022;219(6):962–972. doi: 10.2214/AJR.22.27729

Financing of Pediatric Home Health Care

- *Policy Statement*

POLICY STATEMENT Organizational Principles to Guide and Define the Child Health Care System and/or Improve the Health of All Children

American Academy of Pediatrics
DEDICATED TO THE HEALTH OF ALL CHILDREN™

Financing of Pediatric Home Health Care: Policy Statement

Carolyn C. Foster, MD, MS, FAAP,[1,2] Renee M. Turchi, MD, MPH, FAAP,[3,4] and the Section on Home Care; and Committee on Child Health Financing

abstract

Home health care is essential for children with chronic conditions and disabilities and children recovering from acute illness, injury, or surgery to ensure their daily health, function, and community participation. The American Academy of Pediatrics advocates for accessible, high-quality pediatric home health care by calling for development of pediatric-specific home health care regulations, eligibility guidance, and pediatric-focused metrics to facilitate high quality and access.

[1]Ann & Robert H. Lurie Children's Hospital of Chicago, Chicago, Illinois; [2]Department of Pediatrics, Northwestern University Feinberg School of Medicine, Chicago, Illinois; [3]Department of Pediatrics, Drexel University College of Medicine, Philadelphia, Pennsylvania; and [4]St. Christopher's Hospital for Children, Philadelphia, Pennsylvania

Address correspondence to: Carolyn C. Foster, MD, MS. Email: ccfoster@luriechildrens.org

Dr Foster and Dr Turchi were each responsible for all aspects of writing and editing the document and reviewing and responding to questions and comments from reviewers and the Board of Directors.

 All authors have filed conflict of interest statements with the American Academy of Pediatrics. Any conflicts have been resolved through a process approved by the Board of Directors. The American Academy of Pediatrics has neither solicited nor accepted any commercial involvement in the development of the content of this publication.

Policy statements from the American Academy of Pediatrics benefit from expertise and resources of liaisons and internal (AAP) and external reviewers. However, policy statements from the American Academy of Pediatrics may not reflect the views of the liaisons or the organizations or government agencies that they represent.

The guidance in this statement does not indicate an exclusive course of treatment or serve as a standard of medical care. Variations, taking into account individual circumstances, may be appropriate.

All policy statements from the American Academy of Pediatrics automatically expire 5 years after publication unless reaffirmed, revised, or retired at or before that time.

To cite: Foster CC, Turchi RM; American Academy of Pediatrics, Section on Home Care; and Committee on Child Health Financing. Financing of Pediatric Home Health Care: Policy Statement. *Pediatrics.* 2025;156(6):e2025073624

INTRODUCTION

Home health care (HHC) is defined as services and supplies delivered in the home to treat health conditions and functional impairments.[1,2] Home is the ideal and most beneficial site of long-term health care for children and serves those with chronic medical conditions, behavioral conditions, and/or disabilities and those with acute illnesses, injury, surgery, developmental delay, or end-of-life health needs.[3–5] Because of the breadth of pediatric health needs at home, direct HHC providers can include physicians, advanced practice providers, registered nurses, licensed practical nurses, certified nursing assistants (CNAs), personal care aides, home health aides, therapists, and family caregivers.

Home health care is particularly relevant for children with medical complexity (CMC) whose chronic conditions and disabilities necessitate intricate medication administration, medical device management, vital sign and symptom monitoring within the home and community, including school.[1,6] Home activities of daily living and therapy also are needed by children with disabilities and behavioral needs for adequate growth, development, and social participation.[1] Table 1 provides examples of pediatric conditions that require HHC.

A common misunderstanding of pediatric HHC is that it exists to support parents, but HHC is medically necessary and legally entitled care for children.[7,8] Federal laws, including the Early and Periodic Screening, Diagnostic, and Treatment (EPSDT) provision, Americans with

TABLE 1. Examples of Pediatric Health Conditions and Disabilities That Necessitate Home Health Care Services

Home Health Care Scenarios	Example Patient Stories	Examples of in-Home Medical and Disability Needs	High-level Example in-Home Care Plans
Trauma recovery	7-y-old previously healthy child in motor vehicle collision with persistent wound	Acute wound care	Weekly visits for 6 weeks to assess wound, assist with dressing changes, until its resolution
Developmental delay	18-mo-old term toddler with mild speech and gross motor delay	Speech and physical therapy	Weekly home visits by early intervention speech and physical therapists until resolution of delays or transition to school-based services
Chronic behavioral health condition	16-y-old adolescent with autism spectrum disorder and intermittent aggressive behaviors	Creation of behavioral health plan to address aggressive episodes including how family and teachers can address and modify behavior	Mobile health crisis team is engaged when needed and behavioral specialist attends school daily and supports adolescent at home after school and during weekend community activities
Short-term post-prematurity care	5-mo-old infant born at 28-week gestation with moderate bronchopulmonary dysplasia and feeding difficulties	Continuous oxygen by nasal cannula and oral feeding followed by nasogastric tube feeding when needed	Daily nursing care at home until infant is weaned off oxygen and feeding fully by mouth
Disability focused condition	19-y-old male young adult with muscular dystrophy with moderate impairments in dressing, toileting, self-feeding, and mobility	Activities of daily living (ADL) support	Morning and after school assistance with ADLs by aide as well as in-home occupational, speech, and physical therapy
Integrated palliative care	12-y-old preteen with advanced cancer or other serious illness experiencing chronic pain and mobility impairment	Pain management, mobility support, and social support	Integration of visits by a palliative care clinician and physical therapist
End-of-life care	12-y-old preteen with advanced cancer or other serious illness with a 6 mo or less prognosis and plan of care focused on comfort at the end of life	Symptom management, care coordination, anticipatory guidance related to dying process, as well as social, spiritual, and bereavement support	Hospice care services potentially blended with home nursing support depending on the needs of the preteen.
Concurrent care	3-y-old child with advanced serious illness with a 6 mo or less prognosis and plan of care including life-prolonging interventions	Pain management, care coordination, medical decision making, and social support	Integration of ambulatory, inpatient, home care, and home hospice services as needed by the child
Life-long disabling complex medical condition	9-y-old child with quadriplegic cerebral palsy, epilepsy, and dysphagia leading to aspiration	Every 4-to-6-hour medication administration through gastrostomy tube, seizure monitoring, tube feeding and pump use, and complete support with activities of daily living including wheelchair transfer and use, and suctioning	Daily and evening nursing shifts in perpetuity
Temporary but high-level medical technology needs	2-y-old child with history of extreme prematurity with severe bronchopulmonary dysplasia requiring invasive home mechanical ventilation and tube feeding	Continuous monitoring, hourly airway suctioning, oxygen titration, tracheostomy care, every 4-to-6 h medication administration, and tube feeding and pump use	24-hour nursing level care with awake caregiver until child is weaned off the ventilator, then care hours are decreased to address lower level of need

Pediatric conditions requiring in-home care, organized from children with the most acute and least complex needs to those with higher-level and longer-term needs.

Disabilities Act (ADA), and Patient Protection and Affordable Care Act (ACA), clearly affirm both governmental and commercial payer legal obligations to ensure children receive care at home or otherwise in the least restrictive setting possible (Table 2). Private duty nursing (PDN), CNA, and personal care services; durable medical equipment (DME); and case management are federally mandated Medicaid EPSDT benefits necessary to "correct and ameliorate" a physical or mental condition.[10–12] The ADA and related Olmstead court ruling requires state agencies to administer programs that ensure integration of persons with disability into home- and community-based settings, including PDN.[15–17] In turn, the ACA requires non-grandfathered health plans in the individual and small group markets to cover essential health benefits (EHBs), including rehabilitative and habilitative services.[18,19] The ACA also

TABLE 2. Key Federal Legislation and Court Cases Pertinent to Pediatric Home Health Care

Legislation and/or Court Case	Federal/State Relevance	Pediatric Home Health Care Relevance
Medicare and Medicaid Act, 1965[9] **Early and Periodic Screening, Diagnostic, and Treatment (EPSDT) Program,** 1966[10,11] and **The Omnibus Budget Reconciliation Act,** 1989[12]	Federal laws providing matching funds to state programs that pay for medical services to eligible citizens.	Children enrolled in Medicaid under 21 are entitled to receive and have arranged for them medically necessary home care, including in-home nursing. Under EPSDT, if a health care provider determines a child needs home health care to ameliorate a health condition, state Medicaid programs are required to provide coverage for those services regardless of any existing limits on adult home health care benefits.
Rehabilitation Act, 1973	Federal law that expanded nondiscrimination protections for persons with disabilities. The law states that no qualified individual with a disability shall be excluded from, denied the benefits of, or be subjected to discrimination under any program or activity that either receives federal financial assistance.	Requires "free appropriate public education" (FAPE) to each qualified student with a disability who is in the school district's jurisdiction, regardless of the nature or severity of the disability. Home health care services must be provided in school to allow a child with feeding, nursing or needs to participate fully.
Tax Equity and Fiscal Responsibility Act (TEFRA), 1982[13]	Established the "Katie Beckett" or TEFRA waiver that allows states to provide Medicaid coverage for children who required institutional level of care under 19 y of age.	Provides avenue for children who require institutional level of care living in participating states to access Medicaid coverage, including home health care services and private duty nursing.
Individuals with Disabilities Education Act (IDEA), 1990[14]	Federal law that ensures children with disability receive individualized education plan under Part B. The law also requires individualized family service plan for infants and toddlers with disabilities and developmental delays under part C.	Established early intervention (birth to 3) programs that provide in-home physical, occupational, and speech therapy and other family services.
Americans with Disabilities Act, 1990[15,16] **Olmstead Decision,** 1999[17]	Federal civil rights legislation and reaffirming Supreme Court case affirming that exclusion of individuals with disabilities from community living is discrimination.	Requires public entities, includes state actors, to administer services, programs, and activities in the most integrated setting appropriate to meet the needs of children with disabilities. Home health care recognized service to facilitate community integration for patients with disabling medical conditions.
Affordable Care Act, 2010[18–21]	Established essential health benefits (EHBs) for commercial plans. Health and Human Services (HHS) defines EHBs based on each state's selection of their EHB benchmark plan. Established concurrent care requirement for children under 21 y old with prognosis of 6 mos of less to receive hospice services while also pursuing care that is potentially curative, life-sustaining, and/or life-prolonging.	Home health care is listed an essential health benefit, including in-home rehabilitative or habilitative care. Allows for the integration of home hospice services without disengaging from ongoing medical care for the child.

established a "Concurrent Care for Children" requirement so children with a life-limiting diagnosis could receive curative and/or life-prolonging treatment and hospice care at the same time, including at home.[20,21]

Although the exact population of children receiving HHC is not enumerated, several factors have impacted the scope of pediatric HHC need, especially increasing pediatric survival.[8] One study found approximately 1 in 20 hospitalized children are discharged with HHC services and approximately 1 in 50 are discharged with PDN care.[22,23] Another multistate study found among 5.2 million pediatric Medicaid enrollees, 41 434 (0.8%) had a home health service claim in 2016.[24] Among those users, the level of chronic medical needs varied, with 1 in 4 having no appreciable chronic condition while another 1 in 3 had medical technology dependence. Among this population, in-home services accounted for 25% ($252 million) of the total $1.02 billion Medicaid spent.[24]

Notably, delivering in-home care is less costly than similar in-hospital care, and access to HHC has been associated with overall spending reduction.[25–29] In a matched-cohort study, children who received HHC were less likely to be readmitted to a hospital, had shorter lengths-of-stay, and experienced lower hospital costs than children not receiving HHC.[29] The expansion of HHC for children also presents opportunities for health care system cost savings through prevention of excessive emergency department (ED) utilization and hospitalization.[30]

PROBLEM STATEMENT

Children experience numerous barriers to accessing HHC, including: 1) limited private insurance coverage; 2) limitations as to who can access Medicaid for HHC; 3) limitations on hours allocated for eligible beneficiaries; 4) an insufficient number of trained in-home providers filling authorized shifts; and 5) in-home provider turnover or no-showing for scheduled shifts.[1,26,31–44] One survey of parents reported their children received only a median of 58.4% (interquartile range 31.2%) of approved weekly PDN hours over the past month.[1] The low availability of HHC has been shown to lead to institutionalization in costly acute care hospitals and skilled facilities, while medically stable children await discharge to home and other critically ill children await bed availability.[27,28,42,45–52]

Without their children receiving legally entitled medical services at home from external providers, family caregivers often perform nursing-level tasks unpaid. When families undertake complex medical care themselves, consequences can significantly impair family functioning and quality of life with emotional, financial, and time investment by parents, leading to negative impacts on parental physical health, mental health, and employment.[53–59] A 2016 population-based study found over 5.6 million American children received 1.5 billion hours of unpaid family-provided health care at home, with higher rates of unpaid family caregiving among underresourced racial/ethnic groups.[60,61] Lost earnings from unpaid family medical caregiving were estimated at $18 000/family in 2016–2017.[56] Of particular concern is that families most affected by foregone employment were already of lower income, of Hispanic background, and paying >$5000/y of their child's out-of-pocket costs.[56,60] Given that CMC typically have higher rates of poverty at baseline,[62] insufficient HHC risks worsening social and health disparities by disproportionately affecting underresourced racial and ethnic populations and financially vulnerable families living in urban and rural locations. Scarcity of HHC providers who speak a language other than English also leads to inequitable access for affected children.[32] Children also may not be able to attend school without trained health care provider accompaniment.

Many of these problems occur because no single source of HHC coverage exists. Pediatric HHC coverage routes can include: 1) Medicaid via the EPSDT; 2) ACA exchange plans' EHBs; and 3) private insurance. Within each mechanism, access varies by state for public coverage and by health plans for private coverage.[22,63] Private health insurance plans typically lack benefits for extended HHC services. Many private insurers and Children's Health Insurance Program (CHIP) plans have limited HHC benefits for children, critically limiting their access to those requiring longer-term services.[64] For children who do not access Medicaid through income-based eligibility, other mechanisms exist such as the Tax Equity and Fiscal Responsibility Act (TEFRA) "Katie Beckett" waiver,[13] which provides an avenue to access Medicaid or Medicaid home and community-based waivers (HCBS Waivers 1915(c)) to support long-term care services outside institutions.[31] However, states choose whether to participate in waivers, can limit waiver eligibility, and are allowed to place waiver enrollment caps, resulting in waiting lists for children that can last years.[31,65]

Even when children do access Medicaid, states can define criteria they use to establish the duration and/or scope of a medically necessary benefit. Consequently, state Medicaid agencies differ with respect to eligibility for benefits, duration, and scope of benefits, amount of payment, required provider expertise for service provision, and prior authorization documentation requirements. A lack of agreed upon HHC metrics, standards for eligibility for benefits, and operationalization of "medical necessity" can functionally blunt accountability for provision of HHC under federal law.[48,51]

Another key barrier to access is that Medicaid payments are often less than the total cost of the prescribed service or item, discouraging providers or suppliers to participate in pediatric HHC. Low Medicaid payments for PDN specifically can impede home health agencies' ability to hire skilled nurses to care for CMC and/or incentivizes them to reduce their number of Medicaid-enrolled clients, thereby systematically disadvantaging lower-income children who are statistically more likely from minoritized racial/ethnic backgrounds. Home health care workers are also disproportionately more likely to be female, identify from a minoritized race/ethnicity, and/or are non-native born.[66] As such, HHC's low pay leads to impoverishment within the workforce itself, further exacerbating income inequalities and access gaps.

In addition to service workforce barriers, bundled or prospective payment arrangements for DME disincentivize or delay its coverage, because pediatric-specific equipment is often more expensive, custom-made, and lower volume than adult-sized versions.[67] For example, children with tracheostomies may have difficulties getting adequate monthly supplies for their tracheostomy because of the unique size and paucity of pediatric airway supply manufacturing.[68] Renewal with recurring letters of medical necessity for equipment at frequencies not aligned with long-term care provision adds administrative burden for prescribing providers.[69] Lack of transparent reporting requirements to monitor payment and provision of DME and supplies further erodes payer and agency accountability.

Outsourcing of approvals and care to Medicaid managed care organizations (MCOs) without sufficient oversight has exacerbated HHC access problems because of limited provider networks, burdensome prior authorization procedures, inconsistent guidance regarding medical necessity, inappropriate limit setting, and payments at less than mandated rates. State scope-of-practice variations also impact workforce availability for children by limiting which type of provider can conduct certain care tasks. Although shown to expand workforce size, consumer-directed options and paid family caregiving remain limited in most states for pediatric patients.[70,71]

Access to *qualified* pediatric HHC providers and equipment remains a systemic problem.[1,26,27,36,45–47,72–81] Existing HHC network standards often do not require pediatric-specific training or competencies, including pediatric medical technology, palliative care, and behavioral health. Lack of payment for pediatric evidence-based clinical skills training can be an additional barrier to hire qualified staff.[82,83] Adequate payment for remote patient data monitoring or virtual visits to support HHC providers may prove to be a scalable approach to improve clinical supervision and management, but adequate payment and workflow structure to support these models remain nascent.[84]

Implicit in these policies and practices is the belief that children are not worthy of high-quality, accessible HHC; as a result, most children requiring HHC often do not receive medically necessary care at home.[47,51,55,72,83,85–89] In particular, ableist discrimination within existing policies and practices means that children with disability, especially those with neurologic impairment, do not receive equally necessary life-affirming care as children with other conditions or types of health care needs and may even be unnecessarily segregated in institutions.[90,91] Inadequate HHC also can lead to life-threatening medical complications and serious injury; unnecessary hospital and ED visits; higher health care costs; and excessive family stress, poorer health, and financial hardship.[4,42,44,55,88,92–94] Insufficient HHC can risk children being referred for medical neglect and even removed from their families, despite families providing the best care possible with available resources.[95–100] Over the past several decades, governmental entities and advocacy organizations have undertaken legal challenges under EPSDT and the ADA to enforce pediatric HHC requirements in Washington, Illinois, Texas, Georgia, Louisiana, Missouri, California, and Florida.[101]

CONCLUSION

Pediatric HHC is the delivery of health care in the home to children for their optimal health, highest quality of life, social participation, and end-of-life needs. The number of children who can benefit from home health services continues to increase while medical providers and family members continue to report significant gaps in existing high-quality pediatric HHC services. The American Academy of Pediatrics (AAP) continues to affirm that HHC is an indispensable component of a patient- and family-centered delivery system. To ensure children receive medically necessary HHC, the AAP recommends the following.

RECOMMENDATIONS

Service Determination and Allocation

1. Pediatric HHC should be delivered consistent with a written plan of care developed by the child's medical team in consultation with the family and, as appropriate, the child/youth.
2. Clinicians have the responsibility to prescribe the type, quantity, and intensity of home health services appropriate for the needs of the child. Clinicians should modify prescriptions when there is a change in the child's medical needs, family needs, or plan of care.[101]
3. Any guidance used by states to allocate any type of HHC hours should be transparent and publicly available for providers and patients. Unvalidated service allocation algorithms in lieu of a provider's assessment of a patient's medical need should not be used.

Regulatory Oversight and Assistance

4. The Centers for Medicare and Medicaid Services (CMS) and US Department of Health and Human Services (HHS) should provide clear guidance to assist states to fulfill their obligation to provide coverage of pediatric HHC under the Medicaid Act (EPSDT), ADA, Rehabilitation Act, and ACA. Specifically:
   a. Federal regulations must make clear that state Medicaid programs are obligated to ensure provision of the full breadth of pediatric HHC that children require. If a state has delegated the provision of pediatric HHC to another party such as an MCO, the obligation to ensure receipt of such services remains with the state Medicaid program through proactive, comprehensive monitoring and oversight including data regarding disability status, race/ethnicity, and interpreter services availability.
   b. Guidance of what is "necessary to correct or ameliorate the child's condition," as defined by the Medicaid Act EPSDT provision, should be developed by an interdisciplinary group of pediatric experts and families and informed by an analysis of existing state language, in a manner that considers professional standards of care for children to ensure the full range of HHC under EPSDT for children, regardless of their state of origin or insurance plan.
      i. Federal regulations should additionally clarify whether or how social criteria, such as parental work hours, in addition to a child's medical needs, can be used in determinations of HHC service allocation to avoid worsening health and financial inequalities in patients from marginalized populations.
5. CMS should appoint a federal ombudsman program that works with states to:
   a. Compile and evaluate provider and patient complaints about HHC within Medicaid programs.
   b. Monitor state-level appeals/denials for:
      i. EPSDT-mandated HHC services; and
      ii. Pediatric DME.

c. Track and set standards for missed HHC service shifts and require missed shift mitigation planning.
d. Monitor quality and equity of HHC delivered, including service and equipment errors.
e. Convene working groups of pediatricians, patient-family advocates, and payers to examine the complaints, appeal/denial patterns, and overall utilization (to include acute care, ED care, hospitalizations including readmissions) and make recommendations to safeguard that children's home-based medical needs are met, including within state MCO contracts.

6. Regulations and payment for HHC should be more seamlessly integrated within Medicaid programs to minimize gaps in service and reduce bureaucratic waste for patients transitioning from pediatric to adult care.

Payment and Workforce Development

7. Payment should be adequate to support the skills needed to ensure high-quality HHC and to address income inequities in the HHC workforce. To accomplish this, payment to direct providers should be at levels that attract and retain providers for pediatric HHC and cover overhead costs of clinical management of in-home providers and orders. Payment and benefits should be competitive and flexible to providers with skills sets comparable to hospital settings to care for CMC with medical technology dependence and those needing complex behavioral supports. All payment structures should also cover hospice, concurrent care, and palliative care home visits for pediatric patients.
8. HHS should provide oversight and payments to ensure provider training can include simulation training and continuing education in pediatric competencies and standards, complex medication, and nutrition administration, technological skills, and behavioral health.
   a. Payers also should provide health systems with sufficient payment to cover training of family caregivers prior to discharge home and over time to maintain family caregivers' skillsets to prevent morbidity and mortality.
9. State nursing and related HHC professional boards should review scope of practice laws and their impact on pediatric HHC to assess opportunities for increased delegation and expansion of scope of services whenever safely possible. Boards should consider more licensure and credentialing paths that expand rather than restrict the workforce providing in-home pediatric care, paired with adequate training and oversight, and should support these through federal and state laws and regulations. Closer collaboration between pediatric health care systems and HHC agencies with schooling programs (ie, nursing, allied health programs) could also expand pediatric HHC as a valued professional track.
10. Paid family caregiver programs that include payment of parents (legal guardians) who assume significant and skilled care responsibilities for their children are needed to address unpaid family medical labor. Expansion of programs can be based on successful programs found in Colorado, Arizona, Massachusetts, and other states.[70,71,102] Preparation, training, and support for family caregivers should be available with tuition reimbursement options and waiver of examinations/licensing fees. However, programs should be offered as a *choice* among a robust set of nonfamily program options and should not be required in lieu of nonfamily providers. Patient-families should be meaningfully engaged in their design and oversight. Adequate payment is necessary to avoid exacerbating existing income disparities by participating families.
11. Expansion of optional consumer-directed personal assistance programs, such as "Money Follows the Person"[103,104] programs, are necessary to provide flexibility needed for families to access the care and equipment for their child that suits their families' needs, and all states should be required to participate.
12. To lessen disincentives or barriers to coverage of medically necessary DME, payment for DME should not be bundled into payment for visits or into prospective payment arrangements for intermittent care and should include first-dollar coverage for appropriate and necessary DME. Instead, delivery quality standards should be developed and associated with value-based payments to encourage high-quality and adequate pediatric DME receipt.
13. Interoperability and interfacing of health records should be financially incentivized to support accurate order reconciliation and care plan integration across providers and systems caring for a child, including pediatric health care systems, HHC agencies, and medical supply companies.
14. Letter of medical necessity renewals for payment authorization of children's long-term services should be required only at medically relevant intervals, rather than by acute rehabilitation-based intervals (eg, every 60–90 days). Examples intervals include biyearly, yearly, or after a health status change or caregiver needs/availability (Table 1).
15. Payments should be provided for telemedicine, remote patient monitoring, and other digital health tools that expand oversight and clinical support of HHC providers to improve care quality and bolster workforce participation. Payment should include

coverage of vital sign review and patient symptom monitoring relevant to children at home.

16. All payers should sufficiently pay clinicians for care coordination and case management of children's HHC to ensure comprehensive and continuous care.[17]

Research and Demonstrations

17. CMS should offer opportunities to expand value based and high-quality services for children's HHC. Examples may include funding for innovative models that incorporate specialized training, tiered payment, care integration, virtual provider support, remote patient monitoring, and acute care management (ie, "hospital at home" models).
18. CMS should develop new standardized electronic data structures and regulations specific to pediatric HHC so Medicaid payment information is reproducible, available, and transparent across states and agencies and allows for evaluation of service equity across subpopulations including race/ethnicity, language, and rural/urban locations. CMS should then analyze Medicaid pediatric HHC payment rates and usage across all states to ensure adequate and equitable access, including HHC network adequacy in MCO contracts.
19. CMS, the Agency for Healthcare Research and Quality, and National Institutes of Health should fund clinical and health service research of HHC to improve child and family health outcomes, including access quality-metric development specific to pediatric HHC to support alternative/value-based payment schemes.

LEAD AUTHORS

Carolyn C. Foster, MD, MS, FAAP
Renee M. Turchi, MD, MPH, FAAP

CONTRIBUTORS

Cara L. Coleman, JD, MPH
Heather O'Donnell, MD, MSc

ABBREVIATIONS

ACA: Patient Protection and Affordable Care Act
ADA: Americans with Disabilities Act
AAP: American Academy of Pediatrics
CNA: certified nursing assistant
CHIP: Children's Health Insurance Program
CMC: children with medical complexity
CMS: Centers for Medicare and Medicaid Services
DME: durable medical equipment
ED: emergency department
EHBs: essential health benefits
EPSDT: Early and Periodic Screening, Diagnostic, and Treatment
HHC: home health care
HHS: US Department of Health and Human Services
MCO: managed care organization
PDN: private duty nursing
TEFRA: Tax Equity and Fiscal Responsibility Act

CONFLICT OF INTEREST DISCLOSURE: Dr Foster has disclosures related to: Hello Nurze.

FUNDING: Dr Foster's time was supported by the National Heart, Lung, and Blood Institute (NHLBI) under 1K23HL149829-01A1 for research on care of children with medical complexity. The content is solely the responsibility of the authors and does not necessarily represent the official views of the NHLBI or National Institutes of Health.

Disclosures are reviewed and mitigated through a conflict-of-interest process that consists of reviewing pertinent information which is then used to decide what action is required to maintain content integrity. Disclosures may include salary, wages or other remuneration of any kind (including but not limited to consulting or advising fees, speaking fees, research funding, ownership interests, honoraria, participation in pension or benefit plans or programs or other perquisites, and reimbursement for travel, lodging, and meals) given for services rendered or other activities for which remuneration is received or expected, whether that compensation or other remuneration is paid directly to the individual or to the individual's employer or another third party. A disclosure does not necessarily imply a real or perceived conflict of interest.

Members of Committee on Child Health Financing and the executive committee of the Section on Home Care are required to recuse themselves from participating in the development of policies related to their disclosures.

https://doi.org/10.1542/peds.2025-073624

REFERENCES

1. Foster C, Kaat AJ, Shaunfield S, et al. PediHome: Development of a Family-Reported Measure of Pediatric Home Healthcare Quality. *Acad Pediatr.* 2022;22(8):1510–1519. PubMed doi: 10.1016/j.acap.2022.04.004
2. Guidelines for Pediatric Home Health Care 2nd Edition Direct Textbook. Accessed February 18, 2025. https://www.directtextbook.com/isbn/9781581104394
3. Elias ER, Murphy NA, Liptak GS, et al; Council on Children with Disabilities. Home care of children and youth with complex health care needs and technology dependencies. *Pediatrics.* 2012;129(5):996–1005. PubMed doi: 10.1542/peds.2012-0606
4. Friedman SL, Norwood KW Jr, Norwood KW Jr, et al; COUNCIL ON CHILDREN WITH DISABILITIES. Out-of-Home Placement for Children and Adolescents With Disabilities-Addendum: Care Options for Children and Adolescents With Disabilities and Medical Complexity. *Pediatrics.* 2016;138(6):e20163216. PubMed doi: 10.1542/peds.2016-3216
5. Sobotka SA, Agrawal RK, Msall ME. Prolonged Hospital Discharge for Children with Technology Dependency: A Source of Health Care Disparities. *Pediatr Ann.* 2017;46(10):e365–e370. PubMed doi: 10.3928/19382359-20170919-01
6. Cohen E, Kuo DZ, Agrawal R, et al. Children with medical complexity: an emerging population for clinical and research initiatives. *Pediatrics.* 2011;127(3):529–538. PubMed doi: 10.1542/peds.2010-0910
7. Children's Home Health Care and EPSDT. Lucile Packard Foundation for Children's Health. February 14, 2023. Accessed February 18, 2025. http://lpfch.org/resource/childrens-home-health-care-and-epsdt/
8. Perkins J, Agrawal R. Protecting Rights of Children With Medical Complexity in an Era of Spending Reduction. *Pediatrics.* 2018;141(suppl 3):S242–S249. PubMed doi: 10.1542/peds.2017-1284I
9. Berkowitz E. Medicare and Medicaid: the past as prologue. *Health Care Financ Rev.* 2008;29(3):81–93. PubMed
10. Staff N. Managing the "T" in EPSDT Services – The National Academy for State Health Policy. Accessed February 18, 2025. https://oldsite.nashp.org/managing-t-epsdt-services/
11. Goldstein MM, Rosenbaum S. From EPSDT to EHBs: the future of pediatric coverage design under government financed health insurance. *Pediatrics.* 2013;131(suppl 2):S142–S148. PubMed doi: 10.1542/peds.2013-0252e
12. Gavin NI, Adams EK, Herz EJ. The use of EPSDT and other health care services by children enrolled in Medicaid: the impact of OBRA'89. *Milbank Q.* 1998;76(2):207–250. PubMed doi: 10.1111/1468-0009.00087
13. Semansky RM, Koyanagi C. The TEFRA medicaid eligibility option for children with severe disabilities: a national study. *J Behav Health Serv Res.* 2004;31(3):334–342. PubMed doi: 10.1097/00075484-200407000-00009
14. Lipkin PH, Okamoto J, Norwood KW Jr, et al; Council on Children with Disabilities; Council on School Health. The Individuals With Disabilities Education Act (IDEA) for Children With Special Educational Needs. *Pediatrics.* 2015;136(6):e1650–e1662. PubMed doi: 10.1542/peds.2015-3409
15. Americans with Disabilities Act of 1990, As Amended. ADA.gov. Accessed February 18, 2025. https://www.ada.gov/law-and-regs/ada/
16. Thompson DL, Thomas KR, Fernandez MS. The Americans with Disabilities Act: social policy and worldwide implications for practice. *Int J Rehabil Res.* 1994;17(2):109–121. PubMed doi: 10.1097/00004356-199406000-00002
17. Rosenbaum S, Teitelbaum J, Stewart A. Olmstead v. L.C.: Implications for Medicaid and other publicly funded health services. *Health Matrix.* 2002;12(1):93–138. https://www.researchgate.net/publication/11357338_Olmstead_v_LC_implications_for_Medicaid_and_other_publicly_funded_health_services
18. Essential Health Benefits Standards: Ensuring Quality, Affordable Coverage. CMS. Accessed February 18, 2025. https://www.cms.gov/CCIIO/Resources/Fact-Sheets-and-FAQs/ehb-2-20-2013
19. Information on Essential Health Benefits (EHB) Benchmark Plans | CMS. Accessed February 18, 2025. https://www.cms.gov/marketplace/resources/data/essential-health-benefits
20. Pediatric Concurrent Care. NHPCO. Accessed February 18, 2025. https://www.nhpco.org/palliativecare/pediatrics/pediatric-concurrent-care/
21. American Academy of Pediatrics. Concurrent Care for Children. Accessed February 20, 2025. https://www.aap.org/en/practice-management/medical-home/tools-and-resources-for-medical-home-implementation/medical-home-resources-for-families-and-caregivers/
22. Berry JG, Hall M, Dumas H, et al. Pediatric Hospital Discharges to Home Health and Postacute Facility Care: A National Study.

JAMA Pediatr. 2016;170(4):326–333. PubMed doi: 10.1001/jamapediatrics.2015.4836

23. Foster CC, Kwon S, Whitlow L, et al. Connecting Hospital to Home: Characteristics of and Rehospitalization Rates in Hospitalized Children With Private-Duty Nursing. *Hosp Pediatr.* 2019;9(7):530–537. PubMed doi: 10.1542/hpeds.2018-0282
24. Sobotka SA, Hall DE, Thurm C, Gay J, Berry JG. Home Health Care Utilization in Children With Medicaid. *Pediatrics.* 2022;149(2):e2021050534. PubMed doi: 10.1542/peds.2021-050534
25. Burr BH, Guyer B, Todres ID, Abrahams B, Chiodo T. Home care for children on respirators. *N Engl J Med.* 1983;309(21):1319–1323. PubMed doi: 10.1056/NEJM198311243092112
26. Splaingard ML, Frates RC Jr, Harrison GM, Carter RE, Jefferson LS. Home positive-pressure ventilation. Twenty years' experience. *Chest.* 1983;84(4):376–382. PubMed doi: 10.1378/chest.84.4.376
27. Sobotka SA, Foster C, Lynch E, Hird-McCorry L, Goodman DM. Attributable Delay of Discharge for Children with Long-Term Mechanical Ventilation. *J Pediatr.* 2019;212:166–171. PubMed doi: 10.1016/j.jpeds.2019.04.034
28. Maynard R, Christensen E, Cady R, et al. Home Health Care Availability and Discharge Delays in Children With Medical Complexity. *Pediatrics.* 2019;143(1):e20181951. PubMed doi: 10.1542/peds.2018-1951
29. Gay JC, Thurm CW, Hall M, et al. Home Health Nursing Care and Hospital Use for Medically Complex Children. *Pediatrics.* 2016;138(5):e20160530. PubMed doi: 10.1542/peds.2016-0530
30. Berry JG, Hall M, Neff J, et al. Children with medical complexity and Medicaid: spending and cost savings. *Health Aff (Millwood).* 2014;33(12):2199–2206. PubMed doi: 10.1377/hlthaff.2014.0828
31. Kusma JD, Davis MM, Foster C. Characteristics of Medicaid Policies for Children With Medical Complexity by State: A Qualitative Study. *JAMA Netw Open.* 2022;5(10):e2239270. PubMed doi: 10.1001/jamanetworkopen.2022.39270
32. Foster CC, Morales L, Fawcett AJ, Coleman CL. Access and Quality of Pediatric Home Healthcare: A Systematic Review. *Home Health Care Manag Pract.* 2023;35(4):287–298. doi: 10.1177/10848223231167878
33. Leonard BJ, Brust JD, Choi T. Providing access to home care for disabled children: Minnesota's Medicaid model waiver program. *Public Health Rep.* 1989;104(5):465–472. PubMed
34. Velott DL, Agbese E, Mandell D, et al. Medicaid 1915(c) Home- and Community-Based Services waivers for children with autism spectrum disorder. *Autism.* 2016;20(4):473–482. PubMed doi: 10.1177/1362361315590806
35. Keim-Malpass J, Constantoulakis L, Letzkus LC. Variability In States' Coverage Of Children With Medical Complexity Through Home And Community-Based Services Waivers. *Health Aff (Millwood).* 2019;38(9):1484–1490. PubMed doi: 10.1377/hlthaff.2018.05413
36. Edwards JD, Morris MC, Nelson JE, Panitch HB, Miller RL. Decisions around Long-term Ventilation for Children. Perspectives of Directors of Pediatric Home Ventilation Programs. *Ann Am Thorac Soc.* 2017;14(10):1539–1547. PubMed doi: 10.1513/AnnalsATS.201612-1002OC
37. Adepoju OE, Zhang Y, Phillips CD. Modeling the determinants of Medicaid home care payments for children with special health care needs: A structural equation model approach. *Disabil Health J.* 2014;7(4):426–432. PubMed doi: 10.1016/j.dhjo.2014.05.003
38. Elliott TR, Phillips CD, Patnaik A, et al. Medicaid Personal Care Services and caregivers' reports of children's health: the dynamics of a relationship. *Health Serv Res.* 2011;46(6pt1):1803–1821. PubMed doi: 10.1111/j.1475-6773.2011.01284.x
39. Patnaik A, Elliott TR, Moudouni DM, et al. Severity of children's intellectual disabilities and Medicaid personal care services. *Rehabil Psychol.* 2011;56(4):383–390. PubMed doi: 10.1037/a0025619
40. Baumgardner DJ, Burtea ED. Quality-of-life in technology-dependent children receiving home care, and their families–a qualitative study. *WMJ.* 1998;97(8):51–55. PubMed
41. Nageswaran S, Golden SL. Factors Associated With Stability of Health Nursing Services for Children With Medical Complexity. *Home Healthc Now.* 2017;35(8):434–444. PubMed doi: 10.1097/NHH.0000000000000583
42. Foster CC, Jacob-Files E, Arthur KC, Hillman SA, Edwards TC, Mangione-Smith R. Provider Perspectives of High-Quality Pediatric Hospital-to-Home Transitions for Children and Youth With Chronic Disease. *Hosp Pediatr.* 2017;7(11):649–659. PubMed doi: 10.1542/hpeds.2017-0031
43. Toly VB, Blanchette JE, Musil CM. Mothers caring for technology-dependent children at home: What is most helpful and least helpful? *Appl Nurs Res.* 2019;46:24–27. PubMed doi: 10.1016/j.apnr.2019.02.001
44. Mai K, Davis RK, Hamilton S, Robertson-James C, Calaman S, Turchi RM. Identifying Caregiver Needs for Children With a Tracheostomy Living at Home. *Clin Pediatr (Phila).* 2020;59(13):1169–1181. PubMed doi: 10.1177/0009922820941209
45. Millner BN. Technology-dependent children in New York State. *Bull N Y Acad Med.* 1991;67(2):131–142. PubMed
46. DeWitt PK, Jansen MT, Ward SLD, Keens TG. Obstacles to discharge of ventilator-assisted children from the hospital to home. *Chest.* 1993;103(5):1560–1565. PubMed doi: 10.1378/chest.103.5.1560
47. Jardine E, O'Toole M, Paton JY, Wallis C. Current status of long term ventilation of children in the United Kingdom: questionnaire survey. *BMJ.* 1999;318(7179):295–299. PubMed doi: 10.1136/bmj.318.7179.295
48. Noyes J. Barriers that delay children and young people who are dependent on mechanical ventilators from being discharged from hospital. *J Clin Nurs.* 2002;11(1):2–11. PubMed doi: 10.1046/j.1365-2702.2002.00565.x
49. Noyes J, Godfrey C, Beecham J. Resource use and service costs for ventilator-dependent children and young people in the UK. *Health Soc Care Community.* 2006;14(6):508–522. PubMed doi: 10.1111/j.1365-2524.2006.00639.x
50. Graf JM, Montagnino BA, Hueckel R, McPherson ML. Children with new tracheostomies: planning for family education and common impediments to discharge. *Pediatr Pulmonol.* 2008;43(8):788–794. PubMed doi: 10.1002/ppul.20867

51. Amin R, Sayal A, Syed F, et al. How long does it take to initiate a child on long-term invasive ventilation? Results from a Canadian pediatric home ventilation program. *Can Respir J.* 2015;22(2): 103–108. PubMed doi: 10.1155/2015/107914

52. Weaver MS, Wichman B, Bace S, et al. Measuring the Impact of the Home Health Nursing Shortage on Family Caregivers of Children Receiving Palliative Care. *J Hosp Palliat Nurs.* 2018;20(3):260–265. PubMed doi: 10.1097/NJH.0000000000000436

53. Bourke-Taylor H, Pallant JF, Law M, Howie L. Relationships between sleep disruptions, health and care responsibilities among mothers of school-aged children with disabilities. *J Paediatr Child Health.* 2013;49(9):775–782. PubMed doi: 10.1111/jpc.12254

54. Feeley CA, Turner-Henson A, Christian BJ, et al. Sleep quality, stress, caregiver burden, and quality of life in maternal caregivers of young children with bronchopulmonary dysplasia. *J Pediatr Nurs.* 2014; 29(1):29–38. PubMed doi: 10.1016/j.pedn.2013.08.001

55. Foster CC, Fuentes MM, Wadlington LA, et al. Caregiver and Provider Experiences of Home Healthcare Quality for Children With Medical Complexity. *Home Healthc Now.* 2020;38(3):138–146. PubMed doi: 10.1097/NHH.0000000000000857

56. Foster CC, Chorniy A, Kwon S, Kan K, Heard-Garris N, Davis MM. Children With Special Health Care Needs and Forgone Family Employment. *Pediatrics.* 2021;148(3):e2020035378. PubMed doi: 10.1542/peds.2020-035378

57. Sobotka SA, Lynch E, Quinn MT, Awadalla SS, Agrawal RK, Peek ME. Unmet Respite Needs of Children With Medical Technology Dependence. *Clin Pediatr (Phila).* 2019;58(11–12):1175–1186. PubMed doi: 10.1177/0009922819870251

58. Harrigan RC, Ratliffe C, Patrinos ME, Tse A. Medically fragile children: an integrative review of the literature and recommendations for future research. *Issues Compr Pediatr Nurs.* 2002; 25(1):1–20. PubMed doi: 10.1080/014608602753504829

59. Caicedo C. Health and Functioning of Families of Children With Special Health Care Needs Cared for in Home Care, Long-term Care, and Medical Day Care Settings. *J Dev Behav Pediatr.* 2015; 36(5):352–361. PubMed doi: 10.1097/DBP.0000000000000167

60. Romley JA, Shah AK, Chung PJ, Elliott MN, Vestal KD, Schuster MA. Family-Provided Health Care for Children With Special Health Care Needs. *Pediatrics.* 2017;139(1):e20161287. PubMed doi: 10.1542/peds.2016-1287

61. Data Resource Center for Child & Adolescent Health. National Survey of Children's Health. 2020–21 National Survey of Children's Health Database. Accessed February 18, 2025. https://www.childhealthdata.org/

62. Berry JG, Harris D, Coller RJ, et al. The Interwoven Nature of Medical and Social Complexity in US Children. *JAMA Pediatr.* 2020; 174(9):891–893. PubMed doi: 10.1001/jamapediatrics.2020.0280

63. Rasooly IR, Shults J, Guevara JP, Feudtner C. State Variation in Posthospital Home Nursing for Commercially Insured Medically Complex Children. *Pediatrics.* 2020;146(2):e20192465. PubMed doi: 10.1542/peds.2019-2465

64. Williams E, Published MM. Children with Special Health Care Needs: Coverage, Affordability, and HCBS Access. KFF. October 4, 2021. Accessed February 18, 2025. https://www.kff.org/medicaid/issue-brief/children-with-special-health-care-needs-coverage-affordability-and-hcbs-access/

65. Home & Community-Based Services. 1915(c) | Medicaid. Accessed February 18, 2025. https://www.medicaid.gov/medicaid/home-community-based-services/home-community-based-services-authorities/home-community-based-services-1915c/index.html

66. Baciu A, Negussie Y, Geller A, Weinstein JN, eds. National Academies of Sciences, Engineering, and Medicine, Health and Medicine Division, Board on Population Health and Public Health Practice, Committee on Community-Based Solutions to Promote Health Equity in the United States. In: *Communities in Action: Pathways to Health Equity.* National Academies Press; 2017, https://www.ncbi.nlm.nih.gov/books/NBK425848/. Accessed February 18, 2025.

67. Year C. (CY) 2024 Home Health Prospective Payment System Final Rule (CMS-1780-F) | CMS. Accessed February 18, 2025. https://www.cms.gov/newsroom/fact-sheets/calendar-year-cy-2024-home-health-prospective-payment-system-final-rule-cms-1780-f

68. Sherman J, Zalzal H, Bower K. Equitable Care for Children With a Tracheostomy: Addressing Challenges and Seeking Systemic Solutions. *Health Expect.* 2024;27(4):e14158. PubMed doi: 10.1111/hex.14158

69. Schiff J, Manning L, VanLandeghem K, Langer CS, Schutze M, Comeau M. Financing Care for CYSHCN in the Next Decade: Reducing Burden, Advancing Equity, and Transforming Systems. *Pediatrics.* 2022;149(suppl 7):e2021056150I. PubMed doi: 10.1542/peds.2021-056150I

70. Carter K, Blakely C, Zuk J, Brittan M, Foster C. Employing Family Caregivers: An Innovative Health Care Model. *Pediatrics.* 2022; 149(6):e2021054273. PubMed doi: 10.1542/peds.2021-054273

71. Foster CC, Kwon S, Blakely C, et al. Paying Family Medical Caregivers for Children's Home Healthcare in Colorado: A Working Medicaid Model. *J Pediatr.* 2023;261:113347. PubMed doi: 10.1016/j.jpeds.2022.12.043

72. Hazlett DE. A study of pediatric home ventilator management: medical, psychosocial, and financial aspects. *J Pediatr Nurs.* 1989;4(4):284–294. PubMed

73. Quint RD, Chesterman E, Crain LS, Winkleby M, Boyce WT. Home care for ventilator-dependent children. Psychosocial impact on the family. *AJDC 1960.* 1990;144(11):1238–1241. doi: 10.1001/archpedi.1990.02150350070028

74. Hollingsworth J. Service needs of children with disabilities and their families. *J Paediatr Child Health.* 1992;28(4):283–285. PubMed doi: 10.1111/j.1440-1754.1992.tb02667.x

75. Nelson VS, Carroll JC, Hurvitz EA, Dean JM. Home mechanical ventilation of children. *Dev Med Child Neurol.* 1996;38(8):704–715. PubMed doi: 10.1111/j.1469-8749.1996.tb12140.x

76. Kirk S, Glendinning C. Developing services to support parents caring for a technology-dependent child at home. *Child Care Health Dev.* 2004;30(3):209–218. PubMed doi: 10.1111/j.1365-2214.2004.00393.x

77. Neuss J. Mothers as primary caregivers for their technology dependent child at home: A qualitative study. Published online 2004.

78. Warfield ME, Gulley S. Unmet need and problems accessing specialty medical and related services among children with special

health care needs. *Matern Child Health J.* 2006;10(2):201–216. PubMed doi: 10.1007/s10995-005-0041-3

79. Kuo DZ, Cohen E, Agrawal R, Berry JG, Casey PH. A national profile of caregiver challenges among more medically complex children with special health care needs. *Arch Pediatr Adolesc Med.* 2011; 165(11):1020–1026. PubMed doi: 10.1001/archpediatrics.2011.172
80. Seear M, Kapur A, Wensley D, Morrison K, Behroozi A. The quality of life of home-ventilated children and their primary caregivers plus the associated social and economic burdens: a prospective study. *Arch Dis Child.* 2016;101(7):620–627. PubMed doi: 10.1136/archdischild-2015-309796
81. Andrews MM, Nielson DW. Technology dependent children in the home. *Pediatr Nurs.* 1988;14(2):111–114, 151. PubMed
82. Thrasher J, Baker J, Ventre KM, et al. Hospital to Home: A Quality Improvement Initiative to Implement High-fidelity Simulation Training for Caregivers of Children Requiring Long-term Mechanical Ventilation. *J Pediatr Nurs.* 2018;38:114–121. PubMed doi: 10.1016/j.pedn.2017.08.028
83. Kun SS, Beas VN, Keens TG, Ward SSL, Gold JI. Examining pediatric emergency home ventilation practices in home health nurses: Opportunities for improved care. *Pediatr Pulmonol.* 2015;50(7): 691–697. PubMed doi: 10.1002/ppul.23040
84. Foster C, Schinasi D, Kan K, Macy M, Wheeler D, Curfman A. Remote Monitoring of Patient- and Family-Generated Health Data in Pediatrics. *Pediatrics.* 2022;149(2):e2021054137. PubMed doi: 10.1542/peds.2021-054137
85. Scharer K, Dixon DM. Managing chronic illness: parents with a ventilator–dependent child. *J Pediatr Nurs.* 1989;4(4):236–247. PubMed
86. Kirk S, Glendinning C. Supporting 'expert' parents–professional support and families caring for a child with complex health care needs in the community. *Int J Nurs Stud.* 2002;39(6):625–635. PubMed doi: 10.1016/S0020-7489(01)00069-4
87. Parker G, Spiers G, Cusworth L, Birks Y, Gridley K, Mukherjee S. Care closer to home for children and young people who are ill: developing and testing a model of service delivery and organization. *J Adv Nurs.* 2012;68(9):2034–2046. PubMed doi: 10.1111/j.1365-2648.2011.05893.x
88. Nageswaran S, Golden SL. Improving the Quality of Home Health Care for Children With Medical Complexity. *Acad Pediatr.* 2017; 17(6):665–671. PubMed doi: 10.1016/j.acap.2017.04.019
89. Roque N, Walls N, Vargas-Friere L, Patel A. A QI Approach to Challenges in Home Care for Families of Tracheostomy-Dependent Children. In: *B53. SLEEP DISORDERED BREATHING AND LONG-TERM VENTILATION IN PEDIATRICS.* American Thoracic Society International Conference Abstracts. American Thoracic Society; 2019:A3590–A3590. doi: 10.1164/ajrccm-conference.2019.199.1_MeetingAbstracts.A3590
90. Ames SG, Delaney RK, Houtrow AJ, et al. Perceived Disability-Based Discrimination in Health Care for Children With Medical Complexity. *Pediatrics.* 2023;152(1):e2022060975. PubMed doi: 10.1542/peds.2022-060975
91. Cook S, Mauskar S, Berry JG. Discriminating Against Children With Medical Complexity. *Pediatrics.* 2023;152(1):e2023061604. PubMed doi: 10.1542/peds.2023-061604
92. Berry JG, Goldmann DA, Mandl KD, et al. Health information management and perceptions of the quality of care for children with tracheotomy: a qualitative study. *BMC Health Serv Res.* 2011;11(1): 117. PubMed doi: 10.1186/1472-6963-11-117
93. Nageswaran S, Sebesta MR, Golden SL. Transitioning Children With Medical Complexity From Hospital to Home Health Care: Implications for Hospital-Based Clinicians. *Hosp Pediatr.* 2020; 10(8):657–662. PubMed doi: 10.1542/hpeds.2020-0068
94. Nageswaran S, Golden SL. Home Health Nurse Collaboration in the Medical Neighborhood of Children with Medical Complexity. *Home Healthc Now.* 2016;34(9):507–518. PubMed doi: 10.1097/NHH.0000000000000463
95. Van Horne BS, Moffitt KB, Canfield MA, et al. Maltreatment of Children Under Age 2 With Specific Birth Defects: A Population-Based Study. *Pediatrics.* 2015;136(6):e1504–e1512. PubMed doi: 10.1542/peds.2015-1274
96. Jones L, Bellis MA, Wood S, et al. Prevalence and risk of violence against children with disabilities: a systematic review and meta-analysis of observational studies. *Lancet.* 2012;380(9845):899–907. PubMed doi: 10.1016/S0140-6736(12)60692-8
97. Lightfoot E. Children and Youth with Disabilities in the Child Welfare System: An Overview. *Child Welfare.* 2014;93:23–45.
98. Nowak CB. Recognition and prevention of child abuse in the child with disability. *Am J Med Genet C Semin Med Genet.* 2015;169(4): 293–301. PubMed doi: 10.1002/ajmg.c.31458
99. Slayter E, Springer C. Child welfare-involved youth with intellectual disabilities: pathways into and placements in foster care. *Intellect Dev Disabil.* 2011;49(1):1–13. PubMed doi: 10.1352/1934-9556-49.1.1
100. Watkinson MD, Ehlenbach M, Chung PJ, et al. Interventions in the Home and Community for Medically Complex Children: A Systematic Review. *Pediatrics.* 2023;151(5):e2022058352. PubMed doi: 10.1542/peds.2022-058352
101. Foster CC, Agrawal RK, Davis MM. Home Health Care For Children With Medical Complexity: Workforce Gaps, Policy, And Future Directions. *Health Aff (Millwood).* 2019;38(6):987–993. PubMed doi: 10.1377/hlthaff.2018.05531
102. Honsberger OR Eskedar Girmash. Kate. State Approaches to Reimbursing Family Caregivers of Children and Youth with Special Health Care Needs through Medicaid. NASHP. January 15, 2021. Accessed February 18, 2025. https://nashp.org/state-approaches-to-reimbursing-family-caregivers-of-children-and-youth-with-special-health-care-needs-through-medicaid/
103. Nadash P, Tell EJ, Jansen T. What do Family Caregivers Want? Payment for Providing Care. *J Aging Soc Policy.* 2024;36(4): 547–561. PubMed doi: 10.1080/08959420.2022.2127599
104. Robison J, Porter M, Shugrue N, Kleppinger A, Lambert D. Connecticut's 'Money Follows The Person' Yields Positive Results For Transitioning People Out Of Institutions. *Health Aff (Millwood).* 2015;34(10):1628–1636. PubMed doi: 10.1377/hlthaff.2015.0244

Genetic Evaluation of the Child With Intellectual Disability or Global Developmental Delay

- *Clinical Report*
  - *PPI: AAP Partnership for Policy Implementation See Appendix 1 for more information.*

American Academy of Pediatrics
DEDICATED TO THE HEALTH OF ALL CHILDREN®

AAP Partnership for Policy Implementation

CLINICAL REPORT Guidance for the Clinician in Rendering Pediatric Care

American Academy of Pediatrics

DEDICATED TO THE HEALTH OF ALL CHILDREN™

Genetic Evaluation of the Child With Intellectual Disability or Global Developmental Delay: Clinical Report

Lance H. Rodan, MD,[1,2] Joan Stoler, MD, FAAP,[1] Emily Chen, MD, PhD,[3] Timothy Geleske, MD, FAAP,[4] and the Council on Genetics

abstract

Genetic neurodevelopmental disorders are common in the pediatric population, and establishing a specific diagnosis early provides multiple benefits including prognostication, surveillance for disorder-related complications, accurate recurrence risk, and specific management. This report provides an approach to the genetic evaluation of developmental delay/intellectual disability for the general pediatrician. When possible, genetic testing should be selected by phenotype, and typical distinguishing clinical features to facilitate this are presented. If a specific disorder or group of disorders cannot be ascertained by phenotype, an agnostic (or hypothesis-free) approach is utilized. Recommendations are provided for this agnostic approach based on diagnostic yield and also practical considerations such as test complexity and impact on management. The general guidance in this report for genetic testing does not preclude further evaluation by relevant subspecialists as necessary, including neurologists, developmental pediatricians, and clinical geneticists.

[1]Division of Genetics and Genomics, Boston Children's Hospital, Harvard Medical School, Boston, Massachusetts; [2]Department of Neurology, Boston Children's Hospital, Harvard Medical School, Boston, Massachusetts; [3]Department of Genetics, Kaiser Permanente, San Francisco, California; and [4]Northwestern University Feinberg School of Medicine, Chicago, Illinois

Drs Rodan and Stoler prepared and revised the manuscript. Drs Chen and Geleske revised the manuscript.

FINANCIAL/CONFLICT OF INTEREST DISCLOSURE: The authors have indicated they have no potential conflicts of interest to disclose. All authors have filed conflict of interest statements with the American Academy of Pediatrics. Any conflicts have been resolved through a process approved by the Board of Directors. The American Academy of Pediatrics has neither solicited nor accepted any commercial involvement in the development of the content of this publication.

To cite: Rodan LH, Stoler J, Chen E, et al; American Academy of Pediatrics, Council on Genetics. Genetic Evaluation of the Child With Intellectual Disability or Global Developmental Delay: Clinical Report. *Pediatrics.* 2025;156(1):e2025072219

INTRODUCTION

Global developmental delay (GDD)/intellectual disability (ID) has an estimated global prevalence of 1% to 3%.[1] Further, in pediatric primary care, neurodevelopmental disorders are the most common chronic medical condition, with a combined prevalence of approximately 17%.[2] Neurodevelopmental disorders have a considerable impact at individual, family, and societal levels. Global developmental delay is defined in the *Diagnostic and Statistical Manual of Mental Disorders, 5th Edition* (DSM-5) as the failure to meet expected developmental milestones in several areas of intellectual functioning in an individual younger than 5 years who cannot undergo systematic assessment of intellectual functioning, including children too young to participate in standardized testing. This evaluation necessitates reassessment after a period of time.[3] Intellectual disability is defined in the DSM-5 as significant limitations both in intellectual functioning and in adaptive behavior as expressed in conceptual, social, and practical adaptive skills in individuals 5 years or older.[4] Children with GDD and ID are often first evaluated in the general pediatric setting, so it is pertinent for the general pediatrician to have an initial approach to the evaluation of these patients.

GDD/ID has diverse etiologies, including prenatal injury or developmental disorders (eg, in utero infection, teratogens, toxins, vascular disruption, developmental brain malformations); perinatal/postnatal insult (eg, hypoperfusion injury, asphyxia, infections, trauma, neglect, toxins); and genetic disorders. Genetic disorders account for up to 50% of diagnosed etiologies.[5,6]

Genetic causes can be broadly categorized as:

- chromosomal
- monogenic
- imprinting defects
- oligo/polygenic

Chromosome disorders are commonly associated with GDD/ID. Chromosome disorders may be *numerical*, in which an entire chromosome or multiple chromosomes are added to or missing from the normal pair (eg, trisomy 21), or *structural*, in which a part of a chromosome is deleted (eg, 22q11.2 deletion), duplicated, or rearranged, such as with a translocation. Because chromosome disorders affect multiple contiguous genes, they may also be associated with dysmorphic features, multiple congenital anomalies, and abnormalities of growth.[7] Some chromosome disorders may be inherited from unaffected or more mildly affected parents. Supplementary Table 1 summarizes more common and phenotypically identifiable chromosome disorders. Most chromosome disorders can be identified on chromosome microarray testing, with the main exception being balanced structural chromosome abnormalities, such as translocations and ring chromosomes, which require a karyotype. Some exome sequencing platforms currently offer chromosome (copy number) analysis as well, although sensitivity is lower than with chromosome microarray.

Monogenic disorders are caused by variation in a single gene. There are approximately 20 000 protein-coding genes in the human genome, and more than 1300 causative genes and 1100 candidate genes have thus far been implicated in neurodevelopmental disorders, with this number rapidly increasing.[8] Monogenic disorders may be caused by single nucleotide variants, small insertions or deletions (indels), larger exon-level deletions or duplications, or expansion of an inherently repeating genetic sequence (ie, trinucleotide repeat disorders). Inheritance of monogenic disorders may be X-linked, autosomal dominant, autosomal recessive, or even maternally inherited.[9] Some forms of mitochondrial disorders can be inherited in an autosomal recessive manner, and others are maternally inherited (with rare exceptions).[10] Supplementary Table 2 summarizes a number of phenotypically identifiable monogenic neurodevelopmental disorders. Diagnosis of monogenic disorders can be facilitated by targeted gene testing if the disorder is clinically suspected or can be diagnosed in an agnostic manner with gene panels or exome sequencing.

Mosaicism refers to cell lines with differing genotypes. Mosaicism can involve chromosomes (eg, mosaic Turner syndrome, mosaic trisomy 9) or single genes (eg, *PIK3CA* related overgrowth disorders, McCune-Albright syndrome). The diagnosis of mosaicism may require testing in cultured skin fibroblasts or other affected tissue, because the abnormalities may be difficult to detect or even absent in white blood cells or buccal swab. Pigmentary mosaicism of the skin, typically appearing as a whorled pattern of hypo- or hyperpigmentation following Blaschko lines, can occasionally be a clue to a mosaic disorder.

Imprinting disorders are caused by molecular changes affecting imprinted chromosomal regions and genes. Imprinting refers to the expression of genes in a parent-of-origin specific manner (ie, genes only expressed from either the maternally or paternally inherited allele, but not from both). The prototypical imprinting disorders associated with GDD/ID are Prader-Willi syndrome and Angelman syndrome.[11] A summary of imprinting disorders associated with GDD/ID can be found in Table 1. The genetic diagnosis of imprinting disorders typically requires targeted testing for the specific disorder.

Polygenic disorders are caused by the interaction of a number of genes, with each gene contributing partially to the phenotype. If there are only 2 genes involved, this is termed digenic inheritance. Oligogenic inheritance is when there are several genes involved, less than in polygenic inheritance. Examples of these would be modifier genes in which a second gene variant influences the expression/penetrance of the condition, such as in Bardet Biedl syndrome.[12] In general, polygenic inheritance is difficult to delineate in clinical practice, because the ability to assess the additive or cumulative effects of multiple gene variants on phenotype is limited.

Reasons to Pursue Specific Genetic Diagnosis for GDD/ID

Pursuing genetic diagnosis for GDD/ID allows for accurate prognostication, facilitates surveillance for potential disorder-related complications, provides accurate recurrence risk in families interested in having additional children, and allows for prenatal diagnostic testing and preimplantation genetic diagnosis (PGD). This will also

TABLE 1. Imprinting Disorders Associated With Global Developmental Delay and Intellectual Disability

Disorder	Genetic Etiology	Clinical Features
Angelman syndrome	Abnormal methylation at 15q11.2-q13 (including UBE3A gene) – maternally imprinted	Feeding difficulties, progressive microcephaly, seizures, ataxia/tremulousness, epilepsy behavioral peculiarities (happy disposition, fascination with water), variable developmental delay/intellectual disability[13]
Prader-Willi syndrome	Abnormal methylation of 15q11.2-q13 – paternally imprinted	Severe feeding difficulties in infancy followed by obesity in childhood, severe hypotonia, hypogonadism, short stature, behavioral abnormalities, global developmental delay/intellectual disability[14]
Temple syndrome	Abnormal methylation of 14q32.2 – paternally imprinted	Intrauterine growth restriction, short stature, feeding difficulties in infancy followed by obesity later in childhood, precocious puberty, hypotonia, variable developmental delay/intellectual disability[15]

have reproductive implications for the child him- or herself when they are of reproductive age, as having a genetic diagnosis can help inform their own reproductive decisions. It can directly impact treatment (ie, inborn errors of metabolism) or identify as candidates for future treatments (eg, gene therapy); reduce further unnecessary diagnostic testing; allow access to developmental therapies/services, appropriate disease-specific support networks, or clinical trials; and provide positive psychological impact on parents/caregivers.[16]

The diagnostic yield of genetic testing is influenced by the severity of GDD/ID. In severe ID, as defined in DSM-5, a genetic etiology may be discovered in approximately 80% of cases, whereas in mild ID, the diagnostic yield is closer to 20%.[17] The genetic diagnostic yield is also increased if there are dysmorphic features, congenital anomalies, or neurological comorbidities. The genetic evaluation of GDD and ID requires a thoughtful and systematic evaluation. This evaluation includes a detailed medical history, family history, clinical examination, and use of corollary investigations such as neuroimaging, vision assessment, and hearing assessment.

GDD/ID can be divided into syndromic and nonsyndromic forms. Syndromic refers to clinical features beyond GDD/ID that may suggest a specific disorder or category of disorders, whereas nonsyndromic GDD/ID lacks such features.[18] Up to two-thirds of GDD/ID is considered nonsyndromic.

If the patient has features suggestive of a syndromic form of GDD/ID, when possible, a phenotype-driven diagnostic approach is useful to make the clinical diagnosis or to refer for more targeted genetic testing to improve testing accuracy as well as to save cost and time. When a specific diagnosis is not suspected, or in cases of nonsyndromic GDD/ID, an agnostic, or "hypothesis-free," approach may be utilized.

PHENOTYPE-DRIVEN APPROACH TO DIAGNOSTIC EVALUATION

Following history and examination, the etiology of GDD/ID can be established in up to 17.2% to 34.2% of cases.[19]

Medical History

The evaluation includes taking a full developmental history, including gross motor, fine motor, language, social-emotional, and self-help skills. Developmental delay isolated to the motor domains may suggest a central (eg, brain) or peripheral (eg, neuromuscular) disorder. Abnormalities in language and social domains raises concern for autism spectrum disorder (ASD). Although the genetic etiologies of ASD may overlap with those associated with GDD/ID, the genetic diagnostic approach to ASD will not be covered further in this review.

It is useful to establish the trajectory of the individual's development to assess whether there is developmental regression. Developmental regression may suggest a neurodegenerative disorder or acquired process necessitating a prompt urgent referral to a neurologist and/or geneticist. The diagnostic evaluation for developmental regression will not be covered in this review.

Comorbid behavioral abnormalities are important to elicit in the child with GDD/ID and can suggest a specific diagnosis. For example, severe self-injurious behaviors can be seen in Lesch-Nyhan syndrome and Cornelia-de-Lange syndrome.[20,21] Some genetic disorders are associated with unique behavioral peculiarities, such as fascination with water or crinkly items in Angelman syndrome, skin picking and hyperphagia in Prader-Willi syndrome, midline stereotypies and intense eye contact in Rett syndrome, and episodic hyperventilation and breath-holding in Pitt-Hopkins syndrome.[13,14,22,23]

In addition to the developmental history, it is useful to establish whether there are any additional health concerns. It is often these features that can allow for the differential diagnosis to be narrowed based on phenotype. Additional health concerns can include other neurological symptoms (eg, seizures, movement disorder, weakness, nystagmus, hypotonia, spasticity, dystonia, hyperreflexia, ataxia, focal neurological findings); vision loss; hearing loss; feeding difficulties; organomegaly; and abnormalities of the gastrointestinal, dermatologic, dental, respiratory, cardiovascular, musculoskeletal, or endocrine systems. Occasionally, history of an unusual odor may prompt evaluation for an inborn error of metabolism, such as the maple syrup odor to urine or ear wax in maple syrup urine disease.[24]

Family History

Obtaining a 3-generation pedigree (asking specific questions about siblings, parents, grandparents, aunts, and uncles) provides important information. Additional family history of GDD/ID may suggest a specific mode of inheritance. Absence of other affected individuals may suggest autosomal recessive inheritance, a de novo autosomal dominant disorder, or an X-linked disorder. A history of psychiatric disorders and/or seizures is another potential indicator of genetic disorders in patients with GDD/ID, because some genetic disorders associated with GDD/ID can manifest with psychiatric symptoms and/or epilepsy in other family members as the result of incomplete penetrance and variable expressivity. In addition, psychiatric conditions can indicate genetic predisposition in their children. A family history of premature ovarian failure or ataxia/tremor may suggest fragile X syndrome.[25] A family history of 3 or more miscarriages in an individual may suggest a balanced chromosome rearrangement in a parent, predisposing to an unbalanced structural chromosome abnormality in offspring. Advanced paternal age may suggest a de novo dominant disorder, whereas advanced maternal age (>35 years) may suggest an aneuploidy. In vitro fertilization is associated with an increased risk of imprinting disorders, such as Prader-Willi syndrome and Angelman syndrome.[26,27]

Clinical Examination

Accurate assessment of height, weight, and head circumference is important, because these may inform the differential diagnosis. With respect to head circumference, analysis of growth velocity using a standardized growth curve will identify microcephaly (noting whether the microcephaly is congenital or postnatal), plateauing head circumference, and progressive microcephaly or macrocephaly. It is important to assess weight gain and growth to assess for failure to thrive.

Notation of dysmorphic features and other congenital anomalies, such as limb defects, will indicate the need for referral of the patient to a geneticist for further dysmorphology evaluation. For example, dysmorphic craniofacial features may include abnormal head shape, abnormally spaced or upslanting/downslanting eyes, epicanthal folds, depressed nasal bridge, unusual nasal configuration, long philtrum, and ear abnormalities.

Examination of the skin for neurocutaneous stigmata, such as café au lait macules, other hypo- or hyperpigmented skin regions, or vascular skin markings may indicate specific disorders. Rarely, hair or nail abnormalities also may suggest a specific disorder. A precordial examination may detect a murmur indicative of underlying congenital heart disease. Hepatosplenomegaly can be a feature of genetic overgrowth disorders and some inborn errors of metabolism (eg, lysosomal disorders). Cryptorchidism can be associated with some genetic neurodevelopmental disorders. Vision and hearing screening can also be performed by the pediatrician. A complete neurologic examination may detect abnormalities of muscle tone, weakness, or a movement disorder.

Corollary Testing: Neuroimaging, Vision, Hearing

In children with GDD/ID, evaluation by an ophthalmologist should be considered, both for diagnostic and therapeutic purposes. Retinal and optic nerve abnormalities may provide insight into an underlying genetic disorder. In children with language delay, hearing evaluation is also important. In addition to facilitating treatment, the finding of sensorineural hearing loss may offer a phenotypic clue.[28]

Neuroimaging with magnetic resonance imaging (MRI) is indicated in children with GDD/ID and abnormal head circumference, focal neurological signs or symptoms, seizures, increased tone or developmental regression.[5,29] It may also be considered in moderate to severe GDD/ID, if a specific disorder with abnormal neuroimaging is suspected, or if no etiology is identified following other diagnostic evaluations including genetic studies.[19] Neuroimaging may demonstrate relatively nonspecific findings, such as underrotated hippocampi, abnormally contoured and enlarged ventricles, reduced cerebral volume, delayed myelination, or dysgenesis of corpus callosum. It may also demonstrate more specific structural abnormalities, such as polymicrogyria, lissencephaly, periventricular nodular heterotopia, holoprosencephaly, or cerebellar malformations. There may also be signal abnormalities of the cerebral white matter or basal ganglia that can occasionally suggest a specific disorder based on the pattern.[30] Magnetic resonance spectroscopy may be useful in the evaluation for some inborn errors of metabolism, including disorders of creatine metabolism.[31]

AGNOSTIC APPROACH TO DIAGNOSTIC EVALUATION

If the medical history, family history, clinical examination, and corollary testing do not lead to a suspected diagnosis, then a hypothesis-free algorithmic approach could be pursued. This approach considers diagnostic yield, cost and complexity of the test, and the potential impact of the test results. Previously published agnostic approaches include a prior iteration from the American Academy of Pediatrics (AAP), and recommendations from the American Academy of Neurology (AAN), Canadian Pediatric Society (CPS), and the Treatable Intellectual Disability Endeavor (TIDE) protocol.[1,5,32] The AAP proposes the following updated tiered agnostic approach based on diagnostic yield and practical considerations (see Figure 1). Depending on comfort level, the pediatrician may opt to refer to a geneticist at any point in the genetic diagnostic evaluation. If a geneticist is not available, higher-order evaluation from neurologists

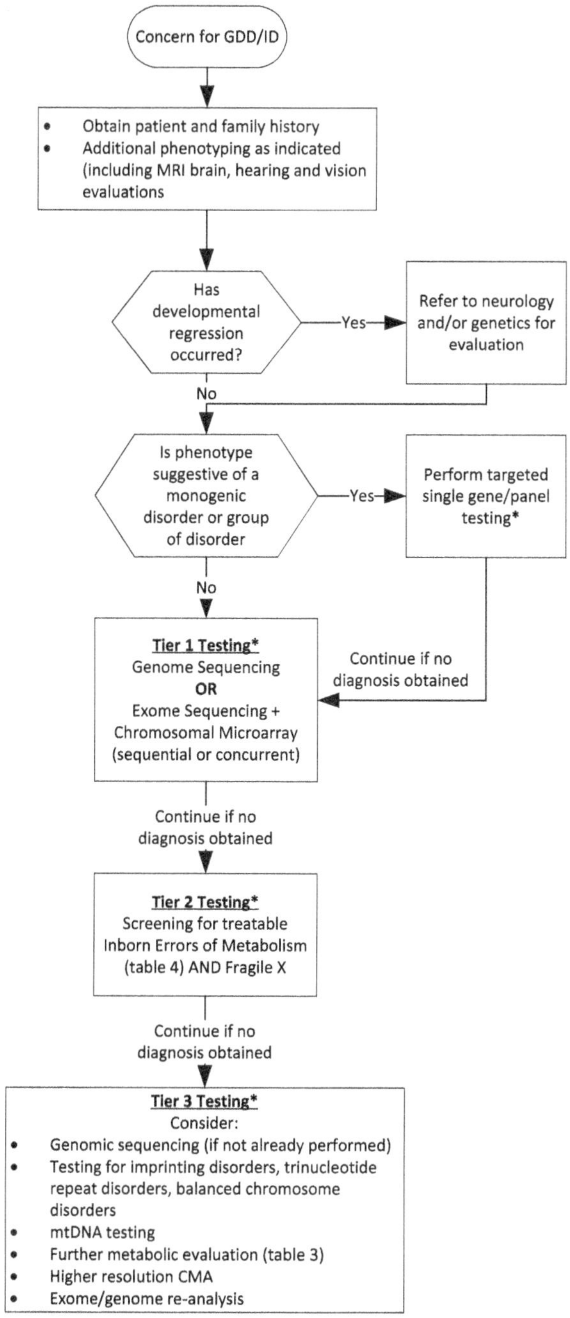

FIGURE 1.
Tiered agnostic approach to diagnostic evaluation.
*Refer to genetics for help with genetic testing.
Abbreviations: CMA, chromosome microarray; GDD, global developmental delay; ID, intellectual disability; MRI, magnetic resonance imaging.

and/or experienced pediatricians including developmental specialists may be considered.

Tier 1: Genome Sequencing or Exome Sequencing + Chromosome Microarray

The American College of Medical Genetics and Genomics (ACMG) recently recommended exome/genome sequencing for pediatric patients with GDD/ID or congenital anomalies as a first- or second-tier test.[33] The AAP recommends exome/genome sequencing as a first-tier test for GDD/ID in most circumstances because of superior diagnostic yield and higher cost-effectiveness if pursued earlier in the diagnostic process. Exome sequencing utilizes high throughput (next generation) sequencing to evaluate the entirety of protein coding exons in the human genome. Some exome sequencing platforms are also able to detect chromosome copy number variation and larger intragenic deletions and duplications (typically 3 exons in size or larger). The reported yield of exome sequencing for GDD/ID ranges from 28% to 43%.[33-35] Genome sequencing is a technique that evaluates almost the entire genome, including intronic and noncoding elements that are not assessed by exome sequencing. It also has the potential to detect copy number variation and structural rearrangements. Genome sequencing has been demonstrated to provide an approximately 10% to 20% higher diagnostic yield than exome sequencing, so it is preferable but currently may be less accessible to providers to order than exome sequencing.[33-35] Genome sequencing may utilize short-read (hundreds of base pairs) or long-read (thousands of base pairs) sequencing. Long-read sequencing has the advantage of being potentially better able to detect structural variations such as large insertions, deletions/duplications, inversions, repeats, translocations, and highly variable or repetitive elements; however, it is more costly and time consuming than short-read sequencing period.[36]

Gene variants reported on exome/genome sequencing are characterized according to the ACMG and the Association for Molecular Pathology (ACMG-AMP) system for variant classification. This classification system utilizes a score based on strict criteria to establishes 5 "classes" of variants: benign, likely benign, variant of unknown significance (VUS), likely pathogenic, and pathogenic.[37] In cases in which the significance of a variant is not definitive (ie, variants that are classified as neither benign nor pathogenic), the clinician must use their best clinical judgement to interpret the clinical significance. Depending on the situation, testing additional affected or unaffected family members for further segregation data may be useful. In addition, there may be a functional test (eg, metabolic testing) or further phenotyping data that can be obtained (eg, specific neuroimaging abnormalities) that can help to confirm or exclude a genetic diagnosis. Finally, the significance of a variant may be reinterpreted over time on the basis of accrued data. Since the interpretation of these results can be challenging, especially when there are variants of uncertain significance, the geneticist should help to provide as much clarification as possible to the family and the pediatrician (who may be asked for their opinion). It must be stressed that in some cases the classification of variants of uncertain significance may change over time.

Pretest genetic counseling should include discussion of variants of uncertain significance and the potential to detect incidental or secondary findings and nonpaternity or nonmaternity. With regard to incidental findings, the ACMG has specified 81 genes that are regarded as clinically actionable, including genes related to increased risk of cancer, cardiomyopathy, cardiac conduction disorders, connective tissue disorders, and metabolic disorders.[38] Pathogenic variants in these genes are included by default in clinical exome reports, although the patient and family may choose to opt out of these findings. There may be implications of such findings on future insurability such as disability, life, and long-term insurance. The diagnostic yield of exome/genome sequencing is improved if a trio sample is sent (proband and both parents), because this can determine de novo variants and can establish the phase of biallelic variants. Limitations of exome/genome sequencing include inability to diagnose repeat disorders and methylation abnormalities.[39] In addition, exome sequencing may have poor coverage of certain genomic regions, reduced sensitivity at detecting intragenic deletions (particularly those less than 3 exons in size) and will not detect balanced chromosome abnormalities. It is also important to note that the laboratory interpretation of exome/genome is very much dependent on the phenotype provided to the laboratory by the ordering clinician. Artificial intelligence is being studied to help with the automation of interpretation of genome sequencing for putative candidate variants.[40] In cases in which the family desires more targeted testing for concern of identifying candidates in less well understood genes, more variants of uncertain significance, or incidental findings, then a focused GDD/ID panel using similar sequencing technology as exome sequencing, but limited to a set of targeted genes, may be utilized. There is no uniformity with such testing, so the specific genes included and methodologies used differ significantly between performing laboratories. One possible benefit, based on the specific laboratory and test utilized, may be improved coverage of the included genes and better detection of intragenic deletions and duplications compared with exome sequencing, but the provider is encouraged to evaluate this on the basis of the specific panel test. In general, targeted GDD/ID panels have a lower diagnostic yield than exome/genome sequencing and are not preferred except in certain situations as noted previously. If a more targeted GDD/ID panel is nondiagnostic, then exome/genome sequencing may be considered next. The involvement of a geneticist or genetic counselor is recommended in these cases to assist in the selection of appropriate testing.

Chromosome Microarray

Genome-wide chromosome microarray (CMA) has been considered a first-line diagnostic test in the evaluation of the child with GDD/ID by the AAP, AAN, CPS, and the ACMG.[1,5,39,41,42] The AAP continues to recommend CMA in the first-tier agnostic evaluation for GDD/ID along with exome sequencing (sequential or concurrent). CMA is a test that quantitatively evaluates for chromosome gains and losses. It can occasionally detect smaller intragenic deletions or duplications. The specific resolution of the CMA varies depending on the platform used. If the CMA utilizes single nucleotide polymorphism (SNP)-based technology, it may also detect genomic regions of homozygosity, which can help to facilitate diagnosis of an autosomal recessive disorder or an imprinted disorder (in cases of uniparental isodisomy). The CMA cannot detect balanced chromosome rearrangements (eg, balanced translocations or balanced ring chromosomes).[16] It is estimated that the diagnostic yield of this test in the child with GDD/ID is between 15% and 20%.[42] Because the CMA screens for copy number variants genome-wide in an unbiased manner, there is the possibility that a CMA may detect copy number variants of uncertain significance, consanguinity, or incidental findings (eg, deletion of a gene implicated in cancer), and so pretest genetic counseling is indicated.

Pretest genetic counseling involves discussion of possible results such as benign, likely benign, pathogenic, likely pathogenic variants, or variants of uncertain significance. The laboratory uses data to determine these classifications, and in some cases, there are not enough data to determine whether a variant is disease causing or not, resulting in designation of a variant of uncertain significance. Identification of carrier status is possible if a deletion is found that includes a gene causing a recessive disorder. Incidental findings such as deletion of a cancer-causing gene may be reported. There may be implications of such findings on future insurability, such as disability, life, and long-term insurance. Areas of homozygosity (in which areas of both copies of the chromosome pair are the same) could indicate possible consanguinity.

Although CMA has a lower diagnostic yield overall than exome/genome sequencing, it can be superior to exome sequencing at detecting chromosome deletions/duplications, including small intragenic copy number variants. CMA also generally has a faster turnaround time and simpler pretest counseling. Pediatricians and other non-geneticist providers may elect to begin with a CMA first on the basis of available resources (eg, access to genetic counselors) and comfort level with genetic testing, while facilitating referral to a geneticist for possible exome/genome sequencing. A CMA may also be performed prior to exome/genome sequencing on the basis of the individual case and patient or clinician preference. Alternatively, CMA can be performed concurrently or following negative exome sequencing for superior coverage of copy number variation. If genome sequencing is initially performed, there is typically adequate evaluation of copy number variation, so CMA can be deferred in most cases.

Tier 2: Fragile X Testing and Metabolic Testing

Fragile X Testing

Fragile X syndrome is caused by *CGG* expansions in the 5′ untranslated region of the *FMR1* gene, and diagnosis required targeted testing that measures repeat length (ie, will *not* be detected on exome/genome sequencing or CMA).[25] Fragile X testing has historically been considered in the first-line agnostic diagnostic evaluation of the male with GDD/ID, including the prior position statements of the AAP, AAN, and CPS.[1,5,28] However, fragile X testing has a diagnostic yield of only approximately 1% in both males and females, and some authors have suggested that it should no longer be included in the first-tier evaluation of GDD/ID in the absence of clinical suspicion.[43] On the basis of the low diagnostic yield, the AAP recommends fragile X testing in the second-tier evaluation in both males and females with apparently nonsyndromic GDD/ID after exome/genome sequencing and CMA. If there are specific clinical features or family history consistent with fragile X syndrome, then it should be pursued earlier in the diagnostic evaluation (see section on phenotype-driven approach).

Screening for Treatable Inborn Errors of Metabolism

Inborn errors of metabolism (IEMs) are monogenic disorders associated with enzymatic defects or abnormal transport of metabolites. They represent the largest *treatable* cause of intellectual disability. With early diagnosis and treatment, there is the potential for improved outcome.

Many newborn screening programs evaluate for a number of IEMs, although the specific disorders screened for and testing methodologies vary based on location. It is also important to distinguish between screening and diagnostic evaluation and potential for missed diagnoses on newborn screening.[44,45]

Karnebeek et al performed a systematic literature review of treatable inborn errors of metabolism presenting with intellectual disability as a predominant feature. They reported 81 total treatable IEMs across 14 different disease categories. Fifty of 81 were diagnosable with routine blood and urine tests, whereas for the remaining disorders, more specialized testing was required, including specific enzyme testing, cerebrospinal fluid studies, or genetic testing.[32]

IEMs often present as syndromic GDD/IDD; however, IEMs may present as nonsyndromic GDD/ID in the earlier stages of illness. Red flags that may suggest an IEM include:

- Developmental regression
- Neurological signs – epilepsy, spasticity, movement disorder
- Multisystem involvement
- Abnormal body odor
- Basic biochemical abnormalities (eg, acidosis, hypoglycemia, etc)
- Abnormal MRI – atrophy, white matter abnormalities, deep gray structures symmetrically affected, abnormal spectroscopy (eg, elevated lactate or glycine, reduced creatine)
- Family history of IEM, or consanguinity

The diagnostic yield of metabolic evaluation in children with GDD/ID has been estimated to be 1% to 5%.[46] Further, this testing has a relatively low cost, prompt turnaround time, and the potential impact on outcome if one of these disorders is identified. The 2014 AAP recommendations[1] and 2018 CPS position statement[5] both suggest metabolic screening in the first tier evaluation of GDD/ID; however, given the very low yield in nonsyndromic GDD/ID, the AAP recommends testing in the second-tier evaluation after exome/genome sequencing and CMA unless there are specific clinical indications of a metabolic disorder (see "red flags" for an IEM and phenotype-driven approach). Further, CMA and exome/genome sequencing will detect most IEMs, including IEMs without clinically measurable biochemical abnormalities. See Table 2 for recommended initial evaluation for *treatable* IEMs. In addition to these specialized biochemical evaluations, general screening with a complete blood cell count, chemistry panel, liver function tests, and thyroid function tests may be considered. A baseline creatine phosphokinase can screen for some genetic muscle disorders (eg, muscular dystrophies, some metabolic myopathies), particularly in individuals with motor delays, hypotonia, and/or weakness (see phenotype-driven approach).

Tier 3 Evaluation

The third tier in the agnostic genetic evaluation for GDD/ID is aimed at identifying genetic etiologies that may have been missed in the first 2 tiers. The third tier includes consideration of: genome sequencing if exome sequencing was previously performed; an imprinting disorder; trinucleotide disorder (which may be missed on panel testing or exome/genome, depending on methodology used); mitochondrial DNA (mtDNA) testing if not included with prior testing; potential further biochemical evaluation for an IEM beyond laboratory tests in tier 2 (see Table 3); karyotype to evaluate for balanced chromosome rearrangements such as ring chromosomes; and broad screening for intragenic deletion/duplications that may have been missed on exome sequencing. The latter may be accomplished with a targeted GDD/ID deletion and duplication panel test, a higher-resolution CMA with specific exon-level coverage of disease-associated genes, or genome sequencing.

If negative, exome/genome sequencing may be clinically reanalyzed every 1 to 2 years following the initial test.[47] Some clinical laboratories offer a one-time complementary reanalysis if requested. It is very important for the ordering clinician to provide any updated phenotype data for the

TABLE 2. Treatable Inborn Errors of Metabolism Associated With Global Developmental Delay and Intellectual Disability for Tier 2 Evaluation

Disorder (Gene)	Clinical Features (Untreated)	Biochemical Evaluation
Phenylketonuria (*PAH*)	Developmental delay/intellectual disability, autism, eczema, reduced skin and hair pigmentation, epilepsy[48]	Plasma amino acids (increased phenylalanine)
Classic homocystinuria (*CBS1*)	Developmental delay/intellectual disability, marfanoid habitus (tall stature, scoliosis, pectus excavatum), eye lens dislocation and/or high myopia, increased risk of thrombosis[49]	Total homocysteine (increased), plasma amino acids (increased methionine)
Organic acidurias	Developmental delay/intellectual disability, metabolic acidosis, hyperammonemia, failure to thrive, epilepsy, movement disorder, metabolic stroke[24]	Urine organic acids, plasma acylcarnitines, ammonia
Urea cycle disorders	Episodes of hyperammonemic encephalopathy, protein aversion[50]	Ammonia, plasma amino acids (abnormal citrulline and/or arginine), urine organic acids (+/− increased orotic acid)
Creatine deficiency syndromes (*AGAT, GAMT, SLC6A8*)	Developmental delay/intellectual disability, autism, epilepsy[51]	Urine creatine/creatinine, plasma creatine, urine and plasma guanidinoacetate
Lesch-Nyhan syndrome (*HPRT1*)	Developmental delay/intellectual disability, autism, spasticity, movement disorder, uric acid nephropathy[20]	Plasma uric acid (increased), urine purine and pyrimidines
Mucopolysaccharidoses	Developmental delay, behavioral abnormalities, coarse facial features, hepatosplenomegaly, ophthalmological findings, orthopedic anomalies (eg, progressive spine deformities)[52]	Urine glycosaminoglycans
Biotinidase deficiency	Developmental delay/regression, hypotonia, ataxia, epilepsy, hearing and vision loss, skin rash, alopecia[53]	Biotinidase enzyme activity (if not included on newborn screening or clinical suspicion)

TABLE 3. Additional Tier 3 Screening Evaluation for Inborn Errors of Metabolism Associated With Global Developmental Delay and Intellectual Disability

Disorder	Clinical Features	Biochemical Evaluation
Congenital disorders of glycosylation (CDG)	Highly variable phenotype, may include developmental delay/intellectual disability, abnormal tone, epilepsy, blood clotting abnormalities (both pro- and antithrombotic), liver disease, lipodystrophy (abnormal fat distribution)[54]	CDG transferrin testing, N-glycans, O-glycans, urine oligosaccharides, and free glycans
Lysosomal disorders	Highly variable phenotype, may include developmental delay/regression, epilepsy, coarse features, hepatosplenomegaly, skeletal anomalies, corneal or retinal abnormalities, hearing loss[55]	Urine mucopolysaccharides, urine oligosaccharides, lysosomal enzyme screening panel
Peroxisomal disorders	Highly variable phenotype, includes developmental delay/regression, hypotonia, epilepsy, neuropathy, craniofacial dysmorphisms, enlarged anterior fontanelle, skeletal abnormalities (eg, rhizomelia, chondrodysplasia punctata), liver disease, renal disease, hearing loss, retinal disease[56]	Plasma very long chain fatty acids, red blood cell plasmalogens
Smith-Lemli-Opitz syndrome (*DHCR7*)	Craniofacial dysmorphisms, short stature, 2/3 toe syndactyly, failure to thrive, microcephaly, congenital heart defects, CAKUT[57]	7-dehydrocholesterol levels
Purine and pyrimidine disorders (other than Lesch-Nyhan syndrome)	Highly variable phenotype, includes developmental delay/regression, movement disorder, epilepsy[58]	Urine purines/pyrimidines
Menkes syndrome (*ATP7A*)	Sparse and wiry hair, pale complexion, lax skin and joints, severe hypotonia, microcephaly, global developmental delay, epilepsy[59]	Serum copper and ceruloplasmin

Abbreviation: CAKUT, congenital anomalies of the kidneys and urinary tract.

reanalysis, because these data may influence the interpretation of the exome/genome sequencing. Some academic centers may also have the capacity for research-based exome reanalysis. The additional diagnostic yield of this iterative approach to exome analysis has been previously demonstrated.[60]

OTHER TESTING

Some genetic neurodevelopmental disorders are associated with abnormal DNA methylation at a single locus (see imprinted disorders discussed previously), whereas other disorders are associated with the abnormal methylation of multiple gene loci. This specific pattern of methylation abnormalities across multiple loci, or "methylation signature," can be syndrome-specific and exploited for diagnostic purposes. Recently, such genome-wide methylation signature testing has become clinically available, although it is still only able to evaluate for a relatively small number of disorders, limiting its utility primarily to the evaluation of variants of uncertain significance in these genes or as a screening evaluation following otherwise nondiagnostic testing as above.[61]

Finally, various facial recognition computer software programs are now available that have been designed to better recognize genetic disorders based on dysmorphology, but it remains to be seen what the clinical utility of such programs is.[62] Also, these facial recognition programs are not routinely available in clinical practice.

ETHICAL ISSUES

There are ethical issues associated with genetic testing, potential harm from genetic testing (privacy concerns, misattributed parentage) and inequities in access to genetic testing. These issues are beyond the scope of this paper and the reader is referred to the AAP policy statement "Ethical and Policy Issues in Genetic Testing and Screening of Children."

CONCLUSIONS/RECOMMENDATIONS

Genetic neurodevelopmental disorders are common in the pediatric population, and it is vital for the general pediatrician to have an approach for their initial evaluation. Establishing a genetic diagnosis early provides multiple benefits. If possible, genetic testing should be selected by phenotype, but in many cases, an agnostic approach may be utilized. The AAP provides recommendations for this agnostic approach based on diagnostic yield and also practical considerations such as test complexity and impact on management. These recommendations for initial testing do not preclude further evaluation by relevant subspecialists as necessary, including neurologists, developmental pediatricians, and clinical geneticists. These recommendations are provided throughout the report and are summarized in Figure 1.

LEAD AUTHORS

Lance H. Rodan, MD
Joan Stoler, MD, FAAP
Emily Chen, MD, PhD
Timothy Geleske, MD, FAAP

COUNCIL ON GENETICS EXECUTIVE COMMITTEE 2024–2025

Samantha Vergano, MD, FAAP (chair)
Ingrid A. Holm, MD, FAAP
Kelly Jones, MD, FAAP
Jennifer Kalish, MD, FAAP
Danielle C. Monteil, MD, FAAP
Amanda Barone Pritchard, MD, FAAP
Sonja A. Rasmussen, MD, MS, FAAP
Bianca Russell, MD, FAAP
Stephanie L. Santoro, MD, FAAP
Pamela Trapane, MD, FAAP
Kathryn Nicole Weaver, MD, FAAP

PARTNERSHIP FOR POLICY IMPLEMENTATION

Juan D. Chaparro, MD, MS, FAAP

LIAISONS

Lynne M. Bird, MD, FAAP - American College of Medical Genetics and Genomics
Steven J. Ralston, MD - American College of Obstetricians & Gynecologists (ACOG)

STAFF

Paul Spire

FUNDING: No external funding.

https://doi.org/10.1542/peds.2025-072219

REFERENCES

1. Moeschler JB, Shevell M, Moeschler JB, et al; Committee on Genetics. Comprehensive evaluation of the child with intellectual disability or global developmental delays. *Pediatrics*. 2014;134(3):e903–e918. PubMed doi: 10.1542/peds.2014-1839
2. Zablotsky B, Black LI, Maenner MJ, et al. Prevalence and trends of developmental disabilities among children in the United States: 2009–2017. *Pediatrics*. 2019;144(4):e20190811. PubMed doi: 10.1542/peds.2019-0811
3. Shevell M, Ashwal S, Donley D, et al; Practice Committee of the Child Neurology Society. Practice parameter: evaluation of the child with global developmental delay: report of the Quality Standards Subcommittee of the American Academy of Neurology and The Practice Committee of the Child Neurology Society. *Neurology*. 2003;60(3):367–380. PubMed doi: 10.1212/01.WNL.0000031431.81555.16
4. Schalock RL, Luckasson RA, Shogren KA. The renaming of mental retardation: understanding the change to the term intellectual

disability. *Intellect Dev Disabil.* 2007;45(2):116–124. PubMed doi: 10.1352/1934-9556(2007)45[116:TROMRU]2.0.CO;2

5. Bélanger SA, Caron J. Evaluation of the child with global developmental delay and intellectual disability. *Paediatr Child Health.* 2018; 23(6): 403–410. DOI: https://doi.org/10.1093/pch/pxy093
6. Srour M, Shevell M. Genetics and the investigation of developmental delay/intellectual disability. *Arch Dis Child.* 2014;99(4):386–389. PubMed doi: 10.1136/archdischild-2013-304063
7. Theisen A, Shaffer LG. Disorders caused by chromosome abnormalities. *Appl Clin Genet.* 2010;3:159–174. DOI: 10.2147/tacg.s8884
8. Kochinke K, Zweier C, Nijhof B, et al. Systematic phenomics analysis deconvolutes genes mutated in intellectual disability into biologically coherent modules. *Am J Hum Genet.* 2016;98(1):149–164. PubMed doi: 10.1016/j.ajhg.2015.11.024
9. Chiurazzi P, Pirozzi F. Advances in understanding - genetic basis of intellectual disability. *F1000 Res.* 2016;5:F1000. PubMed doi: 10.12688/f1000research.7134.1
10. Luo S, Valencia CA, Zhang J, et al. Biparental inheritance of mitochondrial DNA in humans. *Proc Natl Acad Sci U S A.* 2018;115(51):13039–13044. PubMed doi: 10.1073/pnas.1810946115
11. Eggermann T, Perez de Nanclares G, Maher ER, et al. Imprinting disorders: a group of congenital disorders with overlapping patterns of molecular changes affecting imprinted loci. *Clin Epigenetics.* 2015;7(1):123. PubMed doi: 10.1186/s13148-015-0143-8
12. Kousi M, Katsanis N. Genetic modifiers and oligogenic inheritance. *Cold Spring Harb Perspect Med.* 2015;5(6):a017145. PubMed doi: 10.1101/cshperspect.a017145
13. Bird LM. Angelman syndrome: review of clinical and molecular aspects. *Appl Clin Genet.* 2014;7:93–104. PubMed doi: 10.2147/TACG.S57386
14. Angulo MA, Butler MG, Cataletto ME. Prader-Willi syndrome: a review of clinical, genetic, and endocrine findings. *J Endocrinol Invest.* 2015;38(12):1249–1263. DOI: 10.1007/s40618-015-0312-9
15. Ioannides Y, Lokulo-Sodipe K, Mackay DJG, Davies JH, Temple IK. Temple syndrome: improving the recognition of an underdiagnosed chromosome 14 imprinting disorder: an analysis of 51 published cases. *J Med Genet.* 2014;51(8):495–501. PubMed doi: 10.1136/jmedgenet-2014-102396
16. Savatt JM, Myers SM. Genetic testing in neurodevelopmental disorders. *Front Pediatr.* 2021;9:526779. PubMed doi: 10.3389/fped.2021.526779
17. Shaffer LG; American College of Medical Genetics Professional Practice and Guidelines Committee. American College of Medical Genetics guideline on the cytogenetic evaluation of the individual with developmental delay or mental retardation. *Genet Med.* 2005;7(9):650–654. PubMed doi: 10.1097/01.gim.0000186545.83160.1e
18. Kaufman L, Ayub M, Vincent JB. The genetic basis of non-syndromic intellectual disability: a review. *J Neurodev Disord.* 2010;2(4):182–209. PubMed doi: 10.1007/s11689-010-9055-2
19. O'Byrne JJ, Lynch SA, Treacy EP, et al. Unexplained developmental delay/learning disability: guidelines for best practice protocol for first line assessment and genetic/metabolic/radiological investigations. *Ir J Med Sci.* 2016;185(1):241–248. PubMed doi: 10.1007/s11845-015-1284-7
20. Jinnah HA. HPRT1 disorders. In: *GeneReviews [Internet].* University of Washington; 1993–2021. 2000 Sep 25 [Updated 2020 Aug 6]
21. Kline AD, Moss JF, Selicorni A, et al. Diagnosis and management of Cornelia de Lange syndrome: first international consensus statement. *Nat Rev Genet.* 2018;19(10):649–666. PubMed doi: 10.1038/s41576-018-0031-0
22. Weaving LS, Ellaway CJ, Gécz J, Christodoulou J. Rett syndrome: clinical review and genetic update. *J Med Genet.* 2005;42(1):1–7. PubMed doi: 10.1136/jmg.2004.027730
23. Goodspeed K, Newsom C, Morris MA, Powell C, Evans P, Golla S. Pitt-Hopkins syndrome: a review of current literature, clinical approach, and 23-patient case series. *J Child Neurol.* 2018;33(3):233–244. doi: 10.1177/0883073817750490
24. Vaidyanathan K, Narayanan MP, Vasudevan DM. Organic acidurias: an updated review. *Indian J Clin Biochem.* 2011;26(4):319–325. PubMed doi: 10.1007/s12291-011-0134-2
25. Gallagher A, Hallahan B. Fragile X-associated disorders: a clinical overview. *J Neurol.* 2012;259(3):401–413. PubMed doi: 10.1007/s00415-011-6161-3
26. Odom LN, Segars J. Imprinting disorders and assisted reproductive technology. *Curr Opin Endocrinol Diabetes Obes.* 2010;17(6):517–522. PubMed doi: 10.1097/MED.0b013e32834040a3
27. Vermeiden JPW, Bernardus RE. Are imprinting disorders more prevalent after human in vitro fertilization or intracytoplasmic sperm injection? *Fertil Steril.* 2013;99(3):642–651. PubMed doi: 10.1016/j.fertnstert.2013.01.125
28. American Academy of Neurology, Child Neurology Society. *Evaluation of the Child with Global Developmental Delay.* American Academy of Neurology; 2011. Accessed April 9, 2024. https://www.aan.com/globals/axon/assets/2603.pdf
29. Noritz GH, Murphy NA, Murphy NA, et al; Neuromotor Screening Expert Panel. Motor delays: early identification and evaluation. *Pediatrics.* 2013;131(6):e2016–e2027. PubMed doi: 10.1542/peds.2013-1056
30. Ali AS, Syed NP, Murthy GSN, et al. Magnetic resonance imaging (MRI) evaluation of developmental delay in pediatric patients. *J Clin Diagn Res.* 2015;9(1):TC21–TC24. PubMed doi: 10.7860/JCDR/2015/11921.5478
31. Rajvanshi N, Bhakat R, Saxena S, et al. Magnetic resonance spectroscopy in children with developmental delay: time to look beyond conventional magnetic resonance imaging (MRI). *J Child Neurol.* 2021;36(6):440–446. PubMed doi: 10.1177/0883073820978006
32. van Karnebeek CD, Stockler-Ipsiroglu S. Early identification of treatable inborn errors of metabolism in children with intellectual disability: The Treatable Intellectual Disability Endeavor protocol in British Columbia. *Paediatr Child Health.* 2014;19(9):469–471. PubMed doi: 10.1093/pch/19.9.469
33. Manickam K, McClain MR, Demmer LA, et al; ACMG Board of Directors. Exome and genome sequencing for pediatric patients with congenital anomalies or intellectual disability: an

evidence-based clinical guideline of the American College of Medical Genetics and Genomics (ACMG). *Genet Med.* 2021;23(11):2029–2037. PubMed doi: 10.1038/s41436-021-01242-6

34. Srivastava S, Love-Nichols JA, Dies KA, et al. Meta-analysis and multidisciplinary consensus statement: exome sequencing is a first-tier clinical diagnostic test for individuals with neurodevelopmental disorders. *Genet Med.* 2019;21(11):2413–2421. doi: 10.1038/s41436-019-0554-6

35. Ewans LJ, Minoche AE, Schofield D, et al. Whole exome and genome sequencing in mendelian disorders: a diagnostic and health economic analysis. *Eur J Hum Genet.* 2022;30(10):1121–1131. PubMed doi: 10.1038/s41431-022-01162-2

36. Oehler JB, Wright H, Stark Z, Mallett AJ, Schmitz U. The application of long-read sequencing in clinical settings. *Hum Genomics.* 2023;17(1):73–85. PubMed doi: 10.1186/s40246-023-00522-3

37. Riggs ER, Andersen EF, Cherry AM, et al. Technical standards for the interpretation and reporting of constitutional copy-number variants: a joint consensus recommendation of the American College of Medical Genetics and Genomics (ACMG) and the Clinical Genome Resource (ClinGen). *Genet Med.* 2020;22(2):245–257. PubMed doi: 10.1038/s41436-019-0686-8

38. Miller DT, Lee K, Abul-Husn NS, et al; ACMG Secondary Findings Working Group. Electronic address: documents@acmg.net. ACMG SF v3.2 list for reporting of secondary findings in clinical exome and genome sequencing: A policy statement of the American College of Medical Genetics and Genomics (ACMG). *Genet Med.* 2023;25(8):100866. PubMed doi: 10.1016/j.gim.2023.100866

39. Savatt JM, Myers SM. Genetic testing in neurodevelopmental disorders. *Front Pediatr.* 2021;9:526779. DOI: 10.1002/humu.23607

40. De La Vega FM, Chowdhury S, Moore B, et al. Artificial intelligence enables comprehensive genome interpretation and nomination of candidate diagnoses for rare genetic diseases. *Genome Med.* 2021;13(1):153–171. PubMed doi: 10.1186/s13073-021-00965-0

41. Manning M, Hudgins L; Professional Practice and Guidelines Committee. Array-based technology and recommendations for utilization in medical genetics practice for detection of chromosomal abnormalities. *Genet Med.* 2010;12(11):742–745. PubMed doi: 10.1097/GIM.0b013e3181f8baad

42. Miller DT, Adam MP, Aradhya S, et al. Consensus statement: chromosomal microarray is a first-tier clinical diagnostic test for individuals with developmental disabilities or congenital anomalies. *Am J Hum Genet.* 2010;86(5):749–764. PubMed doi: 10.1016/j.ajhg.2010.04.006

43. Borch LA, Parboosingh J, Thomas MA, Veale P. Re-evaluating the first-tier status of fragile X testing in neurodevelopmental disorders. *Genet Med.* 2020;22(6):1036–1039. PubMed doi: 10.1038/s41436-020-0773-x

44. Therrell BL Jr, Padilla CD. Newborn screening in the developing countries. *Curr Opin Pediatr.* 2018;30(6):734–739. PubMed doi: 10.1097/MOP.0000000000000683

45. Fabie NAV, Pappas KB, Feldman GL. The current state of newborn screening in the United States. *Pediatr Clin North Am.* 2019;66(2):369–386. PubMed doi: 10.1016/j.pcl.2018.12.007

46. Tirosh E, Jaffe M. Global developmental delay and mental retardation–a pediatric perspective. *Dev Disabil Res Rev.* 2011;17(2):85–92. PubMed doi: 10.1002/ddrr.1103

47. Ji J, Leung ML, Baker S, Deignan JL, Santani A. Clinical exome reanalysis: current practice and beyond. *Mol Diagn Ther.* 2021;25(5):529–536. PubMed doi: 10.1007/s40291-021-00541-7

48. Mitchell JJ, Trakadis YJ, Scriver CR. Phenylalanine hydroxylase deficiency. *Genet Med.* 2011;13(8):697–707. PubMed doi: 10.1097/GIM.0b013e3182141b48

49. Morris AAM, Kožich V, Santra S, et al. Guidelines for the diagnosis and management of cystathionine beta-synthase deficiency. *J Inherit Metab Dis.* 2017;40(1):49–74. PubMed doi: 10.1007/s10545-016-9979-0

50. Mew NA, Simpson KL, Gropman AL, Lanpher BC, Chapman KA, Summar ML.Urea cycle disorders overview. In: *GeneReviews [Internet].* University of Washington; 1993–2021. 2003 Apr 29 [Updated 2017 Jun 22]

51. Mercimek-Andrews S, Salomons GS. Creatine deficiency syndromes. In: *GeneReviews [Internet].* University of Washington; 1993–2021. 2009 Jan 15 [Updated 2015 Dec 10]

52. Muenzer J. Overview of the mucopolysaccharidoses. *Rheumatology (Oxford).* 2011;50(5)(suppl 5):v4–v12. PubMed doi: 10.1093/rheumatology/ker394

53. Wolf B. Biotinidase deficiency. In: *GeneReviews [Internet].* University of Washington; 1993–2021. 2000 Mar 24 [Updated 2016 Jun 9]

54. Witters P, Morava E. Congenital disorders of glycosylation (CDG): review. *eLS.* November 3, 2016. DOI: 10.1002/9780470015902.a0026783

55. Platt FM, d'Azzo A, Davidson BL, Neufeld EF, Tifft CJ. Lysosomal storage diseases. *Nat Rev Dis Primers.* 2018;4(1):27. PubMed doi: 10.1038/s41572-018-0025-4

56. Braverman NE, D'Agostino MD, Maclean GE. Peroxisome biogenesis disorders: biological, clinical and pathophysiological perspectives. *Dev Disabil Res Rev.* 2013;17(3):187–196. doi: 10.1002/ddrr.1113

57. Nowaczyk MJM, Irons MB. Smith-Lemli-Opitz syndrome: phenotype, natural history, and epidemiology. *Am J Med Genet C Semin Med Genet.* 2012;160C(4):250–262. PubMed doi: 10.1002/ajmg.c.31343

58. Nyhan WL. Disorders of purine and pyrimidine metabolism. *Mol Genet Metab.* 2005;86(1-2):25–33. PubMed doi: 10.1016/j.ymgme.2005.07.027

59. Kaler SG. ATP7A-related copper transport diseases-emerging concepts and future trends. *Nat Rev Neurol.* 2011;7(1):15–29. PubMed doi: 10.1038/nrneurol.2010.180

60. Shashi V, Schoch K, Spillmann R, et al; Undiagnosed Diseases Network. A comprehensive iterative approach is highly effective

in diagnosing individuals who are exome negative. *Genet Med.* 2019;21(1):161–172. PubMed doi: 10.1038/s41436-018-0044-2

61. Cerrato F, Sparago A, Ariani F, et al. DNA Methylation in the diagnosis of monogenic diseases. *Genes (Basel).* 2020;11(4): 355. PubMed doi: 10.3390/genes11040355

62. Dudding-Byth T, Baxter A, Holliday EG, et al. Computer face-matching technology using two-dimensional photographs accurately matches the facial gestalt of unrelated individuals with the same syndromic form of intellectual disability. *BMC Biotechnol.* 2017;17(1):90. PubMed doi: 10.1186/s12896-017-0410-1

Guidance for Caring for Infants and Children With Trisomy 13 and Trisomy 18

- *Clinical Report*

CLINICAL REPORT Guidance for the Clinician in Rendering Pediatric Care

American Academy of Pediatrics

DEDICATED TO THE HEALTH OF ALL CHILDREN™

Guidance for Caring for Infants and Children With Trisomy 13 and Trisomy 18: Clinical Report

Alaina K. Pyle, MD, FAAP,[1,2] Thomas N. George, MD, FAAP,[3] James J. Cummings, MD, FAAP,[4] Naomi T. Laventhal, MD, HEC-C, FAAP,[5] and the Committee on Bioethics; Section on Neonatal-Perinatal Medicine; and Committee on Fetus and Newborn

abstract

Over the last several decades, there has been a steady increase in medical and surgical interventions provided for infants and children with trisomy 13 or trisomy 18 (chromosomal syndromes associated with a range of congenital anomalies and universally severe neurodevelopmental impairment). Despite previous characterizations of these disorders as being uniformly lethal, multiple studies have demonstrated improved morbidity and mortality when indicated interventions, such as cardiac surgery, are performed, and these interventions and their potential risks and benefits can be carefully explored with parents who may wish to pursue them. Although the presence of trisomy 13 or trisomy 18 impacts prognosis for survival and long-term outcomes and cannot be disregarded in complex decision making, there are no ethical justifications for universal, principle-based differential treatment based solely on these genetic diagnoses. Thus, which medical and surgical interventions are offered, denied, or required for patients should be based on the best available evidence and appropriately tailored to the individual's clinical context, should respect the same moral principles as are applied to other children, and should not vary widely between institutions. Pediatric and obstetric clinicians participating in the care of these patients should maintain current knowledge of the literature to provide adequate counseling through a shared decision-making process and offer the broad range of support that is needed for families throughout the continuum of care from the prenatal to postnatal time period and extending throughout the child's life.

[1]University of Connecticut School of Medicine, Farmington, Connecticut; [2]Department of Pediatrics, Division of Neonatology, Connecticut Children's Medical Center, Hartford, Connecticut; [3]Department of Neonatology, Children's Minnesota, Minneapolis, Minnesota; [4]Division of Neonatology, Department of Pediatrics, Albany Medical Center, Albany, New York; and [5]Division of Neonatal-Perinatal Medicine, Department of Pediatrics, Center for Bioethics and Social Sciences in Medicine, University of Michigan, Ann Arbor, Michigan

All authors conceptualized the clinical report. Dr Pyle and Dr Laventhal jointly outlined and drafted the initial manuscript. All authors critically reviewed and revised the manuscript, and responded to peer review questions and comments, and all authors approved the final manuscript as submitted and agree to be accountable for all aspects of the work.

CONFLICT OF INTEREST DISCLOSURE: Dr Cummings has disclosed a financial relationship as an employee of ONY Biotech. Any other disclosures were reviewed and determined not relevant to the work related to "Guidance for Caring for Infants and Children With Trisomy 13 and 18." Disclosures are reviewed and mitigated through a Conflict of Interest process that consists of reviewing pertinent information which is then used to decide what action is required to maintain content integrity. There may be instances where no action is necessary. This process has been approved by the AAP Board of Directors.

To cite: Pyle AK, George TN, Cummings JJ, et al; American Academy of Pediatrics, Committee on Bioethics; Section on Neonatal-Perinatal Medicine; and Committee on Fetus and Newborn. Guidance for Caring for Infants and Children With Trisomy 13 and Trisomy 18: Clinical Report. *Pediatrics.* 2025; 156(2):e2025072719

INTRODUCTION

Historically, trisomy 13 (T13) and trisomy 18 (T18) were viewed as uniformly lethal genetic syndromes.[1] Prenatal counseling for expectant parents whose fetus was found to have T13 or T18 once focused exclusively on options for pregnancy termination or postnatal comfort care, on the presumptive basis that all affected infants died. However, examination of contemporary outcomes for these infants suggests that death in the neonatal period is not universal, particularly for infants who receive intensive medical and surgical care after birth. Although severe cognitive and motor impairment and shortened lifespan are anticipated for all survivors, some infants with these disorders live for 1 year or more, and some attain social and interactive milestones, with positive quality of life noted by their caregivers.[2–4] Care of children with T13 and T18 has become commonplace enough that health surveillance guidelines exist.[5,6]

The purpose of this clinical report is to guide clinicians in the care of infants and children with T13 and T18, with a focus in prenatal and perinatal decision making, based on contemporary principles of pediatric ethics. Trisomy 13 and trisomy 18 are frequently grouped together when discussing the medical and ethical aspects of care. For contexts in which there is considerable similarity, they are referred to as T13/T18 but will be referred to as T13 and T18 separately when differences are discussed. Generally, this clinical report will be applicable to cases of full trisomy or children who manifest a phenotype consistent with complete T13/T18.

ETHICAL BACKGROUND

Which interventions should be offered to infants with T13/T18 has been the source of considerable moral exploration and controversy, with a strong focus in the literature on 2 aspects of care: surgery for congenital heart disease and tracheostomy placement for chronic home mechanical ventilation.[7,8] The ethical themes that emerge in these debates are the same that arise in many other childhood conditions that are accompanied by shortened lifespan, extreme medical complexity, severe disability, or intense resource utilization: moral obligations of beneficence/nonmaleficence, respect for parental authority, just distribution of medical resources, and best interest. Contemporary approaches to values-based shared decision making are also highly salient.

At the heart of the ethical debate about whether life-sustaining interventions (LSIs) such as mechanical ventilation and surgical interventions are appropriate for infants with T13/T18 are the questions of whether the potential benefits of these interventions outweigh their burdens, and who should make that determination. Historically, the basis for withholding these interventions was based on an explicit assumption of futility—T13 and T18 were considered to be uniformly lethal, and painful or expensive treatments were not expected to prevent inevitable death during infancy. T13/T18, however, appear to be prime examples of the "self-fulfilling prophecy" described by Wilkinson, in which high mortality without intervention is used to justify continued nonintervention while failing to recognize that intervention alters the likelihood of mortality.[9] Once it was recognized that surgery for congenital heart disease, mechanical ventilation, airway stabilization via tracheostomy, placement of gastrostomy tubes, and treatment of other surgical conditions could prolong survival for months or years for some infants with T13/T18, attention shifted away from a simple futility claim.

Consideration of neurodevelopmental impairment and quality of life now plays a prominent role in deliberations about provision of LSIs. In contrast to the description of infants burdened by painful conditions and presumed to all die early, as often utilized by clinicians and in medical texts, social media is now replete with images of smiling survivors who experience joy and are beloved children and siblings. This change in imagery drives hope and optimism for many parents of these children, as do data revealing some attainment of developmental milestones.[1,10] As described by Wightman et al, this relational potential provides ethical justification for ongoing LSIs for infants and children with even profound neurodevelopmental limitations.[11] Some families seek to deliver in what are sometimes informally designated by parental support groups as "trisomy-friendly" hospitals or their own local hospitals and actively pursue some or all the interventions that have the potential to prolong their child's life. In contrast, other families conclude that the neurodevelopmental impairment and medical complexity associated with T13/T18 impart an unacceptably poor quality of life and opt for pregnancy termination or comfort care after birth. Still others fall between these poles and choose a more cautious "trial of therapy" with consideration of some therapies but exclusion of others.

On the basis of contemporary outcome data and ethical analyses, we conclude that exclusive comfort care remains a morally acceptable choice that ought to be offered to all parents of infants with confirmed or strongly suspected T13/T18. For families who choose to continue the pregnancy, this diagnosis alone should not categorically preclude offering therapies that could potentially prolong life and/or facilitate hospital discharge. The only exception would be patient-specific factors which exclude treatment on the basis of true physiologic futility (use of the term "futility" in values-sensitive medical decision making is generally discouraged,[12] but here we refer to a therapy that has *no chance* of achieving the stated goal); otherwise, parents of infants with T13/T18 should be informed of the availability of appropriately individualized life-sustaining care and counseled in a fashion similar to other multisystemic genetic syndromes and/or complex medical conditions, in order to fully understand the relevant individual factors, such as gestational age, other comorbidities, or the presence of mosaicism. Like other conditions in which patients or their families may not demand inappropriate treatments, there are limits to what clinicians and hospitals are obligated to provide, and they should follow established processes as described elsewhere.[13]

Recognition of a wider potential range of outcomes, often with the use of some degree of technological support, for infants with T13/T18 has led to a shift toward shared decision making for these infants and children. There is now a more explicit recognition of the plurality of values, spiritual beliefs, and moral norms around care of infants with medical complexity, developmental disability, and shortened lifespan. This has led to considerable attention to T13/T18 in the medical and ethical literature and imparts a need for guidance for pediatric clinicians to offer family-centered and appropriately individualized care to these children. The principle of justice requires consistency in offering or denying specific medical interventions for all children, including those with T13/T18, within and between institutions and geographic areas. Furthermore, there needs to be recognition that implicit bias and structural inequities have the potential to introduce and perpetuate disparities, such as when those families with greater resources are able to travel to a "trisomy-friendly" hospital to access LSIs for their child that would otherwise not be available to them. The well-documented influence of implicit biases around gender, race, ethnicity, socioeconomic status, etc, should not play a role in what is or is not offered to families, and thus, should be assessed prior to meeting with expectant parents.

BRIEF CLINICAL BACKGROUND

Table 1 provides a basic overview of trisomy 13 and trisomy 18. Prior to the availability of fetal ultrasonography and prenatal genetic screening and testing, these syndromes were diagnosed at birth on the basis of hallmark constellations of congenital anomalies and recognized pathognomonic phenotypes among infants with full T13/T18. In resource-abundant health care settings, many of these infants are now identified before birth with noninvasive prenatal screening (NIPS), although the diagnostic certainty for this test may be lower than some parents realize, without subsequent amniocentesis and correlation with specific physical findings.[14]

Trisomy 18 was first described in 1960 and is the second most common chromosomal trisomy syndrome after trisomy 21 among live-born children. It occurs in 3/10 000 live births and occurs 2 to 3 times more often in female than in male live births.[15] Many congenital anomalies are associated with T18, most commonly uteroplacental anomalies; prematurity; neurologic disabilities ranging from general abnormalities of tone and neurodevelopment to persistent, severe issues including seizures; and possible endocrine or hormonal abnormalities; characteristic facies; hand anomalies; and congenital heart disease. T18 has historically been associated with high mortality in the immediate neonatal period and the subsequent year after birth. Approximately 95% of live-born infants with T18 present with full trisomy (with increased risk as maternal age increases), although cases of mosaic and partial T18 have been well described and have more variable clinical presentations.[16,17]

Trisomy 13 was first described in 1957 and occurs in 1.35 in 10 000 live births.[15] Many infants with T13 have major structural central nervous malformations, and all will have significant lifelong neurocognitive problems. Broadly, T13 is characterized by multiple midline anomalies including cleft lip and/or palate, congenital heart disease, scalp defects, and abdominal and pelvic abnormalities. Like T18, T13 is most often associated with a full duplication of the chromosome and increased risk with advanced maternal age, and the mosaic and partial forms have milder presentations.[17]

PRENATAL DIAGNOSIS, CARE COORDINATION, AND DECISION MAKING

There is a robust body of literature exploring the scientific and ethical complexities of prenatal screening and testing, which includes multiple options for all expectant parents

TABLE 1. Important Differences in Epidemiology and Outcomes for T13/18[15,49,62,63]

	Trisomy 18 (Edwards Syndrome)	Trisomy 13 (Patau Syndrome)
Incidence (Note: very high rates of pregnancy terminations in all studies)	3.02 per 10 000 live births (US) 2.6 (International) 4.8 (Europe)	1.35 per 10 000 live births (US) 1.15 (International) 1.9 (Europe)
Liveborn rate	13.5% (US)	18.9% (US)
Survival beyond first week for liveborn infants	52.5%	43.1%
Survival beyond first year for liveborn infants	10–25%[a]	10–25%[a]
Survival beyond 5 y for liveborn infants	12.3%	9.7%
CHD	80–90%	57–80%
Severe CHD	20%	17%

[a] Variable by study/interventions provided.

wishing to screen for aneuploidy. Guidance for specific aspects of prenatal screening and testing is available via other professional organizations such as the American College of Obstetricians and Gynecologists, American College of Medical Genetics, and others.[18–27] Comprehensive obstetric prenatal care ought, in principle, to include appropriate genetic counseling about these various modalities to support informed, values-based decision making. Clinicians from multiple pediatric disciplines who participate in prenatal counseling ought to maintain a basic understanding of these obstetric testing modalities to be able to provide anticipatory guidance about postnatal care (and potentially fetal intervention) and support parental decision making. This basic knowledge does not require comprehensive understanding of the risks and technical aspects of the diagnostic tools, but in some situations, pediatric clinicians may be asked to help parents understand how results of a given test will inform postnatal care and to help develop an appropriate postnatal plan for genetic testing.

Pediatric clinicians might be asked to support expectant parents who are considering pregnancy termination (although limitations in access now exist, making travel necessary or introducing other obstacles for some families pursuing this option), perinatal hospice with comfort care after birth, or pursuit of LSIs. This counseling is an opportunity to dispel the binary assumption that genetic screening and testing before birth are of no value if the pregnancy termination is not a legal option or if the expectant parent has indicated that they would not consider this termination.

Definitive information about fetal aneuploidy has the potential to support families with a plurality of convictions about pregnancy termination and may support a family in planning for the birth of an infant with T13/T18 even if termination would never be considered by the pregnant patient. Examples of uses of this information include developing a plan to share information with siblings, family, friends, and colleagues; choice of delivery hospital; decisions about obstetric care; and preparations for parental leave. Pediatric clinicians, thus, can play a supportive role in helping expectant parents make an informed decision about prenatal testing. Once a diagnosis of T13/T18 is suspected prenatally and the family is considering or planning to continue the pregnancy, a neonatal clinician should meet with the family at the earliest opportunity to provide information and support. This prenatal consultation will ideally involve a shared decision-making process, with the clinician giving accurate data in a nonbiased format and eliciting the family members' personal values and goals.[3,28] Multiple meetings with the family prior to delivery might be necessary to continue providing support and information and to explore any evolution in the choices that have been made by the parents. Expectant parents choosing to continue the pregnancy will need to make various decisions along the way, including specifics on prenatal and perinatal monitoring, which should be based on parental goals of care, and often require a nuanced, individualized plan. Parents who do not desire aggressive LSIs postnatally may choose to have less monitoring ante-/peripartum, although this is not always the case, as a parent's desire to meet their child alive may sometimes drive these choices.[29,30] Coordinated consultation with a perinatal hospice or pediatric palliative care team warrants strong consideration to offer information about comfort care after birth, and, in some cases, to introduce a team that will provide longitudinal support to the family over time, even if life-prolonging interventions are desired. Additional considerations for perinatal care coordination are described in Table 2, including relevant factors for choice of delivery hospital.

Although comfort-focused care is a very important option for postnatal care that should be offered and explained to families, it is no longer ethical to neglect to discuss other options, given that these are not universally lethal disorders. For some parents, a "trial of therapy" approach offers the opportunity to treat reversible, common, short-term causes of neonatal respiratory distress unrelated to the underlying disorder, such as transient tachypnea of the newborn, and to offer short-term support for primary respiratory difficulties, giving the family time to meet their infant alive after delivery. The "trial of therapy" approach also can provide time to confirm the diagnosis and assess the presence and severity of any associated anomalies such as congenital heart disease. This trial can be limited to the delivery room or can extend to neonatal intensive care unit (NICU) admission; the discussion can focus on which interventions will be provided, function around a certain length of time, or be contingent around completion of the postnatal evaluation. Examples of interventions that might be initiated in a trial of therapy are provided in Table 3.

The plan, after being confirmed by the family, should be carefully documented in the medical record, available at the time of delivery, and modified as needed on an ongoing basis. The potential process of redirection of care and withdrawal of LSIs after initial resuscitation should still be sensitively discussed prenatally with those families who are considering LSIs, to provide an advance foundation of knowledge. Some families might initially desire maximal therapy and then wish to transition to comfort care after a period of time for a variety of reasons, such as the infant clinically worsening or not responding adequately to interventions, additional medical or surgical complications arising, laboratory confirmation of the T13/T18 diagnosis, etc. Palliative care or perinatal hospice teams can play a vital role in preparing families for the possible loss of their infant in the neonatal period; institutions without these specialized services may rely on social work, spiritual care, or other institutional and community resources to provide this support. Examples of typical bereavement activities and support are identified in Table 4.

TABLE 2. Considerations for Perinatal Care Coordination

Make a plan for coordination of subspeciality consultation, based on center/family preferences and staff availability		• In all cases, if there is potential for multiple surgeries by multiple surgical specialties, prioritize "whole child" approach, considering interdependence of procedures and complicating factors • Consider appropriate timing of consultation with perinatal hospice/palliative care and other supportive services individualized to hospital resources • Consider identifying a designated, longitudinal health professional (social worker, nurse, case manager, etc) to provide support and care coordination
Option 1	Sequential – expectant parents have individual meetings with relevant subspecialists	• Coordinate consultations on a single day, with planned breaks • Consider multidisciplinary/interprofessional meeting in advance to align recommendations • Consider use of telemedicine modalities if transportation or child care are challenges for the family
Option 2	Integrated – expectant parents meet with multiple specialists together	• Monitor total number of individuals required, with attention to parental preferences and needs • Identify appropriate space for meeting ahead of time
Obstetric considerations	Desired antenatal screening and testing	• Grounded in parental goals of care
	Mode of delivery	• Distinguish maternal and fetal indications for cesarean delivery
	Choice of delivery hospital	• What medical resources are necessary to provide care to the infant that aligns with the goals of care (advanced medical resources, necessary clinical service lines, availability of perinatal hospice/pediatric palliative care)? • What value do the expectant parents place on delivering with the primary obstetrician at the "home hospital" and what are the risks of neonatal transfer and parental separation? • What are the geographic and practical considerations for the family? • For families planning to deliver at a referral center, is a "back-up" plan necessary in the event of preterm or precipitous delivery? • What communication is necessary with the home/community hospital?
Postnatal considerations	Plan for confirmatory testing	• Cord blood vs neonatal specimen; cord blood is potentially less invasive but risks maternal cell contamination; a neonatal specimen potential requires significant blood volume and requires venipuncture, arterial puncture, or umbilical vessel catheterization • Understand institutional norms for postnatal consultation with genetics • Consider evaluation of associated anomalies such as congenital cardiac disease, to guide decision making

TABLE 3. Trial of Therapy Interventions

Examples of respiratory interventions in the delivery room that might be appropriate for a time- or condition-limited "trial of therapy"
Continuous positive airway pressure (CPAP)
Positive pressure ventilation (PPV)
Laryngeal mask airway (LMA)
Endotracheal intubation
Examples of tests and procedures that parents might wish to complete before redirection of care
Confirmatory genetic testing
Echocardiogram
Radiologic evaluation of gastrointestinal tract anomalies
When invasive or noninvasive mechanical ventilation is initiated in the delivery room – assessment of spontaneous respiratory effort
Airway evaluation

Excellent perinatal care for infants with T13/T18, regardless of the family's goals of care, depends on good communication between and within clinical teams both before and after delivery. Components of such communication include clear and specific documentation that is readily

TABLE 4. Bereavement Activities

Memory making	Handprints/footprints Photography Heartbeat recordings Locks of hair and other keepsakes Memory books/boxes
Decedent support	Funeral home arrangements Autopsy and postmortem evaluation Notification of family and community
Family support	Child life specialists for siblings and young family members Perinatal loss support for parents and family

accessible in the medical record, a structured "time out" prior to delivery, closed-loop communication throughout the resuscitation, and opportunities for debriefing after resuscitation.

POSTNATAL DIAGNOSIS

In some cases, T13/T18 is only recognized and diagnosed after birth; this can occur when the expectant parent has no or limited prenatal care or if there was an intentional choice not to pursue genetic screening tests or detailed fetal ultrasonography. In some cases, the diagnosis might be suspected on the basis of prenatal findings, but the parents prefer to pursue confirmation after birth. Finally, some obstetric or fetal factors, such as obstacles to good imaging or mild fetal phenotype, might result in failure to recognize findings consistent with T13/T18 before birth. Cases of unexpected T13/T18 might be recognized by identification of the classic phenotype or by targeted evaluation for the cause of unexpected respiratory failure or congenital anomalies. Table 2 describes options for procuring a specimen for genetic testing. Consultation with a geneticist can support making a provisional clinical diagnosis and selection of the appropriate testing.

In most cases, pursuit of LSIs while seeking diagnostic confirmation of T13/T18 is appropriate. Withdrawing or withholding LSIs solely on the basis of an unconfirmed suspicion of T13/T18 is rarely justifiable. However, withholding or withdrawing life-sustaining care might be ethically appropriate based on the prognosis associated with *confirmed* anomalies for which comfort care is routinely offered, such as certain forms of severe congenital heart disease, or following identification of uniformly lethal conditions. Referral for consultation with a palliative care team need not wait for diagnostic confirmation.

CONGENITAL HEART DISEASE

There is a high prevalence of congenital cardiac disease in patients with T13/T18 (57–80% of infants with T13[31] and 80–90% of infants with T18[16]), a portion of whom may benefit from corrective or palliative surgery, either in the immediate postnatal period or over the first few months of life, for example, in the setting of a large ventricular septal defect, very common among infants with T18,[32–34] as congestive heart failure develops despite maximal medical management. Multiple studies have demonstrated potential benefit for cardiac surgery in patients with T13/T18, albeit with higher peri- and postoperative mortality.[35–38] Studies suggest that infants requiring mechanical ventilation preoperatively have the poorest outcome and are likely to continue to require mechanical ventilation long-term.[39] Extracorporeal membrane oxygenation (ECMO) is used after some cardiac surgeries (distinct from intraoperative cardiopulmonary bypass), although rarely for patients with T13/T18. It is appropriate to consider ECMO for this population as it is for other surgical candidates, with counseling provided to parents about the increased risk of morbidity and mortality.[40] ECMO has been used successfully for infants with T13/T18 with potentially reversible noncardiac indications such as meconium aspiration syndrome, with comparable outcomes to general pediatric ECMO; thus, the presence of T13/T18 may be considered as one of the relevant factors in assessing for ECMO candidacy but is not a contraindication in isolation.[41,42] In some cases, patients are offered palliative rather than corrective surgery to allow for discontinuation of prostaglandin infusion (used to maintain ductal patency for ductal dependent lesions), support discharge to home, or reduce symptoms of congestive heart failure.

It is important for the medical team to discuss the range of options openly and transparently. Given variation between institutions about which procedures are offered for infants with T13/T18 and congenital heart disease, some parents might request hospital transfer for a second opinion if the birth hospital is not offering corrective or palliative surgery for their infant. To avoid this odyssey and support consistency within and between hospitals, decisions about whether to offer or withhold congenital heart disease surgery for infants with T13/T18 should be made on the basis of transparent, clearly articulated institutional standards, medical information about the specific patient, and available evidence published about outcomes following surgery, as they are for any other patients with congenital heart disease. In 2024, the American Association for Thoracic Surgery published guidance based on available evidence and expert consensus advising that surgical decision making should "not be based solely on the presence of trisomy but, instead, should be made on a case-by-case basis, considering both the severity of the baby's heart disease as well as the presence of other anomalies."[43] This structured approach to decision making has the potential to reassure parents that their infants have not been excluded from desired information as a result of biased opinions about future disability, outdated approaches to T13/T18, or what some parents perceive to be discrimination against their infants on the basis of arbitrary rules because of the genetic diagnosis.

NONCARDIAC SURGICAL INTERVENTION IN THE NEONATAL PERIOD AND BEYOND

Infants with T13/T18 often have congenital anomalies and diagnoses that require consideration for noncardiac surgeries in the neonatal period. Decisions to proceed with these surgeries should be guided by the goals for care that are developed with the family, with the understanding that these goals might evolve in the neonatal period. Examples of diagnoses needing more urgent attention in the neonatal period include esophageal atresia with or without tracheoesophageal fistula, imperforate anus, omphalocele, gastroschisis, congenital diaphragmatic hernia, and myelomeningocele.

Given the known feeding challenges among infants with T13/T18, even in the absence of gastrointestinal anomalies, gastrostomy tube placement is one of the more common surgical procedures considered in the neonatal period.[5,44] Gastroesophageal reflux, also common among infants with T13/T18, may complicate decision making about the approach to feeding these infants.[16] Although this might be considered early in the hospital course in coordination with other surgeries, infants can be supported with nasogastric feedings until later in the hospital stay while other medical issues are addressed; discharge home with nasogastric (or nasojejunal) feedings can be considered if appropriate support is in place, with consideration for transition to g-tube feedings if longer-term survival becomes more likely. Alternatively, withdrawal or withholding of medically provided nutrition may be offered in limited circumstances and is often done with involvement of an institutional ethics committee.

Other surgical procedures might be indicated with the goal of providing comfort for the infant and moving care forward, such as bronchoscopy for the assessment and possible treatment of airway issues that are more prevalent in patients with T13/T18,[16,45] or a ventriculoperitoneal shunt if an infant has symptomatic severe ventriculomegaly. The decision to expose an infant to surgical intervention in the neonatal period—urgently or electively—should balance the risks of causing harm with the benefits of surgery, given the higher surgical morbidity and mortality in infants with T13/T18. Families should be counseled that surgical intervention in this population is associated with prolonged hospital stay and increased risks with anesthesia and intubation.[45,46]

CONTINUED CARE IN THE NICU AND BEYOND

Five to forty percent of infants with T13/T18 survive to 1 month of age, depending on their comorbid conditions, level of intervention, gestational age, sex, as well as other factors that are not yet well understood.[46–50] When parents desire all available interventions and the infant survives the first few days of life, many additional decisions will likely need to be made. For the 5% to 15% of infants who survive to 1 year of age, evidence suggests that they could survive for years, even occasionally into their 20s, typically utilizing some degree of medical and/or technological support.[47] There is currently insufficient evidence to differentiate long-term survivors prenatally from those with early mortality, making prognostication challenging, although mosaicism likely provides some survival benefit, and multiple or severe anomalies and prematurity are known to increase the risk for early mortality.[51]

A small proportion of children with T13/T18 will survive the initial neonatal period but require ongoing mechanical ventilation despite maximal medical interventions, often because of a combination of central apnea and airway anomalies, which are much more common in this population.[16] For families who wish to continue LSIs, open and clear discussions about potential placement of a tracheostomy tube ideally begin early in the hospital course, to support informed decision making. The significant lengthening of the hospital stay, need for home nursing care, and risks associated with long-term home ventilation must be carefully explained to these families, as it is with other children who meet indications for tracheostomy. Additionally, the baseline increased surgical risk for children with T13/T18 must be discussed during the consent process, as well as the mixed data around anticipated benefits of long-term mechanical ventilation in this population.[36] Epilepsy-related apnea can occur in this population, so consultation with pediatric neurology, use of electroencephalography, and antiepileptic agents should be considered for those infants exhibiting apnea potentially consistent with seizures or those with central nervous system abnormalities known to increase risk for seizures, after discussion of the risks and benefits with parents.[52,53]

Discharge planning for infants with T13/T18 must be individualized to the infant's specific medical needs, goals of care, and practical considerations such as distance from relevant specialists and family and community resources. To optimize care for this medically complex population, it is important to ensure a smooth transition from the NICU to an outpatient medical home, so the family will continue to have support, as there are likely to be new circumstances that may require ongoing discussions about goals of care.[54] Guidelines for this population were published by Kepple et al, which offer detailed screening recommendations to be used throughout childhood.[5,6] Generally, infants with T13/T18 should receive routine anticipatory guidance and childhood vaccinations.[16] Routine health maintenance, including vaccinations and health screenings, should not be withheld solely on the basis of a diagnosis of T13/T18 and should be based on the family's goals of care. Condition-specific growth curves are available in print[55] as well as online through Support Organization for Trisomy, or SOFT.[56] For those practicing obstetric and neonatal care, there are specific growth curves for 22 weeks' gestation through term.[57] For infants who have not had access to nirsevimab, palivizumab should be considered for any patients with T13/T18 during respiratory syncytial virus season, even if they do not meet respiratory or cardiac criteria, if there is evidence of decreased ability to clear secretions because of their increased risk for complications.[5,16,58]

Important components of discharge planning are described in Table 5. The outpatient plan should be reviewed and clarified regularly before presentation in an acute crisis whenever possible, and provided in writing to the family, in case the parents need to call for emergency

TABLE 5. Discharge Planning
Important Steps in Discharge Planning for Infants with T13/18
Administer appropriate vaccinations
Complete other routine newborn interventions such as newborn screen, hearing screen, car seat education
Consider cardiopulmonary resuscitation (CPR) training for parents
Communicate with designated primary care physician – provide Kepple guidelines[5]
Ensure ongoing decision support is available for the family, ideally with establishment of an outpatient medical home
Provide written information for local emergency medical services and emergency department, consider advance communication
Depending on goals of care, designate code status in accordance with state law (review during reversible illness, surgical procedures, and as needed)
Clarify the role of outpatient hospice, when available
Establish home health care services, as medically indicated and desired by family

care or bring the child into the hospital. Follow-up of these care plans often falls to the pediatrician or subspecialists caring for the patient because of a dearth of pediatric palliative and hospice care clinicians in most communities. For families who live remote from a pediatric medical home (the ideal locus of care for patients with complex health needs), anticipatory communication by the discharging inpatient team with the local emergency department or emergency medical services dispatch may be helpful. Recognition of the plurality of approaches to care of infants with T13/T18 requires time for dissemination, particularly for nonpediatric clinicians. Presentation for emergency care to hospitals with limited experience caring for children with T13/T18 may lead to clinicians' moral distress and delays in appropriate care for these patients.

ORGANIZATIONAL CONSIDERATIONS

Unnecessary Practice Variation

Variability within clinical practice is inevitable, as the art of medicine meets the need for individualized care, particularly when the evidence base is not fully settled for the best approach to a medical problem. When there is controversy between clinicians or centers, this can lead to unjust variation around critical medical decisions, which can cause confusion and distress for families and drive disparities in care. Recently demonstrated differences in likelihood of undergoing surgery among Hispanic and publicly insured infants with T18 and congenital heart disease highlight the importance of continued attention to potential disparities in decision making for these infants.[59] It is advisable for hospitals that provide care for newborn infants to have an established guideline for management of patients with T13/T18 regarding whether LSIs are offered at their institution in addition to offering comfort care. This guideline should be clearly communicated with families prior to delivery so they may seek care elsewhere, if the pathway they desire is not offered at that center. All reasonable efforts should be made to assist families to find other centers for a second opinion, if they seek care beyond that which is offered or available at the initial hospital.

Clinician Moral Distress

Some clinicians might experience moral distress in caring for infants with T13/T18, given the high-stakes nature of medical decisions for these children, the plurality of values and beliefs about care of these children, and the evolution of care in this space. Organizations have an obligation to anticipate and respond to moral distress for the health care team by providing education as well as open discussions and regular, multidisciplinary debriefings, ideally guided by trained professionals such as palliative care, ethicists, social workers, or psychologists, as available in different institutions. If the medical team and family cannot come to an agreement, a hospital-based ethics committee can serve as an excellent resource for mediation.

News Media and Social Media

The evolution of the internet and social media has markedly changed the practice of medicine, in both positive and negative ways. Linking together families who have children with rare diseases such as T13/T18 can provide a type of emotional support that would otherwise be nearly impossible. Robust research involving parental perspectives has also been made possible via partnerships with some of these online groups, such as that done by Janvier et al as well as Farlowe et al.[2,60,61] One downside to this online network can be a bias toward discussing more positive outcomes, which can skew the perception of other families and potentially alter the choices they make for their own child. Social media campaigns for patients with complex medical care and bioethical quandaries have become increasingly widespread and deeply affecting—highly publicized cases of contested care continue to fuel heated debate. The organizational response to cases that make local, national, or international news must balance the imperative to protect patient privacy (regardless of what information the family has chosen to make public), the institution's reputation, such that they are able to continue to provide excellent care for their existing and future patients, and the safety and well-being of health professionals involved in the care. Structured debriefs and event review adhering to the general principles of quality assurance is advisable in the aftermath of a highly contentious or publicized case.

AREAS FOR FUTURE RESEARCH

As medical and surgical capabilities change over time, evidence-based understanding of contemporary outcomes of children with T13/T18 should inform anticipatory guidance and decision making over the lifespan of these children. Continued empirical study of these patients' short- and long-term outcomes is bolstered by exploring quality of life, family experience, and other outcomes, as measured objectively and subjectively by those who know them best—their families. Accurate, individualized prognostication will only be possible as more data are gathered and published about which risk factors predict survival or morbidity and which factors can be ameliorated.

SUMMARY RECOMMENDATIONS

1. Which medical and surgical interventions are offered, denied, or required for patients with T13/T18 should be based on best available evidence and appropriately tailored to the individual's clinical context, should respect the same moral principles as are applied to other children, and should not vary widely between institutions, with transparent, clearly articulated institutional guidelines and referral to other institutions made available when parents desire interventions that are not offered at their current location.
2. Clinicians from multiple pediatric disciplines who participate in prenatal counseling should maintain up-to-date, basic understanding of prenatal testing modalities to be able to provide anticipatory guidance about postnatal care and support parental decision making.
3. Although exclusive comfort care remains a morally acceptable choice that should be offered to all parents of infants with confirmed or strongly suspected T13/T18, this diagnosis alone does not justify unilaterally withholding therapies that have the prospect of prolonging life or facilitating hospital discharge; unless patient-specific factors exclude treatment on the basis of physiological futility, parents of infants with T13/T18 should be informed of the availability of appropriately individualized life-sustaining care and counseled in a fashion similar to other genetic syndromes and complex medical conditions.
4. Regardless of the goals of care, infants with known or suspected T13/T18 should, whenever possible, be delivered in hospitals with the resources to provide timely, comprehensive, and compassionate care that supports the family's goals, to avoid unnecessary postnatal separation of infants and their parents.
5. In most cases, when an evaluation for *postnatally* diagnosed T13/T18 is under way, pursuit of life-sustaining treatment while seeking diagnostic confirmation is appropriate. Withdrawing or withholding life-sustaining care based *solely* on an unconfirmed suspicion of T13/T18 is rarely justifiable.
6. Regardless of the goals of care, hospital discharge of infants and children with T13/T18 requires thoughtful care coordination, anticipatory guidance, and directed communication to support the family in their own community.
7. Routine health maintenance, including vaccinations and health screenings, should not be withheld solely based on a diagnosis of T13/T18 and should be provided in a manner consistent with the family's goals of care.
8. Long-term survivors with T13/T18 typically have complex medical needs that require ongoing care coordination and potential intervention based on best available evidence. Comprehensive care of children with T13/T18, thus, requires iterative exploration and clarification of parents' goals to support personalized decision making.
9. Contemporary, just, evidence-based care of infants with T13/T18 and their families requires continued investigation and reporting of clinical and social outcomes.

LEAD AUTHORS

Alaina K. Pyle, MD, FAAP
Thomas N. George, MD, FAAP
James J. Cummings, MD, FAAP
Naomi T. Laventhal, MD, MA, FAAP

COMMITTEE ON BIOETHICS

Naomi Tricot Laventhal, MD, MA, FAAP, Chairperson
Gina Marie Geis, MD, FAAP
Carrie Morgan Henderson, MD, FAAP
Deborah Susan Loeff, MD, FAAP
Kelly N. Michelson, MD, MPH, FAAP
Mary Anne Ott, MD, MA, FAAP
Sara Taub, MD, FAAP

CONSULTANT

Nanette Elster, JD, MPH – *Legal Consultant*

LIAISONS

Douglas S. Diekema, MD, MPH, FAAP – *American Board of Pediatrics*
Maria McGee, MD, MPH – *American Academy of Child and Adolescent Psychiatry*
Kavita Shah Arora, MD – *American College of Obstetricians and Gynecologists*

STAFF

Anjie Emanuel, MPH

SECTION ON NEONATAL-PERINATAL MEDICINE

Munish Gupta, MD, FAAP, Chairperson
Clara Hyun-Jung Song, MD, FAAP, Chairperson-elect

James Scott Barry, MD, FAAP
Alexis S. Davis, MD, FAAP
Dmitry Dukhovny, MD, MPH, FAAP
Scott Davis Duncan, MD, FAAP
Brian Paul Hackett, MD, FAAPJohn D. Loyd, MD, MPH, FAAP
Craig Alan Nankervis, MD, FAAP
Ravi Mangal Patel, MD, MSc, FAAP
Joshua Erin Petrikin, MD, FAAP
Michael Alan Posencheg, MD, FAAP
Shetal Indravadan Shah, MD, FAAP
Wendy L. Timpson, MD, FAAP

PAST MEMBER:

Thomas N. George, MD, FAAP

LIAISONS

Danielle Ehret, MD, MPH, FAAP – *Vermont Oxford Network (VON)*
Luann Jones – *National Association of Neonatal Nurses*
Judette Louis – *Society for Maternal Fetal Medicine*
Ashley Marie Lucke, MD, FAAP – *Committee on Fetus and Newborn*

STAFF

Jim Couto, MA

COMMITTEE ON FETUS AND NEWBORN

Eric Christopher Eichenwald, MD, FAAP, Chairperson
Namasivayam Ambalavanan, MD, FAAP
Charleta Guillory, MD, FAAP
Mark Hudak, MD, FAAP
David Alan Kaufman, MD, FAAP
Camilia Rivera Martin, MD, FAAP
Margaret Graham Kemper Parker, MD, FAAP
Arun Kumar Pramanik, MD FAAP
Kelly Cant Wade, MD, FAAP

PAST MEMBER:

James Cummings, MD, FAAP

LIAISONS

Timothy Jancelewicz, MD, FAAP Section on Surgery
Michael Narvey, MD, FAAP, Canadian Paediatric Society
Stacy Beck, MD, American College of Obstetricians and Gynecologists
Lisa Grisham, APRN, NNP-BC, National Association of Neonatal Nurses

STAFF

Jim Couto, MA

Clinical reports from the American Academy of Pediatrics benefit from expertise and resources of liaisons and internal (AAP) and external reviewers. However, clinical reports from the American Academy of Pediatrics may not reflect the views of the liaisons or the organizations or government agencies that they represent.

The guidance in this report does not indicate an exclusive course of treatment or serve as a standard of medical care. Variations, taking into account individual circumstances, may be appropriate.

All clinical reports from the American Academy of Pediatrics automatically expire 5 years after publication unless reaffirmed, revised, or retired at or before that time.

FUNDING: No external funding.

https://doi.org/10.1542/peds.2025-072719

REFERENCES

1. Koogler TK, Wilfond BS, Ross LF. Lethal language, lethal decisions. *Hastings Cent Rep.* 2003;33(2):37–41. PubMed doi: 10.2307/3528153
2. Janvier A, Farlow B, Barrington KJ. Parental hopes, interventions, and survival of neonates with trisomy 13 and trisomy 18. *Am J Med Genet C Semin Med Genet.* 2016;172(3):279–287. PubMed doi: 10.1002/ajmg.c.31526
3. Kosho T, Kuniba H, Tanikawa Y, Hashimoto Y, Sakurai H. Natural history and parental experience of children with trisomy 18 based on a questionnaire given to a Japanese trisomy 18 parental support group. *Am J Med Genet A.* 2013;161A(7):1531–1542. PubMed doi: 10.1002/ajmg.a.35990
4. Wu J, Springett A, Morris JK. Survival of trisomy 18 (Edwards syndrome) and trisomy 13 (Patau Syndrome) in England and Wales: 2004–2011. *Am J Med Genet A.* 2013;161A(10):2512–2518. PubMed doi: 10.1002/ajmg.a.36127
5. Kepple JW, Fishler KP, Peeples ES. Surveillance guidelines for children with trisomy 18. *Am J Med Genet A.* 2021;185(4):1294–1303. PubMed doi: 10.1002/ajmg.a.62097
6. Kepple JW, Fishler KP, Peeples ES. Surveillance guidelines for children with trisomy 13. *Am J Med Genet A.* 2021;185(5):1631–1637. PubMed doi: 10.1002/ajmg.a.62133
7. Kochan M, Cho E, Mercurio M, Greco M, Savarese AM, Falck A. Disagreement about surgical intervention in Trisomy 18. *Pediatrics.* 2021;147(1):e2020010686. PubMed doi: 10.1542/peds.2020-010686

8. Neubauer K, Boss RD. Ethical considerations for cardiac surgical interventions in children with trisomy 13 and trisomy 18. *Am J Med Genet C Semin Med Genet.* 2020;184(1):187–191. PubMed doi: 10.1002/ajmg.c.31767
9. Wilkinson D. The self-fulfilling prophecy in intensive care. *Theor Med Bioeth.* 2009;30(6):401–410. PubMed doi: 10.1007/s11017-009-9120-6
10. Bruns DA. Developmental status of 22 children with trisomy 18 and eight children with trisomy 13: implications and recommendations. *Am J Med Genet A.* 2015;167A(8):1807–1815. PubMed doi: 10.1002/ajmg.a.37102
11. Wightman A, Kett J, Campelia G, Wilfond BS. The relational potential standard: rethinking the ethical justification for life-sustaining treatment for children with profound cognitive disabilities. *Hastings Cent Rep.* 2019;49(3):18–25. PubMed doi: 10.1002/hast.1003
12. Kon AA, Davidson JE. Retiring the term futility in value-laden decisions regarding potentially inappropriate medical treatment. *Crit Care Nurse.* 2017;37(1):9–11. PubMed doi: 10.4037/ccn2017234
13. Bosslet GT, Pope TM, Rubenfeld GD, et al; American Thoracic Society ad hoc Committee on Futile and Potentially Inappropriate Treatment; American Thoracic Society; American Association for Critical Care Nurses; American College of Chest Physicians; European Society for Intensive Care Medicine; Society of Critical Care. An Official ATS/AACN/ACCP/ESICM/SCCM Policy Statement: Responding to Requests for Potentially Inappropriate Treatments in Intensive Care Units. *Am J Respir Crit Care Med.* 2015;191(11):1318–1330. PubMed doi: 10.1164/rccm.201505-0924ST
14. Mladenka C. Noninvasive prenatal screening using cell-free DNA. *J Am Assoc Nurse Pract.* 2022;34(6):789–791. PubMed doi: 10.1097/JXX.0000000000000710
15. Mai CT, Isenburg JL, Canfield MA, et al; National Birth Defects Prevention Network. National population-based estimates for major birth defects, 2010–2014. *Birth Defects Res.* 2019;111(18):1420–1435. PubMed doi: 10.1002/bdr2.1589
16. Cereda A, Carey JC. The trisomy 18 syndrome. *Orphanet J Rare Dis.* 2012;7(1):81. PubMed doi: 10.1186/1750-1172-7-81
17. Jones KL, Jones MC, del Campo M. *Smith's Recognizable Patterns of Human Malformation.* 8th ed. Elsevier; 2022.
18. American College of Obstetricians and Gynecologists. Access to Genetic Testing Position Statement: Position Statement. Accessed August 21, 2022. https://www.acog.org/clinical-information/policy-and-position-statements/position-statements/2018/access-to-genetic-testing
19. American College of Obstetricians and Gynecologists. NIPT Summary of Recommendations. Accessed August 21, 2022. https://www.acog.org/advocacy/policy-priorities/non-invasive-prenatal-testing/current-acog-guidance
20. American College of Obstetricians and Gynecologists. Prenatal Diagnostic Testing for Genetic Disorders - Practice Bulletin. Accessed August 21, 2022. https://www.acog.org/clinical/clinical-guidance/practice-bulletin/articles/2016/05/prenatal-diagnostic-testing-for-genetic-disorders
21. American College of Obstetricians and Gynecologists. Screening for Fetal Chromosomal Abnormalities - Practice Bulletin. Accessed August 21, 2022. https://www.acog.org/clinical/clinical-guidance/practice-bulletin/articles/2020/10/screening-for-fetal-chromosomal-abnormalities
22. American College of Obstetricians and Gynecologists. Legal Considerations in Genetic Screening and Testing: Three Case Studies - Legal Opinion. Accessed August 21, 2022. https://www.acog.org/clinical/clinical-guidance/committee-opinion/articles/2020/04/legal-considerations-in-genetic-screening-and-testing-three-case-studies
23. American College of Obstetricians and Gynecologists. Microarrays and Next-Generation Sequencing Technology: The Use of Advanced Genetic Diagnostic Tools in Obstetrics and Gynecology - Committee Opinion. Accessed August 21, 2022. https://www.acog.org/clinical/clinical-guidance/committee-opinion/articles/2016/12/microarrays-and-next-generation-sequencing-technology-the-use-of-advanced-genetic-diagnostic-tools-in-obstetrics-and-gynecology
24. American College of Obstetricians and Gynecologists. Counseling About Genetic Testing and Communication of Genetic Test Results - Committee Opinion Accessed August 21, 2022. https://www.acog.org/clinical/clinical-guidance/committee-opinion/articles/2017/04/counseling-about-genetic-testing-and-communication-of-genetic-test-results
25. American College of Obstetricians and Gynecologists. Ethical Issues in Genetic Testing - Committee Opinion. Accessed August 21, 2022. https://www.acog.org/clinical/clinical-guidance/committee-opinion/articles/2008/06/ethical-issues-in-genetic-testing
26. Benn P, Borell A, Chiu R, et al. Position statement from the Aneuploidy Screening Committee on behalf of the Board of the International Society for Prenatal Diagnosis. *Prenat Diagn.* 2013;33(7):622–629. PubMed doi: 10.1002/pd.4139
27. Gregg AR, Skotko BG, Benkendorf JL, et al. Noninvasive prenatal screening for fetal aneuploidy, 2016 update: a position statement of the American College of Medical Genetics and Genomics. *Genet Med.* 2016;18(10):1056–1065. PubMed doi: 10.1038/gim.2016.97
28. Kukora SK, Boss RD. Values-based shared decision-making in the antenatal period. *Semin Fetal Neonatal Med.* 2018;23(1):17–24. PubMed doi: 10.1016/j.siny.2017.09.003
29. Dotters-Katz SK, Carlson LM, Johnson J, et al. Management of pregnancy and survival of infants with trisomy 13 or trisomy 18. *Am J Perinatol.* 2016;33(12):1121–1127. PubMed doi: 10.1055/s-0036-1585580
30. Dotters-Katz SK, Kuller JA, Grace MR, Laifer SA, Strauss RA. Management considerations for ongoing pregnancies complicated by trisomy 13 and 18. *Obstet Gynecol Surv.* 2016;71(5):295–300. PubMed doi: 10.1097/OGX.0000000000000304
31. Carey JC. Trisomy 18 and Trisomy 13 Syndromes. *Management of Genetic Syndromes.* 2010:807–823.
32. Musewe NN, Alexander DJ, Teshima I, Smallhorn JF, Freedom RM. Echocardiographic evaluation of the spectrum of cardiac anomalies associated with trisomy 13 and trisomy 18. *J Am Coll Cardiol.* 1990;15(3):673–677. PubMed doi: 10.1016/0735-1097(90)90644-5
33. Balderston SM, Shaffer EM, Washington RL, Sondheimer HM. Congenital polyvalvular disease in trisomy 18: echocardiographic

diagnosis. *Pediatr Cardiol.* 1990;11(3):138–142. PubMed doi: 10.1007/BF02238843

34. Van Praagh S, Truman T, Firpo A, et al. Cardiac malformations in trisomy-18: a study of 41 postmortem cases. *J Am Coll Cardiol.* 1989;13(7):1586–1597. PubMed doi: 10.1016/0735-1097(89)90353-7
35. Costello JP, Weiderhold A, Louis C, et al. A contemporary, single-institutional experience of surgical versus expectant management of congenital heart disease in trisomy 13 and 18 patients. *Pediatr Cardiol.* 2015;36(5):987–992. PubMed doi: 10.1007/s00246-015-1109-5
36. Graham EM. Infants with trisomy 18 and complex congenital heart defects should not undergo open heart surgery. *J Law Med Ethics.* 2016;44(2):286–291. PubMed doi: 10.1177/1073110516654122
37. Kosiv KA, Long J, Lee HC, Collins RT II. A validated model for prediction of survival to 6 months in patients with trisomy 13 and 18. *Am J Med Genet A.* 2021;185(3):806–813. PubMed doi: 10.1002/ajmg.a.62044
38. Peterson JK, Kochilas LK, Catton KG, Moller JH, Setty SP. Long-term outcomes of children with trisomy 13 and 18 after congenital heart disease interventions. *Ann Thorac Surg.* 2017;103(6):1941–1949. PubMed doi: 10.1016/j.athoracsur.2017.02.068
39. Cooper DS, Riggs KW, Zafar F, et al. Cardiac surgery in patients with trisomy 13 and 18: an analysis of The Society of Thoracic Surgeons Congenital Heart Surgery Database. *J Am Heart Assoc.* 2019;8(13):e012349. PubMed doi: 10.1161/JAHA.119.012349
40. Furlong-Dillard JM, Amula V, Bailly DK, Bleyl SB, Wilkes J, Bratton SL. Use of extracorporeal membrane oxygenation and mortality in pediatric cardiac surgery patients with genetic conditions: a multicenter analysis. *Pediatr Crit Care Med.* 2017;18(9):850–858. PubMed doi: 10.1097/PCC.0000000000001225
41. Alore EA, Fallon SC, Thomas JA, Vogel AM. Outcomes after extracorporeal life support cannulation in pediatric patients with trisomy 13 and trisomy 18. *J Surg Res.* 2021;257:260–266. PubMed doi: 10.1016/j.jss.2020.07.036
42. Hollis T, Cashen K, Rycus P. 1129: EXTRACORPOREAL MEMBRANE OXYGENATION USE IN NEONATES AND CHILDREN WITH TRISOMY 13 AND TRISOMY 18. *Crit Care Med.* 2015;43(12):284. doi: 10.1097/01.ccm.0000474960.49340.fc
43. St Louis JD, Bhat A, Carey JC, et al. The American Association for Thoracic Surgery (AATS) 2023 Expert Consensus Document: recommendation for the care of children with trisomy 13 or trisomy 18 and a congenital heart defect. *J Thorac Cardiovasc Surg.* 2024;167(5):1519–1532. PubMed doi: 10.1016/j.jtcvs.2023.11.054
44. Nelson KE, Hexem KR, Feudtner C. Inpatient hospital care of children with trisomy 13 and trisomy 18 in the United States. *Pediatrics.* 2012;129(5):869–876. PubMed doi: 10.1542/peds.2011-2139
45. Birmingham EE, Stucke AG, Diaz CD. Anesthesia for children with complete trisomy 18 (Edwards syndrome): a cohort review of 84 anesthesia encounters in nine patients. *Paediatr Anaesth.* 2021;31(4):419–428. PubMed doi: 10.1111/pan.14131
46. Acharya K, Leuthner SR, Zaniletti I, et al; Palliative Care and Ethics Focus Group of the Children's Hospital Neonatal Consortium (CHNC). Medical and surgical interventions and outcomes for infants with trisomy 18 (T18) or trisomy 13 (T13) at children's hospitals neonatal intensive care units (NICUs). *J Perinatol.* 2021;41(7):1745–1754. PubMed doi: 10.1038/s41372-021-01111-9
47. Nelson KE, Rosella LC, Mahant S, Guttmann A. Survival and surgical interventions for children with trisomy 13 and 18. *JAMA.* 2016;316(4):420–428. PubMed doi: 10.1001/jama.2016.9819
48. Dereddy NR, Pivnick EK, Upadhyay K, Dhanireddy R, Talati AJ. Neonatal hospital course and outcomes of live-born infants with trisomy 18 at two tertiary care centers in the United States. *Am J Perinatol.* 2017;34(3):270–275. PubMed doi: 10.1055/s-0036-1586753
49. Goel N, Morris JK, Tucker D, et al. Trisomy 13 and 18-prevalence and mortality-a multi-registry population based analysis. *Am J Med Genet A.* 2019;179(12):2382–2392. PubMed doi: 10.1002/ajmg.a.61365
50. Inoue H, Matsunaga Y, Sawano T, et al. Survival outcomes of very low birth weight infants with trisomy 18. *Am J Med Genet A.* 2021;185(11):3459–3465. PubMed doi: 10.1002/ajmg.a.62466
51. Acharya K, Leuthner S, Clark R, Nghiem-Rao TH, Spitzer A, Lagatta J. Major anomalies and birth-weight influence NICU interventions and mortality in infants with trisomy 13 or 18. *J Perinatol.* 2017;37(4):420–426. PubMed doi: 10.1038/jp.2016.245
52. Fukasawa T, Kubota T, Tanaka M, et al. Apneas observed in trisomy 18 neonates should be differentiated from epileptic apneas. *Am J Med Genet A.* 2015;167A(3):602–606. PubMed doi: 10.1002/ajmg.a.36929
53. Taira R, Inoue H, Sawano T, et al. Management of apnea in infants with trisomy 18. *Dev Med Child Neurol.* 2020;62(7):874–878. PubMed doi: 10.1111/dmcn.14403
54. Kuo DZ, Houtrow AJ; COUNCIL ON CHILDREN WITH DISABILITIES. Recognition and management of medical complexity. *Pediatrics.* 2016;138(6):e20163021. PubMed doi: 10.1542/peds.2016-3021
55. Baty BJ, Blackburn BL, Carey JC. Natural history of trisomy 18 and trisomy 13: I. Growth, physical assessment, medical histories, survival, and recurrence risk. *Am J Med Genet.* 1994;49(2):175–188. PubMed doi: 10.1002/ajmg.1320490204
56. SOFT. Support Organization for Trisomy. Accessed April 18, 2022. https://trisomy.org/
57. Boghossian NS, Horbar JD, Murray JC, Carpenter JH; Vermont Oxford Network. Anthropometric charts for infants with trisomies 21, 18, or 13 born between 22 weeks gestation and term: the VON charts. *Am J Med Genet A.* 2012;158A(2):322–332. PubMed doi: 10.1002/ajmg.a.34423
58. Brady MT, Byington CL, Davies HD, et al; American Academy of Pediatrics Committee on Infectious Diseases; American Academy of Pediatrics Bronchiolitis Guidelines Committee. Updated guidance for palivizumab prophylaxis among infants and young children at increased risk of hospitalization for respiratory syncytial virus infection. *Pediatrics.* 2014;134(2):415–420. PubMed doi: 10.1542/peds.2014-1665
59. Mizrahi M, Well A, Gottlieb EA, et al. Trisomy 18: disparities of care and outcomes in the state of Texas between 2009 and 2019. *Cardiol Young.* 2023;33(11):2328–2333. PubMed doi: 10.1017/S1047951123000215

60. Janvier A, Farlow B, Barrington KJ, Bourque CJ, Brazg T, Wilfond B. Building trust and improving communication with parents of children with trisomy 13 and 18: a mixed-methods study. *Palliat Med.* 2020;34(3):262–271. PubMed doi: 10.1177/0269216319860662

61. Janvier A, Farlow B, Wilfond BS. The experience of families with children with trisomy 13 and 18 in social networks. *Pediatrics.* 2012;130(2):293–298. PubMed doi: 10.1542/peds.2012-0151

62. Meyer RE, Liu G, Gilboa SM, et al; National Birth Defects Prevention Network. Survival of children with trisomy 13 and trisomy 18: a multi-state population-based study. *Am J Med Genet A.* 2016;170A(4):825–837. PubMed doi: 10.1002/ajmg.a.37495

63. Springett A, Wellesley D, Greenlees R, et al. Congenital anomalies associated with trisomy 18 or trisomy 13: a registry-based study in 16 European countries, 2000–2011. *Am J Med Genet A.* 2015;167A(12):3062–3069. PubMed doi: 10.1002/ajmg.a.37355

Guidance for the Primary Care Provider in Identifying Infants With Biliary Atresia by 2–4 Weeks of Life

- *Clinical Report*
  - *PPI: AAP Partnership for Policy Implementation*
    See Appendix 1 for more information.

American Academy of Pediatrics
DEDICATED TO THE HEALTH OF ALL CHILDREN®

AAP Partnership for Policy Implementation

CLINICAL REPORT Guidance for the Clinician in Rendering Pediatric Care

American Academy of Pediatrics

DEDICATED TO THE HEALTH OF ALL CHILDREN™

Guidance for the Primary Care Provider in Identifying Infants With Biliary Atresia by 2–4 Weeks of Life: Clinical Report

Sanjiv Harpavat, MD, PhD, FAAP,[1] Susan W. Aucott, MD, FAAP,[2] Saul J. Karpen, MD, PhD, FAAP,[3] Benjamin L. Shneider, MD, FAAP,[4] Kasper Wang, MD, FAAP,[5] and the SECTION ON GASTROENTEROLOGY, HEPATOLOGY, AND NUTRITION; COMMITTEE ON FETUS AND NEWBORN; SECTION ON SURGERY

abstract

This report helps pediatric primary care providers quickly identify infants with biliary atresia, which has the potential to improve outcomes and reduce need for liver transplant. The strategy is intended to be used between 2 and 4 weeks of life at the "By 1 month" well-child visit in the Bright Futures/American Academy of Pediatrics "Recommendations for Preventive Pediatric Health Care." The strategy involves examining every infant's eye color, stool color, and prior laboratory results to determine whether measurement of a direct or conjugated bilirubin level is warranted.

[1]Division of Gastroenterology, Hepatology, and Nutrition, Department of Pediatrics, Baylor College of Medicine and Texas Children's Hospital, Houston, Texas; [2]Division of Neonatal-Perinatal Medicine, Department of Pediatrics, The Johns Hopkins University School of Medicine and Greater Baltimore Medical Center, Baltimore, Maryland; [3]Chief Scientific Officer, Stravitz-Sanyal Institute for Liver Disease and Metabolic Health, Virginia Commonwealth University School of Medicine, Richmond, Virginia; [4]Division of Gastroenterology, Hepatology, and Nutrition, Department of Pediatrics, Baylor College of Medicine and Texas Children's Hospital, Houston, Texas; and [5]Division of Pediatric Surgery, Department of Surgery, University of Toronto Temerty Faculty of Medicine and The Hospital for Sick Children, Toronto, Ontario

Dr. Harpavat, Dr. Aucott, Dr. Karpen, Dr. Shneider, and Dr. Wang conceptualized the clinical report; Dr. Harpavat drafted the initial manuscript; Dr. Harpavat, Dr. Aucott, Dr. Karpen, Dr. Shneider, and Dr. Wang reviewed and revised the manuscript; Dr. Lehmann developed the final version of the algorithm; and Dr. Harpavat, Dr. Aucott, Dr. Karpen, Dr. Shneider, and Dr. Wang approved the final manuscript as submitted and agree to be accountable for all aspects of the work.

To cite: Harpavat S, Aucott SW, Karpen SJ, et al; American Academy of Pediatrics, Section on Gastroenterology, Hepatology, and Nutrition; Committee on Fetus and Newborn; Section on Surgery. Guidance for the Primary Care Provider in Identifying Infants With Biliary Atresia by 2–4 Weeks of Life: Clinical Report. *Pediatrics.* 2025;155(3):e2024070077

BACKGROUND

A critical period in biliary atresia (BA) is the time between birth and treatment with the Kasai portoenterostomy. Ideally, infants are treated before 30 to 45 days of life to achieve the best outcomes.[1–3] In practice, however, infants are treated on average after 60 days of life in the United States.[4–7] Delays arise because BA can be asymptomatic initially. When symptoms do develop, the 1 in 8000 to 18 000 affected newborn infants each year are difficult to distinguish from the 65% of healthy newborn infants with benign causes of jaundice.[4,8] In part because of these delays, BA outcomes remain poor, with BA accounting for 60% of liver transplants in infants younger than 1 year and 30% of all liver transplants in children.[9]

Pediatric primary care providers (PCPs) have a unique opportunity to improve outcomes by identifying BA during the first well-child visits. This clinical report provides a strategy to be used between 2 and 4 weeks of life at the "By 1 month" well-child visit in the Bright Futures/American Academy of Pediatrics (AAP) "Recommendations for Preventive Pediatric Health Care" (also called the periodicity schedule).[10] The strategy involves examining every infant's eye color, stool color, and prior

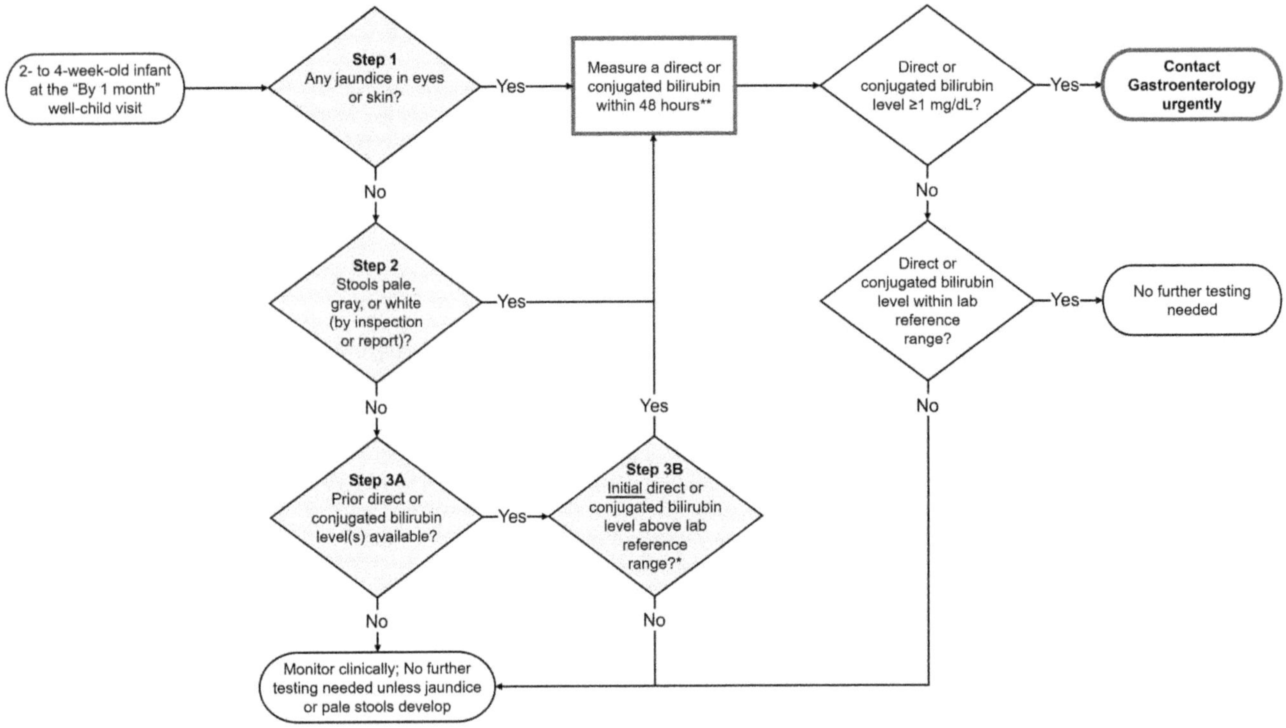

FIGURE 1.

A strategy for the routine well-child visit between 2 and 4 weeks of life. The strategy involves measuring a direct or conjugated bilirubin level in infants based on eye color, stool color, and prior direct or conjugated bilirubin results.

* Before 2 weeks of life, values are interpreted using the reference range specific to the laboratory performing the test (do not use a fixed cut-off or a bilirubin ratio).

** A measurement may not be needed if either of the following is true:
(a) Any prior direct or conjugated bilirubin value was within the laboratory's derived reference range.
(b) Prior direct or conjugated bilirubin values were all abnormal but both (i) less than or equal to the initial value *and* (ii) <1 mg/dL.

laboratory results to determine whether drawing a direct or conjugated bilirubin level is warranted (Figure 1).

STRATEGY

Step 1. Do the Eyes (or Skin) Appear Jaundiced to Any Degree, Beyond 2 Weeks of Life?

Jaundice beyond 2 to 3 weeks of life warrants consideration of testing for direct or conjugated bilirubin levels, according to joint recommendations from North American and European pediatric gastroenterology societies (see "Billing and Scheduling Considerations" below for a discussion on timing).[7] Jaundice is the key physical examination finding, because other signs—such as hepatomegaly and splenomegaly—may be absent in early stages of BA.

If the answer to Step 1 is "No," the strategy proceeds to Step 2 because an infant could still have BA. For example:

- ***Jaundice may not be present yet.*** In early stages, infants with BA may not have visible color changes in the eyes or skin. Visible signs can be lacking even though serum direct or conjugated bilirubin levels are elevated.[11]
- ***Jaundice may not be noticed.*** Certain infants may be vulnerable to a less careful examination because of an assumption that skin assessment is unreliable in infants who have skin with more melanin (importantly, at least one study challenges this assumption; see "Future Directions" section below). To help prevent missed cases, this report emphasizes the importance of assessing eye color, rather than just skin color, for jaundice.

Step 2. Are the Stools Pale, Gray, or White, by Inspection or a Caregiver's Report?

Pale, gray, or white stools at any time warrant consideration of testing for direct or conjugated bilirubin levels. Lighter stools occur in BA and other liver diseases when conjugated bilirubin in bile fails to reach the intestine and color the stools.

If the answer to Step 2 is "No," the strategy proceeds to Step 3 because an infant could still have BA. For example:

- ***The stools have not changed color yet.*** The transition to pale, gray, or white stools occurs over time in BA. Approximately 77% of infants with BA have pale, gray, or white stools at 30 days of life.[12] This proportion increases to 84% and 97% at 45 and 60 days of life, respectively.[13]
- ***A change in stool color may not be noticed.*** To avoid this, stool color can be assessed in multiple ways,

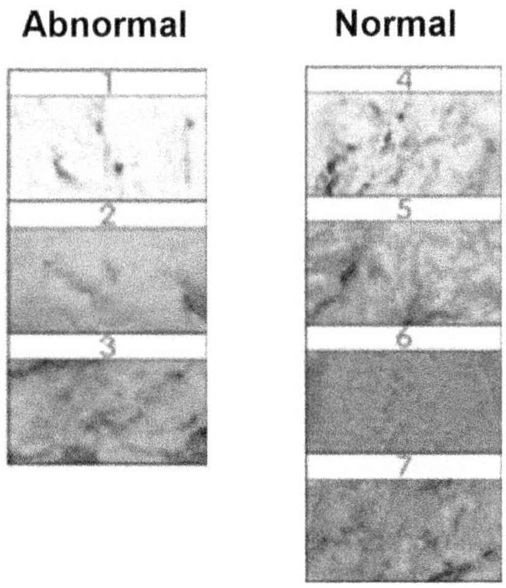

FIGURE 2.
Abnormal and normal stool color (Adapted from Chen SM, et al 2006[14]). Pale stools develop over time in BA as a result of biliary obstruction.

including (i) asking parents about stool color; (ii) inspecting stools at the clinic visit; (iii) reviewing pictures of stool color; (iv) comparing stool color to the "stool color card;" and/or (v) assessing stool color with a phone app such as PopòApp (Figure 2 shows images from a sample stool color card).[14,15]

Step 3. (A) Were Direct or Conjugated Bilirubin Levels Checked Previously? (B) If Yes, Was the *Initial* Value Above the Laboratory's Range?

A previously "high" direct or conjugated bilirubin level warrants consideration of repeat testing. To determine whether previous values were "high," prior laboratory results must be reviewed from the newborn inpatient unit and/or outpatient setting. Many infants have total bilirubin levels checked in accordance with AAP recommendations to assess risk for bilirubin encephalopathy.[16] Alongside total bilirubin, levels of direct or conjugated bilirubin are often measured.

The most important result is the *initial* direct or conjugated bilirubin level, which will be "high" in BA starting at birth.[11,17,18] "High" is defined as exceeding the laboratory's derived reference range, even if only by 0.1 mg/dL (Figure 1, footnote *). In the period before 2 weeks of life, "high" is not defined by exceeding a fixed cut-off or exceeding a bilirubin ratio (see Appendix for further discussion of interpreting initial values).[11,17]

If answers to questions in Step 3A or 3B are "No," skin and stool color should continue to be monitored because an infant could still have BA. For example:

- ***A previous direct or conjugated bilirubin level may not have been obtained.*** This can occur if risk for bilirubin encephalopathy was assessed by (i) total bilirubin levels alone, without also measuring direct or conjugated bilirubin levels; or (ii) transcutaneous measurements, which provide no information about direct or conjugated bilirubin levels.
- ***A direct or conjugated bilirubin level is compared to the wrong reference range.*** For interpreting levels drawn before 2 weeks of life, using the correct reference range is critical. Reference ranges for direct or conjugated bilirubin are laboratory-specific and can vary widely across hospitals (in one multicenter study, the derived reference ranges for participating hospitals varied from 0.0–0.2 mg/dL to 0.0–0.7 mg/dL).[19] As a result, in rare instances, a level may be high but incorrectly reported as normal if the laboratory used a borrowed —rather than derived—reference range (see Appendix for further discussion of deriving reference ranges).[20]

Exceptions to Measuring a Direct or Conjugated Bilirubin Level at 2 To 4 Weeks of Life

Based on the strategy in Figure 1, jaundiced eyes, pale stools, or a high initial laboratory result warrants consideration of testing for direct or conjugated bilirubin levels. However, a blood draw can possibly be avoided if levels checked earlier in the newborn inpatient unit or outpatient setting are available (Figure 1, footnote **). Infants for whom a blood test can be avoided have 1 of the following:

- ***Any prior direct or conjugated bilirubin level that was normal.*** In this instance, normal is defined as within the laboratory-derived reference range (normal is not defined with fixed cut-offs or bilirubin ratios in this early time period). Infants with normal levels are unlikely to have BA. This is because direct or conjugated bilirubin levels are above the reference range in BA starting at birth.[11,17]
- ***Prior direct or conjugated bilirubin levels that were all abnormal but equivalent or decreasing over time.*** In this instance, equivalent or decreasing is defined as both (i) less than or equal to the initial level; *and* (ii) <1 mg/dL. Infants with levels decreasing over time are unlikely to have BA. This is because direct or conjugated bilirubin levels increase over the first few weeks of life in BA before plateauing.[21]

Interpreting a Direct or Conjugated Bilirubin Level Measured at 2 To 4 Weeks of Life

Upon drawing a direct or conjugated bilirubin level, a value ≥1 mg/dL warrants urgent consultation with a pediatric gastroenterologist. The pediatric gastroenterologist will interpret the values and may recommend the following to evaluate for BA:

- ***Perform additional testing***. The pediatric gastroenterologist may ask only for the direct or conjugated bilirubin to be re-checked, to confirm the initial abnormal result. In

TABLE 1. Possible Activities in the First 3 Bright Futures/AAP Periodicity Schedule Patient Encounters to Identify Infants With BA

Bright Futures/ AAP Encounter	Provider Type	Activities
—	Newborn inpatient unit (*Infrastructure improvements*)	• Ensure that hospital laboratories derive their own direct or conjugated bilirubin reference ranges • Order direct or conjugated bilirubin along with any serum total bilirubin measurements • Build an efficient communication pipeline with outpatient PCPs
"Newborn"	Newborn inpatient unit	• Communicate any direct or conjugated bilirubin results to the outpatient PCP • Consider consulting a pediatric gastroenterologist when the first direct or conjugated bilirubin level is ≥1 mg/dL and subsequent levels rising
"3–5 days"	Outpatient PCP	• Remind parents to monitor for pale stools • Review prior direct or conjugated bilirubin results to identify high values • Schedule the "By 1 month" well-child visit • Consider consulting a pediatric gastroenterologist (if not already done) for an initial direct or conjugated bilirubin result of ≥1 mg/dL and subsequent levels rising
"By 1 month"	Outpatient PCP	• Apply the strategy in Figure 1 to determine if a direct or conjugated bilirubin level should be measured

other cases, the pediatric gastroenterologist may ask for more tests such as liver enzymes or an abdominal ultrasound. However, ordering liver enzymes or an abdominal ultrasound before consulting a pediatric gastroenterologist is not recommended, because normal results could be falsely reassuring and delay referrals.[22,23]

- ***Refer to gastroenterology.*** The pediatric gastroenterologist may prefer to see the patient in an outpatient setting before ordering further testing. An urgent referral should be made, and the infant's family should understand the importance of not missing the appointment. Ideally the infant is seen by pediatric gastroenterology within 5 days.
- ***Send to emergency department.*** In some cases, the pediatric gastroenterologist may elect to expedite the evaluation with an inpatient admission. To do this, the pediatric gastroenterologist may ask that the infant be sent to the emergency department to begin the process.

If the direct or conjugated bilirubin level is <1 mg/dL but above the reference interval at 2 to 4 weeks of life, urgent consultation with a pediatric gastroenterologist is not needed. These infants are unlikely to have BA. This is because direct or conjugated bilirubin levels in BA increase to ≥1 mg/dL over the first few weeks of life.[17,21] Possible next steps include monitoring clinically, and no further testing is needed unless signs such as jaundice or pale stools develop.

BILLING AND SCHEDULING CONSIDERATIONS

The strategy outlined in this report may require separately identifiable work in addition to what is performed during the routine 2- to 4-week well-child visit. For example, using this strategy may involve more time and/or more complex decision making. In these instances, separate evaluation and management services may be able to be reported, in accordance with *Current Procedural Terminology* (CPT) guidelines and payer policies.

From a scheduling perspective, the Bright Futures/AAP periodicity schedule allows PCPs to decide the timing of this well-child visit (in contrast, timings for the "3–5 day" and "2-month" well-child visits are specified).[10] Scheduling the visit at 2 weeks will help identify infants with BA earlier and help ensure that treatment with the Kasai portoenterostomy occurs before 30 days of life. However, an earlier visit may result in more infants being tested, because in one study 34% of healthy predominantly breastfed infants still appeared jaundiced at 3 weeks of life.[24] In contrast, scheduling the visit at 4 weeks may result in fewer healthy infants tested but may miss an opportunity for earlier treatment.

ACTIVITIES BEFORE THE "BY 1 MONTH" WELL-CHILD VISIT

The first 2 patient encounters in the Bright Futures/AAP periodicity schedule—the "Newborn" and "3- to 5-day" encounters—can also be used to help identify infants with BA (Table 1). The "Newborn" encounter occurs before hospital discharge. This visit can be used to review direct or conjugated bilirubin levels and to consult a pediatric gastroenterologist in special cases, such as when levels are already ≥1 mg/dL and increasing. The "3–5 day" encounter occurs shortly after discharge. It can be used to (i) remind parents to look for pale stools; (ii) review prior direct or conjugated bilirubin levels; and (iii) schedule a date for the "By 1 month" well-child visit. At the "3–5 day" encounter, a pediatric gastroenterologist can also be consulted in special cases, such as when levels are already ≥1 mg/dL and increasing.

In addition, health care providers in the newborn inpatient unit can help by:

- ***Ensuring their laboratories derive reference ranges.*** Each hospital should establish its own reference range for direct or conjugated bilirubin levels (see Appendix for further discussion of deriving reference ranges). Accurate reference ranges will ensure that all high direct or conjugated bilirubin levels are recognized.

- ***Consider adding direct or conjugated bilirubin testing when serum total bilirubin testing is performed.*** As mentioned earlier, many centers measure at least 1 serum total bilirubin level via heel stick or venipuncture to assess risk for bilirubin encephalopathy. Direct or conjugated bilirubin levels can be measured from the same heel stick or venipuncture sample, without needing an additional blood draw (future studies are needed to determine whether cord blood can also be used to identify BA).
- ***Communicating with outpatient PCPs.*** In the outpatient setting, there is limited time to search through discharge summaries or call birth hospitals to obtain direct or conjugated bilirubin results. Newborn inpatient providers could help by clearly documenting high levels and/or directly informing PCPs about abnormal results.

FUTURE DIRECTIONS

A future goal is to develop a universal screening strategy for BA, which would address the AAP goal of eliminating health disparities arising from current practice. Multiple studies have reported that Hispanic and non-Hispanic Black infants with BA are referred later than non-Hispanic white infants.[5,22,25,26] One potential reason is that some families miss well-child visits after infants are discharged from the hospital for reasons related to social determinants of health. Another potential reason is that identification of some infants is hindered by an implicit bias, which assumes that visually assessing skin color in individuals who have skin with more melanin is unreliable. When formally examined in one study, jaundice was recognized equally in Black and white infants.[27]

There are at least 2 promising options for a universal screening strategy. The first option is the stool color card program, which screens infants for pale stools. The stool color card program has been implemented successfully in several locations, including regions in Japan, Taiwan, provinces in Canada, and Switzerland.[12,13,28–31] The second option is newborn direct or conjugated bilirubin screening before hospital discharge.[32–35] The strategy has been implemented in parts of the United States.[19,36–38] Both strategies have been associated with earlier ages of treatment with the Kasai portoenterostomy, and future implementation studies will examine how well they can be integrated into standard pre-existing newborn management protocols.

SUMMARY

PCPs can identify infants who may have BA at 2 to 4 weeks of life, using a strategy at the "By 1 month" well-child visit in the Bright Futures/AAP periodicity schedule. The strategy involves measuring a direct or conjugated bilirubin level based on an infant's eye color, stool color, and prior laboratory results. By identifying infants earlier, PCPs have a unique opportunity to improve outcomes and help reduce the tremendous liver transplant burden of BA.

APPENDIX: PRINCIPLES OF BILIRUBIN MEASUREMENTS

The body excretes heme by converting it to bilirubin, which is measured in 3 forms:

- ***Unconjugated bilirubin.*** Unconjugated bilirubin is made in the spleen by removing iron from heme molecules. Unconjugated bilirubin is water insoluble and cannot be excreted without further modification. Unconjugated bilirubin levels increase in the neonatal period during the process of normal fetal red blood cell/fetal hemoglobin turnover. Excessively high unconjugated bilirubin levels are thought to cause bilirubin encephalopathy, which can be prevented by following AAP phototherapy guidelines.[16]
- ***Conjugated bilirubin.*** Conjugated bilirubin is made in the liver by modifying unconjugated bilirubin to become water soluble. Conjugated bilirubin then dissolves in bile and flows through bile ducts into the intestine for excretion (conjugated bilirubin derivatives give stool its characteristic color). In BA, conjugated bilirubin cannot leave the liver because the bile ducts are obstructed. Instead, conjugated bilirubin accumulates in blood and can be detected at birth.
- ***Delta bilirubin.*** Delta bilirubin is made when conjugated bilirubin binds to albumin. Delta bilirubin only forms in pathological situations, when conjugated bilirubin accumulates chronically in the blood. Clearance of delta bilirubin follows the half-life of albumin.[39] Delta bilirubin levels are measured with the direct, but not conjugated, assay (see below).

Clinical questions related to measuring these bilirubin forms include:

Why Do Some Laboratories Report "Direct" and Others Report "Conjugated" Bilirubin Levels?

Direct and conjugated bilirubin levels are used interchangeably but are not exactly the same (Appendix Table 1).[40,41] Both direct and conjugated assays measure conjugated bilirubin. In addition, the direct assay measures delta bilirubin as well as small amounts of unconjugated bilirubin. As a result, the direct assay always produces slightly higher results than the conjugated assay. The direct assay is used by more laboratories in the United States, although the direct assay results are sometimes incorrectly reported as "conjugated bilirubin."

Appendix Table 1. Differences Between Direct Bilirubin and Conjugated Bilirubin Tests

	Direct Bilirubin Test	Conjugated Bilirubin Test
Bilirubin form detected	• Conjugated bilirubin • Delta bilirubin • Unconjugated bilirubin (small amount)	• Conjugated bilirubin
Assay type	• Enzymatic with the diazo reagent	• Direct spectrophotometry
Advantages	• Widely available	• Measures only conjugated bilirubin
Limitations	• Measures delta and some unconjugated bilirubin • Differs across machines, so laboratory-derived reference ranges are needed	• Not widely available
Other tests performed with the same/similar assay	• Total bilirubin (includes conjugated, delta, and unconjugated bilirubin) • Indirect bilirubin (calculated by subtracting direct from total bilirubin)	• Unconjugated bilirubin • No equivalent of total bilirubin; sometimes estimated as conjugated plus unconjugated bilirubin

Why Should Fixed Cut-Offs Not Be Used Before 2 Weeks of Life?

The first direct or conjugated bilirubin levels in BA—although elevated—may be only slightly higher than the reference range and still below 1 mg/dL.[11,17,18] For this reason, levels measured before 2 weeks of life are interpreted with laboratory-specific reference ranges (see below for a discussion on how reference ranges are derived). After 2 weeks of life, levels in BA will have increased sufficiently and can be interpreted using the fixed 1 mg/dL cut-off.

Why Should Bilirubin Ratios Not Be Used Before 2 Weeks of Life?

Using bilirubin ratios in the first days of life will miss infants with BA.[11,17] Bilirubin ratios are calculated by dividing the direct or conjugated level by the total level. Bilirubin ratios are often used to evaluate infants with elevated direct or conjugated bilirubin levels, to distinguish between non-liver causes (such as increased red blood cell destruction, ratio <0.2) versus liver causes (ratio ≥0.2). However, in one study, bilirubin ratios were ≥0.2 before 48 hours of life in only 21% of newborn infants later diagnosed with BA.[11] Bilirubin ratios may be more useful for identifying BA when used at later time periods.

How Do Laboratories Derive Reference Ranges?

Each hospital laboratory should derive its own direct bilirubin or conjugated bilirubin reference range. This is especially important for the direct assay, which can vary with slight changes in pH, temperature, and/or reaction times that occur across laboratories.[40] To derive reference ranges, laboratories can follow standard procedures of measuring serum from 120 newborn infants and designating the middle 95% of values (2.5^{th}–97.5^{th} percentiles) as normal.[42]

LEAD AUTHORS

Sanjiv Harpavat, MD, PhD, FAAP
Susan Aucott, MD, FAAP
Saul Karpen, MD, PhD, FAAP
Benjamin Shneider, MD, FAAP
Kasper Wang, MD, FAAP

SECTION ON GASTROENTEROLOGY, HEPATOLOGY, AND NUTRITION EXECUTIVE COMMITTEE, 2021–2022

Mitchell B. Cohen, MD, FAAP, Chairperson
David Brumbaugh, MD, FAAP
Jennifer L. Dotson, MD, FAAP
Sanjiv Harpavat, MD, PhD, FAAP
Jenifer R. Lightdale, MD, FAAP, Immediate Past Chairperson
Daniel Mallon, MD, FAAP
Maria M. Oliva-Hemker, MD, FAAP

STAFF

Debra L. Burrowes, MHA

COMMITTEE ON FETUS AND NEWBORN, 2021–2022

Eric C. Eichenwald, MD, FAAP, Chairperson
Charletta Guillory, MD, FAAP
Ivan Leslie Hand, MD, FAAP
Mark L. Hudak, MD, FAAP
David Alan Kaufman, MD, FAAP
Camilia Rivera Martin, MD, FAAP
Margaret Graham Kemper Parker, MD, FAAP
Arun Kumar Pramanik, MD, FAAP
Kelly Cant Wade, MD, FAAP

STAFF

Jim Couto, MA

SECTION ON SURGERY EXECUTIVE COMMITTEE, 2021–2022

Andrew Davidoff, MD, FAAP, Chairperson
Elizabeth Beierle, MD, FAAP
Gail E. Besner, MD, FAAP, Immediate Past Chairperson
Marybeth Browne, MD, FAAP

Cynthia D. Downard, MD, FAAP
Kenneth Gow, MD, FAAP
Saleem Islam, MD, FAAP
Danielle Walsh, MD, FAAP

STAFF

Vivian Thorne

PARTNERSHIP FOR POLICY IMPLEMENTATION

Christina Jung, MD, FAAP
Christoph U. Lehmann, MD, FAAP

STAFF

Kymika Okechukwu

ACKNOWLEDGEMENT

The authors would like to acknowledge Debra L. Burrowes, staff liaison to the AAP Section on Gastroenterology, Hepatology and Nutrition, for providing instrumental guidance through the permissions, drafting, and review process. The clinical report represents one of Ms. Burrowes' last projects in her 17 year tenure with the AAP.

ABBREVIATIONS

AAP: American Academy of Pediatrics
BA: biliary atresia
PCP: primary care provider

Clinical reports from the American Academy of Pediatrics benefit from expertise and resources of liaisons and internal (AAP) and external reviewers. However, clinical reports from the American Academy of Pediatrics may not reflect the views of the liaisons or the organizations or government agencies that they represent.

The guidance in this report does not indicate an exclusive course of treatment or serve as a standard of medical care. Variations, taking into account individual circumstances, may be appropriate.

All clinical reports from the American Academy of Pediatrics automatically expire 5 years after publication unless reaffirmed, revised, or retired at or before that time.

CONFLICT OF INTEREST DISCLOSURE: The authors have indicated they have no potential conflicts of interest to disclose.

FUNDING: No external funding.

https://doi.org/10.1542/peds.2024-070077

REFERENCES

1. Schreiber RA, Barker CC, Roberts EA, et al. Biliary atresia: the Canadian experience. *J Pediatr.* 2007;151(6):659–665, 665.e1. doi: 10.1016/j.jpeds.2007.05.051
2. Serinet MO, Wildhaber BE, Broué P, et al. Impact of age at Kasai operation on its results in late childhood and adolescence: a rational basis for biliary atresia screening. *Pediatrics.* 2009; 123(5):1280–1286. doi: 10.1542/peds.2008-1949
3. Tessier MEM, Shneider BL. 60 Days in Biliary Atresia: A Historical Dogma Challenged. *Clin Liver Dis (Hoboken).* 2020;15(Suppl 1): S3–S7. doi: 10.1002/cld.843
4. Jimenez-Rivera C, Jolin-Dahel KS, Fortinsky KJ, Gozdyra P, Benchimol EI. International incidence and outcomes of biliary atresia. *J Pediatr Gastroenterol Nutr.* 2013;56(4):344–354. doi: 10.1097/MPG.0b013e318282a913
5. Shneider BL, Brown MB, Haber B, et al. A multicenter study of the outcome of biliary atresia in the United States, 1997 to 2000. *J Pediatr.* 2006;148(4):467–474. doi: 10.1016/j.jpeds.2005.12.054
6. Hopkins PC, Yazigi N, Nylund CM. Incidence of Biliary Atresia and Timing of Hepatoportoenterostomy in the United States. *J Pediatr.* 2017;187:253–257. doi: 10.1016/j.jpeds.2017.05.006
7. Fawaz R, Baumann U, Ekong U, et al. Guideline for the Evaluation of Cholestatic Jaundice in Infants: Joint Recommendations of the North American Society for Pediatric Gastroenterology, Hepatology, and Nutrition (NASPGHAN) and the European Society for Pediatric Gastroenterology, Hepatology,. *J Pediatr Gastroenterol Nutr.* 2017;64(1):154–168. doi: 10.1097/MPG.0000000000001334
8. Maisels MJ. Jaundice in healthy newborns-redefining physiologic jaundice. *West J Med.* 1988;149(4):451.
9. Mysore KR, Shneider BL, Harpavat S. Biliary Atresia as a Disease Starting In Utero: Implications for Treatment, Diagnosis, and Pathogenesis. *J Pediatr Gastroenterol Nutr.* 2019;69(4):396–403. doi: 10.1097/MPG.0000000000002450
10. 2022 Recommendations for Preventive Pediatric Health Care. *Pediatrics.* 2022;150(1). doi: 10.1542/PEDS.2022-058044
11. Harpavat S, Finegold MJ, Karpen SJ. Patients with biliary atresia have elevated direct/conjugated bilirubin levels shortly after birth. *Pediatrics.* 2011;128(6):e1428–33. doi: 10.1542/peds.2011-1869
12. Gu YH, Yokoyama K, Mizuta K, et al. Stool color card screening for early detection of biliary atresia and long-term native liver survival: a 19-year cohort study in Japan. *J Pediatr.* 2015;166(4): 897–902.e1. doi: 10.1016/j.jpeds.2014.12.063

13. Hsiao CH, Chang MH, Chen HL, et al. Universal screening for biliary atresia using an infant stool color card in Taiwan. *Hepatology*. 2008;47(4):1233–1240. doi: 10.1002/hep.22182

14. Chen SM, Chang MH, Du JC, et al. Screening for biliary atresia by infant stool color card in Taiwan. *Pediatrics*. 2006;117(4): 1147–1154. doi: 10.1542/peds.2005-1267

15. Angelico R, Liccardo D, Paoletti M, et al. A novel mobile phone application for infant stool color recognition: An easy and effective tool to identify acholic stools in newborns. *J Med Screen*. 2021;28(3):230–237. doi: 10.1177/0969141320974413

16. Kemper AR, Newman TB, Slaughter JL, et al. Clinical Practice Guideline Revision: Management of Hyperbilirubinemia in the Newborn Infant 35 or More Weeks of Gestation. *Pediatrics*. 2022;150(3). doi: 10.1542/PEDS.2022-058859

17. Liao FM, Chang KC, Wu JF, Chen HL, Ni YH, Chang MH. Direct Bilirubin and Risk of Biliary Atresia. *Pediatrics*. 2022;149(6). doi: 10.1542/PEDS.2021-053073

18. Kastenberg ZJ, Deneau MR, O'Brien EA, et al. Fractionated Bilirubin Among 252,892 Utah Newborns With and Without Biliary Atresia: A 15-year Historical Birth Cohort Study. *J Pediatr*. Published online January 2023. doi: 10.1016/J.JPEDS.2022.12.041

19. Harpavat S, Garcia-Prats JA, Anaya C, et al. Diagnostic Yield of Newborn Screening for Biliary Atresia Using Direct or Conjugated Bilirubin Measurements. *JAMA*. 2020;323(12):1141–1150. doi: 10.1001/jama.2020.0837

20. Harpavat S, Devaraj S, Finegold MJ. An infant with persistent jaundice and a normal newborn direct bilirubin measurement. *Clin Chem*. 2015;61(2):330–333. doi: 10.1373/clinchem.2014.223115

21. Terui K, Higashimoto Y, Saito E, et al. Diagnosis of biliary atresia can not be excluded by declining trend of serum direct bilirubin. *Pediatr Rep*. 2013;5:73–75. doi: 10.4081/pr.2013.e17

22. Harpavat S, Lupo PJ, Liwanag L, et al. Factors Influencing Time-to-diagnosis of Biliary Atresia. *J Pediatr Gastroenterol Nutr*. 2018; 66(6):850–856. doi: 10.1097/MPG.0000000000001887

23. Hwang SM, Jeon TY, Yoo SY, Choe YH, Lee SK, Kim JH. Early US findings of biliary atresia in infants younger than 30 days. *Eur Radiol*. 2018;28(4):1771–1777. doi: 10.1007/s00330-017-5092-5

24. Maisels MJ, Clune S, Coleman K, et al. The natural history of jaundice in predominantly breastfed infants. *Pediatrics*. 2014;134(2). doi: 10.1542/PEDS.2013-4299

25. Lee H, Lewis J, Schoen BT, Brand T, Ricketts RR. Kasai portoenterostomy: Differences related to race. *J Pediatr Surg*. 2001;36(8): 1196–1198. doi: 10.1053/jpsu.2001.25761

26. Raval MV, Dzakovic A, Bentrem DJ, Reynolds M, Superina R. Trends in age for hepatoportoenterostomy in the United States. *Surgery*. 2010;148(4):785–791; discussion 791-2. doi: 10.1016/j.surg.2010.07.028

27. Keren R, Tremont K, Luan X, Cnaan A. Visual assessment of jaundice in term and late preterm infants. *Arch Dis Child Fetal Neonatal Ed*. 2009;94(5). doi: 10.1136/adc.2008.150714

28. Wildhaber BE. Screening for biliary atresia: Swiss stool color card. *Hepatology*. 2011;54(1):367–368; author reply 369. doi: 10.1002/hep.24346

29. Woolfson JP, Schreiber RA, Butler AE, et al. Province-wide Biliary Atresia Home Screening Program in British Columbia: Evaluation of First 2 Years. *J Pediatr Gastroenterol Nutr*. 2018;66(6):845–849. doi: 10.1097/MPG.0000000000001950

30. Tseng JJ, Lai MS, Lin MC, Fu YC. Stool color card screening for biliary atresia. *Pediatrics*. 2011;128(5):e1209–15. doi: 10.1542/peds.2010-3495

31. Lin JS, Chen SCC, Lu CL, Lee HC, Yeung CY, Chan WT. Reduction of the ages at diagnosis and operation of biliary atresia in Taiwan: A 15-year population-based cohort study. *World J Gastroenterol*. 2015; 21(46):13080–13086. doi: 10.3748/wjg.v21.i46.13080

32. Keffler S, Kelly DA, Powell JE, Green A. Population screening for neonatal liver disease: a feasibility study. *J Pediatr Gastroenterol Nutr*. 1998;27(3):306–311. Accessed May 11, 2015. http://www.ncbi.nlm.nih.gov/pubmed/9740202

33. Powell JE, Keffler S, Kelly DA, Green A. Population screening for neonatal liver disease: potential for a community-based programme. *J Med Screen*. 2003;10(3):112–116. doi: 10.1258/096914103769010996

34. Harpavat S, Ramraj R, Finegold MJMJ, et al. Newborn Direct or Conjugated Bilirubin Measurements As a Potential Screen for Biliary Atresia. *J Pediatr Gastroenterol Nutr*. 2016;62(6): 799–803. doi: 10.1097/MPG.0000000000001097

35. Noorulla F, Dedon R, Maisels MJ. Association of Early Direct Bilirubin Levels and Biliary Atresia Among Neonates. *JAMA Netw Open*. 2019;2(10):e1913321. doi: 10.1001/jamanetworkopen.2019.13321

36. Harpavat S, Garcia-Prats JA, Shneider BL. Newborn Bilirubin Screening for Biliary Atresia. *N Engl J Med*. 2016;375(6):605–606. doi: 10.1056/NEJMc1601230

37. Guthery SL, Deneau M, Christensen R, et al. Fractionated Bilirubin in >250,000 Utah Newborns Confirms Conjugated or Direct Bilirubin is Elevated in the Newborn Period in Biliary Atresia: Implications for Newborn Screening. *Hepatology*. 2019;70(S1): 54–55A.

38. Rabbani T, Guthery SL, Himes R, Shneider BL, Harpavat S. Newborn Screening for Biliary Atresia: a Review of Current Methods. *Curr Gastroenterol Rep*. 2021;23(12):28. doi: 10.1007/S11894-021-00825-2

39. Ye W, Rosenthal P, Magee JC, Whitington PF, Childhood Liver Disease Research and Education Network. Factors Determining δ-Bilirubin Levels in Infants With Biliary Atresia. *J Pediatr Gastroenterol Nutr*. 2015;60(5):659–663. doi: 10.1097/MPG.0000000000000690

40. Doumas BT, Wu TW. The measurement of bilirubin fractions in serum. *Crit Rev Clin Lab Sci*. 1991;28(5-6):415–445. doi: 10.3109/10408369109106872

41. Davis AR, Rosenthal P, Escobar GJ, Newman TB. Interpreting conjugated bilirubin levels in newborns. *J Pediatr*. 2011;158(4): 562–565.e1. doi: 10.1016/j.jpeds.2010.09.061

42. CSLI. *EP28-A3c: Defining, Establishing, and Verifying Reference Intervals in the Clinical Laboratory; Approved Guideline—Third Edition*. EP28-A3c ed. Clinical and Laboratory Standards Institute; 2008.

Health Supervision for Children With 22q11.2 Deletion Syndrome

- *Clinical Report*
  - *PPI: AAP Partnership for Policy Implementation See Appendix 1 for more information.*

American Academy of Pediatrics
DEDICATED TO THE HEALTH OF ALL CHILDREN®

AAP Partnership for Policy Implementation

CLINICAL REPORT Guidance for the Clinician in Rendering Pediatric Care

American Academy of Pediatrics

DEDICATED TO THE HEALTH OF ALL CHILDREN™

Health Supervision for Children With 22q11.2 Deletion Syndrome: Clinical Report

Angela E. Scheuerle, MD, FAAP,[1] Timothy A. Geleske, MD, FAAP,[2] Nadia Merchant, MD, FAAP,[3] Paula C. Goldenberg, MD, FAAP,[4,5] and the Council on Genetics

22q11.2 deletion syndrome is the most frequent chromosomal microdeletion syndrome, with an estimated frequency of about 1/4000 in children younger than 1 year. Associated features in neonates and infants are conotruncal heart defects, interrupted aortic arch type B, cleft palate, hypocalcemia (which can present as seizures), feeding problems, developmental delay, and immune system abnormalities. Older children, adolescents, and adults may have neurocognitive impairments and/or speech disorders. Psychiatric diagnoses are more common than in the general population. Newborn infants may have a positive newborn screening for severe combined immunodeficiency (SCID). Genetic diagnosis is confirmed by chromosome microarray. This document is intended to provide guidance for health care providers to help identify individual patients at high risk of developing serious sequelae and to enable intervention before complications develop.

INTRODUCTION

The condition now known as 22q11.2 (Note: This is read and pronounced as "twenty-two Q one-one-point-two") deletion syndrome (22q11.2DS) has a prevalence of ~ 1/4000 live births and is likely undercounted.[1] Until the common deletion was established in the early 1990s as the cause of a range of medical conditions,[2] the full extent of the syndrome was unrecognized. The phenotype is broad, ranging from physically unremarkable with mild intellectual disabilities to seriously affected with congenital heart defect, other major malformations, thymic and parathyroid abnormalities, significant neurocognitive impairments, and risk for psychiatric disorders. As a result, the same condition was described by various authors who were seeing one collection of features but not the whole spectrum. Thus, there have been multiple names assigned: DiGeorge syndrome, velocardiofacial syndrome, conotruncal anomaly face

abstract

[1]*University of Texas Southwestern Medical Center, Dallas, Texas;* [2]*Northwestern University Feinberg School of Medicine, Chicago, Illinois;* [3]*University of Texas Southwestern Medical Center, Dallas, Texas;* [4]*Massachusetts General Hospital, Boston, Massachusetts; and* [5]*Harvard Medical School, Boston Massachusetts*

Drs Scheuerle, Geleske, Merchant, and Goldberg were directly involved in the planning, researching, and writing of this report, approved the final manuscript as submitted, and agree to be accountable for all aspects of the work. Drs. Geleske and Scheuerle were members of the Council on Genetics Executive Committee at the time this guidance was proposed.

FINANCIAL/CONFLICT OF INTEREST DISCLOSURE: Dr Paula Goldenberg has disclosed a nonfinancial relationship with the 22q11 Family Foundation as an advisory board member. Any other disclosures were reviewed and determined not relevant to the work related to "Health Supervision for Children With 22q11.2 Deletion Syndrome." Disclosures are reviewed and mitigated through a Conflict-of-Interest process that consists of reviewing pertinent information which is then used to decide what action is required to maintain content integrity. There may be instances where no action is necessary. This process has been approved by the AAP Board of Directors.

Clinical reports from the American Academy of Pediatrics benefit from expertise and resources of liaisons and internal (AAP) and external reviewers. (Continued)

To cite: Scheuerle AE, Geleske TA, Merchant N, et al; American Academy of Pediatrics, Council on Genetics. Health Supervision for Children With 22q11.2 Deletion Syndrome: Clinical Report. *Pediatrics.* 2025;156(2):e2025072717

syndrome, autosomal dominant Opitz G/BBB syndrome, Cayler cardiofacial syndrome, and others.[3] These are now all subsumed under the more appropriate and accurate name of 22q11.2DS. The patient support group website is 22q.org and the established multidisciplinary clinics are called "22q clinics."

The term DiGeorge syndrome is used differently across specialties and institutions. Experts recommend that the diagnosis of DiGeorge syndrome be limited to those patients with normal cytogenetic testing who have clinical features of the condition.[4]

DIAGNOSIS

Neonatal Period

The presenting clinical features depend on the severity of the phenotype. Severe congenital heart defects, such as tetralogy of Fallot or truncus arteriosus, may be identified prenatally by ultrasonography or shortly after birth because of murmur or cardiovascular compromise. The classic cardiovascular abnormality—a type B interrupted aortic arch (IAA-B)—may be asymptomatic until the ductus arteriosus closes. Universal complex congenital heart defect (CCHD) point-of-service screening potentially can identify these and other asymptomatic neonates. Regardless of presentation, diagnosis of a conotruncal heart defect or IAA-B in a newborn infant should prompt investigation for the 22q11.2 deletion. Genetics consultation is appropriate for any child with a conotruncal heart defect, particularly if there are additional malformations or other features of 22q11.2DS.

Newborn screening (NBS) for severe combined immunodeficiency (SCID)[5] and conditions associated with severe T-cell lymphopenia is currently performed in 50 states plus the District of Columbia and Puerto Rico. The method of this screening is to detect T-cell receptor excision circles (TRECs), small circular DNA fragments that are released during maturation and specification of T lymphocytes. Although the NBS for TRECs was designed to identify SCID, it can detect several syndromes, including 22q11.2DS, associated with severe T-cell lymphopenia.

22q11.2DS can manifest with a wide variety of structural malformations and functional problems including cleft palate, vertebral abnormalities, laryngotracheoesophageal abnormalities, thymic aplasia or hypoplasia, upper and lower intestinal malformations, genitourinary tract anomalies, hypoparathyroidism or hypocalcemia, feeding problems, velopharyngeal incompetence, speech delays, and global developmental delay. Some of these combinations might not immediately suggest a specific diagnosis but would certainly bring the child to medical attention and should precipitate a genetic evaluation.

Infancy and Childhood

Physically and immunologically healthy children with 22q11.2DS are most likely to present with developmental delay and growth impairment or short stature.[6] Children with these nonspecific problems are more at risk of a diagnostic odyssey before final diagnosis. The short stature is not related to feeding problems and in only a minority of cases is it attributable to abnormalities of growth hormone. Developmental delays in general and speech/articulation disorders in particular may be the most prominent presenting feature in childhood. Various neurocognitive problems can be present, and approximately 20% of patients manifest autism spectrum disorders.[4,7]

Adolescence

Children born before 2010 would not have had NBS that included SCID/TREC, so they may present with an otherwise unexplained history of frequent common infections. Intellectual disability and speech problems continue in this group. Also present is an increased risk of psychiatric disorders, particularly psychosis, schizophrenia, and depression. Frank schizophrenia has been diagnosed in about 25% of patients, and up to 60% of adult patients have some degree of psychiatric disorder.[4] Although unusual, genital anomalies such as hematometrocolpos can present in adolescent girls as a manifestation of 22q11.2DS.[8]

GENETIC TESTING AND COUNSELING

The 22q11.2 region has 8 low copy number repeats (LCRs) identified linearly by letters A through H (Figure 1). These are, as the name implies, repeated and similar DNA sequences. The presence of the LCRs leads to abnormal chromosome recombination in meiosis and, thus, deletion or duplication of the stretch of DNA between any 2 LCRs.

The most common genotype, in approximately 85% of patients, is a recurrent deletion of 2.54 megabases (Mb)

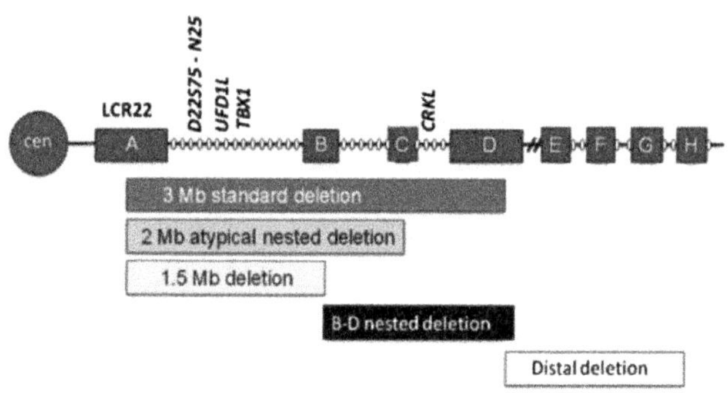

FIGURE 1.
The 22q11.2 region. Reprinted with permission from McDonald-McGinn DM, Hain HS, Emanuel BS, et al. 22q11.2 deletion syndrome. In: Adam MP, Ardinger HH, Pagon RA, et al, eds. *GeneReviews*. University of Washington; 1993–2021. https://www.ncbi.nlm.nih.gov/books/NBK1523/.

between LCRs A and D (Note: 1 megabase = 1 million base pairs). This deletion includes approximately 40 genes. The remaining patients have definable deletions between LCRs A and B, A and C, B and D, or C and D.[4] About 5% of patients have a smaller 1.5 Mb deletion that is nested within the common deletion. An estimated 7% of patients have overlapping or adjoining small deletions. There are reciprocal duplications, and the features of duplication patients are similar to those in the deletion patients.

Prenatal Screening

Noninvasive prenatal screening using cell-free DNA from a maternal blood sample is now widely used. Some laboratories include screening for 22q11.2DS in their offered tests. It is important to remember that this is not a diagnostic test and that the positive predictive value of this screen is about 50% (CI: 28.9–75.6).[9] If the cell-free DNA analysis is screen positive for an increased risk of 22q11.2DS, it should be confirmed by direct cytogenetic testing of the fetus via amniocentesis or testing the infant after delivery. A negative cell-free DNA screen should not rule out the possibility of diagnosis if the fetus or infant otherwise has a concerning phenotype.

Chromosome Microarray

Chromosome microarray technology, as it is currently used, will identify all deletions in patients. This test is the preferred one.[10] It will identify deletions in areas not covered by other methods as well as complex rearrangements of the 22q11.2 region. This test can identify the corresponding duplication syndromes and diagnose (or rule out) other copy number variants. Chromosome microarrays are widely available. The test can be performed prenatally via chorionic villus sampling or amniocentesis and postnatally using blood or buccal sample.

Fluorescent In Situ Hybridization

Fluorescent in situ hybridization (FISH) for 22q11.2DS is used to identify the presence or absence of a stretch of DNA sequence just distal to LCR A (see Figure 1). It will detect 90% to 92% of the deletions in the patients. FISH is unlikely to identify duplications. It can be useful for testing parents and other family members once a diagnosis is established in the initial patient but only if the deletion is in the region covered by the FISH probe.

It should be noted that the "nickname" for the 22q11.2DS FISH probe is the "DiGeorge probe," and the eponym is often used by laboratories in their reports. This name should not be interpreted as the child having a particular phenotype, nor should it precipitate a diagnosis of DiGeorge syndrome rather than 22q11.2DS.

Redundancy of Testing

Postnatal testing of any sort is unnecessary if the diagnosis is prenatally established by chorionic villus or amniotic fluid sampling. Likewise, FISH and microarray are redundant. It is not cost-effective to pursue both: microarray is sufficient and preferred.

Karyotype

Routine chromosome analysis is inadequate to diagnosis 22q11.2DS. In order for a deletion to be visible by light microscopy, it must be 4 to 5 Mb in size. The standard 22q11.2DS deletion is about half that, so it is not visible by routine chromosome analysis.

Family Testing and Counseling

The majority (>90%) of patients with 22q11.2DS are the first affected individual in their family. The deletion occurs in the egg or sperm prior to fertilization. Some parents who are clinically unaffected may wish to be tested to confirm; this testing can be accomplished using FISH in most families. When neither parent has the deletion, the pediatrician should counsel that their recurrence risk—their likelihood of having another child with 22q11.2DS—is 1%.

Ten percent of patients inherited the deletion from an affected parent. Whether a parent is affected or not may be observable based on interaction and routine evaluation, with the caveat that the phenotype can be very mild. An affected parent may not have come to direct medical attention because of the minimal problems and absence of structural anomalies. Expanded questioning may reveal that the parent needed assistance in school, had palatal surgery because of velopharyngeal incompetence, or lives with depression. Other children in the family may have features suggestive of 22q11.2DS warranting testing of them.

22q11.2DS is an autosomal-dominant condition. A person with the deletion has a 50% risk of passing it on, regardless of how affected they are. The pediatrician should counsel parents who have the deletion that their risk of having another affected child is 50% with each pregnancy. Further, the parent(s) of all affected children should be counseled that this will be the child's risk of having an affected offspring in the future. It is important to convey that the severity of the condition can vary widely within a family: a mildly affected parent can have a severely affected child.

Summary of Diagnosis and Confirmatory Testing and Counseling Testing

- 22q11.2DS is the most frequent chromosomal microdeletion syndrome, with an estimated frequency of about 1/4000 in children younger than 1 year.
- Presentation varies by age. Neonates and infants are more likely to have the diagnosis made by abnormal

NBS for SCID or the presence of malformations. Older children, adolescents, and adults are more likely to have the diagnosis made because of neurocognitive impairments and speech disorders.
- Newborn infants with 22q11.2DS may screen positive for SCID on the state NBS, even in the absence of physical malformations.
- Diagnosis of any conotruncal heart defect or interrupted aortic arch type B (IAA-B) should prompt a chromosome microarray to evaluate for 22q11.2DS.
- Diagnosis is best made by chromosome microarray performed prenatally on an amniocentesis sample or via a blood or buccal sample postnatally.
- Other family members can be studied by FISH if the identified deletion can be detected with this method.
- When neither parent has the deletion, their chance of having a second affected child is estimated at 1%.
- A person affected with 22q11.2DS has a 50% chance of passing it on to a child of either sex. An affected parent should be counseled about this risk.

IMMUNOLOGIC MANIFESTATIONS AND MANAGEMENT

22q11.2DS is characterized in part by thymic abnormalities and immunodeficiencies. The thymus may be congenitally absent or may have been surgically removed during repair of a heart defect, but even patients with an intact thymus can manifest immunodeficiency. Typically, the impact is mild, resulting in reduced T-cell numbers and low immunoglobulin (Ig) IgA and IgM. The most significant deficiencies improve by 2 years of age in most patients, although older children may continue to have low IgA and IgM and can manifest other immunodeficiencies. There is some genotype:phenotype correlation. Patients with the most common deletions, those involving the genome segment between LCRA and LCRB and resulting in deletion of one copy of the *TBX1* gene, had significantly lower CD3 and CD4 T-lymphocyte counts than those with the nested or distal deletions (see Figure 1).[4]

Initial Evaluation

Positive NBS for SCID should prompt evaluation for 22q11.2DS by chromosome microarray in addition to other appropriate follow-up testing relevant to the abnormal screen.[11] Once a diagnosis of 22q11.2DS is confirmed in a neonate or infant, all persons caring for the patient should presume the presence of an immunodeficiency until full evaluation can be completed. This presumption means minimizing infectious exposures, administering influenza vaccinations and respiratory syncytial virus prophylaxis, withholding all live-virus vaccines, and using cytomegalovirus-negative irradiated blood products.[12] A second treatment with respiratory syncytial virus prophylaxis should be considered in older children age 8 through 19 months based on existing AAP guidance.[13]

Complete blood cell (CBC) count with differential should be performed at the time of diagnosis. Low absolute lymphocyte count should prompt evaluation of T-lymphocyte and B-lymphocyte subsets and referral to immunology as appropriate. More detailed immunologic evaluation, if indicated, should include flow cytometry, measurement of tetanus and antibodies to gauge presence and strength of seroconversion, and assessment of T-lymphocyte function.[1,14]

Recurrent Infections

T-lymphocyte immunodeficiency does not appear to translate into increased parasitic infection, and most pediatric patients do not require directed management of an immunodeficiency. However, antibody dysfunctions can impair responsiveness to bacterial and viral infections.[15] Patients of all ages who have 22q11.2DS have multiple anatomic and physiologic predispositions to upper and lower respiratory tract infections. There is a propensity for recurrent or persistent otitis media, sinusitis, and pneumonia. The infectious agents are most likely those common in the population and local community; standard management regimens should be used. For patients in whom the infections are severe, are impacting other functions such as weight gain, or that may complicate (or be complicated by) structural anomalies, referral to immunology may be warranted. More aggressive management of persistent or recurrent infections can include prophylactic antibiotics, intravenous immunoglobulin therapy, or thymic transplantation.[4]

Vaccine Considerations

As with any potentially immunocompromised individual, infants identified to have lymphocyte abnormalities should not be given live-virus vaccines without further immunology evaluation. If immunologic abnormalities were found in infancy and there have been no clinical concerns, repeat immunologic evaluation consisting of flow cytometry, measurement of tetanus IgG, and assessment of T-lymphocyte function should be performed prior to administration of live-virus vaccines.[1,10] For measles, mumps, rubella, and varicella vaccinations, assessment parameters have been suggested: 1) CD4 $\geq$ 400 cells/mm^3; 2) CD8 $\geq$ 200 cells/mm^3; 3) tetanus IgG protective 3+ weeks after the third dose; and 4) $CD45RA^+CD3^+/4^+\% > CD45RO^+CD3^+/4^+\%$. A patient meeting all 4 criteria may be considered for live-virus vaccination.[10]

Non-live ("killed" or inactivated) vaccines and influenza vaccination are recommended and should be administered. Infantile COVID-19 vaccination should be administered as recommended by the Centers for Disease Control and Prevention on the schedule appropriate for an immunocompromised or immunocompetent individual.[16] Other vaccine types should be administered on the AAP-recommended schedule.[17]

Autoimmune Disease

Autoimmune diseases, particularly juvenile idiopathic arthritis, are as much as twenty times more common in the 22q11.2DS population than in the general population. The incidence of idiopathic thrombocytopenic purpura is 200 times more common in patients with 22q11.2DS.[12] Patients with autoimmune disorders can have persistent T-cell lymphopenia and IgA deficiency. Other autoimmune conditions associated with 22q11.2DS are Graves disease (hyperthyroidism), hypothyroidism, vitiligo, hemolytic anemia, autoimmune neutropenia, aplastic anemia, and celiac disease.[12]

Summary and Recommendations About Immunologic Manifestations

- Recognize that a positive NBS for SCID includes other conditions of T-cell lymphopenia and may indicate a diagnosis of 22q11.2DS.
- Once a diagnosis of 22q11.2DS is confirmed, presume that the patient has an immunodeficiency until appropriate evaluation can be completed. Specifically:
    - Minimize infectious exposure
    - Withhold live-virus vaccines
    - Administer influenza and other age-appropriate non-live-virus vaccines
    - Administer respiratory syncytial virus (RSV) prophylaxis
    - Use cytomegalovirus (CMV)-negative, irradiated blood products if transfusion is necessary
- At the time of diagnosis of 22q11.2DS, order CBC to check for absolute lymphocyte count.
- Refer to immunology for further evaluation and management.
- Recognize that patients with 22q11.2DS have anatomic and functional deficiencies that predispose to infection, even in the absence of an immunodeficiency.
- Treatment of community-acquired infections should be treated with standard medications and protocols.
- Be aware that patients with 22q11.2DS have an increased risk of autoimmune disorders, particularly juvenile idiopathic arthritis and idiopathic thrombocytopenic purpura.

CARDIOVASCULAR MANIFESTATIONS AND MANAGEMENT

22q11.2DS is the second most common genetic cause of congenital heart disease (CHD) with neurocognitive impairments after Down syndrome/trisomy 21.[3] Conversely, patients with 22q11.2DS represent a large proportion of neonates with CHD.[18,19] Before addition of SCID to newborn screening, heart malformations were responsible for bringing the largest portion of these children to medical attention. Although it is likely that 60% to 80% of patients with 22q11.2DS have a cardiac malformation, the actual prevalence of CHD in the 22q11.2DS is not known and estimates vary with the age of diagnosis.[14] Approximately 70% to 80% of neonates and infants presenting with 22q11.2DS have significant cardiac defects. This proportion decreases to 30% in children older than 2 years at the time of syndrome diagnosis.[5,14]

Conotruncal Heart Defects

Conotruncal heart defects, affecting the great arteries and outflow tract of the heart, are the most common congenital cardiac malformations in 22q11.2DS and represent the main cause of mortality in children with 22q11.2DS.[3,20] Interrupted aortic arch type B (IAA-B) is almost exclusively associated with 22q11.2DS, and it should be considered the underlying diagnosis of this malformation until proven otherwise. IAA-B is a division of the aorta between the left common carotid artery and the left subclavian artery. Other conotruncal defects common in 22q11.2DS are tetralogy of Fallot, truncus arteriosus, atrioventricular canal, and transposition of the great arteries.[3,5,14,21]

A wide variety of aortic arch anomalies can be present: cervical aortic arch, double aortic arch with or without a vascular ring, right-sided aortic arch, and abnormal origin of the subclavian arteries, including both aberrant and isolated subclavian arteries.[13,14,22] The pulmonary arteries can be discontinuous, hypoplastic, or stenotic, and there can be major aortopulmonary collaterals.[3,12,13,15] The semilunar valves can be bicuspid, severely dysplastic, insufficient, or stenotic.[18] Despite the known association between 22q11.2DS and conotruncal anomalies, it should be recognized that any heart defect is possible and 22q11.2DS should be considered regardless of the type of cardiac malformation if there are other concerning features.

Cardiac Management

Management of associated congenital heart malformations follows standard approaches to diagnosis and repair, although associated anomalies can complicate the anatomy and surgical treatment.[3,17] Surgical timing and technique are dependent, as with all patients, on the cardiac phenotype and are tailored to the needs of the patient. Ductal-dependent lesions are typically corrected in the first few days of life.[17] In cases with hypoplastic or absent pulmonary arteries, a palliative repair may be required, followed by definitive surgical repair at a later time.[17]

In general, cardiac patients with 22q11.2DS do not experience higher mortality after surgical intervention compared with patients without the diagnosis who have similar cardiac anomalies. Patients with 22q11.2DS, however, may experience more perioperative management difficulties with a more complicated postoperative course.[3,14,16,17] Depending on the patient, factors contributing to surgical and perioperative management complexities may include depressed immune function, pulmonary vascular reactivity, hypocalcemia, bronchomalacia and bronchospasm, presence of a laryngeal web, and a tendency to airway bleeding.[17] Calcium concentrations should be monitored and supplemented as needed. Immune deficiency is not always clearly defined before surgery, and some compromise of the immune system should be presumed with consideration of antibiotic prophylaxis and CMV-negative, irradiated blood products.[1,17,23]

Lifetime surveillance for cardiac sequelae is indicated for patients with major CHD who have undergone repair. Patients with 22q11.2DS who have cardiac anomalies are at increased risk well into adulthood for residual valve lesions and outflow tract obstruction, ventricular dysfunction, arrhythmias, heart failure, aortic root dilatation, and bacterial endocarditis.[3,24–26] Pediatricians should evaluate cardiac status, including trustworthy measurements of blood pressure, at every visit.

Because of the common association between 22q11.2DS and congenital heart disease, it is recommended that chromosome microarray be sent in a patient of any age (including in utero) in the presence of IAA-B, tetralogy of Fallot, truncus arteriosus, or conoventricular septal defect, as well as those with an isolated aortic arch anomaly.[27] In older infants and children in whom 22q11.2DS is diagnosed because of noncardiac manifestations, cardiac evaluation is recommended to identify those with noncyanotic lesions and isolated aortic arch anomalies such as vascular rings.[5]

Summary of Cardiovascular Manifestations

- 22q11.2DS diagnostic testing should be performed on patients of any age who have interrupted aortic arch type B (IAA-B), truncus arteriosus, tetralogy of Fallot, ventricular septal defect with aortic arch anomaly, isolated aortic arch anomaly, or any congenital heart malformation with additional features of 22q11.2DS.
- Neonates with known or suspected 22q11.2DS should have an immediate cardiac evaluation including an echocardiogram.
- Infants and older children in whom 22q11.2 deletion is diagnosed on the basis of noncardiac signs and symptoms should have a cardiac evaluation.
- Patients with 22q11.2DS undergoing cardiac surgery should be presumed to have a compromised immune system, whether formally diagnosed or not. Management should include:
  - Antibiotic prophylaxis
  - CMV-negative, irradiated blood products
- Perioperative hypocalcemia is a risk in all patients regardless of whether or not there is a history of hypocalcemia. Pre- and postoperative calcium concentrations should be monitored during hospitalization with supplementation as necessary.
- Lifetime cardiac surveillance, including trustworthy measurement of blood pressure, is indicated at all primary care visits for patients who have undergone surgery because of the risk of residual complications.

ENDOCRINOLOGIC MANIFESTATIONS AND MANAGEMENT

Hypocalcemia and Hypoparathyroidism

Hypocalcemia attributable to hypoparathyroidism is one of the cardinal features of 22q11.2DS, as described by Angelo DiGeorge in 1965.[28] Hypoparathyroidism and hypocalcemia are present in 17% to 60% of persons with 22q11.2DS, most typically in the neonatal period.[4] These problems are frequently transient in children but can become more significant in adults. Overall lifetime prevalence of hypocalcemia has been reported in up to 80.4% of individuals with 22q11.2DS.[23,29,30] Hypocalcemia results from aplasia or hypoplasia of the parathyroid glands.[31]

Hypocalcemia and hypoparathyroidism can vary in severity and presentation. Hypoparathyroidism may be transient at times of physiologic stress if there is a sufficient supply of parathyroid hormone (PTH) at baseline, but not at a level adequate for times of increased metabolic needs, such as surgery or febrile illness. Transient hypoparathyroidism may persist lifelong and may be found in patients of all ages; therefore, routine screening of both total calcium and PTH is important (Table 1).[22]

Parents and patients should be educated about symptoms of hypocalcemia, and calcium concentrations should be monitored at least as frequently as indicated in Table 1. Those with cardiac conditions or acute illnesses should be tested more often as necessary.[32] Hypocalcemia can present as new-onset seizures, fatigue, emotional irritability, paresthesia, muscle cramps, jitteriness, tremors, rigidity, and/or prolonged QT interval.

Diagnosis of hypocalcemia, or presence of any of the concerning symptoms, should be further investigated with workup including serum calcium, albumin, phosphate, magnesium, PTH, vitamin D (25-OH-D), and urine calcium/creatinine. Hypoparathyroidism manifests as low calcium, with an elevated phosphate and inappropriately low PTH. It is important to evaluate 25-OH-D concentration, because this may be abnormal even without hypoparathyroidism. It is recommended that calcium concentrations be checked every 3 to 6 months during the first year of life, then annually thereafter into adulthood. Calcium concentrations should be evaluated preoperatively, postoperatively, and during severe illness because of the risk of transient hypoparathyroidism during times of increased metabolic needs.[1]

Symptomatic hypocalcemia and hypocalcemic seizures often are initially treated with parenteral calcium along with oral calcitriol and calcium supplementation. Parenteral calcium should be infused slowly per current guidelines to avoid cardiac dysfunction and extravasation

TABLE 1. Summary of 22q11.2 Deletion Syndrome-Specific Health Supervision Guidance

	At Diagnosis Any Age	Before Live-Virus Vaccine	Infancy (0–12 mo)	Early Childhood (1–5 y)	Late Childhood (6–11 y)	Adolescence (12–18 y)	Adult (>18 y)	Comment
All Patients								
Laboratory Testing								
Chromosome microarray	X		X					
Total calcium	X		Every 3–6 mo	Annually	Annually	Annually	Annually	1) If calcium reading is low, repeat and evaluate further with PTH, phosphorous, magnesium, albumin, creatinine, vitamin D (25-OH-D), and urine calcium/creatinine. If total calcium is low and ionized calcium normal, check albumin to determine corrected calcium. 2) Check calcium and PTH pre- and post-operatively. 3) If the patient is on calcium/calcitriol supplementation, check calcium and spot urine calcium/creatinine ratio every 3–4 mo regardless of calcium concentration.
Parathyroid hormone (PTH)	X		X	Annually	Annually	Annually	Annually	Other testing as needed if calcium is low.
Thyroid-stimulating hormone (TSH)& free T4	X		X	Annually	Annually	Annually	Annually	Check if growth velocity decreases.
CBC with differential	X		X	Annually	Annually	Annually	Annually	
Flow cytometry (lymphocyte phenotype)		X	X					Decreased absolute lymphocyte count necessitates referral to immunology. Irradiated blood products until immune function is confirmed or normalized. Evaluate immunity before live-virus vaccines.
T-cell function		X	X					
Tetanus and HiB immune globulins		X	X					
Referrals/Diagnostic Evaluations								
Cardiology (echocardiogram, EKG)	X		X					Follow-up as indicated by cardiology.
Genetics	X		X			For mature patient, counseling as needed.	For adult patient, counseling as needed	Counsel about diagnosis. Test other family members as indicated.
Audiology/hearing test	X		X	X	X	prn	prn	
Renal ultrasound	X		X					
Palatal competency evaluation	X		X (feeding, nasal regurgitation)	X (voice/speech quality)	X (voice/speech quality)	X (voice/speech quality)	X (voice/ speech quality)	
Developmental assessment/ therapy	X		X	X	School performance	School performance		Speech/language and motor assessment before age 1 y with appropriate and rapid referrals for therapy.
Ophthalmology			As needed	Refraction by 3 y	As needed	As needed		

(Continued on next page)

TABLE 1. Summary of 22q11.2 Deletion Syndrome-Specific Health Supervision Guidance (Continued)

	At Diagnosis Any Age	Before Live-Virus Vaccine	Infancy (0–12 mo)	Early Childhood (1–5 y)	Late Childhood (6–11 y)	Adolescence (12–18 y)	Adult (>18 y)	Comment
Spinal x-rays			Evaluate for vertebral anomalies	6-view cervical spine films after age 4		Evaluate for scoliosis if indicated by clinical examination		Anterior/posterior, lateral, extension, open mouth, and skull base films done after ossification about age 4 y and/or prior to any procedure requiring intubation or neck hyperextension and/or contact sports or gymnastics.
Ongoing								
Growth assessment			Growth velocity and weight:length	Growth velocity and weight: length	Growth velocity and weight: length	Growth velocity and weight: length		Use 22q11.2 deletion-specific growth charts. Slowing of linear growth should include endocrinologic evaluation.
Feeding assessment			X	As needed	As needed	As needed	As needed	
Dental				Semiannual	Semiannual	Semiannual	Semiannual	Evaluate for and treat enamel hypoplasia and caries.
Psychiatry/psychology				Evaluate changes in behavior, emotional state, and thinking	Evaluate changes in behavior, emotional state, and thinking	Additionally assess risky/ addictive behaviors	Additionally assess risky/ addictive behaviors	
Additional Referrals as Needed								
Gynecologic services						X	X	Menstrual cycle management and contraceptives: Note that female genitourinary malformations are a recognized component of 22q11.2 deletion syndrome. Delayed menses in the presence of otherwise normal puberty should be investigated for anatomic abnormalities (as well as pregnancy).
Hematology			Indication: Easy bleeding or bruising					
Nephrology			Indication: Primary or secondary abnormal renal function or renal-based hypertension					
Neurology			Indication: Seizures or symptoms of cord compression					
Rheumatology			Indication: Symptoms of arthritis (limb pain, stiffness, swelling) or suspicion of other autoimmune disease					

leading to necrosis. Asymptomatic or chronic hypocalcemia is treated with oral calcitriol and calcium supplementation. Hypomagnesemia may also contribute to the problem; thus, magnesium supplementation is indicated for those with hypomagnesemia.[25]

Vitamin D supplementation and a calcium-rich diet based on recommended daily intake for age should be emphasized from infancy to adulthood. For those with transient or persistent hypoparathyroidism, maintenance therapy is 1,25-dihydroxyvitamin D (calcitriol), with or without calcium supplementation, based on standard replacement for those with hypoparathyroidism.[27] The goal of treatment is to maintain a low-normal calcium concentration since calcium supplementation can lead to high urinary losses of calcium and renal calculi formation. In patients requiring supplementation, it is important to monitor for hypercalciuria with spot urinary calcium and calcium/creatinine ratio when measuring blood calcium every 3 to 4 months and to consider intermittent renal ultrasonography.[1] For patients with structural renal anomalies, such as renal agenesis or dysplastic kidney, lower calcium doses may be needed. Referral to a pediatric endocrinologist and/or pediatric nephrologist should be arranged at the time of diagnosis if there is any concern about hypo- or hypercalcemia and for subsequent management.[27]

Osteopenia/Osteoporosis

Hypocalcemia and other comorbidities may predispose to osteopenia and/or osteoporosis.[25] Vitamin D and a calcium-rich diet based on recommended daily intake for age, along with physical activity, should be stressed for bone health.

Thyroid

Children and adults with 22q11.2DS have thyroid abnormalities that can present at any age. It has been reported that up to 20% may have hypothyroidism and 5% may have hyperthyroidism.[1] There are reported cases of congenital hypothyroidism, autoimmune hypothyroidism (Hashimoto disease) and hyperthyroidism (Graves disease). Management is standard thyroid replacement or antithyroid therapy as indicated.[27] Baseline screening with thyroxine (T4) and thyroid stimulating hormone (TSH) should be performed in all patients, and there should be annual screening via TSH.[1]

Summary and Recommendations About Endocrinologic Manifestations

- Any symptomatic presentation of hypocalcemia should prompt an urgent evaluation for hypoparathyroidism including measurements of total calcium, ionized calcium, PTH, phosphate, 25-OH-D, and magnesium.
- Check total calcium concentrations every 3 to 6 months during infancy, then every 1 to 2 years thereafter.
- Check total calcium concentrations preoperatively, postoperatively, and during severe illness.
- Symptomatic hypocalcemia is managed acutely via intravenous infusion of calcium along with standard oral replacement of calcium and calcitriol.
- Long-term management of hypocalcemia has the goal of maintaining a low-normal calcium concentration to avoid complications of hypercalciuria.
- For patients receiving calcium supplementation, check spot urinary calcium and calcium/creatinine ratio when measuring blood calcium.
- Obtain baseline renal ultrasonogram and consider intermittent renal ultrasonography if receiving calcium supplementation.
- Perform annual screening for thyroid abnormalities with treatment as indicated.
- Using 22q11.2DS-specific growth charts, monitor weight and growth velocity closely during infancy and then weight, height, and BMI annually. (See Growth section below.)

CRANIOFACIAL MANIFESTATIONS AND MANAGEMENT

Palatal Abnormalities

22q11.2DS is the most common cause of syndromic palatal anomalies. Conversely, palate problems occur in two thirds to three quarters of patients with 22q11.2DS.[3,4,19,33] Palatal abnormalities may be structural, such as a frank or submucous cleft palate or velopharyngeal disproportion (short palate), a functional problem such as hypotonia of the velopharyngeal musculature, or a combination.[26,34,35] Orofacial clefts are typically addressed in early childhood using treatments that are, in general, the same as for any child with clefts. Referral should be made to otolaryngology, craniofacial plastic surgery, and/or oral maxillofacial surgery with expertise in surgical correction of palatal defects. Repair can improve feeding and speech and reduce incidence of otitis and sinusitis.[3]

The most common palatal abnormality is muscle weakness of the palate or velum, either alone or in combination with a submucosal cleft, resulting in velopharyngeal insufficiency (VPI).[19] In infancy, this can manifest as persistent/recurrent nasal regurgitation of formula. With development of verbal language, weakness of the velopharyngeal muscles leads to hypernasal speech from abnormal nasal resonance and nasal emissions (air escaping through the nasal passage with speech). Other communication problems common in 22q11.2DS include speech/language delay and related disorders, and these continue into the school-aged years in at least half of patients.[36] Children with 22q11.2DS should be referred to speech pathology for evaluation and therapy. This evaluation will help differentiate those who have structural abnormalities requiring surgical intervention.[37]

By 4 to 6 years of age, the patient typically has sufficient speech development to allow for an individualized surgical management plan.[19,38] The goals of VPI surgery are to normalize or at least mitigate hypernasality, nasal emission, and pressure-associated deficits in consonant production.[39] Patients who have already had a speech evaluation should have structural abnormalities evaluated by video nasopharyngeal endoscopy or multiview videofluoroscopy. Patients should be referred to otolaryngology or craniofacial plastic surgery for these evaluations.[19,33,40]

Therapy and surgery for VPI in patients with 22q11.DS are similar to those in persons with nonsyndromic cleft palate and VPI; however, it is often more difficult to treat with worse surgical outcomes, higher revision rates, and inferior postoperative speech outcomes.[19,41–44] Mechanical improvement does not necessarily correspond to an improvement in speech or in language use[38]: only a third of patients achieve normal speech after surgery. Other congenital and acquired anatomic abnormalities can impact speech and language development.[1,45]

Obstructive Sleep Apnea

Obstructive sleep apnea (OSA) can occur for a variety of reasons, including but not limited to congenital malformations of the upper respiratory tract, laryngomalacia, hypotonia, and recurrent infection. Management of (OSA can be problematic. Addressing OSA by removal of the tonsils and/or adenoids may increase rather than decrease the air leak through the nasopharynx, thus making speech worse.[1,46] Persistent problems despite speech therapy and surgical intervention should prompt more detailed workup and appropriate referral or re-referral to otolaryngology or craniofacial plastic surgery.

Chronic/Secretory Otitis Media

Structural abnormalities of the ears can be present ranging from various minor anomalies of the external ear to true microtia and anotia. Auricular anomalies are common and patients with 22q11.2DS have high rates of otitis media and chronic sinusitis attributable to underlying immune deficiencies, recurrent upper respiratory tract infections, and palatal abnormalities resulting in eustachian tube dysfunction.[38,47] The need for myringotomy tubes is considered likely in most patients. Nasopharyngeal reflux can contribute to persistent otorrhea with myringotomy tubes in place as well as acute and chronic sinusitis in older children and adolescents.[19,48]

Hearing Loss

Hearing loss of any type—conductive, sensorineural, or mixed—occurs in approximately two thirds of patients with 22q11.2DS.[43] Conductive loss is the most common of these, often associated with palatal anomalies and recurrent otitis media.[49] Sensorineural hearing loss and mixed hearing loss may be secondary to cochlear dysplasia. Ossicular chain damage has also been reported.[45,50] Management of hearing loss should be tailored to the needs of the patient using standard modalities.

Summary and Recommendations About Craniofacial Manifestations

- Assess for nasal regurgitation at diagnosis and through infancy (0–1 year) and for hypernasal speech and speech quality during early childhood (1–5 years). Abnormality should prompt referral to otolaryngology or craniofacial plastic surgery.
- Cleft palate cases require evaluation and management by a cleft palate/craniofacial team.
- Formal audiology assessment at diagnosis, infancy (0–1 year), preschool (0–5 years), late childhood (6–11 years), and then as needed in adolescence and adulthood. Brain stem evoked response should be performed on children of any age who cannot perform behavioral hearing tests. Note that newborn hearing screening, unless performed as a full, sedated auditory brainstem response, is insufficient.
- Patients with hearing loss should be assessed for hearing aid needs and referred for services through early intervention, the school district, or private providers.
- Speech-language evaluation should be performed at diagnosis or at the first sign of delay or disorder, with referral to ongoing therapy as indicated.
- Head and neck anatomy should be thoroughly evaluated prior to surgical interventions.

GASTROINTESTINAL PROBLEMS AND GROWTH CONCERNS

Gastrointestinal Problems

Gastrointestinal problems have been reported in 58% to 65% of patients.[26,51] The common features are dysphagia, abdominal pain, gastroesophageal reflux and esophageal dysmotility, and chronic constipation.

Dysphagia is present in around 30% of patients. Dysphagia can be presaged by the presence of polyhydramnios during the affected pregnancy. As many as 14% of fetuses have gastrointestinal ultrasonographic findings, including suggestions of tracheoesophageal fistula.[52] On the basis of modified barium swallow studies, pharyngoesophageal dysmotility is a major contributor to dysphagia. Therefore, it is important to evaluate the feeding status and, if there are concerns, refer for studies such as modified barium swallow.[53] Dysphagia often precipitates enteral feeding with nasogastric and/or gastronomy tube placement (5%–16%). Of patients who transition to complete oral feeding regimens, 95% do so by 4.5 years of age.[26] In patients with 22q11.2DS who have persistent choking during feeding, recurrent pulmonary infections or respiratory distress, or reactive airway disease, aspiration should be considered as a potential etiology.[26] Feeding difficulties may also occur as a result of a vascular ring or congenital diaphragmatic hernia.[26]

Chronic constipation affects 35% of patients. Celiac disease is more common than in the general population. Structural bowel anomalies including intestinal malrotation, Hirschsprung disease, and imperforate anus are more common compared with the general population.[26] Cholelithiasis has been reported in 19.2% of a cohort of adults with 22q11.2DS, among whom 12.8% required cholecystectomy by a median age of 27.5 years.[54]

Growth and Obesity

Short stature and poor weight gain are a common finding during infancy in patients with 22q11.2DS, especially in those with congenital cardiac conditions, feeding difficulties, recurrent infections, and structural bowel anomalies.[55] Growth restriction during infancy is *not* typically attributable to growth hormone deficiency, although it can occur. It is important to identify and treat thyroid disease, because this can impact linear growth. Final adult height is reported in the low-normal range of mid-parental height. Therefore, the pediatrician should monitor prepubertal and pubertal growth velocity along with onset of puberty on the appropriate growth charts.[51,56] Growth charts specific to 22q11.2DS from birth to age 20 years have been published[57] and are available online at no cost (https://doi.org/10.1002/ajmg.a.35485).

Conversely, obesity has been reported in up to 35% of adults with 22q11.2DS. Because the onset is often during childhood, it is necessary to recognize risk factors. Patients with 22q11.2DS are genetically predisposed to short stature. There is also an emphasis on weight gain during infancy, with less attention to linear growth, which may later be a risk factor for obesity. It is important to monitor weight verses length/height and to emphasize healthy lifestyle with diet and exercise.[1] In some patients, medically managed weight loss, pharmaceutical treatment, or surgery may be considered.[58]

Summary and Recommendations About Gastrointestinal Problems and Growth Concerns

- Carefully evaluate feeding status of infants, and consider further evaluation for dysphagia with modified barium swallow and/or other studies.
- Patients with persistent choking during feeding, recurrent pulmonary infections or respiratory distress, or reactive airway disease should be evaluated for aspiration.
- Dysphagia, chronic constipation, and gastroesophageal reflux are not uncommon.
- Using 22q11.2DS-specific growth charts, monitor weight, height, weight-for-height, and growth velocity closely during infancy, childhood, and through puberty.
- Adjust caloric intake for best weight-for-height. Do not use weight alone as a measure of growth, as individuals with 22q11.2DS are predisposed to short stature.

NEURODEVELOPMENTAL MANIFESTATIONS AND MANAGEMENT

All persons with 22q11.2DS have some degree of neurologic impairment, although the spectrum is broad and impairments may be limited to manageable learning problems. In infancy, this can manifest either as seizures or as generalized hypotonia. The hypotonia, in turn, can impact multiple aspects of development including feeding, speech, and attainment of motor milestones.

Seizures

Seizures in a neonate are most often provoked seizures attributable to hypocalcemia and will respond to appropriate electrolyte management. Hypocalcemic seizures can happen at any age, even in patients without a history of either calcium abnormalities or seizures. Thus, evaluation of calcium concentration should be a part of the immediate investigation in any patient with 22q11.2DS presenting with seizures.

An early study of seizures in patients with 22q11.2DS showed that 7% of the studied population had apparently unprovoked seizures, with more than expected meeting criteria for a diagnosis of generalized epilepsy.[59] The type of seizure and precipitating events are generally consistent with those seen in the general population from the most severe generalized tonic-clonic seizures to absence or focal impaired awareness seizures. Seizures can manifest as confusion, memory loss, or recurrent or fixed hallucinations, and in patients with baseline neurocognitive impairments, the fact that they are seizures may be missed.[22] Pediatricians should include seizure evaluation or referral to neurology for any patient with 22q11.2DS who has an acute change in neurologic function, even in the absence of clinically recognizable seizures.

Brain malformations such as cortical dysplasia, polymicrogyria, and periventricular heterotopia can increase the risk of seizure development. Functional magnetic resonance imaging (MRI) has shown reduction in brain volumes with white matter loss.[4] Patients with new-onset seizures not related to hypocalcemia should have MRI and electroencephalography (EEG) performed to evaluate seizure type and possible etiology. Studies to date indicate that routine anticonvulsant therapy is useful in treatment.[22]

Developmental Delay and Intellectual Disability

Children with 22q11.2DS have delays that can impact any or all areas of development.[6] The mean age of walking is 18 months. Fine motor delays are present. Depending on the published study, mean developmental indices and IQ tend to fall in the range of 60 to 80. One study of preschoolers' language development using Wechsler preschool and Primary Scale of Intelligence (WPPSI-R) showed that measured full-scale IQ was 78 ± 12. IQ was 78 ± 12 for performance and 81 ± 13 for verbal. In the language category specifically, 20% fell in the average range while 46% and 34% were mildly and significantly delayed, respectively.[4] As mentioned in other sections, speech and language delay or disorder can be a function of orofacial anatomy, hearing loss, neurocognitive impairments, or any combination thereof. The delays involve both expressive and receptive language, with the former generally being more impacted.

This distribution of neurocognitive function as measured by IQ—about one third each in the average, mildly impaired, and significantly impaired ranges—has been shown in studies of school-aged and older patients. There are, however, areas of relative strength. Patients with 22q11.2DS tend to be better at concrete tasks such as rote learning, reading decoding, and spelling. Deficits in executive function are common in patients with 22q11.2DS. These deficits can be negatively impacted by psychosis.[60] Patients with 22q11.2DS have more problems in the abstract areas of memory, such as verbal, working, and visual-spatial; mathematics; and nonverbal processing.[4] Identifying these patterns allows developmental therapies to be more adequately targeted to the needs of the patients. Clinicians should refer for appropriate developmental assessments. These assessments can be performed by individual therapists or specialists in neurodevelopmental testing.

As with trisomy 21/Down syndrome, there is limited correlation between degree of physical involvement and the impact on neurocognitive development. Patients with severe congenital heart malformations requiring surgery in the neonatal period and those with significant brain malformations are at higher risk of neurologic impairments than patients without these malformations. There is otherwise no basis for predicting a particular patient's neurocognitive prognosis.

Mental Health

Psychiatric conditions are commonly seen in individuals with 22q11.2DS. In addition, many children and teenagers have behavioral difficulties and problems with social skills and risk being victims of bullying.[61] Anxiety and attention-deficit/hyperactivity disorder (ADHD) each occur in about a third of patients, with codiagnosis in some. Anxiety can decrease concentration and potentially be misdiagnosed as ADHD. Autism spectrum disorder (ASD) is seen; however, there is significant overlap with other psychiatric diagnoses. For example, repetitive questions and restrictive behaviors are commonly seen in patients with 22q11.2DS,[62] and these might be considered manifestations of ASD when that may not be an accurate diagnosis for the patient. Clinicians should consider a broad differential. Clinicians are encouraged to use standardized assessment tools and multiple modalities (eg, parent interview and direct observation) when assessing patients with concern for ASD. The AAP provides an overview of diagnostic options and testing instruments useful in evaluation of ASD.[63]

Other common psychiatric conditions include depressive disorders, which can be diagnosed across the lifespan from childhood (2%) to adulthood (16%). Bipolar disorder is much less common, in the range of 4% in adulthood. Childhood-onset psychosis, including childhood schizophrenia, is less common than in adults with 22q11.2DS but more common than in the general population (2%).[64] The risk increases in adolescents and young adults to 25% to 30%.[50] During adolescence and early adulthood, clinicians should screen for symptoms of hallucinations and delusions at all primary care visits. Early intervention for psychosis is associated with improved outcomes.[65]

Patients with 22q11.2DS typically respond to standard treatments such as cognitive behavioral therapy, applied behavior analysis (ABA) therapy for individuals with ASD, and medication regimens as one would use in the general population.

Summary and Recommendations About Neurodevelopmental Manifestations

- Total and ionized calcium concentrations should be checked and treatment initiated as indicated in any patient with 22q11.2DS who has new-onset seizures. This testing should be performed regardless of age and history of calcium status.
- Patients with acute or short-term changes in awareness or other cognitive function should be evaluated for seizures.
- Otherwise standard evaluation with brain MRI and EEG is indicated in patients with seizures. Treatment with standard antiseizure medicines and antiepileptic protocols is useful in treatment of seizures not related to hypocalcemia.
- Hypotonia is an almost universal finding and impacts multiple areas of development.
- In general, persons with 22q11.2DS are more functional in areas of concrete thinking and receptive language than in abstract thinking and expressive language. Neuropsychiatric or educational testing can identify a patient's specific areas of strength and weakness to allow for tailoring of therapies.
- Anxiety occurs in about a third (36%) of children with 22q11.2DS. Anxiety should be managed with standard medications or other therapies.
- ASD is more common than in the general population, but some features of generalized neurocognitive impairment can be overinterpreted as ASD, so specialized evaluation is recommended.

- Screen for symptoms of hallucinations and delusions at all primary care visits. Any report of hallucinations should be investigated.

MEDICAL HOME

Patients with 22q11DS require a medical home[66] prepared to manage patients with the potential for multiple medical concerns and a wide degree of severity. Each patient should have appropriate ongoing management individualized to their comorbidities, with ongoing guideline management recommendations. As a general concept, this is no different from any other child; however, the medical home must be sufficiently trained to recognize, address, and manage the potential complexities of patients with 22q11.2DS. The medical home is the model for providing high-quality, comprehensive primary care usually implemented by a primary care provider. Other providers such as complex care clinics, geneticists, or 22q centers may serve as the medical home if they provide, in addition to specialty care, comprehensive primary care.

Summary and Recommendations for a Medical Home

- Perform surveillance for medical conditions common in patients with 22q11.2DS including routine laboratory and imaging studies.
- Management of vaccinations with attention to possible need to delay live-virus vaccines.
- Referral to and coordination of appropriate specialty care for the patient either as individual specialists or a multidisciplinary 22q clinic.
- Monitor developmental milestones with rapid referral for developmental assessment and appropriate therapies and/or special education services.
- Psychoeducational testing every 2 to 3 years for patients with learning disabilities or intellectual disability until at least age 22.
- Screening for psychiatric conditions such as anxiety, ADHD, depression, and psychosis during well-child examinations, with a low threshold for therapy or psychiatry referral.

TRANSITION TO ADULTHOOD

It is recommended that youth with 22q11.2DS and their parent(s) or guardian(s) have ongoing discussions regarding 22q11.2DS so they can be knowledgeable of their health care needs and risks. It is also important for clinicians not to neglect risky behaviors and vulnerability during the time of adolescence, including sexuality and sexually transmitted infections. There should be heightened awareness for patients with neurocognitive impairments. Some features of 22q11.2DS can impact pubertal development. Typical pubertal development should be expected, and any deviation from that should be investigated.

All patients with 22q11.2DS should have an understanding of the risk of having a child also affected by 22q11.2DS (50% with each pregnancy) as well as options for family planning to reduce this genetic risk, if desired. Community supports (home, family, support groups) as well as broader organization and social media groups (see Table 2 for support groups and resources) are available.

Pediatricians may continue to provide primary care during early adult years. There should be a plan for transition to adult primary care and specialists to continue the appropriate medical home in adult medicine. Particular attention should be paid to continuation of adult cardiology care in the patients with congenital heart anomalies. Transition to adult providers should happen progressively (rather than all at once) for patients with multiple specialty providers unless there is availability of a targeted adult/internal medicine-based 22q11.2DS clinic. The AAP provides support in considering needs during patient transition to adult medicine.[67] The organization Got Transition also provides guidance.

For patients with intellectual disability, the pediatrician should counsel the parent(s) or legal guardian(s) to consider ongoing guardianship if indicated. The degrees of oversight include full guardianship, medical proxy, financial oversight, group home independent living, and others. Social services can help establish what might be most appropriate for a given family. This plan should be established before the patient's 18th birthday. Discussion should include establishing wills and special needs trusts for the patient as well as identifying an alternate legal guardian. It should be recommended that the parents(s) or guardian(s) apply for Supplemental Security Income (SSI) assistance when the patient with 22q11.2DS reaches age 18 years, if not before, and that they contact Developmental Disability Services and identify relevant vocational training and a supportive environment such as day habilitation and/or independent living programs.

For higher-functioning individuals in secondary education or employment, neuropsychological evaluation can support the family in obtaining appropriate accommodations. The patient and guardian(s) can identify and request disability services in college or at the workplace.

One quarter to one third of adult patients with 22q11.2DS manifest mental health problems, particularly psychosis and schizophrenia.[60] The highest risk of development of psychosis is in adolescence and during the transition to young adulthood. If the patient is not already under psychiatric management, it is recommended that the pediatrician obtain neuropsychological evaluation for the patient at 21 years of age, prior to transition to adult physicians.

TABLE 2. Support Groups and Resources

US Based	Europe Based
International 22q11.2 Deletion Syndrome Foundation, Inc PO Box 2269 Cinnaminson, NJ 08077 Phone: 877-739-1849 (toll free) Email: info@22q.org www.22q.org	*Max Appeal* 15 Meridian Avenue Stourbridge West Midlands DY8 1049 United Kingdom Phone: 0800 389 1049 (toll free) Email: info@maxappeal.org.uk http://www.maxappeal.org.uk
The 22q Family Foundation 725 Clubhouse Drive Aptos, CA 95003 Phone: 831-200-4227 Email: info@22qfamiyfoundation.org 22qfamilyfoundation.org	*European Society for Immunodeficiencies (ESID) Registry* Dr. Gerhard Kindle University Medical Center Freiburg Centre of Chronic Immunodeficiency Engesserstr. 4 79106 Freiburg Germany Phone: 49-761-270-34450 Email: esid-registry@uniklinik-freiburg.de http://ESIISD.org/Working-Parties/Registry-Working-Party
National Library of Medicine Genetics Home Reference 22q11.2 deletion syndrome	
NCBI Genes and Disease DiGeorge syndrome	
Chromosome 22 Central c/o Murney Rinholm 7108 Partinwood Drive Fuquay-Varina, NC 27526 Phone: 919-567-8167 Email: usinfo@c22c.org http://www.c22c.org	
Chromosome Disorder Outreach (CDO) PO Box 724 Boca Raton, FL 33429-0724 Phone: 561-395-4252 (Family Helpline) Email: info@chromodisorder.org http://www.chromodisorder.org	

Summary and Recommendations for Transition to Adulthood

- Patients with 22q11.2DS should be counseled that their risk of having an affected child is 50% with each pregnancy and that the child may not have the same features as the parent. An active plan to transition patients to adult medicine should be made, and this should happen progressively, rather than concurrently, across specialties.
- If the patient is not already under care of psychiatry, a neuropsychological evaluation should be performed prior to transition.
- The parent(s) or guardians(s) should be counseled about establishing ongoing guardianship, which, if necessary, should be established before the patient turns 18 years old.
- The clinician should discuss with the parent(s) or guardians(s) the usefulness of establishing wills and trusts as well as identifying an alternate guardian for the patient.
- The clinician should make the parent(s) or guardians(s) aware of resources through their state health department, SSI, and Developmental Disability Services and that there may be local resources available for additional adult care.

OTHER

Patients with 22q11.2DS have a small but increased risk of other internal malformations that may require monitoring and/or management. There is also the potential that deletion of one allele of an included gene, particularly *TANGO2*, will unmask a recessive condition that requires additional management.

Genitourinary Anomalies

Structural abnormalities of the genitourinary tract occur in a significant minority of patients with 22q11.2DS,[26] and renal ultrasonography is indicated for all patients at the time of diagnosis. The majority of genitourinary anomalies are found in the urinary tract and can include hydronephrosis, multicystic dysplastic kidney, and renal agenesis. (Apparent unilateral renal agenesis at birth can be secondary to earlier involution of a multicystic dysplastic kidney.) Genital anomalies are ascertained more commonly in males, with cryptorchidism and hypospadias each being reported in 4% of the male patient population.[4] Female genital malformations may not be identified until puberty, with persistence of primary amenorrhea or hematometrocolpos.[7]

Strabismus and Refractory Errors

Patients with 22q11.2DS are not at increased risk of strabismus or refractive errors compared with the general population, and these should have standard management. There is a higher incidence of eyelid and globe abnormalities, most of which do not require intervention. Cataract and coloboma have been documented.[4]

Spine Anomalies

Scoliosis is a relatively common feature of 22q11.2DS, but meta-analysis revealed a wide spread of prevalence rates—0.6% to 60%—making it difficult to know whether this exceeds the risk to the unaffected population. Of more concern are cervical spine abnormalities including specifically an open arch of the first cervical vertebra and malformations of the second. One report of flexion-extension radiographs showed increases segmental motion of the cervical vertebrae in 56% of those studied. There has not been a formal recommendation for flexion/extension radiographs in patients with 22q11.2DS[4]; however, these should be performed in early childhood or may be considered prior to procedures requiring intubation or prior to participation in contact sports.

Thrombocytopenia

Within the 22q11.2 locus is the gene *GP1BB*. This gene encodes an integral component of the platelet receptor that binds von Willebrand factor. The normal function is to promote and recruit platelet binding to damaged endothelium.[68] It appears that deletion of one allele of *GP1BB* leads to macrothrombocytopenia and an increased bleeding risk in patients with 22q11.2DS. Thrombocytopenia may be present even in patients who do not have a history of unusual bleeding or bruising.

Loss of function of both *GP1BB* alleles causes Bernard-Soulier syndrome (BSS). This is a lifelong autosomal recessive bleeding disorder that usually presents in neonates. Patients have macrothrombocytopenia and a prolonged bleeding time. In patients with 22q11.2DS who manifest BSS, testing of the remaining allele for pathogenic variant(s) should be performed.[64]

Cancer Predisposition

A variety of blood-based and solid tumor malignancies have been reported in patients with 22q11.2DS. The overall prevalence of all types of cancer is estimated at 6%. There is not a predisposition to a particular type or manifestation of cancer. Leukemias are not related to the presence of macrothrombocytopenia.[64]

Metabolic Encephalopathy and Arrhythmia

A patient with 22q11.2DS manifesting metabolic crisis, arrhythmia, rhabdomyolysis, or seizures (other than hypocalcemic seizures) should be referred for genetics consultation and evaluated for *TANGO2*-related metabolic encephalopathy and arrhythmia. This is an autosomal-recessive condition resulting from deficiency or malfunction of both copies of *TANGO2*. One allele is typically deleted in 22q11.2DS. As long as the opposite allele is functional, there is no consequence. However, if there is loss of function of the remaining allele, the condition will manifest in addition to the standard 22q11.2DS phenotype. More information may be found in the publication by Miyake et al.[69]

LEAD AUTHORS

Angela E. Scheuerle, MD, FAAP
Timothy A. Geleske, MD, FAAP
Nadia Merchant, MD, FAAP
Paula C. Goldenberg, MD, FAAP

However, clinical reports from the American Academy of Pediatrics may not reflect the views of the liaisons or the organizations or government agencies that they represent.

The guidance in this report does not indicate an exclusive course of treatment or serve as a standard of medical care. Variations, taking into account individual circumstances, may be appropriate.

All clinical reports from the American Academy of Pediatrics automatically expire 5 years after publication unless reaffirmed, revised, or retired at or before that time.

FUNDING: No external funding.

https://doi.org/10.1542/peds.2025-072717

REFERENCES

1. Bassett AS, McDonald-McGinn DM, Devriendt K, et al; International 22q11.2 Deletion Syndrome Consortium. Practical guidelines for managing patients with 22q11.2 deletion syndrome. *J Pediatr.* 2011;159(2):332–9.e1. PubMed doi: 10.1016/j.jpeds.2011.02.039
2. Driscoll DA, Budarf ML, Emanuel BS. A genetic etiology for DiGeorge syndrome: consistent deletions and microdeletions of 22q11. *Am J Hum Genet.* 1992;50(5):924–933. PubMed
3. McDonald-McGinn DM, Sullivan KE, Marino B, et al. 22q11.2 deletion syndrome. *Nat Rev Dis Primers.* 2015;1(1):15071. PubMed doi: 10.1038/nrdp.2015.71
4. McDonald-McGinn DM, Hain HS, Emanuel BS, et al. 22q11.2 Deletion syndrome. In: Adam MP, Ardinger HH, Pagon RA, et al, ed. *GeneReviews.* University of Washington; 2020:1993–2021.
5. The Screening, Technology And Research in Genetics (STAR-G) Project. SCID (Severe Combined Immunodeficiency). Accessed May 28, 2025. https://www.newbornscreening.info/scid-severe-combined-immunodeficiency/
6. Cancrini C, Puliafito P, Digilio MC, et al; Italian Network for Primary Immunodeficiencies. Clinical features and follow-up in patients with 22q11.2 deletion syndrome. *J Pediatr.* 2014;164(6):1475–80.e2. PubMed doi: 10.1016/j.jpeds.2014.01.056
7. Swillen A, McDonald-McGinn D. Developmental trajectories in 22q11.2 deletion. *Am J Med Genet C Semin Med Genet.* 2015;169(2):172–181. PubMed doi: 10.1002/ajmg.c.31435
8. Scheuerle A. Teenager with uterine didelphys, absent kidney and 22q11.2 deletion. *Am J Med Genet A.* 2008;146A(6):800–801. PubMed doi: 10.1002/ajmg.a.32224
9. Dar P, Jacobsson B, Clifton R, et al. Cell-free DNA screening for prenatal detection of 22q11.2 deletion syndrome. *Am J Obstet Gynecol.* 2022;227(1)79e1–79e11. PubMed doi: 10.1016/j.ajog.2022.01.002
10. Miller DT, Adam MP, Aradhya S, et al. Consensus statement: chromosomal microarray is a first-tier clinical diagnostic test for individuals with developmental disabilities or congenital anomalies. *Am J Hum Genet.* 2010;86(5):749–764. PubMed doi: 10.1016/j.ajhg.2010.04.006
11. American College of Medical Genetics. Newborn Screening ACT sheet: Severe Combined Immunodeficiency (SCID) and Condition Associated with T Cell Lymphopenia. Accessed December 8, 2023. https://www.acmg.net/PDFLibrary/SCID.pdf
12. Habel A, Herriot R, Kumararatne D, et al. Towards a safety net for management of 22q11.2 deletion syndrome: guidelines for our times. *Eur J Pediatr.* 2014;173(6):757–765. PubMed doi: 10.1007/s00431-013-2240-z
13. American Academy of Pediatrics. AAP Recommendations for the Prevention of RSV Disease in Infants and Children. Red Book Online. Accessed April 22, 2025. https://publications.aap.org/redbook/resources/25379/AAP-Recommendations-for-the-Prevention-of-RSV
14. Mustillo PJ, Sullivan KE, Chinn IK, et al. Clinical practice guidelines for the immunological management of chromosome 22q11.2 deletion syndrome and other defects in thymic development. *J Clin Immunol.* 2023;43(2):247–270. PubMed doi: 10.1007/s10875-022-01418-y
15. Sullivan KE, McDonald-McGinn D, Driscoll DA, Emanuel BS, Zackai EH, Jawad AF. Longitudinal analysis of lymphocyte function and numbers in the first year of life in chromosome 22q11.2 deletion syndrome (DiGeorge syndrome/velocardiofacial syndrome). *Clin Diagn Lab Immunol.* 1999;6(6):906–911. PubMed doi: 10.1128/CDLI.6.6.906-911.1999
16. Centers for Disease Control and Prevention. 2024–2025 COVID-19 Vaccination Guidance for People 6 Months of Age and Older. Accessed May 28, 2025. https://www.cdc.gov/vaccines/covid-19/downloads/covid-19-immunization-schedule-ages-6months-older.pdf
17. American Academy of Pediatrics. Immunization schedules. In: Red Book Online. Accessed December 8, 2023. https://publications.aap.org/redbook/pages/Immunization-Schedules
18. Goldmuntz E. 22q11.2 deletion syndrome and congenital heart disease. *Am J Med Genet C Semin Med Genet.* 2020;184(1):64–72. PubMed doi: 10.1002/ajmg.c.31774
19. Peyvandi S, Lupo PJ, Garbarini J, et al. 22q11.2 deletions in patients with conotruncal defects: data from 1,610 consecutive cases. *Pediatr Cardiol.* 2013;34(7):1687–1694. PubMed doi: 10.1007/s00246-013-0694-4
20. Repetto GM, Guzmán ML, Delgado I, et al. Case fatality rate and associated factors in patients with 22q11 microdeletion syndrome: a retrospective cohort study. *BMJ Open.* 2014;4(11):e005041. PubMed doi: 10.1136/bmjopen-2014-005041

21. Carotti A, Digilio MC, Piacentini G, Saffirio C, Di Donato RM, Marino B. Cardiac defects and results of cardiac surgery in 22q11.2 deletion syndrome. *Dev Disabil Res Rev.* 2008;14(1):35–42. PubMed doi: 10.1002/ddrr.6

22. Marino B, Digilio MC, Toscano A, et al. Anatomic patterns of conotruncal defects associated with deletion 22q11. *Genet Med.* 2001; 3(1):45–48. PubMed doi: 10.1097/00125817-200101000-00010

23. McDonald-McGinn DM, Sullivan KE. Chromosome 22q11.2 deletion syndrome (DiGeorge syndrome/velocardiofacial syndrome). *Medicine (Baltimore).* 2011;90(1):1–18. PubMed doi: 10.1097/MD.0b013e3182060469

24. John AS, McDonald-McGinn DM, Zackai EH, Goldmuntz E. Aortic root dilation in patients with 22q11.2 deletion syndrome. *Am J Med Genet A.* 2009;149A(5):939–942. PubMed doi: 10.1002/ajmg.a.32770

25. Warnes CA, Williams RG, Bashore TM, et al. ACC/AHA 2008 guidelines for the management of adults with congenital heart disease: a report of the American College of Cardiology/American Heart Association Task Force on Practice Guidelines (Writing Committee to Develop Guidelines on the Management of Adults With Congenital Heart Disease). Developed in Collaboration With the American Society of Echocardiography, Heart Rhythm Society, International Society for Adult Congenital Heart Disease, Society for Cardiovascular Angiography and Interventions, and Society of Thoracic Surgeons. *J Am Coll Cardiol.* 2008;52(23): e143–e263. PubMed doi: 10.1016/j.jacc.2008.10.001

26. Fung WL, Butcher NJ, Costain G, et al. Practical guidelines for managing adults with 22q11.2 deletion syndrome. *Genet Med.* 2015;17 (8):599–609. PubMed doi: 10.1038/gim.2014.175

27. Pierpont ME, Brueckner M, Chung WK, et al; American Heart Association Council on Cardiovascular Disease in the Young; Council on Cardiovascular and Stroke Nursing; and Council on Genomic and Precision Medicine. Council on Cardiovascular and Stroke Nursing; and Council on Genomic and Precision Medicine. Genetic basis for congenital heart disease: revisited: a scientific statement from the American Heart Association. *Circulation.* 2018;138(21):e653–e711. PubMed doi: 10.1161/CIR.0000000000000606

28. DiGeorge AM. Discussions on a new concept of the cellular basis of immunity. *J Pediatr.* 1965;67(5):907–908. doi: 10.1016/S0022-3476(65)81796-6

29. Cheung EN, George SR, Costain GA, et al. Prevalence of hypocalcaemia and its associated features in 22q11·2 deletion syndrome. *Clin Endocrinol (Oxf).* 2014;81(2):190–196. PubMed doi: 10.1111/cen.12466

30. Campbell IM, Sheppard SE, Crowley TB, et al. What is new with 22q? An update from the 22q and You Center at the Children's Hospital of Philadelphia. *Am J Med Genet A.* 2018;176(10):2058–2069. PubMed doi: 10.1002/ajmg.a.40637

31. Weinzimer SA. Endocrine aspects of the 22q11.2 deletion syndrome. *Genet Med.* 2001;3(1):19–22. PubMed doi: 10.1097/00125817-200101000-00005

32. Garabédian M. Hypocalcemia and chromosome 22q11 microdeletion. *Genet Couns.* 1999;10(4):389–394. PubMed

33. Jackson O, Crowley TB, Sharkus R, et al. Palatal evaluation and treatment in 22q11.2 deletion syndrome. *Am J Med Genet A.* 2019;179(7):1184–1195. PubMed doi: 10.1002/ajmg.a.61152

34. McDonald-McGinn DM, LaRossa D, Goldmuntz E, et al. The 22q11.2 deletion: screening, diagnostic workup, and outcome of results; report on 181 patients. *Genet Test.* 1997;1(2):99–108. PubMed doi: 10.1089/gte.1997.1.99

35. Rouillon I, Leboulanger N, Roger G, et al. Velopharyngoplasty for noncleft velopharyngeal insufficiency: results in relation to 22q11 microdeletion. *Arch Otolaryngol Head Neck Surg.* 2009;135(7): 652–656. PubMed doi: 10.1001/archoto.2009.64

36. Solot CB, Gerdes M, Kirschner RE, et al. Communication issues in 22q11.2 deletion syndrome: children at risk. *Genet Med.* 2001;3(1): 67–71. PubMed doi: 10.1097/00125817-200101000-00015

37. Naran S, Ford M, Losee JE. What's new in cleft palate and velopharyngeal dysfunction management? *Plast Reconstr Surg.* 2017;139 (6):1343e–1355e. PubMed doi: 10.1097/PRS.0000000000003335

38. Kirschner RE, Baylis AL. Surgical considerations in 22Q11.2 deletion syndrome. *Clin Plast Surg.* 2014;41(2):271–282. PubMed doi: 10.1016/j.cps.2013.12.002

39. Baylis AL, Shriberg LD. Estimates of the prevalence of speech and motor speech disorders in youth with 22q11.2 deletion syndrome. *Am J Speech Lang Pathol.* 2019;28(1):53–82. PubMed doi: 10.1044/2018_AJSLP-18-0037

40. Ryan AK, Goodship JA, Wilson DI, et al. Spectrum of clinical features associated with interstitial chromosome 22q11 deletions: a European collaborative study. *J Med Genet.* 1997;34(10):798–804. PubMed doi: 10.1136/jmg.34.10.798

41. Failla S, You P, Rajakumar C, Dworschak-Stokan A, Doyle PC, Husein M. Characteristics of velopharyngeal dysfunction in 22q11.2 deletion syndrome: a retrospective case-control study. *J Otolaryngol Head Neck Surg.* 2020;49(1):54. PubMed doi: 10.1186/s40463-020-00451-4

42. Widdershoven JC, Stubenitsky BM, Breugem CC, MinkvanderMolen AB. Outcome of velopharyngoplasty in patients with velocardiofacial syndrome. *Arch Otolaryngol Head Neck Surg.* 2008;134(11):1159–1164. PubMed doi: 10.1001/archotol.134.11.1159

43. Kennedy WP, Mudd PA, Maguire MA, et al. 22q11.2 Deletion syndrome and obstructive sleep apnea. *Int J Pediatr Otorhinolaryngol.* 2014;78(8):1360–1364. PubMed doi: 10.1016/j.ijporl.2014.05.031

44. Losken A, Williams JK, Burstein FD, Malick D, Riski JE. An outcome evaluation of sphincter pharyngoplasty for the management of velopharyngeal insufficiency. *Plast Reconstr Surg.* 2003;112(7): 1755–1761. PubMed doi: 10.1097/01.PRS.0000090720.33554.8B

45. Dyce O, McDonald-McGinn D, Kirschner RE, Zackai E, Young K, Jacobs IN. Otolaryngologic manifestations of the 22q11.2 deletion syndrome. *Arch Otolaryngol Head Neck Surg.* 2002;128(12):1408–1412. PubMed doi: 10.1001/archotol.128.12.1408

46. Solot CB, Sell D, Mayne A, et al. Speech-language disorders in 22q11.2 deletion syndrome: best practices for diagnosis and management. *Am J Speech Lang Pathol.* 2019;28(3):984–999. PubMed doi: 10.1044/2019_AJSLP-16-0147

47. Verheij E, Kist AL, Mink van der Molen AB, et al. Otologic and audiologic findings in 22q11.2 deletion syndrome. *Eur Arch Oto-Rhino-Laryngol.* 2017;274(2):765–771. PubMed doi: 10.1007/s00405-016-4365-y

48. Spruijt NE, Vorstman JA, Kon M, Mink van der Molen AB. Self-reported speech problems in adolescents and young adults with 22q11.2 deletion syndrome: a cross-sectional cohort study. *Arch Plast Surg.* 2014;41(5):472–479. PubMed doi: 10.5999/aps.2014.41.5.472

49. Digilio MC, Pacifico C, Tieri L, Marino B, Giannotti A, Dallapiccola B. Audiological findings in patients with microdeletion 22q11 (di George/velocardiofacial syndrome). *Br J Audiol.* 1999;33(5):329–333. PubMed doi: 10.3109/03005369909090116

50. Verheij E, Derks LSM, Stegeman I, Thomeer HGXM. Prevalence of hearing loss and clinical otologic manifestations in patients with 22q11.2 deletion syndrome: a literature review. *Clin Otolaryngol.* 2017;42(6):1319–1328. PubMed doi: 10.1111/coa.12874

51. Giardino G, Cirillo E, Maio F, et al. Gastrointestinal involvement in patients affected with 22q11.2 deletion syndrome. *Scand J Gastroenterol.* 2014;49(3):274–279. PubMed doi: 10.3109/00365521.2013.855814

52. Schindewolf E, Khalek N, Johnson MP, et al. Expanding the fetal phenotype: prenatal sonographic findings and perinatal outcomes in a cohort of patients with a confirmed 22q11.2 deletion syndrome. *Am J Med Genet A.* 2018;176(8):1735–1741. PubMed doi: 10.1002/ajmg.a.38665

53. Eicher PS, McDonald-Mcginn DM, Fox CA, Driscoll DA, Emanuel BS, Zackai EH. Dysphagia in children with a 22q11.2 deletion: unusual pattern found on modified barium swallow. *J Pediatr.* 2000;137(2):158–164. PubMed doi: 10.1067/mpd.2000.105356

54. Bassett AS, Chow EW, Husted J, et al. Clinical features of 78 adults with 22q11 deletion syndrome. *Am J Med Genet A.* 2005;138(4):307–313. PubMed doi: 10.1002/ajmg.a.30984

55. Guzman ML, Delgado I, Lay-Son G, Willans E, Puga A, Repetto GM. Growth in Chilean infants with chromosome 22q11 microdeletion syndrome. *Am J Med Genet A.* 2012;158A(11):2682–2686. PubMed doi: 10.1002/ajmg.a.35525

56. Levy-Shraga Y, Gothelf D, Goichberg Z, et al. Growth characteristics and endocrine abnormalities in 22q11.2 deletion syndrome. *Am J Med Genet A.* 2017;173(5):1301–1308. PubMed doi: 10.1002/ajmg.a.38175

57. Tarquinio DC, Jones MC, Jones KL, Bird LM. Growth charts for 22q11 deletion syndrome. *Am J Med Genet A.* 2012;158A(11):2672–2681. PubMed doi: 10.1002/ajmg.a.35485

58. Hampl SE, Hassink SG, Skinner AC, et al. Clinical practice guideline for the evaluation and treatment of children and adolescents with obesity. *Pediatrics.* 2023;151(2):e2022060640. PubMed doi: 10.1542/peds.2022-060640

59. Kao A, Mariani J, McDonald-McGinn DM, et al. Increased prevalence of unprovoked seizures in patients with a 22q11.2 deletion. *Am J Med Genet A.* 2004;129A(1):29–34. PubMed doi: 10.1002/ajmg.a.30133

60. Gur RE, McDonald-McGinn DM, Moore TM, et al. Psychosis spectrum features, neurocognition and functioning in a longitudinal study of youth with 22q11.2 deletion syndrome. *Psychol Med.* 2023;53(14):6763–6772. PubMed doi: 10.1017/S0033291723000259

61. Mayo D, Bolden KA, Simon TJ, Niendam TA. Bullying and psychosis: the impact of chronic traumatic stress on psychosis risk in 22q11.2 deletion syndrome - a uniquely vulnerable population. *J Psychiatr Res.* 2019;114:99–104. PubMed doi: 10.1016/j.jpsychires.2019.04.011

62. Uljarević M, McCabe KL, Angkustsiri K, Simon TJ, Hardan AY. Interrelationship between cognitive control, anxiety and restricted and repetitive behaviors in children with 22q11.2 deletion syndrome. *Autism Res.* 2019;12(12):1737–1744. PubMed doi: 10.1002/aur.2194

63. Hyman SL, Levy SE, Myers SM, et al; COUNCIL ON CHILDREN WITH DISABILITIES, SECTION ON DEVELOPMENTAL AND BEHAVIORAL PEDIATRICS. Identification, evaluation, and management of children with autism spectrum disorder. *Pediatrics.* 2020;145(1):e20193447. PubMed doi: 10.1542/peds.2019-3447

64. Schneider M, Debbané M, Bassett AS, et al; International Consortium on Brain and Behavior in 22q11.2 Deletion Syndrome. Psychiatric disorders from childhood to adulthood in 22q11.2 deletion syndrome: results from the International Consortium on Brain and Behavior in 22q11.2 Deletion Syndrome. *Am J Psychiatry.* 2014;171(6):627–639. PubMed doi: 10.1176/appi.ajp.2013.13070864

65. Albert N, Melau M, Jensen H, Hastrup LH, Hjorthøj C, Nordentoft M. The effect of duration of untreated psychosis and treatment delay on the outcomes of prolonged early intervention in psychotic disorders. *NPJ Schizophr.* 2017;3(1):34–41. PubMed doi: 10.1038/s41537-017-0034-4

66. American Academy of Pediatrics. National Resource Center for Patient/Family-Centered Medical Home. Medical Home. Accessed December 8, 2023. https://medicalhomeinfo.aap.org/Pages/default.aspx

67. White PH, Cooley WC; TRANSITIONS CLINICAL REPORT AUTHORING GROUP; AMERICAN ACADEMY OF PEDIATRICS; AMERICAN ACADEMY OF FAMILY PHYSICIANS; AMERICAN COLLEGE OF PHYSICIANS. Supporting the health care transition from adolescence to adulthood in the medical home. *Pediatrics.* 2018;142(5):e20182587. PubMed doi: 10.1542/peds.2018-2587

68. Lambert MP, Arulselvan A, Schott A, et al. The 22q11.2 deletion syndrome: cancer predisposition, platelet abnormalities and cytopenias. *Am J Med Genet A.* 2018;176(10):2121–2127. PubMed doi: 10.1002/ajmg.a.38474

69. Miyake CY, Burrage L, Glinton K, et al. TANGO2 deficiency. In: Adam MP, Feldman J, Mirzaa GM, et al, eds. *GeneReviews.* University of Washington; 1993–2023. Accessed December 8, 2023. https://www.ncbi.nlm.nih.gov/books/NBK476443//

Home Health Care of Children, Adolescents and Young Adults With Complex Medical Needs

- *Clinical Report*

CLINICAL REPORT Guidance for the Clinician in Rendering Pediatric Care

American Academy of Pediatrics

DEDICATED TO THE HEALTH OF ALL CHILDREN™

Home Health Care of Children, Adolescents and Young Adults With Complex Medical Needs: Clinical Report

Elaine Lin, MD, FAAP,[1] Garey Noritz, MD, FAAP, FACP,[2] Council on Children With Disabilities; Section on Home Care

abstract

The majority of children, adolescents, and young adults with complex medical needs, especially those who use life-sustaining equipment, are cared for at home by their families and community. Home health care is an essential service that supports families to be able to safely care for their children outside of the hospital, and the medical home serves as the hub to help coordinate and communicate between providers and families. It is essential that pediatric health care providers develop and implement an interdisciplinary and coordinated plan of care that addresses the child's ongoing health care needs. The goal is to ensure that each child remains healthy, thrives, and obtains optimal medical home and developmental supports that promote ongoing care at home. Discharge planning from long-term hospitalizations and rehabilitation for this population can be a complicated process that requires a deliberate, multistep approach. This clinical report presents an approach to addressing the needs of children with complex medical needs and their families in the home environment and supporting the transitions between hospital and home.

[1]*Complex Care, Division of General Pediatrics, Boston Children's Hospital, Harvard Medical School, Boston, Massachusetts; and* [2]*Nationwide Children's Hospital, The Ohio State University College of Medicine, Columbus, Ohio*

All authors participated in conception, design, drafting, and critical revision of the clinical report and approved the final manuscript as submitted.

To cite: Lin E, Noritz G; American Academy of Pediatrics, Council on Children With Disabilities; Section on Home Care. Home Health Care of Children, Adolescents and Young Adults With Complex Medical Needs: Clinical Report. *Pediatrics.* 2025; 156(3):e2025073171

INTRODUCTION

Enormous advances in neonatal, pediatric, and surgical care have led to the survival of a greater number of children and youth with complex medical needs who are cared for at home.[1] The issues faced by these children and their families are often lifelong and may include significant developmental/behavioral, feeding, and respiratory problems, often needing technology assistance. Many of these children have intellectual disabilities, physical impairments, and sensory deficits that require specialized therapeutic and educational interventions that may be delivered at home. The overarching goal of home health care is to optimize each child's health and function through the provision of comprehensive, cost-effective, family-centered health care rendered in a nurturing home environment while minimizing recurrent or prolonged hospitalizations. Caring for children with complex chronic conditions at home can be challenging to pediatric health care providers but successful and rewarding when care is provided in the context of a coordinated, family-centered, and comprehensive medical home. Pediatric health care providers include pediatricians, other physicians, and nonphysician clinicians treating children and adolescents and young adults.

Home health care services are federally mandated under the Early and Periodic Screening, Diagnosis and Treatment (EPSDT) benefits for children enrolled in Medicaid, including the Children's Health Insurance Program (CHIP). Pediatric health care providers may need to help the family access appropriate home health care services "when necessary to correct or ameliorate a mental or physical illness or condition."[2] Many private insurance plans do not adequately cover home health care services, and families must often find other ways to gain coverage through Medicaid waiver programs or other mechanisms.

In contrast to the past, when many children with disabilities were placed in congregate care settings, today most children, even with medical complexity, are cared for at home with their families.[3,4] The US Supreme Court decision in 1999 in *Olmstead vs L.C.* led to the requirement for states to provide services that allow children and adults with disabilities to live at home in their communities rather than in institutions.[5] Congregate care is still an important option in some situations, but families must always be presented with the option to care for their child at home with adequate support to prepare them for success.[6–8]

Children and youth with special health care needs are defined as those who "have or are at increased risk of having a chronic physical, developmental, behavioral, or emotional condition and who also require health and related services of a type or amount beyond that required by children generally."[9] More than 15 million children in the United States meet this definition.[10,11] A subset of children, adolescents, and young adults with special health care needs has been termed "children with medical complexity" (CMC), as defined by substantial health care needs, multiple chronic conditions, functional limitations often associated with technology dependence, and high health care use, including home health care.[12] Depending on the definition and algorithm used to define CMC, the prevalence of this population is between 1% to 11% of children and adolescents.[13] "Technology dependency" refers to the use of medical devices without which—if they were to fail or be discontinued—adverse health consequences and hospitalization would likely follow.[14] Examples include mechanical ventilators, wheelchairs, mobility devices, ventricular shunts, intravenous catheters, oxygen delivery, tracheostomy tubes, enteral feeding devices, colostomy bags, and urinary catheters. The multifaceted medical, developmental, and psychosocial needs of children with such a diverse group of diagnoses typically require the expertise of many pediatric subspecialists and related health care providers in a coordinated system of care.[15,16]

Home health care can include a wide range of health care professionals such as private duty and intermittent nursing, home and personal care aides, trained caregivers, therapists, and behavioral or mental health specialists (Table 1). The medical needs and conditions, as well as the psychosocial situation, help determine the type of home health care and skill level needed by the home health care provider. Children who use life-sustaining equipment need a more advanced skill set as their care routine involves frequent clinical assessments and complex medication or feeding regimens. The medical home and primary care provider (PCP) are often responsible for helping to coordinate this care including initiating referrals, prescribing and reviewing orders, and advocating for the appropriate level of service.[17] Of note, the term primary care provider (PCP) is used throughout this report and recognizes that in addition to pediatricians, other clinicians may care for children with medical complexity, including family physicians and nurse practitioners or physician assistants. Although some CMC receive care through complex care programs at tertiary care centers or academic children's hospitals, most families require a local, community PCP to provide primary care and care coordination support.[18] Care coordination is defined as a patient- and family-centered, assessment-driven, team-based activity designed to meet the needs of children and youth while enhancing the caregiving capabilities of families.[19] A team-based approach to care that enhances communication and care coordination is often the best way to support families and pediatric health care providers.[20]

As the acuity of hospitalized children has increased over time, so too has the severity and complexity of the unresolved medical conditions present on discharge.[21] Children are now frequently sent home to continue or complete interventions that previously would have occurred in hospitals. They are discharged with complex medical interventions, including oxygen, tracheostomies with or without ventilators, enteral feeding tubes, wound care and wound vacuums, intravenous infusions, dialysis, and complex medication regimens. Home health care for children with technology assistance accounts for more than 70% of all pediatric home health care spending.[22] Arranging home health care is an integral part of the discharge process for families and can help reduce caregiver burden and stress.[23,24]

Disparities in health care utilization are known to exist in CMC based on geographic location (urban vs rural) and race and ethnicity.[25] The intersection of social drivers of health and medical complexity is of growing interest; because

TABLE 1. Overview of Home Health Care Services[a]

Type of Home Health Care Provider	Background/Training needed	Skills or Tasks Performed
Private duty nurse	Registered nurse (RN) or licensed practical nurse	Administration of medications (including intravenous [IV] medications), IV nutrition or enteral tube feedings; monitoring vital signs and performing clinical assessments; providing respiratory care (ventilator care, suctioning, chest physiotherapy, nebulizer treatments); performing ostomy or catheter care
Intermittent skilled nurse	Registered nurse or licensed practice nurse	Short-term visits (often to support a transitional period and reinforce education) that include monitoring vital signs, performing clinical assessment and care plan review; medication or equipment teaching; administration of medications, IV nutrition, or enteral tube feeding; providing respiratory care; performing ostomy or catheter care
Personal care assistant	Training program and competency required in most states	Bathing, dressing, meal preparation, medication reminders, mobility assistance
Home health aide/attendant or certified nursing assistant	Training program and competency required with licensing	Personal care, ambulation assistance, assistance with medication administration, simple health care tasks as an extension of nursing or therapy services (taking vital signs)
Paid family caregiver	Family member who has received formal or informal training	Often perform personal care, unskilled care and skilled tasks of private duty nursing delegated by an RN
Respite care worker	Training and certification may be required in some states	Provide short-term relief to primary caregiver(s); may or may not be able to perform medical tasks based on background
Habilitative service therapists	Completion of therapy-specific education and certification	Provide therapy-specific evaluation and treatment (ie, physical therapy, speech therapy, etc)
Other home health care workers Examples: respiratory therapists, mental health specialists	Training and certification based on specialty	Variable

[a] Definition, allowable skills, and intervention may vary by state. Some of these providers may be independently contracted by families or through an agency.

psychosocial barriers can exacerbate health inequities,[26] pediatric health care providers need to recognize this and advocate for equitable access and care. Medical complexity, in and of itself, is a driver of health inequity, and advocating for value-based, risk-adjusted payment structures may help practices with additional resources to support care coordination for these families.[27]

The focus of this report is on the medical aspects of pediatric home health care and is intended to provide an easily accessible resource for pediatric health care providers caring for children, adolescents, and young adults with complex medical needs (referred to as CMC in this report). Other vital types of home care, such as newborn home visiting and behavioral or mental health supports at home, will not be covered in this report. A deeper discussion of the financial aspects of pediatric home health care can be found in the American Academy of Pediatrics (AAP) policy statement, "Financing of Pediatric Home Health Care."[28]

Part I of this report discusses how to optimally supervise home health care for children with medical complexity through a medical home. Part II offers guidance on the hospital discharge of these children to home.

PART I: CARING FOR CHILDREN AND YOUTH WITH MEDICAL COMPLEXITY AT HOME

Pediatric home health care includes services from a range of health care professionals including nurses, personal care assistants, and therapists. Table 1 provides an overview of the different home health care providers, the typical background, and training needed as well as typical skills and tasks. Pediatric health care providers should familiarize themselves with the available services in their area and the scope of practice allowed for each home health care provider as this may vary considerably. A pediatric health care provider, who may be a PCP or a pediatric medical subspecialist, is responsible for reviewing the plan of care and ensuring home health care services are being appropriately and safely provided. For simplicity, an approach to caring for children with complex health care needs at home can be divided into the following main areas: (1) identifying the basic medical issues; (2) identifying the needs and goals of the patient and family; (3) identifying developmental and educational needs; (4) establishing the role of the medical home and care coordination; and (5) maintaining ongoing home health care needs.

Identifying the Basic Medical Issues

CMC often have multiple organ systems affected, and having an organized, systematic approach that addresses each system helps to define their home health care needs. Nutrition is one of the most basic medical needs of every child. Many children with complex health care needs are unable to meet their nutritional requirements orally and rely on enteral or parenteral supports. At every visit, it is important to assess each child's growth by using readily available standardized growth curves and using a consistent measuring approach at subsequent visits.[29] For children who cannot stand independently, a length measuring board or wheelchair scale or having the patient held by the parent and measuring knee height or arm span may be needed to measure growth more accurately.[30] Specific growth curves exist such as those for children with Down syndrome, prematurity, or cerebral palsy, although most guidelines recommend using standard growth charts for follow-up.[31]

It is important to consider the route of feeding as well as its safety and efficacy. Specialized feeding and swallowing evaluations, including videofluoroscopic studies, may be indicated to best determine the method of feeding. Oral health assessment and care in this population is also important to consider, because there is a higher risk of dental caries and oral hygiene issues that can pose high infection risks.[32] Alternative options to oral intake include enteral feeding via gastrostomy tube, nasogastric tube, jejunal or nasojejunal tubes, or parenteral feeding via intravenous catheter. Some children require specialized formulas, such as elemental or higher-calorie formulas, or supplements to increase the caloric or nutritional density of the diet. A balanced intake of fiber and fluid is recommended for optimal bowel motility. Elimination disorders, which can be exacerbated by immobility, can be managed with careful attention to regular bowel and bladder emptying, facilitated with optimized nutrition and hydration, regular bowel programs including rectal stimulants and other medications, enemas, bladder irrigations, and intermittent catheterization as needed. The need for consultations with dietitians, gastroenterologists, or bowel management or motility specialists is determined by the child's feeding tolerance, nutritional status, and related concerns (eg, gastroesophageal reflux disease, dysmotility, vitamin deficiencies, constipation).

Respiratory issues can be frequent and often life-limiting challenges for children and youth with special health care needs.[33] Chronic lung disease may follow preterm delivery or result from chronic aspiration of feedings and secretions in children with neurologic disabilities. Children with neuromuscular conditions that cause restrictive lung disease, such as muscular dystrophy, or preterm infants with severe bronchopulmonary dysplasia may need ventilator assistance (via noninvasive bilevel positive airway pressure or via tracheostomy with mechanical ventilation).[34] Oxygen supplementation and pulse oximetry monitoring are frequently needed for children with neurologic impairments, lung disease, or complex congenital heart disease. Airway issues related to upper airway obstruction in children with craniofacial anomalies or severe neuromuscular disorders may necessitate use of noninvasive positive pressure support or placement of a tracheostomy, often with continuous or intermittent ventilator support. Children may frequently be prescribed bronchodilators or long-term inhaled or systemic steroids. Other interventions such as regular mechanical airway clearance using a high-frequency chest wall oscillation vest or mechanical cough assist device may be used. Children with respiratory impairments benefit from ongoing input from pediatric pulmonologists in conjunction with their PCP as part of the medical home model.[34] Preventive care is a priority, including the provision of pneumococcal, COVID-19, and annual influenza vaccines for at-risk children and their families and caregivers as well as respiratory syncytial virus (RSV) prophylaxis and RSV vaccine. The most up-to-date recommendations for these vaccinations can be found through the American Academy of Pediatrics immunization schedule, which is updated annually.

CMC frequently receive complex medication regimens, sometimes with dozens of medication doses per day.[35] All medications have the potential for adverse effects, and the use of multiple medications increases the risk of drug–drug interactions.[36] All prescribing physicians are responsible for understanding a patient's medication regimen, and although challenging, it is essential that the PCP and all specialists maintain the current medication list to support holistic, rather than fragmented, prescribing. When possible, addition of a clinical pharmacist who can help prevent polypharmacy, monitor for interactions and side effects, and assist when drug shortages become an issue to the care team is extremely helpful. It is important that medication organization be discussed with families to avoid medication errors, especially when multiple caregivers are involved.[35] Pediatric health care providers advise safe storage of medications, especially controlled substances, which should be locked securely. These actions facilitate timely refills, reduce risks of medication errors, and allow pediatric health care providers to regularly monitor for and address potential drug interactions.

Immobility can lead to secondary conditions in children with physical disabilities. Limited mobility and impaired sensation associated with some conditions can put children at risk for skin breakdown. Pediatric health care providers and home health care providers need to vigilantly avoid and otherwise identify and address early threats to skin integrity, such as decubitus ulcers over pressure points, stoma sites, insensate areas, the perineum and other areas with moisture, particularly the posterior occiput, sacrum, ischium, and heels.[37,38] Immobility and lack of weight bearing also contributes to osteoporosis and increases the risk of pathologic fractures.[39] A pediatric rehabilitation medicine specialist or physical therapist, in conjunction with the PCP, may recommend bracing and range-of-motion exercises to prevent musculoskeletal contractures and deformities for children with medical disabilities. These may be implemented by both home health care providers and families. Children may benefit from home occupational and physical therapy for the establishment of exercise regimens and to help decide on appropriate equipment to optimize mobility and minimize complications (eg, hospital beds, bathing equipment, wheelchairs).

Pain in children with medical complexity is common and may be caused by orthopedic, gastrointestinal, neurologic, or other issues. Aside from the negative effects of pain on the child, irritability and discomfort can be distressing to families and home health care providers. It may be challenging to determine whether there is an underlying medical issue causing pain that requires intervention, particularly in a child with limited communication abilities.[40] Validated and reliable measures can be useful in assessing pain in children with cognitive impairments, such as the r-FLACC (revised-Face, Legs, Activity, Cry, and Consolability) Scale[41] and the Individualized Number Rating Scale.[42] Consultations with palliative care providers might further benefit children with chronic pain and the families who care for them.[43] Pediatric health care providers may be called on to evaluate the child to evaluate for basic pediatric problems, such as otitis media, or constipation. Early identification of these issues may avoid unnecessary emergency department visits or hospitalizations. Less obvious problems, such as urinary tract infections, kidney stones, dental issues, or pathologic fractures, may be contributing to discomfort and need to be considered and treated. Algorithms for these assessments have been published and validated.[44]

Identifying The Needs and Goals of the Patient and Family

Family-centered care is a critical component of the medical home for children, adolescents, and young adults with complex health care needs. Pediatric health care providers can periodically assess the needs and goals of the family, in addition to caregiver skill and comfort in rendering care, particularly when life-sustaining equipment is present, and offer opportunities to refresh or extend skills to other close relatives or caregivers. Involving the patients and families is essential to care coordination and communication across medical and nonmedical systems to provide optimal support.[15] It is important that the primary coordinator of care be identified; parents often assume this role without adequate support and spend hours on care coordination, which can result in forgone medical care, lost wages, and less family time.[45] Family caregivers have the most insight on the realities of care and services at home and creating a trusting relationship is critical to success.[46] A shared decision-making approach is used in discussions with families regarding what services and interventions will be put in place to best support patients and caregivers. For adolescents and young adults who may be able to direct their own care, it is important to elicit needs and goals from the patient directly. Pediatric health care providers have regular, collaborative conversations with the families regarding met and unmet home health care staffing, equipment, and transportation needs. To minimize the gaps and support families to receive adequate home health care services, some states have adopted paid family caregiving models in which parents or relatives can be compensated financially for the care they provide to their CMC.[47] Pediatric health care providers can familiarize themselves with what is available in their state and educate families on options for home health care services.

It is important to recognize the needs of parents in their roles as long-term caregivers as well as the unique needs of siblings of children with complex health care needs and disabilities with appropriate referrals to community agencies (Table 2). Families and pediatric health care providers need to partner in care planning and proactive discussions regarding their child's prognosis, including explicit statement of family preferences regarding resuscitation status and end-of-life care.[48,49] Community-based pediatric palliative care and hospice care can help support this shared decision-making process with the pediatric health care providers and can be initiated at any time based on family's goals and preferences.[50,51] Formal and informal opportunities for respite care can be identified and accessed whenever possible.

TABLE 2. Examples of Community Organizations Families Might Find Helpful

Type of Agency	Examples
Family support	Family Voices, Courageous Parent Network, Parent to Parent Information Centers
Benefits programs	Medicaid, Supplemental Security Income, Developmental Disabilities Administration, Social Security Administration
Disease-specific organizations	Cerebral palsy organizations, muscular dystrophy organizations, Spina Bifida Association, National Down Syndrome Society, Sickle Cell Society, Autism Society of America, National Family Association for DeafBlind
Adaptive sports and recreational programs	Special Olympics, American Association of Adaptive Sports Programs
Advocacy and legal support	American Association of People with Disabilities, Special Needs Alliance, National Center for Medical Legal Partnership
Home based palliative care programs	Pediatric Palliative Care Network; academic institution-affiliated programs
Respite care programs	Ryan's House, George Mark House, Crescent Cove, A Rosie Place for Children
Other	Make a Wish, A Kid Again

The presence of a child with complex medical and developmental needs associated with technology assistance and long-term home health care certainly affects the physical and emotional health and well-being of the child, their parents, siblings, and other family members.[49,52,53] Siblings of children with disabilities may demonstrate behavioral problems or academic struggles, as they often assume caregiving responsibilities and may have unmet needs for parental attention and support.[54,55] Family vacations may be canceled or postponed, parental attendance at important school or sports events may not occur, and sometimes even serious medical symptoms in the "well" sibling may go unattended. Siblings may sometimes be called on to assume caregiving roles for which they have not been appropriately trained or are not developmentally prepared. Pediatric health care providers can assist these children and their families by being cognizant of these issues, seeing the well siblings for separate appointments where they can receive individualized attention, and sometimes meeting privately with the siblings to allow them to express their feelings. Because children with disabilities are at increased risk of abuse and neglect, pediatric health care providers need to be particularly attentive to child–family interactions and sensitive to early indications of maltreatment.[56] In some instances, family support services and counseling are indicated.[57]

Identifying Developmental and Educational Needs

Many CMC have developmental and physical disabilities that affect their overall health and development. If developmental disabilities are suspected on the basis of history, underlying diagnosis, or developmental screening results, it is critical to advocate that children receive appropriate educational and related assessments and services. Community agencies that provide developmental care include early intervention for children from birth to 3 years of age and adaptive educational programs that often include medically based habilitative therapies for older children.[58,59] Specialized referrals may be needed for children who are deaf/hard of hearing or blind/low vision. Referrals for individualized habilitative services often require prescriptions from PCPs, particularly when coverage is requested for medically based (as opposed to educationally based) therapeutic services, and pediatric health care providers may need to advocate for these services.[60] The ideal educational environment is one that is least restrictive and in which children can maximize their potential while remaining safe. Individualized education programs (IEPs) and 504 plans may include the provision of medical care (eg, enteral feedings, airway suctioning, medication administration) to maintain the health and safety of the child while in school. Pediatric health care providers can contribute important medical information to help school administration decide the appropriate accommodations are being provided for the child to receive free appropriate public education. Some states may provide these educational services in nontraditional settings such as day rehabilitation programs or medical day cares.

Community services are critical to families, as they offer developmental programs (eg, early intervention programs),[61] educational services, and recreational opportunities.[62] Programs of adaptive sports and recreation, specialized vacation camps, and community-based religious or cultural services offer additional opportunities for child and family participation in their communities.

Establishing the Role of the Medical Home and Care Coordination

Although pediatric health care providers cannot be experts in every chronic condition of childhood, it is important that they update their knowledge regarding the individual children and youth with special health care needs in their practices. By reviewing the literature and consulting with specialists, PCPs can gain the needed expertise to manage and coordinate care. Depending on the unique medical needs of the child and the available community resources, medical home providers may be either a general pediatric clinician, a pediatric clinician who specializes in care of children with medical complexity, or a pediatric subspecialist such as a pulmonologist. As the population of children with medical complexity grows, new models of care for this population have emerged rapidly. These models of care may be primary care centered, consultative/comanagement based, or episode based.[63] Helping families identify who their primary medical home is can be critical in facilitating communication and coordination of care.

Medical homes support coordination and integration of care among families of CMC, home health care providers, and community systems, including emergency medical services and utility companies.[64] This care coordination, which is mandated by Medicaid through EPSDT, along with other supports and services, is often the main pillar of care delivery for children with special health care needs. Care management services through hospital, government, or insurance agencies may be integrated into primary care settings to support pediatric health care providers in the care of children with special health care needs.[15,63]

Pediatric health care providers need to consider their own access to care managers, social workers, community health workers, dietitians, and other support staff members who contribute substantially to the care of children and youth with special health care needs. Multidisciplinary care teams that are disease specific, such as spina bifida or craniofacial teams, allow for efficient and coordinated care delivery, and PCPs may partner with them to provide comprehensive care. Pediatric palliative care programs that can address unmet physical, emotional, social, and spiritual needs for families can be considered as they help support care coordination and family education. These programs not only address issues surrounding potential end-of-life scenarios but also help address symptom burden, improve overall quality of life, and reduce time spent in the hospital.[65–67] Pediatric residency and fellowship programs may need to reassess the training experiences for their residents so that future pediatricians have the needed expertise and comfort in providing medical homes for all children, including those with medical complexity, disabilities, and complex home health care needs.[68,69]

The medical home office visit for children and youth with special health care needs, particularly with technology assistance, needs to be carefully orchestrated in terms of the frequency, duration, and content of visits. It can be useful to provide separate chronic condition management visits and well-child visits or schedule longer-than-routine visits, because acute issues often crowd out much-needed time for routine pediatric care. Accessibility, as defined by the Americans with Disabilities Act, is an important part of being able to provide care to this population.[70] Accommodations may include larger examination rooms and accessible examination tables that allow for transfer from a wheelchair. Designations within the electronic health record may indicate environmental or behavioral preferences of patients to attempt to accommodate each child's individual physical and developmental needs.

Telehealth has played a large role in providing more opportunities for care coordination that are convenient and effective for families.[71,72] Home monitoring devices and other innovative technologies may allow families to avoid traveling for office visits as well as emergency department visits and hospitalizations.[73,74] As technology continues to advance, the integration of telehealth into primary and specialty care services and care management will be critical in efforts to maintain continuous services, reduce unnecessary emergency department utilization, readmissions to the hospital, and other potential complications. Adequate payment for telehealth and remote monitoring services is also needed for pediatric health care providers to continue to offer this type of care to families.

A systematic method of communication among all providers needs to be established so that critical information is available during and after office visits. Electronic health records are increasingly used for this purpose, but they are often difficult to access by PCPs outside the specialty system. A detailed problem list and care plan, including the names and contact information for consulting specialists and home health care providers, needs to be regularly updated in the medical record. The medical home should also maintain a record of medications and refills, the preferred pharmacy, home health care orders, referrals, and letters of medical necessity.[14] Access to an emergency information form is important for the medical home as well as the families.[75] Patient portals within the electronic health record are being increasingly used to facilitate provider and patient/caregiver communication and centralized storage of the important information mentioned above for families.

Home visits by pediatric health care providers can offer a safe and efficient alternative to traditional office visits.[76] Visits can be made as part of well-child or urgent care, for management of chronic problems, to assist in transition home from the inpatient setting, or to perform home and psychosocial assessments. Home visits can be billed for as a distinct visit type and should be adequately paid for by payers.

Each individual medical home needs to address payment for direct and indirect services rendered. A major disincentive in the current system of care is the lack of physician compensation for time invested in phone management, care coordination, completion of home health care orders and recertifications, management of medication refills, and letters of medical necessity, although some public and private payers are starting to cover care coordination.[77] As payment reform continues to evolve, it is important to develop pediatric risk adjustment factors so that PCPs are incentivized to (and not discouraged from) caring for children with complex health care needs. PCPs can familiarize themselves with what their local payers may pay for non–face-to-face care coordination activities and interactions, including telehealth and maintaining and updating the integrated plan of care for children who receive home health care. Children with complex health care needs and disabilities may be insured by Medicaid instead of or in addition to private insurance companies, and adequate payment for the time and effort to support high-quality care integration for home health care services should be recognized and paid to the medical home practices by all payers.

Maintaining Ongoing Home Health Care Needs

Most CMC have chronic conditions associated with complete and irreversible dependence on technology. Consequently, they may require lifelong home health care services. The provision of uninterrupted home health care is threatened by national nursing shortages, limitations in the availability of skilled pediatric nurses, and lack of funding.[78] Pediatric equipment is not universally available. Pediatric health care providers need to provide frequent updates on orders, letters of medical necessity, and prior authorizations. These sometimes require "peer to peer evaluations" with medical staff at the insurance company. Thus, home health care services are carefully monitored and maintained to provide continuous access to children and youth with special health care needs and their families. Table 3 lists issues that are important to monitor for children who are receiving home health care.

Transitioning from pediatric to adult care health care providers also requires careful planning. Many families will continue to need home health care support as children age

TABLE 3. Issues Related to Ongoing Monitoring of Home Health Care
1. Regular review of home health care discharge plan to determine whether goals are being met or have changed
2. Child assessment
a. Physical condition
b. Appropriateness of current home health care hours and service type
c. Developmental and educational issues
d. Advance care planning
3. Family assessment
a. Strengths
b. Problem identification
c. Changes
d. Family–provider communications
e. Adequacy of current services
4. Financial
a. Paperwork
b. Policy benefit changes
c. Family financial changes
d. Adequate coverage
5. Equipment/supplies/medications
a. Identification and tracking of current needs
b. Prescriptions written
c. Justification letters
6. Diagnostics ordered with appropriate interventions made, and referrals to specialists as needed
7. Follow-up appointments made
a. To primary care provider
b. To specialists
c. Coordination of appointments and procedures whenever possible
d. Communication with subspecialists and home health care providers in a timely way so that the child's changing needs are being addressed

out of educational programs and may spend more time at home. The AAP, the American College of Physicians, and the American Academy of Family Physicians recommend in the clinical report, "Supporting the Health Care Transition From Adolescence to Adulthood in the Medical Home,"[79] initial discussions to transition to adult care can happen as early as 12 years of age, because it is an ongoing process with multiple aspects. For children with complex health care needs, it is important to identify the adult hospital system that will assume their care, and many centers have set up transition clinics or programs that facilitate both outpatient and inpatient transition. PCPs need to consider primary and subspecialty care, behavioral and mental health supports, housing, and community integration including vocational programs.

Home health care eligibility and allotted hours will be reassessed with transfer to adult Medicaid plans or any other insurance or waiver services. To plan for this change, documentation of nursing care and scheduled tasks and time it takes to do various care tasks can be helpful to support the types of service and hours needed for care. Resources are available to families to identify home health companies, coordinate assessments and advocate for families' needs. For young adults who may be able to direct their home health care providers, it is important that they learn how to manage their home environment and navigate the health care system.

Families need to consider guardianship,[80] financial planning, and establishment of a will or trust as part of the transition to adult care. In order to maintain continuous access to home health care and durable medical equipment services, families need to familiarize themselves with insurance age limitations that may vary by payer and state. Most adult health care systems still lack adequate infrastructure and the workforce to care for young adults with medical complexity, which is why starting the process early and preparing families for these challenges is essential.[81]

PART II: TRANSITIONING FROM HOSPITAL TO HOME HEALTH CARE AND VICE VERSA

This part of the report is directed primarily at the inpatient team who is discharging a CMC to home, as well as the child's specialists, who are usually located at one or more medical centers. In addition to physicians, the discharging team may include nurse or social work care coordinators, therapists, dietitians, and others; where needed, the team may reach out to community agents as well, such as public health nurses and local emergency services. There are 6 main issues that need to be addressed by the discharging inpatient team (Table 4). These issues include: (1) establishing a partnership with the family and specialty and acute care providers to identify family and community resources available to support the transition process; (2) training the family and other home health care providers; (3) assisting in the selection of a home care agency and/or providers of supplies and equipment; (4) arranging educational and developmental services; (5) identifying the medical home and verifying that it is able to provide medical home services including care coordination; and (6) optimizing insurance coverage at home. Ideally, discharge planning will commence in a timely way, preferably as soon as the child is admitted, and the PCP will be given the opportunity to participate throughout the process and be paid adequately for their services by the child's insurance.[82]

Transportation on discharge is accomplished most safely with an individualized approach using the principles outlined in the AAP clinical report "Transporting Children With Special Health Care Needs."[83] In addition, if the family has decided to implement any limitations on care such as a "do not resuscitate" order, the local emergency medical services can be contacted to relay these wishes. The family needs to have copies of these orders available in the home.

TABLE 4. Issues Related to Planning for Home Health Care Before Discharge From the Hospital
A. Evaluating child, child's family, home, and community
1. Child
a. Child is medically stable for home health care
2. Family
a. Family desires to have child at home
b. Family has learned the necessary skills
c. Family has considered palliative care and end-of-life care options
3. Home
a. Assessing home safety and accessibility
(1) Structure
(2) Electrical (eg, 3-pronged plugs, 220-V line)[a]
(3) Access (eg, bathroom and ramps)
(4) Heat, hot water, clean water supply
(5) Air conditioning
(6) Driveway/road accessibility
(7) Other (eg, snow removal)
(8) Telephone access[b]
4. Community
a. Community health nurse
b. Home health care nurses
c. Therapists (eg, physical and occupational therapy)
d. Ambulance/emergency medical services
e. Specialty care
f. Medical supply vendors
g. Pharmacist
h. School/early intervention program
i. Counseling
j. Support group(s)
k. Palliative and hospice care if desired
B. Finding a medical home
1. PCP
2. Roles and communication network
3. Patient summary
a. Plan for emergency care
b. Medications
c. Equipment
d. Disposable supplies
e. Advance care plan, out of hospital do-not-resuscitate order, where appropriate
C. Training the home caregivers
1. Training schedule
2. Actual care with supervision (trial home health care)
D. Arranging home health care nursing and developmental/educational services
1. Nursing care coverage is outlined
2. Alternative plans are made if nursing care is not available
3. Arrangements with school or preschool programs for ongoing educational needs
E. Finding home health care agencies and vendors for supplies and equipment
F. Insurance coverage
1. Verify that adequate coverage will be provided
2. Pursue alternative or additional coverage and benefits such as Medicaid waiver program and Supplemental Security Income (SSI)
3. Evaluate ability of family to pay for uncovered care (eg, transportation, electricity)

[a] Secondary power generators may be necessary; local power companies and emergency providers should be alerted on hospital discharge to help prioritize responsiveness to emergencies.
[b] Arrangements should be made with telephone companies to prevent interrupted services. Internet services may also be required, especially for those parents with hearing impairment who cannot easily communicate via telephone.

Evaluating the Child, Family, Home, and Community

Each child should be evaluated to determine whether they are medically stable for care at home. Although there is no clear definition of "stability" given the numerous underlying and complex issues involved, ideally the child would have no major changes made to the medical regimen for a reasonable period of time, such that subsequent changes can happen on an outpatient basis. The child does not need to be on a "final goal" feeding, respiratory, or other regimen, but the family needs to be comfortable providing the care at this point in the home and progressing to the "usual" care with support from the medical home.

The needs, preferences, and resources of families of children with medical complexity should be evaluated well in advance of hospital discharge.[84] Families need to be made aware of and provided all available resources to transition their child home to best support their decision making. The home may be evaluated through an interdisciplinary approach to confirm that it is an adequate, safe, and accessible environment. Consideration of individual and cultural expectations families may have in caring for a CMC at home is important. Home ventilation, in particular, can be accomplished successfully but is a significant strain on caregivers.[85]

Architectural barriers, including the ability to accommodate equipment such as wheelchairs, lift systems, hospital beds, and other medical equipment, must be considered as part of the ordering process. Local emergency medical services, as well as heating and electrical providers, could be alerted by families or PCPs to the specialized needs in homes of children with high medical complexity and fragility. Arrangements for uninterrupted power in homes of children with life-sustaining equipment may include the prioritization by utility companies for immediate restoration of services in the event of disruptions.[86] Some families may be able to obtain power generators through insurance or self-pay. Safe, accessible, and predictable means of transporting the child and essential equipment and supplies should be established. At a minimum, the family needs access to a telephone so that they can activate emergency services. Broadband access and telehealth equipment may assist the family and team to maintain the patient safely at home, and pilot programs have demonstrated the safety and cost-effectiveness of deploying these services from the health system.[87] Striving for health equity is an important focus while advocating for access to services to minimize ongoing disparities in health care.[88]

Training the Home Caregivers

Before the child's discharge, the caregivers (usually the parents but often the grandparents or other family and friends) will require appropriate training to be able to care for the child at home. Caregivers should be taught and should demonstrate competency in the care and use of the devices that support the child at home. These frequently include enteral feeding tubes, tracheostomy tubes, respiratory treatments and supports (eg, nebulizers, ventilators), wound care, intravenous line care, and medication management. Cardiopulmonary resuscitation (CPR) training is generally advisable. In addition to teaching the home caregivers how to render care, teaching assessment skills is also essential. For example, it is important to know not only *how* to suction or change a tracheostomy tube but also *when and why* a child needs this intervention. Home caregivers also need to have a clear understanding of when and how to contact the PCP or specialist when problems arise. Family preferences need to be considered when developing care regimens, including timings for feeding and medication administration. Hospital schedules of administering enteral feedings or medications constantly around the clock indefinitely are unsustainable and not clinically necessary. Near the end of a prolonged hospitalization, some hospitals recommend or require that the parents stay overnight for 1 to 2 days before discharge, allowing them to render all the child's care independently but with the support of hospital staff for questions and problem solving before the discharge.[89] Parents must demonstrate competency in the use of monitors that may be used in the home in preparation of transitioning from hospital to home. Many children's hospitals also have patient and family advisory councils that may include caregivers who serve as educators and support to families as they transition from hospital to home. Standardized criteria for caregiver competencies and ongoing demonstration of skills are needed.

Arranging Home Health Care Services

CMC are entitled to home health care services, and states are mandated to provide this service to allow these children to transition safely to their homes and communities.[78] Children who require intensive respiratory supports, such as those with tracheostomy and ventilator dependencies associated with high suctioning requirements, are likely to require private duty home nursing rather than brief and periodic skilled nursing visits. A nationwide shortage of qualified pediatric registered nurses and licensed practical nurses often complicates and delays discharge, as does ensuring coverage by insurance for such support.[90,91] CMC and their families who reside in areas with limited nursing and community resources have unique needs that require exploring alternative solutions such as programs where caregivers can select their own home health care provider (often called consumer direct care). Parents should be actively involved in determining the child's care plan to confirm that the plan is feasible from their perspective in the context of their daily life and community. For example, parents who work outside the home often elect to have home nursing during the day, whereas other families elect to have night-time nursing so that they can sleep. Pediatric health care providers can help advocate for paid family caregiving as well as increased payments in order to improve the situation for families. Families and pediatric health care providers need to have contingency plans that are responsive to unanticipated interruptions in caregiving, such as the nurse canceling a shift because of illness. In one survey of families receiving home-based palliative care services, nearly 40% of approved nursing hours went unstaffed, leaving families to provide these nursing hours themselves.[92] Partnering with legal advocates to collectively advocate is one method for pediatric health care providers to help address these limitations.

Arranging Providers for Supplies and Durable Medical Equipment

Many large pediatric centers now have care coordinators or discharge planners (usually registered nurses or social workers) who arrange for home equipment such as oxygen, respiratory technologies, enteral feeding supplies, intravenous medications, specialized enemas, urinary catheters, and other durable medical equipment (DME) before discharge. The prescription of DME that supports safe and effective transfers, such as specialized beds, bath seats, lift systems, and adaptive car seats, can be completed collaboratively with interdisciplinary providers before hospital discharge.[93] The child's insurance coverage usually dictates which DME providers may be accessed, further influenced by geographic considerations. Early and meticulous discharge planning is essential to ensure the appropriate supplies are ordered and delivered in a timely way so that they can be readily available for training of caregivers and use on discharge. Once the patient is home, the PCP may be called on to help troubleshoot or order additional supplies.

Arranging Developmental and Educational Services

Ensuring a smooth transition to educational and therapy services at discharge is essential to optimize each child's medical, developmental, and functional outcomes. Frequent and consistent communication between PCPs and early intervention and other therapy providers is an important part of the process. For school-aged children, it is important for a member of the care team to communicate with the school, including the school nurse, to plan for appropriate educational, therapeutic, and medical services before discharge from the hospital.[59] For children requiring care for their tracheostomy tube or enteral feedings in school, training of the school personnel by hospital personnel can be considered before patient discharge.

Working With the Medical Home

For patients who already have a PCP, it is critical to work with that provider as the patient approaches discharge, especially if there have been important changes in care or status, such as the identification of new chronic illnesses, addition of new technology, or change in goals of care. The PCP needs the information and resources to effectively resume care of the patient. If there is not already a PCP, it is important that one be identified prior to discharge.

A discharge summary transmitted to the PCP is a *minimum* expectation; a verbal or electronic conversation between the inpatient team and PCP can be extremely helpful in ensuring the continuity of care and treatment. It is incumbent on the discharging service to confirm that the family has enough medication and supplies until they can see the PCP, and the family can be counseled about which questions and issues need to be discussed with the specialists and which can be directed to the PCP.

Providing comprehensive medical home health care to CMC in the primary care setting can be challenging because of time, financial, and logistical constraints, and not every PCP will be able to invest the time and energy that this responsibility demands. The PCP clinic's ability to coordinate care for the patient needs to be confirmed before discharge.[94] Comanagement with specialty care providers can help support the PCPs in treating the child's conditions as well as optimizing community support services. A detailed and immediately accessible care plan should be developed jointly by the family, medical team, and care coordinators, with continuous updates as indicated. Plans should include treatment interventions that the family implements when the child is both sick and well and who to contact when further care is needed. Confirming the family's language of choice and using methods they identify as helpful for learning, such as pictures or charts, is important. The PCP for children with complex conditions and disabilities who receive home health care support should be provided with a comprehensive discharge summary that includes details of all the issues and events of the hospitalization and an accurate list of medications, therapies, equipment, and services that have been arranged before the discharge.[95] It is critical that the PCP know how to communicate with other subspecialists involved in the child's care and how frequently the child will need visits with other habilitative service providers and therapists.[15]

Proactively planning for "sick days" may increase the caregivers' competence and confidence in managing acute issues at home, decreasing the likelihood that emergency or hospital care will be needed. Common scenarios for which planning may be helpful could include management of fever, upper respiratory symptoms, vomiting or diarrhea, increased seizures, or equipment malfunction.[96]

It is helpful if the team and family discuss various methods of communication and when to use them. Care plans need to include under which circumstances they need to call or send a secure portal message, whether the message will go to the PCP or the specialist, and when they need to activate emergency medical services.

Insurance Coverage for Care at Home

As home health care is essential medical care for children with chronic conditions and disability, the AAP has released a policy statement, "Financing of Pediatric Home Health Care,"[28] which outlines legal and financial requirements for home health care and needed reforms to support that all families can access this type of care. Frequently, third-party payers fail to cover the costs of specialized pediatric private duty home health care, leading to delayed or even canceled hospital discharges for children with complex, chronic conditions and technology assistance.[28,77,97] Lack of coverage for home nursing or extended therapeutic services is not uncommon. Families may seek secondary insurance coverage through Medicaid to cover costs denied by primary commercial payers. Some children may be eligible for Medicaid waivers, which can augment the amount of care children can get at home.

Families often face financial hardship related to extensive medical bills from lengthy hospitalizations as well as lost revenue related to the need to reduce employment outside of the home.[98] Some children with disabilities are eligible for Supplemental Security Income (SSI) benefits, which may help meet the financial demands.[99] The newer model of paying family caregivers or the care they provide can help mitigate these financial challenges.[100]

Vice-versa: Transitioning From Home to Hospital

Admissions (and readmissions) of CMC who have home nursing to the inpatient hospital are common. In one study, cumulative all-cause rehospitalization rates were 18% by 30 days, 62% by 365 days, and 87% within 2 years; the median rehospitalization frequency was 3 per patient. The most common reasons for unplanned rehospitalization were infection (41%) and device complication (10%).[101]

The clinical observations of both the family and home nurse can be vital to understanding the process that is requiring acute care, and both may be sought.[102] They are vital members of the child's care team when in the hospital.

Given the high frequency of rehospitalization, it is important for the family, home nursing staff, and medical home to expect this will happen. They tend to have an up-to-date care plan, especially the most recent medication regimen. Families often keep a "go bag" packed with essential medical supplies, clothing, and toiletries for both the child and the caregiver(s).

SUMMARY AND CONCLUSIONS

CMC represent a significant percentage of hospitalized pediatric patients and are being discharged to home with an ever-expanding range of complex medical and life sustaining equipment. Medical homes for children with complex medical needs can coordinate a team of providers toward the overarching goal of optimizing each child's health, development, and well-being. Pediatric health care providers must understand the complexities of the child's underlying conditions, including ongoing medical and developmental needs, family needs, and available home health care and community resources. Disease-specific clinical guidelines exist for patients with certain more common diseases, which may help PCPs with clinical care. Medical homes may need to adopt routine practices and individualize their approaches to best orchestrate the multifaceted needs of CMC, their parents and families, and health care systems. A systematic approach to pediatric care with explicit care coordination, family-centered care, and advanced planning supports the best outcomes and provides the most rewarding experiences for children and youth with complex medical needs, their families, and providers.

Recommendations

- All pediatric health care providers who care for CMC, including children requiring technology assistance, should familiarize themselves with the child's underlying conditions, including ongoing medical and developmental needs, family needs, and available home health care and community resources. This familiarity is necessary for both ongoing outpatient care and arranging care at transition out and into the hospital.
- Care coordination by the PCP (and their team) is an essential part of the medical home for children with complex health care needs, and identifying best communication methods with families, specialists, and home health care providers is critical.
- Pediatric health care providers should be aware of and take advantage of mechanisms to be paid for non–face-to-face services that improve care in the home for children.
- The medical home should strive to keep an up-to-date care plan and medication list as well as contact information for members of the child's care team, including specialists and community services. When transitioning between inpatient and outpatient care, medical home and home health care providers should be provided with the discharge summary that includes this vital information.
- Developmental and educational supports including therapy and services to address disabilities delivered at home are an important aspect of care and should be continually reassessed.
- Home health care is an important aspect of health care delivery when transitioning from pediatric to adult care. Families should work closely with their child's care team to identify long-term health care needs and start the process of transition early.
- Inpatient pediatric health care providers and their teams should identify the medical needs of the child, involved specialists in the care team, as well as medication and equipment needs and arrange for appropriate home health care service, therapies, and vendors at hospital discharge.
- Prior to discharge, the inpatient team should assess family needs including psychosocial, financial, and environmental barriers, which are critical to supporting and training families on their child's care at home. Families should be trained on medications and medical equipment and provided with contact information on who to call for which concerns.
- Pediatric health care providers should be aware of ongoing changes to coverage of home health services and advocate, when possible, for the appropriate and maximal level of service to support families to care for their CMC at home and in the community.

LEAD AUTHORS

Elaine Lin, MD, FAAP
Garey Noritz, MD, FAAP, FACP

COUNCIL ON CHILDREN WITH DISABILITIES EXECUTIVE COMMITTEE, 2024–2025

Garey Noritz, MD, FAAP, FACP, Chairperson
Rishi Agrawal, MD, MPH, FAAP
Deanna S. Bell, MD, FAAP
Jessica E. A. Foster, MD, MPH, FAAP
Ellen Fremion, MD, FAAP, FACP
Sheryl Frierson, MD, MEd, FAAP
Michelle Melicosta, MD, MPH, MSc, FAAP
Barbara S. Saunders, DO, FAAP
Siddharth Srivastava, MD, FAAP
Jilda Vargus-Adams, MD, MSc, FAAP
Katharine E. Zuckerman, MD, MPH, FAAP

PAST COUNCIL ON CHILDREN WITH DISABILITIES EXECUTIVE COMMITTEE MEMBERS

Dennis Z. Kuo, MD, MHS, FAAP, Immediate Past Chairperson

LIAISONS

Jennifer Walton, MD, FAAP – *Section on Developmental and Behavioral Pediatrics*
Matthew Sadof, MD, FAAP – *Section on Home Care*
Allysa Ware, PhD, MSW – *Family Voices*
Rajapillai Pillai, PhD – *Section on Pediatric Trainees*

STAFF

Alex Kuznetsov

SECTION ON HOME CARE EXECUTIVE COMMITTEE, 2024–2025

Elaine P. Lin, MD, FAAP, Chairperson
Carolyn Foster, MD, FAAP
Amy J. Houtrow, MD, PhD, MPH, FAAP
Patrick Jones, MD, MA, FAAP
Matthew Sadof MD, FAAP
Edwin Simpser, MD, FAAP

LIAISONS

Andrea Reitzel, Family Liaison

STAFF

Heather Fitzpatrick, MPH

ABBREVIATIONS

CHIP: Children's Health Insurance Program
CMC: children with medical complexity
EPSDT: Early and Period Screening, Diagnosis and Treatment
PCP: primary care provider

FINANCIAL/CONFLICT OF INTEREST DISCLOSURE: The authors have indicated they do not have a financial relationship relevant to this article to disclose.

FUNDING: No external funding.

https://doi.org/10.1542/peds.2025-073171

REFERENCES

1. Perrin JM. Health services research for children with disabilities. *Milbank Q*. 2002;80(2):303–324. PubMed doi: 10.1111/1468-0009.t01-1-00005
2. Early and Periodic Screening, Diagnosis, and Treatment (EPSDT) of Individuals Under Age 21. 42 CFR Part 441 Subpart B. Last amended December 4, 2024. Accessed December 10, 2024. https://www.ecfr.gov/current/title-42/chapter-IV/subchapter-C/part-441/subpart-B
3. Rosenbaum S, Wilensky S, Allen K. *EPSDT at 40: Modernizing a Pediatric Health Policy to Reflect a Changing Health Care System*. Center for Healthcare Strategies; 2008. Accessed December 10, 2024. https://www.chcs.org/resource/epsdt-at-40-modernizing-a-pediatric-health-policy-to-reflect-a-changing-health-care-system/
4. Goldstein MM, Rosenbaum S. From EPSDT to EHBs: the future of pediatric coverage design under government financed health insurance. *Pediatrics*. 2013;131(suppl 2):S142–S148. PubMed doi: 10.1542/peds.2013-0252e
5. *Olmstead v L.C.*, 527 US 581 (1999)
6. Friedman SL, Norwood KW Jr, Norwood KW Jr, et al; COUNCIL ON CHILDREN WITH DISABILITIES. Out-of-home placement for children and adolescents with disabilities—addendum: care options for children and adolescents with disabilities and medical complexity [reaffirmed February 2019, reaffirmed November 2024]. *Pediatrics*. 2016;138(6):e20163216. PubMed doi: 10.1542/peds.2016-3216
7. Americans with Disabilities Act. 42 USC §12101 (1990)
8. Rosenbaum S, Teitelbaum J, Stewart A. Olmstead v. L.C.: implications for Medicaid and other publicly funded health services. *Health Matrix*. 2002;12(1):93–138. PubMed
9. McPherson M, Arango P, Fox H, et al. A new definition of children with special health care needs. *Pediatrics*. 1998;102(1 Pt 1):137–140. PubMed doi: 10.1542/peds.102.1.137
10. Kogan MD, Strickland BB, Newacheck PW. Building systems of care: findings from the National Survey of Children With Special Health Care Needs. *Pediatrics*. 2009;124(suppl 4):S333–S336. PubMed doi: 10.1542/peds.2009-1255B
11. Maternal and Child Health Bureau, Health Resources and Services Administration. Children and Youth with Special Health Care Needs. Accessed December 10, 2024. https://mchb.hrsa.gov/sites/default/files/mchb/programs-impact/nsch-data-brief-children-youth-special-health-care-needs.pdf
12. Cohen E, Kuo DZ, Agrawal R, et al. Children with medical complexity: an emerging population for clinical and research initiatives. *Pediatrics*. 2011;127(3):529–538. PubMed doi: 10.1542/peds.2010-0910
13. Leyenaar JK, Schaefer AP, Freyleue SD, et al. Prevalence of children with medical complexity and associations with health care

utilization and in-hospital mortality. *JAMA Pediatr.* 2022;176(6): e220687. PubMed doi: 10.1001/jamapediatrics.2022.0687

14. Feudtner C, Villareale NL, Morray B, Sharp V, Hays RM, Neff JM. Technology-dependency among patients discharged from a children's hospital: a retrospective cohort study. *BMC Pediatr.* 2005; 5(1):8. PubMed doi: 10.1186/1471-2431-5-8
15. Turchi RM, Antonelli RC, Norwood KW Jr, et al; Council on Children with Disabilities and Medical Home Implementation Project Advisory Committee. Patient- and family-centered care coordination: a framework for integrating care for children and youth across multiple systems [reaffirmed April 2023]. *Pediatrics.* 2014;133(5):e1451–e1460. PubMed doi: 10.1542/peds.2014-0318
16. McLellan SE, Mann MY, Scott JA, Brown TW. A blueprint for change: guiding principles for a system of services for children and youth with special health care needs and their families. *Pediatrics.* 2022;149(suppl 7):e2021056150C. PubMed doi: 10.1542/peds.2021-056150C
17. Fratantoni K, Raisanen JC, Boss RD, et al. The pediatric home health care process: perspectives of prescribers, providers, and recipients. *Pediatrics.* 2019;144(3):e20190897. PubMed doi: 10.1542/peds.2019-0897
18. Antonelli RC, Turchi RM. Care management for children with medical complexity: integration is essential. *Pediatrics.* 2017;140(6): e20172860. PubMed doi: 10.1542/peds.2017-2860
19. Antonelli R, McAllister J, Popp J.Making Care Coordination a Critical Component of the Pediatric Health System: a Multidisciplinary Framework. The Commonwealth Fund; May 21, 2009. Accessed December 10, 2024. https://www.commonwealthfund.org/publications/fund-reports/2009/may/making-care-coordination-critical-component-pediatric-health
20. Katkin JP, Kressly SJ, Edwards AR, et al; TASK FORCE ON PEDIATRIC PRACTICE CHANGE. Guiding principles for team-based pediatric care [reaffirmed December 2023]. *Pediatrics.* 2017;140(2): e20171489. PubMed doi: 10.1542/peds.2017-1489
21. Simon TD, Berry J, Feudtner C, et al. Children with complex chronic conditions in inpatient hospital settings in the United States. *Pediatrics.* 2010;126(4):647–655. PubMed doi: 10.1542/peds.2009-3266
22. Sobotka SA, Hall DE, Thurm C, Gay J, Berry JG. Home health care utilization in children with Medicaid. *Pediatrics.* 2022;149(2): e2021050534. PubMed doi: 10.1542/peds.2021-050534
23. Kuo DZ, Cohen E, Agrawal R, Berry JG, Casey PH. A national profile of caregiver challenges among more medically complex children with special health care needs. *Arch Pediatr Adolesc Med.* 2011; 165(11):1020–1026. PubMed doi: 10.1001/archpediatrics.2011.172
24. Edelstein H, Schippke J, Sheffe S, Kingsnorth S. Children with medical complexity: a scoping review of interventions to support caregiver stress. *Child Care Health Dev.* 2017;43(3):323–333. PubMed doi: 10.1111/cch.12430
25. Ming DY, Jones KA, White MJ, et al. Healthcare utilization for Medicaid-insured children with medical complexity: differences by sociodemographic characteristics. *Matern Child Health J.* 2022;26(12):2407–2418. PubMed doi: 10.1007/s10995-022-03543-x
26. Berry JG, Harris D, Coller RJ, et al. The interwoven nature of medical and social complexity in US children. *JAMA Pediatr.* 2020; 174(9):891–893. PubMed doi: 10.1001/jamapediatrics.2020.0280
27. Kuo DZ, Goudie A, Cohen E, et al. Inequities in health care needs for children with medical complexity. *Health Aff (Millwood).* 2014; 33(12):2190–2198. PubMed doi: 10.1377/hlthaff.2014.0273
28. Simpser E, Hudak ML, Okun AL, et al; SECTION ON HOME CARE, COMMITTEE ON CHILD HEALTH FINANCING. Financing of pediatric home health care [reaffirmed June 2022]. *Pediatrics.* 2017; 139(3):e20164202. PubMed doi: 10.1542/peds.2016-4202
29. Marchand V, Motil KJ; NASPGHAN Committee on Nutrition. Nutrition support for neurologically impaired children: a clinical report of the North American Society for Pediatric Gastroenterology, Hepatology, and Nutrition. *J Pediatr Gastroenterol Nutr.* 2006;43(1):123–135. PubMed doi: 10.1097/01.mpg.0000228124.93841.ea
30. Cirillo DM, Hart SK, Reich RR, Mason TM. Height measures: evaluating alternatives to standing height in the ambulatory setting. *Clin J Oncol Nurs.* 2018;22(5):529–533. PubMed doi: 10.1188/18.CJON.529-533
31. Romano C, van Wynckel M, Hulst J, et al. European Society for Paediatric Gastroenterology, Hepatology and Nutrition guidelines for the evaluation and treatment of gastrointestinal and nutritional complications in children with neurological impairment. *J Pediatr Gastroenterol Nutr.* 2017;65(2):242–264. PubMed doi: 10.1097/MPG.0000000000001646
32. Sarvas E, Webb J, Landrigan-Ossar M, et al; SECTION ON ORAL HEALTH; COUNCIL ON CHILDREN WITH DISABILITIES; SECTION ON ANESTHESIOLOGY AND PAIN MEDICINE. Council on Children With Disabilities; Section on Anesthesiology and Pain Medicine. Oral health care for children and youth with developmental disabilities: Clinical report. *Pediatrics.* 2024;154(2):e2024067603. PubMed doi: 10.1542/peds.2024-067603
33. Marpole R, Blackmore AM, Gibson N, Cooper MS, Langdon K, Wilson AC. Evaluation and management of respiratory illness in children with cerebral palsy. *Front Pediatr.* 2020;8:333. PubMed doi: 10.3389/fped.2020.00333
34. Sterni LM, Collaco JM, Baker CD, et al; ATS Pediatric Chronic Home Ventilation Workgroup. An official American Thoracic Society clinical practice guideline: Pediatric chronic home invasive ventilation. *Am J Respir Crit Care Med.* 2016;193(8):e16–e35. PubMed doi: 10.1164/rccm.201602-0276ST
35. Feinstein JA, Friedman H, Orth LE, et al. Complexity of medication regimens for children with neurological impairment. *JAMA Netw Open.* 2021;4(8):e2122818–e2122818. PubMed doi: 10.1001/jamanetworkopen.2021.22818
36. Feinstein JA, Feudtner C, Kempe A. Adverse drug event-related emergency department visits associated with complex chronic conditions. *Pediatrics.* 2014;133(6):e1575–e1585. PubMed doi: 10.1542/peds.2013-3060
37. Delmore B, Deppisch M, Sylvia C, Luna-Anderson C, Nie AM. Pressure injuries in the pediatric population: a national pressure ulcer advisory panel white paper. *Adv Skin Wound Care.* 2019; 32(9):394–408. PubMed doi: 10.1097/01.ASW.0000577124.58253.66

38. Freundlich K. Pressure injuries in medically complex children: a review. *Children (Basel)*. 2017;4(4):25. PubMed doi: 10.3390/children4040025

39. Weber DR. Bone health in childhood chronic disease. *Endocrinol Metab Clin North Am*. 2020;49(4):637–650. PubMed doi: 10.1016/j.ecl.2020.07.002

40. Hauer J, Houtrow AJ, Feudtner C, et al; SECTION ON HOSPICE AND PALLIATIVE MEDICINE, COUNCIL ON CHILDREN WITH DISABILITIES. Pain assessment and treatment in children with significant impairment of the central nervous system [reaffirmed November 2021]. *Pediatrics*. 2017;139(6):e20171002. PubMed doi: 10.1542/peds.2017-1002

41. Malviya S, Voepel-Lewis T, Burke C, Merkel S, Tait AR. The revised FLACC observational pain tool: improved reliability and validity for pain assessment in children with cognitive impairment. *Paediatr Anaesth*. 2006;16(3):258–265. PubMed doi: 10.1111/j.1460-9592.2005.01773.x

42. Solodiuk JC, Scott-Sutherland J, Meyers M, et al. Validation of the Individualized Numeric Rating Scale (INRS): a pain assessment tool for nonverbal children with intellectual disability. *Pain*. 2010;150(2):231–236. PubMed doi: 10.1016/j.pain.2010.03.016

43. Schwantes S, O'Brien HW. Pediatric palliative care for children with complex chronic medical conditions. *Pediatr Clin North Am*. 2014;61(4):797–821. PubMed doi: 10.1016/j.pcl.2014.04.011

44. Morse BL, Solodiuk JC, Greco CD, Mauskar S, Hauer J. Initial validation of GRASP: a differential diagnoses algorithm for children with medical complexity and an unknown source of pain. *Hosp Pediatr*. 2020;10(8):633–640. PubMed doi: 10.1542/hpeds.2019-0322

45. Vasan A, Kyle MA, Venkataramani AS, Kenyon CC, Fiks AG. Inequities in time spent coordinating care for children and youth with special health care needs. *Acad Pediatr*. 2023;23(8):1526–1534. PubMed doi: 10.1016/j.acap.2023.03.002

46. Hoover CG, Coller RJ, Houtrow A, Harris D, Agrawal R, Turchi R. Understanding caregiving and caregivers: supporting children and youth with special health care needs at home. *Acad Pediatr*. 2022;22(2S):S14–S21. PubMed doi: 10.1016/j.acap.2021.10.007

47. Carter K, Blakely C, Zuk J, Brittan M, Foster C. Employing family caregivers: an innovative health care model. *Pediatrics*. 2022;149(6):e2021054273. PubMed doi: 10.1542/peds.2021-054273

48. HarnEnz Z, Vermilion P, Foster-Barber A, Treat L; HarnEnz Z. Vermilion P, Foster-Barber A, Treat L. Pediatric neuropalliative care. *Handb Clin Neurol*. 2023;191:157–184. doi: 10.1016/B978-0-12-824535-4.00015-X

49. Henderson CM, Boss RD. Establishing goals of care in serious and complex pediatric illness. *Pediatr Clin North Am*. 2024;71(1):71–82. PubMed doi: 10.1016/j.pcl.2023.08.008

50. Kaye EC, Rubenstein J, Levine D, Baker JN, Dabbs D, Friebert SE. Pediatric palliative care in the community. *CA Cancer J Clin*. 2015;65(4):316–333. PubMed doi: 10.3322/caac.21280

51. Yu JA, Schenker Y, Maurer SH, Cook SC, Kavlieratos D, Houtrow A. Pediatric palliative care in the medical neighborhood for children with medical complexity. *Fam Syst Health*. 2019;37(2):107–119. PubMed doi: 10.1037/fsh0000414

52. Teicher J, Moore C, Esser K, et al. The experience of parental caregiving for children with medical complexity. *Clin Pediatr (Phila)*. 2023;62(6):633–644. PubMed doi: 10.1177/00099228221142102

53. Bogetz JF, Munjapara V, Henderson CM, et al. Home mechanical ventilation for children with severe neurological impairment: Parents' perspectives on clinician counselling. *Dev Med Child Neurol*. 2022;64(7):840–846. PubMed doi: 10.1111/dmcn.15151

54. O' Brien I, Duffy A, Nicholl H. Impact of childhood chronic illnesses on siblings: a literature review. *Br J Nurs*. 2009;18(22):1358–1365, 1360–1365. PubMed doi: 10.12968/bjon.2009.18.22.45562

55. Frankel H, Matiz LA, Friedman S. Siblings of children with medical complexity—a vulnerable population in the medical home. *J Health Care Poor Underserved*. 2022;33(2):702–713. PubMed doi: 10.1353/hpu.2022.0057

56. Azzopardi C, Cohen E, Pépin K, Netten K, Birken C, Madigan S. Child welfare system involvement among children with medical complexity. *Child Maltreat*. 2022;27(2):257–266. PubMed doi: 10.1177/10775595211029713

57. Legano LA, Desch LW, Messner SA, et al; COUNCIL ON CHILD ABUSE AND NEGLECT; COUNCIL ON CHILDREN WITH DISABILITIES. Maltreatment of children with disabilities. *Pediatrics*. 2021;147(5):e2021050920. PubMed doi: 10.1542/peds.2021-050920

58. Duby JC; American Academy of Pediatrics Council on Children With Disabilities. Role of the medical home in family-centered early intervention services. *Pediatrics*. 2007;120(5):1153–1158. PubMed doi: 10.1542/peds.2007-2638

59. Lipkin PH, Okamoto J, Norwood KW Jr, et al; Council on Children with Disabilities; Council on School Health. The Individuals With Disabilities Education Act (IDEA) for children with special educational needs [reaffirmed October 2019; new reaffirmation pending and will update prior to publication]. *Pediatrics*. 2015;136(6):e1650–e1662. PubMed doi: 10.1542/peds.2015-3409

60. Houtrow A, Murphy N, Kuo DZ, et al; COUNCIL ON CHILDREN WITH DISABILITIES. Prescribing physical, occupational, and speech therapy services for children with disabilities [reaffirmed July 2023]. *Pediatrics*. 2019;143(4):e20190285. PubMed doi: 10.1542/peds.2019-0285

61. Adams RC, Tapia C, Murphy NA, et al; Council on children with disabilities. Early intervention, IDEA Part C services, and the medical home: collaboration for best practice and best outcomes [reaffirmed April 2024]. *Pediatrics*. 2013;132(4):e1073–e1088. PubMed doi: 10.1542/peds.2013-2305

62. Carbone PS, Smith PJ, Lewis C, LeBlanc C; American Academy of Pediatrics, Council on Children With Disabilities, Council on Sports Medicine and Fitness. Promoting the participation of children and adolescents with disabilities in sports, recreation, and physical activity. *Pediatrics*. 2021;148(6):e2021054664. PubMed doi: 10.1542/peds.2021-054664

63. Pordes E, Gordon J, Sanders LM, Cohen E. Models of care delivery for children with medical complexity. *Pediatrics*. 2018;141(suppl 3):S212–S223. PubMed doi: 10.1542/peds.2017-1284F

64. Hoffman A, Larson IA. Primary care preparation for children with medical complexity for emergency encounters in the community. *Pediatr Ann.* 2018;47(3):e102–e105. PubMed doi: 10.3928/19382359-20180221-02

65. Hammer NM, Bidstrup PE, Brok J, et al. Home-based specialized pediatric palliative care: a systematic review and meta-analysis. *J Pain Symptom Manage.* 2023;65(4):e353–e368. PubMed doi: 10.1016/j.jpainsymman.2022.12.139

66. Bertrand A, Veyet V, Goy F, Cervos M, Schell M. Pediatric palliative care at home by Home Care Unit: how home nurses feel? *Support Care Cancer.* 2022;30(3):2091–2099. PubMed doi: 10.1007/s00520-021-06623-w

67. Bower KA, Lau M, Short R, Lawrence S, Beauchamp-Walters J, Marc-Aurele K. Impact of home-based pediatric palliative care on hospital and emergency department utilization at a single institution. *J Palliat Med.* 2022;25(2):301–306. PubMed doi: 10.1089/jpm.2021.0307

68. Huth K, Newman L, Glader L. Core curricular priorities in the care of children with medical complexity: a North American modified Delphi study. *Acad Pediatr.* 2020;20(4):558–564. PubMed doi: 10.1016/j.acap.2020.01.014

69. Houtrow AJ, Garcia AM, Edinger J, Akamagwuna U. Disability competent care in pediatric milestones. *JAMA Pediatr.* 2024;178(8):835–837. PubMed doi: 10.1001/jamapediatrics.2024.1555

70. Uppal P, Donohue PK, Seltzer RR. Home modifications for children with medical complexity: untapped potential for improving care. *Pediatrics.* 2022;150(6):e2022058346. PubMed doi: 10.1542/peds.2022-058346

71. Notario PM, Gentile E, Amidon M, Angst D, Lefaiver C, Webster K. Home-based telemedicine for children with medical complexity. *Telemed J e-Health.* 2019;25(11):1123–1132. PubMed doi: 10.1089/tmj.2018.0186

72. McKissick HD, Cady RG, Looman WS, Finkelstein SM. The impact of telehealth and care coordination on the number and type of clinical visits for children with medical complexity. *J Pediatr Health Care.* 2017;31(4):452–458. PubMed doi: 10.1016/j.pedhc.2016.11.006

73. Nkoy F, Stone B, Hofmann M, et al. Home-monitoring application for children with medical complexity: a feasibility trial. *Hosp Pediatr.* 2021;11(5):492–502. PubMed doi: 10.1542/hpeds.2020-002097

74. Kaushik R. Telehealth and children with medical complexity. *Pediatr Ann.* 2024;53(3):e74–e81. PubMed doi: 10.3928/19382359-20240109-01

75. Callahan JM, Baldwin S, Bodnar C, et al; COMMITTEE ON PEDIATRIC EMERGENCY MEDICINE; COUNCIL ON CLINICAL INFORMATION TECHNOLOGY; COUNCIL ON CHILDREN AND DISASTERS; AMERICAN COLLEGE OF EMERGENCY PHYSICIANS, PEDIATRIC EMERGENCY MEDICINE COMMITTEE. Council on Clinical Information Technology; Council on Children and Disasters; American College of Emergency Physicians, Pediatric Emergency Medicine Committee. Access to critical health information for children during emergencies: emergency information forms and beyond. *Pediatrics.* 2023;151(3):e2022060970. PubMed doi: 10.1542/peds.2022-060970

76. Lin E, Scharbach K, Liu B, et al. A multidisciplinary home visiting program for children with medical complexity. *Hosp Pediatr.* 2020;10(11):925–931. PubMed doi: 10.1542/hpeds.2020-0093

77. Schiff J, Manning L, VanLandeghem K, Langer CS, Schutze M, Comeau M. Financing care for CYSHCN in the next decade: reducing burden, advancing equity, and transforming systems. *Pediatrics.* 2022;149(suppl 7):e2021056150I. PubMed doi: 10.1542/peds.2021-056150I

78. Foster CC, Agrawal RK, Davis MM. Home health care for children with medical complexity: workforce gaps, policy, and future directions. *Health Aff (Millwood).* 2019;38(6):987–993. PubMed doi: 10.1377/hlthaff.2018.05531

79. White PH, Cooley WC; TRANSITIONS CLINICAL REPORT AUTHORING GROUP; AMERICAN ACADEMY OF PEDIATRICS; AMERICAN ACADEMY OF FAMILY PHYSICIANS; AMERICAN COLLEGE OF PHYSICIANS. Supporting the Health Care Transition From Adolescence to Adulthood in the Medical Home [published correction in Pediatrics. 2019;143(2):e20183610]. *Pediatrics.* 2018;142(5):e20182587. PubMed doi: 10.1542/peds.2018-2587

80. Turchi RM, Kuo DZ, Rusher JW, et al; COUNCIL ON CHILDREN WITH DISABILITIES; COMMITTEE ON MEDICAL LIABILITY AND RISK MANAGEMENT. Committee on Medical Liability and Risk Management. Considerations for alternative decision-making when transitioning to adulthood for youth with intellectual and developmental disabilities: policy statement. *Pediatrics.* 2024;153(6):e2024066841. PubMed doi: 10.1542/peds.2024-066841

81. Ziemann M, Salsberg E, McManus M, White P, Schmidt A. *Strengthening the Adult Primary Care Workforce to Support Young Adults with Medical Complexity Transitioning to Adult Health Care.* Fitzhugh Mullan Institute for Health Workforce Equity, George Washington University; 2023. Accessed December 10, 2024. https://www.gwhwi.org/uploads/4/3/3/5/43358451/yamc_workforce_final_report_may2023__05.02.23_.pdf

82. Nageswaran S, Sebesta MR, Golden SL. Transitioning children with medical complexity from hospital to home health care: implications for hospital-based clinicians. *Hosp Pediatr.* 2020;10(8):657–662. PubMed doi: 10.1542/hpeds.2020-0068

83. O'Neil J, Hoffman B, Agran PF, et al; COUNCIL ON INJURY, VIOLENCE, AND POISON PREVENTION. Transporting children with special health care needs. *Pediatrics.* 2019;143(5):e20190724. PubMed doi: 10.1542/peds.2019-0724

84. Edwards JD, Panitch HB, Nelson JE, Miller RL, Morris MC. Decisions for long-term ventilation for children. Perspectives of family members. *Ann Am Thorac Soc.* 2020;17(1):72–80. PubMed doi: 10.1513/AnnalsATS.201903-271OC

85. Seear M, Kapur A, Wensley D, Morrison K, Behroozi A. The quality of life of home-ventilated children and their primary caregivers plus the associated social and economic burdens: a prospective study. *Arch Dis Child.* 2016;101(7):620–627. PubMed doi: 10.1136/archdischild-2015-309796

86. Seltzer RR, Thompson BS, Feudtner C. The daunting problem of medical complexity and housing instability. *Pediatrics.* 2020;146(1):e20193284. PubMed doi: 10.1542/peds.2019-3284

87. Foster CC, Steltzer M, Snyder A, et al. Integrated multimodality telemedicine to enhance in-home care of infants during the interstage period. *Pediatr Cardiol.* 2021;42(2):349–360. PubMed doi: 10.1007/s00246-020-02489-7

88. Houtrow A, Martin AJ, Harris D, et al. Health equity for children and youth with special health care needs: a vision for the future. *Pediatrics.* 2022;149(suppl 7):e2021056150F. PubMed doi: 10.1542/peds.2021-056150F

89. Gillen JK, Morris MC. Preparing families of technology-dependent children for emergencies. *Hosp Pediatr.* 2019;9(11):874–879. PubMed doi: 10.1542/hpeds.2019-0091

90. Sobotka SA, Foster C, Lynch E, Hird-McCorry L, Goodman DM. Attributable delay of discharge for children with long-term mechanical ventilation. *J Pediatr.* 2019;212:166–171. PubMed doi: 10.1016/j.jpeds.2019.04.034

91. Maynard R, Christensen E, Cady R, et al. Home health care availability and discharge delays in children with medical complexity. *Pediatrics.* 2019;143(1):e20181951. PubMed doi: 10.1542/peds.2018-1951

92. Weaver MS, Wichman B, Bace S, et al. Measuring the impact of the home health nursing shortage on family caregivers of children receiving palliative care. *J Hosp Palliat Nurs.* 2018;20(3):260–265. PubMed doi: 10.1097/NJH.0000000000000436

93. Sneed RC, May WL, Stencel C. Policy versus practice: comparison of prescribing therapy and durable medical equipment in medical and educational settings. *Pediatrics.* 2004;114(5):e612–e625. PubMed doi: 10.1542/peds.2004-1063

94. Wise PH. The future pediatrician: the challenge of chronic illness. *J Pediatr.* 2007;151(5)(suppl):S6–S10. PubMed doi: 10.1016/j.jpeds.2007.08.013

95. Kind AJH, Smith MA. Advances in patient safety documentation of mandated discharge summary components in transitions from acute to subacute care. In: Henriksen K, Battles JB, Keyes MA, Grady ML, eds. *Advances in Patient Safety: New Directions and Alternative Approaches (Vol 2: Culture and Redesign).* Agency for Healthcare Research and Quality (US); 2008.

96. Larrow A, Doshi A, Fisher E, et al. Empowering pediatric palliative homecare patients and caregivers with symptom management plans. *J Pain Symptom Manage.* 2022;64(4):340–348. PubMed doi: 10.1016/j.jpainsymman.2022.06.015

97. Kuo DZ, Comeau M, Perrin JM, et al. Moving from spending to investment: a research agenda for improving health care financing for children and youth with special health care needs. *Acad Pediatr.* 2022;22(2S):S47–S53. PubMed doi: 10.1016/j.acap.2021.11.009

98. Foster CC, Chorniy A, Kwon S, Kan K, Heard-Garris N, Davis MM. Children with special health care needs and forgone family employment. *Pediatrics.* 2021;148(3):e2020035378. PubMed doi: 10.1542/peds.2020-035378

99. Council on Children With Disabilities. From the American Academy of Pediatrics: Policy statements–Supplemental Security Income (SSI) for children and youth with disabilities [reaffirmed February 2015, reaffirmed August 2021]. *Pediatrics.* 2009;124(6):1702–1708. PubMed doi: 10.1542/peds.2009-2557

100. Brittan MS, Chavez C, Blakely C, Holliman BD, Zuk J. Paid family caregiving for children with medical complexity. *Pediatrics.* 2023;151(6):e2022060198. PubMed doi: 10.1542/peds.2022-060198

101. Foster CC, Kwon S, Whitlow L, et al. Connecting hospital to home: characteristics of and rehospitalization rates in hospitalized children with private-duty nursing. *Hosp Pediatr.* 2019;9(7):530–537. PubMed doi: 10.1542/hpeds.2018-0282

102. Nkoy F, Stone B, Sheng X, Murphy N. High parental concern in children with medical complexity: an early indicator of illness. *Hosp Pediatr.* 2023;13(3):250–257. PubMed doi: 10.1542/hpeds.2022-006876

Human Trafficking and Exploitation of Children and Adolescents

- *Policy Statement*

POLICY STATEMENT Organizational Principles to Guide and Define the Child Health Care System and/or Improve the Health of All Children

American Academy of Pediatrics

DEDICATED TO THE HEALTH OF ALL CHILDREN™

Human Trafficking and Exploitation of Children and Adolescents: Policy Statement

Jordan Greenbaum, MD,[1] Dana Kaplan, MD,[2] Nia Bodrick, MD, MPH,[3] the Council on Child Abuse and Neglect; and the Section on Global Health

abstract

Trafficking of children and adolescents for labor and sexual exploitation is associated with significant adverse physical and mental health implications. Pediatricians and other health care professionals may encounter affected patients who present with infections, injuries, posttraumatic stress disorder, suicidality, or a variety of other health and mental health conditions. The health sector response requires a public health approach based on scientific research using an equity and social justice lens, community participatory strategies, and rigorous study designs, including implementation science, which build a solid evidence base. It should include training for pediatric clinicians (eg, pediatricians, other physicians, and nonphysician clinicians treating children and adolescents) to recognize possible signs of exploitation and to intervene using a culturally responsive, community-centered, sensitive, trauma-informed, rights-based, and patient-centered approach. The health sector response should include a multidisciplinary approach to the provision of service, with clinicians working with a diverse group of professionals in the community to assist children and adolescents at risk for trafficking and exploitation. Advocacy is needed for legislation and policies that promote child rights and victim/survivor services for all children and adolescents, regardless of immigration status. The health sector should support policies that address the social drivers of health, which influence the vulnerability to human trafficking. This policy statement outlines major issues regarding public policy, medical education, research, and collaboration in the area of child labor and sex trafficking/exploitation and provides recommendations for future work.

[1]International Centre for Missing and Exploited Children, Alexandria, Virginia; [2]Division of Child Abuse and Neglect, Department of Pediatrics, Staten Island University Hospital, Staten Island, New York; and [3]Division of General and Community Pediatrics, Children's National Hospital, Washington, District of Columbia

Address correspondence to: Jordan Greenbaum, MD.
Email: vg5893@hotmail.com

All authors contributed to the writing and editing of the document.

CONFLICT OF INTEREST DISCLOSURE: The authors have indicated they do not have a financial relationship relevant to this article to disclose.

To cite: Greenbaum J, Kaplan D, and Bodrick N; American Academy of Pediatrics, the Council on Child Abuse and Neglect; Section on Global Health. Human Trafficking and Exploitation of Children and Adolescents: Policy Statement. *Pediatrics.* 2025;156(1):e2025072214

INTRODUCTION

Children and adolescents experiencing trafficking in human beings and exploitation (THB/E) for labor and/or sex routinely are deprived of their rights to basic needs, including health, dignity, respect, and safety from violence and exploitation, as outlined in the United Nations Convention on the Rights of the Child.[1] In this policy statement, the term "children and adolescents" is used to describe individuals younger than 18 years, although many national and international terms refer to this age group as "child/children") (eg, "child trafficking"). Although laws and conventions[2,3] may restrict the definition of "child" to those younger than 18 years, many issues and recommendations outlined in this statement also apply to young adults.

Child labor exploitation occurs when a child is treated unfairly in the context of work[4]; labor trafficking occurs when a person uses force, fraud, or coercion to compel the minor to work.[3] Child labor THB/E in the United States (US) occurs in various industries,[5,6] including domestic servitude, construction, forced peddling settings (eg, door-to-door magazine sales), illicit activities, agriculture, health and beauty services, and hotel and restaurant businesses.[7–15] Common settings outside the US include begging, fishing, domestic work, manufacturing, and armed conflict.[16–19]

According to US federal law, child sex trafficking involves commercial sex acts (sexual activity for which there is an exchange of something of value) with individuals younger than 18 years.[3,20] Demonstration of force, fraud, or coercion is unnecessary, as is the movement of trafficked persons across borders. The commercial sexual exploitation of children (CSEC) is closely related, involving "crimes of a sexual nature committed against juvenile victims for financial or other economic reasons...."[21] CSEC may occur online/offline, may involve transactional sex, may include monetary enticement, and may occur in the context of business travel and tourism. It also includes cases of mail-order-bride trade/early forced marriage, production of child sexual abuse material (CSAM, formerly called "child pornography"), live-stream sexual acts (wherein an online buyer directs the child to engage in sexual activities in real time, in front of a webcam), and performing in sexual venues.[21] Image-based sexual abuse and exploitation of children (IBSEAC)[22] includes production of sexual images by adults, peers, and victims with nonconsensual or consensual (but illegal) distribution. It includes "sextortion" (inducing an individual to send sexual images/videos, then blackmailing them for money or other items of value).[23]

Major methodologic challenges hinder child THB/E prevalence estimates, as do the relative scarcity of robust antitrafficking ecosystems that can identify impacted individuals, and the paucity of validated screening tools for special populations.[7,21,24,25] The International Labour Organization estimated that more than 3.3 million children and adolescents were involved in forced labor globally in 2021 (including 1.9 million in CSEC).[17] Accurate statistics on the US prevalence of child THB/E are similarly challenging.[26] Four recent studies of runaway and homeless youth suggest that rates of sex trafficking range from 6.5% to 25.8%, whereas labor trafficking ranges from 4.6% to 54.2%.[27–30] In 2021, the National Human Trafficking Resource Center (NHTRC) hotline received reports of 10 360 unique cases (incidents) of potential THB/E, including 136 possible child labor trafficking cases and 2078 possible sex trafficking cases.[31] This likely represents a small portion of US THB/E. In a nationally representative sample of young adults (18–28 years), prevalence rates of online commercial sexual exploitation and sextortion were 1.7% and 3.5%, respectively.[32] Girls, transgender and gender-fluid youth had higher rates than cisgender males; 13- to 17-year-olds were at highest risk.

The United States is a "destination" country for THB/E, and statistics from 2021 indicate that the leading "origin" countries for federally identified victims (all ages, all types of trafficking) were the United States, Mexico, and Honduras.[33] The production of CSAM is a vast global phenomenon: the internet Watch Foundation identified 255 588 URLs (webpages) containing CSAM or links to images in 2022, originating from countries worldwide.[34]

Factors at the individual, community, and societal levels contribute to THB/E vulnerability globally[17] (see Table 1). Children in the custody of government child welfare agencies, notably in the United States, are at increased risk, which may be partially related to co-existence of other risk factors such as a history of sexual abuse, and family dysfunction.[9,53] Attitudes and practices that marginalize populations (eg, systemic racism, colonialization, and xenophobia) limit economic and social opportunities, restrict health care access, condone persecution, and increase the risk of THB/E.[17,33,35,36,54–61]

Massive population displacement often involves children and adolescents, including unaccompanied minors (UMs).[59,60,62] Individuals and families may flee war, community or familial violence, persecution, poverty, natural disasters, or other major crises. UMs are at significant risk for THB/E,[17,61,63] given their age, absence of adult supervision, lack of knowledge pertaining to host language/culture, need to repay debt or support family, and precarious legal status.[6,15,64]

Global pandemics, as observed during the COVID-19 pandemic of 2020, increase the risk for THB/E, especially involving those already at risk for exploitation.[37,38,65–68] Increases in unemployment, poverty, homelessness, and illness or death of caregivers contribute to THB/E vulnerability.[33,64,69–75]

Access to the internet continues to expand. As of 2019, 95% of US children 3 to 18 years old had home internet access.[76] COVID-19 led to increased use in response to social isolation requirements.[77] Concurrently, exploiters use the internet to recruit, groom, sexually abuse[78–80] and extort,[81,82] produce/distribute CSAM,[72] manage THB/E

TABLE 1. Factors Contributing to Vulnerability to Child Trafficking[5–9,19,30,35–52]

Individual	Family	Community	Societal
2SLGBTQIA+ identifying	Poverty	Tolerance of sexual/labor exploitation	Gender-based violence and discrimination
Abuse/neglect	Unemployment	Weather-related and geophysical disasters	Cultural beliefs/stigma that facilitate marginalization, systemic discrimination
Sexual exploitation	Intrafamilial violence and dysfunction	Community violence	Weak recognition of child rights, labor rights, weak labor governance
Substance misuse	Forced migration	Community upheaval	Political/social upheaval
Homeless/runaway/thrown out of home	Intolerance of 2SLGBTQIA+ identifying	Lack of community resources/ support	Pandemics
Untreated mental health conditions	Family health needs	Lack of awareness of trafficking practices	Global climate change
Behavioral problems	Undocumented immigration status		Attitudes that condone labor exploitation/ trafficking (eg, focus on cheap material goods and cheap labor)
Involvement with legal system			Glorification of child commercial sexual exploitation
Involvement with child protective services system (especially foster care)			
Lack of documentation (immigration, birth certificate, etc)			
Unaccompanied status, including immigrant and refugee children and adolescents			
Member of group facing discrimination (eg, AI/AN/I, 2SLGBTQIA+, BIPOC)			
Presence of disability			

2SLGBTQIA+ indicates two-spirit, lesbian, gay, bisexual, transgender, queer and/or questioning, intersex, asexual, or other; AI/AN/I, American Indian/Alaska Native/Indigenous; BIPOC, Black, Indigenous, and people of color.

financial transactions,[33] and arrange live-stream sex acts for global buyers.[83] Resources on internet safety, including legal protections, are widely available (AAP's Center of Excellence on Social Media and Youth Mental Health),[84,85] although outcome/impact studies are needed.[84,85]

Global climate change may increase THB/E vulnerability.[39,40,86–88] Drought, sudden storms, flooding, and slow-onset coastline erosion may drive agriculturally dependent families to migrate, exposing children and adolescents to the risk of THB/E as described earlier.[17,60] In 2020, weather events displaced 30 million individuals.[40] Massive individual losses and demand for cheap labor accompany severe weather events and lay a foundation for THB/E.[40,89,90]

Although evidence suggests that legal residents experiencing sex THB/E in the United States are likely to seek medical attention during their period of exploitation,[91,92] those without legal documentation and individuals trafficked in foreign countries around the world (US citizens and others) may have limited access to health care.[93,94] It is important for pediatric clinicians in any country to appropriately recognize and respond to THB/E (see AAP clinical report on labor and sex trafficking).[41]

Increasingly, THB/E is being viewed through a public health lens focusing on, raising public awareness,[95] prevention, identification of risk and protective factors, resilience and recovery, rigorous scientific research, and development of a multidisciplinary response.[54,75,96–104] Pediatric clinicians play a critical role in advocating for public health efforts to combat and prevent THB/E.[105]

EXISTING FRAMEWORK

Current Legislation

In the United States, THB/E involves the criminal justice and child protective systems at federal and state levels. The Trafficking Victims Protection Act (TVPA) of 2000,[3] recognizes THB/E as a federal crime and offers protection; multiple reauthorizations have expanded its scope.[106–108] In the 2008 William Wilberforce Trafficking Victims Protection Reauthorization Act (TVPRA),[106] special provisions were added to protect unaccompanied minor migrant children. These include mandatory screening for possible THB/E and persecution in the home country. To date, all 50 states and the District of Columbia have passed legislation making THB/E a felony offense. Information on these and related laws is available from the AAP Committee on State Government Affairs as well as Shared Hope International.

Foreign national children and adolescents in the United States who are identified as having experienced THB/E may be eligible for various special visas that allow them to remain temporarily in the United States and receive federal assistance. Health professionals may refer patients who they suspect have experienced THB/E to the Office of Trafficking in Persons (https://www.acf.hhs.gov/otip/victim-assistance/child-eligibility-letters/request-assistance). Referrals to pro-bono immigration attorneys or organizations providing immigration legal assistance are also helpful.

The 2014 Preventing Sex Trafficking and Strengthening Families Act (Pub L No. 113–183) requires that state child welfare agencies develop procedures to identify and serve individuals under their care or supervision who may have experienced THB/E. The Justice for Victims of Trafficking Act of 2015[20] requires that states include sex THB/E in their definitions of child abuse, although not all states have laws requiring mandatory reporting when the alleged perpetrator of sex THB/E is not the parent/caregiver. Criminal sanctions were additionally expanded to include persons who patronize/solicit individuals younger than 18 years for commercial sex acts. The Act provides federal grant incentives for states to pass comprehensive Safe Harbor Laws to eliminate a punitive approach to individuals who engaged in illegal activity related to their exploitation, and to instead provide immunity, diversion, and/or mandatory referral for services.[109]

The United Nations Convention on the Rights of the Child (UNCRC) safeguards children from violence, exploitation, and abuse. Although the United States signed the agreement in 1995, it is the only nation not to ratify it, endorsing the principles without legal commitment.[1] Opponents of ratification assert that the Convention conflicts with some US laws regarding privacy and family rights, that it is an ineffective mechanism for protecting child rights, and that it undermines US sovereignty.[110] The AAP commits to advocate for policies that conform to the principles of the United Nations Convention on the Rights of the Child and supports US ratification.

HEALTH SECTOR ROLE IN COMBATTING THB/E

Research continues to demonstrate the need for clinician training for recognition and care of patients who experience THB/E.[111–113] In a study of pediatric clinicians at an academic children's hospital, 62.8% of participants reported they had never received education on THB/E. [114] Multiple training curricula are available[115–120] however, outcomes research is needed.[118,121–123]

An AAP clinical report on child THB/E provides detailed information on the trauma-informed health care response,[41] and online training is available.[124] A set of core competencies for a THB/E response in health care/behavioral health systems provides further guidance to professionals, health care organizations, and training programs.[125] Of critical importance is the need to protect patient privacy and safety when documenting sensitive information in the medical record. Individuals who have experienced THB/E have valid concerns regarding potential access to the record by traffickers, caregivers and others who may harm the patient, and they may also fear staff bias and discrimination by those discovering stigmatizing data such as substance misuse, commercial sexual exploitation and undocumented immigration status. Strategies to protect patient privacy and promote safety include granular metadata and segmentation that is incorporated into all facets of the EHR, and clinician transparency with patients regarding information to be included in the record. A thorough discussion of the privacy and confidentiality issues associated with THB/E and guidance regarding documentation of sensitive patient information is available.[126–128] Comprehensive clinical guidelines on pediatric THB/E are critical[41,125] and resources exist to help clinicians and health administrators design tailored clinical protocols for their organizations.[129–131]

Pediatric THB/E screening tools specifically designed for health settings are limited, especially for young children, and lack validation for individuals with significant intellectual disabilities, migrant populations, or American Indian/Alaska Native/Indigenous (AI/AN/I) patients. Most do not screen for labor THB/E.[132–135] Universal education and resource strategies tend to focus on sexual and domestic violence.[136,137] The development of validated, brief, trauma-informed screening tools and universal education resources addressing all forms of THB/E are needed across diverse at-risk populations.

Prevention initiatives for THB/E can encompass various strategies including promoting healthy and safe relationships, child sexual abuse prevention, internet safety, and providing information on THB/E, labor rights, and risk reduction.[103–105,137–140] The AAP *Bright Futures: Guidelines for Health Supervision of Infants, Children, and Adolescents* includes anticipatory guidance recommendations for patients from newborn infants to 21 years of age.[141] However, these recommendations do not provide specific guidance on THB/E. There is relatively limited evaluation of THB/E prevention efforts,[142] and outcomes research is needed. Consideration should be given to integrating THB/E prevention into existing, evidence-based child sexual abuse prevention programs.[139]

RESEARCH

Evidence-based research on THB/E remains relatively limited[143] with an overall low level of rigor.[144] Large gaps exist, particularly regarding special subpopulations; the impact of cultural beliefs/practices; biases/systemic racism and colonialism as they impact individuals of color; exploitation of child migrants; and child labor trafficking. Evaluation studies of treatment models are also lacking.[101,144,145]

The vast majority of THB/E research is focused on cisgender female individuals and on people experiencing sex trafficking.[146] Many studies on THB/E publish aggregate results for adults and children/adolescents,[147–149] male and female individuals,[150] or individuals from multiple countries of origin.[71] Some merge individuals victimized by various forms of THB/E.[91] Aggregated data may preclude identification of findings specific to children and adolescents or subpopulations.

The limited[42,151–154] research on male individuals experiencing THB/E may indirectly reinforce societal beliefs that boys cannot be victimized, exacerbate the under recognition of exploitation and restricted services for this population,[155] and fuel the tendency to treat males as offenders rather than as individuals needing services.[156]

Research remains limited regarding the THB/E experiences of individuals identifying as 2SLGBTQIA+, although their increased risk of abuse, violence, homelessness, and exploitation has been documented.[28,67,157,158] Research exploring similarities and differences in the experiences and health needs of specific populations of 2SLGBTQIA+ individuals is needed.

Our knowledge of the prevalence of THB/E, risk factors, experiences and related needs of affected AI/AN/I children and adolescents is minimal.[35,159,160] Sexual exploitation is associated with oil rigging sites, uranium mines and with casinos on AI/AN/I tribal territory.[159,161,162] A national inquiry into missing and murdered Indigenous women and girls in Canada emphasizes the need to focus on vulnerabilities and needs of AI/AN/I children and adolescents as well as protective factors that are critical in designing culturally relevant prevention and intervention efforts.[163]

Labor THB/E has not received the same public attention as sex THB/E[164] and there is a dearth of research in the United States.[6,10] Researching child employment, child labor, hazardous child labor, forced child labor, and trafficking is challenging due to subtleties of identifying and differentiating between these phenomena.[165]

Systemic racism, deeply held implicit biases, the effects of colonialism, and widespread social and health inequities increase risk for THB/E in BIPOC populations and hinder access to assistance for those experiencing THB/E.[35,54,166] Research is needed to elucidate conditions that condone and promote continued discrimination and to facilitate positive cultural change.

Burgeoning research of online child sexual exploitation includes studies on risk, prevalence, offender characteristics, and prevention.[22,32,81,167,168] Studies published by nongovernmental organizations (eg, "gray literature") supplement research published in peer-reviewed journals.[158,169,170]

EXTERNAL COLLABORATION

Multidisciplinary collaboration in the investigation and treatment of child abuse has become the standard in the United States,[171–173] and similar collaborations are evolving globally.[174,175] These collaborations involve work with other health professionals as well as professionals from legal, child welfare, education, law enforcement, immigration, and victim/survivor services. However, pediatric clinicians seeking to report cases and obtain services for patients often lack knowledge of available community partners or The National Human Trafficking Resource Center (1-888-373-7888),[112,176,177] and education is needed.[178]

CONCLUSIONS

Major issues exist regarding public policy, medical education, research, and collaboration in the areas of child THB/E. There are needs for victim/survivor advocacy; increased victim/survivor services; training for health professionals; and research on THB/E.

RECOMMENDATIONS

The following recommendations apply to AAP chapters and to all individual health care professionals serving children and adolescents, including but not limited to physicians, nurses, advanced practice clinicians, dentists, behavioral health professionals, social workers, and trainees in these fields.

Public Policy

1. The AAP advocates for prevention of THB/E and respect for fundamental children's rights.
2. Support relevant state, federal, and global anti-trafficking policies that address the following

Access to Services, Including Health Care

- Increase equitable access to direct services for all children and adolescents impacted by THB/E (online and offline), regardless of immigration status, race/ethnicity, abilities, gender identity, etc.
- Increase interagency collaboration.
- Improve THB/E screening and universal education in health care settings.
- Provide continuous financial coverage for physical and mental health expenses for individuals impacted by THB/E regardless of immigration status.[179]
- Increase availability of pediatric examiners trained in THB/E and trauma-informed care, especially in rural areas.
- Ensure access to family planning and reproductive health services irrespective of immigration status, promoting harm reduction strategies for those experiencing THB/E.
- Advocate for 2SLGBTQIA+ children, adolescents, and adults who experience THB/E, ensuring access to physical and psychosocial health services to all.
- Increase protection and assistance to migrant children and adolescents during[164,180] and after migration; increase access to free/low-cost medical homes; expand post-release services for unaccompanied minors (UMs),

facilitate screening, and improve access to immigration legal services.[181]

Child Labor

- Combat child labor THB/E globally.[17] This includes legislation, international treaties, memoranda of understanding, and other agreements to:
  - protect children and adolescents in all occupational sectors;
  - ensure monitoring and enforcement of child labor laws;
  - train labor inspectors to detect and respond to labor violations that may represent THB/E;
  - promote fair and ethical recruitment of adults and children for employment;
  - ensure respect for the rights of all migrants regardless of immigration status;
  - incorporate THB/E prevention, recognition, and response measures into all levels of humanitarian crisis responses and disaster risk reduction strategies[182];
  - require industries to take appropriate measures to ensure that all workers are protected from adverse health and safety consequences;
  - improve data collection regarding national and global child labor THB/E.

Risk and Prevention

- Support efforts to address social drivers of health and economic factors linked to vulnerability factors for THB/E.
- Support legislation addressing systemic racism and bias/discrimination against populations.[36]
- Address climate change and its impact on children's vulnerability to THB/E.
- Facilitate primary prevention of child THB/E through education of children and adolescents, caregivers, child welfare professionals, and clinicians. These efforts should be informed by rigorous research incorporating the views of young people.[183,184] Include school programs and extend efforts to reach nonattenders. Explore opportunities to integrate internet safety and THB/E prevention into evidence-based programs on healthy relationships.[32,139]

Legal Protection

- Protect individuals <18 years who have experienced any type of THB/E from prosecution for related offenses, emphasizing treatment and services.
- Prevent detention of migrant children and adolescents and separation from their families, as this increases the vulnerability to THB/E.
- Increase legal access to cross-border migration so UMs and families do not need to rely on smugglers.

3. Facilitate a public health approach to THB/E[102] that embraces culturally responsive, rights-based, trauma-informed, and child-centered care.[41]

Medical Education

1. Advocate for:
   A. Standardized pediatric clinician training on THB/E, including:
      - Prevention, recognition, assessment, treatment, follow-up and referral for community services.[125]
      - A trauma-informed, culturally responsive, and rights-based approach[41];
      - Awareness of THB/E involving caregivers, young adults, and specific high-risk populations.
      - Guidance on identifying referral pathways to immigration attorneys and organizations that assist foreign-born patients with obtaining visas and benefits.
      - Use of strategies to address social drivers of health and connecting patients to community resources.
      - Advocate for patient-informed and appropriate documentation of sensitive health information and use of THB/E ICD-10 codes in the health record in ways that protect the safety and privacy of patients.[126,127,185] This includes granular metadata and segmentation that is incorporated into all facets of the record, and age-appropriate transparency with patients regarding who may have access to sensitive information. Patients should be empowered to make decisions regarding data documentation, while ensuring safe and appropriate ongoing care, and adherence to existing laws and policies.[128]
      - Education mitigating implicit/explicit bias and discrimination at individual and systemic levels.[186,187]

   B. Provide timely medical education on THB/E at the trainee level.

   C. Promote financial support, development, and global dissemination of culturally appropriate, trauma-informed curricula and clinical management guidance for pediatric clinicians addressing THB/E.

Research

1. Advocate for research addressing:
   - THB/E prevalence;
   - Protective and resilience factors;
   - The intersection of THB/E with specific populations (eg, males, 2SLGBTQIA+ individuals, individuals with disabilities, those in the custody of the state, etc);
   - Effective implementation of trauma-informed care into a busy health care setting[188];
   - Effectiveness of telehealth encounters in identifying/screening for THB/E;

- Impact of:
  - telehealth resources on service provision;
  - prevention initiatives, screening tools and universal education resources, and harm reduction strategies;
  - integration/reintegration services.

2. Facilitate research using an equity lens, rigorous designs including implementation science, and community-based strategies informed by individuals with lived experience.[143,144]
3. Advocate for centralized surveillance and data collection on THB/E using clearly operationalized definitions.

Collaboration

1. Advocate for pediatric clinicians to join community multidisciplinary teams combating THB/E, educating team members about survivors' health needs and facilitating services to enhance the well-being of trafficked persons.
2. Encourage pediatric clinicians to promote public awareness of THB/E and advocate for increased service provision. This may involve supporting education initiatives, advocating for anti-trafficking legislation, and working with the media to counteract inaccurate representations that sensationalize and stereotype human trafficking.
3. Advocate for pediatric clinicians to identify local service providers and establish "warm hand-off" referral mechanisms, aiding patients in contacting referral organizations before leaving the health facility. Pediatric clinicians in small practices may collaborate with local/state task forces, the National Human Trafficking Resource Center (1-888-3737-888), or nongovernmental organizations (eg, International Organization for Migration) in areas where there is an absence of community partnerships.
4. Advocate for trauma-informed, patient-centered, and culturally responsive health care to recognize and respond to suspected THB/E.

LEAD AUTHORS

Jordan Greenbaum, MD
Dana Kaplan, MD, FAAP
Nia Bodrick, MD, MPH, FAAP

ACKNOWLEDGMENTS

The authors would like to thank Hanni Stoklosa, MD, MPH, HEAL Trafficking, Harvard Medical School, for her input and review of the policy statement.

ABBREVIATIONS

THB/E: trafficking in human beings and exploitation
CSAM: child sexual abuse materials
AAP: American Academy of Pediatrics
ACE: adverse childhood experience
BIPOC: Black, Indigenous, and other people of color
AI/AN/I: American Indian/Alaska Native/Indigenous
HEAL (Trafficking): Health, Education, Advocacy & Linkage
IBCSAE: image-based child sexual abuse/exploitation
ICD: International Classification of Diseases

2SLGBTQIA+: two-spirit, lesbian, gay, bisexual, transgender, queer and/or questioning, intersex, asexual, or other

PATH: Physicians Against the Trafficking of Humans
TVPA: Trafficking Victims Protection Act

FUNDING: No external funding.

Accepted for Publication Date: April 25, 2025

https://doi.org/10.1542/peds.2025-072214

REFERENCES

1. United Nations. Human Rights, Office of the High Commissioner for Human Rights. Convention on the Rights of the Child. 1990. Accessed April 14, 2024. https://www.ohchr.org/en/instruments-mechanisms/instruments/convention-rights-child
2. United Nations. Protocol to prevent, suppress and punish trafficking in persons especially women and children, supplementing the United Nations convention against transnational organized crime. 2000. Accessed April 14, 2024. https://www.ohchr.org/en/instruments-mechanisms/instruments/protocol-prevent-suppress-and-punish-trafficking-persons
3. Trafficking Victims Protection Act. Pub L No 106–386 (2000). 22 USC 78. Accessed December 30, 2019. https://uscode.house.gov/view.xhtml?path=/prelim@title22/chapter78&edition=prelim
4. Oxford Languages and Google. Definition of 'exploitation'. Accessed October 12, 2022. https://www.google.com/search?q=definition+of+exploitation&rlz=1C1CHBF_enUS978US978&oq=definition+of+exploitation&aqs=chrome.69i57j0i512l6j0i22i30l2j0i15i22i30.4128j1j7&sourceid=chrome&ie=UTF-8
5. Kaufka Walts K. Child labor trafficking in the United States: a hidden crime. *Soc Incl (Lisboa)*. 2017;5(2):59–68. doi: 10.17645/si.v5i2.914.
6. Farrell A, Dank M, Kaufka Walts K, Hansson C, Hughes A, Neal C. Understanding the trafficking of children for the purposes of labor in the United States. 2024. Accessed May 4, 2024. https://www.ojp.gov/pdffiles1/nij/grants/308903.pdf
7. Letsie NC, Lul B, Roe-Sepowitz D. An eight-year analysis of child labor trafficking cases in the United States: Exploring characteristics, and patterns of child labor trafficking. *Child Abuse Negl*. 2021;121(1):105265. PubMed doi: 10.1016/j.chiabu.2021.105265
8. Gibbs DA, Aboul-Hosn S, Kluckman MN. Child labor trafficking within the US: a first look at allegations investigated by Florida's child welfare agency. *J Hum Traffick*. 2020;6(4):435–449. doi: 10.1080/23322705.2019.1594551.
9. Gibbs DA, Henninger AM, Tueller SJ, Kluckman MN. Human trafficking and the child welfare population in Florida. *Child Youth Serv Rev*. 2018;88:1–10. doi: 10.1016/j.childyouth.2018.02.045.
10. Greenbaum J, Sprang G, Recknor F, Harper NS, Titchen K. Labor trafficking of children and youth in the United States: A scoping review. *Child Abuse Negl*. 2022;131:105694. PubMed doi: 10.1016/j.chiabu.2022.105694
11. Hopper EK, Gonzalez LD. A comparison of psychological symptoms in survivors of sex and labor trafficking. *Behav Med*. 2018;44(3):177–188. PubMed doi: 10.1080/08964289.2018.1432551
12. Koegler E, Howland W, Gibbons P, Teti M, Stoklosa H. "When her visa expired, the family refused to renew it," intersections of human trafficking and domestic violence: qualitative document analysis of case examples from a major Midwest city. *J Interpers Violence*. 2022;37(7–8):NP4133–NP4159. PubMed doi: 10.1177/0886260520957978
13. Koegler E, Mohl A, Preble K, Teti M. Reports and victims of sex and labor trafficking in a major Midwest metropolitan area, 2008–2017. *Public Health Rep*. 2019;134(4):432–440. PubMed doi: 10.1177/0033354919854479
14. Márquez YI, Deblinger E, Dovi AT. The value of trauma-focused cognitive behavioral therapy (TF-CBT) in addressing the therapeutic needs of trafficked youth: a case study. *Cogn Behav Pract*. 2020;27(3):253–269. doi: 10.1016/j.cbpra.2019.10.001.
15. National Human Trafficking Resource Center. Child Labor Trafficking in the United States. 2015. Accessed April 23, 2025. https://cwlibrary.childwelfare.gov/permalink/01CWIG_INST/10a03se/alma991000865979707651
16. Cockbain E, Bowers K. Human trafficking for sex, labour and domestic servitude: how do key trafficking types compare and what are their predictors? *Crime Law Soc Change*. 2019;72(1):9–34. doi: 10.1007/s10611-019-09836-7.
17. International Labour Organization, Walk Free, International Organization for Migration. *Global Estimates of Modern Slavery: Forced Labour and Forced Marriage*. International Labour Organization; 2022.
18. Polaris. Landscape Analysis: Human Trafficking for the Purpose of Labor Exploitation in Mexico. 2018. Accessed October 13, 2022. https://polarisproject.org/resources/landscape-analysis-human-trafficking-for-the-purpose-of-labor-exploitation-in-mexico/
19. UNICEF. Children recruited by armed forces or armed groups. 2021. Accessed October 13, 2022. https://www.unicef.org/protection/children-recruited-by-armed-forces

20. US Government. Justice for Victims of Trafficking Act of 2015. Pub L No. 114–22. Accessed on July 15, 2023. https://www.congress.gov/114/plaws/publ22/PLAW-114publ22.pdf

21. Institute of Medicine, National Research Council. *Confronting Commercial Sexual Exploitation and Sex Trafficking of Minors in the United States*. National Academies Press; 2013.

22. Finkelhor D, Turner H, Colburn D, Mitchell K, Mathews B. Child sexual abuse images and youth produced images: The varieties of Image-based Sexual Exploitation and Abuse of Children. *Child Abuse Negl*. 2023;143:106269. PubMed doi: 10.1016/j.chiabu.2023.106269

23. Patchin JW, Hinduja S. Sextortion among adolescents: results from a national survey of U.S. youth. *Sex Abuse*. 2020;32(1): 30–54. PubMed doi: 10.1177/1079063218800469

24. Stransky M, Finkelhor D. *How Many Juveniles are Involved in Prostitution in the U.S.?* Crimes Against Children Research Center, University of New Hampshire; 2008.

25. Schroeder E, Edgemon TG, Aletraris L, Kagotho N, Clay-Warner J, Okech D. A review of prevalence estimation methods with human trafficking populations. *Public Health Rep*. 2022;137(1_suppl) (suppl):46S–52S. PubMed doi: 10.1177/00333549211044010

26. Franchino-Olsen H, Chesworth BR, Boyle C, et al. The prevalence of sex trafficking of children and adolescents in the United States: a scoping review. *Trauma Violence Abuse*. 2022;23(1):182–195. PubMed doi: 10.1177/1524838020933873

27. Chisolm-Straker M, Singer E, Rothman EF, et al. Building RAFT: trafficking screening tool derivation and validation methods. *Acad Emerg Med*. 2020;27(4):297–304. PubMed doi: 10.1111/acem.13888

28. Greeson JKP, Treglia D, Wolfe DS, Wasch S. Prevalence and correlates of sex trafficking among homeless and runaway youths presenting for shelter services. *Soc Work Res*. 2019;43(2):91–100. doi: 10.1093/swr/svz001.

29. Mostajabian S, Santa Maria D, Wiemann C, Newlin E, Bocchini C. Identifying sexual and labor exploitation among sheltered youth experincing homelessness: a comparison of screening methods. *Int J Environ Res Public Health*. 2019;16(3):363–378. PubMed doi: 10.3390/ijerph16030363

30. Wright ER, LaBoy A, Tsukerman K, et al. The prevalence and correlates of labor and sex trafficking in a community sample of youth experiencing homelessness in Metro-Atlanta. *Soc Sci*. 2021;10(2):32. doi: 10.3390/socsci10020032.

31. National Human Trafficking Hotline Data Report: 1/1/2021-12/31/2021. Accessed April 10, 2024. https://polarisproject.org/wp-content/uploads/2020/07/Polaris-Analysis-of-2021-Data-from-the-National-Human-Trafficking-Hotline.pdf

32. Finkelhor D, Turner H, Colburn D. Prevalence of online sexual offenses against children in the US. *JAMA Netw Open*. 2022;5(10): e2234471. PubMed doi: 10.1001/jamanetworkopen.2022.34471

33. US Department of State. Trafficking in Persons Report: July 2022. 2022. Accessed July 22, 2022. https://www.state.gov/reports/2022-trafficking-in-persons-report/

34. Internet Watch Foundation. Annual Report: 2022. Accessed on April 10, 2024. https://annualreport2022.iwf.org.uk/

35. Farley M, Deer S, Golding JM, et al. The prostitution and trafficking of American Indian/Alaska Native women in Minnesota. *Am Indian Alsk Native Ment Health Res*. 2016;23(1):65–104. PubMed doi: 10.5820/aian.2301.2016.65

36. Chang KSG, Tsang S, Chisolm-Straker M. Child trafficking and exploitation: Historical roots, preventive policies, and the Pediatrician's role. *Curr Probl Pediatr Adolesc Health Care*. 2022;52(3):101167. PubMed doi: 10.1016/j.cppeds.2022.101167

37. United Nations Office on Drugs and Crime. Impact of the Covid-19 pandemic on trafficking in persons: Preliminary findings and messaging based on rapid stocktaking. 2020. Accessed December 21, 2020. https://www.un.org/ruleoflaw/wp-content/uploads/2020/05/Thematic-Brief-on-COVID-19-EN-ver.21.pdf

38. Peterman A, Potts A, O'Donnell M, et al. Pandemics and violence against women and children: Working paper 528. 2020. Accessed December 21, 2020. Available at: https://www.cgdev.org/publication/pandemics-and-violence-against-women-and-children

39. Sheu JC, Torres MIM, Gordon MR, Nguyen PT, Coverdale JH. Potential impact of climate change on human trafficking: a narrative review. *J Nerv Ment Dis*. 2021;209(5):324–329. PubMed doi: 10.1097/nmd.0000000000001312

40. Internal Displacement Monitoring Centre. Global report on internal displacement; Grid 2021: Internal displacement in a changing climate. 2021. Accessed October 15, 2022. https://www.internal-displacement.org/global-report/grid2021/

41. Greenbaum J, Kaplan D, Young J; COUNCIL ON CHILD ABUSE AND NEGLECT; COUNCIL ON IMMIGRANT CHILD AND FAMILY HEALTH. Clinical report: Exploitation, labor and sex trafficking of children and adolescents: health care needs of patients. *Pediatrics*. 2023; 151(1):e2022060416. PubMed doi: 10.1542/peds.2022-060416

42. Saewyc EM, Shankar S, Pearce LA, Smith A. Challenging the stereotypes: unexpected features of sexual exploitation among homeless and street-involved boys in western Canada. *Int J Environ Res Public Health*. 2021;18(11):5898. PubMed doi: 10.3390/ijerph18115898

43. Hornor G, Hollar J, Landers T, Sherfield J. Healthcare use and case characteristics of commercial sexual exploitation of children: teen victims versus high-risk teens. *J Forensic Nurs*. 2023;19(3): 160–169. PubMed doi: 10.1097/jfn.0000000000000402

44. Kafafian M, de Vries I, Farrell A, Goldfarb S, Bouchard E. Understanding factors associated with re-referral of youth for commercial sexual exploitation. *Child Abuse Negl*. 2021;117: 105092. PubMed doi: 10.1016/j.chiabu.2021.105092

45. Gezie LD, Yalew AW, Gete YK, Samkange-Zeeb F. Exploring factors that contribute to human trafficking in Ethiopia: a socio-ecological perspective. *Global Health*. 2021;17(1):76. PubMed doi: 10.1186/s12992-021-00725-0

46. Wood LCN. Child modern slavery, trafficking and health: a practical review of factors contributing to children's vulnerability and the potential impacts of severe exploitation on health. *BMJ Paediatr Open*. 2020;4(1):e000327. PubMed doi: 10.1136/bmjpo-2018-000327

47. Dank M, Yahner J, Madden K, et al. *Surviving the Streets of New York: Experiences of LGBTQ Youth, YMSM, YWSW Engaged in Survival Sex.* Urban Institute; 2015.

48. Greenbaum J. Child labor and sex trafficking. *Pediatr Rev.* 2021; 42(12):639–654. PubMed doi: 10.1542/pir.2020-001396

49. Franchino-Olsen H, Martin SL, Halpern CT, Preisser JS, Zimmer C, Shanahan M. Adolescent experiences of violence victimizations among minors who exchange sex/experience minor sex trafficking. *J Interpers Violence.* 2022;37(17–18):NP16277–NP16301. PubMed doi: 10.1177/08862605211021967

50. Reid JA. Sex Trafficking of girls with intellectual disabilities: an exploratory mixed methods study. *Sex Abuse.* 2018;30(2): 107–131. PubMed doi: 10.1177/1079063216630981

51. Kiss L, Fotheringhame D, Kyegombe N, et al. Paper: violence, abuse and exploitation among trafficked women and girls: a mixed-methods study in Nigeria and Uganda. *BMC Public Health.* 2022; 22(1):794. PubMed doi: 10.1186/s12889-022-13021-2

52. Fortuna LR, Porche MV. Upholding the human rights and well-being of refugee children through effective clinical care. *Child Adolesc Psychiatr Clin N Am.* 2024;33(2):111–124. a International Centre for Missing and Exploited Children, Alexandria, Virginia b Division of Child Abuse and Neglect, Department of Pediatrics, Staten Island University Hospital, Staten Island, New York c Division of General and Community Pediatrics, Children's National Hospital, Washington, District of Columbia. PubMed doi: 10.1016/j.chc.2023.09.003

53. Greeson JKP, Treglia D, Wolfe DS, Wasch S, Gelles RJ. Child welfare characteristics in a sample of youth involved in commercial sex: An exploratory study. *Child Abuse Negl.* 2019;94:104038. PubMed doi: 10.1016/j.chiabu.2019.104038

54. Cook MC, Le PD, García JJ. Addressing racism in the domestic minor sex trafficking of black girls: the role of public health critical race praxis. *Public Health Rep.* 2022;137(1_suppl) (suppl):10S–16S. PubMed doi: 10.1177/00333549211058735

55. Stepanikova I, Oates GR. Perceived discrimination and privilege in health care: the role of socioeconomic status and race. *Am J Prev Med.* 2017;52(1S1)(suppl 1):S86–S94. PubMed doi: 10.1016/j.amepre.2016.09.024

56. Pierce AS. Shattered hearts (full report): The commercial sexual exploitation of American Indian women and girls in Minnesota. *First Annual Interdisciplinary Conference on Human Trafficking.* 2009. Accessed February 25, 2020. https://digitalcommons.unl.edu/humtraffconf/26/

57. Buller AM, Pichon M, McAlpine A, Cislaghi B, Heise L, Meiksin R. Systematic review of social norms, attitudes, and factual beliefs linked to the sexual exploitation of children and adolescents. *Child Abuse Negl.* 2020;104:104471. PubMed doi: 10.1016/j.chiabu.2020.104471

58. Fehrenbacker AE, Musto J, Hoefinger H, et al. Transgender people and human trafficking: intersectional exclusion of transgender migrants and people of color from anti-trafficking protection in the United States. *J Hum Traffick.* 2020;6(4):182–194. doi: http://dx.doi.org/10.1080/23322705.2020.1690116

59. United Nations High Commissioner for Refugees. Children on the run: Unaccompanied children leaving Central America and Mexico and the need for international protection. 2014. Accessed April 14, 2024. https://www.unhcr.org/us/children-run#:~:text=UNHCR's%20latest%20report%2C%20Children%20on,recommendations%20for%20a%20way%20forward

60. Garin E, Beise J, Hug L, You D. UNICEF. Uprooted: The growing crisis for refugee and migrant children. Accessed April 14, 2024. https://data.unicef.org/resources/uprooted-growing-crisis-refugee-migrant-children/

61. US Senate, Permanent Subcommittee on Investigations, Committee on Homeland Security and Government Affairs. Protecting Unaccompanied Alien Children from Trafficking and Other Abuses: The Role of the Office of Refugee Resettlement. 2016. Accessed May 17, 2021. https://www.hsgac.senate.gov/imo/media/doc/Majority%20&%20Minority%20Staff%20Report%20-%20Protecting%20Unaccompanied%20Alien%20Children%20from%20Trafficking%20and%20Other%20Abuses%202016-01-282.pdf

62. International Centre for Migration Policy Development. Targeting vulnerabilities: the impact of the Syrian war and refugee situation on trafficking in persons: A study of Syria, Turkey, Lebanon, Jordan and Iraq. 2015. Accessed March 17, 2022. https://respect.international/wp-content/uploads/2021/07/Targeting-Vulnerabilities-The-Impact-of-the-Syrian-War-and-Refugee-Situation-on-Trafficking-in-Persons-Briefing-Paper.pdf

63. Chester H, Lummert N, Mullooly A. Child victims of human trafficking: Outcomes and service adaptation within the U.S. Unaccompanied Refugee Minor programs. 2015. Accessed April 23, 2025. https://www.usccb.org/offices/anti-trafficking-program/child-victims-human-trafficking

64. International Labour Organization, United Nations Children's Fund. COVID-19 and Child Labour: A Time of Crisis, A Time to Act. 2020. Accessed April 23, 2025. https://www.ilo.org/publications/covid-19-and-child-labour-time-crisis-time-act

65. Ratzan SC, Kimball S, Rauh L, Sommariva S. *CUNY New York City Covid-19 Survey Week 2.* 2020. Accessed April 23, 2025. https://sph.cuny.edu/life-at-sph/news/2020/03/23/covid-19-survey-week-2/

66. Tai DBG, Shah A, Doubeni CA, Sia IG, Wieland ML. The disproportionate impact of COVID-19 on racial and ethnic minorities in the United States. *Clin Infect Dis.* 2021;72(4):703–706. PubMed doi: 10.1093/cid/ciaa815

67. Hogan KA, Roe-Sepowitz D. LGBTQ+ homeless young adults and sex trafficking vulnerability. *J Hum Traffick.* 2023;9:63–78. doi: 10.1080/23322705.2020.1841985.

68. Human Rights Campaign Foundation. The lives and livelihoods of many in the LGBTQ+ community are at risk amidst Covid-19 crisis. 2020. Accessed October 14, 2022. https://www.hrc.org/resources/the-lives-and-livelihoods-of-many-in-the-lgbtq-community-are-at-risk-amidst-covid-19-crisis

69. Todres J, Diaz A. COVID-19 and Human trafficking-the amplified impact on vulnerable populations. *JAMA Pediatr.* 2021;175(2): 123–124. PubMed doi: 10.1001/jamapediatrics.2020.3610

70. UNICEF. WePROTECT Global Alliance, World Health Organization, United Nations Office on Drugs and Crime, World Childhood

Foundation, et al. Covid-19 and its implications for protecting children online. 2020. Accessed April 14, 2024. https://wwwend-violenceorg/sites/default/files/paragraphs/download/COVID-19%20and%20its%20implications%20for%20protecting%20children%20online_Final%20%28003%29pdf

71. Europol. Exploiting isolation: Offenders and victims of online child sexual abuse during the Covid-19 pandemic: June 19, 2020. Accessed April 14, 2024. https://www.europol.europa.eu/publications-events/publications/exploiting-isolation-offenders-and-victims-of-online-child-sexual-abuse-during-covid-19-pandemic

72. Interpol. Threats and trends: Child sexual exploitation and abuse: Covid-19 impact. 2020. Accessed November 10, 2020. https://www.interpol.int/content/download/15611/file/COVID19%20-%20Child%20Sexual%20Exploitation%20and%20Abuse%20threats%20and%20trends.pdf

73. Office for Democratic Institutions and Human Rights. UN Women. Guidance: Addressing emerging human trafficking trends and consequences of the Covid-19 pandemic. Accessed August 28, 2020. https://www.osce.org/files/f/documents/2/a/458434_3.pdf

74. Rojanaworarit C, El Bouzaidi S. International labour trafficking: A neglected social origin of COVID-19. *Lancet Reg Health West Pac.* 2021;8:100121. PubMed doi: 10.1016/j.lanwpc.2021.100121

75. Greenbaum J, Stoklosa H, Murphy L. The public health impact of Coronavirus disease on human trafficking. *Front Public Health.* 2020;8:561184. PubMed doi: 10.3389/fpubh.2020.561184

76. National Center for Education Statistics. Children's internet access at home. U.S. Department of Education, Institute of Education Sciences. Accessed October 14, 2022. https://nces.ed.gov/programs/coe/indicator/cch/home-internet-access

77. McClain C, Vogels EA, Perrin A, Sechopoulos S, Rainie L; PEW Research Center. The internet and the pandemic. 2021. Accessed October 15, 2022. https://www.pewresearch.org/internet/2021/09/01/the-internet-and-the-pandemic/

78. Ly T, Murphy L, Fedoroff JP. Understanding online child sexual exploitation offenses. *Curr Psychiatry Rep.* 2016;18(8):74. PubMed doi: 10.1007/s11920-016-0707-0

79. Merdian HL, Moghaddam N, Boer DP, et al. Fantasy-driven versus contact-driven users of child sexual exploitation material: offender classification and implications for their risk assessment. *Sex Abuse.* 2018;30(3):230–253. PubMed doi: 10.1177/1079063216641109

80. Teixeira SA, Taquette SR. Violence and unsafe sexual practices in adolescents under 15 years of age. *Rev Assoc Med Bras.* 2010;56(4):440–446. PubMed doi: 10.1590/s0104-42302010000400017

81. Wolak J, Finkelhor D, Walsh W, Treitman L. Sextortion of minors: characteristics and dynamics. *J Adolesc Health.* 2018;62(1):72–79. PubMed doi: 10.1016/j.jadohealth.2017.08.014

82. Hong S, Lu N, Wu D, Jimenez DE, Milanaik RL. Digital sextortion: Internet predators and pediatric interventions. *Curr Opin Pediatr.* 2020;32(1):192–197. PubMed doi: 10.1097/mop.0000000000000854

83. Child Rights Resource Centre. Webcam child sex tourism: Becoming Sweetie: A novel approach to stopping the global rise of webcam child sex tourism. Terre des hommes; 2013. Accessed April 14, 2024. https://resourcecentre.savethechildren.net/document/webcam-child-sex-tourism-becoming-sweetie-novel-approach-stopping-global-rise-webcam-child/

84. King G, Bui T, Dedeaux J, Ahlers-Schmidt CR, Harris K. Trends in internet safety education by healthcare providers. *Kans J Med.* 2021;14(3):273–276. PubMed doi: 10.17161/kjm.vol14.14805

85. American Academy of Pediatrics. Center of excellence on social media and youth mental health. 2024. Accessed April 10, 2024. Available at https://www.aap.org/en/patient-care/media-and-children/center-of-excellence-on-social-media-and-youth-mental-health/

86. Uddin R, Philipsborn R, Smith D, Mutic A, Thompson LM. A global child health perspective on climate change, migration and human rights. *Curr Probl Pediatr Adolesc Health Care.* 2021;51(6):101029. PubMed doi: 10.1016/j.cppeds.2021.101029

87. Coverdale J, Balon R, Beresin EV, et al. Climate change: a call to action for the psychiatric profession. *Acad Psychiatry.* 2018;42(3):317–323. PubMed doi: 10.1007/s40596-018-0885-7

88. Intergovernmental Panel on Climate Change. Climate change 2022: Mitigtion of climate change. Accessed October 17, 2022. https://www.ipcc.ch/report/ar6/wg3/

89. Geissler R. Hurricanes & human trafficking: Natural disasters highlight the vulnerability of America's farm workers. Human Trafficking Institute; 2022. Accessed October 14, 2022. https://traffickinginstitute.org/hurricanes-human-trafficking-natural-disasters-highlight-the-vulnerability-of-americas-farm-workers/

90. Hepburn S, Simon RJ. Hidden in plain sight: Human trafficking in the United States. *Gend Issues.* 2010;27:1–26. doi: 10.1007/s12147-010-9087-7.

91. Baldwin S, Eisenman D, Sayles J, Ryan G, Chang K. Identification of human trafficking victims in health care settings. *Health and Human Rights,* Harvard University; 2011. Accessed September 21, 2013. https://www.hhrjournal.org/2013/08/20/identification-of-human-trafficking-victims-in-health-care-setting/

92. Lederer L, Wetzel C. The health consequences of sex trafficking and their implications for identifying victims in healthcare facilities. *Ann Health Law.* 2014;23:61–91.

93. Albright K, Greenbaum J, Edwards SA, Tsai C. Systematic review of facilitators of, barriers to, and recommendations for healthcare services for child survivors of human trafficking globally. *Child Abuse Negl.* 2020;100:104289. PubMed doi: 10.1016/j.chiabu.2019.104289

94. Garg A, Panda P, Neudecker M, Lee S. Barriers to the access and utilization of healthcare for trafficked youth: A systematic review. *Child Abuse Negl.* 2020;100:104137. PubMed doi: 10.1016/j.chiabu.2019.104137

95. Houston-Kolnik JD, Soibatian C, Shattell MM. Advocates' experiences with media and the impact of media on human trafficking advocacy. *J Interpers Violence.* 2020;35(5–6):1108–1132. PubMed 10.1177/0886260517692337

96. Robichaux K, Torres MIM. The role of social determinants in caring for trafficked patients: A public health perspective on human trafficking. *Bull Menninger Clin.* 2022;86(suppl A):8–17. PubMed doi: 10.1521/bumc.2022.86.suppA.8

97. Violence Prevention Alliance, World Health Organization. Violence Prevention Alliance. The VPA approach. Accessed April 14, 2024. https://www.who.int/groups/violence-prevention-alliance/approach

98. Greenbaum J. A public health approach to global child sex trafficking. *Annu Rev Public Health.* 2020;41(1):481–497. PubMed doi: 10.1146/annurev-publhealth-040119-094335

99. Forni G, Pietronigro A, Tiwana N, et al. Little red riding hood in the social forest. Online grooming as a public health issue: a narrative review. *Ann Ig.* 2020;32(3):305–318. PubMed doi: 10.7416/ai.2020.2353

100. Such E, Walton E, Bonvoisin T, Stoklosa H. Modern slavery: a global public health concern. *BMJ.* 2019;364:l838. PubMed doi: 10.1136/bmj.l838

101. Rothman EF, Stoklosa H, Baldwin SB, Chisolm-Straker M, Kato Price R, Atkinson HG; HEAL Trafficking. Public health research priorities to address US human trafffficking. *Am J Public Health.* 2017;107(7):1045–1047. PubMed doi: 10.2105/ajph.2017.303858

102. Gallo M, Thinyane H. Sentinel surveillance and centring prevention in anti-trafficking policy and response. *J Modern Slavery.* 2929; 5(1):1–24.

103. Alpert EJ, Chin SE. Human trafficking: perspectives on prevention. In: Chisolm-Straker M, Stoklosa H, eds. *Human Trafficking is a Public Health Issue: A Paradigm Expansion in the Unites States.* Springer; 2017:379–400.

104. Duger A. Focusing on prevention: the social and economic rights of children vulnerable to sex trafficking. *Health Hum Rights.* 2015; 17(1):E114–E123. PubMed

105. Greenbaum VJ, Titchen K, Walker-Descartes I, Feifer A, Rood CJ, Fong HF. Multi-level prevention of human trafficking: The role of health care professionals. *Prev Med.* 2018;114:164–167. PubMed doi: 10.1016/j.ypmed.2018.07.006

106. US Government. William Wilberforce Trafficking Victims Protection Reauthorization Act. Pub L No. 110–457 (2008)

107. US Government. Trafficking Victims Protection Reauthorization Act. Pub L No. 109–164 (2005)

108. US Government. Trafficking Victims Protection Reauthorization Act. Pub L No. 108–193 (2003)

109. Green B, Gies SV, Healy EB, Bobnis A. Safe Harbor Laws: Changing the Legal Response to Minors Involved in Commercial Sex, Phase 3. The *Qualitative Analysis.* Development Services Group Inc; 2019.

110. Congressional Research Service, The United Nations Convention on the Rights of the Child. 2015. Accessed April 11, 2024. https://crsreports.congress.gov/product/pdf/R/R40484/25#:~:text=Bush%20Administrations%20played%20significant%20roles,advice%20and%20consent%20to%20ratification

111. Miller CL, Chisolm-Straker M, Duke G, Stoklosa H. A framework for the development of healthcare provider education programs on human trafficking part three: recommendations. *J Hum Traffick.* 2020;6(4):425–434. 10.1080/23322705.2019.1635342.

112. Bechtel K, Passmore S, Kondis J, Walker Descartes I, Adewusi A, Greenbaum V. Training experiences of emergency department providers in the recognition of child trafficking. *Pediatr Emerg Care.* 2022;38(2):e988–e992. PubMed doi: 10.1097/pec.0000000000002511

113. Nordstrom BM. Multidisciplinary human trafficking education: inpatient and outpatient healthcare settings. *J Hum Traffick.* 2022;8(2):184–194. 10.1080/23322705.2020.1775049.

114. Titchen KE, Kuelbs C, Rhee KE, You H. Physician understanding of youth labor and sex trafficking: a need for training. *J Pediatr Adolesc Gynecol.* 2023;36(2):226–227. 10.1016/j.jpag.2023.01.080.

115. Ahn R, Alpert EJ, Purcell G, et al. Human trafficking: review of educational resources for health professionals. *Am J Prev Med.* 2013; 44(3):283–289. PubMed doi: 10.1016/j.amepre.2012.10.025

116. Talbott JMV, Dutcher JS, Pougnier CA, Calvin SL, Roe-Sepowitz D, Kling JM. Review of published curriculum on sex trafficking for undergraduate medical trainees. *Am J Prev Med.* 2020;58(4): 604–611. PubMed doi: 10.1016/j.amepre.2019.11.013

117. Salami T, Boland G, Hari C, Hegarty I, Williams K. Digital training in the wake of a pandemic: Using technology to train health care professionals in the identification of human trafficking victims. *Bull Menninger Clin.* 2022;86(suppl A):18–33. PubMed doi: 10.1521/bumc.2022.86.suppa.18

118. Lee H, Geynisman-Tan J, Hofer S, Anderson E, Caravan S, Titchen K. The impact of human trafficking training on healthcare professionals' knowledge and attitudes. *J Med Educ Curric Dev.* 2021;8:23821205211016523. PubMed doi: 10.1177/23821205211016523

119. Trafficking HEAL; Laboratory to Combat Human Trafficking. Assessment tool for healthcare provider human trafficking training. 2018. Accessed September 4, 2020. https://healtrafficking.org/2018/12/assessment-tool-for-health-care-provider-human-trafficking-training/

120. HEAL Trafficking Education and Training Committee. Introductory training on human trafficking for U.S. health care professionals: Essential content. 2018. Accessed September 4, 2020. https://healtrafficking.org/wp-content/uploads/2018/04/Essential-Components-for-a-Health-Professional-Trafficking-Training.pdf

121. Powell C, Dickins K, Stoklosa H. Training US health care professionals on human trafficking: where do we go from here? *Med Educ Online.* 2017;22(1):1267980. PubMed doi: 10.1080/10872981.2017.1267980

122. Donahue S, Schwien M, LaVallee D. Educating emergency department staff on the identification and treatment of human trafficking victims. *J Emerg Nurs.* 2019;45(1):16–23. PubMed doi: 10.1016/j.jen.2018.03.021

123. Fraley HE, Aronowitz T, Stoklosa HM. Systematic review of human trafficking educational interventions for health care providers. *West J Nurs Res.* 2020;42(2):131–142. PubMed doi: 10.1177/0193945919837366

124. National Human Trafficking Training and Technical Assistance Center. SOAR Online training. Administration for Children and Families, Office on Trafficking in Persons; 2023. Accessed July 22, 2023. https://nhttac.acf.hhs.gov/soar/soar-for-individuals/soar-online

125. National Human Trafficking Training and Technical Assistance Center, US Department of Health and Human Services. HEAL Trafficking, International Centre for Missing and Exploited Children, National Association of Pediatric Nurse Practitioners. Core competencies for human trafficking response in health care and behavioral health systems. 2021. Accessed January 13, 2025. https://www.napnap.org/wp-content/uploads/CoreCompetencies_Infographic_FINAL-508-Complete.pdf

126. Greenbaum J, Garrett A, Chon K, Bishop M, Luke J, Stoklosa H. Principles for safe implementation of ICD codes for human trafficking. *J Law Med Ethics.* 2021;49(2):285–289. PubMed doi: 10.1017/jme.2021.40

127. Greenbaum J, McClure RC, Stare S, et al. Documenting ICD codes and other sensitive information in electronic health records: guidelines for healthcare professionals who encounter patients with a history of human trafficking or other forms of violence. 2021. Accessed March 27, 2021. https://www.icmec.org/healthportal-resources/topic/research-and-resources-child-sexual-abuse-exploitation-and-trafficking/guidelines-protocols-for-child-sexual-abuse-exploitation-trafficking/

128. Dufendach KR, Lehmann CU, Spooner SA; COUNCIL ON CLINICAL INFORMATION TECHNOLOGY. Special requirements of electronic health record systems in pediatrics: Clinical report. *Pediatrics.* 2024;154(4):e2024068509. PubMed doi: 10.1542/peds.2024-068509

129. International Centre for Missing and Exploited Children. Human Trafficking Toolkit. 2022. Accessed August 18, 2022. https://www.icmec.org/healthportal-resources/topic/human-trafficking-toolkit/

130. Trafficking HEAL. Hope for Justice. HEAL Trafficking and Hope for Justice's Protocol Toolkit for Developing a Response to Victims of Human Trafficking in Health Care Settings. Accessed March 8, 2022. https://www.healtrafficking.org/resources/protocol-toolkit

131. International Centre for Missing and Exploited Children. A 'how-to' guide to develop a healthcare protcol for responding to child trafficking/exploitation. Accessed April 14, 2024. https://www.icmec.org/healthportal-resources/topic/research-and-resources-child-sexual-abuse-exploitation-and-trafficking/resources-to-accompany-the-e-learning-course-a-how-to-guide-to-develop-healthcare-protocol-for-responding-to-child-trafficking/

132. Chang KSG, Lee K, Park T, Sy E, Quach T. Using a clinic-based screening tool for primary care providers to identify commercially sexually exploited children. *J Appl Res Child.* 2015;6(1):6. doi: 10.58464/2155-5834.1235.

133. Greenbaum VJ, Dodd M, McCracken C. A short screening tool to identify victims of child sex trafficking in the health care setting. *Pediatr Emerg Care.* 2018;34(1):33–37. PubMed doi: 10.1097/pec.0000000000000602

134. Hurst IA, Abdoo DC, Harpin S, Leonard J, Adelgais K. Confidential screening for sex trafficking among minors in a pediatric emergency department. *Pediatrics.* 2021;147(3):e2020013235. PubMed doi: 10.1542/peds.2020-013235

135. Kaltiso SO, Greenbaum VJ, Agarwal M, et al. Evaluation of a screening tool for child sex trafficking among patients with high-risk chief complaints in a pediatric emergency department. *Acad Emerg Med.* 2018;25(11):1193–1203. PubMed doi: 10.1111/acem.13497

136. Bair-Merritt MH, Lewis-O'Connor A, Goel S, et al. Primary care-based interventions for intimate partner violence: a systematic review. *Am J Prev Med.* 2014;46(2):188–194. PubMed doi: 10.1016/j.amepre.2013.10.001

137. Futures Without Violence. *Prevent, Assess, and Respond: A Domestic Violence Toolkit for Health Centers and Domestic Violence Programs.* National Health Resource Center on Domestic Violence; 2017.

138. Quayle E. Prevention, disruption and deterrence of online child sexual exploitation and abuse. *ERA Forum.* 2020;21:429–447.

139. Finkelhor D, Walsh K, Jones L, Mitchell K, Collier A. Youth internet safety education: Aligning programs with the evidence base. *Trauma Violence Abuse.* 2021;22(5):1233–1247. PubMed doi: 10.1177/1524838020916257

140. Ybarra ML, Mitchell KJ, Finkelhor D, Wolak J. Internet prevention messages: targeting the right online behaviors. *Arch Pediatr Adolesc Med.* 2007;161(2):138–145. PubMed doi: 10.1001/archpedi.161.2.138

141. Hagan JF, Shaw JS, Duncan PM, eds. *Bright Futures: Guidelines for Health Supervison of Infants, Children, and Adolescents (Pocket Guide).* 4th ed. American Academy of Pediatrics; 2017.

142. Rothman EF, Farrell A, Paruk J, Bright K, Bair-Merritt M, Preis SR. Evaluation of a multi-session group designed to prevent commercial sexual exploitation of minors: the "My Life My Choice" curriculum. *J Interpers Violence.* 2021;36(19–20):9143–9166. PubMed doi: 10.1177/0886260519865972

143. Sprang G, Stoklosa H, Greenbaum J. The public health response to human trafficking: a look back and a step forward. *Public Health Rep.* 2022;137(1_suppl)(suppl):5S–9S. PubMed doi: 10.1177/00333549221085588

144. Kim BE, Dierkhising CB, De Leon J, Sandoval J, Brissett A, Bounds D. Evaluation of services for the commercial sexual exploitation of children and youth: a scoping review. *Trauma Violence Abuse.* 2023;24(5):3236–3250. PubMed doi: 10.1177/15248380221126185

145. Hainaut M, Thompson KJ, Ha CJ, Herzog HL, Roberts T, Ades V. Are screening tools for identifying human trafficking victims in healthcare settings validated? A scoping review. *Public Health Rep.* 2022;137(1_suppl)(suppl):63S–72S. PubMed doi: 10.1177/00333549211061774

146. Oram S, Stöckl H, Busza J, Howard LM, Zimmerman C. Prevalence and risk of violence and the physical, mental, and sexual health problems associated with human trafficking: systematic review. *PLoS Med.* 2012;9(5):e1001224. PubMed doi: 10.1017/s2045796016000135

147. Raymond JG, Hughes DM. Sex Trafficking of Women in the United States: International and Domestic Trends. US Department of Justice; 2001. Accessed April 23, 2025. https://www.ncjrs.gov/pdffiles1/nij/grants/187774.pdf

148. Raphael J, Reichert J, Powers M. Pimp control and violence: domestic sex trafficking of Chicago women and girls. *Women*

Crim Justice. 2010;20(1–2):89–104. doi: 10.1080/089744510036 41065.

149. Zimmerman C, Yun K, Shvab I, Watts C, Trappolin L. *Treppete Mea. The Health Risks and Consequences of Trafficking in Women and Adolescents: Findings from a European Study.* London School of Hygiene and Tropical Medicine; 2003.

150. Turner-Moss E, Zimmerman C, Howard LM, Oram S. Labour exploitation and health: a case series of men and women seeking post-trafficking services. *J Immigr Minor Health*. 2014;16(3):473–480. PubMed doi: 10.1007/s10903-013-9832-6

151. Moss C, Smith SJ, Kim K, et al. A global systematic scoping review of literature on the sexual exploitation of boys. *Child Abuse Negl*. 2023;142(Pt 2):106244. PubMed doi: 10.1016/j.chiabu.2023.106244

152. Moynihan M, Mitchell K, Pitcher C, Havaei F, Ferguson M, Saewyc E. A systematic review of the state of the literature on sexually exploited boys internationally. *Child Abuse Negl*. 2018;76:440–451. PubMed doi: 10.1016/j.chiabu.2017.12.003

153. Hohendorff JV, Habigzang LF, Koller SH. "A boy, being a victim, nobody really buys that, you know?": Dynamics of sexual violence against boys. *Child Abuse Negl*. 2017;70:53–64. PubMed doi: 10. 1016/j.chiabu.2017.05.008

154. Hounmenou C. An initial exploration of prostitution of boys in the West African region. *Child Abuse Negl*. 2017;69:188–200. PubMed doi: 10.1016/j.chiabu.2017.04.027

155. ECPAT USA. And Boys Too: An ECPAT-USA discussion paper about the lack of recognition of the commercial sexual exploitation of boys in the United States. 2013 Accessed April 14, 2024. https://www.wcsap.org/sites/default/files/uploads/webinars/Commercial_Sexual_Exploitation_Boys/And_Boys_Too.pdf

156. Finkelhor D, Ormrod R. Prostitution of juveniles: Patterns from NIBRS. *Juvenile Justice Bulletin*. US Department of Justice; 2004. Accessed March 13, 2021. https://www.researchgate.net/publication/237780561_Prostitution_of_Juveniles_Patterns_From_NIBRS

157. Corliss HL, Goodenow CS, Nichols L, Austin SB. High burden of homelessness among sexual-minority adolescents: findings from a representative Massachusetts high school sample. *Am J Public Health*. 2011;101(9):1683–1689. PubMed doi: 10.2105/ajph.2011. 300155

158. THORN, Benenson Strategy Group. LGBTQ+ youth perspectives: How LGBTQ+ youth are navigating exploration and risks of sexual exploitation online: Findings from 2022 qualitative and quantitative research among 13–20-year-olds. THORN, Benenson Strategy Group; 2023. Accessed April 23, 2025. https://info.thorn.org/hubfs/Research/Thorn_LGBTQ+YouthPerspectives_June2023_FNL.pdf

159. Goodwin GL; US Government Accountability Office. Human Trafficking Investigations in Indian Country or Involving Native Americans and Actions Needed to Better Report on Victims Served. 2017. Accessed November 9, 2023. https://www.gao.gov/assets/gao-17-762t.pdf

160. Kingsley C, Mark M. Sacred Lives: Canadian aboriginal children and youth speak out about sexual explotation. Human Resources Development Canada; 2013. Accessed April 14, 2024. https://publications.gc.ca/site/eng/9.698389/publication.html

161. Sethi A. Domestic sex trafficking of Aboriginal girls in Canada: issues and implications. *First Peoples Child Family Rev.* 2007;3(3): 57–71. Accessed April 23, 2025 https://fpcfr.com/index.php/FPCFR/article/view/50

162. National Indian Gaming Commission, Bureau of Indian Affairs, Department of Homeland Security, Department of Treasury. Human Trafficking Response Guide for the Tribal Gaming and Hospitality Industry. 2023. Accessed November 9, 2023. https://www.dhs.gov/sites/default/files/2024-06/240618_bc_tribal_gaming_hospitality_toolkit.pdf

163. Commision of the National Inquiry Into Missing and Murdered Indigenous Women and Girls. Reclaiming Power and Place: Volume 2: A Supplementary Report. 2019. Accessed November 9, 2023. https://www.mmiwg-ffada.ca/final-report/

164. Walker V. UC Committe for Refugees and Immigrants. Policy brief: Crossing for a future: Children migrating through the Darien Gap. August 8, 2023. Accessed August 9, 2023. https://sway.office.com/jBjEJCKlbBbellVs?ref=email

165. International Labour Office. *Making progress against child labour: Global estimates and trends 2000–2012.* International Programme on the Elimination of Child Labour/International Labour Office; 2013.

166. Chisolm-Straker M. Hisotrical context matters: health research, health care and bodies of color in the United States. In: Chisolm-Straker M, Chon K, eds. *The Historical Roots of Human Trafficking: Informing Primary Prevention of Commercialized Violence*. Springer; 2021:257–278.

167. Greenbaum J, Rood CJ. Human trafficking and sexual exploitation via electronic media. In: Laskey A, Sirotnak A, eds. *Child Abuse: Medical Diagnosis and Management*. 4th ed. American Academy of Pediatrics; 2020:725–764.

168. Wolak J, Finkelhor D. Are crimes by online predators different from crimes by sex offenders who know youth in-person? *J Adolesc Health*. 2013;53(6):736–741. PubMed doi: 10.1016/j.jadohealth.2013.06.010

169. ECPAT. INTERPOL. Towards a Global Indicator on Unidentified Victims in Child Sexual Exploitation Material: Technical Report. 2018. Accessed March 13, 2021. https://www.ecpat.org/wp-content/uploads/2018/02/Technical-Report-TOWARDS-A-GLOBAL-INDICATOR-ON-UNIDENTIFIED-VICTIMS-IN-CHILD-SEXUAL-EXPLOITATION-MATERIAL.pdf

170. THORN. Sextortion: Summary of Findings from a 2017 Survey of 2,097 Survivors. 2019. Accessed June 22, 2023. https://www.thorn.org/wp-content/uploads/2019/12/Sextortion_Wave2Report_121919.pdf

171. Miller A, Rubin D. The contribution of children's advocacy centers to felony prosecutions of child sexual abuse. *Child Abuse Negl*. 2009;33(1):12–18. PubMed doi: 10.1016/j.chiabu.2008.07.002

172. Wolfteich P, Loggins B. Evaluation of the children's advocacy center model: Efficiency, legal and revictimization outcomes. *Child Adolesc Social Work J*. 2007;24:333–352. doi: 10.1007/s10560-007-0087-8.

173. National Children's Alliance website. Accessed April 14, 2024. https://www.nationalchildrensalliance.org/

174. Macias Konstantopoulos WL, Munroe D, Purcell G, Tester K, Burke TF. The commercial sexual exploitation and sex trafficking of minors in the Boston metropolitan area: experiences and challenges faced by front-line providers and other stakeholders. *J Appl Res Child.* 2015;6(1):4. doi: 10.58464/2155-5834.1242.

175. Isaac R, Solak J, Giardino A. Health care providers' training needs related to human trafficking: maximizing the opportunity to effectively screen and intervene. *J Appl Res Child.* 2011;2(1):8. doi: 10.58464/2155-5834.1029.

176. Polaris Project. National Human Trafficking Resource Center. Accessed April 23, 2025. https://polarisproject.org/national-human-trafficking-hotline/

177. Trafficking HEAL. Anti-trafficking nongovernmental organizations. Accessed April 14, 2024. https://healtrafficking.org/non-governmental-organizations/

178. Greenbaum J, Crawford-Jakubiak JE; Committee on Child Abuse and Neglect. Child sex trafficking and commercial sexual exploitation: health care needs of victims. *Pediatrics.* 2015;135(3):566–574. PubMed doi: 10.1542/peds.2014-4138

179. Kusma JD, Raphael JL, Perrin JM, Hudak ML; COMMITTEE ON CHILD HEALTH FINANCING. Medicaid and the Children's Health Insurance Program: optimization to promote equity in child and young adult health. *Pediatrics.* 2023;152(5):e2023064088. PubMed doi: 10.1542/peds.2023-064088

180. UNICEF. Harrowing journeys: Children and youth on the move across the Mediterranean Sea, at risk of trafficking and exploitation. Accessed April 14, 2024. https://data.unicef.org/resources/harrowing-journeys/

181. Linton JM, Green A; COUNCIL ON COMMUNITY PEDIATRICS. Providing care for children in immigrant families. *Pediatrics.* 2019;144(3):e20192077. PubMed doi: 10.1542/peds.2019-2077

182. Stoklosa H, Burns CJ, Karan A, et al. Mitigating trafficking of migrants and children through disaster risk reduction: insights from the Thailand flood. *Int J Disaster Risk Reduct.* 2021;60:102268. doi: 10.1016/j.ijdrr.2021.102268.

183. Ojeda M, Dodaj A, Sesar K, Del Rey R. "Some voluntarily and some under pressure": Conceptualization, reasons, attitudes, and consequences of sexting among adolescents. *Telemat Inform.* 2022;75:101891. doi: 10.1016/j.tele.2022.101891.

184. Patchin JW, Hinduja S. It is time to teach safe sexting. *J Adolesc Health.* 2020;66(2):140–143. PubMed doi: 10.1016/j.jadohealth.2019.10.010

185. American Hospital Association. Factsheet: ICD-10-CM Coding for Human Trafficking. 2018. Accessed August 1, 2019. https://www.aha.org/factsheet/2018-factsheet-icd-10-coding-human-trafficking

186. Barnert E, Kelly M, Godoy S, Abrams LS, Bath E. Behavioral health treatment "Buy-in" among adolescent females with histories of commercial sexual exploitation. *Child Abuse Negl.* 2020;100:104042. PubMed doi: 10.1016/j.chiabu.2019.104042

187. Barnert E, Kelly M, Godoy S, Abrams LS, Rasch M, Bath E. Understanding commercially sexually exploited young women's access to, utilization of, and engagement in health care: "Work around what I need.". *Womens Health Issues.* 2019;29(4):315–324. PubMed doi: 10.1016/j.whi.2019.02.002

188. American Academy of Pediatrics. Professional tools and resources for trauma-informed care. Accessed April 14, 2024. https://www.aap.org/en/patient-care/trauma-informed-care/professional-tools-resources/

Increasing Access to Antiretroviral Therapy for the Prevention and Treatment of HIV in Infants, Children, and Youth in the United States

- *Policy Statement*

POLICY STATEMENT Organizational Principles to Guide and Define the Child Health Care System and/or Improve the Health of All Children

American Academy of Pediatrics
DEDICATED TO THE HEALTH OF ALL CHILDREN™

Increasing Access to Antiretroviral Therapy for the Prevention and Treatment of HIV in Infants, Children, and Youth in the United States: Policy Statement

Rosemary Olivero, MD, FAAP, FPIDS,[1,2] Susan Gillespie, MD, PHD, FAAP,[3] and the Committee on Pediatric and Adolescent HIV

[1]Section of Pediatric Infectious Diseases, Corewell Health Helen DeVos Children's Hospital, Grand Rapids, Michigan; [2]Department of Pediatrics and Human Development, Michigan State College of Human Medicine, Lansing, Michigan; and [3]Department of Pediatrics, Division of Immunology, Allergy and Retrovirology, Baylor College of Medicine, Houston, Texas

Drs Olivero and Gillespie completed all elements of the revision of this policy statement. Both authors contributed to the design, writing, and literature review of this policy statement and performed all edits and approval of recommended edits from other AAP committee members.

FINANCIAL/CONFLICT OF INTEREST DISCLOSURE: Dr Olivero has disclosed a non-financial relationship as an owner with Inspired Biometrics; a financial relationship as a stockholder with Gilead and Moderna. Any other disclosures were reviewed and determined not relevant to the work related to "Increasing Access to Antiretroviral Therapy for the Prevention and Treatment of HIV in Infants, Children, and Youth in the United States." Disclosures are reviewed and mitigated through a Conflict-of-Interest process that consists of reviewing pertinent information which is then used to decide what action is required to maintain content integrity. There may be instances where no action is necessary. This process has been approved by the AAP Board of Directors.

To cite: Olivero R, Gillespie S; American Academy of Pediatrics, Committee on Pediatric and Adolescent HIV. Increasing Access to Antiretroviral Therapy for the Prevention and Treatment of HIV in Infants, Children, and Youth in the United States: Policy Statement. *Pediatrics.* 2025;156(2): e2025072718

abstract

Although significant progress has been made in prevention and treatment of HIV in the United States, nationally and globally, infants and children younger than 13 years have less access to optimal antiretroviral therapy compared with youth (13–24 years) and adults, which can negatively affect health outcomes for those with HIV. Despite youth having nearly as many antiretroviral options for HIV management as adults, optimal HIV management in youth is challenged by psychosocial and structural barriers that result in poor access to HIV prevention and care. Significant barriers remain in providing equitable access to optimal HIV treatment and prevention services in the pediatric population.

BACKGROUND

Epidemiology, Prognosis, and Outcome of HIV in Infants, Children, and Youth

Without treatment, HIV infection is characterized by progressive immune suppression, leading to AIDS, with opportunistic infections (OIs) and other significant morbidities causing death. Antiretroviral therapy (ART) has changed the prognosis and outcome in infants, children, and youth with HIV. Since the mid-1990s, when triple-drug ART became standard of care, children on ART have improved survival and are less likely to experience OIs, complications of HIV, or AIDS-related death.[1–4] Compared with youth and adults, infants and children have limited access to optimal ART, which narrows options for effective HIV treatment. Table 1 describes the epidemiology of HIV in infants, children, and youth.

Prevention

Most children acquire HIV vertically. Without ART or other interventions, the risk of perinatal transmission in the United States was approximately 25%.[5] The risk of perinatal transmission was reduced to <1% to 2% when ART was used during pregnancy, viral loads were consistently undetectable during pregnancy and delivery, infants received appropriate neonatal antiretroviral (ARV) prophylaxis, and breastfeeding was avoided.[6,7]

Timely identification of HIV infection in pregnancy is critical for ensuring appropriate ART during pregnancy and delivery. Communication and coordination of care between obstetricians and neonatologists/pediatricians is essential to ensure timely initiation of risk-adapted ART in neonates with HIV exposure.

Counseling regarding infant feeding has evolved to acknowledge that the risk of HIV transmission during lactation can also be reduced to <1% with ART postpartum. US Department of Health and Human Services (HHS) perinatal guidelines encourage patient-centered counseling and shared decision making to support the decision of individuals with HIV to exclusively breastfeed, provided that the breastfeeding parent is receiving ART and has a consistently undetectable viral load. Pediatricians should be aware of national HHS perinatal and pediatric HIV treatment and prevention guidelines,[8,9] guidance from the American Academy of Pediatrics (AAP),[6] and state policies on HIV screening in pregnancy.

Youth are most likely to acquire HIV through sex. Pediatricians play a key role in preventing HIV infection by providing risk reduction counseling and offering routine HIV testing and prophylaxis to adolescent and young adult patients.[10] Adolescents at high risk for HIV acquisition (including pregnant youth) should be offered HIV preexposure prophylaxis (PrEP). HIV postexposure prophylaxis (PEP) should be prescribed following high-risk exposures.[10,11] Pediatricians should be aware of laws on consent and privacy surrounding sexual health care, which vary by state.[12,13]

Timely Identification of Infants, Children, and Youth with HIV

Timely diagnosis of HIV allows for optimal management of HIV, including early initiation of ART. The Centers for Disease Control and Prevention,[14] US Public Health Service, and AAP[15] recommend universal and routine HIV screening of youth in health care settings at least once, and more frequently if a person is at increased risk of contracting HIV, including those who are sexually active, engage in intravenous drug use, or are being tested for sexually transmitted infections.[10,15] HIV testing is encouraged for immigrant children newly arriving to the United States (including international adoptees and refugees).

Early initiation of ART has several health benefits, including reducing the risk of AIDS, OIs, comorbidities, and death; preserving health, growth, development, and quality of life; and for youth who are sexually active, preventing sexual transmission of HIV.[16–20] Early treatment of HIV in infants has been shown to significantly improve infant survival and neurocognitive outcomes.[21–25] After a person receives an HIV diagnosis, it is critical to expedite care with a specialist in HIV for counseling and prompt initiation of ART. Pediatricians should leverage patient-centered approaches to linking youth with HIV to care as outlined in the HHS guidelines.[8,26]

STATEMENT OF PROBLEM

ARV medications are prescribed as single agents or in combination for HIV prevention and always in combination for treatment of HIV in infants, children, and youth. Pediatricians should be aware of potential barriers to optimal prevention or treatment options for persons with HIV exposure or infection. The following sections present optimal ARVs for neonatal and infant HIV prophylaxis and treatment (priority 1); optimal ARV formulations for child HIV treatment (priority 2); optimal ARV formulations, patient engagement, and multidisciplinary care for youth HIV treatment (priority 3); and strategies to remove barriers to HIV

TABLE 1. Epidemiology of HIV in Infants, Children, and Youth

HIV in Infants	HIV in Children	HIV in Youth
In 2019, the United States met its 2012 goals[7] for the elimination of HIV among newborn infants, achieving an incidence of <1 case per 100 000 live births and perinatal transmission rate of <1%.[51] These elimination goals were accomplished despite persistent racial and ethnic disparities.[51] To achieve elimination of HIV among children, there must be recognition of the interrelated social and structural conditions that form a web of factors influencing health outcomes of the birthing person and infant.[52]	As of 2019, an estimated 1669 children (younger than 13 y) were living with HIV in the United States,[53] and annual perinatal HIV transmissions decreased to fewer than 100 transmissions per year since 2010.	Youth (13–24 y) with HIV include those who acquired HIV early in life (usually perinatally) and later in life (most commonly through sexual activity). In 2021, youth accounted for 19% (6927) of the 36 136 new HIV diagnoses in the United States; 51.5% were diagnosed in Black youth, 88% were in males, and 93% were in gay, bisexual, and other (including transgender) men who have sex with men.[54]

prevention and care services for all infants, children, and youth (priority 4).

Priority 1: Optimal ARVs for Neonatal and Infant HIV Prophylaxis and Treatment

Most ARV use in neonates in the United States is for prevention of perinatal transmission of HIV. High-risk perinatal exposures require multiple ARVs as prophylaxis or treatment (either as early presumptive treatment or treatment for a confirmed perinatal HIV infection). A limited number of ARVs are available for prophylaxis and treatment of HIV in neonates and infants. Table 2 provides an overview of ARVs available for use in neonates and challenges associated with the use of each ARV.

A challenge when providing multiple ARVs for neonatal HIV prophylaxis (including extended prophylaxis when infants are breastfed by persons with HIV) or treatment is that neonates change weight rapidly, and frequent dosing changes and medical visits are required in the neonatal period. Dosing information for neonates is limited. For some ARVs, dosing is based on pharmacokinetic modeling studies. Some ARVs recommended for neonatal and infant use by the World Health Organization may only be prescribed off-label in the United States. Neonatal and infant HIV treatment may be complex and require expert consultation for prescribing optimal ART. Because zidovudine is currently the only ARV with safety and dosing information for infants born before 30 weeks' gestation, in extremely preterm neonates with high-risk HIV exposures (eg, unsuppressed viral load in the birthing parent), there is inadequate safety and dosing information to inform a recommendation for a 2- or 3-drug regimen for prophylaxis or treatment regimens.

TABLE 2. Antiretroviral Medications Approved or Recommended for Neonatal HIV Prophylaxis and/or Treatment

Antiretroviral Medication	Recommended for HIV Prophylaxis and/or Treatment	Lowest Gestational Age With Dosing Guidance Available	Challenges With Use
Zidovudine	Prophylaxis, treatment	<30 weeks	Anemia and neutropenia can occur; intravenous dosing available in neonates and infants not able to take enteral medications; dosing adjustment start at 4 weeks' postgestational age for neonates with confirmed HIV infection.
Nevirapine[a]	Prophylaxis, treatment	32 weeks[b]	Complex prescribing recommendations that vary on the basis of gestational age, birth weight, whether the drug is being prescribed for prophylaxis or treatment, and whether other ARVs are being prescribed; low threshold to development of resistance; potential for development of hepatotoxicity; for treatment, transition to an integrase strand inhibitor is recommended by US Department of Health and Human Services (HHS) at 4 weeks of age.
Lamivudine[a]	Prophylaxis, treatment	≥32 weeks	Anemia and neutropenia can occur; dosing, administration, and concentration differs between 2 brand name products; low threshold to development of resistance.
Raltegravir	Prophylaxis, treatment	≥37 weeks	Need to prepare oral solution from granules requiring immediate administration; complex dosing adjustments required at 1 week of age; timing of first dose may need to be delayed if birthing parent was receiving raltegravir; for treatment, transition to dolutegravir is recommended by at 4 weeks of age.
Emtricitabine	Treatment	≥37 weeks	Limited use and access in the United States.
Lopinavir-ritonavir[c]	Treatment	42 weeks' postmenstrual age	Pronounced bitter taste; gastrointestinal side effects and related poor weight gain commonly reported; should not be used in neonates <14 d of age (and <42 weeks' postmenstrual age) given serious and fatal adverse reactions with liquid formulation have occurred; for treatment, transition to an integrase strand inhibitor is recommended by HHS at 4 weeks of age; not recommended for use with polyurethane feeding tubes because of potential incompatibility.
Abacavir[a,b,d,e]	Treatment	≥37 weeks	Testing for HLA-B5*701 recommended before use.
Dolutegravir[a]	Treatment	N/A	May be used in infants ≥4 weeks of age and weighing ≥3 kg; dispersed tablet; must administer within 30 min of mixing with liquid.
Maraviroc	Treatment	≥37 weeks	Dosing varies if used with cytochrome P450 3A inhibitors (eg, protease inhibitors); limited use and access in the United States.

[a] Not approved by US Food and Drug Administration in neonates.
[b] Dosing for certain gestational ages extrapolated by pharmacokinetic modeling.
[c] Recommended only by the World Health Organization (not reflected in US-based perinatal guidelines).
[d] No longer recommended in US-based HHS perinatal or pediatric guidelines.
[e] HHS recommended for use in neonates in special circumstances only.

Zidovudine is the only ARV available in intravenous formulation for use in preterm or medically complex neonates who cannot take enteral medications.

When caring for an infant born to a person with multidrug-resistant HIV (MDR-HIV, an HIV strain that contains mutations that cause reduced susceptibility to multiple ARVs),[27–29] the limited selection of ARVs in neonates poses challenges to develop a safe and effective ARV regimen for infant prophylaxis or treatment, which may increase the risk of transmission of MDR-HIV to those infants.[30] Infants with HIV may also develop MDR-HIV from inadequate ART adherence because of incorrect dosing and/or administration, poor palatability, or adverse effects (Table 2). Resistance to ARVs may occur in neonates because of the relatively low barrier to developing resistance to some ARVs used in neonates. An additional risk factor for infants contracting MDR-HIV, especially outside of the United States, is ongoing exposure to breastfeeding, especially by persons receiving ART who have uncontrolled viremia.[31,32] Novel modalities, such as the use of broadly neutralizing antibodies and long-acting ARVs, are being investigated to decrease risk of transmission of MDR-HIV (as well as non-MDR-HIV) as prophylaxis for breastfed infants of people with HIV.[30,33]

Select ARVs used for neonatal HIV prophylaxis may also be prescribed for extended prophylaxis in people with HIV who breastfeed their infants.[9] Infant ART must be frequently adjusted for rapid changes in weight and length in this growth period. Caregivers of infants taking ARVs often encounter administration and palatability challenges that can preclude optimal medication adherence. The development of compounds that can block the bitter taste of certain medications is in process; such "universal bitter-blockers" would be an important adjunct to optimize adherence to selected ARV formulations with poor palatability.[34,35] For infants with MDR-HIV, the ARVs in Table 2 should be considered for infant HIV treatment in consultation with an expert in managing MDR-HIV. Although there are additional ARVs in use for adults with MDR-HIV (including the capsid inhibitor lenacapavir, the second-generation nonnucleoside reverse transcriptase inhibitor doravirine, and monoclonal antibodies), the limited market for infant MDR-HIV treatments may preclude research and development of such agents for infants.[36]

There are fewer optimal ARV preparations for treatment of HIV in infants compared with children, youth, and adults. Available ARV formulations for infants pose challenges to caregivers in preparation, storage, and administration. Liquid medications and granules have specific distribution, storage, and supply chain requirements to ensure medication integrity. Many ARVs used in infants require twice-daily dosing. Currently, there are no fixed-dose ARV combinations for use in infants. Frequent dosing changes, especially for multiple medications, increase risks for dosing errors, which can provide sub- or supratherapeutic ARV exposure and can prompt development of ARV resistance and toxicities, respectively. Infant HIV management can be medically intensive for caregivers, often requiring use of labeled/marked syringes, refrigeration, and attention to the appropriate administration of each ARV as liquids, granules, or chewable tablets. Use of weight-band dosage tables for infant ARVs can simplify dosing strategies and may reduce the frequency of medical visits. There remains a significant need for development of more ARV preparations, fixed-dose combinations (FDCs), long-acting ARVs, and broadly neutralizing antibody therapy, possibly administered through new drug delivery technologies, to allow for more safe, convenient, and comprehensive prevention and treatment of HIV in infants.[37–39]

Priority 2: Optimal ARV Formulations for Child HIV Treatment

Significant progress has been made in the development of safe, well-tolerated ARVs for children with HIV. ARVs developed for adults often initially have no pharmacokinetic/pharmacodynamic data and toxicity information for prepubescent children, which may differ widely from adult data. There has historically been a significant lag, in years or decades, between ARV approval in adults to subsequent research and development for that specific ARV for use in pediatrics.[38] The lag between adult and pediatric ARV research, development, and approval can cause difficulty in selecting optimal ART for a child whose HIV has specific ARV resistance mutations or who has medical complexity, obesity, contraindications to certain ARVs, and/or drug interactions between ARVs and commonly used medications in pediatrics, including psychiatric and anticonvulsant medications.

Table 3 lists ARVs recommended for children who cannot swallow pills and how ARVs should be prepared for use in children. Several ARVs listed in Table 3 have specific considerations for children receiving medications via gastrostomy tubes. Some ARV formulations have poor palatability, and several ARVs approved for use in children require 2 doses per day, making consistent use of the prescribed regimen more difficult. Intermittent supply shortages from ARV manufacturers also jeopardize continuity of ART for children. Until they reach an age where youth or adult formulations and dosing are used, growing children require dose adjustments of their ARVs, which adds complexity and intensiveness to their HIV care. As in infant HIV management, use of ARV weight-band dosage tables in children can simplify dosing strategies and reduce the frequency of medical visits, and development of more FDCs (including in dispersible tablet formulations), long-acting ART, and broadly neutralizing antibody therapy and use of new drug delivery technologies would simplify the medical intensity of childhood HIV treatment for children and caregivers.[37–39]

TABLE 3. Antiretroviral Medications Approved or Recommended for HIV Treatment in Children Who Cannot Swallow Pills

Antiretroviral Medication	Preparation Type	Challenges With Dosing and Administration
Zidovudine	Solution	
Nevirapine	Solution	Dosing is based on body surface area; dosing may vary based on other ARVs being prescribed.
Lamivudine	Solution	Dosing, administration, and concentration differs between 2 brand name products; low threshold to development of resistance.
Raltegravir	Chewable tablet Granules for oral suspension	Film-coated tablets, chewable tablets, and oral suspension are not interchangeable; need to prepare oral solution from granules requiring immediate administration.
Emtricitabine	Solution	
Efavirenz	Capsule that can be opened	Ideally taken on an empty stomach and before bedtime; sleep disturbance and central nervous system side effects are common; opened capsules have a peppery taste; opened capsules ideally should be mixed in age-appropriate soft food, and mixing in milk or formula should only be considered for young infants who cannot reliably consume solid foods and should also be used in caution in those receiving medications through a gastrostomy tube; in this case, the entire capsule content should be gently mixed into 2 teaspoons of room-temperature milk or formula in a small container, drawing up the mixture into a 10 mL syringe, and administered; after administration, an additional 2 teaspoons of formula or milk should be added to the empty mixing container, stirred, and then administered.
Dolutegravir	Dispersible tablet	Tablet is dispersed with water and must be administered within 30 min of mixing and with additional swirling of cup with water and swallowing.
Lopinavir-ritonavir	Solution	Pronounced bitter taste; gastrointestinal side effects and poor weight gain commonly reported; not recommended for use with polyurethane feeding tubes because of potential incompatibility.
Abacavir	Solution	
Pediatric FDC of abacavir, lamivudine, and dolutegravir (Triumeq PD)	Dissolvable tablet	Tablet is dissolved by adding water and must be administered within 30 min of preparation, followed by an additional swirling of water to the dosing cup and swallowing.
Atazanavir (with or without ritonavir)	Powder	Powder must be mixed with food or beverage before taking; palatability of ritonavir oral solution is poor; powder may be mixed with a beverage such as 30 mL of milk or water in a small drinking cup, mixed with a spoon, then administered; an additional 15 mL of beverage should then be added to the cup, mixed, and then administered by mouth or gastrostomy tube.
Tenofovir disoproxil fumarate	Powder	Dose is measured with a dosing scoop, mixed with soft food that does not require chewing, and swallowed immediately to avoid bitter taste; cannot be mixed in liquid to administer.

Priority 3: Optimal ARV Formulations, Patient Engagement, and Multidisciplinary Care for Youth HIV Treatment

Treatment of HIV in youth has become simplified by availability of effective and well-tolerated ART regimens with higher barriers to drug resistance. Most ARVs approved in adults, as separate ARVs and FDCs, are approved for use in those who are at least 12 years old and weigh at least 25 or 35 kg, depending on the ARV or FDC. The first complete ART regimen available as 2 injections of cabotegravir and rilpivirine, administered monthly or every 2 months, has now been approved for use in virologically suppressed adolescents 12 years old weighing at least 35 kg who have no history of relevant drug resistance mutations. Poor medication adherence has been reported in approximately half of adolescents with HIV.[40] This population must be prioritized for research and development of ARVs that do not require daily oral dosing such as other long-acting injectable ARVs, and ARVs delivered intramuscularly, subcutaneously, or through biodegradable or nonbiodegradable implants. Delivery systems that combine long-acting ARVs with contraceptives would be of particular benefit in youth capable of becoming pregnant. Youth with HIV also should be prioritized in development of ART regimens that can accommodate specific pharmacokinetic challenges such as obesity or concomitant use of contraceptive, psychiatric, and/or anti-tuberculosis medications. Further drug development is also needed to meet the needs of adolescents with MDR-HIV, because the single monoclonal antibody for use in MDR-HIV, ibalizumab, is only approved for use in adults.

The landscape of ARVs prescribed in youth is rapidly evolving, and pediatric HIV specialists are faced with maintaining competency in optimal ART management in this population; generally, ART should be managed in consultation with a pediatric and/or adult HIV expert. Pediatric HIV specialists have opportunities to receive timely education on updated recommendations and approvals for ARVs in youth, which will allow for optimal treatment of this population with the best tolerated medications. Pediatric HIV specialists should monitor for changes in HHS guidelines for treatment of HIV in youth.[8,9,26,41] Pediatricians should be aware of the National Clinician Consultation Center,[41] which can be used when urgent HIV clinical or treatment concerns arise. General pediatricians should be familiar with current and evolving recommendations and options to provide PrEP to youth, including the approval by the US Food and Drug Administration of long-acting injectable cabotegravir and rilpivirine for those 12 years and older weighing at least 35 kg.[10,42,43]

When compared with younger children and adults older than 25 years, youth with HIV have worse clinical outcomes at each step of the HIV care continuum (ie, HIV diagnosis, linkage to HIV care, retention in care, achievement of viral suppression, and maintenance of viral suppression).[44–46] Viral suppression is lower in this age group because of poor adherence to ART, and mortality is 6 to 12 times higher in US youth with perinatally acquired HIV compared with age-, sex- and race-matched controls in the general population. Barriers to ART adherence and optimal HIV-related medical care include factors that need to be addressed at individual, psychosocial, and structural levels. Strategies to improve and support adherence include providing psychosocial support, addressing challenges related to the ART regimen, and optimizing health care delivery through youth-friendly services.[26]

Youth may become sexually active during this developmental period, highlighting the need for youth with HIV to understand the role of virologic suppression for both their own health and reducing the risk of HIV transmission to sexual partners.

Priority 4: Remove Barriers to HIV Prevention and Care Services for All Infants, Children, and Youth

Despite progress made in prevention and treatment of pediatric HIV infection, significant gaps remain in access to HIV prevention, testing, and treatment services. Pediatricians should recognize the potential for systemic barriers, including poverty and racism,[47,48] to interfere with optimal HIV care, particularly for youth, in whom psychosocial, behavioral, and environmental factors can undermine adherence to ART needed for successful HIV care.[49]

Comprehensive HIV treatment services must be provided to all US infants, children, and youth with HIV, regardless of immigration status, health insurance coverage, socioeconomic status, or the circumstances of their families and caregivers. Pediatricians must be aware of resources available to uninsured children, including the Ryan White HIV/AIDS Program and its AIDS Drug Assistance Program (Table 4). In the event of a disaster, pediatricians should

TABLE 4. Resources for Medical Providers in Caring for Children With Barriers to Insurance and Medical Care Payment

Title	URL	Summary
HIV.gov - Paying for HIV care and treatment	https://www.hiv.gov/hiv-basics/staying-in-hiv-care/hiv-treatment/paying-for-hiv-care-and-treatment	Provides links to resources to support payment for HIV care.
Medicaid and Children's Health Insurance Program (CHIP)	https://www.healthcare.gov/medicaid-chip/getting-medicaid-chip/	Children's Medicaid is a health care program for children in low-income families. CHIP is a health care program for children without health insurance whose families earn too much to get Medicaid but cannot afford health insurance.
Children and youth with special health care needs (CYSHCN)	https://mchb.hrsa.gov/programs-impact/focus-areas/children-youth-special-health-care-needs-cyshcn	Program for children who have or are at increased risk for chronic physical, developmental, behavioral, or emotional conditions. They also require health and related services of a type or amount beyond that required by children generally.
Ryan White HIV/AIDS Program (RWHAP), Part D	https://ryanwhite.hrsa.gov/about/parts-and-initiatives/part-d-swic	RWHAP Part D grant recipients provide outpatient family-centered primary and specialty medical care and support services for low-income women, infants, children, and youth with HIV.
AIDS Drug Assistance Program (ADAP), Ryan White Part B	https://ryanwhite.hrsa.gov/about/parts-and-initiatives/part-b-adap	A federal program administered by the HRSA HIV/AIDS Bureau that covers medication costs for people with HIV.
Pharmaceutical company patient assistance programs (PAPs)	https://targethiv.org/library/CPAPA	A PAP is a program run by, or in association with, pharmaceutical companies to provide free or low-cost medications to people with low incomes who do not qualify for any other insurance or assistance programs, such as Medicaid, Medicare, or ADAPs. Each individual company has different eligibility criteria for enrollment in their patient assistance program.

be aware of federal guidance regarding management of persons with HIV who have been displaced, including which ARVs may be temporarily substituted.[50] This management should ideally occur in consultation with a clinician experienced in pediatric HIV care and ART.

Although the market for development of novel ART for use in infants and children in the United States is relatively small, HIV disproportionately affects children in poverty from minoritized groups. Advocacy is needed for governments and funding agencies to prioritize inclusion of infants, children, and youth in clinical trials on optimal ART in these age groups. Advocacy efforts should be developed to address structural barriers to inclusion of children with HIV and the mistrust that underprivileged sectors may feel toward the medical system.

Although optimal ART has been shown to be an effective public health strategy for reducing HIV transmission, morbidity, and mortality, significant barriers remain in providing access to HIV prevention services. Prevention of HIV among people of childbearing age will decrease the number of children exposed to HIV perinatally. Prevention of new infections among youth should be prioritized through increased testing and wider access to PrEP, including long-acting oral and injectable medications.

RECOMMENDATIONS

The AAP recommends the following to address barriers and limitations in the treatment and prevention of HIV among infants, children, and youth.

1. Optimize ARVs for **neonate and infant** HIV prophylaxis and treatment.
   - Develop ARVs that can be used in preterm and low birth weight neonates and infants.
   - Develop ARV formulations that are easily administered, are palatable, are well-tolerated, and have high barriers to resistance.
   - Simplify ARV dosing from the neonatal period through infancy and reduce medical visits through use of weight-band dosage tables.
   - Increase the number of ARVs for infant prophylaxis and treatment, particularly in infants whose birthing parent has MDR-HIV.
2. Optimize ARV formulations for **childhood** HIV treatment.
   - Expand research and development to facilitate more timely approval of ARVs for use in children.
   - Simplify ARV dosing and reduce medical visits in child HIV management with weight-band dosage tables. Increase availability of FDCs for use in children.
   - Facilitate medication adherence among children by developing tolerable and palatable medication formulations including dispersible tablets, chewable tablets, and FDCs for children.
   - Develop alternative delivery systems for use in children, including injectable long-active ARVs and skin patches.
   - Increase ARV drug options for children with MDR-HIV.
3. Optimize ARV formulations, patient engagement, and multidisciplinary care for **youth** HIV treatment.
   - Include youth in adult ARV clinical trials to allow more timely approval of ARVs in youth.
   - Support adherence to ART by developing optimal HIV drugs, including daily single tablet regimens that are well tolerated with a high barrier to resistance; long-acting or extended-release for both prevention and treatment of HIV; and ART regimens that can be safely used without interacting with other medications (contraception and psychiatric medications).
   - Increase knowledge, access, and uptake of PrEP in youth.
   - Increase support for optimal engagement in care and ART adherence by providing youth-friendly support, addressing and mitigating racism, reducing stigma around sexual orientation and gender identity, and addressing social and structural determinants affecting health care.
   - Increase ARV drug options for youth with MDR-HIV.
4. Remove barriers to HIV prevention and care services for all.
   - Increase routine HIV screening and prevention services for youth.
   - Decrease barriers to financing HIV-related care and ART.
   - Increase support for optimal ART adherence using a patient- and family-centered approach.
   - Provide access to HIV prevention and treatment services regardless of immigration status or insurance coverage, with special attention on mitigating structural racism and health disparities.
   - Increase awareness of resources available to uninsured children.

LEAD AUTHORS

Rosemary Olivero, MD, FAAP
Susan Gillespie, MD, PHD, FAAP

COMMITTEE ON PEDIATRIC AND ADOLESCENT HIV, 2022–2023

Natella Yurievna Rakhmanina, MD, PhD, FAAP
Lisa Abuogi, MD, MS, FAAP
Susan Gillespie, MD, PhD
Jennifer Jao, MD, MPH, FAAP
Anne Neilan, MD, MPH, FAAP

Rosemary Olivero, MD, FAAP
Julia Rosebush, DO, FAAP
George Siberry, MD, MPH, FAAP

CONSULTANT

Athena P. Kourtis, MD, PhD, MPH, FAAP, Consultant – Committee on Infectious Diseases

STAFF

Heather Stob

ABBREVIATIONS

ARV: antiretroviral [medication]
ART: antiretroviral therapy
HHS: US Department of Health and Human Services
MDR-HIV: multidrug-resistant HIV
OI: opportunistic infection
PEP: postexposure prophylaxis
PrEP: preexposure prophylaxis

Policy statements from the American Academy of Pediatrics benefit from expertise and resources of liaisons and internal (AAP) and external reviewers. However, policy statements from the American Academy of Pediatrics may not reflect the views of the liaisons or the organizations or government agencies that they represent.

The guidance in this statement does not indicate an exclusive course of treatment or serve as a standard of medical care. Variations, taking into account individual circumstances, may be appropriate.

All policy statements from the American Academy of Pediatrics automatically expire 5 years after publication unless reaffirmed, revised, or retired at or before that time.

FUNDING: No external funding.

https://doi.org/10.1542/peds.2025-072718

REFERENCES

1. Brady MT, Oleske JM, Williams PL, et al; Pediatric AIDS Clinical Trials Group219/219C Team. Declines in mortality rates and changes in causes of death in HIV-1-infected children during the HAART era. *J Acquir Immune Defic Syndr.* 2010;53(1):86–94. PubMed doi: 10.1097/QAI.0b013e3181b9869f
2. Kapogiannis BG, Soe MM, Nesheim SR, et al. Mortality trends in the US Perinatal AIDS Collaborative Transmission Study (1986–2004). *Clin Infect Dis.* 2011;53(10):1024–1034. PubMed doi: 10.1093/cid/cir641
3. Mirani G, Williams PL, Chernoff M, et al; IMPAACT P1074 Study Team. Changing Trends in Complications and Mortality Rates Among US Youth and Young Adults With HIV Infection in the Era of Combination Antiretroviral Therapy. *Clin Infect Dis.* 2015;61(12):1850–1861. PubMed doi: 10.1093/cid/civ687
4. Nesheim SR, Balaji A, Hu X, Lampe M, Dominguez KL. Opportunistic illnesses in children with HIV infection in the United States, 1997–2016. *Pediatr Infect Dis J.* 2021;40(7):645–648. PubMed doi: 10.1097/INF.0000000000003154
5. Davis SF, Byers RH Jr, Lindegren ML, Caldwell MB, Karon JM, Gwinn M. Prevalence and incidence of vertically acquired HIV infection in the United States. *JAMA.* 1995;274(12):952–955. PubMed doi: 10.1001/jama.1995.03530120044039
6. Chadwick EG, Ezeanolue EE, Hsu KK-C, et al; COMMITTEE ON PEDIATRIC AIDS. Evaluation and management of the infant exposed to HIV in the United States. *Pediatrics.* 2020;146(5):e2020029058. PubMed doi: 10.1542/peds.2020-029058
7. Nesheim S, Taylor A, Lampe MA, et al. A framework for elimination of perinatal transmission of HIV in the United States. *Pediatrics.* 2012;130(4):738–744. PubMed doi: 10.1542/peds.2012-0194
8. Panel on Antiretroviral Therapy and Medical Management of Children Living with HIV. *Guidelines for the Use of Antiretroviral Agents in Pediatric HIV Infection.* Department of Health and Human Services. Accessed June 9, 2025. https://clinicalinfo.hiv.gov/en/guidelines/pediatric-arv
9. National Institutes of Health. Clinicalinfo.HIV.gov. Recommendations for the Use of Antiretroviral Drugs During Pregnancy and Interventions to Reduce Perinatal HIV Transmission in the United States. Accessed June 9, 2025. https://clinicalinfo.hiv.gov/en/guidelines/perinatal/recommendations-arv-drugs-pregnancy-overview
10. Hsu KK, Rakhmanina NY. Adolescents and young adults: the pediatrician's role in HIV testing and pre- and postexposure HIV prophylaxis. *Pediatrics.* 2022;149(1):e2021055207. PubMed doi: 10.1542/peds.2021-055207
11. US Public Health Service, Centers for Disease Control and Prevention, National Center for HIV/AIDS, Viral Hepatitis, STD, and TB Prevention, Division of HIV/AIDS Prevention, Preexposure Prophylaxis Work Group. Preexposure prophylaxis for the prevention of HIV infection in the United States – 2021 update : a clinical

practice guideline. Published December 2021. Accessed June 9, 2025. https://stacks.cdc.gov/view/cdc/112360

12. Maslyanskaya S, Alderman EM. Confidentiality and consent in the care of the adolescent patient. *Pediatr Rev.* 2019;40(10):508–516. PubMed doi: 10.1542/pir.2018-0040

13. Sharko M, Jameson R, Ancker JS, Krams L, Webber EC, Rosenbloom ST. State-by-state variability in adolescent privacy laws. *Pediatrics.* 2022;149(6):e2021053458. PubMed doi: 10.1542/peds.2021-053458

14. Branson BM, Handsfield HH, Lampe MA, et al; Centers for Disease Control and Prevention (CDC). Revised recommendations for HIV testing of adults, adolescents, and pregnant women in health-care settings. *MMWR Recomm Rep.* 2006;55(RR-14):1–17; quiz CE1–CE4. PubMed

15. Richerson JE, Simon GR, Abularrage JJ, et al; Committee On Practice and Ambulatory Medicine; Bright Futures Periodicity Schedule Workgroup. 2017 recommendations for preventive pediatric health care. *Pediatrics.* 2017;139(4):e20170254. PubMed doi: 10.1542/peds.2017-0254

16. Grinsztejn B, Hosseinipour MC, Ribaudo HJ, et al; HPTN 052-ACTG Study Team. Effects of early versus delayed initiation of antiretroviral treatment on clinical outcomes of HIV-1 infection: results from the phase 3 HPTN 052 randomised controlled trial. *Lancet Infect Dis.* 2014;14(4):281–290. PubMed doi: 10.1016/S1473-3099(13)70692-3

17. Lundgren JD, Babiker AG, Gordin F, et al; INSIGHT START Study Group. Initiation of antiretroviral therapy in early asymptomatic HIV infection. *N Engl J Med.* 2015;373(9):795–807. PubMed doi: 10.1056/NEJMoa1506816

18. Danel C, Moh R, Gabillard D, et al; TEMPRANO ANRS 12136 Study Group. A trial of early antiretrovirals and isoniazid preventive therapy in Africa. *N Engl J Med.* 2015;373(9):808–822. PubMed doi: 10.1056/NEJMoa1507198

19. Severe P, Juste MA, Ambroise A, et al. Early versus standard antiretroviral therapy for HIV-infected adults in Haiti. *N Engl J Med.* 2010;363(3):257–265. PubMed doi: 10.1056/NEJMoa0910370

20. Wyl V, Gianella S, Fischer M, et al; Swiss HIV Cohort Study-SHCS. Early antiretroviral therapy during primary HIV-1 infection results in a transient reduction of the viral setpoint upon treatment interruption. *PLoS One.* 2011;6(11):e27463. PubMed doi: 10.1371/journal.pone.0027463

21. Crowell CS, Huo Y, Tassiopoulos K, et al; PACTG 219C Study Team and the Pediatric HIVAIDS Cohort Study (PHACS). Early viral suppression improves neurocognitive outcomes in HIV-infected children. *AIDS.* 2015;29(3):295–304. PubMed doi: 10.1097/QAD.0000000000000528

22. Crowell CS, Malee KM, Yogev R, Muller WJ. Neurologic disease in HIV-infected children and the impact of combination antiretroviral therapy. *Rev Med Virol.* 2014;24(5):316–331. PubMed doi: 10.1002/rmv.1793

23. Lewis-de Los Angeles CP, Alpert KI, Williams PL, et al; Pediatric HIV/AIDS Cohort Study (PHACS). Deformed subcortical structures are related to past HIV disease severity in youth with perinatally acquired HIV infection. *J Pediatric Infect Dis Soc.* 2016;5(suppl 1):S6–S14. PubMed doi: 10.1093/jpids/piw051

24. Sanford R, Ances BM, Meyerhoff DJ, et al. Longitudinal trajectories of brain volume and cortical thickness in treated and untreated primary human immunodeficiency virus infection. *Clin Infect Dis.* 2018;67(11):1697–1704. PubMed doi: 10.1093/cid/ciy362

25. Goetghebuer T, Haelterman E, Le Chenadec J, et al; European Infant Collaboration group. Effect of early antiretroviral therapy on the risk of AIDS/death in HIV-infected infants. *AIDS.* 2009;23(5):597–604. PubMed doi: 10.1097/QAD.0b013e328326ca37

26. Department of Health and Human Services. Guidelines for the Use of Antiretroviral Agents in Adults and Adolescents Living with HIV. Accessed May 29, 2025. https://clinicalinfo.hiv.gov/sites/default/files/guidelines/documents/adult-adolescent-arv/guidelines-adult-adolescent-arv.pdf

27. Brennan-Benson P, Pakianathan M, Rice P, et al. Enfurvitide prevents vertical transmission of multidrug-resistant HIV-1 in pregnancy but does not cross the placenta. *AIDS.* 2006;20(2):297–299. PubMed doi: 10.1097/01.aids.0000200535.02232.1b

28. Desai N, Mathur M. Selective transmission of multidrug resistant HIV to a newborn related to poor maternal adherence. *Sex Transm Infect.* 2003;79(5):419–421. PubMed doi: 10.1136/sti.79.5.419

29. Wensing AM, Boucher CA, van Kasteren M, van Dijken PJ, Geelen SP, Juttmann JR. Prevention of mother-to-child transmission of multidrug resistant HIV-1 using maternal therapy with both enfuvirtide and tipranavir. *AIDS.* 2006;20(10):1465–1467. PubMed doi: 10.1097/01.aids.0000233587.94961.4f

30. Boyce CL, Sils T, Ko D, et al. Maternal human immunodeficiency virus (HIV) drug resistance is associated with vertical transmission and is prevalent in infected infants. *Clin Infect Dis.* 2022;74(11):2001–2009. PubMed doi: 10.1093/cid/ciab744

31. Fogel JM, Mwatha A, Richardson P, et al. Impact of maternal and infant antiretroviral drug regimens on drug resistance in HIV-infected breastfeeding infants. *Pediatr Infect Dis J.* 2013;32(4):e164–e169. PubMed doi: 10.1097/INF.0b013e31827f44ee</jrn>

32. John-Stewart G, Mbori-Ngacha D, Ekpini R, et al; Ghent IAS Working Group on HIV in Women Children. Breast-feeding and transmission of HIV-1. *J Acquir Immune Defic Syndr.* 2004;35(2):196–202. PubMed doi: 10.1097/00126334-200402010-00015

33. Dugdale CM, Ufio O, Alba C, et al. Cost-effectiveness of broadly neutralizing antibody prophylaxis for HIV-exposed infants in sub-Saharan African settings. *J Int AIDS Soc.* 2023;26(1):e26052. PubMed doi: 10.1002/jia2.26052

34. Andrews D, Salunke S, Cram A, et al. Bitter-blockers as a taste masking strategy: a systematic review towards their utility in pharmaceuticals. *Eur J Pharm Biopharm.* 2021;158:35–51. PubMed doi: 10.1016/j.ejpb.2020.10.017

35. World Health Organization. Global Accelerator for Paediatric Formulations Network (GAP-f). Accessed March 10, 2023. https://www.who.int/initiatives/gap-f

36. Penazzato M, Gnanashanmugam D, Rojo P, et al; Paediatric Antiretroviral Working Group (PAWG). Optimizing research to speed up availability of pediatric antiretroviral drugs and

formulations. *Clin Infect Dis.* 2017;64(11):1597–1603. PubMed doi: 10.1093/cid/cix194

37. Penazzato M, Townsend CL, Rakhmanina N, et al; PADO4 participants. Prioritising the most needed paediatric antiretroviral formulations: the PADO4 list. *Lancet HIV.* 2019;6(9):e623–e631. PubMed doi: 10.1016/S2352-3018(19)30193-6

38. Penazzato M, Townsend CL, Sam-Agudu NA, et al; PADO-HIV 5 participants. Advancing the prevention and treatment of HIV in children: priorities for research and development. *Lancet HIV.* 2022; 9(9):e658–e666. PubMed doi: 10.1016/S2352-3018(22)00101-1

39. Rome Action Plan. Paediatric HIV & TB: Rome Action Plan. Accessed March 10, 2023. https://www.paediatrichivactionplan.org/updates

40. Taddeo D, Egedy M, Frappier JY. Adherence to treatment in adolescents. *Paediatr Child Health.* 2008;13(1):19–24. PubMed doi: 10.1093/pch/13.1.19

41. AIDS Education & Training Center Program. National Clinician Consultation Center. Accessed March 8, 2023. https://aidsetc.org/aetc-program/national-clinician-consulation-center

42. Clement ME, Kofron R, Landovitz RJ. Long-acting injectable cabotegravir for the prevention of HIV infection. *Curr Opin HIV AIDS.* 2020;15(1):19–26. PubMed doi: 10.1097/COH.0000000000000597

43. US Food and Drug Administration. FDA Approves First Injectable Treatment for HIV Pre-Exposure Prevention. December 20, 2021. Accessed December 11, 2022. https://www.fda.gov/news-events/press-announcements/fda-approves-first-injectable-treatment-hiv-pre-exposure-prevention

44. Kapogiannis BG, Koenig LJ, Xu J, et al; Adolescent Medicine Trials Network for HIV/AIDS Interventions. The HIV continuum of care for adolescents and young adults attending 13 urban US HIV care centers of the NICHD-ATN-CDC-HRSA SMILE Collaborative. *J Acquir Immune Defic Syndr.* 2020;84(1):92–100. PubMed doi: 10.1097/QAI.0000000000002308

45. Zanoni BC, Mayer KH. The adolescent and young adult HIV cascade of care in the United States: exaggerated health disparities. *AIDS Patient Care STDs.* 2014;28(3):128–135. PubMed doi: 10.1089/apc.2013.0345

46. Rojo P, Carpenter D, Venter F, Turkova A, Penazzato M. The HIV drug optimization agenda: promoting standards for earlier investigation and approvals of antiretroviral drugs for use in adolescents living with HIV. *J Int AIDS Soc.* 2020;23(suppl 5):e25576. PubMed doi: 10.1002/jia2.25576

47. Cotton NK, Shim RS. Social determinants of health, structural racism, and the impact on child and adolescent mental health. *J Am Acad Child Adolesc Psychiatry.* 2022;61(11):1385–1389. PubMed doi: 10.1016/j.jaac.2022.04.020

48. Trent M, Dooley DG, Dougé J; Section On Adolescent Health; COUNCIL ON COMMUNITY PEDIATRICS; COMMITTEE ON ADOLESCENCE. The impact of racism on child and adolescent health. *Pediatrics.* 2019;144(2):e20191765. PubMed doi: 10.1542/peds.2019-1765

49. Martinez J, Chakraborty R, Chakraborty R, et al; American Academy of Pediatrics Committee on Pediatric Aids. Psychosocial support for youth living with HIV. *Pediatrics.* 2014;133(3):558–562. PubMed doi: 10.1542/peds.2013-4061

50. Clinical Info HIV.gov. Guidance for Non-HIV-Specialized Providers Caring for Persons with HIV Who Have Been Displaced by Disasters (such as a Hurricane). Updated September 17, 2021. Accessed March 21, 2025. https://clinicalinfo.hiv.gov/en/guidelines/archived-guidelines/guidelines-caring-persons-hiv-disaster-areas

51. Lampe MA, Nesheim SR, Oladapo KL, Ewing AC, Wiener J, Kourtis AP. Achieving elimination of perinatal HIV in the United States. *Pediatrics.* 2023;151(5):e2022059604. PubMed doi: 10.1542/peds.2022-059604

52. Crear-Perry J, Correa-de-Araujo R, Lewis Johnson T, McLemore MR, Neilson E, Wallace M. Social and structural determinants of health inequities in maternal health. *J Womens Health (Larchmt).* 2021;30(2):230–235. PubMed doi: 10.1089/jwh.2020.8882

53. Centers for Disease Control and Prevention. HIV Surveillance Report. May 24, 2022. Accessed May 29, 2025. https://www.cdc.gov/nchhstp/director-letters/2020-hiv-surveillance-report.html

54. Centers for Disease Control and Prevention. HIV Surveillance Report: Diagnoses of HIV Infection in the United States and Dependent Areas, 2021. May 1, 2023. Accessed May 29, 2025. https://stacks.cdc.gov/view/cdc/149071

Management of Food Allergy in Schools

- *Clinical Report*

CLINICAL REPORT Guidance for the Clinician in Rendering Pediatric Care

American Academy of Pediatrics

DEDICATED TO THE HEALTH OF ALL CHILDREN™

Management of Food Allergy in Schools: Clinical Report

Scott H. Sicherer, MD, FAAP,[1] Sonja O'Leary, MD, FAAP,[2] Michael Pistiner, MD, MMSc, FAAP,[3] Julie Wang, MD, FAAP,[1] and the Section on Allergy and Immunology; and the Council on School Health

abstract

This clinical report updates and replaces a 2010 clinical report from the American Academy of Pediatrics that addressed food allergy management in schools. Food allergy affects up to 10% of children, and anaphylaxis is estimated to occur in 1 in 15 schools per year. School food allergy management requires strategies to reduce the risk of ingestion of the allergen as well as procedures to recognize and treat allergic reactions and anaphylaxis. The role of the pediatrician or pediatric primary care clinician may include diagnosing and documenting a potentially life-threatening food allergy; prescribing self-administered epinephrine to individual patients or for general use in a school (stock/unassigned epinephrine); educating children, parents, and school personnel on prevention, recognition, and management of allergic reactions to food; and working with schools in developing plans to reduce the risk of anaphylaxis and to implement emergency treatment in the event of a reaction. This clinical report highlights the role of the pediatrician and primary care clinician in managing students with food allergies.

INTRODUCTION

Food allergy affects up to 10% of school-aged children; reactions may be severe (42%) and life-threatening (anaphylaxis).[1,2] This clinical report updates and replaces a previous report from the American Academy of Pediatrics (AAP) on this topic.[3] Subsequent to the publication of the prior report, the Centers for Disease Control and Prevention (CDC) published "Voluntary Guidelines for Managing Food Allergies in Schools and Early Care and Education Programs," which provides comprehensive guidance for management.[4] Table 1 summarizes key recommendations from the CDC guidelines. In addition, some state laws now encourage or require schools to have unassigned (stock) epinephrine auto-injectors (EAIs) for emergency use. The AAP published several clinical reports relevant to food allergy and anaphylaxis management that supersede the previous

[1]*Division of Allergy and Immunology, Department of Pediatrics, Jaffe Food Allergy Institute, Icahn School of Medicine at Mount Sinai, New York, New York;* [2]*Department of Pediatrics, University of Colorado, Denver Health, School and Community Programs, Denver, Colorado; and* [3]*MassGeneral Hospital for Children, Harvard Medical School, Boston, Massachusetts*

Drs Sicherer, O'Leary, Pistiner, and Wang contributed to the identification and incorporation/interpretation of the literature used to compose the report and assisted in drafting, reviewing, and editing the manuscript. All authors approve of the final manuscript.

FINANCIAL/CONFLICT OF INTEREST DISCLOSURE: Dr Sicherer had disclosures related to: the American Academy of Allergy, Asthma, and Immunology; Elsevier; Food Allergy Research and Education; HAL Allergy; the Immune Tolerance Network; the International Association for Food Protein Enterocolitis; the International FPIES Association; Johns Hopkins University Press; the National Institute of Allergy and Infectious Diseases; Pfizer; Regeneron; and Up to Date. Dr O'Leary had disclosures related to: Dohme, Merck, and Sharp. Dr Pistiner had disclosures related to: Aimmune Therapeutics; the Allergy Asthma Network; the Allergy Home and Allergy Certified Training; the American Academy of Allergy, Asthma, and Immunology; the American College of Allergy, Asthma, and Immunology; Anjo AI; Aquestive; ARS Pharmaceuticals; the Asthma and Allergy Foundation of America; Boston Scientific Corporation; Bryn; DBV Technologies; the Egg Nutrition Center; Food Allergy Research and Education; Foodgraph; Kaleo; Kenvue; the National Peanut Board; and Novartis. Dr Wang had disclosures related to: Aimmune Therapeutics; ALK Abello; DBV Technologies; Hoffman La Roche/Genentech; Jubilant; National Institute of Allergy and Infectious Diseases; Novartis; Regeneron; and Up to Date. Disclosures are reviewed and mitigated through a conflict-of-interest process that consists of reviewing pertinent information which is then used to decide what action is required to maintain content integrity. (Continued)

To cite: Sicherer SH, O'Leary S, Pistiner M, et al; American Academy of Pediatrics, Section on Allergy and Immunology; Council on School Health. Management of Food Allergy in Schools: Clinical Report. *Pediatrics.* 2025;156(6):e2025073168

TABLE 1. Key Priority Areas Emphasized in the CDC Voluntary Guidelines for Managing Food Allergy in Schools

Category	Advice
Daily food allergy management for the individual student	• Identify students with food allergy • Develop a plan for managing and preventing food-allergic reactions in individual students through an Emergency Care Plan (Food Allergy Action Plan) • Support students in managing their food allergies
Allergic emergency preparedness	• Establish emergency communication within school grounds and with local emergency medical services • Ensure that staff have rapid access to epinephrine devices • Ensure appropriate epinephrine utilization for allergic emergencies and notification of emergency medical services • Establish roles of each staff member in preparation for a food allergy emergency • Prepare for food allergy reactions in children without a prior history of food allergies • Document the food allergy emergency response
Food allergy staff training/professional development	• Provide general food allergy training for the entire staff • Provide in-depth training for staff with frequent contact with students with food allergies • Provide specialized training for staff who routinely manage the health of students with food allergies
Food allergy education for the school community (students and their family)	• Teach all students, both with and without food allergy, about food allergy and school policy • Teach all parents, both with and without children with food allergy, about food allergy and school policy
Creation of "healthy and safe educational environment"	• Create an environment that is as safe as possible from exposure to food allergen • Develop policies and procedures to prevent cross contact of food allergen • Work with outside groups to follow food allergy policies when utilizing school building/grounds • Create a positive psychosocial culture with goals to reduce bullying and social isolation • Promote awareness and understanding

school food allergy clinical report,[5,6] and the National Academies of Sciences, Engineering, and Medicine[7] and professional organizations have published guidance for school management of food allergy, including an evidence-based practice guideline.[8,9] This updated clinical report utilizes these resources and additional studies to provide pediatricians and primary care clinicians with the information necessary to counsel patients, families, school personnel, and policy makers on effective food allergy management practices. Discussion of the roles and responsibilities of the school physician is beyond the scope of this clinical report, but the AAP has published a policy statement on these roles.[10]

DOCUMENTATION OF FOOD ALLERGY

An accurate diagnosis of food allergy is needed before a management plan can be developed. National guidelines on food allergy diagnosis are available.[11] The pediatrician or pediatric primary care clinician may wish to work with an allergist to optimize diagnosis. The following are key points of note:

- Although any food may trigger an allergic reaction, most serious reactions are attributable to peanut, tree nuts (eg, cashew, walnut, etc), milk, egg, soy, wheat, fish, shellfish, and sesame.[11,12]
- Reactions may include anaphylaxis, which, in rare cases, may be fatal.[13]
- Establishing a food allergy diagnosis includes a clinical history consistent with IgE-mediated allergy (eg, urticaria, wheezing with onset shortly after ingestion) and confirmation of the relevant allergen with testing (eg, allergy skin-prick tests or food-specific serum immunoglobulin E [IgE] testing). Although increasingly large (more reactive) skin tests and elevated levels of food-specific IgE antibodies correlate with increased risk of allergy, an isolated positive test alone is not diagnostic, and tests do not reliably predict severity.[11] Clinician-supervised oral food-challenge testing may be needed to confirm a diagnosis. Confirmation of a diagnosis is beneficial, because food-allergen avoidance and management of allergic reactions create significant burdens for patients and their families in all aspects of the child's life, including school, after-school programs, and camps. Diagnosis is reviewed in another AAP clinical report.[14]

SCHOOL NOTIFICATION AND WRITTEN PLANS

The child's primary care physician/clinician or allergist plays a key role in communicating the diagnosis and authorizing treatment, typically by providing a signed allergy and anaphylaxis emergency plan, described below. Additional opportunities for the child's primary care physician/clinician or allergist regarding communication about diagnosis, treatment, and management of allergic risks include discussion with the family regarding food allergy care (such as developmentally appropriate avoidance strategies), prescriptions for epinephrine devices for home and school, and assistance with creating school plans (individualized health care plan [IHP]) for effective management and communication with the school team, if needed.

Allergy and Anaphylaxis Emergency Plans

A universal individualized written allergy and anaphylaxis emergency plan (available in English and Spanish) has been developed by the AAP, as described in a clinical report that details utilization,[6] although other formats are used.[15] The plan can be embedded into the provider's electronic health record (EHR) for ease of completing and signing yearly. A copy of the plan may be kept by the parent/caregiver, school office(s)/health or nursing office, and the student, if appropriate. The written plan provides individualized guidance and treatment authorization but is not a sole means of imparting the full scope of anaphylaxis recognition and management. Additional education about food allergy and anaphylaxis can provide context (as described below, Emergency Management). In addition, the individualized emergency plan can inform a school-wide Emergency Action Plan, identifying exact locations of individual and stock epinephrine devices, local emergency medical services contacts, current parent/guardian contact information, and specific interventions necessary to meet state and district rules and laws (see School Emergency Management, below).

Individualized Health Care Plans and 504 Plans

The CDC recommends a team approach to managing food allergy in schools.[4] This partnership includes the child with food allergy, parents/guardians, school staff, school nurse, and the child's health care providers. The primary role of the pediatrician or primary care clinician is to provide documentation of the allergy and a treatment plan by providing an individualized written food allergy and anaphylaxis emergency plan. When the school receives a written allergy and anaphylaxis emergency plan, this may provide a basis for the student's IHP. In most cases, the student-specific written allergy and anaphylaxis emergency plan is sufficient for documentation of allergy and authorization of treatment. The IHP is a nursing document that may be created by a school nurse, or school health service provider as permitted, that contains a management plan with preventive procedures for day-to-day management in the school. The student's IHP is typically developed by the school nurse in collaboration with the family, primary care clinician, and other school personnel. The IHP can be revised by the nurse according to the child's needs on the basis of age and developmental stages. Schools may establish a core team responsible for food allergy management to ensure that reasonable and nondiscriminatory avoidance plans are in place, that an emergency treatment plan is reviewed and practiced periodically, that people are designated and trained to recognize and treat anaphylaxis, etc, whether for the individual student or schoolwide.

Students with food allergy are protected by federal civil rights laws, including Free Appropriate Public Education under Section 504, to access education in the least restrictive environment. A 504 Plan, which is available under a federal civil rights law, Section 504 of the Rehabilitation Act of 1973, applies to any school that receives federal money (ie, all public schools and many private schools) and applies to a variety of health conditions, including a life-threatening food allergy. Section 504 allows the school to create a 504 Plan, a written management plan of accommodations for the individual student, allowing the student to participate safely and equally alongside peers during all normal facets of the school day. In addition, Section 504 provides legal recourse for students and their families when they and the school are unable to come to terms on educational plans based on health care needs through normal channels. Schoolwide approaches and policies often address food allergy resulting in a safe environment for all of the children with food allergies. An IHP can be used to individualize needs, if necessary. Development of a 504 Plan can also be considered on an individual basis, if needed, to ensure protections. Development of written management materials by the school for parents/students may require attention to language or reading level barriers and developmental stages.

LAWS REGARDING MANAGEMENT AND STOCK EPINEPHRINE

Federal and state laws provide parameters by which schools can care for students with food allergy and other potentially life-threatening allergies. Although federal laws are universally applicable, state laws and regulations regarding the management of food allergies and anaphylaxis in schools are wide ranging and vary by state. These laws can range from regulations that apply to a specific element of allergy care (eg, self-carry of epinephrine devices) to more comprehensive laws. Schools may also have their own policies about medication administration. Pediatric health care clinicians can also advocate for patients and students by supporting common sense legislation that support students with potentially life-threatening allergies. Table 2 reviews selected federal and state laws applicable to food allergy management, and the reader is referred to another AAP policy statement on the role of the school physician regarding laws applicable to that role.[10]

Stock Epinephrine

Stock ("unassigned") epinephrine refers to epinephrine devices that have not been prescribed to a particular person and can be used in emergencies to treat those with undiagnosed food allergies as well as those with a confirmed allergy who do not have access to their epinephrine devices or need additional doses.[16] A 2021 evidence-based guideline discusses the benefits of child care centers and schools stocking unassigned epinephrine.[9] The guidance points out that in 15% to 31% of cases, students treated with epinephrine have no prior history of allergy and, in settings with stock epinephrine, a median of 49% of reactions were

TABLE 2. Selected Federal and State Laws Applicable to Food Allergy Management

	Law	Explanation
Federal laws	Section 504 of the Rehabilitation Act of 1973	This law protects the rights of all students to a free and appropriate public education of students with disabilities, including food allergy (US Department of Education (https://www2.ed.gov/about/offices/list/ocr/504faq.html). A 504 Plan is a written, enforceable agreement ensuring the implementation of adequate policies, procedures, and protocols to support the student with food allergy.
	USDA regulations 7 CFR Part 15b	Substitutions must be available for meals for students whose medical condition (ie, food allergy) restricts their diet. Substitutions are made by the school when a licensed physician provides documentation identifying a student's disability (ie, food allergy), the major life activity impacted by their medical condition (ie, eating), the food allergen that need to be avoided, and foods that replace them.
	Family Education Rights and Privacy Act (FERPA)	FERPA is a federal law that pertains to the protection of a student's education records, including private health information. According to FERPA, such information including that pertinent to food allergy shall only be shared with those that are necessary to protect the safety of the student.
	American Disabilities Act of 1990 and ADA Amendments of 2008	These protect the civil rights of individuals, including students with disabilities. A disability is currently defined as a person with an impairment that can, at certain times, substantially limit a major life activity. In the case of food allergy, the major life activities can be eating and the possibility of trouble breathing that may occur at the time of an allergic reaction due to ingestion of the food allergen. Unlike Section 504 of the Rehabilitation Act of 1973, these apply to some private schools that do not receive federal funding.
	The FDA Food Safety Modernization Act 2011	The law required the Department of Health and Human Services and the Department of Education, to develop voluntary guidelines for schools and early childhood education programs to manage food allergies and severe allergic reactions in children, resulting in the release of the Voluntary Guidelines for Managing Food Allergies in Schools and Early Care and Education Programs.
	School Access to Emergency Epinephrine Act 2013	This law incentivizes states that pass legislation that supports stock epinephrine in schools. States that develop these policies are given preference for federal asthma education grants. The law encourages states to pass their own laws mandating that schools within that state stock epinephrine.
State laws	Medication administration	All states allow for the administration of epinephrine to students with known allergy although there is variation in requirements for delegation and designation to appropriately trained unlicensed assistive personnel when a school nurse is not immediately available. Importantly, some states only allow for the administration of epinephrine and do not allow unlicensed assistive personnel to administer antihistamine or other medication.
	Self-carry and self-administration	Most states have laws that allow for self-carriage and/or self-administration of epinephrine. Elements may include written authorization for self-carriage and/or administration, from school nurse and/or prescriber, and demonstration of ability to self-administer.
	Stock epinephrine laws	Most states have laws that address undesignated (stock) epinephrine. These laws essentially support the ability for designated school personnel to administer epinephrine to a person without a prior history of anaphylaxis known to the school and extend epinephrine availability to those without a prior diagnosis or student specific epinephrine at school. There is wide variability in laws from state to state that may cover some or all elements including the availability of undesignated epinephrine including the acquisition, prescription, storage, and distribution of epinephrine. Laws also apply to the administration, including designation and training in addition to added liability protection beyond those covered by Good Samaritan laws. Additional variation regards required vs voluntary policy supporting stock epinephrine.
	School policy and staff training	Some states have requirements for having a school food allergy management policy and/or requirements for some degree of staff training. These laws range from limited scope (ie, stock epinephrine) to more comprehensive policies that address prevention of reactions in addition to dealing with allergic emergencies. Although comprehensive state guidelines in some states and the federal guidelines are now available that address both policy and staff training, few states require school adoption.

treated with an unassigned device. In 2013, the School Access to Emergency Epinephrine Act was signed into law, which provides financial incentives for states to pass laws that require K-12 schools to have stock epinephrine on hand. These laws differ by state, and some states require, while others allow, an option that K-12 schools maintain stock epinephrine. Without stock epinephrine, there have been situations in which schools have used assigned epinephrine for those without a prior diagnosis who were experiencing anaphylaxis. The 2021 guidelines[9] suggest that, when laws permit, child care centers and schools stock unassigned epinephrine instead of requiring personal epinephrine device (conditional recommendation; very low certainty of evidence). However, at this time, accomplishing this recommendation is likely limited by various financial and practical factors such as funding, school size, and numbers of affected children. State laws may affect the pediatrician's ability or need to prescribe stock epinephrine (additional information can be requested by emailing stgov@aap.org).

Additional considerations for the pediatric health care clinician include:

- Stock epinephrine prescriptions must be written by a licensed medical professional, and rules vary by state. Schools have asked physicians in private and/or academic practice, the school district's physician or chief medical officer (if there is one), or the county or state's senior-most medical officer to provide the prescriptions.
- Benefits of stock epinephrine may include expanding availability for those unable to afford or provide personal devices and to those without a known diagnosis.
- Challenges to implementation may include costs, training, acceptability, and supportive laws as well as the need to monitor and replace expired or used medication.
- Provisions may be made to ensure campus-wide coverage and coverage for field trips (perhaps utilizing stock and/or individual epinephrine as available/feasible). Devices are best stored in accessible, unlocked secure locations, laws permitting.[17]
- Whether or not stock epinephrine is implemented, in addition to the school nurse, school personnel can be trained to administer epinephrine. Regardless of who can administer epinephrine, education on food allergies and anaphylaxis can be provided (for example, by school nurses or through educational resources) to all school staff including cafeteria workers, sports staff, and bus drivers. The content of any required epinephrine training for school staff varies by state.
- State laws have been enacted that protect schools, school nurses, and, in some cases, prescribers from liability concerns. Schools may choose not to implement stock epinephrine policies without liability protections for the school and school nurses, and it may be difficult for the school to obtain epinephrine without liability protections for the prescriber. Liability protections may vary by state and other laws.
- A number of states have passed "entity laws," which permit venues to stock undesignated epinephrine in case of an anaphylactic emergency. These public entities include colleges/universities, day camps, child care centers, and public venues.

RISK REDUCTION STRATEGIES

Avoidance of allergen ingestion is the cornerstone of management and is reviewed in multiple guidelines.[4,7–9,11] Key points that may be helpful to the clinician, especially those collaborating with schools and districts, providing advice to parents and schools are as follows.

- Reading ingredient labels and working to reduce the risk of cross-contact of allergens during food preparation is good practice.
  - Strict avoidance is important, because it is possible for exposure to small amounts of allergen to trigger severe allergic reactions.[18,19]
- The primary route of allergen exposure causing severe allergic reactions is by oral ingestion.
  - Avoidance of shared cups/utensils/cookware is important, because food cross-contamination with allergen can trigger reactions.
  - Products that have precautionary allergen advisory labels (eg, "may contain" or "made in a facility that processes") could contain allergen levels that can trigger allergic reactions in some children.[18,20]
- Allergen exposures through skin contact or inhalation are unlikely to trigger severe allergic reactions[21–25]; however:
  - In some cases, allergic reactions can be triggered by inhalation of actively aerosolized food allergens, such as boiling or steaming food in close proximity of the individual with food allergy. Therefore, participation in school cooking activities involving known allergens may pose a risk for some students with food allergy.
  - Some art or science supplies may contain hidden allergens that can trigger allergic reactions,[27] such as paste, finger paint, play dough, and animal feeds (may contain nuts and seeds). Alternative activities or substitute materials could be used when students with severe food allergy or young children prone to hand-mouth transfer are involved.
  - The CDC guidelines encourage children to wash hands before and after handling or consuming food.[4]
- In one study, nearly a quarter of reactions occurred during special celebrations, such as a birthday party,[27] so vigilance is important, especially when there is a break from routine school activities, such as occurs with after-school programs.
  - Alternative approaches could include: nonfood treats (movie, storytelling, coloring, games), having prearranged safe food treats, including shelf-stable packaged treats, and/or discussing activities with parents to identify substitute approaches.
- Conventional cleaning agents can be used to remove allergens from hands and surfaces. Hand washing using soap and water or commercial wipes is effective; however, water alone or antibacterial hand sanitizer will leave residual allergen. Studies also demonstrate that cleaning surfaces with common household products effectively reduces detectable allergen to below levels reported to trigger objective symptoms.[18,19,23,25]

- The CDC voluntary guidelines and others[4,8] suggest strict "no food sharing" policies and policies of no eating on the school bus (except if necessary for medical reasons) and having a means of communication on the bus.
- Restrictions on allergens require careful consideration. There are some contradictory views.
  - The CDC voluntary guidelines recommend consideration for designated "allergy-friendly" seating arrangements during meals or in some classroom settings that may add supervision and distance children from specific allergens.[4]
  - Some schools have implemented directed allergen "bans" for classrooms, in designated areas, or schoolwide. There are few studies examining the effectiveness of allergen restrictions in schools on reducing allergic reactions. Schoolwide peanut restrictions do not result in elimination of peanuts in the school.[28,29] Schoolwide restrictions also do not prevent allergic reactions. One study suggests that peanut-free tables resulted in lower rates of epinephrine administration.
  - Despite the approaches mentioned above, recent practice guidelines suggest that schools not prohibit specific foods site-wide (conditional recommendation; very low certainty of evidence).[9] These guidelines, with the same level of evidence, suggest that child care centers and schools not establish allergen-restricted zones (ie, peanut-free classrooms, tables) except in special circumstances, such as when students lack developmental capacity to self-manage because of young age or impairments (see additional information below regarding early education and child care settings). These recommendations consider potential social isolation and other negative effects of allergen restrictions against the potential benefits.
  - Managing food allergy in young children and students who are intellectually or developmentally challenged/impaired can be challenging, because they are unable to identify potential allergens, more often have hand-mouth transfer habits (ie, thumb sucking), and are less able to verbalize symptoms of an allergic reaction.[31] For these students, increased school staff oversight and additional precautions may be helpful to minimize risk of allergen exposures and support rapid identification of allergic symptoms.
- As part of a comprehensive plan for managing food allergy, the CDC recommends that school staff be trained on allergen avoidance.[4] Training might be provided by school nurses, trained school staff, pediatricians and other health care professionals, or online modules. Staff who have frequent contact with students with food allergies or provide food may benefit from more detailed training that covers label reading and risks of cross contact in food preparation to identify food allergens and strategies for allergen removal. It is good practice to communicate the needs of students with food allergy to substitute teachers. School nurses and nutrition service personnel are key for coordination and implementation of these plans.[4,32,33]

SCHOOL EMERGENCY MANAGEMENT

According to the CDC guidelines,[4] all staff at a school with a student with food allergy should be trained to recognize anaphylaxis and to begin the emergency protocol. Recent evidence-based guidelines also support that child care centers and schools implement food allergy training for staff (on prevention, recognition, and treatment) and require families to provide written emergency plans.[9] Many families do not provide allergy information to schools, so the guidelines suggest schools implement site-wide food allergy and anaphylaxis protocols to be ready for any student with known or unknown allergies. Studies demonstrate that school staff training on food allergy and anaphylaxis can have a positive impact on staff confidence and attitudes, reducing allergic reactions in schools, and improving rates of student-specific epinephrine devices.[34,35]

Training objectives and processes can vary across the country as states and school districts create differing policies or guidelines for these trainings, which are often coordinated through the school nurse. Some key suggestions include:

- Annual training.
- Assessment of staff confidence and competence.
- Employ CPR and First Aid training.
- Implement a debriefing to identify areas of improvement, further training needs, etc, following an allergic reaction.
- Documentation of the event using district guidelines. Schools may look at food allergy outcomes (like the number of allergic reactions that occur) and strive to improve yearly. Schools may be encouraged to report the occurrence to the primary care provider so that they can include the event in the medical record in their medical home.
- Key points (not mentioned above) that are important in anaphylaxis training include:
  - Anaphylaxis can occur without skin symptoms such as hives.
  - Epinephrine is the only life-saving drug for anaphylaxis.
  - Antihistamines are adjunctive therapies to treat an allergic reaction but cannot be depended on to treat anaphylaxis.
  - Inhaled bronchodilators may be given for respiratory reactions but must not be depended on to treat anaphylaxis.
  - There are proper ways to administer epinephrine. Multiple types of epinephrine devices are marketed.

Trainer dummy devices and online videos can aid in training.
  - Epinephrine devices are sensitive to extremes in temperature, and storage conditions are relevant. They expire, so monitoring is required (there is typically relevant residual potency in an expired unit if it needs to be used if there is no alternative).
  - It should be emphasized that epinephrine is generally safe and there is no contraindication for using it in suspected anaphylaxis (ie, when in doubt, give epinephrine).
  - Parents, caregivers, and school staff can be advised that common adverse effects of epinephrine are usually transient and mild (eg, tremor, tachycardia, flushing/paleness).

In addition to all staff training, staff members who will work with a particular student can review and understand that child's life-threatening allergies and emergency plan, including whether that student self-carries an epinephrine device. Additional points that may be helpful to the clinician in advising parents and schools:

- Anaphylaxis recognition is necessary for effective management. Recent school guidelines suggest that child care or school personnel administer epinephrine when anaphylaxis is suspected rather than as a universal approach for any allergic reaction (ie, mild symptoms) or for an ingestion of an allergen without symptoms (conditional recommendation; very low certainty of evidence).[9] However, special circumstances are noted where epinephrine should be administered nonetheless:
  - Uncertain whether anaphylaxis is occurring.
  - A student with known allergy has impaired consciousness.
  - If the written allergy and anaphylaxis emergency plan advises to give epinephrine with mild or no symptoms in specific circumstances.
- Anaphylaxis is likely if any of the following 3 situations are observed[36]:
  1. Acute onset (minutes to several hours from exposure) of symptoms with involvement of the skin and/or mucosal tissue (eg, generalized hives, pruritus or flushing, swollen lips/tongue/uvula) and signs or symptoms of either respiratory compromise (eg, dyspnea, wheeze/bronchospasm, stridor, reduced peak expiratory flow, hypoxemia) and/or reduced blood pressure or associated symptoms of end-organ dysfunction (eg, hypotonia, syncope, incontinence); or
  2. Two or more of the following occur rapidly after exposure to a likely allergen for that patient: involvement of the skin/mucosal tissue; respiratory compromise; reduced blood pressure or associated symptoms; or persistent gastrointestinal tract symptoms (eg, crampy abdominal pain, vomiting);

  or
  3. Decreased blood pressure after exposure to a known allergen for that patient (within minutes to several hours).
- Individuals experiencing severe anaphylaxis may benefit from being in the supine position as there have been some cases of fatalities associated with raising to the upright position. These cases of "empty-ventricle syndrome" attributable to blood pooling in the legs during anaphylactic shock were reported in adults. Children more often experience respiratory compromise during anaphylaxis and may not tolerate being supine, in which case the recovery position—lying on one's side—may be preferable. This position would also be preferred for children who are vomiting.
- As students mature and become increasingly independent adolescents, self-carrying of emergency medication and self-treatment can be discussed (although prompt access to epinephrine in addition to any carried device should be provided, and an adult should ultimately be responsible for administration). A survey of pediatric allergists found that most expect students to be able to recognize symptoms of anaphylaxis and demonstrate use of an epinephrine auto-injector with a trainer by 9 to 11 years of age, and self-carrying and self-administering an epinephrine auto-injector is expected by 12 to 14 years of age.[38]
- Readiness for self-administration and/or self-carrying can be assessed by the pediatric health care provider for each student with input from the family and school. Decisions may take into consideration both student-specific factors (ie, maturity, competence) and school-specific factors (ie, size of the school, availability of trained staff). Some students may be deemed ready for self-carry in school before they are able to self-administer; re-assessment and review of self-management skills may be performed periodically. Adolescents are not always consistent in self-carrying,[39,40] and they can be encouraged and trained to have their epinephrine devices available at all times.
  - In the event of a reaction, trained school staff should still have epinephrine available and be ultimately responsible for administration of epinephrine, because in emergency situations, the student may be too symptomatic or distressed to self-administer medication or may not have their epinephrine device easily accessible.
- The most common location of allergic reactions at school is the classroom (79%), followed by lunchrooms (12%), but reactions are also reported to occur during outdoor recess and on field trips.[27] Therefore, it is good practice to have emergency medications and trained personnel available during all school-sponsored activities.

- Food protein-induced enterocolitis syndrome[41] is a form of non-IgE mediated food allergy in which the primary symptoms are severe vomiting and possible hypotension/lethargy starting about 2 hours following ingestion of the trigger foods. Unlike anaphylaxis, treatment does not involve epinephrine but may require intravenous hydration and other emergency management interventions. Emergency management typically requires transfer to an emergency department for care, and details can be provided in the Emergency Action Plan or other medical documentation.

SOCIAL AND EMOTIONAL CONCERNS

Children with food allergy may experience a negative impact on quality of life, anxiety and teasing, harassment, or bullying.[42–44] Students and even teachers have been identified as perpetrators of food allergy-related harassment and bullying. Students should be encouraged to report bullying, and anti-bullying programs can be implemented. General education about food allergy for students and staff may promote peer support. The implementation of allergen mitigation strategies can be sensitive to the psychosocial needs of children with food allergies. For example, the child with food allergy must be able to participate in school activities with accommodations if needed (eg, celebrations with safe snacks or alternatives to food rewards without identifying the child with food allergy as the reason for these approaches).

SPECIAL CONSIDERATIONS FOR EARLY EDUCATION, CHILD CARE, AND CAMP SETTINGS

Toddlers and younger students in various child care settings may need extra supervision and restrictions to keep them from ingesting allergens. Younger children may not understand their allergy and may take unsafe food from others. Children 2 to 5 years of age put hands or objects in their mouth up to 40 times an hour, increasing the risk of exposure to allergens if they are in reach.[46] Mitigation strategies may, therefore, include hand cleaning before and following meals/snacks and specified times for meals where there is increased supervision for preventing children from sharing foods or scattering foods outside of designated areas that can be cleaned after the meal.

Toddlers and younger students may also present a challenge for identifying allergic reactions. Infants and toddlers may not report symptoms, and the allergic reaction may not be identified until the symptoms are more advanced. Staff can be taught to recognize the unique ways that young children may demonstrate their allergic symptoms including: putting their hands in their mouths, scratching their tongues, changes in voice, and slurring words. They may also describe the food as "spicy" or their tongue as "hot," "burning," "tingling," "itchy," being "poked," "hairy," or "heavy." They may say that their mouth is "funny," that their throat has "something stuck in it" like a "bump" or "frog."

Many children with food allergies attend summer camps/programs. A majority of camps have children with food allergies attending, and in a survey study, 24% reported cases of anaphylaxis treated with epinephrine, but less than half had individualized emergency plans.[47] The majority (60%) of campers with food allergy do not provide the camp with epinephrine devices.[48] Pediatric health care clinicians can encourage families to provide camps with emergency plans and epinephrine devices, in addition to asthma and other medications.

SPECIAL CONSIDERATIONS FOR ADOLESCENTS

Adolescents may be at higher risk of fatal food-induced anaphylaxis because of risk-taking behaviors in acquiring safe foods (ie, not reading labels, not asking questions about food ingredients, risk of cross contact, etc) and delays in treatment of anaphylaxis.[10,12,39] General school education about food allergy may be helpful. Attention can be focused to education of this age group about identifying safe foods and avoidance of unintentional allergen ingestion (label reading, no food sharing, caution about intimate kissing when a partner recently ingested the allergen, etc) and acquiring safe foods from restaurants or others (discussion of cross contact and hidden ingredients). Adolescents can also be educated about self-recognizing and promptly treating allergic reactions and how to notify others about an allergic reaction.

SUMMARY

Numerous strategies are needed to ensure a safe educational environment for children with food allergies. The pediatrician and primary care clinician play an important role in contributing to the management of children with food allergies in child care and school settings. Consultation with a board-certified allergist-immunologist can help to secure a diagnosis and provide directed treatments and advice.[49] Through collaboration among the pediatric clinician, students, families, school nurses, allergists, and school staff, appropriate plans can be achieved for ensuring safe and effective management of food allergies.

In summary, the pediatrician or pediatric primary care clinician can support food allergy management in school or child care settings by:

- Ensuring an appropriate diagnosis of food allergy[11,14];
- Providing individualized documentation of allergy and anaphylaxis risks and management using a written allergy and anaphylaxis emergency plan[5,6];
- Prescribing epinephrine devices for anaphylaxis management; and
- Being a resource to patients, families, and schools in providing evidence-based advice on food allergy management.

LEAD AUTHORS

Scott H. Sicherer, MD, FAAP
Sonja O'Leary, MD, FAAP
Michael Pistiner MD, MMSc, FAAP
Julie Wang, MD, FAAAP

SECTION ON ALLERGY AND IMMUNOLOGY EXECUTIVE COMMITTEE, 2021–2022

Julie Wang, MD, FAAP, Chairperson
Theresa Bingemann, MD, FAAP
John A. Bird, MD, FAAP
Carla McGuire Davis, MD, FAAP
Vivian Pilar Hernandez-Trujillo, MD, FAAP
Elizabeth C. Matsui, MD, FAAP, Immediate Past Chairperson
Jordan S. Orange, MD, PhD, FAAP
Michael Pistiner, MD, MMSc, FAAP

LIAISONS

Todd A. Mahr, MD, FAAP – American College of Allergy, Asthma, and Immunology
Paul V. Williams, MD, FAAP – American Academy of Allergy, Asthma, and Immunology

STAFF

Pia Daniels, MPH, PMP
Debra L. Burrowes, MHA

COUNCIL ON SCHOOL HEALTH EXECUTIVE COMMITTEE, 2021–2022

Sonja C. O'Leary, MD, FAAP, Chairperson
Sara Bode, MD, FAAP, Chairperson-Elect
Marti Baum, MD, FAAP
Katherine A. Connor, MD, MSPH, FAAP
Emily Frank, MD, FAAP
Erica Gibson, MD, FAAP
Viju Jacob, MD, FAAP
Marian Larkin, MD, FAAP
Yuri Okuizumi-Wu, MD, FAAP
Ryan Padrez, MD, FAAP
Heidi Schumacher, MD, FAAP

LIAISONS

Anna Goddard, PhD, APRN, CPNP-PC – School-Based Health Alliance
Kate King, DNP, RN, MSN – National Association of School Nurses
Erika Ryst, MD – American Academy of Child and Adolescent Psychiatry

STAFF

Carolyn McCarty, PhD
Address correspondence to Scott H. Sicherer, MD, FAAP. E-mail: scott.sicherer@mssm.edu

ABBREVIATIONS

AAP: American Academy of Pediatrics
CDC: Centers for Disease Control and Prevention
IgE: immunoglobulin E
IHP: Individualized Health Care Plan

Disclosures may include salary, wages, or other remuneration of any kind (including but not limited to consulting or advising fees, speaking fees, research funding, ownership interests, honoraria, participation in pension or benefit plans or programs or other perquisites, and reimbursement for travel, lodging, and meals) given for services rendered or other activities for which remuneration is received or expected, whether that compensation or other remuneration is paid directly to the individual or to the individual's employer or another third party. For this clinical report, an additional review was conducted to confirm the absence of bias prior to publication. Members of executive committees of the Section on Allergy and Immunology and the Council on School Health are required to recuse themselves from participating in the development of policies related to their disclosures.

FUNDING: No external funding.

Clinical reports from the American Academy of Pediatrics benefit from expertise and resources of liaisons and internal (AAP) and external reviewers. However, clinical reports from the American Academy of Pediatrics may not reflect the views of the liaisons or the organizations or government agencies that they represent.

The guidance in this report does not indicate an exclusive course of treatment or serve as a standard of medical care. Variations, taking into account individual circumstances, may be appropriate.

All clinical reports from the American Academy of Pediatrics automatically expire 5 years after publication unless reaffirmed, revised, or retired at or before that time.

https://doi.org/10.1542/peds.2025-073168

REFERENCES

1. Gupta RS, Warren CM, Smith BM, et al. The public health impact of parent-reported childhood food allergies in the United States. *Pediatrics*. 2018;142(6):e20181235. PubMed doi: 10.1542/peds.2018-1235
2. Gupta RS, Warren CM, Smith BM, et al. Prevalence and severity of food allergies among US adults. *JAMA Netw Open*. 2019;2(1):e185630. PubMed doi: 10.1001/jamanetworkopen.2018.5630
3. Sicherer SH, Mahr T; American Academy of Pediatrics Section on Allergy and Immunology. Management of food allergy in the school setting. *Pediatrics*. 2010;126(6):1232–1239. PubMed doi: 10.1542/peds.2010-2575
4. Centers for Disease Control and Prevention. Voluntary Guidelines for Managing Food Allergies in Schools and Early Care and Education Programs. US Department of Health and Human Services; 2013. Accessed July 16, 2025. https://www.cdc.gov/school-health-conditions/media/pdfs/20_316712-a_fa_guide_508tag.pdf
5. Sicherer SH, Simons FER, Mahr TA, et al; SECTION ON ALLERGY AND IMMUNOLOGY. Epinephrine for first-aid management of anaphylaxis. *Pediatrics*. 2017;139(3):e20164006. PubMed doi: 10.1542/peds.2016-4006
6. Wang J, Sicherer SH, Matsui E, et al; SECTION ON ALLERGY AND IMMUNOLOGY. Guidance on completing a written allergy and anaphylaxis emergency plan. *Pediatrics*. 2017;139(3):e20164005. PubMed doi: 10.1542/peds.2016-4005
7. Sicherer SH, Allen K, Lack G, Taylor SL, Donovan SM, Oria M. Critical issues in food allergy: a National Academies Consensus Report. *Pediatrics*. 2017;140(2):e20170194. PubMed doi: 10.1542/peds.2017-0194
8. Wang J, Bingemann T, Russell AF, Young MC, Sicherer SH. The allergist's role in anaphylaxis and food allergy management in the school and childcare setting. *J Allergy Clin Immunol Pract*. 2018;6(2):427–435. PubMed doi: 10.1016/j.jaip.2017.11.022
9. Waserman S, Cruickshank H, Hildebrand KJ, et al. Prevention and management of allergic reactions to food in child care centers and schools: Practice guidelines. *J Allergy Clin Immunol*. 2021;147(5):1561–1578. PubMed doi: 10.1016/j.jaci.2021.01.034
10. Devore CD, Wheeler LS, Allison M, et al; Council on School Health; American Academy of Pediatrics. Role of the school physician. *Pediatrics*. 2013;131(1):178–182. PubMed doi: 10.1542/peds.2012-2995
11. Boyce JA, Assa'ad A, Burks AW, et al; NIAID-Sponsored Expert Panel. Guidelines for the diagnosis and management of food allergy in the United States: report of the NIAID-sponsored expert panel. *J Allergy Clin Immunol*. 2010;126(6)(suppl):S1–S58. PubMed doi: 10.1016/j.jaci.2010.10.008
12. Warren CM, Chadha AS, Sicherer SH, Jiang J, Gupta RS. Prevalence and severity of sesame allergy in the United States. *JAMA Netw Open*. 2019;2(8):e199144. PubMed doi: 10.1001/jamanetworkopen.2019.9144
13. Pouessel G, Turner PJ, Worm M, et al. Food-induced fatal anaphylaxis: From epidemiological data to general prevention strategies. *Clin Exp Allergy*. 2018;48(12):1584–1593. PubMed doi: 10.1111/cea.13287
14. Sicherer SH, Wood RA, Sicherer SH, et al; American Academy of Pediatrics Section On Allergy And Immunology. Allergy testing in childhood: using allergen-specific IgE tests. *Pediatrics*. 2012;129(1):193–197. PubMed doi: 10.1542/peds.2011-2382
15. Mercer RD, Jones CJ, Smith HE. Reviewing the content and design of anaphylaxis management plans published in English. *J Allergy Clin Immunol Pract*. 2017;5(5):1288–1294. doi: 10.1016/j.jaip.2017.06.032 e2.
16. Russell AF, Bingemann TA, Cooke AT, et al. The Need for Required Stock Epinephrine in All Schools: A Work Group Report of the AAAAI Adverse Reactions to Foods Committee. *J Allergy Clin Immunol Pract*. 2023;11(4):1068–1082.e1. PubMed doi: 10.1016/j.jaip.2022.12.047
17. Tanner A, Clarke C. Epinephrine Policies and Protocols Guidance for Schools: Equipping School Nurses to Save Lives. *NASN Sch Nurse*. 2016;31(1):13–22. PubMed doi: 10.1177/1942602X15607604
18. Zhu J, Pouillot R, Kwegyir-Afful EK, Luccioli S, Gendel SM. A retrospective analysis of allergic reaction severities and minimal eliciting doses for peanut, milk, egg, and soy oral food challenges. *Food Chem Toxicol*. 2015;80:92–100. PubMed doi: 10.1016/j.fct.2015.02.023
19. Chu DK, Baumert JL, Taylor SL, et al. Peanut allergen reaction thresholds during controlled food challenges in 2 Canadian randomized studies (Canada-ARM1 and PISCES). *J Allergy Clin Immunol Pract*. 2021;9(6):2524–2526. doi: 10.1016/j.jaip.2021.02.009 e2.
20. Ford LS, Taylor SL, Pacenza R, Niemann LM, Lambrecht DM, Sicherer SH. Food allergen advisory labeling and product contamination with egg, milk, and peanut. *J Allergy Clin Immunol*. 2010;126(2):384–385. NOT IN FILE. doi: 10.1016/j.jaci.2010.05.034
21. Simonte SJ, Ma S, Mofidi S, Sicherer SH. Relevance of casual contact with peanut butter in children with peanut allergy. *J Allergy Clin Immunol*. 2003;112(1):180–182. PubMed doi: 10.1067/mai.2003.1486
22. Wainstein BK, Kashef S, Ziegler M, Jelley D, Ziegler JB. Frequency and significance of immediate contact reactions to peanut in peanut-sensitive children. *Clin Exp Allergy*. 2007;37(6):839–845. PubMed doi: 10.1111/j.1365-2222.2007.02726.x
23. Perry TT, Conover-Walker MK, Pomés A, Chapman MD, Wood RA. Distribution of peanut allergen in the environment. *J Allergy Clin Immunol*. 2004;113(5):973–976. PubMed doi: 10.1016/j.jaci.2004.02.035
24. Johnson RM, Barnes CS. Airborne concentrations of peanut protein. *Allergy Asthma Proc*. 2013;34(1):59–64. PubMed doi: 10.2500/aap.2013.34.3622
25. Brough HA, Makinson K, Penagos M, et al. Distribution of peanut protein in the home environment. *J Allergy Clin Immunol*. 2013;132(3):623–629. NOT IN FILE. doi: 10.1016/j.jaci.2013.02.035
26. Roberts G, Golder N, Lack G. Bronchial challenges with aerosolized food in asthmatic, food-allergic children. *Allergy*. 2002;57(8):713–717. PubMed doi: 10.1034/j.1398-9995.2002.03366.x

27. Sicherer SH, Furlong TJ, DeSimone J, Sampson HA. The US Peanut and Tree Nut Allergy Registry: characteristics of reactions in schools and day care. *J Pediatr.* 2001;138(4):560–565. PubMed doi: 10.1067/mpd.2001.111821

28. Nguyen-Luu NU, Ben-Shoshan M, Alizadehfar R, et al. Inadvertent exposures in children with peanut allergy. *Pediatr Allergy Immunol.* 2012;23(2):133–139. PubMed doi: 10.1111/j.1399-3038.2011.01235.x

29. Banerjee DK, Kagan RS, Turnbull E, et al. Peanut-free guidelines reduce school lunch peanut contents. *Arch Dis Child.* 2007; 92(11):980–982. PubMed doi: 10.1136/adc.2006.113118

30. Bartnikas LM, Huffaker MF, Sheehan WJ, et al. Impact of school peanut-free policies on epinephrine administration. *J Allergy Clin Immunol.* 2017;140(2):465–473. PubMed doi: 10.1016/j.jaci.2017.01.040

31. Simons FE, Sampson HA. Anaphylaxis: Unique aspects of clinical diagnosis and management in infants (birth to age 2 years). *J Allergy Clin Immunol.* 2015;135(5):1125–1131. PubMed doi: 10.1016/j.jaci.2014.09.014

32. Pistiner M, Devore CD, Schoessler S. School food allergy and anaphylaxis management for the pediatrician–extending the medical home with critical collaborations. *Pediatr Clin North Am.* 2015; 62(6):1425–1439. PubMed doi: 10.1016/j.pcl.2015.07.016

33. Holmes BW, Sheetz A, Allison M, et al; COUNCIL ON SCHOOL HEALTH. Role of the school nurse in providing school health services. *Pediatrics.* 2016;137(6):e20160852. PubMed doi: 10.1542/peds.2016-0852

34. Tsuang A, Atal Z, Demain H, Patrick K, Pistiner M, Wang J. Benefits of school nurse training sessions for food allergy and anaphylaxis management. *J Allergy Clin Immunol Pract.* 2019;7(1):309–311. doi: 10.1016/j.jaip.2018.05.015 e2.

35. Chokshi NY, Patel D, Davis CM. Long-term increase in epinephrine availability associated with school nurse training in food allergy. *J Allergy Clin Immunol Pract.* 2015;3(1):128–130. PubMed doi: 10.1016/j.jaip.2014.09.015

36. Sampson HA, Muñoz-Furlong A, Campbell RL, et al. Second symposium on the definition and management of anaphylaxis: summary report–Second National Institute of Allergy and Infectious Disease/Food Allergy and Anaphylaxis Network symposium. *J Allergy Clin Immunol.* 2006;117(2):391–397. PubMed doi: 10.1016/j.jaci.2005.12.1303

37. Pumphrey RS. Fatal posture in anaphylactic shock. *J Allergy Clin Immunol.* 2003;112(2):451–452. PubMed doi: 10.1067/mai.2003.1614

38. Simons E, Sicherer SH, Simons FE. Timing the transfer of responsibilities for anaphylaxis recognition and use of an epinephrine auto-injector from adults to children and teenagers: pediatric allergists' perspective. *Ann Allergy Asthma Immunol.* 2012; 108(5):321–325. PubMed doi: 10.1016/j.anai.2012.03.004

39. Warren CM, Zaslavsky JM, Kan K, Spergel JM, Gupta RS. Epinephrine auto-injector carriage and use practices among US children, adolescents, and adults. *Ann Allergy Asthma Immunol.* 2018;121(4):479–489.e2. PubMed doi: 10.1016/j.anai.2018.06.010

40. Robinson M, Koplin JJ, Field MJ, et al; SchoolNuts Investigators. SchoolNuts Investigators. Patterns of carriage of prescribed adrenaline autoinjectors in 10- to 14-year-old food-allergic students: a population-based study. *J Allergy Clin Immunol Pract.* 2019;7(2):437–443. PubMed doi: 10.1016/j.jaip.2018.06.025

41. Nowak-Wegrzyn A, Chehade M, Groetch ME, et al. International consensus guidelines for the diagnosis and management of food protein-induced enterocolitis syndrome: executive summary-workgroup report of the Adverse Reactions to Foods Committee, American Academy of Allergy, Asthma & Immunology. *J Allergy Clin Immunol.* 2017;139(4):1111–1126. doi: 10.1016/j.jaci.2016.12.966 e4.

42. Shemesh E, Annunziato RA, Ambrose MA, et al. Child and parental reports of bullying in a consecutive sample of children with food allergy. *Pediatrics.* 2013;131(1):e10–e17. PubMed doi: 10.1542/peds.2012-1180

43. Herbert L, Shemesh E, Bender B. Clinical management of psychosocial concerns related to food allergy. *J Allergy Clin Immunol Pract.* 2016;4(2):205–213. PubMed doi: 10.1016/j.jaip.2015.10.016

44. Bingemann T, Herbert LJ, Young MC, et al. Deficits and opportunities in allergists' approaches to food allergy-related bullying. *J Allergy Clin Immunol Pract.* 2020;8(1):343–345. e2.

45. Lieberman JA, Weiss C, Furlong TJ, Sicherer M, Sicherer SH. Bullying among pediatric patients with food allergy. *Ann Allerg Asthma Im.* Oct 2010;105(4):282–286. NOT IN FILE. doi: 10.1016/j.anai.2010.07.011

46. Tulve NS, Suggs JC, McCurdy T, Cohen Hubal EA, Moya J. Frequency of mouthing behavior in young children. *J Expo Anal Environ Epidemiol.* 2002;12(4):259–264. PubMed doi: 10.1038/sj.jea.7500225

47. Schellpfeffer NR, Leo HL, Ambrose M, Hashikawa AN. Camp leadership perspectives on food allergy-related anaphylaxis events and training for camp staff: a national survey of summer camps. *J Allergy Clin Immunol Pract.* 2020;8(4):1247–1252. doi: 10.1016/j.jaip.2019.11.014 e1.

48. Schellpfeffer NR, Leo HL, Ambrose M, Hashikawa AN. Food Allergy Trends and Epinephrine Autoinjector Presence in Summer Camps. *J Allergy Clin Immunol Pract.* 2017;5(2):358–362. PubMed doi: 10.1016/j.jaip.2016.10.018

49. Leung D, Schatz M; American Academy of Allergy, Asthma & Immunology. Consultation and referral guidelines citing the evidence: how the allergist-immunologist can help. *J Allergy Clin Immunol.* 2006;117(2)(Suppl Consultation):S495–S523. PubMed doi: 10.1016/j.jaci.2005.10.047

Medical vs Nonmedical Immunization Exemptions for Child Care and School Attendance

- *Policy Statement*

POLICY STATEMENT Organizational Principles to Guide and Define the Child Health Care System and/or Improve the Health of All Children

American Academy of Pediatrics

DEDICATED TO THE HEALTH OF ALL CHILDREN™

Medical vs Nonmedical Immunization Exemptions for Child Care and School Attendance: Policy Statement

Jesse M. Hackell, MD, FAAP,[1] Kyle Brothers, MD, PhD, FAAP,[2] Sara Bode, MD, FAAP,[3] Lisa M. Costello, MD, MPH, FAAP,[4] Lisa M. Kafer, MD, FAAP, Sean T. O'Leary, MD, MPH, FAAP,[5] and the Committee on Practice and Ambulatory Medicine; Committee on Infectious Diseases; Committee on State Government Affairs; and Council on School Health

Routine childhood immunizations against infectious diseases are an integral part of our public health infrastructure. They provide direct protection to the immunized individual and indirect protection to children and adults unable to be immunized by reducing spread of vaccine-preventable diseases in the community. All 50 states, the District of Columbia, and Puerto Rico have regulations requiring proof of immunization as a condition for child care and school attendance as a public health strategy to protect children in these settings and to secondarily serve as a mechanism to promote timely immunization of children by their caregivers. Although all states and the District of Columbia have mechanisms to exempt school attendees from specific immunizations for medical reasons, the majority also have a heterogeneous collection of regulations and laws that allow nonmedical reasons for exemption. The American Academy of Pediatrics (AAP) supports certification of immunization to attend child care and school as a sound means of providing a safe environment for attendees and employees of these settings. The AAP also supports medically indicated exemptions to specific immunizations as determined for each individual child. The AAP advocates for the elimination of nonmedical exemptions from immunizations as contrary to optimal individual and public health.

BACKGROUND

Principles of Childhood Immunization and Community Protection

Childhood immunization is one of the greatest accomplishments of modern medicine. In the United States, for children born from 1994–2023, data

abstract

[1]Department of Pediatrics, New York Medical College, Valhalla, New York; [2]Norton Children's Research Institute Affiliated with the University of Louisville School of Medicine, Louisville, Kentucky; [3]Nationwide Children's Hospital, Columbus, Ohio; [4]Department of Pediatrics, West Virginia University School of Medicine, Morgantown, West Virginia; and [5]Department of Pediatrics, University of Colorado School of Medicine, Aurora, Colorado

All authors participated in conception, design, drafting, and critical revision of the clinical report and approved the final manuscript as submitted.

FINANCIAL/CONFLICT OF INTEREST DISCLOSURE: The authors have indicated they do not have a financial relationship relevant to this article to disclose.

Policy statements from the American Academy of Pediatrics benefit from expertise and resources of liaisons and internal (AAP) and external reviewers. However, policy statements from the American Academy of Pediatrics may not reflect the views of the liaisons or the organizations or government agencies that they represent.

To cite: Hackell JM, Brothers K, Bode S, et al; American Academy of Pediatrics, Committee on Practice and Ambulatory Medicine; Committee on Infectious Diseases; Committee on State Government Affairs; and Council on School Health. Medical vs Nonmedical Immunization Exemptions for Child Care and School Attendance: Policy Statement. *Pediatrics.* 2025;156(2):e2025072714

analysis and modeling suggest that routine childhood immunization will have prevented approximately 500 million cases of illness, 32 million hospitalizations, and 1.1 million deaths, eventually saving $540 billion in direct costs and $2.7 trillion in societal costs.[1]

Certain infants, children, and adolescents cannot safely receive certain vaccines because of age or specific health conditions, and some vaccinated individuals may not develop immunity despite appropriate immunization. These individuals benefit from the effectiveness of immunizations through high rates of vaccination in their community. When nearly all individuals for whom a vaccine is not contraindicated have been appropriately immunized, the risk of illness or spread of a contagious vaccine-preventable infectious agent to those who do not have the direct benefit of immunization is minimized. Although there is variation in levels of immunization required to generate community-wide protection specific to each disease and vaccine, the Healthy People 2030 goals seek to immunize at least 90% of the eligible population.[2] Certain highly contagious diseases, such as pertussis and measles, require a population immunization rate of ≥95% to prevent sustained community transmission.

Immunizations as a Condition for School Attendance

Each of the 50 states, the District of Columbia, and Puerto Rico have established conditions, including receipt of immunizations, which must be met by attendees of child care centers and public schools, and nearly all have laws covering private schools as well.[3] Some states allow local discretion, although the majority set these conditions at the state level. These policies are designed to protect children attending child care and school from vaccine-preventable diseases (VPDs) by creating a learning environment with a very high rate of immunization. In addition, vocational schools, colleges, and universities also have made immunization a condition of attendance and participation in activities. In addition to primary disease prevention and preventing in-school spread to susceptible children of VPDs, these policies may also serve to prevent spread of disease to school staff members as well as transmission of disease from the school to susceptible individuals at home, including immunocompromised individuals and infants too young to have been immunized. Implementation of these conditions also serves as a public health benefit by providing a strong incentive for parents and families to immunize their children according to the schedule recommended by the Centers for Disease Control and Prevention and the American Academy of Pediatrics (AAP). Public health data show setting and enforcing these conditions for child care and/or school entry result in increased community immunization rates[4] and decreased incidence of VPDs.[5,6] Pediatricians partnering with school nurses and administration to ensure equitable and timely access to vaccination for students prior to school entry plays an important role in keeping children healthy and in promoting daily school attendance.[7]

Medical Exemptions From Immunization

Although there are fairly consistent standards for immunizations across the United States, every state, the District of Columbia, and Puerto Rico have allowances permitting school attendance without certain vaccines for medically indicated reasons. Examples of such include allergy to a vaccine component, previous significant adverse reaction to a vaccine or its components, or other underlying health condition such as immunosuppression in an organ transplant recipient.[8] Almost half of states have laws that distinguish between temporary and permanent medical contraindications,[3] with nearly another half of these states requiring annual or more frequent health care provider recertification for the medical exemptions. Because only a very small proportion of children have medical conditions prohibiting specific immunizations,[9] medically indicated exemptions, when granted appropriately, typically do not have a significant impact on overall community vaccination coverage.

Nonmedical Exemptions From Immunization

As of this writing, 5 states (CA, CT, ME, NY, and WV) have laws that accept only medical exemptions from immunizations. Mississippi had a similar law, but in April 2023, a federal court required the state health department to include provisions for a religious exemption, to avoid having the entire school vaccination law struck down.[10,11] Forty-five states allow religious beliefs to be used as a basis for an exemption, and 15 states allow "personal beliefs," "philosophical," or "conscientious objection" exemptions. Although nearly ubiquitous, nonmedical exemption regulations are quite heterogeneous from state to state in terms of how they are granted, used, and maintained.[3] Some states explicitly exclude "philosophical" and "personal belief" exemptions and define these as not falling under the scope of religious exemptions. More than half of the states can exclude unimmunized students during outbreaks, epidemics, or emergencies, and more than one-quarter of the states require parents to provide an affidavit confirming either a religious or another nonmedical justification in applying for a nonmedical school immunization exemption. A number of states, such as Michigan,[1] have laws requiring parent/guardian education by health departments or health care providers about the benefits of vaccines and the risks and consequences of not receiving recommended childhood immunizations. These requirements have resulted in a decline in the total number of exemptions requested and approved.[1]

Exemptions Based on Religious Beliefs

Among the major world religious traditions, none include scriptural or doctrinal guidelines that preclude adherents from being vaccinated.[12] In fact, the leaders of some religious groups have highlighted that vaccination can be one important way to protect oneself and one's neighbors and have thus suggested that there is a moral or religious obligation to seek vaccination.[13] Importantly, however, religious belief is one area where we see the richness of human diversity being expressed. Perspectives on vaccines might be drawn from religious traditions that developed independently of the major world religions as well as from the diverse denominational perspectives that exist within major religions.[14] Just as with other types of doctrines, those related to vaccines might even be developed by small communities or individuals in ways that are completely independent from antecedent scriptural or doctrinal traditions but are, nonetheless, thought of as "religious" commitments by those who hold them.[15,16]

In the face of such complexity, it can be extraordinarily difficult to interpret what is meant when a perspective on vaccination is asserted to have a religious dimension. State legislatures are rightly reticent to enact public policies that are perceived to interfere with the exercise of religion. However, in practice, nonmedical exceptions based on religious belief can substantially limit the public health value of vaccine requirements for school attendance. There is no practicable way for schools or other involved community partners to distinguish fairly among religious or other nonmedical claims. State-level policies that differentiate among these types of claims serve only to introduce opportunities for uneven application, which in turn leads inevitably to disparities in immunization coverage and schools that are less safe.

PUBLIC HEALTH EFFECTS OF IMMUNIZATION EXEMPTIONS

Exemption Rates and VPD Incidence

Legislation establishing immunization standards as a condition for school entry increases immunization rates and dramatically decreases the incidence of VPDs.[17] Examples of these include immunization against measles and chickenpox. Likewise, higher rates of immunization exemptions in communities correlate with higher rates of vaccine-preventable illnesses and disease outbreaks, such as pertussis and measles.[18–21]

Although overall rates of many immunizations have increased or remained steady over the past 10 years, recent studies show that unvaccinated children are often geographically clustered within communities[20] with higher rates of immunization exemption. This clustering reflects the fact that families with similar sociocultural beliefs often live near each other or attend the same schools, which results in population clusters within larger communities with significantly lower immunization rates that are insufficient to prevent spread of disease within those communities. This phenomenon results in a greater likelihood of disease outbreaks when a vaccine-preventable illness is introduced into these communities. Outbreaks that start in communities with low vaccination coverage have the potential to spread beyond those communities into other communities with low vaccination coverage or into the broader population, particularly for diseases like measles, varicella, and pertussis.

Exemption Rates and State Legal Requirements

States with less stringent restrictions on nonmedical exemptions and those that grant permanent medical exemptions have significantly higher vaccine exemption rates than those states with more rigorous rules or those that only grant exemptions that require regular review.[21]

States that permit nonmedical exemptions have had steady increases in the number of exemptions over time, with the national rate of exemption gradually increasing as well, reaching 3% in the 2022–23 school year.[3,9] Religious exemptions have increased for states that do not offer other types of nonmedical exemptions but have, through regulatory language, broadly defined religion for the purposes of obtaining vaccine exemption. The ease of requirements to obtain nonmedical exemptions can have a significant impact on the rate of exemptions and immunizations.[22] It should also be noted that nonmedical exemptions erode the safety of school environments, and heterogeneous implementation of these policies across states and locales creates a confusing legal environment for children, parents, and pediatricians.[23]

JUSTIFICATION FOR IMMUNIZATION REQUIREMENTS

Legal Justification for the AAP Policy Statement

The legal dynamics surrounding immunization conditions for school attendance and exemptions from those conditions are extraordinarily complex and evolving quickly as a result of both new state legislative initiatives and challenges to them.[24] A comprehensive consideration of the legal issues and case law relevant to this topic are beyond the scope of this policy statement, but it is important to highlight a few key legal issues that underpin the AAP policy. There are numerous court rulings that place school safety above the interests of individual parents where immunizations are concerned. In *Jacobson v Massachusetts* (1905),[25] the court found legislative vaccine mandates to be constitutional as a means of protecting public health and public safety. In *Zucht v King* in 1922, the Supreme Court upheld a local ordinance requiring vaccination as a condition for school attendance.[26] In the 1944 case *Prince v Commonwealth of Massachusetts*, the court ruled that the constitutional rights of religion or parenthood were not beyond limitation and that states had the authority to protect the welfare of children and the community. Although the specific case was with regard to child labor laws, the court extended its language to encompass both religious and personal activities such that, "The right to practice religion freely does not include liberty to expose the community or the child to communicable disease or the latter to ill health or death."[27] Since these rulings, there have been numerous challenges to state and local immunization rules (eg, *Workman v Mingo County Schools, Phillips v City of New York, Love et al v Department of Education et al)*. These challenges to state school vaccination laws are rarely successful, but new challenges continue to be filed in many areas and remain a threat to maintaining high vaccination coverage in the United States.

Ethical Justification for the AAP Policy Statement

There are a wide array of ethical considerations relevant to policy on exemptions to immunization conditions for school attendance. These include ethical topics typically associated with medical ethics, such as personal autonomy and parental authority, as well as concepts associated with public health ethics, like communal responsibility and equity.[28] Although a comprehensive discussion of these issues is beyond the scope of this policy statement, it is important to highlight some ethical arguments that ground the AAP policy on nonmedical exemptions.

One important consideration is parental authority, which recognizes the rights of parents to make decisions for their children, including health decisions.[29] An important feature of parental authority is that it is constrained in a variety of ways. For example, parental authority implies not only a right for parents to make decisions for their child but also a responsibility for parents to advance their children's interests and to make decisions that do not harm them.[30] Balancing parental authority with factors like the state's interest in protecting school communities is, of course, a matter of intense public interest. Ideally, the state's interest in protecting school communities should be exercised in a way that protects the family's other interests as much as possible and that constrains parental authority as little as possible.[31] Immunization conditions for school attendance offer a reasonable strategy for striking this balance. Unlike an outright vaccine mandate, this policy permits parents some leeway in exercising their authority over health decisions for their children. An obvious drawback of such a policy is that the children in these families are not able to benefit from group educational contexts. This drawback not only carries consequences for the children, since the benefits of in-person school attendance are well established,[7] but also for parents who often depend on schools for free and reduced lunch and for supervision of their children during the workday. In addition, the ability of families to adapt financially and logistically to not being able to send their child to school varies widely based on their available resources. The AAP acknowledges the challenges that such a policy can create for some families.

Even recognizing these difficult trade-offs, making certification of vaccination a condition for in-person school attendance remains the only way to maintain a safe school environment *and* protect parental authority. Although nonmedical exemptions might seem like reasonable accommodation to lessen the challenges that some families face, the fact is that exemptions are a deeply problematic tool for addressing these challenges. They inevitably lead to school environments becoming less safe, especially for children unable to be protected by vaccination, and they cannot be applied in a way that ensures that these trade-offs are managed in an equitable way. Although there are certainly families who would value having the option to decline vaccines and also send their children to school, nonmedical exemptions threaten the safety of the entire school community and shift the burden of protecting their children to the parents of children who are medically fragile, immunocompromised, or unable to receive immunizations for medical reasons. These parents depend on the state to ensure that school environments are as safe as possible for their children. Fundamentally, policies that make immunization a uniform condition of school attendance and permit only medical exemptions are an equitable choice and strike the optimal balance between parental authority and public safety for all children.

CONCLUSIONS

Making immunizations a condition for child care and school attendance is an effective means of protecting people from VPDs, both directly by vaccination and indirectly via community-wide protection. Making sure children are vaccinated at the start of the school year can also have a beneficial effect on the timeliness of immunization. Because medically recognized contraindications for specific individuals from specific vaccines exist, there continues to be a place for legitimate medical exemptions to immunization. However, exempting children for nonmedical reasons from immunizations is problematic for medical, public health, and ethical reasons and creates unnecessary risk to both individuals and communities.

RECOMMENDATIONS

1. The AAP supports laws and regulatory measures that require certification of immunization as a condition of attending child care and school as a sound means of providing a safe environment for students and staff of these settings.
2. The AAP supports equitable, timely access to vaccination to ensure consistent in-person schooling and avoid exclusion because of lack of access through a safety net of vaccine services including the medical home, public health, and school health programs.
3. The AAP supports medically indicated exemptions to specific immunizations as determined for each

individual student. The AAP further recommends that all pediatric health care providers understand bona fide reasons for granting medical exemptions, as detailed in the *Red Book*,[32] only grant exemptions when medically justified, and recertify the need for these exemptions on a regular basis.

4. The AAP recommends that all states, territories, and the District of Columbia eliminate all nonmedical exemptions from immunizations as a condition of school attendance. In addition, states and territories should develop policies to ensure that any medical exemptions are appropriate and evidence based.
5. The AAP recommends that pediatricians continue to counsel their families who request nonmedical exemptions and that they not participate in vetting or endorsing applications for nonmedical exemptions from immunization as a condition of attending child care and school. In addition, such vetting or endorsing should not be required by schools or other authorities.
6. The AAP recommends that all child care centers, schools, and other covered entities comply with state laws and regulations requiring current and accurate documentation of appropriate immunization status and appropriate medical exemptions of attendees and students and that state departments of health and education enforce these laws and regulations on a uniform and equitable basis.
7. The AAP recommends that the appropriate public health authorities provide communities with information about immunization rates in child care centers, schools, and other covered entities to a) determine whether there are risks of outbreaks of vaccine-preventable diseases on the basis of this information; and b) offer parents information about the safety of individual child care centers and schools.

LEAD AUTHORS

Jesse M. Hackell, MD, FAAP
Kyle Brothers, MD, PhD, FAAP
Sara Bode, MD, FAAP
Lisa M. Costello, MD, MPH, FAAP
Lisa Kafer, MD, FAAP
Sean T. O'Leary, MD, MPH, FAAP

COMMITTEE ON PRACTICE AND AMBULATORY MEDICINE, 2024–2025

Carolyn Cleary, MD, FAAP
Mona Doss Roberts, DO, MA, FAAP
Elizabeth Hawse, MD, FAAP
Cailly Howell-McLean, MD, FAAP
Lisa M. Kafer, MD, FAAP
Tomitra Latimer, MD, FAAP
Robert Wiskind, MD, FAAP

LIAISONS

Seth Kaplan, MD, FAAP, Section on Administration and Practice Management

PAST COMMITTEE ON PRACTICE AND AMBULATORY MEDICINE CONTRIBUTORS

Jesse M. Hackell, MD, FAAP
Yvette Almendarez, MD, FAAP
Alisa Skatrud, MPA, Family Liaison

STAFF

Mackenzie Magnus MBA, MPH

COMMITTEE ON INFECTIOUS DISEASES, 2024–2025

Sean T. O'Leary, MD, MPH, FAAP, Chairperson
James D. Campbell, MD, MS, FAAP, Vice Chairperson
Monica I. Ardura, DO, MSCS, FAAP
Kristina A. Bryant, MD, FAAP, *Red Book Online* Team Lead
Mary T. Caserta, MD, FAAP
Claudia Espinosa, MD, MSc, FAAP
Robert W. Frenck, Jr., MD, FAAP
C. Mary Healy, MD
Chandy C. John, MD, MS, FAAP
Aaron M. Milstone, MD, MHS, FAAP
Angela L. Myers, MD, MPH, FAAP
Pia S. Pannaraj, MD, MPH, FAAP
Adam J. Ratner, MD, MPH, FAAP, *Red Book* Associate Editor
José R. Romero, MD, FAAP
Matthew Zahn, MD, FAAP

EX OFFICIO

David W. Kimberlin, MD, FAAP – *Red Book* Editor
Ritu Banerjee, MD, PhD, FAAP – *Red Book* Associate Editor
Elizabeth D. Barnett MD, FAAP– *Red Book* Associate Editor
Ruth Lynfield, MD, FAAP - *Red Book* Associate Editor

LIAISONS

Amina Ahmed, MD, FAAP, American Thoracic Society
Michelle Barton, MD, Canadian Paediatric Society
Lisa M. Kafer, MD, FAAP, Committee on Practice Ambulatory Medicine
Denee Moore, MD, American Academy of Family Physicians
Jennifer L. Thompson, MD, American College of Obstetricians and Gynecologists
Juan P. Torres, MD, PhD, Sociedad Latinoamericana de Infectología Pediátrica

STAFF

Gillian Gibbs, MPH

COMMITTEE ON STATE GOVERNMENT AFFAIRS, 2024–2025

Lisa Marie Costello, MD, MPH, FAAP
Lisa A. Gwynn, DO, MPH, MBA, FAAP
Dena K. Wisner Hubbard, MD, FAAP
Morissa Jean Ladinsky, MD, FAAP
Honorable Richard J. Pan, MD, MPH, FAAP
Lauren Wilson, MD, FAAP

PAST COMMITTEE ON STATE GOVERNMENT AFFAIRS CONTRIBUTORS

Pam K. Shaw, MD, FAAP
Cindy W. Christian, MD, FAAP

STAFF

Ian Van Dinther

COUNCIL ON SCHOOL HEALTH EXECUTIVE COMMITTEE, 2024–2025

Sara Bode, MD, FAAP, Chairperson
Marian Larkin, MD, FAAP, Chairperson-elect
Katherine A. Connor, MD, MSPH, FAAP
Emily Frank, MD, FAAP
Ronald Vincent Marino, DO, MPH, FAAP
Tracie Newman, MD, MPH, FAAP
Yuri Okuizumi-Wu, MD, FAAP
Ryan Padrez, MD, FAAP
Anjali Rao, MD, FAAP
Michelle Shankar, MD, MHS, FAAP
Elizabeth Zmuda, DO, FAAP

LIAISONS

Ana Caskin, MD, School-Based Health Alliance
Lynn Nelson, RN, National Association of School Nurses
Kristie Ladegard, MD, American Academy of Child and Adolescent Psychiatry

STAFF

Carolyn Lullo McCarty, PhD

ABBREVIATIONS

AAP: American Academy of Pediatrics
VPD: vaccine-preventable disease

The guidance in this statement does not indicate an exclusive course of treatment or serve as a standard of medical care. Variations, taking into account individual circumstances, may be appropriate.

All policy statements from the American Academy of Pediatrics automatically expire 5 years after publication unless reaffirmed, revised, or retired at or before that time.

FUNDING: No external funding.

https://doi.org/10.1542/peds.2025-072714

REFERENCES

1. Zhou F, Jatlaoui TC, Leidner AJ, et al. Health and economic benefits of routine childhood immunizations in the era of the Vaccines for Children Program—United States, 1994–2023. *MMWR Morb Mortal Wkly Rep.* 2024;73(31):682–685. PubMed doi: 10.15585/mmwr.mm7331a2
2. US Department of Health and Human Services, Office of Disease Prevention and Health Promotion. Vaccination - Healthy People 2030. Published 2022. Accessed October 31, 2024. https://health.gov/healthypeople/objectives-and-data/browse-objectives/vaccination
3. Centers for Disease Control and Prevention. State School Immunization Requirements and Vaccine Exemption Laws. Published February 2022. https://www.cdc.gov/phlp/docs/school-vaccinations.pdf
4. Davis MM, Gaglia MA. Associations of daycare and school entry vaccination requirements with varicella immunization rates. *Vaccine.* 2005;23(23):3053–3060. PubMed doi: 10.1016/j.vaccine.2004.10.047
5. Ernst KC, Pogreba-Brown K, Rasmussen L, Erhart LM. The effect of policy changes on hepatitis A vaccine uptake in Arizona children, 1995–2008. *Public Health Rep.* 2011;126(suppl 2):87–96. PubMed doi: 10.1177/00333549111260S211
6. Lopez AS, Kolasa MS, Seward JF. Status of school entry requirements for varicella vaccination and vaccination coverage 11 years after implementation of the varicella vaccination program. *J Infect Dis.* 2008;197(suppl 2):S76–S81. PubMed doi: 10.1086/522139
7. Allison MA, Attisha E, Lerner M, et al; COUNCIL ON SCHOOL HEALTH. The link between school attendance and good health. *Pediatrics.* 2019;143(2):e20183648. PubMed doi: 10.1542/peds.2018-3648
8. Centers for Disease Control and Prevention. Contraindications and Precautions: General Best Practices for Immunization. Updated July 25, 2024. Accessed October 31, 2024. https://www.cdc.gov/vaccines/hcp/imz-best-practices/contraindications-precautions.html
9. Seither R, Yusuf OB, Dramann D, Calhoun K, Mugerwa-Kasujja A, Knighton CL. Coverage with selected vaccines and exemption from

school vaccine requirements among children in kindergarten—United States, 2022–23 school year. *MMWR Morb Mortal Wkly Rep.* 2023;72(45):1217–1224. PubMed doi: 10.15585/mmwr.mm7245a2

10. Mississippi State Department of Health. Position Statement of the Mississippi State Board of Health. July 14, 2023. Accessed October 31, 2024. https://msdh.ms.gov/page/resources/19957.pdf
11. Exemptions Permitted for State Childcare and School (K–12) Immunization Requirements as of May 2024. Accessed October 31, 2024. https://www.immunize.org/official-guidance/state-policies/vaccine-requirements/exemptions-childcare-school/
12. Grabenstein JD. What the world's religions teach, applied to vaccines and immune globulins. *Vaccine.* 2013;31(16):2011–2023. PubMed doi: 10.1016/j.vaccine.2013.02.026
13. The Associated Press. On COVID vaccinations, Pope says health care is a "moral obligation." *NPR.* January 10, 2022. Accessed October 31, 2024. https://www.npr.org/2022/01/10/1071785531/on-covid-vaccinations-pope-says-health-care-is-a-moral-obligation
14. Kuru O, Chan MS, Lu H, Stecula DA, Jamieson KH, Albarracín D. Religious affiliation and philosophical and moral beliefs about vaccines: a longitudinal study. *J Health Psychol.* 2022;27(13):3059–3081. PubMed doi: 10.1177/13591053221082770
15. Slone J. *Theological Incorrectness.* Oxford University Press; 2007.
16. Preston JL, Khan A. Comparing the influence of intellectual humility, religiosity, and political conservatism on vaccine attitudes in the United States, Canada, and the United Kingdom. *Public Underst Sci.* 2024;33(3):343–352. PubMed doi: 10.1177/09636625231191633
17. Diekema DS. Personal belief exemptions from school vaccination requirements. *Annu Rev Public Health.* 2014;35(1):275–292. PubMed doi: 10.1146/annurev-publhealth-032013-182452
18. Phadke VK, Bednarczyk RA, Salmon DA, Omer SB. Association between vaccine refusal and vaccine-preventable diseases in the United States. *JAMA.* 2016;315(11):1149–1158. PubMed doi: 10.1001/jama.2016.1353
19. Atwell JE, Van Otterloo J, Zipprich J, et al. Nonmedical vaccine exemptions and pertussis in California, 2010. *Pediatrics.* 2013;132(4):624–630. PubMed doi: 10.1542/peds.2013-0878
20. Hill HA, Elam-Evans LD, Yankey D, Singleton JA, Kolasa M. National, state, and selected local area vaccination coverage among children aged 19–35 months—United States, 2014. *MMWR Morb Mortal Wkly Rep.* 2015;64(33):889–896. PubMed doi: 10.15585/mmwr.mm6433a1
21. Blank NR, Caplan AL, Constable C. Exempting schoolchildren from immunizations: states with few barriers had highest rates of nonmedical exemptions. *Health Aff (Millwood).* 2013;32(7):1282–1290. PubMed doi: 10.1377/hlthaff.2013.0239
22. Stadlin S, Bednarczyk RA, Omer SB. Medical exemptions to school immunization requirements in the United States–association of state policies with medical exemption rates (2004–2011). *J Infect Dis.* 2012;206(7):989–992. PubMed doi: 10.1093/infdis/jis436
23. Kass NE. An ethics framework for public health. *Am J Public Health.* 2001;91(11):1776–1782. PubMed doi: 10.2105/AJPH.91.11.1776
24. Network for Public Health Law. The Legal Landscape of Religious Exemptions to School Vaccination Requirements. Published June 7, 2024. Accessed August 28, 2024. https://www.networkforphl.org/news-insights/the-legal-landscape-of-religious-exemptions-to-school-vaccination-requirements/
25. *Jacobson v Massachusetts*, 197 U.S. 11 (1905)
26. *Zucht v King*, 260 U.S. 174 (1922)
27. *Prince v Massachusetts*, 321 U.S. 158 (1944)
28. Coughlin SS. How many principles for public health ethics? *Open Public Health J.* 2008;1(1):8–16. PubMed doi: 10.2174/1874944500801010008
29. Friedman Ross L. *Children, Families, and Health Care Decision Making.* Clarendon Press; 2004.
30. Navin MC, Wasserman JA, Diekema DS, Pope TM. Limits on parental discretion in medical decision-making: pediatric intervention principles converge. *Perspect Biol Med.* 2024;67(2):277–289. PubMed doi: 10.1353/pbm.2024.a929023
31. Hendrix KS, Sturm LA, Zimet GD, Meslin EM. Ethics and childhood vaccination policy in the United States. *Am J Public Health.* 2016;106(2):273–278. PubMed doi: 10.2105/AJPH.2015.302952
32. American Academy of Pediatrics. Discussing vaccines with patients and parents. In: Kimberlin DW, Banerjee R, Barnett ED, Sawyer MH, eds. *Red Book: 2024 Report of the Committee on Infectious Diseases.* American Academy of Pediatrics; 2024:25–38.

New and Evolving Dimensions in the Pediatrician-Family-Patient Relationship: Maintaining and Managing Boundaries

- *Clinical Report*

CLINICAL REPORT Guidance for the Clinician in Rendering Pediatric Care

American Academy of Pediatrics
DEDICATED TO THE HEALTH OF ALL CHILDREN™

New and Evolving Dimensions in the Pediatrician-Family-Patient Relationship: Maintaining and Managing Boundaries: Clinical Report

Douglas J. Opel, MD, MPH, FAAP,[1,2] Douglas S. Diekema, MD, MPH, FAAP,[1,2] and the Committee on Bioethics

abstract

Maintaining and managing boundaries in relationships with patients and their family members remains extremely important for the practicing pediatrician. Technological innovations that facilitate communication and information sharing, such as social media, have created new dimensions within the pediatrician-family-patient relationship. Shifts in patient and family expectations of the medical profession that have occurred over time, such as a greater desire among patients and families to have increased access to their pediatrician, also present novel challenges to traditional professional boundaries. Further, social and political issues that have bearing on the practice of medicine have raised questions about pediatricians' role as advocates for individual patients and child health within the pediatrician-family-patient relationship. The 2009 AAP policy statement, "Pediatrician-Family-Patient Relationships: Managing the Boundaries," offers guidance for pediatricians in navigating several key scenarios regarding professional boundaries, including accepting gifts, dual relationships, and romantic relationships with patients or caregivers. Since the content in this 2009 policy statement remains relevant, the intent of this clinical report is to complement the 2009 statement and provide guidance for navigating new and evolving dimensions of the traditional pediatrician-family-patient relationship, including advocacy within the pediatric clinical encounter, self-disclosure, and social media relationships with patients or caregivers.

[1]Treuman Katz Center for Pediatric Bioethics and Palliative Care, Seattle Children's Research Institute, Seattle, Washington; and [2]Department of Pediatrics, University of Washington School of Medicine, Seattle, Washington

Address correspondence to Douglas J. Opel, MD, MPH, FAAP. Email: douglas.opel@seattlechildrens.org

Drs Opel and Diekema participated in all phases of this manuscript development, including literature review, conceptualization and drafting of the report, and revisions, and both authors approved the final manuscript as submitted and agree to be accountable for all aspects of the work.

FINANCIAL/CONFLICT OF INTEREST DISCLOSURE: The authors have indicated they have no potential conflicts of interest to disclose.

To cite: Opel DJ, Diekema DS; American Academy of Pediatrics, Committee on Bioethics. New and Evolving Dimensions in the Pediatrician-Family-Patient Relationship: Maintaining and Managing Boundaries: Clinical Report. *Pediatrics.* 2025;156(1):e2025072215

INTRODUCTION

There is an inherent power differential in the pediatrician-family-patient relationship. Pediatricians, like other physicians, hold power over patients (and their families) because of the diagnostic and treatment knowledge and skills they possess as well as the privileged socioeconomic and educational status they experience.[1] Some patients and their families may also first meet a pediatrician at a time of illness, which can further create a sense of powerlessness and vulnerability. This power differential underscores the essential role of trust in the pediatrician-family-patient relationship.

Boundaries within the pediatrician-family-patient relationship primarily exist to prevent the exploitation of the patient's or family's dependency on the pediatrician, to maintain patient safety, and to protect the trust necessary for a healthy and healing relationship with the pediatrician. Accordingly, boundaries in the medical profession have been defined as "the parameters that describe the limits to the fiduciary relationship in which one person (a patient) entrusts his or her welfare to another (the physician)."[2] Boundaries, in essence, denote limits and separation. They can help protect and respect space, attitudes, and experience.

Abuse of these parameters signifies a lack of respect for the patient and family and their vulnerability. It can be damaging to a patient's intrinsic moral worth or dignity, ability to trust, and physical and emotional well-being. In fact, central to considerations of whether an action constitutes an abuse of power within the pediatrician-family-patient relationship is the degree to which the action compromises a pediatrician's fiduciary responsibilities to the patient and family, including the preservation of the patient's and family's trust, respect, and dignity.

Boundaries within the pediatrician-family-patient relationship also serve to protect a pediatrician's objectivity. Objectivity is recognized as "intrinsic to the healing end of medicine" and "necessary for proper diagnosis and treatment."[3(p87)] Several biases and cognitive shortcuts can contribute to a loss of objectivity and cause a disregard or discounting of certain aspects of the clinical evaluation,[4,5] threatening the accuracy and soundness of a pediatrician's clinical judgment and placing the patient at risk of physical or emotional harm. Although there is a place in medicine for emotion and sentiment—compassion is an essential virtue in medicine—these must exist in tension with objectivity to ultimately achieve the goals of medicine.[3]

Breaches of professional boundaries within the pediatrician-family-patient relationship exist on a continuum.[6] At one end of the continuum are minor breaches, or boundary crossings. Boundary crossings are nonexploitative; carry only a small potential for having a negative effect on a pediatrician's responsibilities toward preserving patient trust, respect, or dignity; and have a low risk of physical or emotional harm to the patient. In addition, there is minimal risk that a pediatrician's objectivity is compromised. An activity that could be characterized as a boundary crossing may even be associated with some benefits. Therefore, boundary crossings may be justifiable in certain circumstances when their perceived benefits outweigh their potential risks; however, potential boundary crossings should always be carefully scrutinized and promptly reflected on regarding their impact on the patient's trust and vulnerability as well as the pediatrician's objectivity. At the other end of the continuum are major breaches of the pediatrician-family-patient relationship. Major breaches, or boundary violations, represent an exploitation of the power imbalance and are not acceptable, as they significantly compromise a patient's trust, respect, or dignity; undermine or call into question the capacity for objectivity; and/or carry a high risk of physical or emotional harm to the patient. Avoiding boundary violations is fundamental to the practice of medicine.[7]

CASE STUDIES

The 2009 policy statement, "Pediatrician-Family-Patient Relationships: Managing the Boundaries," offers guidance for pediatricians in navigating several key scenarios regarding professional boundaries, including accepting gifts, dual relationships, and romantic relationships with patients or caregivers. That guidance remains relevant today. This current clinical report complements the 2009 policy statement by providing additional guidance for navigating new and evolving dimensions of the traditional pediatrician-family-patient relationship: issues related to advocacy, self-disclosure, and social media.

Advocacy

To advocate is "to defend or serve (a cause) through action" or "support, recommend, or speak in favor of a person or thing."[8] Advocacy is a process in which stakeholders make their voices heard on issues that affect their lives or the lives of others. Advocacy by physicians can manifest in many ways within and outside the clinical setting.[9] For instance, advocacy by pediatricians within the clinical setting can include ensuring quick access to subspecialty consultation for a patient in need of further diagnostic work-up or ensuring access for all non-English–speaking patients at one's practice by improving interpreter access. Advocacy by pediatricians outside the clinical setting can be similarly diverse, including, for example, improving voting access in a local community or lobbying a state legislature to impose taxes on sugar-sweetened beverages.

Physicians have obligations to advocate within the clinical setting to provide high-quality care to their patients, such as advocacy to improve systems of care that impact patient outcomes. These obligations to advocate can extend beyond issues pertinent to individual patients or groups of patients and include issues affecting the health of populations.[9] This broader obligation to advocate for population health follows from society's social contract with the medical profession: in exchange for "monopoly use of knowledge, practice autonomy, and the right to self-regulate... the medical profession is expected to promote society's health."[9] Although some argue that such advocacy is not mandatory[10] or may simply be aspirational as it becomes more distant from factors that directly influence an individual's health,[9] responsibilities to advocate for societal health have been integrated into the medical profession. The American Medical Association's 7th Principle in its Code of Ethics states "a physician shall recognize a responsibility to participate in activities contributing to the improvement of the community and the betterment of public health."[11] Similarly, the American Academy of Pediatrics Committee on Bioethics states that pediatricians have responsibilities "to address issues of advocacy for child health and the effective use of health care and public health resources."[12]

What is less clear, however, is the appropriateness of advocating for issues related to societal health (or, more specifically, pediatric population health or public health) *within* an individual patient-family clinical encounter. Consider the following scenario:

> Your pediatric colleague is about to see her first patient of the day. Before she leaves the doctor's room, she puts on her white coat. You notice a pin on her white coat that reads United for Kids: We Shall Overcome.

Wearing a pin with the intent to make its message visible to others is a form of advocacy. In this scenario, wearing a *United for Kids: We Shall Overcome* pin—a modification of the 1960s era pin associated with the civil rights movement that employed the words "United: We Shall Overcome" surrounding an image of interracial shaking hands—can be an opportunity to draw attention to racially motivated violence against historically marginalized communities and raise awareness of structural racism in US society, including its effect on the health of children of color.[13] It can also communicate solidarity and allyship. Therefore, wearing a *United for Kids: We Shall Overcome* pin in the clinical setting could be viewed as an opportunity for physicians to fulfill their obligations to advocate for child and public health.

Whether or not this scenario represents a breach of the pediatrician-family-patient relationship depends on its potential to 1) exploit the power differential in the pediatrician-family-patient relationship and compromise a patient's (or their family's) trust, respect, or dignity; 2) undermine or call into question the physician's capacity for objectivity; and/or 3) carry a risk of physical or emotional harm to the patient. It is unlikely that wearing such a pin compromises a physician's capacity for objectivity. On the contrary, it may signal a commitment to being more attentive to disrupting individual- and system-level biases within the health care encounter. Though wearing such a pin may carry some risk of emotional trauma to patients or families that have experienced racism or suffered from generational trauma from systemic racism, it can also be a powerful way to communicate solidarity and allyship with patients.

It may be argued, however, that wearing such a pin will make some patients or families uncomfortable by exploiting the power differential between physicians and patients/families and generating the perception that patients or their families must adopt the same position taken by the physician if they want to remain patients. However, the salience of this argument depends on the message being conveyed and the physician's intent. Conveying messages within a clinical encounter that reflect consensus positions within pediatrics on issues related to an individual's health or pediatric population health and that are intended to educate the patient or family about such issues are an appropriate form of advocacy within the pediatrician-family-patient relationship, whether communicated in conversation or on a pin. A pin that reads *United for Kids: We Shall Overcome* is this type of message: it is a positively valenced message about overcoming racial injustice and discrimination that is in alignment with a consensus AAP position.[11] Messages that are directly related to the health of the individual patient in the encounter are most appropriate, but given physicians' responsibilities to also promote societal health, messages that are discernibly pertinent to consensus positions within pediatrics related to population health or public health more generally also represent an appropriate form of physician advocacy within the clinical encounter. As such, pins that read FluVaccine✓,[13,14] Protect our Children: End Gun Violence,[15] or Clean Air: It's Up to Us,[16] would also be appropriate. Messages that do not clearly relate to the health of the individual patient in the encounter or to pediatric population health or public health more generally and/or in which there is not professional consensus on an issue with some relationship to pediatric population health or public health (eg, Blue or Vote) have potential to exploit the power differential within the pediatrician-family-patient relationship. As such, messages with these characteristics should generally be avoided. In the current polarized environment in which several medical issues have been politicized, such actions require particular attention.

Wearing a *United for Kids: We Shall Overcome* pin in a clinical encounter is, therefore, a justifiable means to fulfilling physician obligations to promote societal health by combating racism. Racism is an important societal issue for which there is professional consensus regarding its effects on child and public health. There is the potential that wearing a *United for Kids: We Shall Overcome* pin will have a direct positive impact on individual patients and caregivers by visibly advocating against racism while carrying low risk of undermining a physician's capacity for objectivity.

Consider another scenario:

> A pediatrician has formed a coalition of doctors, bicyclists, and child advocates in her community with the public health goal to increase child helmet use while biking. During a well-child visit with a 6-year-old, she mentions to the patient's mother that her coalition is sponsoring a free helmet giveaway at the local YMCA the following weekend.

Communicating this sponsored event to the caregiver in this scenario is an appropriate form of advocacy, because it relates to a consensus position on an issue of child or public health regarding the importance of bike helmet use for injury prevention,[17] it is rooted in the physician's obligation to promote the child's health and public health, and it has the potential to positively impact the health of the individual patient in the encounter (who is at an age where he may be learning to ride a bike). Given the physician's intent to promote the individual child's health, and assuming there is no financial conflict of interest for the pediatrician (it is important to note here that *selling* bike helmets or other health-related products in the office would require separate consideration, given that it "presents a financial conflict of interest, risks placing undue pressure on the patient, and threatens to erode patient trust and undermine the primary obligation of physicians to serve the interests of their patients before their own"[18]), conveying information about this event has little potential to exploit the power differential in the pediatrician-family-patient relationship or undermine or call into question the capacity for objectivity. It also represents an effort to minimize, not heighten, the risk of physical or emotional harm to the patient. This form of advocacy, therefore, does not breach pediatrician-family-patient boundaries.

Self-Disclosure

Physician disclosure of information about themselves during a clinical encounter with patients is controversial. Physician self-disclosure can expend valuable time during the encounter and shift the focus of the encounter from the patient's needs to the physician.[19] In addition, physician self-disclosure is often non sequitur and unrelated to any discussion in the encounter.[19] The impact of physician self-disclosure on outcomes such as patient satisfaction[20–23] and compliance with medical recommendations[24,25] remains unclear.

Physician self-disclosure can also expose patients to physician biases and vulnerabilities that may undermine trust in the relationship as well as a physician's ability to be objective.[26] This, in turn, can increase the risk of harming a patient. For these reasons, "personal disclosure related to social, cultural, religious, or other demographics" is considered by some to be a boundary crossing.[27]

It is important, however, to recognize the potential benefits of physician self-disclosure in a clinical encounter. Self-disclosure can deepen therapeutic relationships with patients, build trust and rapport, communicate a shared humanity, and be an effective means in which to respond to suffering.[26,28–30] In particular, physicians who have, themselves, at one time been patients—and for pediatricians, perhaps their child has been a patient—have an opportunity through self-disclosure to provide "insight... [gained] in one role from the experiences [had] in another."[28] This type of self-disclosure about an illness or a health care experience, even something as ordinary as a pediatrician's experience having their own child vaccinated,[31] can convey a shared understanding and empathy with patients that has the potential to have a positive impact on the individual patient's health and/or the pediatrician-family-patient relationship.

As such, the appropriateness of physician self-disclosure in a clinical encounter hinges on several factors. One such factor is the physician's intent. Self-disclosure done with the intent to benefit the patient by building trust and rapport is more easily justifiable.[28] Important here, however, is not only being truthful with oneself about intent—it can be easy to disguise motives that are selfish rather than altruistic[26]—but also balancing this intent with insight into its impact, namely how the self-disclosure may be received by the patient, as well as how it may affect one's capacity to remain objective. If there were uncertainty around intent for disclosing information about oneself in a clinical encounter, it would be prudent not to do so.

A second factor is the context in which self-disclosure is used. Self-disclosure should not be used indiscriminately, gratuitously, or without tact. It is important to match delivery of information in a clinical encounter to the preferences of the patient or caregiver. If the patient or family is interested in the physician's personal perspective or self-disclosure seems consistent with the patient's or family's communication preferences, it may be appropriate when utilized in small, measured amounts and in ways clearly connected to the patient's benefit. Physician self-reflection is required to know how much to share and when to limit further disclosure as it no longer is for the patient's benefit.

Consider the following two dialogues between a physician and an adolescent patient (modified from real encounters[19]):

Dialogue 1

Patient: I'm six feet, and the nurse just told me I was 204 pounds on check-in.

Physician: Is that up a little bit for you weight-wise?

Patient: ... it might be up a few pounds ... I used to be 190 pounds during football season... I just haven't ...

Physician: See, 'cause I'm weighing more like 172, 173, and I'm six foot ... and I don't play football like you but I do still run.... I'm still doing the 5 and 10 and 15Ks. The half-marathons and ...

Patient: So ... I'm 30 pounds heavier than you?

Physician: Right now, yeah.

Dialogue 2

Physician: ... I live with it myself.

Patient: Oh, you're kidding me?

Physician: Absolutely.

Patient: So what I'm saying to you is ... what you have? The exact same thing?

Physician: Exactly.

Patient: Oh, my gosh!

Physician: Exactly.

Patient: What a coincidence.

Physician: Basically ... the acids in the stomach are coming back up. That's the reflux. And that really irritates the lining of the esophagus.

The self-disclosure by the physician in Dialogue 1 is non sequitur and shifts the focus of the encounter from the patient to the physician. Although the physician is, perhaps, intending to utilize self-disclosure to develop rapport, the physician instead insinuates competition with the patient. This potentially undermines any attempt at building rapport in a way that benefits the patient. This self-disclosure, therefore, constitutes a boundary crossing of the pediatrician-family-patient relationship.

In Dialogue 2, however, it is more apparent how the physician's use of self-disclosure may benefit the patient. Her self-disclosure may deepen the therapeutic relationship with her patient, for instance, by communicating a shared humanity and experience around the patient's recent diagnosis. The self-disclosure is also not used gratuitously but rather to help communicate empathy and share information about the diagnosis with the patient. If the physician in this scenario does not believe her self-disclosure undermines her capacity to remain objective and is consistent with the communication preferences of the patient, this type of self-disclosure is appropriate and does not represent a breach of the pediatrician-family-patient relationship.

Social Media

Today, 9 in 10 Americans use the internet,[32] and the majority of Americans have looked for health information online.[33] Social media has also become a staple of American life,[34] with nearly half all adults in a recent survey stating it is appropriate to contact their physician about a health issue through social media.[35] Although this accessibility and use carries with it the potential to promote health equity, health-related social media may also exacerbate disparities if its design and content do not account for user group factors, such as socioeconomic status, health literacy, culture, and social media access.[36] It is nevertheless clear that the democratization of scientific and medical knowledge through increased accessibility to online health and medical information has transformed the role of patients and caregivers in the pediatrician-family-patient relationship.[37] Compared with past generations, today's patients and caregivers are accustomed to new ways of social interaction and communication and have new expectations regarding physician availability and accessibility of health information.

These new expectations create challenges for the pediatrician-family-patient relationship. One particular challenge is responding to friend requests from patients or caregivers. Consider the following scenario, adapted from a published narrative[38]:

> You were the primary oncology attending for an adolescent patient who died a few years ago. She was your patient for several years before her death, and you had become close with her and her parents. However, you were not present when she died in the hospital and did not get a chance to speak with her parents afterwards. You wonder frequently how the parents are doing, but avoid contacting them out of respect for their privacy. To your surprise, 2 years after her daughter's death, the mother sends a friend request to your personal social media page.

As discussed in the clinical report "Ethical Considerations in Pediatrician's Use of Social Media,"[39] accepting friend requests on personal social media accounts from patients or their caregivers blurs traditional pediatrician-family-patient boundaries. Foremost, entering into a social media relationship with a patient or caregiver is akin to having a dual relationship with them: one that is professional, as the patient's doctor, and the other, that is more personal over social media. This social media relationship may involve the patient or caregiver having access to other elements of the physician's personal social media profile and posts (and vice versa), which creates the potential for exposing patients and caregivers to physician biases and vulnerabilities that may undermine a physician's ability to be objective and increase the risk of harming a patient. For this reason, accepting friend requests from current patients or their families represents, at a minimum, a boundary crossing in the pediatrician-family-patient relationship. When it is difficult to avoid this breach, such as may be the case for pediatricians who are one of only a few pediatric practitioners in a rural community (where they may have relationships that have developed outside of the office with people for whom they also provide a medical home), it is critical that pediatricians remain cognizant of the potential risks it carries for patients and families in their practice and strive to minimize those risks.

One way to minimize these risks is to have a public professional social media profile in addition to a private personal profile.[40] Professional social media profiles can be means to share information about the physician's professional interests and experiences and educate patients regarding specific health topics. These professional profiles can also provide some limited information about physician personal interests. Physician professional social media profiles that contained educational information or professional information with some limited "healthy" personal information (eg, personal interests in hiking and reading), in fact, were perceived by patients as professional.[41,42] Accepting friend requests from current patients made to a physician's professional profile can be an appropriate way to connect patients to this information while upholding commitments to preserve patients trust and physician objectivity by maintaining professionalism standards.

In the above case, however, the parent making the friend request is the parent of a past patient. Accepting friend requests of family members of past patients to personal social media profiles can be an "opportunity and a privilege" to learn from family members, convey support and compassion, and empower their voice.[38] Given there is no ongoing professional relationship, there is also no risk of undermining a physician's objectivity in the care of the patient. However, given the past professional relationship between the physician and the patient, there is some potential that the parents may perceive some elements of the physician's social media profile or posts as incongruous with their conception of and experience with the physician. This, in addition to the power differential between pediatrician and family that still exists, could have a negative impact for families, such as complicating their bereavement. Therefore, physicians should not initiate friend requests of patients or families and should only accept friend requests of family members of past patients to personal social media profiles after serious consideration of the potential risks. Accepting friend request of family members of past patients is perhaps best done through a professional social media profile.

RECOMMENDATIONS

1. Boundary breaches exist on a continuum. Physicians should only consider taking actions that constitute minor breaches, or boundary crossings, after assessing their potential risks and benefits and determining that the action is likely to result in a net benefit for the patient and pediatrician-family-patient relationship. Boundary violations are major breaches and should be avoided as they significantly compromise a patient's trust, respect, or dignity; undermine or call into question the capacity for objectivity; and/or carry a risk of physical or emotional harm to the patient.
2. Advocacy within the clinical encounter is most justifiable when the advocacy message is child-focused and represents a consensus issue on pediatric population health or public health and clearly relates to and seeks to promote the health of the individual patient in the encounter.
3. Physician self-disclosure within the clinical encounter can expose patients to physician biases and vulnerabilities that may undermine patient trust in the physician and compromise a physician's ability to be objective. However, physician self-disclosure may also deepen therapeutic relationships with patients and communicate a shared humanity. Use of self-disclosure within the clinical encounter is appropriate when done with the intent to benefit the patient and when utilized in small, measured amounts and in ways clearly connected to the patient's benefit.
4. Accepting social media friend requests from current patients or their families on physician *personal* social media accounts represents at a minimum a boundary crossing in the pediatrician-family-patient relationship, although it may be acceptable if the request comes from families of former patients. Accepting friend requests from current patients or families through physician *professional* social media accounts can be an appropriate way to connect with patients while maintaining professionalism standards and upholding commitments to preserve patients trust and physician objectivity.

LEAD AUTHORS

Douglas J. Opel, MD, MPH, FAAP
Douglas S. Diekema, MD, MPH, FAAP

COMMITTEE ON BIOETHICS, 2022–2023

Naomi Tricot Laventhal, MD, FAAP, Chairperson
Gina Marie Geis, MD, FAAP
Carrie Henderson, MD, FAAP
Deborah S. Loeff, MD, FAAP
Mary A. Ott MD, MA, FAAP
Sara Taub, MD, FAAP

FORMER COMMITTEE MEMBER

Douglas J. Opel, MD, MPH, FAAP

LIAISONS

Maria de Brito McGee, MD, – *American Academy of Child and Adolescent Psychiatry*
Douglas S. Diekema, MD, MPH, FAAP – *American Board of Pediatrics*
Kavita S. Arora, MD, MBE, MS– *American College of Obstetricians and Gynecologists*
Nanette Elster, JD, MPH – *Legal Consultant*

STAFF

Anjie Emanuel, MPH

The guidance in this report does not indicate an exclusive course of treatment or serve as a standard of medical care. Variations, taking into account individual circumstances, may be appropriate.

The guidance in this document does not necessarily reflect the views or opinions of liaisons or the organizations or government agencies they represent.

All clinical reports from the American Academy of Pediatrics automatically expire 5 years after publication unless reaffirmed, revised, or retired at or before that time.

FUNDING: No external funding.

https://doi.org/10.1542/peds.2025-072215

REFERENCES

1. Brody H. *The Healer's Power.* Yale University Press; 1992.
2. Gabbard GO, Nadelson C. Professional boundaries in the physician-patient relationship. *JAMA.* 1995;273(18):1445–1449. PubMed doi: 10.1001/jama.1995.03520420061039
3. Pellegrino ED, Thomasma DC. *The Virtues in Medical Practice.* Oxford University Press; 1993.
4. Rinke ML, Singh H, Heo M, et al. Diagnostic errors in primary care pediatrics: Project RedDE. *Acad Pediatr.* 2018;18(2):220–227. PubMed doi: 10.1016/j.acap.2017.08.005
5. Redelmeier DA. Improving patient care. The cognitive psychology of missed diagnoses. *Ann Intern Med.* 2005;142(2):115–120. PubMed doi: 10.7326/0003-4819-142-2-200501180-00010
6. Gutheil TG, Gabbard GO. The concept of boundaries in clinical practice: theoretical and risk-management dimensions. *Am J Psychiatry.* 1993;150(2):188–196. PubMed doi: 10.1176/ajp.150.2.188
7. American Medical Association. Code of Medical Ethics: Physician Self-Regulation. Accessed March 21, 2023. https://code-medical-ethics.ama-assn.org/chapters/professional-self-regulation
8. Moulding NT, Silagy CA, Weller DP. A framework for effective management of change in clinical practice: dissemination and implementation of clinical practice guidelines. *Qual Health Care.* 1999; 8(3):177–183. PubMed doi: 10.1136/qshc.8.3.177
9. Gruen RL, Pearson SD, Brennan TA. Physician-citizens–public roles and professional obligations. *JAMA.* 2004;291(1):94–98. PubMed doi: 10.1001/jama.291.1.94
10. Huddle TS, Maletz KK. Physician involvement with politics-obligation or avocation? *Virtual Mentor.* 2011;13(11):757–764. PubMed doi: 10.1001/virtualmentor.2011.13.11.ccas2-1111
11. Americal Medical Association. *Code of Medical Ethics: Physicians and the Health of the Community.* American Medical Association; 2016.
12. Fallat ME, Glover J; American Academy of Pediatrics, Committee on Bioethics. Professionalism in pediatrics: statement of principles. *Pediatrics.* 2007;120(4):895–897. PubMed doi: 10.1542/peds.2007-2229
13. Trent M, Dooley DG, Dougé J; SECTION ON ADOLESCENT HEALTH; COUNCIL ON COMMUNITY PEDIATRICS; COMMITTEE ON ADOLESCENCE. The impact of racism on child and adolescent health. *Pediatrics.* 2019;144(2):e20191765. PubMed doi: 10.1542/peds.2019-1765
14. Committee on Infectious Diseases. Recommendations for prevention and control of influenza in children, 2023-2024: Policy statement. *Pediatrics.* 2024;154(4):e2024068507. PubMed doi: 10.1542/peds.2024-068507
15. Lee LK, Fleegler EW, Goyal MK, et al; American Academy of Pediatrics, Council on Injury, Violence, and Poison Prevention. Firearm-related injuries and deaths in children and youth: injury prevention and harm reduction. *Pediatrics.* 2022;150(6): e2022060070. PubMed doi: 10.1542/peds.2022-060070
16. COUNCIL ON ENVIRONMENTAL HEALTH. Global climate change and children's health. *Pediatrics.* 2015;136(5):992–997. PubMed doi: 10.1542/peds.2015-3232
17. American Academy of Pediatrics. Committee on Injury and Poison Prevention. Bicycle helmets. *Pediatrics.* 2001;108(4):1030–1032. PubMed doi: 10.1542/peds.108.4.1030
18. Americal Medical Association. AMA Code of Medical Ethics: 9.6.4 - Sale of Health-Related Products from Physicians' Offices. Accessed August 31, 2023. https://code-medical-ethics.ama-assn.org/ethics-opinions/sale-health-related-products
19. McDaniel SH, Beckman HB, Morse DS, Silberman J, Seaburn DB, Epstein RM. Physician self-disclosure in primary care visits: enough about you, what about me? *Arch Intern Med.* 2007; 167(12):1321–1326. PubMed doi: 10.1001/archinte.167.12.1321
20. Beach MC, Roter D, Rubin H, Frankel R, Levinson W, Ford DE. Is physician self-disclosure related to patient evaluation of office visits? *J Gen Intern Med.* 2004;19(9):905–910. PubMed doi: 10.1111/j.1525-1497.2004.40040.x
21. Zink KL, Perry M, London K, et al. "Let me tell you about my..." Provider self-disclosure in the emergency department builds patient rapport. *West J Emerg Med.* 2017;18(1):43–49. PubMed doi: 10.5811/westjem.2016.10.31014
22. McLean M, Steinauer J, Schmittdiel J, Chan P, Dehlendorf C. Provider self-disclosure during contraceptive counseling. *Contraception.* 2017;95(2):161–166. PubMed doi: 10.1016/j.contraception.2016.08.010
23. Norling Holmes G, Grant Harrington N, Parrish AJ. Exploring the relationship between pediatrician self-disclosure and parent satisfaction. *Commun Res Rep.* 2010;27(4):365–369. doi: 10.1080/08824096.2010.518922.
24. Frank E, Breyan J, Elon L. Physician disclosure of healthy personal behaviors improves credibility and ability to motivate. *Arch Fam Med.* 2000;9(3):287–290. PubMed doi: 10.1001/archfami.9.3.287

25. Donahue K, Hendrix K, Sturm L, Zimet G. Provider communication and mothers' willingness to vaccinate against human papillomavirus and influenza: a randomized health messaging trial. *Acad Pediatr.* 2018;18(2):145–153. PubMed doi: 10.1016/j.acap.2017.07.007

26. Curran KA. Too much information–the ethics of self-disclosure. *N Engl J Med.* 2014;371(1):8–9. PubMed doi: 10.1056/NEJMp1404119

27. Chen JA, Rosenberg LB, Schulman BJ, Alpert JE, Waldinger RJ. Reexamining the call of duty: teaching boundaries in medical school. *Acad Med.* 2018;93(11):1624–1630. PubMed doi: 10.1097/ACM.0000000000002305

28. Opel DJ. Physician, patient, parent: where exactly is the line? *Hastings Cent Rep.* 2012;42(6):14–18. PubMed doi: 10.1002/hast.83

29. Wales J. Last song—sharing humanity while maintaining boundaries. *N Engl J Med.* 2019;381(20):1894–1895. PubMed doi: 10.1056/NEJMp1907600

30. Schiff GD. A piece of my mind. Crossing boundaries–violation or obligation? *JAMA.* 2013;310(12):1233–1234. PubMed doi: 10.1001/jama.2013.276133

31. Lepere K, Etsekson N, Opel DJ. Provider self-disclosure during the childhood vaccine discussion. *Clin Pediatr (Phila).* 2019;58(6):691–695. PubMed doi: 10.1177/0009922818817828

32. Pew Research Center. *Internet/Broadband Fact Sheet.* Pew Research Center; 2019.

33. Pew Research Center. The internet and Health. 2013. Accessed December 18, 2019. https://www.pewresearch.org/internet/2013/02/12/the-internet-and-health/

34. Pew Research Center. Social Media Fact Sheet. 2019. Accessed April 25, 2021. https://www.pewresearch.org/internet/fact-sheet/social-media/

35. American Osteopathic Association. Survey Finds Patients Want to be Friends with their Physicians on Social Media. Accessed April 25, 2021. https://osteopathic.org/2018/05/14/survey-finds-patients-want-to-be-friends-with-their-physicians-on-social-media/

36. Rivera-Romero O, Gabarron E, Miron-Shatz T, Petersen C, Denecke K. Social media, digital health literacy, and digital ethics in the light of health equity. *Yearb Med Inform.* 2022;31(1):82–87. PubMed doi: 10.1055/s-0042-1742503

37. Tan SS, Goonawardene N. Internet health information seeking and the patient-physician relationship: a systematic review. *J Med Internet Res.* 2017;19(1):e9. PubMed doi: 10.2196/jmir.5729

38. Caruso Brown AE. Porous Boundaries. *JAMA.* 2017;317(24):2487–2488. PubMed doi: 10.1001/jama.2017.1589

39. Macauley R, Elster N, Fanaroff JM; COMMITTEE ON BIOETHICS, COMMITTEE ON MEDICAL LIABILITY AND RISK MANAGEMENT. Ethical considerations in pediatricians' use of social media. *Pediatrics.* 2021;147(3):e2020049685. PubMed doi: 10.1542/peds.2020-049685

40. American Medical Association. AMA Code of Medical Ethics; 2.3.2. Professionalism in the Use of Social Media. Accessed March 18, 2023. https://code-medical-ethics.ama-assn.org/ethics-opinions/professionalism-use-social-media

41. Clyde JW, Domenech Rodríguez MM, Geiser C. Medical professionalism: an experimental look at physicians' Facebook profiles. *Med Educ Online.* 2014;19:23149. PubMed doi: 10.3402/meo.v19.23149

42. Maben-Feaster RE, Stansfield RB, Opipari A, Hammoud MM. Evaluating patient perspectives of provider professionalism on twitter in an academic obstetrics and gynecology clinic: patient survey. *J Med Internet Res.* 2018;20(3):e78. PubMed doi: 10.2196/jmir.8056

Newborn Screening for Critical Congenital Heart Disease: A New Algorithm and Other Updated Recommendations

- *Clinical Report*
  - *PPI: AAP Partnership for Policy Implementation See Appendix 1 for more information.*

American Academy of Pediatrics
DEDICATED TO THE HEALTH OF ALL CHILDREN®

AAP Partnership for Policy Implementation

CLINICAL REPORT Guidance for the Clinician in Rendering Pediatric Care

American Academy of Pediatrics

DEDICATED TO THE HEALTH OF ALL CHILDREN™

Newborn Screening for Critical Congenital Heart Disease: A New Algorithm and Other Updated Recommendations: Clinical Report

Matthew E. Oster, MD, MPH, FAAP,[1] Nelangi M. Pinto, MD,[2] Arun K. Pramanik, MD, FAAP,[3,4] Allison Markowsky, MD, MSHS, FAAP,[5] Bryanna N. Schwartz, MD, MPH, FAAP,[5] Alex R. Kemper, MD, MPH, MS, FAAP,[6] Lisa A. Hom, RN, Esq,[5] Gerard R. Martin, MD, FAAP[5]; and the SECTION ON CARDIOLOGY AND CARDIAC SURGERY; SECTION ON HOSPITAL MEDICINE; COMMITTEE ON FETUS AND NEWBORN

abstract

Critical congenital heart disease (CCHD) screening was added to the US Recommended Uniform Screening Panel in 2011 and adopted by all US states and territories by 2018. In addition to reviewing key developments in CCHD screening since the initial American Academy of Pediatrics (AAP) endorsement in 2011, this clinical report provides 3 updated recommendations. First, a new AAP algorithm has been endorsed for use in CCHD screening. Compared with the original AAP algorithm from 2011, this new algorithm a) has a passing oxygen saturation threshold of ≥95% in both pre- and post-ductal measurements; and b) has only 1 retest instead of 2 for infants who did not pass the first screen. Second, to continue to improve screening, state newborn screening programs should collect a recommended minimum uniform dataset to aid in surveillance and monitoring of the program. Finally, stakeholders should be educated on the limitations of screening, the significance of non-CCHD conditions, and the importance of protocol adherence. Future directions of CCHD screening include improving overall sensitivity and implementing methods to reduce health inequities. It will remain critical that the AAP and its chapters and members work with health departments and hospitals to achieve awareness and implementation of these recommendations.

[1]Children's Healthcare of Atlanta, Emory University School of Medicine, Atlanta, Georgia; [2]Primary Children's Hospital, University of Utah School of Medicine, Salt Lake City, Utah; [3]Seattle Children's Hospital/University of Washington, Seattle, Washington; [4]Louisiana State University Health, Shreveport, Louisiana; [5]Children's National Hospital, The George Washington University School of Medicine and Health Sciences, Washington, District of Columbia; and [6]Division of Primary care Pediatrics, Nationwide Children's Hospital, Columbus, Ohio

Address correspondence to: Matthew E. Oster, MD, MPH, FAAP. Email: osterm@kidsheart.com

All authors discussed the recommendations and contributed to the final manuscript.

CONFLICT OF INTEREST DISCLOSURES: The authors have indicated they have no potential conflicts of interest to disclose.

FUNDING: No external funding.

To cite: Oster ME, Pinto NM, Pramanik AK, et al; American Academy of Pediatrics, Section on Cardiology and Cardiac Surgery, Section on Hospital Medicine, Committee on Fetus and Newborn. Newborn Screening for Critical Congenital Heart Disease: A New Algorithm and Other Updated Recommendations: Clinical Report. *Pediatrics.* 2025;155(1): e2024069667

INTRODUCTION AND BACKGROUND

In 2011, critical congenital heart disease (CCHD) screening was added to the US Recommended Uniform Screening Panel, with the endorsement of the American Academy of Pediatrics (AAP), to help detect those heart conditions that typically present with hypoxemia and require intervention in the first year of life.[1–3] State newborn screening programs reviewed and implemented CCHD screening policies with adoption of CCHD screening in all states and territories by July 2018.[4] Newborn CCHD screening using pulse oximetry plays an important role in the timely identification of children with CCHD, in conjunction with other screening modalities such as prenatal ultrasonography, physical examinations, and genetic testing in high-risk cases.

Implementation of CCHD screening using pulse oximetry has been a landmark success in public health. Since 2011, CCHD screening has proven to decrease infant mortality,[5] to be cost-effective,[6] and to save resources.[7] However, several opportunities remain to improve the implementation and effectiveness of CCHD screening. This clinical report reviews key developments in CCHD screening since the initial AAP endorsement in 2011, provides recommendations for improving this important public health program, and identifies future areas of improvement for CCHD screening.

DEVELOPMENTS IN CCHD SCREENING

Updated Evidence on Benefits of Screening

When CCHD screening was added to the US Recommended Uniform Screening Panel, several studies had demonstrated screening to be effective.[8,9] However, uncertainties remained regarding its implementation on a broad scale, including the degree to which it would decrease morbidity and mortality and its effect on resource utilization. Many of these issues have now been addressed.

First, the implementation of CCHD screening policies at the state level is associated with decreased infant mortality and decreased emergency hospitalizations attributable to CCHD.[5] Abouk et al found that, compared with prior periods and compared with states that did not have screening policies, early infant deaths from CCHD decreased by 33% after states implemented mandatory CCHD screening. Beyond mortality, Sakai-Bizmark et al used a similar methodologic approach to demonstrate that states with mandatory CCHD screening policies saw decreases in the rates of emergency hospitalizations attributable to CCHD compared with states that did not have such policies.[10] These findings reinforced implementation of screening policies at the state level rather than as an optional medical test at the hospital level.

Second, initially concerns existed about the costs and resource utilization of CCHD screening.[11] In a cost survey and time and motion study conducted in New Jersey, Peterson et al found that the estimated time per newborn screening was 9.1 minutes, at a cost of $14.19 (in 2011 US dollars), with costs decreasing with the use of reusable sensors.[12] When the improvements in mortality were considered, it was estimated that the cost of CCHD screening for life-year gained was $12,000.[6] Fortunately, widespread CCHD screening did not result in increased resource utilization. In an Oregon study, researchers found that the use of neonatal echocardiography decreased, not increased, after the introduction of CCHD screening using pulse oximetry.[7] Similarly, a study using data from the Healthcare Cost and Utilization Project Statewide Inpatient Databases[13] found no significant increase, and potentially a decrease, in the use of neonatal echocardiography.

A secondary benefit of CCHD screening using pulse oximetry is the detection of hypoxemic conditions other than CCHD. The CCHD screening algorithm endorsed by the AAP had a goal of detecting a core set of congenital heart conditions that may lead to poor outcomes if not detected promptly[14] (Table 1). However, there are a number of non-CCHD conditions with hypoxemia that have been identified via this screening program.[14] An infant who fails screening because of a low oxygen level is more likely to have one of the non-CCHD conditions than a CCHD core condition.[15] Although these may be considered false positives for the core set of conditions, patients with these noncardiac conditions detected by pulse oximetry screening (eg, sepsis, pneumonia, persistent pulmonary hypertension of newborn) may also benefit from identification and treatment in a timely manner. Early identification of these non-CCHD conditions may lead to fewer infant deteriorations in the newborn nursery during the first days of life.[15] Indeed, when the treatment of an identified non-CCHD condition leads to the resolution of hypoxemia, further cardiac workup may not be necessary.[14]

Diverging Algorithms

Although CCHD screening is now universal in US neonates, it has not been implemented in a uniform manner,

Table 1. Conditions Detected via Screening for Critical Congenital Heart Disease (CCHD) Using Pulse Oximetry

Core Conditions (CCHD)	Coarctation of the aorta Double outlet right ventricle Ebstein's anomaly Hypoplastic left heart syndrome Interrupted aortic arch Pulmonary atresia Single ventricle (not otherwise specified) Tetralogy of Fallot Total anomalous pulmonary venous return D-Transposition of the great arteries Tricuspid atresia Truncus arteriosus Other critical cyanotic lesions not otherwise specified
Secondary Conditions (non-CCHD)	Hemoglobinopathy Hypothermia Infection, including sepsis Lung disease (congenital or acquired) Non-critical congenital heart defect Persistent pulmonary hypertension Other hypoxemic condition not otherwise specified

Reprinted with permission from Oster ME, Aucott SW, Glidewell J, et al. Lessons learned from newborn screening for critical congenital heart defects. *Pediatrics*. 2016;137(5):e20154573

particularly regarding the algorithm used to interpret pulse oximetry readings. Almost all states and territories use the algorithm recommended by the AAP in 2011,[3,11] with some states specifically mandating the of use the algorithm endorsed by the AAP.[14] Other states (eg, New Jersey) instituted an algorithm with a slight modification: instead of requiring the right hand OR the lower extremity to have a saturation of ≥95%, the New Jersey algorithm requires *both* to meet this criterion.[16] Finally, in Tennessee, it is recommended to start with only the lower extremity. If the saturation in the lower extremity is ≥97%, the result is considered "pass"; if <97%, it is recommended to test the right hand and proceed with using the algorithm endorsed by the AAP.[17] Each of these algorithms has various advantages and disadvantages with regards to sensitivity, specificity, ease of use, and costs.[14]

Special Circumstances and Exceptions

As outlined in the AAP 2011 policy statement on CCHD screening, CCHD screening targets healthy-appearing newborn infants in the newborn nursery. In special settings, such as the neonatal intensive care unit (NICU), areas of high altitude, or out-of-hospital birth settings, the screening guidelines may not be as applicable. The applicability of the CCHD screening policy has been questioned and even legislated in infants outside the intended targeted population.[18]

Infants in the NICU frequently have lower oxygen saturations than healthy newborn infants because of lung disease associated with preterm birth or as a result of underlying conditions.[19] Proposed modifications to aid in CCHD screening in the NICU setting include that screening **be performed after the child has been weaned off oxygen**, even if this delays screening well beyond the standard 24-hours-of-life timeframe.[20] If weaning to room air prior to discharge is not possible, then echocardiography is warranted and screening with pulse oximetry is unnecessary, unless required by state law.

Similarly, many infants undergo echocardiography between birth and the intended CCHD screening for a reason other than a failed CCHD screen. In such cases, formal CCHD screening is unnecessary, unless required by state law.[18]

High altitude affects CCHD screening, particularly when using pulse oximetry at elevations above 6800 feet (approximately 2100 meters). However, even lower elevations may affect screening.[21–25] In infants screened at higher altitude, the mean oxygen saturation is lower than in infants screened at sea level, with the difference becoming more pronounced at higher elevation.[26,27] The use of the standard threshold in high elevations can lead to an increase in false-positive results. Limited studies at higher elevations have evaluated lowering the saturation needed to pass and/or administering oxygen via an oxygen hood to increase the potential oxygen saturation level during screening.[28,29] However, more studies are needed to determine which modifications are needed at various elevations.

For children born outside the hospital setting, there are unique CCHD screening challenges regarding the timing, equipment, process, and follow-up testing. Successful home-birth CCHD screening programs have been implemented in the United States and abroad.[30–33] These programs typically adapted their processes to fit the needs of the population served by performing screening earlier than 24 hours and adjusting the timing of repeat screening. These modifications may result in marginal increase in the false-positive rate for CCHD but also an increase in the diagnosis of respiratory and infectious illnesses.[34]

Algorithm Implementation and Electronic Health Record (EHR) Integration

Despite adoption of CCHD screening by all states and territories, tracking and reporting implementation compliance has been challenging and incomplete. For programs that have reported or published compliance data, implementation rates have been variable, with many opportunities for improvement.[35,36] Health information technology and clinical decision support have been shown to improve health care process measures and the quality and efficacy of newborn screening programs.[37–40] One study showed that utilizing an EHR-driven automated screening protocol for CCHD was effective in achieving a high screening compliance (98.9%) prior to discharge and reducing the days to CCHD diagnosis.[41] Automated orders and clinical decision support integrated into the EHR have been shown to standardize practice, reduce delays and gaps in screening, and minimize time to subsequent action for failed screens.

FUTURE AREAS FOR IMPROVEMENT

Despite the success of CCHD screening pulse oximetry, there remains opportunity for improvement. First, although pulse oximetry is useful in detecting conditions that typically present with hypoxia, it is less ideal in detecting CCHDs that have normal oxygen saturation levels.[42] The sensitivity to detect certain lesions such as coarctation of the aorta can be as low as 21%.[43,44] Attempts have been made to increase the sensitivity of CCHD screening by using methods such as adding perfusion index, but such efforts have had unacceptably high false-positive rates.[45] Future efforts that build on the capabilities of pulse oximetry waveforms, utilize existing technology in a new way, or create new detection technologies through innovation are needed to improve the sensitivity of CCHD screening.[46–48]

Second, CCHD screening using pulse oximetry has the potential to address disparities and improve equity in care, but future studies are needed to determine its true effect. Despite improvements in prenatal detection of CCHD, prenatal detection rates remain under 60% in many areas of the United States. One study demonstrated that lower socioeconomic status was associated with decreased prenatal diagnosis for transposition of the great arteries and hypoplastic left heart syndrome.[49] Other studies also demonstrated an association between lower prenatal detection rate and poverty, rural residence, and public/governmental insurance.[50,51] Given the widespread use of CCHD screening in birthing hospitals and its relative simplicity compared to prenatal ultrasonographic screening in terms of technical skills and equipment required, it can serve as a final safety net prior to discharge to identify infants with CCHD that may not have been detected during prenatal screening or by clinical assessment in the newborn nursery. To ensure that this safety net is effective, there must also be equitable access to care, including echocardiograms.[52] There may be a role for telemedicine to facilitate care in areas without immediate access to pediatric subspeciality care. Finally, there are concerns that the accuracy of pulse oximetry to detect hypoxemia may differ based on skin pigmentation.[53] Future study is needed to ensure that any potential disparities in the performance of pulse oximetry testing are mitigated.

CONCLUSIONS AND RECOMMENDATIONS

After more than 10 years of experience and evaluation, this clinical report provides recommended updates to CCHD screening by simplifying the screening algorithm, improving data collection efforts, and adding education of providers. These recommendations are summarized in Table 2.

Algorithm

The AAP is endorsing a new simplified CCHD screening algorithm published in 2020.[4] There are 2 important changes in the new algorithm as compared to the initial CCHD screening algorithm from the AAP published in 2011 (Figure 1).

First, the lower limit of an acceptable oxygen saturation should be ≥95% in *BOTH* the pre- *AND* post-ductal measurements. Studies showed that allowing the saturation to be 95% in *either* the right arm *OR* a lower extremity can lead to confusion and misinterpretation.[54] Modifying the algorithm with this requirement does not have a clinically significant effect on retesting rates.[16,55]

Second, **there should be only 1 retest for indeterminate results**, instead of 2. In the past, an infant who had not passed after 2 attempts was considered as having failed screening. The 2 retests in the past were intended to decrease the false-positive rate and the burden on the health care system of potentially unnecessary echocardiography. However, the fear of an increased burden on the health care systems did not materialize, and many infants who fail the screening test may have clinically important disease other than CCHD.[7,15] Modeling studies have demonstrated that removing the second retest has a minimal effect on the false-positive rate.[56,57]

The recommended changes to the algorithm simplify the screening process, potentially decreasing error rates in the interpretation of the algorithm and reducing the time to conduct a screening. There may be a slight increase in the false-positive rate, but it is balanced by the potential for identifying other clinically important disease. Finally, the recommended changes would not be expected to decrease the sensitivity of screening, because all infants who would have failed under the 2011 algorithm would also fail under the new algorithm. The revised algorithm may potentially increase the screen's sensitivity, although more studies are needed to fully assess the effect. Initial provider opinions of the changes to the algorithm have been positive.[58]

Table 2. Recommendations to Improve Newborn Screening for Critical Congenital Heart Disease (CCHD) Using Pulse Oximetry

Area	Recommendation	Rationale
Algorithm	1. Lower limit of an acceptable oxygen saturation should be ≥95% in *both* the pre- AND post-ductal measurements	• Less confusion and misinterpretation • Potentially increased sensitivity without a clinically significant impact on retesting rates
	2. Only 1 retest following an indeterminate result	• Shorter time to recognition of CCHD • Potentially increased sensitivity without a clinically significant impact on retesting rates
Clinical condition	3. Newborn should not be on supplemental oxygen	• Avoids false negative screening
Data collection	4. Use of the recommended minimum dataset	• Improved ability to monitor and assess the impact of CCHD screening
	5. Linkage of newborn screening programs with birth defects monitoring programs and vital records	• Allow states and territories to detect false negative results from screening and to identify opportunities to improve the screening process
Education	6. Limitations of screening	• Recognition that CCHD may still be present in a child that has "passed" CCHD screening
	7. Identification of disease other than CCHD	• Identification of hypoxemic conditions other than CCHD
	8. Enhanced efforts to use health information technology and optimization of electronic health records	• Streamlined implementation of CCHD screening • Improved compliance with CCHD screening

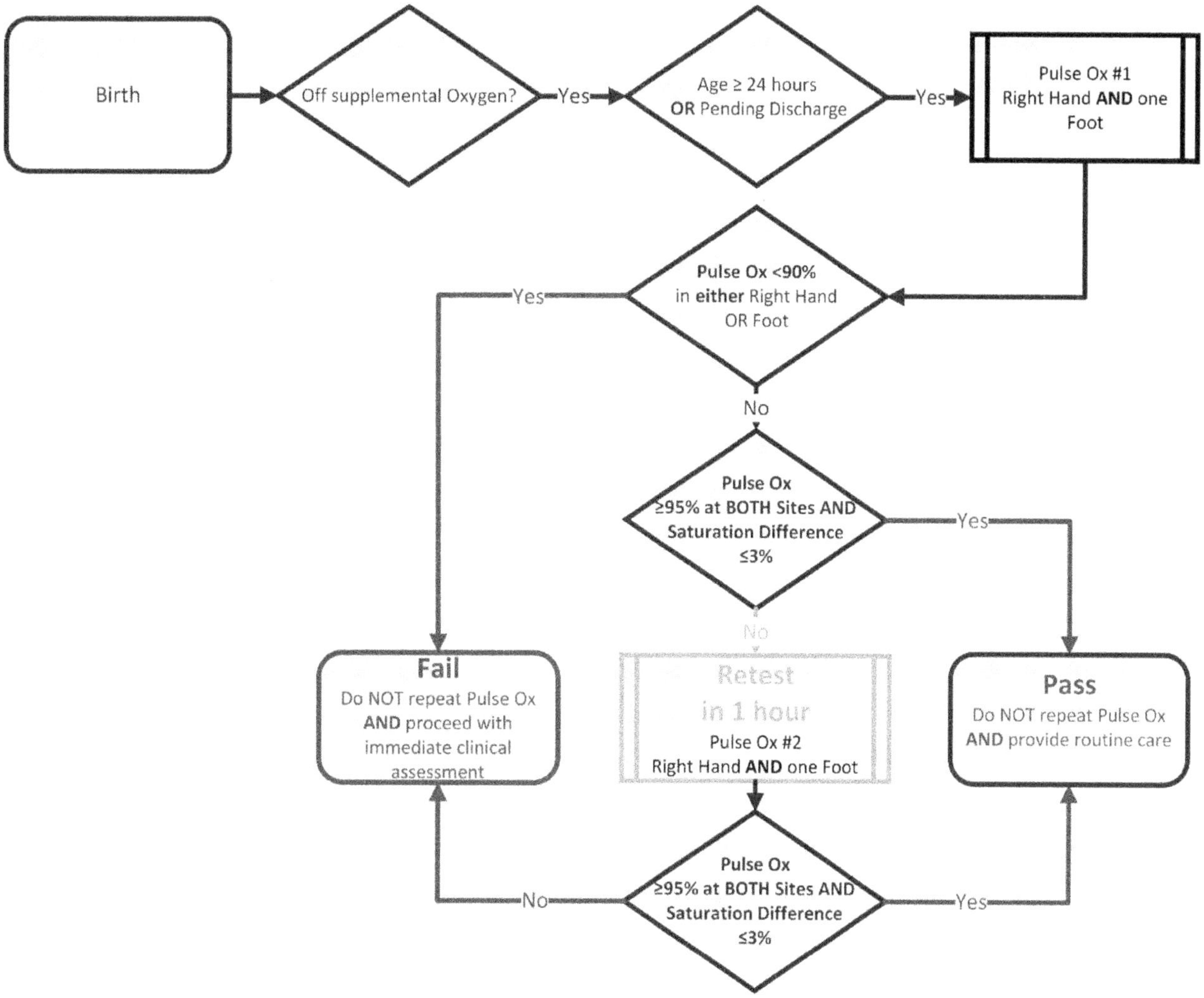

FIGURE 1.
Recommended algorithm for newborn screening for critical congenital heart disease using pulse oximetry

Clinical Condition

Although prior guidelines made it clear that CCHD screening should apply to asymptomatic term infants, clarification is needed to state that the child should be in room air. Thus, **during CCHD screening, infants should either have no respiratory support or any such respiratory support should have an FiO2 of 21%.**

Data Collection

With CCHD screening being a state-implemented public health program, there are notable differences in the program data collection and quality improvement efforts by each state.[18,59] The lack of standardized data collection efforts hinders the ability to truly assess the effect of CCHD screening on a national level. The national adoption of a previously identified uniform dataset for CCHD screening surveillance would overcome some of these obstacles.[14,60] As such, **state public health programs should adopt a common uniform dataset for CCHD screening oversight** (Table 3). This dataset should ideally be created using electronic data sharing to minimize burden on hospitals and states; as electronic medical records vary in content and capability, universal sharing of all data elements may not be possible. Such data could prove useful both by ensuring quality in the implementation of CCHD screening and by informing future research to improve the sensitivity and specificity of CCHD screening.

Furthermore, although some states are able to link their newborn screening efforts with vital records and birth defects monitoring programs, this process is not standardized and not all states have birth defect programs.[61] Automatic data exchanges with birth defect programs allow states to identify cases missed by newborn screening (detect false-negative results), match identified cases from screening (verify true positives), and to engage in outcomes

TABLE 3. Elements to Consider for an Optimal Dataset for Surveillance of Screening for Critical Congenital Heart Disease (CCHD)

Recommended Core Elements	• Age (in hours) at screen • Demographic characteristics as defined by newborn screening program • Pulse oximetry saturation levels for each screen (pre- and post-ductal) • Screening outcome (pass/fail) • For failed screens: ∘ Presence and type of CCHD condition identified, if any ∘ Presence of non-CCHD condition identified, if any
Additional Elements to Consider	• Setting (newborn nursery, neonatal intensive care unit, home, other) • Results of echocardiogram, if performed • Prenatal diagnosis status • Long-term outcomes (survival to ages 1, 5, 10 years and adulthood, morbidity, neurodevelopment, comorbidities, other)

Adapted from Oster ME, Aucott SW, Glidewell J, et al. Lessons learned from newborn screening for critical congenital heart defects. *Pediatrics*. 2016;137(5):e20154573

analysis and long-term follow-up. Strengthening relationships and data exchange with vital records departments can aid in understanding the denominator, confirming that all eligible infants are screened, and assessing any gaps in screening of eligible infants. Data linkages will aid detection of disparities based on race/ethnicity or education level. Therefore, **state newborn screening public health programs are recommended to implement data exchanges with birth hospitals**. This will require funding to strengthen infrastructure, improve data collection and data interoperability, and allow for quality improvement efforts at the state level.[14]

Education

At a 2018 stakeholders meeting to address successes, challenges, and opportunities for CCHD screening, education was identified as a key area of emphasis.[4] Specifically, there were 3 key topic areas of recommended education for pediatricians, pediatric hospitalists, neonatologists, pediatric cardiologists, nurses, other hospital staff, policy makers, and families: (1) limitations of screening; (2) importance of CCHD to identify non-cardiac diseases; and (3) protocol adherence. First, CCHD screening using pulse oximetry is only one tool to identify newborns with CCHD. Because of the nature of the test and the characteristics of certain types of CCHD, the sensitivity of CCHD screening using pulse oximetry is currently 50% to 76%.[44] Therefore, **all stakeholders should be educated that CCHD should *not* be ruled out based on the results of screening with pulse oximetry alone.**[62] Second, even when CCHD has been ruled out, pulse oximetry can detect other relevant disease[14,15] (Table 1). **In the child who fails CCHD screening using pulse oximetry but in whom CCHD is not present, providers should continue to evaluate for other reasons for hypoxemia, particularly if it persists.** Finally, despite 10+ years of experience with CCHD screening since it was added to the US Recommended Uniform Screening Panel, compliance with CCHD screening has been inadequate.[35] **Enhanced efforts to use clinical decision support tools in the electronic health record should be explored to facilitate implementation and compliance with CCHD screening.**

LEAD AUTHORS

Matthew E. Oster, MD, MPH, FAAP
Nelangi M. Pinto, MD
Arun K. Pramanik, MD, FAAP
Allison Markowsky, MD, MSHS, FAAP
Bryanna N. Schwartz, MD, MPH, FAAP
Alex R. Kemper, MD, MPH, MS, FAAP
Lisa A. Hom, RN, Esq
Gerard R. Martin, MD, FAAP

COMMITTEE ON FETUS AND NEWBORN, 2022–2023

Eric Eichenwald, MD, Chairperson
Namasivayam Ambalavanan, MD
Charleta Guillory, MD
Mark Hudak, MD
David Kaufman, MD
Camilia Martin, MD
Ashley Lucke, MD
Margaret Parker, MD
Arun Pramanik, MD
Kelly Wade, MD

LIAISONS

Timothy Jancelewicz, MD – AAP Section on Surgery
Michael Narvey, MD – Canadian Paediatric Society
Russell Miller, MD – American College of Obstetricians and Gynecologists
RADM Wanda Barfield, MD, MPH – Centers for Disease Control and Prevention
Lisa Grisham, APRN, NNP-BC – National Association of Neonatal Nurses

STAFF

Jim Couto, MA

PARTNERSHIP FOR POLICY IMPLEMENTATION

Christoph U. Lehmann, MD, FAAP

ACKNOWLEDGEMENTS

The authors wish to acknowledge Amy Gaviglio for her review and insights related to the collection of CCHD screening data.

ABBREVIATIONS

AAP: American Academy of Pediatrics
CCHD: critical congenital heart disease
NICU: neonatal intensive care unit.

Clinical reports from the American Academy of Pediatrics benefit from expertise and resources of liaisons and internal (AAP) and external reviewers. However, clinical reports from the American Academy of Pediatrics may not reflect the views of the liaisons or the organizations or government agencies that they represent.

The guidance in this report does not indicate an exclusive course of treatment or serve as a standard of medical care. Variations, taking into account individual circumstances, may be appropriate.

All clinical reports from the American Academy of Pediatrics automatically expire 5 years after publication unless reaffirmed, revised, or retired at or before that time.

Accepted for Publication Date: October 22, 2024

https://doi.org/10.1542/peds.2024-069667

REFERENCES

1. Sebelius K. Interagency Coordinating Committee on Newborn and Child Screening (ICC): Screening for Congenital Heart Disease: A Federal Plan of Action. Summary of Federal Activities. Health Resources and Services Administration. September 21, 2011. Accessed February 6, 2019. https://www.hrsa.gov/sites/default/files/hrsa/advisory-committees/heritable-disorders/reports-recommendations/response-congenital-cyanotic.pdf
2. Centers for Disease Control and Prevention. Critical Congenital Heart Defects. Published January 7, 2020. Accessed August 21, 2023. https://www.cdc.gov/heart-defects/
3. American Academy of Pediatrics, Section on Cardiology and Cardiac Surgery. Endorsement of Health and Human Services recommendation for pulse oximetry screening for critical congenital heart disease. *Pediatrics*. 2012;129(1):190–192. doi: 10.1542/peds.2011-3211
4. Martin GR, Ewer AK, Gaviglio A, et al. Updated strategies for pulse oximetry screening for critical congenital heart disease. *Pediatrics*. 2020;146(1):e20191650. doi: 10.1542/peds.2019-1650
5. Abouk R, Grosse SD, Ailes EC, Oster ME. Association of us state implementation of newborn screening policies for critical congenital heart disease with early infant cardiac deaths. *JAMA*. 2017;318(21):2111–2118. doi: 10.1001/jama.2017.17627
6. Grosse S, Peterson C, Abouk R, Glidewell J, Oster M. Cost and cost-effectiveness assessments of newborn screening for critical congenital heart disease using pulse oximetry: a review. *Int J Neonatal Screen*. 2017;3(4):34. doi: 10.3390/ijns3040034
7. Cave AT, Lowenstein SA, McBride C, Michaud J, Madriago EJ, Ronai C. Pulse oximetry screening and critical congenital heart disease in the state of oregon. *Clin Pediatr (Phila)*. 2021;60(6-7):290–297. doi: 10.1177/00099228211008704
8. de-Wahl Granelli A, Wennergren M, Sandberg K, et al. Impact of pulse oximetry screening on the detection of duct dependent congenital heart disease: a Swedish prospective screening study in 39 821 newborns. *BMJ*. 2009;338(jan08 2):a3037–a3037. doi: 10.1136/bmj.a3037
9. Riede FT, Wörner C, Dähnert I, Möckel A, Kostelka M, Schneider P. Effectiveness of neonatal pulse oximetry screening for detection

of critical congenital heart disease in daily clinical routine—results from a prospective multicenter study. *Eur J Pediatr.* 2010;169(8):975–981. doi: 10.1007/s00431-010-1160-4

10. Sakai-Bizmark R, Kumamaru H, Marr EH, et al. Pulse oximetry screening: association of state mandates with emergency hospitalizations. *Pediatr Cardiol.* 2023;44(1):67–74. doi: 10.1007/s00246-022-03027-3
11. Kemper AR, Mahle WT, Martin GR, et al. Strategies for implementing screening for critical congenital heart disease. *Pediatrics.* 2011;128(5):e1259–1267. doi: 10.1542/peds.2011-1317
12. Peterson C, Grosse SD, Oster ME, Olney RS, Cassell CH. Cost-effectiveness of routine screening for critical congenital heart disease in us newborns. *Pediatrics.* 2013;132(3):e595–e603. doi: 10.1542/peds.2013-0332
13. Sakai-Bizmark R, Kumamaru H, Webber EJ, et al. Effect of newborn screening for critical CHD on healthcare utilisation. *Cardiol Young.* 2020;30(8):1157–1164. doi: 10.1017/S1047951120001742
14. Oster ME, Aucott SW, Glidewell J, et al. Lessons learned from newborn screening for critical congenital heart defects. *Pediatrics.* 2016;137(5):e20154573–e20154573. doi: 10.1542/peds.2015-4573
15. Singh A, Rasiah SV, Ewer AK. The impact of routine predischarge pulse oximetry screening in a regional neonatal unit. *Arch Dis Child - Fetal Neonatal Ed.* 2014;99(4):F297–F302. doi: 10.1136/archdischild-2013-305657
16. Garg LF, Van Naarden Braun K, Knapp MM, et al. Results from the new jersey statewide critical congenital heart defects screening program. *Pediatrics.* 2013;132(2):e314–e323. doi: 10.1542/peds.2013-0269
17. Mouledoux J, Guerra S, Ballweg J, Li Y, Walsh W. A novel, more efficient, staged approach for critical congenital heart disease screening. *J Perinatol.* 2017;37(3):288–290. doi: 10.1038/jp.2016.204
18. Glidewell J, Olney RS, Hinton C, et al. State legislation, regulations, and hospital guidelines for newborn screening for critical congenital heart defects - United States, 2011–2014. *MMWR Morb Mortal Wkly Rep.* 2015;64(23):625–630.
19. Manja V, Mathew B, Carrion V, Lakshminrusimha S. Critical congenital heart disease screening by pulse oximetry in a neonatal intensive care unit. *J Perinatol.* 2015;35(1):67–71. doi: 10.1038/jp.2014.135
20. Van Naarden Braun K, Grazel R, Koppel R, et al. Evaluation of critical congenital heart defects screening using pulse oximetry in the neonatal intensive care unit. *J Perinatol.* 2017;37(10):1117–1123. doi: 10.1038/jp.2017.105
21. Ravert P, Detwiler TL, Dickinson JK. Mean oxygen saturation in well neonates at altitudes between 4498 and 8150 feet. *Adv Neonatal Care.* 2011;11(6):412–417. doi: 10.1097/ANC.0b013e3182389348
22. Han LM, Klewer SE, Blank KM, Seckeler MD, Barber BJ. Feasibility of pulse oximetry screening for critical congenital heart disease at 2643-foot elevation. *Pediatr Cardiol.* 2013;34(8):1803–1807. doi: 10.1007/s00246-013-0716-2
23. Wright J, Kohn M, Niermeyer S, Rausch CM. Feasibility of critical congenital heart disease newborn screening at moderate altitude. *Pediatrics.* 2014;133(3):e561–e569. doi: 10.1542/peds.2013-3284
24. Samuel TY, Bromiker R, Mimouni FB, et al. Newborn oxygen saturation at mild altitude versus sea level: implications for neonatal screening for critical congenital heart disease. *Acta Paediatr.* 2013;102(4):379–384. doi: 10.1111/apa.12155
25. Rao S, Goens MB, Myers OB, Sebesta EA. Pulse oximetry screening for detection of congenital heart defects at 1646 m in Albuquerque, New Mexico. *Cardiol Young.* 2020;30(12):1851–1855. doi: 10.1017/S1047951120002899
26. Crocker ME, Hossen S, Goodman D, et al. Effects of high altitude on respiratory rate and oxygen saturation reference values in healthy infants and children younger than 2 years in four countries: a cross-sectional study. *Lancet Glob Health.* 2020;8(3):e362–e373. doi: 10.1016/S2214-109X(19)30543-1
27. Guo F, Tang S, Guo T, Bartell S, Detrano R. Revised threshold values for neonatal oxygen saturation at mild and moderate altitudes. *Acta Paediatr.* 2020;109(2):321–326. doi: 10.1111/apa.14962
28. Lueth E, Russell L, Wright J, et al. A novel approach to critical congenital heart disease (cchd) screening at moderate altitude. *Int J Neonatal Screen.* 2016;2(3):4. doi: 10.3390/ijns2030004
29. Hoffman JIE. Pulse oximetry in neonates at high altitudes: a modified Colorado protocol. *Cardiol Young.* 2020;30(2):177–179. doi: 10.1017/S1047951119003330
30. Cawsey MJ, Noble S, Cross-Sudworth F, Ewer AK. Feasibility of pulse oximetry screening for critical congenital heart defects in homebirths. *Arch Dis Child - Fetal Neonatal Ed.* 2016;101(4):F349–F351. doi: 10.1136/archdischild-2015-309936
31. Miller KK, Vig KS, Goetz EM, Spicer G, Yang AJ, Hokanson JS. Pulse oximetry screening for critical congenital heart disease in planned out of hospital births and the incidence of critical congenital heart disease in the Plain community. *J Perinatol.* 2016;36(12):1088–1091. doi: 10.1038/jp.2016.135
32. Narayen IC, Blom NA, Bourgonje MS, et al. Pulse oximetry screening for critical congenital heart disease after home birth and early discharge. *J Pediatr.* 2016;170:188–192.e1. doi: 10.1016/j.jpeds.2015.12.004
33. Williams KB, Horst M, Hollinger EA, Freedman J, Demczko MM, Chowdhury D. Newborn pulse oximetry for infants born out-of-hospital. *Pediatrics.* 2021;148(4):e2020048785. doi: 10.1542/peds.2020-048785
34. Narayen IC, Blom NA, van Geloven N, et al. Accuracy of pulse oximetry screening for critical congenital heart defects after home birth and early postnatal discharge. *J Pediatr.* 2018;197:29–35.e1. doi: 10.1016/j.jpeds.2018.01.039
35. Siefkes H, Kair LR, Saarinen A, Lakshminrusimha S. Inadequacies of hospital-level critical congenital heart disease screening data reports: implications for research and quality efforts. *J Perinatol.* 2021;41(7):1611–1620. doi: 10.1038/s41372-020-00783-z
36. John C, Phillips J, Hamilton C, Lastliger A. Implementing universal pulse oximetry screening in west virginia: findings from year one. *W V Med J.* 2016;112(4):42–46.

37. Downing GJ, Zuckerman AE, Coon C, Lloyd-Puryear MA. Enhancing the quality and efficiency of newborn screening programs through the use of health information technology. *Semin Perinatol.* 2010;34(2):156–162. doi: 10.1053/j.semperi.2009.12.005

38. Bright TJ, Wong A, Dhurjati R, et al. Effect of clinical decision-support systems: a systematic review. *Ann Intern Med.* 2012; 157(1):29–43. doi: 10.7326/0003-4819-157-1-201207030-00450

39. Pandya C, Sabatka S, Kettinger M, et al. Using electronic medical record system to improve compliance with national guidelines for comprehensive distress screening in cancer patients. *J Clin Oncol.* 2018;36(30_suppl):309–309. doi: 10.1200/JCO.2018.36.30_suppl.309

40. Choudhary D, Brown B, Khawar N, Narula P, Agdere L. Implementation of electronic medical record template improves screening for complications in children with type 1 diabetes mellitus. *Pediatr Health Med Ther.* 2020;11:219–223. doi: 10.2147/PHMT.S233998

41. Zarouni SA, Mheiri NMA, Blooshi KA, et al. Impact of an electronic medical record-based automated screening program for critical congenital heart disease: Emirates Health Services, United Arab Emirates. *BMC Med Inform Decis Mak.* 2022;22(1):165. doi: 10.1186/s12911-022-01900-y

42. Mahle WT, Newburger JW, Matherne GP, et al. Role of pulse oximetry in examining newborns for congenital heart disease: a scientific statement from the aha and aap. *Pediatrics.* 2009;124(2): 823–836. doi: 10.1542/peds.2009-1397

43. Lannering K, Bartos M, Mellander M. Late diagnosis of coarctation despite prenatal ultrasound and postnatal pulse oximetry. *Pediatrics.* 2015;136(2):e406–e412. doi: 10.1542/peds.2015-1155

44. Ailes EC, Gilboa SM, Honein MA, Oster ME. Estimated number of infants detected and missed by critical congenital heart defect screening. *Pediatrics.* 2015;135(6):1000–1008. doi: 10.1542/peds.2014-3662

45. Siefkes H, Kair L, Tancredi DJ, et al. Oxygen saturation and perfusion index-based enhanced critical congenital heart disease screening. *Am J Perinatol.* 2020;37(02):158–165. doi: 10.1055/s-0039-1685445

46. Clausen H, Norén E, Valtonen S, Koivu A, Sairanen M, Liuba P. Evaluation of circulating cardiovascular biomarker levels for early detection of congenital heart disease in newborns in sweden. *JAMA Netw Open.* 2020;3(12):e2027561. doi: 10.1001/jamanetworkopen.2020.27561

47. Sorensen MW, Sadiq I, Clifford GD, Maher KO, Oster ME. Using pulse oximetry waveforms to detect coarctation of the aorta. *Biomed Eng OnLine.* 2020;19(1):31. doi: 10.1186/s12938-020-00775-2

48. Troisi J, Cavallo P, Richards S, et al. Noninvasive screening for congenital heart defects using a serum metabolomics approach. *Prenat Diagn.* 2021;41(6):743–753. doi: 10.1002/pd.5893

49. Krishnan A, Jacobs MB, Morris SA, et al. Impact of socioeconomic status, race and ethnicity, and geography on prenatal detection of hypoplastic left heart syndrome and transposition of the great arteries. *Circulation.* 2021;143(21):2049–2060. doi: 10.1161/CIRCULATIONAHA.120.053062

50. Peiris V, Singh TP, Tworetzky W, Chong EC, Gauvreau K, Brown DW. Association of socioeconomic position and medical insurance with fetal diagnosis of critical congenital heart disease. *Circ Cardiovasc Qual Outcomes.* 2009;2(4):354–360. doi: 10.1161/CIRCOUTCOMES.108.802868

51. Hill GD, Block JR, Tanem JB, Frommelt MA. Disparities in the prenatal detection of critical congenital heart disease. *Prenat Diagn.* 2015;35(9):859–863. doi: 10.1002/pd.4622

52. Kochilas LK, Lohr JL, Bruhn E, et al. Implementation of critical congenital heart disease screening in minnesota. *Pediatrics.* 2013;132(3):e587–e594. doi: 10.1542/peds.2013-0803

53. Ruppel H, Makeneni S, Faerber JA, et al. Evaluating the accuracy of pulse oximetry in children according to race. *JAMA Pediatr.* 2023;177(5):540–543. doi: 10.1001/jamapediatrics.2023.0071

54. Oster ME, Kuo KW, Mahle WT. Quality improvement in screening for critical congenital heart disease. *J Pediatr.* 2014;164(1):67–71.e2. doi: 10.1016/j.jpeds.2013.08.044

55. Kochilas LK, Menk JS, Saarinen A, Gaviglio A, Lohr JL. A comparison of retesting rates using alternative testing algorithms in the pilot implementation of critical congenital heart disease screening in minnesota. *Pediatr Cardiol.* 2015;36(3):550–554. doi: 10.1007/s00246-014-1048-6

56. Diller CL, Kelleman MS, Kupke KG, Quary SC, Kochilas LK, Oster ME. A modified algorithm for critical congenital heart disease screening using pulse oximetry. *Pediatrics.* 2018;141(5). doi: 10.1542/peds.2017-4065

57. Schwartz BN, Hom LA, Von Kohorn I, et al. Newborn pulse oximetry screening at a community hospital: an 8-year experience. *Pediatrics.* 2021;148(3):e2020049847. doi: 10.1542/peds.2020-049847

58. Walters JC, Zhang X, Hokanson JS. Providers' attitudes to proposed changes in the critical congenital heart disease screening algorithm. *Pediatr Cardiol.* Published online March 4, 2022. doi: 10.1007/s00246-022-02858-4

59. Glidewell J. Actions in support of newborn screening for critical congenital heart disease—United States, 2011–2018. *MMWR Morb Mortal Wkly Rep.* 2019;68. doi: 10.15585/mmwr.mm6805a3

60. Martin GR, Beekman RH, Mikula EB, et al. Implementing recommended screening for critical congenital heart disease. *Pediatrics.* 2013;132(1):e185–e192. doi: 10.1542/peds.2012-3926

61. Case AP, Miller SD, McClain MR. Using state birth defects registries to evaluate regional critical congenital heart disease newborn screening. *Birth Defects Res.* 2017;109(18):1414–1422. doi: 10.1002/bdr2.1108

62. Oster ME, Colarusso T, Glidewell J. Screening for critical congenital heart disease: a matter of sensitivity. *Pediatr Cardiol.* 2013; 34(1):203–204. doi: 10.1007/s00246-012-0582-3

Patent Ductus Arteriosus in Preterm Infants

- *Clinical Report*

CLINICAL REPORT Guidance for the Clinician in Rendering Pediatric Care

American Academy of Pediatrics

DEDICATED TO THE HEALTH OF ALL CHILDREN™

Patent Ductus Arteriosus in Preterm Infants

Namasivayam Ambalavanan, MD,[1] Susan W. Aucott, MD,[2] Arash Salavitabar, MD,[3] Victor Y. Levy, MD,[4] and the Committee on Fetus and Newborn and Section on Cardiology and Cardiac Surgery

Despite extensive research in basic science and in clinical settings with thousands of infants over decades, uncertainty and controversy persist regarding the significance, assessment, and management of the patent ductus arteriosus (PDA) in preterm infants, resulting in substantial variability in clinical approach. This clinical report aims to succinctly review the available evidence to guide evaluation and treatment of preterm infants with prolonged ductal patency. Delayed closure of the PDA is common in preterm infants, particularly at more extreme immaturity. Echocardiography is essential for confirming the presence of a PDA and assessing hemodynamic significance. Medical closure of a PDA using ibuprofen or acetaminophen is an option for a hemodynamically significant PDA (hsPDA). Recent data from multiple clinical trials indicate the lack of benefits of prophylactic or early (<2 weeks of age) medical closure of PDA as compared with expectant management, and they are, therefore, not recommended. There are insufficient data to support firm recommendations on management of infants with an hsPDA beyond 2 weeks of age as relative benefits and risks of expectant management with close monitoring, attempted pharmacologic closure, or procedural (transcatheter/surgical) closure have not been adequately defined. Many clinicians attempt medical closure of an hsPDA beyond 2 weeks of age. If the hsPDA persists despite medical therapy (or if medical therapy is contraindicated), such infants may be considered for either transcatheter closure or surgical ligation. In recent years, surgical closure of the PDA has become less frequent, and transcatheter closure is more common in many centers. Although there are known adverse effects of an hsPDA, there is a lack of evidence to guide management, necessitating equipoise regarding treatment options and timing and a need for trials that can expand the available body of evidence, especially regarding long-term cardiopulmonary and neurodevelopmental outcomes.

abstract

[1]*University of Alabama at Birmingham, Birmingham, Alabama;* [2]*Division of Neonatology, Greater Baltimore Medical Center, Baltimore, Maryland;* [3]*Nationwide Children's Hospital, Columbus, Ohio; and* [4]*Phoenix Children's Hospital, Phoenix, Arizona*

Drs Levy, Salavitabar, Aucott, and Ambalavanan conceptualized and designed the manuscript, edited for content and reviewed and revised the manuscript. All authors approved the final manuscript as submitted and agree to be accountable for all aspects of the work.

FINANCIAL/CONFLICT OF INTEREST DISCLOSURE: The authors have indicated they have no potential conflicts of interest to disclose.

FUNDING: No external funding.

https://doi.org/10.1542/peds.2025-071425

To cite: Ambalavanan N, Aucott SW, Salavitabar A, et al; American Academy of Pediatrics, Committee on Fetus and Newborn and Section on Cardiology and Cardiac Surgery. Patent Ductus Arteriosus in Preterm Infants. *Pediatrics.* 2025; 155(5):e2025071425

CLINICAL EPIDEMIOLOGY, PHYSIOLOGY, AND NATURAL HISTORY OF THE PATENT DUCTUS ARTERIOSUS

In term infants, the ductus arteriosus normally constricts after birth and becomes functionally closed in 90% by 48 hours of age, in nearly all by 96 hours of age, and further delayed in preterm infants.[1] More immature infants have a more pronounced delay, with the ductus remaining open at 4 days of age in approximately 10% of infants born at 30 through 37 weeks' gestation, 80% of those born at 25 through 28 weeks' gestation, and >90% of those born at 24 weeks' gestation.[2] By day 7 after birth, those rates decline to approximately 2%, 65%, and 87%, respectively.

Spontaneous closure is likely in infants born at >28 weeks' gestation (73%),[3] in those with birth weight >1000 g (94%),[4] and in the few infants born at 26 to 29 weeks' gestation who do not have respiratory distress syndrome (RDS; 93%).[5] In the PDA-TOLERATE study, 40% of infants born at less than 28 weeks' gestation had no PDA or minimal respiratory impact from their PDA in the first 2 weeks of life.[6] Rates of later spontaneous ductal closure among smaller, less mature infants with RDS from placebo arms of controlled trials demonstrate that spontaneous ductal closure in these infants is quite frequent. In the Trial of Indomethacin Prophylaxis in Preterms (TIPP), which included infants with birth weight from 500 to 999 g, 50% of placebo recipients never developed clinical signs of a PDA.[7] In a trial of early vs late indomethacin treatment of infants born at 26 through 31 weeks' gestation in whom PDA was confirmed by echocardiography on day 3, the ductus closed spontaneously by 9 days of age in 78% of those randomized to late intervention.[8] As conservative management has become more prevalent, the majority of infants (90%) born at less than 26 weeks' gestation have been found to have spontaneous closure of the ductus, with closure occurring at a median of 36 weeks' postmenstrual age (PMA).[9] Of infants discharged home with persistent patent ductus, 50% will go on to close spontaneously by 9 months of age (approximately 49 weeks' PMA) and 80% will close by 2 years of age.[10] The hemodynamic significance of the PDA during that time is unclear and has not been well studied.

While the ductus remains open, blood typically flows left-to-right from the aorta into the pulmonary arteries. As pulmonary vascular resistance declines in the initial days after birth, there is an augmented diversion of aortic blood flow into the pulmonary circulation, known as the "ductal steal." This phenomenon results in additional blood flow through the lungs, predisposing to the development of pulmonary congestion, pulmonary edema, and exacerbated respiratory failure. The diversion of blood flow from the systemic circulation may surpass compensatory increases in total cardiac output, resulting in compromised perfusion of vital organs such as the bowel, kidney, and brain. Prolonged patency is associated with numerous adverse outcomes, including prolonged assisted ventilation and higher rates of death, bronchopulmonary dysplasia (BPD), pulmonary hemorrhage, necrotizing enterocolitis (NEC), impaired renal function, intraventricular hemorrhage (IVH), periventricular leukomalacia (PVL), and cerebral palsy (CP).[11] However, the precise extent to which these adverse outcomes are attributable to the hemodynamic consequences of ductal patency vs comorbid conditions resulting from extreme prematurity has not been defined. These associations prompted the hypothesis that intervention to close the ductus might prevent or reduce the severity of these complications seen more commonly in prematurity. The widespread adoption of interventions designed to achieve early closure of the ductus in preterm infants ensued with the anticipation that this hypothesis would be substantiated. The efficacy of these interventions is discussed subsequently.

ASSESSMENT OF HEMODYNAMIC SIGNIFICANCE

To date, an accurate and precise definition of a "hemodynamically significant" PDA (hsPDA) remains elusive. The hemodynamic effects of a large left-to-right shunt associated with a PDA may be evident by physical examination, echocardiography, or serum biomarkers.

In addition to the presence of a classic continuous murmur at the left sternal border, affected infants may have an increased precordial impulse and clinical signs of a widened pulse pressure, such as prominent or bounding arterial pulses, or palpable pulses in the palms of the hands. Nevertheless, these findings are nonspecific and have been found to be unreliable predictors of the presence of an hsPDA. Some infants may present with clinical evidence of pulmonary overflow (persistent or increased need for respiratory support) or systemic hypoperfusion (hypotension, renal dysfunction, feeding intolerance). These clinical features usually prompt clinicians to perform echocardiography to evaluate for a PDA.

Neonatal echocardiography has a critical role for PDA diagnosis and evaluation of therapeutic responses.[12] Defining an hsPDA involves careful determination of: (1) PDA shunt assessment and its impact on the systemic and pulmonary circulations; (2) myocardial and mitral valve function evaluation, especially in the context of the potential for myocardial ischemia secondary to impaired coronary artery perfusion; and (3) clinically relevant characteristics that modify the effects a shunt may have to an already compromised milieu.[13]

Pulmonary overcirculation, systemic hypoperfusion, and characterization of the duct itself, including diameter and Doppler flow pattern, are typically evaluated and considered when examining the ductus. Echocardiographic measurements that are indicative of pulmonary overcirculation and left heart volume overload include left atrial-to-aortic root ratio (LA:Ao), left ventricular end-diastolic diameter, mitral valve E/A (early passive filling to late

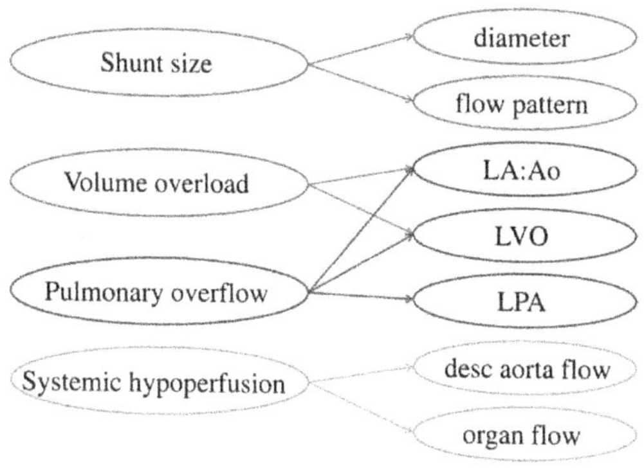

Figure 1.
Echocardiographic indicators of an hsPDA. For each echocardiogram, consider evaluating the size of the shunt, the extent of volume overload, the degree of pulmonary overflow, and the magnitude of systemic hypoperfusion. PDA shunt size can be estimated using the diameter and flow pattern through the PDA. Volume overload can be determined by calculating the left atrial (LA) to aortic (Ao) ratio (LA:Ao) and the left ventricular output (LVO). Pulmonary overflow can be evaluated by the LA:Ao, LVO, and by the end-diastolic velocity in the left pulmonary artery (LPA). Systemic hypoperfusion can be assessed by flow in the descending aorta (desc aorta flow) and flow to organs, such as in the cerebral, renal, or splanchnic arteries. Copyright © 2019 Shepherd JL, Noori S.[12] Published by Tech Science Press. This work is licensed under a Creative Commons Attribution 4.0 International License, which permits unrestricted use, distribution, and reproduction in any medium, provided the original work is properly cited.

Table 1. A Suggested Definition of a Hemodynamically Significant PDA (hsPDA): a Combination of Clinical and Echocardiographic Parameters

Clinical criteria (should fulfill 2 of 4 criteria)	1. High CPAP/NIMV with high FiO_2 or moderate or high ventilator settings at any FiO_2
	2. Hypotension needing a vasopressor
	3. Persistent oliguria or renal dysfunction
	4. Abdominal distension, feeding intolerance, poor growth despite optimization of nutrition, or history of NEC
AND	
Echocardiographic criteria (should fulfill at least one criterion)	1. Minimum PDA diameter >1.5 mm
	2. Unrestrictive left to right transductal flow (PDA Vmax <2 m/s)
	3. Left sided volume overload (≥moderate LA or LV enlargement)
	4. Decreased, absent, or reversed end-diastolic flow in abdominal descending aorta

CPAP indicates continuous positive airway pressure; FiO_2, fraction of inspired oxygen; LA, left articular; LV, left ventricular; NIMV, noninvasive mechanical ventilation; Vmax, maximum velocity.

active phase velocities), and isovolumic relaxation time (IVRT).[13] Mitral regurgitation may occur in some infants with a large PDA shunt.

Echocardiography and color Doppler ultrasonography can be used to assess the effect of hsPDA on end-organ perfusion and function (Figure 1). In the presence of a PDA in very low birth weight infants, the superior mesenteric artery has been associated with a smaller diameter, greater systolic velocity, lower diastolic velocity, and higher resistivity and pulsatility indices, as compared with those without a PDA.[14] Some infants with a PDA may also have absent or reversed end-diastolic flow in the superior mesenteric artery consistent with a steal effect and lower values of portal vein diameter and flow.[14] It was previously thought that the PDA would only exert negative effects on the blood flow of post-ductal vessels; however, a persistent PDA was also associated with reversed diastolic flow in the brachiocephalic artery[15] and with reduced middle cerebral artery blood flow velocity[16] indicating that preductal flow may also be impaired.

Myocardial performance is an essential component of assessing hsPDA. The diastolic dysfunction that is common in preterm infants with a PDA may increase adverse effects of increased pulmonary blood flow, emphasizing the importance of considering LV diastolic function in the definition of hemodynamic significance.[13,17]

Antenatal and perinatal clinical factors, such as lower gestational ages, growth restriction, lack of antenatal steroids, and other adverse perinatal events may contribute to adverse effects associated with a PDA. Therefore, determination of an hsPDA must not only include echocardiographic markers of shunt volume and right ventricular and left ventricular function but must also incorporate important clinical characteristics such as gestational age, postnatal age, and clinical evidence of pulmonary overflow or systemic hypoperfusion.

Table 1 provides a definition of an hsPDA that may be appropriate for most preterm infants.

Biomarkers have been used alone and in combination with echocardiography to diagnose ductal significance. B-type natriuretic peptide (BNP) and amino-terminal pro-B-type natriuretic peptide (NT-proBNP) have moderate accuracy in identifying hemodynamic significance of a PDA and may possibly be helpful in selecting infants for echocardiography, although nonspecific.[18] However, studies evaluating the diagnostic accuracy of BNP and NT-proBNP vary by assay characteristics and infant characteristics, and local validation of these tests is required before routine use.[18]

EVIDENCE FOR BENEFITS AND RISKS OF TREATMENT

Since the early reports of feasibility of surgical closure[19] and efficacy of nonsteroidal anti-inflammatory drugs (NSAIDs) for medical treatment of PDA,[20,21] results have been reported from multiple randomized trials of various medical and surgical therapies for PDA. A recent overview of 16 Cochrane Systematic Reviews combined data from

138 randomized clinical trials and 11 856 preterm infants.[22] Of the 16 Cochrane Reviews, 6 reported on prophylactic interventions, including pharmacological prophylaxis, prophylactic surgical ligation, and nonpharmacologic interventions (chest shielding during phototherapy and fluid restriction), and 9 reported on intervention for symptomatic PDA, including pharmacotherapy, surgical ligation, and adjunct therapies (use of furosemide and dopamine in combination with indomethacin).[22] The Grading of Recommendations Assessment, Development, and Evaluation (GRADE) approach[23] which is a systematic process of grading the quality of evidence and strength of recommendations was used to assess the quality of evidence in Cochrane Reviews, which will be discussed further in this section.

Prophylactic Interventions

Prophylactic interventions (those not guided by knowledge of PDA status) have included the use of indomethacin,[24] ibuprofen,[25] and acetaminophen[26] in preterm infants during the first 3 days after birth, and prophylactic surgical ligation in 1 study.[27,28] The Cochrane Review of prophylactic intravenous indomethacin reports on 19 trials with 2872 infants.[24] Indomethacin reduced symptomatic PDA (typical relative risk [RR], 0.44; 95% confidence interval [CI], 0.38–0.50), PDA surgical ligation (RR, 0.51; 95% CI, 0.37–0.71), and severe IVH (RR, 0.66; 95% CI, 0.53–0.82) but did not significantly change mortality (RR, 0.96; 95% CI, 0.81–1.12), BPD (RR, 1.06; 95% CI, 0.92–1.22), NEC (RR, 1.09; 95% CI, 0.82–1.46), or death/severe neurodevelopmental disability at 18 months to 3 years of age (RR, 1.02; 95% CI, 0.90–1.15)[24] (level of evidence: 1A).[29] For ibuprofen, there have been 9 trials (n = 1070) comparing prophylactic ibuprofen (intravenous or oral) with placebo/no intervention or indomethacin. It was noted that ibuprofen reduced the risk of a PDA by day 3 or 4 (RR, 0.39; 95% CI, 0.31–0.48), rescue treatment with cyclooxygenase-2 (COX) inhibitors (RR, 0.17; 95% CI, 0.11–0.26), and surgical ligation (RR, 0.46; 95% CI, 0.22–0.96), and possibly the risk of severe IVH (RR, 0.67; 95% CI, 0.45–1.00) (moderate-quality evidence), but with increased risk of oliguria (RR, 1.45; 95% CI, 1.04–2.02) (high-quality evidence).[25] No differences were noted for mortality or BPD.[25] Acetaminophen (paracetamol) has been evaluated in 27 studies enrolling 2278 infants, with acetaminophen (either alone or in combination) compared with no intervention, placebo, or other agents (indomethacin or ibuprofen).[26] Acetaminophen was more effective than placebo (RR, 0.27; 95% CI, 0.18–0.42; low certainty evidence) but has little to no difference compared with indomethacin or ibuprofen in failure of ductal closure after a single course (moderate certainty), or on all-cause mortality during hospital stay.[26] The single randomized trial of prophylactic PDA ligation was performed in the presurfactant and preantenatal steroid era, and had a limited sample size (44 extremely low birth weight infants randomly assigned to receive standard treatment and 40 randomly assigned to undergo prophylactic ligation).[28] It was found that infants in the prophylactic PDA ligation group had a lower risk of severe NEC, but no differences in mortality, BPD, severe IVH, or retinopathy of prematurity (ROP) were noted.[28]

In summary, these results suggest that the use of prophylactic indomethacin, ibuprofen, or acetaminophen is associated with a lower risk of a symptomatic PDA and with less severe IVH (for indomethacin and ibuprofen) but with no effects on mortality or BPD (level of evidence: 1A).[29]

Pharmacologic Therapy for Symptomatic PDA

Overall, all available prostaglandin inhibitor drugs (indomethacin, ibuprofen, and acetaminophen) are very effective in symptomatic PDA closure compared with no therapy (indomethacin: RR, 0.30; 95% CI, 0.23–0.38; 10 randomized controlled trials [RCTs], 654 infants; high-certainty evidence; ibuprofen: RR, 0.62; 95% CI, 0.44–0.86; 2 RCTs, 206 infants; moderate-certainty evidence; acetaminophen: RR, 0.35; 95% CI, 0.23–0.53; 2 RCTs, 127 infants; low-certainty evidence)[22] (level of evidence: 1A).[29] Ibuprofen used intravenously at the standard dose of 10 mg/kg followed by 2 doses of 5 mg/kg at 24-hour intervals may be preferred as it is as effective as indomethacin for PDA closure (typical failure rate, 1.07; 95% CI, 0.92–1.24; moderate quality evidence) and has a significantly better safety profile than indomethacin with lower risk of NEC (RR, 0.68; 95% CI, 0.49–0.94; number needed to benefit, 25; moderate quality evidence), trend toward less intestinal perforation (RR, 0.48 95% CI, 0.20–1.14), and less oliguria (RR, 0.28; 95% CI, 0.14–0.54; NNTB 11; moderate quality evidence).[30] A systematic review and meta-analysis of placebo, indomethacin, ibuprofen, and acetaminophen for closure of a hemodynamically significant PDA evaluated 68 RCTs of 4802 infants comparing 14 different variations of indomethacin, ibuprofen, or acetaminophen.[31] The overall PDA closure rate was 67.4%, and a high dose of oral ibuprofen (15 mg/kg to 20 mg/kg followed by 2 doses of 7.5 mg/kg to 10 mg/kg at 24-hour intervals) was associated with a higher odds of PDA closure compared with standard dose of intravenous ibuprofen (odds ratio [OR], 3.59; 95% credible interval 1.64–8.17; absolute risk difference, 199; 95–258 more per 1000 infants) or standard indomethacin (RR, 2.35; 95% CI, 1.08–53.1; absolute risk difference, 124; 14–188 more per 1000 infants). However, this high-dose regimen has not been adequately evaluated in extremely preterm infants (<29 weeks' gestation) as the sample size of such infants has been very limited and its efficacy and safety in this population is not known.[30,32]

A recent Cochrane Review assessed the effectiveness and safety of early treatment (defined as treatment initiated by 7 days of age) or very early treatment (treatment initiated by 72 hours of age) vs expectant management for a hemodynamically significant PDA and found that early or very early treatment did not decrease mortality and did not impact the rates of BPD, severe IVH, NEC, or surgical ligation while increasing exposure to NSAIDs.[33]

The efficacy and safety of repeat courses of medications if the initial course fails to close the PDA has not been adequately investigated in RCTs. Observational studies suggest that a second course may increase the closure rate, but a third course is less likely to lead to closure, and that adverse effects are rare with additional courses[34,35] (level of evidence: 2B).[29] There is no evidence to indicate that dual medication (combination) therapy improves the rate of successful PDA closure or clinical outcomes[36] (level of evidence: 1A).[29]

However, even though these medical therapies are frequently effective in closing the PDA, improvements in hospital and longer-term outcomes including all-cause mortality, BPD, NEC, or moderate/severe neurodevelopmental impairment have not been demonstrated[22] (level of evidence: 1A).[29] Although the reasons are not clear, it is possible that some of the benefits in improved hemodynamics with a closed PDA may be balanced by adverse effects of NSAIDs on the lung.[37–40] It is also possible that closing the PDA only affects specific outcomes and endotypes of neonatal disease, which may not have been the ones evaluated in studies or may not be able to be fully captured. For example, prolonged PDA exposure was associated with pulmonary hypertension in infants with BPD,[41] but such clinical phenotyping and endotyping of neonatal disorders has not been performed for PDA management. Adverse effects may also potentially occur in other organs such as the brain, although these effects may be more relevant to prenatal exposure[42] and not with postnatal exposure or in preterm infants.[43,44] A single center retrospective cohort study suggests that a highly targeted approach to PDA using very early hemodynamic screening, a comprehensive scoring system, and a physiology-based approach is associated with survival free of severe IVH,[45] but this approach has to be evaluated further.

Conservative (Expectant) Management

With increasing concerns of exposure to these medications without clear benefit, conservative or expectant management, defined as the practice of tolerating the presence of a persistent PDA that does not appear to be hemodynamically significant and allowing a delayed spontaneous closure, has become common. Numerous reports after this change in management suggest that this approach is safe[46–48] but are retrospective, and do not address the question of which infants may most benefit from this strategy and which infants could benefit from intervention. A retrospective review of a California Perinatal Quality Care Collaborative (CPQCC) found that neonatal intensive care unit (NICU)-specific reduced use of COX inhibitors was associated with lower rates of BPD in infants weighing more than 1000 g but not in those weighing less than 750 g in whom there was an association of reduced use of COX inhibitors with increased mortality.[49] A similar retrospective multicenter study in the Pediatrix Clinical Data Warehouse at 259 NICUs summarized data on 78 105 infants. The between-year reductions in the NICU-specific proportion treated with indomethacin or ibuprofen/ligation were associated with concurrent increases in local mortality but with reduced BPD among infants weighing 400–749 g and decreased pulmonary hemorrhage in larger infants.[50] A recent systematic review by Hundscheid et al[51] compared conservative management with any other active treatment (either prophylactic or nonprophylactic pharmacological or surgical therapy), in 12 cohort studies and 4 RCTs, encompassing 41 804 and 720 patients, respectively. It was noted that the cohort studies demonstrated a higher risk of mortality (RR, 1.34; 95% CI, 1.12–1.62) but lower BPD (RR, 0.85; 95% CI, 0.77–0.93), IVH (RR, 0.88; 95% CI, 0.83–0.95), and ROP (RR, 0.47; 95% CI, 0.28–0.79) with conservative management, while the meta-analysis of the RCTs did not reveal any significant differences between conservative and active treatment.[51]

To address the question prospectively, there have been some recent randomized trials. The PDA-TOLERATE Trial[6] randomly assigned 202 preterm infants born at <28 weeks' gestation with a moderate-to-large PDA between 6 and 14 days of age to early routine treatment (ERT) with either indomethacin, ibuprofen, or acetaminophen (with indomethacin backup if the PDA failed to constrict after the initial treatment) or conservative treatment(CT), with open-label (rescue) treatment for those infants in either group with hemodynamically significant PDA. Although infants in the conservative management arm were more likely to receive open-label therapy, especially in those infants born at <26 weeks' gestation, no significant differences were noted in the primary outcome of ligation or presence of a PDA at discharge (ERT 32% vs conservative treatment 39%) or any of the secondary outcomes of NEC (ERT 16% vs conservative treatment 19%), BPD (ERT 49% vs conservative treatment 53%) or BPD/death (ERT 58% vs conservative treatment 57%).[6] A trend for higher death was noted in the early routine therapy group (ERT 19% vs conservative treatment 10%; RR, 1.9; 95% CI, 0.92–3.8). In addition, among infants who were born at ≥26 weeks' gestational age, those receiving ERT took significantly longer to achieve enteral feeding of 120 mL/kg/d (ERT 14 days vs CT 6 days) and had significantly higher incidence of late-onset non-coagulase-negative *Staphylococcus* bacteremia (ERT 24% vs CT 6%) and death (ERT 16% vs CT 2%).[6]

The BeNeDuctus Trial[52] randomly assigned 273 infants born at <28 weeks' gestational age with PDA (>1.5 mm with left to right shunting at 24–72 hours of age) to receive either expectant management or early ibuprofen therapy received at a median postnatal age of 63 hours (range, 55–70 hours), with the primary outcome being a composite of NEC, moderate/severe BPD, and/or death at 36 weeks' PMA. Open-label treatment was considered if prespecified criteria were met for clinical or echocardiogram findings of heart failure associated with a clinically significant left-to-right shunt. The primary outcome occurred in 63 of 136 infants (46.3%) in the expectant management group and in 87 of 137 (63.5%) in the early ibuprofen group (absolute risk difference, −17.2 percentage points; upper boundary of the one-sided 95% CI, −7.4; $P<.001$ for noninferiority). No significant differences were noted in rates of NEC (17.6% expectant vs 15.3% ibuprofen) and death (14.0% expectant vs 18.2% ibuprofen) although there was an increase in BPD in the ibuprofen group (33.3% expectant vs 50.9% ibuprofen; absolute risk difference, −17.6%; 95% CI, −30.2 to −5.0).[52]

The Baby-OSCAR trial evaluated early treatment (≤72 hours after birth) with ibuprofen for a large PDA (≥1.5 mm diameter with pulsatile flow) in extremely preterm infants (23 weeks' to 28 weeks, 6 days' gestational age) and randomly assigned 326 infants to receive ibuprofen and 327 to receive placebo.[53] Death or moderate/severe BPD occurred in 69.2% of the ibuprofen group and 63.5% of the placebo group (adjusted risk ratio, 1.09; 95% CI, 0.98–1.20; $P=.1$), with death occurring in 13.6% of the ibuprofen group and 10.3% of the placebo group (adjusted risk ratio, 1.32; 95% CI, 0.92–1.90), demonstrating no reduction in death or BPD in infants.[53]

Studies on this topic have left several unanswered questions. First, hemodynamic significance has not been fully evaluated in most RCTs to date. Second, most RCTs enrolled infants soon after birth (when spontaneous closure is more likely), and it is not known whether a more selective approach enrolling only infants at later time points would show different results. It is possible that the PDA trial (NCT03456336) currently under way in the Eunice Kennedy Shriver NICHD Neonatal Research Network with a planned enrollment of 836 infants would provide important data in this regard. With these important limitations not yet accounted for, there has not been clear evidence that early (1–2 weeks of age) pharmacologic closure of PDA helps to improve outcomes of extreme prematurity.

Therefore, selective treatment of infants born at or before 28 weeks' gestation, who are at highest risk of PDA, may remain an option beyond 2 weeks' postnatal age. Deferral of early treatment in infants without hemodynamic compromise may allow avoidance of treatment of those in whom spontaneous closure occurs without compromising the potential efficacy of future medical treatment. Deferring early procedural closure in the PDA that is not hemodynamically significant may have similar advantages, avoiding a procedure in many infants in whom the ductus closes without treatment. The duration of such watchful expectancy needs to be determined and more evidence is needed to determine an optimal treatment strategy.

Surgical Closure

Surgical closure of the PDA is accomplished very predictably either by a clip application or by ligation and has had low morbidity and mortality even in very preterm infants for many decades.[54,55] There have been no recent randomized studies comparing surgical closure to medical therapies, with the Cochrane Review[56] including only 1 study from 1983.[57] In this trial, Gersony et al[57] compared surgical ligation to indomethacin, and found that surgical closure was more effective at closing the ductus (1% failure vs 30% failure with indomethacin), but with no differences in mortality or BPD, NEC, or IVH, although pneumothorax and ROP were more common in the surgical ligation group.

Although surgical closure is effective in achieving rapid and complete ductal closure, it may sometimes be followed by severe hemodynamic and respiratory collapse, requiring marked escalation in supportive intensive care.[58] The risk of this complication appears to decline substantially over the first 6 weeks after birth.[59] Complications of surgical closure include pneumothorax,[60] wound infection,[60] paresis of the left vocal cord[61,62] or diaphragm,[63] chylothorax,[64] and risk of scoliosis.[65] In addition, infants who undergo surgical ligation have been found to be more likely to develop BPD,[66,67] ROP,[67] and neurodevelopmental impairment.[67–69] Because of these risks and the risks of anesthesia and transfer from the NICU to the operating room, surgical closure is often reserved for infants who have a persistent PDA despite medical therapy (usually after 2 or more failed courses) or in whom medical therapy is contraindicated. From 2006 to 2015 in a large multicenter database evaluating 61 250 infants born between 23 and 30 weeks' gestation from 280 NICUs in the United States, the rates of surgical closure of PDA decreased from 8.4% to 2.9% ($P<.001$), accompanied by a decrease in the diagnosis of PDA (79% of sites), use of indomethacin or ibuprofen from 32% to 18% ($P<.001$) and a decrease in overall mortality without increases in any measured morbidity.[70] In another large multicenter database study from 2014 to 2021, evaluating 64 580 infants born between 22 and 30 weeks' gestation, 24 028 (37.2%) were diagnosed with a PDA.[71] The percentage of infants receiving any procedural closure of the PDA decreased from 4.4% in 2014 (4.36% surgical; 0.02% transcatheter closure) to 1.9% (0.84% surgical; 1.05% transcatheter closure) in 2021 ($P<.001$ for all comparisons), with transcatheter occlusion surpassing surgical ligation in 2021.[71] These data suggest that many centers had shifted to a more conservative approach in recent years, with fewer evaluations for PDA and subsequent decreases in medical and surgical management and with more frequent transcatheter as compared with surgical closure.

Transcatheter Closure of PDA

In 1966, Portsmann was the first to successfully close a PDA by a transcatheter method and reported subsequently that this approach was successfully used in 56 of 62 patients with no mortality and minimal morbidity.[72] Since then, there has been a constant pursuit to perform PDA closure at a younger age and smaller size to treat presumed associated deleterious physiologic effects. Transcatheter closure has classically been the procedure of choice for definitive PDA occlusion in adults, children, and infants weighing >6 kg and has become a first-line intervention for much smaller patients in many institutions as devices and techniques have improved and developed. In a recent large multicenter study, the number of sites offering transcatheter closure increased from 5 of 274 (1.8%) in 2014–2015 to 35 of 276 (12.7%) in 2020–2021, while centers offering surgical ligation decreased from 112/274 (40.9%) to 54/276 (19.6%) ($P<.0001$).[71]

In a meta-analyses of percutaneous PDA closure during infancy that included 38 studies through 2015, Backes et al[73] reported a technical success of percutaneous PDA closure of 92% (95% CI, 89–95), with clinically significant adverse event incidence of 10% (95% CI, 7.8-12.5).[73] Patients specifically <6 kg in weight who had a PDA device closure were studied from the IMPACT (Improving Pediatric and Adult Congenital Treatments) NCDR Registry and had a 94.3% procedural success rate among 73 hospitals during 2011–2015.[74] There was a 2.4% incidence of device embolization requiring retrieval and 3.5% incidence of acute arterial occlusion in that study. A meta-analysis of percutaneous PDA closure through 2020 in 373 infants weighing ≤1.5 kg by Bischoff et al[75] found that technical success was 96% (93–98), with overall adverse effect incidence of 27% (17–38) and major adverse event of 8% (5–10), with 5 deaths related to the procedure (4 in infants weighing <0.8 kg). Importantly, experience has grown exponentially since that time in smaller and more preterm infants and with that has come greater procedural success and safety.[76] The above study periods included limited percutaneous device choices and there has since been an increase in the availability of devices to address the unique ductal morphology of preterm infants, and there have been increasing levels of expertise in such procedures by interventional teams in smaller and less mature infants.[76] The successful technique of solely utilizing femoral venous access for PDA device closure and with echocardiographic guidance was described by Zahn et al,[77] thus eliminating the risk of arterial occlusion and even potentially eliminating the need for contrast administration in a small pilot group of preterm infants with off-label use of the Amplatzer Vascular Plug II (AVP II [Abbott Structural Heart, Plymouth, MN]) device. This was followed by a single-institution report of this approach of implanting the AVP II device with 88% success rate in 24 patients.[78] With the prior device limitations, several uncommon but important challenges of left pulmonary artery (LPA) and aortic obstruction occurred, emphasizing the need for tools designed for the extremely low weight and preterm population.

The Amplatzer Piccolo Occluder received FDA approval in 2019 and became the first device approved for PDA closure in patients weighing ≥700 g.[79] A single-arm, prospective, multicenter, nonrandomized study to evaluate the Amplatzer Piccolo Occluder in patients weighing ≥700 g evaluated 200 patients in 9 centers, with 100 patients weighing ≤2 kg (and 33 weighing ≤1 kg).[79] The implant success rate was 95.5% (191/200) overall, and 99% in those weighing ≤2 kg.[79] The primary effectiveness endpoint of PDA closure at 6-month follow-up was achieved in 99.4% of implanted patients, but 4 patients had a primary safety endpoint (2 transfusions, 1 hemolysis, and 1 aortic obstruction), and 5 patients (all weighing ≤2 kg) had worsening nonclinically evident tricuspid regurgitation. There was one instance of device-related aortic obstruction. Intraprocedural device embolization occurred in 5 patients (3 weighing <2 kg), all of which were successfully retrieved and replaced during the same procedure. There was no branch pulmonary artery obstruction. The 3-year follow-up of this study showed no new complications and no device or procedure-related deaths.[80] Although 2 patients had elevated LPA velocity by echocardiography of >2.5 m/s, both resolved with somatic growth and without intervention. Of the 5 patients with worsened tricuspid regurgitation, one had a nonprocedure-related mortality, one was withdrawn from the study for a device not being placed following initial device retrieval, and the other 3 have not required interventions on their tricuspid valves. All successfully closed PDAs that were followed to completion remained closed.

A recent cohort study using the IMPACT Registry of 1587 attempted PDA closures in infants weighing ≤2 kg (nearly all weighing >700 g) from 2016–2021, showing a significant increase in the distribution of percutaneous PDA device closures during the 2019–2021 time period, as compared with 2016–2019.[81] This study reported a 3% incidence of technical failure with a 5.5% incidence of the composite outcome of technical failure and/or major adverse event.[81] The most common major adverse event included device embolization requiring retrieval (1.3%) and unplanned cardiac or vascular surgery (1.3%).[81] The incidence of the composite outcome was associated with the use of arterial access (OR, 5.25; 95% CI, 2.3–12.01; $P<.001$), which has been largely abandoned by most institutions for this weight range; in addition, the composite outcome was associated with annual hospital volume of percutaneous PDA closures in infants weighing ≤2 kg (for higher volume: OR, 0.51; 95% CI, 0.28–0.93; $P=.03$), with similar rates of procedural failure across weight categories.[81]

A recent C3PO (Congenital Cardiac Catheterization Project on Outcomes) Registry study focusing on PDA device closure in infants weighing <2.5 kg from 2019–2020 showed a 98.7% success rate among 300 cases with a median weight of 1.0 kg (0.7–2.4) at 13 institutions.[82] There was a 1.7% incidence of level 4/5 adverse events (AEs), including device malposition causing aortic obstruction (n = 2) and respiratory arrest (n = 2). There was 1 death 12 hours postprocedure in the setting of urosepsis and "postligation syndrome." The 5.6% incidence of level 3 AEs include a 1.3% (n = 4) incidence of device embolization; these were all retrieved successfully during the same procedure. Age and weight at the time of catheterization were not significantly associated with AEs. This study's timeframe corresponds with the approval of the Piccolo Occluder, although an off-label device (Micro Vascular Plug [Medtronic, Minneapolis, MN]) was used first in 20% of cases and showed that patients who had the Micro Vascular Plug as the first device had a higher likelihood of failed device placement (OR, 12.9; $P = .028$).

The challenges to using transcatheter or surgical closure strategies are establishing the appropriate timing, the selection of patients, and the experience and expertise within each center. Although there are no randomized trials comparing transcatheter and surgical closure, there are some data from observational studies, although data from the most immature infants (born at 22–23 weeks' gestational age) are very limited. Ogando et al[83] in Spain performed a retrospective cohort study of 25 very low weight preterm infants undergoing percutaneous closure using the Piccolo Occluder (then named the Amplatzer Duct Occluder-II-Additional Sizes [ADO-II-AS]) to 28 matched infants (for gestational age, birth weight, and procedure weight) with surgical closure from 2011–2016. There was quicker improvement in the pulmonary status in the percutaneous closure group and a higher morbidity in the surgical closure group with a high rate of recurrent laryngeal nerve palsy (17%).[83] There were 2 device embolizations, which were successfully retrieved and replaced during the same procedure. Unfortunately, the majority of the remainder of studies comparing percutaneous to surgical treatment were performed prior to the availability and approval of the Amplatzer Piccolo Occluder as well as widespread use of a sole transvenous approach with echocardiographic guidance. Kim et al[84] compared 33 infants receiving device closure to 39 infants with surgical closure during 2014–2017 period and noted that infants undergoing surgical ligation were younger and smaller and required more preoperative support, but the procedure time was shorter for surgical ligation, with fewer complications. The procedural charges were higher for percutaneous closure, driven by device charge and catheterization room utilization.[84] Regan et al[85] compared 64 infants undergoing transcatheter closure to 83 matched surgical cases. PDA closure was successful in all cases, with 4 deaths in catheter group (6.3%) vs 10 (12%) in the surgical group ($P = .24$), and with a shorter duration of mechanical ventilation after catheterization (median 3 vs 5 days, $P = .04$).[85] Kuntz et al[86] compared trends and outcomes for surgical (n = 175) vs transcatheter (n = 503) PDA closure at US Children's Hospitals. Surgical patients were younger (0.1 vs 0.53 years; $P < .001$) and more premature (60% vs 20.3%; $P < .001$), with higher rates of comorbidity. When only preterm infants (n = 102 for catheter vs 105 for surgical ligation) were compared, infants surgically ligated were more likely to be mechanically ventilated, and for longer, with a longer hospital stay (adjusted difference in medians, 4 days; 95% CI, 1.7–6.3 days; $P < .001$) and postoperative length of stay (adjusted difference in medians, 3 days; 95% CI, 1.1–4.9 days; $P = .002$).[86]

Advances in the percutaneous device closure of the PDA have led to its widespread adoption among many institutions with a congenital interventional cardiology team as a viable treatment option for preterm infants. With the approval of the Amplatzer Piccolo Occluder and advanced technical approaches, safety and efficacy have improved. If there is no transcatheter or surgical closure available at a center, decisive treatment of hsPDAs failing medical therapy (or in whom it is contraindicated) requires transfer to centers with expertise in such procedures. Development of collaborative, multidisciplinary teams who can assess the regional availability of procedural closure along with the risks and benefits of patient transfer may be required to best determine the timing and eligibility of intervention. It is likely that the availability of such specialized care and procedures may not be easily accessible or available, resulting in potential inequities in health care delivery. Although procedural outcomes have been shown in registry-based and multicenter clinical studies, it is important to determine whether closing the PDA by transcatheter approaches improves short-term clinical outcomes (initial hospital mortality, BPD, NEC, ROP, etc) or longer-term outcomes (neurodevelopmental impairment). The ongoing Percutaneous Intervention Vs Observational Trial of Arterial Ductus in Low Birth Weight Infants (PIVOTAL) (NCT05547165) will yield useful data in this regard.

Adjunct and Other Medical Nonpharmacological Therapies

Expectant management of the PDA includes management of fluid, electrolyte, and nutrition status, and support of the cardiac, circulatory, and respiratory systems that may be impacted by the PDA. These frequently include restriction of fluid intake, diuresis, and use of higher end-expiratory pressures and permissive hypercapnia.[87]

Restricted water intake in preterm infants has been shown to increase postnatal weight loss (overall weighted mean difference, 1.94% of birth weight; 95% CI, 0.82–3.07) and significantly reduce the risks of PDA (RR, 0.52; 95% CI, 0.37–0.73; number needed to treat, 7; range, 5–14) and NEC (RR, 0.43; 95% CI, 0.21–0.87; NNT, 20; range, 11–100), with trends for reduction in BPD (RR, 0.85; 95% CI, 9.63–1.14), IVH (RR, 0.74; 95% CI, 0.48–1.14), and death (RR, 0.81; 95% CI, 0.54–1.23).[88] Hence, there is some evidence that early fluid restriction may reduce the incidence of a PDA; however, this evidence is based on trials that are from several decades ago and may not be generalizable to current practices and more immature infants. There is no evidence that fluid restriction is helpful following the diagnosis of a hemodynamically significant PDA. Fluid restriction after diagnosis negatively affects energy intake and growth.[89] A reduction of fluid intake from 145 ± 15 to 108 ± 10 mL/kg/d did not change respiratory variables, FiO_2, blood gas values, PDA diameter, blood flow velocities (in the PDA, left pulmonary artery, or descending aorta), or LA/Ao ratio but reduced flow in the superior vena cava significantly (105 ± 40 to 61 ± 25 mL/kg/min, $P < .001$) and lowered blood flow velocity in the superior mesenteric artery.[90] It may be optimal to limit fluid restriction to a minimum of 120 to 130 mL/kg/d after the first week, to limit such adverse effects of over-restricted fluid intake.

Diuresis is often induced with furosemide in an attempt to reduce pulmonary edema associated with a hemodynamically significant PDA. However, loop diuretics such as furosemide (but not thiazides) also increase renal prostaglandin E_2 production in vitro[91] and cause PDA dilatation in vivo in neonatal rats.[92] Early prophylactic use of furosemide in a small randomized trial led to more rapid postnatal weight loss and a higher heart rate but with a trend toward a higher prevalence of PDA (40% in furosemide group with PDA vs 24% in placebo group; $P = .09$).[93] Hence, there is a concern over the use of loop diuretics in PDA and a lack of consensus.[94] However, the use of concomitant furosemide did not reduce the efficacy of acetaminophen in closing the PDA,[95] and a recent large retrospective cohort study showed that exposure to furosemide was actually associated with decreased odds of PDA treatment (OR, 0.72; 95% CI, 0.65–0.79),[96] suggesting that although prophylactic use of furosemide may not be appropriate, it may be useful in management in the setting of pulmonary edema.

Respiratory management using higher end-expiratory pressures and permissive hypercapnia may potentially reduce left-to-right shunting in the setting of a PDA.[87] However, these management strategies based on respiratory physiology have not been adequately studied.

CLINICAL TRIAL OPPORTUNITIES

Additional research is needed to address 2 broad questions related to prolonged ductal patency in preterm infants. First, the relationship between measures of hemodynamic significance and increased risks for both very prolonged patency and adverse clinical outcomes, such as BPD, pulmonary hypertension, or neurodevelopmental impairment, needs to be established, with additional focus on the optimal timing and method of achieving closure. Second, well-designed and meticulously executed intervention trials, for which the endpoints are clinically important long-term outcomes in addition to short-term physiologic changes, and not simply rates of ductal closure and adverse procedural events, are essential. In these trials, both treatment arms must be unambiguously defined so that the superior strategy can be replicated in clinical practice and evaluated against alternatives in future trials. If it is not feasible to forego use of rescue treatment in the control (placebo or late-treatment) arm, strict criteria for both a required time interval and diagnostic thresholds for such treatment are essential. Long-term follow up with assessment of neurodevelopmental outcomes would further guide treatment. Without clear demonstration that adverse outcomes can be averted by medical, surgical, or transcatheter closure of the ductus, the hypothesis that ductal patency is causal with respect to those outcomes remains unproven.

RECOMMENDATIONS

For Clinical Practice

1. Prophylactic medical interventions (those not guided by knowledge of PDA status) are not recommended at any age or birth weight for the purpose of reducing the risk of a symptomatic PDA, as there are no effects on mortality, BPD, or neurodevelopmental impairment (level of evidence: 1A).[29]
2. Early fluid restriction may reduce the incidence of a PDA (level of evidence: 1A).[29] However, such data are from several decades ago and may not be generalizable to current practices and extremely preterm infants. There is no evidence that fluid restriction is helpful following diagnosis of a hemodynamically significant PDA (level of evidence: 2B).[29] Furosemide may be useful as an adjunct in management (level of evidence: 2B).[29] Ventilator management strategies have not been adequately studied for firm recommendations.
3. Very early (<72 hours of age) or early (<7 to 14 days of age) routine treatment to induce PDA closure (regardless of hemodynamic significance) in preterm infants, either medically, via transcatheter, or surgically, is able to close the ductus but does not improve outcomes and is not recommended (level of evidence: 1A).[29] Conservative management in this age group may let infants avoid medical therapy or procedural exposure (either surgical or transcatheter closure), allowing spontaneous delayed closure without risk of increased adverse outcomes. It is likely that the presence of a

PDA is a marker for more extreme immaturity and a biomarker for worse outcomes, but treatments to close the PDA may not significantly impact such outcomes.

4. There are insufficient data for recommendations on management of infants with a hemodynamically significant PDA beyond 2 weeks of age. Benefits and risks of watchful expectancy with close monitoring, attempted medical closure, transcatheter closure, or surgical ligation of the hemodynamically significant PDA have not been adequately defined. The duration of watchful expectancy needs to be determined and more evidence is needed to determine an optimal treatment strategy.
5. It is considered reasonable to attempt pharmacologic closure of a hemodynamically significant PDA beyond 2 weeks of age (ibuprofen as a preferred agent, although acetaminophen or indomethacin are acceptable alternatives) (level of evidence: 5).[29]
6. If the hsPDA persists beyond 2 weeks of age despite pharmacologic therapy of up to 2 courses (or if medical therapy is contraindicated), such infants may be considered for either transcatheter closure or surgical ligation (level of evidence: 4).[29]

For Further Study

1. The role of more selective use of medical therapies for inducing PDA closure, both for defined higher-risk infants in the first 2 postnatal weeks (perhaps by early hemodynamic screening or other targeting), or for older infants in whom the PDA remains patent (whether hemodynamically significant or not), remains uncertain and is currently the subject of ongoing studies. There is a lack of evidence to guide management, necessitating equipoise regarding treatment options and support for parents to permit enrollment of their infants in trials that can expand the available body of evidence, especially regarding long-term cardiopulmonary and neurodevelopmental outcomes.
2. Increasing numbers of infants currently undergo transcatheter closure while surgical ligation of PDA has declined in recent years. Transcatheter closure is very effective in closing the PDA but the risks, benefits, and longer term outcomes need to be adequately defined, and the eligibility and optimal timing for transcatheter interventions need to be better understood before firm recommendations can be developed (level of evidence: 4).[29]

LEAD AUTHORS

Namasivayam Ambalavanan, MD
Susan W. Aucott, MD
Arash Salavitabar, MD
Victor Y. Levy, MD

COMMITTEE ON FETUS AND NEWBORN, 2023–2024

Eric Eichenwald, MD, Chairperson
Namasivayam Ambalavanan, MD
Charleta Guillory, MD
Mark Hudak, MD
David Kaufman, MD
Camilia Martin, MD
Ashley Lucke, MD
Margaret Parker, MD
Arun Pramanik, MD
Kelly Wade, MD

LIAISONS

Timothy Jancelewicz, MD – AAP Section on Surgery
Michael Narvey, MD – Canadian Paediatric Society
Russell Miller, MD – American College of Obstetricians and Gynecologists
RADM Wanda Barfield, MD, MPH – Centers for Disease Control and Prevention
Lisa Grisham, APRN, NNP-BC – National Association of Neonatal Nurses

STAFF

Jim Couto, MA

SECTION ON CARDIOLOGY AND CARDIAC SURGERY EXECUTIVE COMMITTEE, 2022–2023

Stuart Berger, MD, FAAP – Chair
Christopher Scott Snyder MD, FAAP – Immediate Past Chair
Laurie Bertanyi Armsby, MD, FAAP
Carlos M. Mery, MD, FAAP
Jonathan Johnson, MD FAAP
Fred "Rusty" Rodriguez, MD, FAAP
Jeffrey Vergales, MD, FAAP
Juan Villafane, Jr, MD, FAAP
Markus Renno, MD, MPH, FAAP – Early Career Representative
Andrew Headrick, MD, FAAP – Trainee Representative
Dean S. Karahalios, DO, FAAP – Trainee Representative

STAFF

Vivian Thorne

ACKNOWLEDGMENT

We acknowledge the contributions of Dr William E. Benitz and the former members of the Committee on Fetus and Newborn for their work on the previous version of this clinical report (Benitz WE; American Academy of Pediatrics, Committee on Fetus and Newborn. Patent ductus arteriosus in preterm infants. *Pediatrics.* 2016;137[1]:e20153730).

ABBREVIATIONS

BPD: bronchopulmonary dysplasia
COX: cyclooxygenase-2
ERT: early routine treatment
hsPDA: hemodynamically significant patent ductus arteriosus
NT-proBNP: amino-terminal pro-B-type natriuretic peptide
PDA: patent ductus arteriosus
RCT: randomized controlled trial
RDS: respiratory distress syndrome
ROP: retinopathy of prematurity

REFERENCES

1. Gentile R, Stevenson G, Dooley T, Franklin D, Kawabori I, Pearlman A. Pulsed Doppler echocardiographic determination of time of ductal closure in normal newborn infants. *J Pediatr.* 1981;98(3):443–448. PubMed doi: 10.1016/S0022-3476(81)80719-6
2. Clyman RI, Couto J, Murphy GM. Patent ductus arteriosus: are current neonatal treatment options better or worse than no treatment at all? *Semin Perinatol.* 2012;36(2):123–129. PubMed doi: 10.1053/j.semperi.2011.09.022
3. Koch J, Hensley G, Roy L, Brown S, Ramaciotti C, Rosenfeld CR. Prevalence of spontaneous closure of the ductus arteriosus in neonates at a birth weight of 1000 grams or less. *Pediatrics.* 2006;117(4):1113–1121. PubMed doi: 10.1542/peds.2005-1528
4. Nemerofsky SL, Parravicini E, Bateman D, Kleinman C, Polin RA, Lorenz JM. The ductus arteriosus rarely requires treatment in infants > 1000 grams. *Am J Perinatol.* 2008;25(10):661–666. PubMed doi: 10.1055/s-0028-1090594
5. Reller MD, Rice MJ, McDonald RW. Review of studies evaluating ductal patency in the premature infant. *J Pediatr.* 1993;122(6):S59–S62. PubMed doi: 10.1016/S0022-3476(09)90044-0
6. Clyman RI, Liebowitz M, Kaempf J, et al; PDA-TOLERATE (PDA: TO LEave it alone or Respond And Treat Early) Trial Investigators. PDA-TOLERATE Trial: An Exploratory Randomized Controlled Trial of Treatment of Moderate-to-Large Patent Ductus Arteriosus at 1 Week of Age. *J Pediatr.* 2019;205:41–48.e6. PubMed doi: 10.1016/j.jpeds.2018.09.012
7. Schmidt B, Davis P, Moddemann D, et al; Trial of Indomethacin Prophylaxis in Preterms Investigators. Long-term effects of indomethacin prophylaxis in extremely-low-birth-weight infants. *N Engl J Med.* 2001;344(26):1966–1972. PubMed doi: 10.1056/NEJM200106283442602
8. Van Overmeire B, Van de Broek H, Van Laer P, Weyler J, Vanhaesebrouck P. Early versus late indomethacin treatment for patent ductus arteriosus in premature infants with respiratory distress syndrome. *J Pediatr.* 2001;138(2):205–211. PubMed doi: 10.1067/mpd.2001.110528
9. de Carvalho Nunes G, Wutthigate P, Simoneau J, Beltempo M, Sant'Anna GM, Altit G. Natural evolution of the patent ductus arteriosus in the extremely premature newborn and respiratory outcomes. *J Perinatol.* 2022;42(5):642–648. PubMed doi: 10.1038/s41372-021-01277-2
10. Weber SC, Weiss K, Bührer C, Hansmann G, Koehne P, Sallmon H. Natural History of Patent Ductus Arteriosus in Very Low Birth Weight Infants after Discharge. *J Pediatr.* 2015;167(5):1149–1151. PubMed doi: 10.1016/j.jpeds.2015.06.032
11. Benitz WE. Treatment of persistent patent ductus arteriosus in preterm infants: time to accept the null hypothesis? *J Perinatol.* 2010;30(4):241–252. PubMed doi: 10.1038/jp.2010.3
12. Shepherd JL, Noori S. What is a hemodynamically significant PDA in preterm infants? *Congenit Heart Dis.* 2019;14(1):21–26. PubMed doi: 10.1111/chd.12727
13. El-Khuffash A, Levy PT, Gorenflo M, Frantz ID III. The definition of a hemodynamically significant ductus arteriosus. *Pediatr Res.* 2019;85(6):740–741. PubMed doi: 10.1038/s41390-019-0342-7
14. Cavalcanti LS, da Costa E Silva EJ, Falbo AR, et al. Serial Doppler velocimetry of mesenteric and portal flow in very-low-birth-weight preterm neonates with and without patent ductus arteriosus. *Pediatr Radiol.* 2020;50(8):1107–1114. PubMed doi: 10.1007/s00247-020-04689-y
15. Breatnach CR, Franklin O, McCallion N, El-Khuffash A. The Effect of a Significant Patent Ductus Arteriosus on Doppler Flow Patterns of Preductal Vessels: An Assessment of the Brachiocephalic Artery. *J Pediatr.* 2017;180:279–281.e1. PubMed doi: 10.1016/j.jpeds.2016.09.029
16. Weir FJ, Ohlsson A, Myhr TL, Fong K, Ryan ML. A patent ductus arteriosus is associated with reduced middle cerebral artery blood flow velocity. *Eur J Pediatr.* 1999;158(6):484–487. PubMed doi: 10.1007/s004310051125
17. Bischoff AR, Stanford AH, Aldoss O, et al. Left ventricular function before and after percutaneous patent ductus arteriosus closure in preterm infants. *Pediatr Res.* 2023;94(1):213–221. PubMed doi: 10.1038/s41390-022-02372-6
18. Gokulakrishnan G, Kulkarni M, He S, et al. Brain natriuretic peptide and N-terminal brain natriuretic peptide for the diagnosis of haemodynamically significant patent ductus arteriosus in preterm neonates. *Cochrane Database Syst Rev.* 2022;12(12):CD013129. PubMed doi: 10.1002/14651858.CD013129.pub2
19. Gupta JM, Van Vliet PK, Fisk GC, Wright JS. Ductus ligation in respiratory distress syndrome. *J Thorac Cardiovasc Surg.* 1972;63(4):642–647. PubMed doi: 10.1016/S0022-5223(19)41882-5
20. Friedman WF, Hirschklau MJ, Printz MP, Pitlick PT, Kirkpatrick SE. Pharmacologic closure of patent ductus arteriosus in the premature infant. *N Engl J Med.* 1976;295(10):526–529. PubMed doi: 10.1056/NEJM197609022951003
21. Heymann MA, Rudolph AM, Silverman NH. Closure of the ductus arteriosus in premature infants by inhibition of prostaglandin synthesis. *N Engl J Med.* 1976;295(10):530–533. PubMed doi: 10.1056/NEJM197609022951004
22. Mitra S, de Boode WP, Weisz DE, Shah PS. Interventions for patent ductus arteriosus (PDA) in preterm infants: an overview of Cochrane Systematic Reviews. *Cochrane Database Syst Rev.* 2023;4(4):CD013588. PubMed doi: 10.1002/14651858.CD013588.pub2

23. Group GW. Handbook for grading the quality of evidence and the strength of recommendations using the GRADE approach (updated October 2013). Published 2013. Accessed June 10, 2023. http://gdt.guidelinedevelopment.org/app/handbook/handbook.html

24. Fowlie PW, Davis PG, McGuire W. Prophylactic intravenous indomethacin for preventing mortality and morbidity in preterm infants. *Cochrane Database Syst Rev.* 2010;2010(7):CD000174. PubMed doi: 10.1002/14651858.CD000174.pub2

25. Ohlsson A, Shah SS. Ibuprofen for the prevention of patent ductus arteriosus in preterm and/or low birth weight infants. *Cochrane Database Syst Rev.* 2020;1(1):CD004213. PubMed doi: 10.1002/14651858.CD004213.pub5

26. Jasani B, Mitra S, Shah PS. Paracetamol (acetaminophen) for patent ductus arteriosus in preterm or low birth weight infants. *Cochrane Database Syst Rev.* 2022;12:CD010061. PubMed doi: 10.1002/14651858.CD010061.pub5

27. Mosalli R, Alfaleh K. Prophylactic surgical ligation of patent ductus arteriosus for prevention of mortality and morbidity in extremely low birth weight infants. *Cochrane Database Syst Rev.* 2008;2008(1):CD006181. PubMed doi: 10.1002/14651858.CD006181.pub2

28. Cassady G, Crouse DT, Kirklin JW, et al. A randomized, controlled trial of very early prophylactic ligation of the ductus arteriosus in babies who weighed 1000 g or less at birth. *N Engl J Med.* 1989;320(23):1511–1516. PubMed doi: 10.1056/NEJM198906083202302

29. Oxford Centre for Evidence-based Medicine—Levels of Evidence. 2009. Accessed June 9, 2023. https://www.cebm.ox.ac.uk/resources/levels-of-evidence/oxford-centre-for-evidence-based-medicine-levels-of-evidence-march-2009

30. Ohlsson A, Walia R, Shah SS. Ibuprofen for the treatment of patent ductus arteriosus in preterm or low birth weight (or both) infants. *Cochrane Database Syst Rev.* 2020;2(2):CD003481. PubMed doi: 10.1002/14651858.CD003481.pub8

31. Mitra S, Florez ID, Tamayo ME, et al. Association of Placebo, Indomethacin, Ibuprofen, and Acetaminophen With Closure of Hemodynamically Significant Patent Ductus Arteriosus in Preterm Infants: A Systematic Review and Meta-analysis. *JAMA.* 2018;319(12):1221–1238. PubMed doi: 10.1001/jama.2018.1896

32. Dani C, Vangi V, Bertini G, et al. High-dose ibuprofen for patent ductus arteriosus in extremely preterm infants: a randomized controlled study. *Clin Pharmacol Ther.* 2012;91(4):590–596. PubMed doi: 10.1038/clpt.2011.284

33. Mitra S, Scrivens A, von Kursell AM, Disher T. Early treatment versus expectant management of hemodynamically significant patent ductus arteriosus for preterm infants. *Cochrane Database Syst Rev.* 2020;12(12):CD013278. PubMed doi: 10.1002/14651858.CD013278.pub2

34. Olgun H, Ceviz N, Kartal İ, et al. Repeated Courses of Oral Ibuprofen in Premature Infants with Patent Ductus Arteriosus: Efficacy and Safety. *Pediatr Neonatol.* 2017;58(1):29–35. PubMed doi: 10.1016/j.pedneo.2015.04.017

35. Richards J, Johnson A, Fox G, Campbell M. A second course of ibuprofen is effective in the closure of a clinically significant PDA in ELBW infants. *Pediatrics.* 2009;124(2):e287–e293. PubMed doi: 10.1542/peds.2008-2232

36. Shah SD, Makker K, Zhang M, Harnett S, Aziz KB, Hudak ML. Dual medication therapy (acetaminophen and ibuprofen) for the management of patent ductus arteriosus in preterm infants: a systematic review and meta-analysis. *J Perinatol.* 2022;42(12):1654–1661. PubMed doi: 10.1038/s41372-022-01500-8

37. Wright CJ, McCulley DJ, Mitra S, Jensen EA. Acetaminophen for the patent ductus arteriosus: has safety been adequately demonstrated? *J Perinatol.* 2023;43(10):1230–1237. PubMed doi: 10.1038/s41372-023-01697-2

38. Chen X, Han D, Wang X, et al. Vascular and pulmonary effects of ibuprofen on neonatal lung development. *Respir Res.* 2023;24(1):39. PubMed doi: 10.1186/s12931-023-02342-4

39. Dobrinskikh E, Sherlock LG, Orlicky DJ, et al. The developing murine lung is susceptible to acetaminophen toxicity. *Am J Physiol Lung Cell Mol Physiol.* 2021;320(5):L969–L978. PubMed doi: 10.1152/ajplung.00072.2021

40. Chen X, Qiu X, Sun P, et al. Neonatal ibuprofen exposure and bronchopulmonary dysplasia in extremely premature infants. *J Perinatol.* 2020;40(1):124–129. PubMed doi: 10.1038/s41372-019-0444-4

41. Gentle SJ, Travers CP, Clark M, Carlo WA, Ambalavanan N. Patent Ductus Arteriosus and Development of Bronchopulmonary Dysplasia-associated Pulmonary Hypertension. *Am J Respir Crit Care Med.* 2023;207(7):921–928. PubMed doi: 10.1164/rccm.202203-0570OC

42. Ji Y, Azuine RE, Zhang Y, et al. Association of Cord Plasma Biomarkers of In Utero Acetaminophen Exposure With Risk of Attention-Deficit/Hyperactivity Disorder and Autism Spectrum Disorder in Childhood. *JAMA Psychiatry.* 2020;77(2):180–189. PubMed doi: 10.1001/jamapsychiatry.2019.3259

43. Alemany S, Avella-García C, Liew Z, et al. Prenatal and postnatal exposure to acetaminophen in relation to autism spectrum and attention-deficit and hyperactivity symptoms in childhood: Meta-analysis in six European population-based cohorts. *Eur J Epidemiol.* 2021;36(10):993–1004. PubMed doi: 10.1007/s10654-021-00754-4

44. Srajer A, Roychoudhury S, Tang S, et al. Postnatal acetaminophen exposure and neurodevelopmental outcomes at 18–21 months corrected gestational age in preterm infants <29 weeks gestation: a retrospective cohort study. *Pediatr Res.* 2024;96(2):388–394. PubMed doi: 10.1038/s41390-023-02901-x

45. Giesinger RE, Rios DR, Chatmethakul T, et al. Impact of Early Hemodynamic Screening on Extremely Preterm Outcomes in a High-Performance Center. *Am J Respir Crit Care Med.* 2023;208(3):290–300. PubMed doi: 10.1164/rccm.202212-2291OC

46. Chock VY, Punn R, Oza A, et al. Predictors of bronchopulmonary dysplasia or death in premature infants with a patent ductus arteriosus. *Pediatr Res.* 2014;75(4):570–575. PubMed doi: 10.1038/pr.2013.253

47. Mirea L, Sankaran K, Seshia M, et al; Canadian Neonatal Network. Treatment of patent ductus arteriosus and neonatal mortality/morbidities: adjustment for treatment selection bias. *J Pediatr.* 2012;161(4):689–94.e1. PubMed doi: 10.1016/j.jpeds.2012.05.007

48. Janz-Robinson EM, Badawi N, Walker K, Bajuk B, Abdel-Latif ME, Neonatal Intensive Care Units N; Neonatal Intensive Care Units Network. Neurodevelopmental Outcomes of Premature Infants Treated for Patent Ductus Arteriosus: A Population-Based Cohort Study. *J Pediatr.* 2015;167(5):1025–32.e3. PubMed doi: 10.1016/j.jpeds.2015.06.054

49. Hagadorn JI, Bennett MV, Brownell EA, Payton KSE, Benitz WE, Lee HC. Covariation of Neonatal Intensive Care Unit-Level Patent Ductus Arteriosus Management and In-Neonatal Intensive Care Unit Outcomes Following Preterm Birth. *J Pediatr.* 2018;203: 225–233.e1. PubMed doi: 10.1016/j.jpeds.2018.07.025

50. Hagadorn JI, Shaffer ML, Tolia VN, Greenberg RG. Covariation of changing patent ductus arteriosus management and preterm infant outcomes in Pediatrix neonatal intensive care units. *J Perinatol.* 2021;41(10):2526–2531. PubMed doi: 10.1038/s41372-021-01170-y

51. Hundscheid T, Jansen EJS, Onland W, Kooi EMW, Andriessen P, de Boode WP. Conservative Management of Patent Ductus Arteriosus in Preterm Infants-A Systematic Review and Meta-Analyses Assessing Differences in Outcome Measures Between Randomized Controlled Trials and Cohort Studies. *Front Pediatr.* 2021;9:626261. PubMed doi: 10.3389/fped.2021.626261

52. Hundscheid T, Onland W, Kooi EMW, et al; BeNeDuctus Trial Investigators. Expectant Management or Early Ibuprofen for Patent Ductus Arteriosus. *N Engl J Med.* 2023;388(11):980–990. PubMed doi: 10.1056/NEJMoa2207418

53. Gupta S, Subhedar NV, Bell JL, et al; Baby-OSCAR Collaborative Group. Trial of Selective Early Treatment of Patent Ductus Arteriosus with Ibuprofen. *N Engl J Med.* 2024;390(4):314–325. PubMed doi: 10.1056/NEJMoa2305582

54. Palder SB, Schwartz MZ, Tyson KR, Marr CC. Management of patent ductus arteriosus: a comparison of operative v pharmacologic treatment. *J Pediatr Surg.* 1987;22(12):1171–1174. PubMed doi: 10.1016/S0022-3468(87)80730-3

55. Alexander F, Chiu L, Kroh M, Hammel J, Moore J. Analysis of outcome in 298 extremely low-birth-weight infants with patent ductus arteriosus. *J Pediatr Surg.* 2009;44(1):112–117; disscusion 117. PubMed doi: 10.1016/j.jpedsurg.2008.10.019

56. Malviya MN, Ohlsson A, Shah SS. Surgical versus medical treatment with cyclooxygenase inhibitors for symptomatic patent ductus arteriosus in preterm infants. *Cochrane Database Syst Rev.* 2013;2013(3):CD003951. PubMed doi: 10.1002/14651858.CD003951.pub3

57. Gersony WM, Peckham GJ, Ellison RC, Miettinen OS, Nadas AS. Effects of indomethacin in premature infants with patent ductus arteriosus: results of a national collaborative study. *J Pediatr.* 1983;102(6):895–906. PubMed doi: 10.1016/S0022-3476(83)80022-5

58. Teixeira LS, Shivananda SP, Stephens D, Van Arsdell G, McNamara PJ. Postoperative cardiorespiratory instability following ligation of the preterm ductus arteriosus is related to early need for intervention. *J Perinatol.* 2008;28(12):803–810. PubMed doi: 10.1038/jp.2008.101

59. Teixeira LS, McNamara PJ. Enhanced intensive care for the neonatal ductus arteriosus. *Acta Paediatr.* 2006;95(4):394–403. PubMed doi: 10.1111/j.1651-2227.2006.tb02251.x

60. Warnock A, Szatkowski L, Lakshmanan A, Lee L, Kelsall W. Surgical management of patent ductus arteriosus in pre-term infants - a british paediatric surveillance study. *BMC Pediatr.* 2021;21(1):270. PubMed doi: 10.1186/s12887-021-02734-9

61. Engeseth MS, Olsen NR, Maeland S, Halvorsen T, Goode A, Røksund OD. Left vocal cord paralysis after patent ductus arteriosus ligation: A systematic review. *Paediatr Respir Rev.* 2018;27:74–85. PubMed doi: 10.1016/j.prrv.2017.11.001

62. Orb Q, Dunya G, Padia R, et al. Long-term Outcomes of Vocal Fold Paralysis Following Patent Ductus Arteriosus Ligation in Neonates. *Laryngoscope.* 2023;133(5):1257–1261. PubMed doi: 10.1002/lary.30343

63. Hsu KH, Chiang MC, Lien R, et al. Diaphragmatic paralysis among very low birth weight infants following ligation for patent ductus arteriosus. *Eur J Pediatr.* 2012;171(11):1639–1644. PubMed doi: 10.1007/s00431-012-1787-4

64. Mandhan P, Brown S, Kukkady A, Samarakkody U. Surgical closure of patent ductus arteriosus in preterm low birth weight infants. *Congenit Heart Dis.* 2009;4(1):34–37. PubMed doi: 10.1111/j.1747-0803.2008.00241.x

65. Seghaye MC, Grabitz R, Alzen G, et al. Thoracic sequelae after surgical closure of the patent ductus arteriosus in premature infants. *Acta Paediatr.* 1997;86(2):213–216. PubMed doi: 10.1111/j.1651-2227.1997.tb08871.x

66. Clyman R, Cassady G, Kirklin JK, Collins M, Philips JB III. The role of patent ductus arteriosus ligation in bronchopulmonary dysplasia: reexamining a randomized controlled trial. *J Pediatr.* 2009; 154(6):873–876. PubMed doi: 10.1016/j.jpeds.2009.01.005

67. Kabra NS, Schmidt B, Roberts RS, Doyle LW, Papile L, Fanaroff A, et al. Neurosensory impairment after surgical closure of patent ductus arteriosus in extremely low birth weight infants: results from the Trial of Indomethacin Prophylaxis in Preterms. *J Pediatr.* 2007;150(3):229–234, 234 e221. PubMed doi: 10.1016/j.jpeds.2006.11.039

68. Wickremasinghe AC, Rogers EE, Piecuch RE, et al. Neurodevelopmental outcomes following two different treatment approaches (early ligation and selective ligation) for patent ductus arteriosus. *J Pediatr.* 2012;161(6):1065–1072. PubMed doi: 10.1016/j.jpeds.2012.05.062

69. Bourgoin L, Cipierre C, Hauet Q, et al. Neurodevelopmental Outcome at 2 Years of Age according to Patent Ductus Arteriosus Management in Very Preterm Infants. *Neonatology.* 2016;109(2):139–146. PubMed doi: 10.1159/000442278

70. Bixler GM, Powers GC, Clark RH, Walker MW, Tolia VN. Changes in the Diagnosis and Management of Patent Ductus Arteriosus from 2006 to 2015 in United States Neonatal Intensive Care Units. *J Pediatr.* 2017;189:105–112. PubMed doi: 10.1016/j.jpeds.2017.05.024

71. Shah ZS, Clark RH, Patt HA, Backes CH Jr, Tolia VN. Trends in Procedural Closure of the Patent Ductus Arteriosus among

Infants Born at 22 to 30 Weeks' Gestation. *J Pediatr.* 2023;263: 113716. PubMed doi: 10.1016/j.jpeds.2023.113716

72. Porstmann W, Wierny L, Warnke H, Gerstberger G, Romaniuk PA. Catheter closure of patent ductus arteriosus. 62 cases treated without thoracotomy. *Radiol Clin North Am.* 1971;9(2):203–218. PubMed doi: 10.1016/S0033-8389(22)01768-7
73. Backes CH, Rivera BK, Bridge JA, et al. Percutaneous Patent Ductus Arteriosus (PDA) Closure During Infancy: A Meta-analysis. *Pediatrics.* 2017;139(2):e20162927. PubMed doi: 10.1542/peds.2016-2927
74. Backes CH, Kennedy KF, Locke M, et al. Transcatheter Occlusion of the Patent Ductus Arteriosus in 747 Infants <6 kg: Insights From the NCDR IMPACT Registry. *JACC Cardiovasc Interv.* 2017;10(17): 1729–1737. PubMed doi: 10.1016/j.jcin.2017.05.018
75. Bischoff AR, Jasani B, Sathanandam SK, Backes C, Weisz DE, McNamara PJ. Percutaneous Closure of Patent Ductus Arteriosus in Infants 1.5 kg or Less: A Meta-Analysis. *J Pediatr.* 2021;230: 84–92.e14. PubMed doi: 10.1016/j.jpeds.2020.10.035
76. Backes CH, Hill KD, Shelton EL, et al. Patent Ductus Arteriosus: A Contemporary Perspective for the Pediatric and Adult Cardiac Care Provider. *J Am Heart Assoc.* 2022;11(17):e025784. PubMed doi: 10.1161/JAHA.122.025784
77. Zahn EM, Nevin P, Simmons C, Garg R. A novel technique for transcatheter patent ductus arteriosus closure in extremely preterm infants using commercially available technology. *Catheter Cardiovasc Interv.* 2015;85(2):240–248. PubMed doi: 10.1002/ccd.25534
78. Zahn EM, Peck D, Phillips A, et al. Transcatheter Closure of Patent Ductus Arteriosus in Extremely Premature Newborns: Early Results and Midterm Follow-Up. *JACC Cardiovasc Interv.* 2016; 9(23):2429–2437. PubMed doi: 10.1016/j.jcin.2016.09.019
79. Sathanandam SK, Gutfinger D, O'Brien L, et al. Amplatzer Piccolo Occluder clinical trial for percutaneous closure of the patent ductus arteriosus in patients ≥700 grams. *Catheter Cardiovasc Interv.* 2020;96(6):1266–1276. PubMed doi: 10.1002/ccd.28973
80. Morray BH, Sathanandam SK, Forbes T, et al. 3-year follow-up of a prospective, multicenter study of the Amplatzer Piccolo™ Occluder for transcatheter patent ductus arteriosus closure in children ≥ 700 grams. *J Perinatol.* 2023;43(10):1238–1244. PubMed doi: 10.1038/s41372-023-01741-1
81. Bischoff AR, Kennedy KF, Backes CH, Sathanandam S, McNamara PJ. Percutaneous Closure of the Patent Ductus Arteriosus in Infants ≤2 kg: IMPACT Registry Insights. *Pediatrics.* 2023;152(3): e2023061460. PubMed doi: 10.1542/peds.2023-061460
82. Barry OM, Gudausky TM, Balzer DT, et al. Safety and Short-Term Outcomes for Infants < 2.5 kg Undergoing PDA Device Closure: A C3PO Registry Study. *Pediatr Cardiol.* 2023;44(6):1406–1413. PubMed doi: 10.1007/s00246-023-03147-4
83. Rodríguez Ogando A, Planelles Asensio I, de la Blanca ARS, et al. Surgical Ligation Versus Percutaneous Closure of Patent Ductus Arteriosus in Very Low-Weight Preterm Infants: Which are the Real Benefits of the Percutaneous Approach? *Pediatr Cardiol.* 2018; 39(2):398–410. PubMed doi: 10.1007/s00246-017-1768-5
84. Kim HS, Schechter MA, Manning PB, et al. Surgical Versus Percutaneous Closure of PDA in Preterm Infants: Procedural Charges and Outcomes. *J Surg Res.* 2019;243:41–46. PubMed doi: 10.1016/j.jss.2019.04.069
85. Regan W, Benbrik N, Sharma SR, et al. Improved ventilation in premature babies after transcatheter versus surgical closure of patent ductus arteriosus. *Int J Cardiol.* 2020;311:22–27. PubMed doi: 10.1016/j.ijcard.2020.03.040
86. Kuntz MT, Staffa SJ, Graham D, et al. Trend and Outcomes for Surgical Versus Transcatheter Patent Ductus Arteriosus Closure in Neonates and Infants at US Children's Hospitals. *J Am Heart Assoc.* 2022;11(1):e022776. PubMed doi: 10.1161/JAHA.121.022776
87. Smith A, McNamara PJ, El-Khuffash AF. Non-pharmacological management of a hemodynamically significant patent ductus arteriosus. *Semin Fetal Neonatal Med.* 2018;23(4):245–249. PubMed doi: 10.1016/j.siny.2018.03.008
88. Bell EF, Acarregui MJ. Restricted versus liberal water intake for preventing morbidity and mortality in preterm infants. *Cochrane Database Syst Rev.* 2014;2014(12):CD000503. PubMed doi: 10.1002/14651858.CD000503.pub3
89. Hansson L, Lind T, Wiklund U, Öhlund I, Rydberg A. Fluid restriction negatively affects energy intake and growth in very low birthweight infants with haemodynamically significant patent ductus arteriosus. *Acta Paediatr.* 2019;108(11):1985–1992. PubMed doi: 10.1111/apa.14815
90. De Buyst J, Rakza T, Pennaforte T, Johansson AB, Storme L. Hemodynamic effects of fluid restriction in preterm infants with significant patent ductus arteriosus. *J Pediatr.* 2012;161(3): 404–408. PubMed doi: 10.1016/j.jpeds.2012.03.012
91. Miyanoshita A, Terada M, Endou H. Furosemide directly stimulates prostaglandin E2 production in the thick ascending limb of Henle's loop. *J Pharmacol Exp Ther.* 1989;251(3):1155–1159. PubMed doi: 10.1016/S0022-3565(25)21067-9
92. Toyoshima K, Momma K, Nakanishi T. In vivo dilatation of the ductus arteriosus induced by furosemide in the rat. *Pediatr Res.* 2010; 67(2):173–176. PubMed doi: 10.1203/PDR.0b013e3181c2df30
93. Green TP, Johnson DE, Bass JL, Landrum BG, Ferrara TB, Thompson TR. Prophylactic furosemide in severe respiratory distress syndrome: blinded prospective study. *J Pediatr.* 1988;112(4): 605–612. PubMed doi: 10.1016/S0022-3476(88)80182-3
94. Dudley S, Sen S, Hanson A, El Khuffash A, Levy PT. The role of furosemide and fluid management for a hemodynamically significant patent ductus arteriosus in premature infants. *J Perinatol.* 2022; 42(12):1703–1707. PubMed doi: 10.1038/s41372-022-01450-1
95. Sridharan K, Al Madhoob A, Al Jufairi M, Al Ansari E, Al Marzooq R. Intravenous frusemide does not interact pharmacodynamically with acetaminophen in critically ill preterm neonates with patent ductus arteriosus. *Eur Rev Med Pharmacol Sci.* 2021;25(3):1612–1615. PubMed doi: 10.26355/eurrev_202102_24871
96. Thompson EJ, Greenberg RG, Kumar K, et al. Association between Furosemide Exposure and Patent Ductus Arteriosus in Hospitalized Infants of Very Low Birth Weight. *J Pediatr.* 2018;199: 231–236. PubMed doi: 10.1016/j.jpeds.2018.03.067

Pediatric Acute-Onset Neuropsychiatric Syndrome (PANS)

- *Clinical Report*

CLINICAL REPORT Guidance for the Clinician in Rendering Pediatric Care

American Academy of Pediatrics

DEDICATED TO THE HEALTH OF ALL CHILDREN™

Pediatric Acute-Onset Neuropsychiatric Syndrome (PANS): Clinical Report

Board of Directors

INTRODUCTION AND BACKGROUND

The sudden onset of severe behavioral and neuropsychiatric symptoms in children is a frightening and potentially life-changing situation. The pediatric health care providers and clinicians to whom families turn need guidance on how to accurately diagnose and treat new-onset neuropsychiatric symptoms in children. They need expert guidance about whether these symptoms indicate a diagnosis compatible with pediatric acute-onset neuropsychiatric syndrome (PANS). The cause of PANS is unknown, but it is theorized to be triggered, in some cases, by a recent infection and/or autoimmunity issues (similar to Sydenham chorea, autoimmune encephalitis [AE], and Guillain-Barré syndrome). The condition is challenging from a clinical perspective, because it lacks disease-specific biomarkers, strong evidence for pathogenic causes, and consensus on treatment of clinical symptoms. Further, the evidence base for PANS encompasses multiple subspecialties, including child and adolescent psychiatry, pediatric rheumatology, pediatric neurology, pediatric infectious diseases, pediatric immunology, and developmental-behavioral pediatrics.

Given this complexity, there is a clear need for guidance and advice for pediatric clinicians and the families they serve and support. To that end, with the encouragement of the Board of Directors, the American Academy of Pediatrics (AAP) has developed this clinical report. It focuses primarily on PANS, an umbrella condition that encompasses pediatric autoimmune neuropsychiatric disorders associated with streptococcal infections (PANDAS). Although PANDAS is, by definition, associated with streptococcal infection,[1] it is now considered by many to represent a subset of the larger spectrum of infection-induced acute-onset neuropsychiatric symptoms.[2,3] This clinical report was developed after a comprehensive literature review and analysis of the findings. Because they are limited by the present level of evidence on the topic, the findings are presented as a report rather than a clinical practice guideline. The contents are intended to aid the pediatric health care provider in evaluating, diagnosing, and treating sudden-onset and severe behavioral changes in children that

Address correspondence to: president@aap.org.

CONFLICT OF INTEREST DISCLOSURES: The authors have indicated they have no potential conflicts of interest to disclose.

FUNDING: No external funding.

https://doi.org/10.1542/peds.2024-070334

To cite: American Academy of Pediatrics, Board of Directors. Pediatric Acute-Onset Neuropsychiatric Syndrome (PANS): Clinical Report. *Pediatrics.* 2025;155(3):e2024070334

could indicate potential PANS and in supporting these children and their families.

Expert Panel Process

The AAP leadership formed an expert panel of experienced clinicians to provide their perspectives and guide the development of this clinical report. The expert panel members were recruited from relevant subspecialty areas (eg, rheumatology, neurology, child and adolescent psychiatry, infectious diseases, developmental-behavioral pediatrics, and primary care) and focused on the existing evidence basis associated with PANS. The panel met 3 times to discuss relevant questions and reach consensus on diagnosis, treatment, research needs, and other key issues. These discussions were facilitated by senior leaders of the AAP. To support the expert panel's deliberations, the AAP commissioned an external evidence review of pertinent literature on PANS/PANDAS to gather the comprehensive base of published research. The comprehensive review of the literature was performed in March–April 2020 and included literature in PubMed, the Cumulative Index to Nursing and Allied Health Literature (CINAHL), and PsychInfo databases. The expert panel members also provided additional references for consideration throughout the process. A subsequent review of more recent literature was conducted in June 2023, and new information integrated into the document. The final document was reviewed by expert panel members along with other members with expertise in immunology, mental health, and emergency medicine. It was reviewed and approved by the AAP Board of Directors.

Summary

The AAP recognizes that PANS is likely a valid diagnosis, although the diagnostic process is challenged by a lack of well-accepted evidence to guide the clinician. Much remains unknown about the condition, however. This clinical report explicitly acknowledges the pressing need for research and enrollment of patients in multicenter studies to explore the potential etiology, epidemiology, evaluation, and treatment for PANS. The AAP is committed to working collegially with other physicians and scientists to learn more about this condition and develop a dependable and clear evidence base that supports evaluation, diagnosis, and treatment to address a specific child's symptoms. Until that goal has been reached, the AAP recommends a deliberate and cautious approach, grounded in evidence, and focused on helping children who have the symptoms of possible PANS. The AAP further recommends that the best care for children with potential or diagnosed PANS is provided in a medical home, is family centered, and is delivered by a multidisciplinary team.

SYMPTOMS AND ETIOLOGY

Pediatric Acute-Onset Neuropsychiatric Syndrome (PANS)

PANS is a condition that involves a constellation of psychiatric and neurologic symptoms that present simultaneously and in rapid onset, the cause or causes of which are unknown. Although the cause is still under investigation, the manifestations may follow a recent infection. The acute onset of symptoms can appear similar to both infectious and noninfectious conditions that may have classic features of sudden onset neuropsychiatric symptoms. Although other neuropsychiatric conditions have been associated with infection (Sydenham chorea is a classic example of this paradigm), there are additional noninfectious autoimmune etiologies for acute neuropsychiatric symptoms, such as anti-NMDAR (N-methyl-D-aspartate receptor) autoimmune encephalitis (AE).

PANS was first described as a diagnostic entity in 2012, more than a decade after the description of PANDAS, in order to expand the characterization and broaden the scope of pediatric neuropsychiatric disorders. Although group A beta-hemolytic streptococcal (GAS) infection is a hallmark of PANDAS' description, PANS encompasses other potential instigator events.[4] PANS has the following criteria[5]:

- Unusually abrupt and dramatic onset of obsessive compulsive disorder (OCD) or severely restricted food intake;
- Concurrent, abrupt onset of additional severe neuropsychiatric symptoms from at least 2 of the following 7 categories:
  1. Anxiety;
  2. Emotional lability and/or depression;
  3. Irritability, aggression, and/or severe oppositional behaviors;
  4. Developmental regression;
  5. Deterioration in school performance;
  6. Sensory or motor abnormalities including heightened sensitivity to sensory stimuli, hallucinations, dysgraphia, and complex motor and/or vocal tics; and
  7. Somatic signs and symptoms, including sleep disturbances, enuresis, or urinary frequency that are not better explained by a known neurologic or medical disorder.[2,3]

Again, it is important to note that the most distinctive characteristic of both PANS and PANDAS is the dramatic acuity of onset and short time to peak severity of the cardinal symptom(s) of OCD, tics, or food restriction.

The factors that trigger PANS symptoms are postulated to be multimodal and include psychological trauma, genetic predisposition, and postinfectious autoimmune causes.[6,7] The OCD, tics, and other neuropsychiatric symptoms seen in these patients are theorized to sometimes result from postinfection autoimmunity, similar to Sydenham chorea.[2,8] Infections that have been suggested as triggers of PANS-like symptoms include group A *Streptococcus*, *Mycoplasma pneumoniae*, influenza, and sinusitis.[6] Not all cases of PANS are reported to be triggered by an infection, however, and no single microbe has been associated with the onset of PANS.[9]

As noted, PANS is an umbrella term that subsumes PANDAS. PANDAS' 5 diagnostic criteria include presence of OCD and/or tic disorder; prepubertal onset of symptoms; episodic course characterized by acute, severe onset and dramatic symptom exacerbations; temporal relationship between GAS infection, symptom onset, and exacerbations; and association with neurologic abnormalities (eg, choreiform movements, motor hyperactivity, tics).[1,9] The hypothesis for PANDAS' pathophysiology is that GAS infection in a susceptible host incites the production of antibodies to group A *Streptococcus*, which cross-react with antigens in the basal ganglia, particularly in the caudate nucleus and putamen, through molecular mimicry. This relationship remains unproven based on current evidence.

Historically, research has described this condition as "PANDAS," without differentiating between PANDAS and the more recently defined PANS. Although much of the evidence specifies PANDAS, the findings have relevance to understanding the possible etiology in both that condition and PANS. A 2020 review of articles from 1977 onward noted that children in whom PANDAS was diagnosed had some evidence of alterations within the structures of the central nervous system (CNS), including caudate, putamen, globus pallidus, and striatum. Additionally, autoantibodies that interact with basal ganglia were observed in some patients with PANDAS.[10]

Researchers have used animal models to test for the plausibility of GAS infection causing immunologic abnormalities in the brain, as summarized by Wald.[4] Brimberg and colleagues demonstrated that autoimmune-prone strains of rats immunized with GAS antigen exhibited motor symptoms and compulsive behaviors (grooming, marble-burying) that are similar to those seen in Sydenham chorea and PANDAS and were alleviated by haloperidol and selective serotonin reuptake inhibitors (SSRIs).[11] Examination of the brains of those rats showed autoantibodies deposited in the striatum, thalamus, and frontal cortex. When immunoglobulin G (IgG) was infused from these GAS-exposed rats into naïve rats, the latter demonstrated similar behavioral and motor problems and had IgG deposits in the striatum of their brains.[12] Further evidence comes from a 2018 experiment of Frick and colleagues in which sera from patients with well-characterized PANDAS were infused into the striatum of mice; antibodies from these children were found to be bound to 80% of cholinergic interneurons (which have been implicated in the pathogenesis of tic disorders).[13] After the patients were treated with immune globulin intravenous (IGIV) and their symptoms improved, their sera no longer contained antibodies that had elevated binding to cholinergic interneurons in the mice. Conflicting evidence also exists. Loiselle and colleagues found that sera from patients with PANDAS and Tourette syndrome infused into striata in rats did not induce behavioral changes.[14] Further, Gilbert and colleagues point out that attempts to identify definite autoantibodies in PANDAS have yielded inconsistent results and that there is no association between symptom exacerbations and changes in levels of antineuronal antibodies in patients with PANDAS.[15,16]

The risk factors, diagnostic biomarkers, and biological mechanisms are not clearly established, creating challenges in making a definite diagnosis. The lack of longitudinal high-quality research, consistent diagnostic criteria, and a national database hamper a precise estimation of the prevalence and incidence of PANS.

PANS and Autoimmune Encephalitis

PANS and AE are not the same. The 2 conditions have different diagnostic criteria, treatment recommendations, and testing and diagnostic workups. Children with AE present with acute or subacute (usually less than 3 months) onset of neuropsychiatric symptoms attributable to an underlying abnormal immune response of the CNS.[17] These patients also present with seizures, complex movement disorders, and/or focal neurologic signs on examination. The diagnostic criteria for pediatric seronegative AE require evidence of inflammation within the CNS (ie, by examination of the cerebrospinal fluid or magnetic resonance imaging [MRI]). When a pathogenic antibody (such as NMDAR antibody) is identified in the serum and/or cerebrospinal fluid, patients are described to have seropositive AE, whereas the absence of such an antibody is described as seronegative AE. AE symptoms also persist over time, which differs from the relapsing-remitting course observed with PANS.[17] The vast majority of children with AE demonstrate some degree of cognitive impairment, whereas most children with PANS demonstrate normal cognition on formal testing.[17]

DIAGNOSIS AND RECOMMENDED WORKUP

The diagnosis and workup of PANS/PANDAS is complicated by several issues:

1. There is a lack of clarity about the potential causes of PANS and a broad array of possible causes to be considered.
2. There is no listing of PANS in the *Diagnostic and Statistical Manual of Mental Disorders, Fifth Edition (DSM-V)*, which provides diagnostic criteria for recognized mental health conditions, or the *International Classification of Diseases, 11th Revision (ICD-11)* coding system, which is the global standard for recording health information.

3. PANS is characterized as being a "diagnosis of exclusion," which requires the clinician to rule out many other diseases that may explain the acute onset of symptoms before a diagnosis of PANS can be assigned to the patient.[7,9]
4. The average child experiences multiple infections a year, including a high prevalence of streptococcal infections.
5. Pediatric anxiety and tic disorders occur frequently.

Thus, the patient may face an extensive workup before a diagnosis is made, often based on uncertain causes and without any guidance from widely recognized systems like the *DSM-V* and *ICD-11*. Therefore, it is critical to conduct a thorough patient and family history, physical and psychiatric examination, and a phased laboratory and imaging workup.

When a child presents with one or more of the symptoms that make up the criteria for PANS, it is also critical to remember the ages at which primary psychiatric syndromes tend to first present in the context of normal pediatric development. Anxiety disorders occur in 7.1% of children 3 to 17 years of age,[18] and transient tics may occur in as many as 20% of school-aged children.[19] OCD—a key criterion of PANS—occurs in 1% to 3% of all children and adolescents, although less commonly in younger children compared with adolescents.[20,21] In contrast, disease-related OCD, such as with PANS, occurs more frequently in prepubertal children—an age group with much lower rates of OCD in isolation. Regardless of the child's age, anxiety, tics, and OCD are more likely to be a primary psychiatric disorder that is unrelated to PANS. This consideration will aid pediatric health care clinicians in differentiating PANS from other mental health conditions.

Patient Medical/Psychiatric History and Physical Examination

When assessing a child for potential PANS, pediatric health care providers are encouraged to initially discuss a broad but individually tailored differential diagnosis—including acute-onset OCD or other anxiety disorders, tic disorder, Tourette syndrome, Sydenham chorea, or AE. A complete medical history and review of symptom longevity are required to assess these potential diagnoses.

Patient History and Examination

The patient's medical history and physical examination should address the signs and symptoms characteristic of PANS—including whether they occurred abruptly or over time as well as their duration, severity level, and impact on normal life functioning.[9] This symptomatology is the most important part of the history. The history and examination should assess for signs and symptoms of disorders that must be excluded, including Sydenham chorea, Tourette syndrome, AE, and anorexia nervosa. Although nearly all children with PANS have OCD, the presence of OCD alone should not lead to a PANS workup unless the onset is extremely abrupt. Because children with Tourette syndrome (which is estimated to occur in 0.3% to 0.6% of school-aged children)[18] may have tics in combination with OCD and attention-deficit/hyperactivity disorder (ADHD), they could be confused with children with PANS. The sudden onset of symptoms distinguishes children with PANS from those with Tourette syndrome.

The patient history should thoroughly assess previous mental health problems, because patients with preexisting mental health challenges may have symptoms related to that condition rather than to a new, acute-onset syndrome such as PANS and because patients with PANS frequently have mental health comorbidities including anxiety, ADHD, and autism spectrum disorder. These comorbidities include previous OCD or anxiety (especially separation anxiety), mood disorders, psychological trauma, tic disorders, ADHD, oppositional defiant disorder, and learning issues in school. History of symptomatic pharyngitis (not just asymptomatic carrier status for GAS infection) and other upper respiratory infections should be noted, along with treatment with antibiotics for episodes of symptomatic GAS infections. A review of primary health care and school records is often helpful and may disclose prior neurodevelopmental or neuropsychiatric evaluations and issues that family members might not recognize as being relevant to the current history.

Neurologic Examination

Most children with PANS have a normal neurologic examination except for the presence of tics, inattention, or choreiform finger movements (eg, fine piano-playing movements when the child has arms and hands extended and eyes closed). These choreiform finger movements should be differentiated from more generalized chorea, defined as random-appearing, continuous, involuntary movements (while awake) that can affect the entire body and often include the face and tongue. If present, chorea should prompt the clinician to evaluate the child for Sydenham chorea and AE.[9] Choreiform movements of the hands are often considered "overflow" movements and may be observed in typically developing children who do not have PANS. These movements seem to be a sign of cortical immaturity of systems involved with automatic inhibition, tend to decrease as the child matures, and are reported to be observed more often in children who have learning disorders.[22]

Children with PANS usually have normal cognition, although school performance may deteriorate because of inattentiveness, anxiety, OCD, and/or perfectionism. Assessing the child's actual cognitive abilities includes both a detailed history and neuropsychological examination to identify any specific deficits; this assessment may lead to formal neurocognitive testing if deficits are suspected. More significant cognitive or memory impairment suggests the possibility of AE or other brain disorders.[9]

Psychiatric/Psychological Assessment

A comprehensive evaluation by an experienced child and adolescent psychiatrist or psychologist is necessary to eliminate other disorders that present with similar neuropsychiatric syndromes.[7] If psychiatric evaluation is not available, then assessment by the primary care pediatrician should, at a minimum, focus on the psychiatric and behavioral symptoms seen in PANS.

Family History

The family history may be contributory but is not conclusive either in supporting the diagnosis of PANS or suggesting the presence of other diagnoses. First-degree relatives of patients with PANS have been reported to have increased rates of OCD, tics, acute rheumatic fever, and maternal autoimmune disorders.[9] It is not known whether these conditions suggest a genetic cause of PANS or whether families with these symptoms are more likely to recognize PANS symptoms in their children.

Laboratory and Imaging Workup: A Phased Approach

Extensive workups and testing are not necessary in most cases of suspected PANS. A phased workup is recommended with stop points to mitigate the risk of the child (and family) having to endure an unnecessary major diagnostic odyssey.

Initial Workup

Because it is theorized that *Streptococcus pyogenes* infection or colonization, in conjunction with other factors, may be a trigger for PANS, some have proposed that testing all children with new onset abrupt neuropsychiatric symptoms consistent with PANS undergo a diagnostic test for *S pyogenes* (ie, throat culture, throat swab for *S pyogenes* polymerase chain reaction [PCR] or antigen tests) at the time of the diagnosis. Current recommendations are to perform this test only for children who otherwise are recommended to undergo streptococcal diagnostic tests (those with pharyngitis consistent with streptococcal infection). The only study to address this question is a case series of children at a single site who presented with both new onset abrupt neuropsychiatric symptoms consistent with PANS and some degree of pharyngeal symptoms consistent with GAS pharyngitis. The 12 children who tested positive for GAS were treated with oral antibiotics recommended for symptomatic GAS pharyngitis and were reported to have significant improvement in neuropsychiatric symptoms. Given that these are the only data in support of routinely testing for and treating children found to harbor GAS organisms, since the study had a small sample size, had a select population, included children with pharyngeal findings, and provided no control group for comparison or longer term follow-up, the AAP does not believe the data are strong enough to support universal testing of all cases of acute onset neuropsychiatric symptoms consistent with PANS. The AAP recognizes that there are theoretical analogies between PANS triggered by GAS infection and acute rheumatic fever (ARF) manifested as Sydenham chorea, but without additional empiric evidence of benefit and recognizing the potential for harm, the AAP does not endorse universal GAS testing and subsequent antibiotic treatment of children who are positive. For children who otherwise meet criteria for testing for GAS infection because of signs and symptoms consistent with current recommendations for whom to test, the AAP recommends testing and appropriate treatment. The AAP also endorses and supports further research to evaluate the causes of PANS and the efficacy of interventions to reduce its subsequent morbidity.

Because of well-described problems with sensitivity and specificity, antistreptococcal serologic testing (ie, antistreptolysin O and anti-DNAase B levels) is not recommended to evaluate for GAS infection.[4] Sustained high or low titers are difficult to interpret and do not support a recent episode of GAS infection.

Further Workup

Additional evaluation is recommended when the child displays focal neurologic signs and symptoms or specific signs and symptoms that may indicate the potential for AE, including[17]:

- Symptoms of psychosis (eg, hallucinations, catatonia);
- Persistence of symptoms over months (ie, not relapsing-remitting, which is characteristic of PANS);
- Altered level of consciousness;
- Cognitive impairment (including confusion, aphasia, amnesia, memory deficits) that are not attributable to anxiety, OCD, or depression[23];
- Seizures that are not associated with a preexisting seizure disorder; and
- Movement disorders other than tics, such as chorea, dystonia, tremor, myoclonus, and/or ataxia.

The presence of the above symptoms should lead to additional evaluation, which may include:

- Electroencephalography (EEG);
- Brain MRI with contrast;
- Lumbar puncture with cell count, protein, and glucose measures to evaluate for signs of CNS inflammation as well as auto-antibodies to targets associated with AE (eg, NMDAR, myelin oligodendrocyte glycoprotein);
- Blood tests to evaluate for signs of inflammation (eg, erythrocyte sedimentation rate [ESR], C-reactive

protein [CRP], complete blood cell count [CBC]), thyroid function, antineuronal antibodies, and markers for other systemic autoimmune conditions (such as lupus erythematosus, vasculitis, etc);

- Neurocognitive evaluations; a comparison to any previous evaluations is critical; and
- A complete autoimmune panel of autoantibodies commonly associated with AE.

Tests That Are Not Recommended

Some groups recommend that children with potential PANS have a CBC with differential, ESR, CRP, metabolic panel, and urinalysis.[9] There is no evidence for the utility of these tests in deciding on either diagnosis or treatment; therefore, they should not be routinely performed.[15] In addition, there is no evidence for the following tests; their use is not recommended for diagnosing PANS:

- PCR assay for *Mycoplasma* infection (pharynx): Although some have hypothesized that *M pneumonia* infection may be a cause of PANS, good evidence to support this hypothesis does not exist. In addition, the PCR test result is usually positive only for a few weeks at the beginning of the infection and may also be positive in asymptomatic children.[24,25]
- Antinuclear antibody test: In isolation, this test result may be positive in healthy children, especially at low levels; its high false-positive rate makes the test problematic to use for autoimmune disorder screening.[26] If a positive antinuclear antibody result occurs in the context of systemic signs and symptoms suggestive of rheumatologic disease as well as other positive laboratory markers that indicate inflammation, the patient should be referred to a rheumatologist for consideration of an alternate diagnosis to PANS.
- Cunningham panel: This commercially available set of assays purports to measure levels of biomarkers that are related to autoantibodies to dopamine receptors and other components found in basal ganglia. Current literature documents that the Cunningham panel has very high positive rates among children who are generally healthy and, therefore, very low specificity (eg, 6% for PANS and 10% for PANDAS).[15,27] The panel is not recommended, because results will neither confirm nor eliminate PANS and will not alter planned treatment.
- Workup for other conditions: Myriad other conditions have been mentioned in association with PANS, either for the initial onset or for exacerbations. These include viruses (eg, influenza, Epstein-Barr, herpes simplex, enterovirus, and varicella—all of which are known to have neurologic complications), Lyme disease, sinusitis, dental infections, and gastrointestinal infections. Workups for these conditions are rarely, if ever, helpful. For example, there are only anecdotal case reports that claim an association with sinusitis; these are probably the simultaneous occurrence of a common and an uncommon event. Some advocates recommend workups to rule out AE, neuropsychiatric systemic lupus erythematosus, and acute disseminated encephalomyelitis using EEG, MRI, and lumbar puncture. These conditions have specific clinical presentations that are usually different from PANS. Hence, such a workup should not be performed in a patient being evaluated for PANS unless symptoms of encephalopathy, seizures, myelitis, or other focal neurologic deficits are present or there is overlap of other neuropsychiatric symptoms typical of these syndromes.

Obtaining imaging is not warranted unless CNS or orbital complications are being evaluated.

TREATMENT

Treatment recommendations for PANS are generally grouped into 3 types of interventions[7]: 1) psychiatric and behavioral interventions for OCD, other types of anxiety, tics, or avoidant/restrictive food intake disorder (ARFID); 2) antibiotic treatment for GAS infection; and 3) aggressive therapies for presumed underlying neuroinflammation and autoimmune problems. Treatment is complicated by the fact that there are no well-designed trials that provide evidence-based guidance on treatment for PANS' symptoms—except for specific psychiatric and behavioral symptoms such as OCD, tics, and anxiety that can be seen without PANS. Effective treatments are described below. Families may ask pediatric care providers about other treatments they have heard about, including immunomodulatory therapies. Despite the lack of evidence for these treatments, they are also described in order to fully inform providers who may be considering these unproven treatments for potential PANS. As has been noted throughout this clinical report, more evidence is needed to identify the best possible treatment(s) for children in whom PANS has been diagnosed.

Psychiatric and Behavioral Interventions

There are evidence-based recommendations for psychiatric and behavioral interventions for children with PANS across a spectrum of symptoms observed.[20,21] These treatments include psychosocial; psychiatric; physical therapy/occupational therapy; and other traditional, symptom-based, and function-based interventions. They should be started early in the course of symptoms in children with PANS, whether or not other treatments for infectious agents or immune modulation are being considered or given. In particular, because medications take time to work, especially in children with severe symptoms, it is important not to delay treatment. Treatments for some of the common psychiatric and behavioral problems seen in children with PANS are described below.

Treatment for OCD

OCD is the most common symptom complex in PANS and can be the most troubling. Standard evidence-based behavioral and medication treatments are available. The studies of treatments for OCD were in patients who were referred for OCD that was unrelated to PANS; nonetheless, it is reasonable to expect these treatments will be effective in PANS. In fact, pilot studies suggest that the treatments are effective.[28]

First-line treatment for children with OCD is cognitive behavioral therapy (CBT) and SSRIs, usually sertraline or fluoxetine. The specific type of CBT is exposure and response prevention (ERP), in which the patient is exposed to actual situations, imagined situations, or the sensations associated with the discomfort attributable to those situations and then guided to resist (prevent) performing the compulsions that relieve their anxiety. This exposure is performed on a graded basis from least anxiety-producing to most anxiety-producing.[29] Although both CBT and SSRIs are individually helpful in reducing symptoms, in children, the combination of the 2 has been shown to be more effective than the use of either alone (50% to 70% response in 12 weeks vs 40% for CBT alone and 20% to 30% for SSRIs alone).[30,31] CBT/ERP is also intensive and may involve as much as 14 one-hour visits over 12 weeks; more severe cases may take even longer. Families may face barriers in accessing CBT because of insurance restrictions or shortage of available therapists in their area.

Because SSRIs can cause activation in children (ie, a state of restlessness, lability, agitation, and anxiety), doses begin low and increase slowly with frequent monitoring. Once a therapeutic dose is reached, it may take up to 12 weeks to see a full response.[32] Anecdotal evidence has suggested that children with PANS may be more sensitive to the adverse effects of SSRIs, making parents concerned about SSRI use.[32] It is important for the physician to address and refute any concerns that SSRIs are contraindicated.[32]

In addition to CBT and SSRIs, parent education to "hold the line" and resist giving into or accommodating the child's compulsions (which frequently control the entire family's routines and escalate symptoms) has been shown to decrease OCD symptoms, family disruption, and family conflict.[33]

Treatment for Separation Anxiety

Separation anxiety, which is commonly observed in children with PANS, can severely limit the child's and parent's activities. Parent accommodation of the child's anxiety for a limited time may be helpful, but escalation often occurs. Parent training should be offered to help the caregiver move the child back to normal sleeping arrangements and activities (including school) and to spend time with attachment figures other than parents (such as grandparents and other relatives, nannies, neighbors, and older siblings). CBT may also be helpful and may involve reappraisal of fears and problem-solving practice.[28] Drug therapy is rarely necessary, but for severe cases, clinicians may consider use of an SSRI, especially in older children.

Treatment for Tics

Tics are very common in children with PANS and may range from simple motor tics to complex motor and phonic tics. When a triad of OCD, ADHD, and complex tics occurs, Tourette syndrome should be considered. In most cases, tics are not treated. Treatment may be considered if the tics interfere with the child's functioning or if the child experiences severe embarrassment, teasing, or bullying.[28] Comprehensive behavioral intervention for tics (CBIT) has been shown to be effective. CBIT includes relaxation techniques, inhibition of tics with competing motor movements when the urge is felt (habit-reversal training), and awareness of situational antecedents or consequences of tics that may inadvertently reinforce them.[34] Occasionally, medications are offered, of which the most common are alpha-2 agonists (guanfacine or clonidine). Antipsychotics are also effective, but significant adverse effects preclude their use to suppress tics in most children.

Treatment for Sleep Disturbances

Sleep disturbances are also common in children with PANS. They may be attributable to separation anxiety, OCD bedtime rituals, enuresis, nightmares, or rapid eye movement (REM) sleep behavior disorder.[28] In general, the treatment for sleep disturbances includes counseling and implementation of the principles of good sleep hygiene. Occasionally, melatonin may be helpful. REM sleep behavior disorder consists of the lack of atonia (which is usually a hallmark of REM sleep), nightmares, and flailing of arms and legs that may be reenactment of dreams and are often violent enough to harm anyone who is sleeping with the child.[35,36] There is some indication that SSRIs may be one of the inciting agents, leading parents to be concerned about their use. Most children with REM sleep behavior disorder are not on SSRIs, however.[35,36] If REM sleep behavior disorder is of concern, psychiatry or sleep specialty consultation should be sought.

Treatment for ARFID

Abrupt, dramatic onset of OCD or severely restricted food intake are the cardinal symptoms of PANS; severely restricted food intake may be the only symptom of PANS. Almost all children in whom PANS is diagnosed who have ARFID symptoms also have OCD. In these children, restricted food intake is usually attributable to obsessive fears of contamination, choking, or vomiting and, thus, is an extension of the child's OCD. In a 2015 case series of children diagnosed with PANS, all of the children had OCD; many also had separation anxiety, tics, and symptoms of

ADHD.[37] Two-thirds were restricting food secondary to contamination fears, with some restricting food for fear of choking or vomiting. In addition, the children also reported compulsive ways of preparing food or deciding what foods to restrict and/or refuse. Only a few had concerns about being overweight or body image; when present, these concerns were often concomitant with the fears described above.[37]

Recommended treatment is two-pronged.[28,38] First, a medical assessment should be performed including vital signs, electrocardiogram (EKG), electrolytes, and monitoring for weight loss. In children with significant weight loss, medical treatment may include hospitalization, feeding tubes, and intravenous fluids (if needed for nutrition, hydration, and correction of electrolyte abnormalities). Second, ERP should be offered to address the fears and compulsions with gradual exposure to foods and incremental expansion of diet and intake. SSRIs may also be added to the treatment regimen, similar to the treatment of OCD in children with PANS.[28]

Treatment for Other Psychiatric and Behavioral Symptoms

Children with PANS may have other psychiatric or behavioral symptoms, including irritable or aggressive behavior, mood lability, depression, and/or ADHD. These symptoms may or may not require treatment with behavioral interventions or medications; standard protocols for these problems can be used, in consultation with psychiatry or developmental-behavioral pediatrics.[28]

Antibiotic Treatment for GAS Infection

Children with sudden and abrupt onset of behavioral symptoms of PANS (almost always OCD) with clinical pharyngitis should receive a diagnostic test for GAS infection—a throat culture, a rapid antigen detection test, or a nucleic acid amplification test. If a workup for GAS infection is performed in such patients and the result is positive, the child should be treated with appropriate antibiotics for a 10-day course (usually amoxicillin).[36] In the absence of a positive culture, treatment is not recommended, even if an antistreptococcal antibody test result is positive.[15]

The AAP does not recommend follow-up tests, treatment for longer than 10 days, or prophylaxis if a follow-up test result is positive.[39–41] There is no robust evidence basis for recommendations[2] for long-term treatment with antibiotics for children with documented GAS pharyngitis. Nevertheless, some clinicians institute long-term streptococcal prophylaxis for patients who have either multiple GAS infection-associated exacerbations or are severely affected with symptoms of PANS. This practice may lead clinicians to offer or prescribe long-term antibiotics to children, perhaps for years or until adulthood, without any evidence of its effectiveness. In addition, because there is no evidence-basis for this practice, clinicians may create their own definition of "long-term" (eg, months or years) and select a specific antibiotic based on their own opinion, using some hybrid definition of "long-term" that includes extended treatment for an exacerbation (with or without documented GAS infection) and prophylaxis for future prevention. For a more detailed evaluation of the evidence base for antibiotic treatment, see Sigra, Hesselmark, and Bejerot, "Treatment of PANDAS and PANS: A Systematic Review" (2018).[42] Only 2 studies cited in that review included a placebo arm, both of which found no significant effect from antibiotics.

Other Treatments that are Not Recommended

In the age of the internet, caregivers are likely to search online for solutions and may seek information about the following unproven treatments. Because parents may ask about them, these treatments are described for the pediatric clinician's information.

- Treatment for Lyme Disease: Lyme disease has been suggested as a possible trigger for PANS because of its neuropsychiatric symptoms (including OCD).[2] To-date, however, no clear-cut cases of PANS have been associated with Lyme disease. Testing or treatment for Lyme disease for children with PANS is not recommended at this time.
- Tonsillectomy and/or Adenoidectomy (T&A): T&A has been recommended to decrease incidence of GAS infections. A number of studies have evaluated the impact of T&A on exacerbations of PANS. Although no controlled studies have been conducted, 2 prospective observational studies found no helpful effect on symptom severity.[42] T&A are not recommended treatments for PANS.
- Treatment for Sinusitis and/or Influenza: Although sinusitis and influenza have been labeled as "inciting" agents for PANS, this connection is not supported by evidence. Sinusitis and influenza are common diagnoses in children and, therefore, frequently occur around the time of an initial PANS diagnosis or a subsequent exacerbation.[43] The relationship is most likely coincidental and temporal. Both conditions have well-developed guidelines for diagnosis and treatment that should be followed.[43] Treatment for sinusitis and influenza is not recommended outside of the usual criteria for respiratory disease.

Unfortunately, concerns among patients and families about the influenza vaccine exist (especially the live-virus formulation) because of its anecdotal association with PANS. These fears may lead to concerns about vaccines in general.[2] The AAP has long supported vaccines as one of the most effective medical advances of all time; vaccines are safe, are effective, and save lives. There is no reason to curtail their use in children with PANS. Pediatricians are encouraged to discuss and counter concerns about vaccination, in relationship to causing or exacerbating PANS, whenever they are raised by parents.

- Treatment for *M pneumoniae*: The focus on *M pneumoniae* is primarily because of its association with a number of other neurologic disorders, including encephalitis, transverse myelitis, Guillain-Barré syndrome, acute disseminated encephalitis, choreoathetosis, ataxia, and acute psychosis.[2,44] No well-documented cases connecting *M pneumoniae* and PANS have been described. Because *M pneumoniae* is treated with macrolides, some clinicians have used macrolides (such as azithromycin) to either treat or provide long-term prophylaxis to children with PANS. Until a clear connection to PANS is demonstrated, however, there is no need to treat for *M pneumoniae* outside of the usual criteria for respiratory disease or other known neurologic complications.
- Treatment for Other Viruses and Infections: Treatment for a myriad of other conditions has been mentioned in association with potential PANS, either for the initial onset or for exacerbations. These include treatment for viruses (eg, Epstein-Barr, herpes simplex, enterovirus, and varicella, which are known to have neurologic complications), dental infections, and gastrointestinal infections. It is hard to know what to make of these potential triggers, because they are very common in all children. No treatment for these conditions is indicated at this time for children in whom PANS has been diagnosed.
- Invasive Therapies for Presumed Underlying Neuroinflammation and Autoimmune Problems: Patients and their families may ask about aggressive therapies that have been reported as helpful or recommended by experts and other parents. These may include IGIV; biologics, such as rituximab; immunosuppressives, such as mycophenolate mofetil; and therapeutic plasma exchange (TPE). These immunomodulatory therapies are the most controversial area of treatment for PANS. Some experts recommend their use, especially for children with moderate-to-severe or extreme neuropsychiatric symptoms and impairment of functioning.[45] Many subspecialists and other medical experts are skeptical about the use of immunomodulatory therapies to treat patients with PANS, given the lack of demonstrated evidence of underlying CNS inflammation or autoimmunity for many children in whom PANS has been diagnosed. A 2018 systematic review of treatments for PANS found that the evidence for the benefit of treatments such as nonsteroidal anti-inflammatory drugs (NSAIDs), steroids, IGIV, and TPE was inconclusive because of poor study designs, small numbers of subjects, and conflicting results.[42] The randomized controlled trial (RCT) of treatment with IGIV did not show efficacy for children in whom PANS was diagnosed.[46] Because of the lack of evidence strength for autoimmunity and the potential for adverse effects, including immunocompromise, severe headaches, anaphylaxis, aseptic meningitis, thromboembolic phenomena, hemolysis, renal failure, among other serious reactions,[6,15,45] treatment with invasive immunotherapies is not usually recommended.

Children who have severe and incapacitating symptoms should be evaluated by a neurologist, rheumatologist, or immunologist who has expertise in assessing and treating autoimmune neuropsychiatric conditions. In children with severe and incapacitating neuropsychiatric symptoms, it is more difficult to distinguish PANS from other conditions, because the severity of a predominant symptom may mask other disease manifestations. If the symptoms are severe enough to warrant consideration of intravenous therapies such as IGIV, TPE, or immunosuppressant medications, a thorough workup to exclude other conditions should strongly be considered. The AAP believes that immunomodulatory therapies should only be used in rare cases and only after consultation with a multispecialty team that includes pediatric neurologists and rheumatologists who are experienced in the diagnosis of other conditions (such as AE) and in the use of these medications. These drugs should be administered in pediatric infusion centers/inpatient pediatric centers and not in a general office setting because of the need to monitor patients closely to ensure their safety. Further, these drugs are ideally only used in the context of clinical trials designed to improve our understanding of, and evidence for, effective treatment for PANS.

Despite the lack of compelling evidence to support efficacy in treating PANS, advocacy for IGIV treatment is occurring across the country and becoming more widespread. Several states have passed laws mandating insurance coverage of IGIV for PANS/PANDAS treatment (including Arkansas, Delaware, Illinois, Indiana, Maryland, Minnesota, and New Hampshire). Pediatricians are encouraged to engage with their local chapters to learn more about the situation in their state and community.

Delivering Family-Centered Treatment in the Medical Home

All children—including those with a potential PANS diagnosis—should receive care that is delivered in a medical home and involving a team of caregivers, that is family centered, and that includes resources and support as well as treatment.[47] The AAP acknowledges that there is much to do before all children and families have equal access to the trusted services provided by the medical home.

Medical homes facilitate the creation of team-based partnerships with parents and other caregivers. The trusted relationships and continuity of care provided by the medical home are helpful in supporting parents and children during challenging and frightening health crises—including when children are being evaluated for potential PANS. Clinicians must introduce the family to all of the team members who will be collaborating and communicating with the family about treatment options. Early engagement with partners who form the treatment team is critical to ensure that families get the help and support they need. As described, team members may include—depending on the child's symptoms—the medical home primary care clinician, psychiatry, psychology, neurology, rheumatology, physical therapy, developmental-behavioral pediatrics, and occupational therapy.

> A *medical home* is not a place. It is a way for children and families to receive health care from a primary care provider they know and trust. The health care professional and family work together to make sure children and teens are healthy and know about any special health needs. They respect each other and make decisions as a team. Health care professionals value the family's role as the constant in the child's life.

Providing family-centered care requires clear communication with the family throughout evaluation, diagnosis, and treatment. Family-centered care involves stressing that evaluation for potential PANS is an evolving field and that a definitive diagnosis often cannot be immediately determined (see Diagnosis). Families need to know that the evaluation process can be lengthy because of the time required for psychiatric consultation and laboratory work. Explicit acknowledgement of the ongoing stress of waiting for a diagnosis and treatment determination may help support parents throughout this challenging experience. Family-centered care also includes clearly describing what the treatment process is likely to be (eg, SSRIs and referral for CBT for many cases) and that it will focus on managing symptoms, particularly those causing the most distress to the child. It is useful to reinforce that behavioral treatments will not either interfere with the diagnostic evaluation or hamper the identification of any underlying diagnosis.

Pediatric health care clinicians should also help families by connecting them with information, resources, and support groups about acute-onset psychiatric conditions. The pediatric clinician's role also includes staying in contact and proactively reaching out to families to see how they are doing and what they need and assessing evolving complications (eg, weight loss, poor nutrition, sleep cycle disruption, increasing behavior problems). The pediatric clinician can also help families communicate with institutions to ensure the child gets needed supports, such as accommodations in schools and child care facilities.

Treatment Summary

The opinion of the AAP expert panel is that PANS may be part of a group of conditions that are potentially triggered by infectious agents and/or involve autoimmunity. Best-practice treatment modalities for PANS are not clear at this time, other than consistent use of CBT and SSRIs when OCD and/or anxiety are prominent symptoms. There is a strong evidence base for behavioral and psychiatric treatments for OCD and other neuropsychiatric symptoms; these treatments are effective and should be the first line of therapies when identified in children with concern for PANS. There is also agreement that a short 10-day course of amoxicillin should be administered in children who have a positive test result for GAS throat infection. Otherwise, there is a lack of evidence to support the use of antimicrobial and immunomodulatory agents. Subspecialty consultation should be sought in severe cases. Pediatric health care clinicians are encouraged to describe the evidence quality for effective interventions to families as well as the lack of evidence for unproven treatments that parents may ask about. Providing factual information can help families navigate decisions about potential treatments and rebut the medical misinformation that often circulates on the internet.

SUMMARY AND CONCLUSION

Concerned pediatric health care clinicians and families alike are still learning about PANS. Numerous limitations in the current body of evidence impede the ability to evaluate, diagnose, and treat PANS with confidence; this reality must be clearly and compassionately conveyed to families who are searching for answers. These limitations include the small sample sizes in published studies; the lack of long-term follow-up on outcomes for children in whom PANS has been diagnosed; design limitations, such as the use of predominantly retrospective versus prospective design and parental report versus direct observation; and the paucity of RCTs that eliminate bias and provide evidence about the impact of infectious triggers. There is an urgent need for well-designed, placebo-controlled RCTs to test the efficacy of potential treatment modalities for children affected by PANS. Only when the results of such RCTs are available will we be able to fully understand the prevalence, incidence, risk factors, progression, diagnostic biomarkers, biological mechanisms, and pathophysiological and immune dysregulation mechanisms that characterize this condition. Without well-established and evidence-based treatments for PANS, the situation is challenging. Families are encouraged to partner with subspecialists and clinicians who are experienced in treatment of children with PANS in order to benefit from accurate information that can guide the choice of effective treatment modalities.

Diagnosis of potential PANS involves a thorough patient and family medical history, including psychiatric history for both the child and their family members; physical and psychiatric examination; and a phased laboratory and imaging workup. Pediatric health care providers are encouraged to initially discuss the likelihood of a diagnosis that is broader than PANS—including acute-onset OCD or other anxiety disorders, tic disorder, Tourette syndrome, Sydenham chorea, or AE. A review of symptom longevity is required to assess these possibilities. Initial laboratory workup consists of a diagnostic test for GAS infection (eg, throat culture, a rapid antigen detection test, or a nucleic acid amplification test) when signs of pharyngitis are present. Focal neurologic signs and symptoms and those that indicate the potential for AE require additional evaluation.

Most children with OCD, tics, and/or other neuropsychiatric symptoms likely have conditions unrelated to PANS. Even when PANS is strongly considered, psychosocial, behavioral, and psychiatric therapies are effective and should be first-line therapies for children with PANS. In addition, a 10-day course of amoxicillin or other recommended antibiotic should be administered to children who have a positive test result for an acute, symptomatic GAS throat infection. There is no strong evidence to support the use of other treatments. Subspecialty consultation should be sought when the patient's symptoms are severe.

The AAP strives to ensure that children and their families have access to high-quality and evidence-based care. In the context of potential PANS, care should be provided by a multidisciplinary team; housed within a medical home; and grounded in best practices for mental health, neuropsychiatry, and movement disorders. This goal is not yet a reality for too many children, however. Further, challenges in accessing specialized centers of care for PANS affect which patients can access different types of treatment. These challenges include geography, cost, insurance status, and other factors. The situation raises important questions about equity. Variations in access are likely to skew treatment outcomes and hamper unbiased assessments of various treatments' efficacy. As a result of these factors, consensus statements about PANS/PANDAS—although welcome—have been inconsistent in their recommendations, which has increased confusion and frustration on the part of clinicians and families alike.[42]

Acute symptom onset, including neuropsychiatric and behavioral changes seen in children with PANS, can be very stressful and challenging for families. The pediatricians and pediatric subspecialists of the AAP understand and acknowledge the stresses that these symptoms cause for our families and are committed to simultaneously supporting children and families and seeking a greater understanding of the causes, diagnosis, and potential treatments for PANS. The AAP looks forward to engaging and collaborating with a wide range of partners to address the challenges complicating the field and to meet the goals of robust and unbiased evidence and equitable access to care that will ensure the health and well-being of all children.

ABBREVIATIONS

AAP: American Academy of Pediatrics
ADHD: attention-deficit/hyperactivity disorder
AE: autoimmune encephalitis
ARFID: avoidant/restrictive food intake disorder
CRP: C-reactive protein
CNS: central nervous system
CBT: cognitive behavioral therapy
CBC: complete blood cell count
CBIT: comprehensive behavioral intervention for tics
CINAHL: Cumulative Index to Nursing and Allied Health Literature
DSM-5: *Diagnostic and Statistical Manual of Mental Disorders, Fifth Edition*
EEG: electroencephalography
EKG: electrocardiogram
ERP: exposure and response prevention
ESR: erythrocyte sedimentation rate
GAS: group A beta-hemolytic streptococcal (infection)
IgG: immunoglobulin
IGIV: immune globulin intravenous
MRI: magnetic resonance imaging
NMDAR: N-methyl-D-aspartate receptor
NSAID: nonsteroidal anti-inflammatory drug
OCD: obsessive-compulsive disorder
PANS: pediatric acute-onset neuropsychiatric syndrome
PANDAS: pediatric autoimmune neuropsychiatric disorders associated with streptococcal infections
PCR: polymerase chain reaction
RCT: randomized controlled trial
REM: rapid eye movement
SSRIs: selective serotonin reuptake inhibitors
TPE: therapeutic plasma exchange
T&A: tonsillectomy and/or adenoidectomy

REFERENCES

1. Swedo SE, Leonard HL, Garvey M, et al. Pediatric autoimmune neuropsychiatric disorders associated with streptococcal infections: clinical description of the first 50 cases. *Am J Psychiatry.* 1998;155:264–271.
2. Cooperstock MS, Swedo SE, Pasternack MS, Murphy TK, Consortium PP. Clinical management of pediatric acute-onset neuropsychiatric syndrome: Part III–treatment and prevention of infections. *J Child Adolesc Psychophamacol.* 2017;27: 594–606.

3. Murphy TK, Sajid M, Soto O, et al. Detecting pediatric autoimmune neuropsychiatric disorders associated with *Streptococcus* in children with obsessive-compulsive disorder and tics. *Biol Psychiatry.* 2004;55:61–68.
4. Wald ER. A pediatric infectious disease perspective on pediatric autoimmune neuropsychiatric disorder associated with streptococcal infection and pediatric acute-onset neuropsychiatric syndrome. *Pediatr Infect Dis J.* 2019;38(7):706–709.
5. Swedo SE, Leckman JF, Rose NR. From research subgroup to clinical syndrome: modifying the PANDAS criteria to describe PANS (pediatric acute-onset neuropsychiatric syndrome). *Pediatr Therapeut.* 2012;2:113.
6. British Paediatric Neurology Association. *Consensus Statement on Childhood Neuropsychiatric Presentations, with a Focus on PANDAS/PANS.* British Paediatric Neurology Association; 2021.
7. Swedo SE, Frankovich J, Murphy TK. Overview of treatment of pediatric acute-onset neuropsychiatric syndrome. *J Child Adolesc Psychopharmacol.* 2017;27(7):562–565.
8. Snider LA, Swedo SE. Post-streptococcal autoimmune disorders of the central nervous system. *Curr Opin Neurol* 2003;16(3):359–365.
9. Chang K, Frankovich J, Cooperstock M, et al. PANS Collaborative Consortium. Clinical evaluation of youth with pediatric acute-onset neuropsychiatric syndrome (PANS): recommendations from the 2013 PANS Consensus Conference. *J Child Adolesc Psychopharmacol.* 2015;25(1):3–13.
10. Baj J, Sitarz E, Forma A, Wróblewska K, Karakuła-Juchnowicz H. Alterations in the nervous system and gut microbiota after β-hemolytic *Streptococcus* group A infection-characteristics and diagnostic criteria of PANDAS recognition. *Int J Mol Sci.* 2020;21(4):1476.
11. Brimberg L, Benhar I, Mascaro-Blanco A, et al. Behavioral, pharmacological, and immunological abnormalities after streptococcal exposure: a novel rat model of Sydenham chorea and related neuropsychiatric disorders. *Neuropsychopharmacology.* 2012; 37(9):2076–2087.
12. Lotan D, Benhar I, Alvarez K, et al. Behavioral and neural effects of intra-striatal infusion of anti-streptococcal antibodies in rats. *Brain Behav Immun.* 2014;38:249–262.
13. Frick LR, Rapanelli M, Jindachomthong K, et al. Differential binding of antibodies in PANDAS patients to cholinergic interneurons in the striatum. *Brain Behav Immun.* 2018;69:304–311.
14. Loiselle CR, Lee O, Moran TH, Singer HS. Striatal microinfusion of Tourette syndrome and PANDAS sera: failure to induce behavioral changes. *Mov Disord.* 2004;19(4):390–396.
15. Gilbert DL, Mink JW, Singer HS. A pediatric neurology perspective on pediatric autoimmune neuropsychiatric disorder associated with streptococcal infection and pediatric acute-onset neuropsychiatric syndrome. *J Pediatr.* 2018;199:243–251.
16. Singer HS, Gause C, Morris C, Lopez P, Tourette Syndrome Study Group. Serial immune markers do not correlate with clinical exacerbations in pediatric autoimmune neuropsychiatric disorders associated with streptococcal infections. *Pediatrics.* 2008;121(6): 1198–1205.
17. Cellucci T, Van Mater H, Graus F, et al. Clinical approach to the diagnosis of autoimmune encephalitis in the pediatric patient. *Neural Neuroimmunol Neuroinflamm.* 2020;7(2):e663.
18. Centers for Disease Control and Prevention. *Children's Mental Health—Anxiety and Depression in Children: Get the Facts.* Centers for Disease Control and Prevention; Accessed April 5, 2022. https://www.cdc.gov/childrensmentalhealth/features/anxiety-depression-children.html
19. Scahill L, Specht M, Page C. The prevalence of tic disorders and clinical characteristics in children. *J Obsessive Compuls Relat Disord.* 2014;3(4):394–400.
20. Heyman I, Fombonne E, Simmons H, Ford T, Meltzer H, Goodman R. Prevalence of obsessive-compulsive disorder in the British nationwide survey of child mental health. *Br J Psychiatry.* 2001; 179:324–329.
21. American Academy of Child and Adolescent Psychiatry. *Facts For Families: Obsessive-Compulsive Disorder in Children and Adolescents.* Fact Sheet American Academy of Child and Adolescent Psychiatry; 2018. Accessed April 5, 2022. https://www.aacap.org/AACAP/Families_and_Youth/Facts_for_Families/Layout/FFF_Guide-01.aspx
22. Larson JC, Mostofsky SH, Goldberg MC, Cutting LE, Denckla MB, Mahone EM. Effects of gender and age on motor exam in typically developing children. *Dev Neuropsychol.* 2007;32(1):543–562.
23. Hacohen Y, Wright S, Waters P, et al. Paediatric autoimmune encephalopathies: clinical features, laboratory investigations and outcomes in patients with or without antibodies to known central nervous system autoantigens. *J Neurol Neurosurg Psychiatry.* 2013;84:748–755.
24. Spuesens EB, Fraaij PL, Visser EG, et al. Carriage of *Mycoplasma pneumoniae* in the upper respiratory tract of symptomatic and asymptomatic children: an observational study. *PLoS Med.* 2013;10(5):e1001444.
25. Dorigo-Zetsma JW, Wilbrink B, van der Nat H, Bartelds AI, Heijnen ML, Dankert J. Results of molecular detection of *Mycoplasma pneumoniae* among patients with acute respiratory infection and in their household contacts reveals children as human reservoirs. *J Infect Dis.* 2001;183(4):675–678.
26. Malleson PN, Mackinnon MJ, Sailer-Hoeck M, Spencer CH. Review for the generalist: the antinuclear antibody test in children - when to use it and what to do with a positive titer. *Pediatr Rheumatol Online J.* 2010;8:27.
27. Hesselmark E, Bejerot S. Biomarkers for diagnosis of pediatric acute neuropsychiatric syndrome (PANS) - sensitivity and specificity of the Cunningham panel. *J Neuroimmunol.* 2017;15(312): 31–37
28. Thienemann M, Murphy T, Leckman J, et al. Clinical management of pediatric acute-onset neuropsychiatric syndrome: Part I—psychiatric and behavioral interventions. *J Child Adolesc Psychopharmacol.* 2017;27(7):566–573.
29. Law C, Boisseau CL. Exposure and response prevention in the treatment of obsessive-compulsive disorder: current perspectives. *Psychol Res Behav Manag.* 2019;12:1167–1174.

30. The Pediatric OCD Treatment Study (POTS) Team. Cognitive-behavior therapy, sertraline, and their combination for children and adolescents with obsessive-compulsive disorder: The Pediatric OCD Treatment Study (POTS) randomized controlled trial. *JAMA.* 2004;292(16):1969–1976.

31. Franklin ME, Sapyta J, Freeman JB, et al. Cognitive behavior therapy augmentation of pharmacotherapy in pediatric obsessive-compulsive disorder: the Pediatric OCD Treatment Study II (POTS II) randomized controlled trial. *JAMA.* 2011;306(11):1224–1232.

32. Murphy T, Storch E, Strawser M. Selective serotonin reuptake inhibitor-induced behavioral activation in the PANDAS subtype. *Primary Psychiatry.* 2006;13(8):87–89.

33. Lebowitz ER, Omer H, Hermes H, Scahill L. Parent training for childhood anxiety disorders: The SPACE Program. *Cognitive and Behavioral Practice.* 2014;21(4):456–469.

34. Sukhodolsky DG, Woods DW, Piacentini J, et al. Moderators and predictors of response to behavior therapy for tics in Tourette syndrome. *Neurology.* 2017;88(11):1029–1036.

35. Lloyd R, Tippmann-Peikert M, Slocumb N, Kotagal S. Characteristics of REM sleep behavior disorder in childhood. *J Clin Sleep Med.* 2012;8(2):127–131.

36. Gaughan T, Buckley A, Hommer R, et al. Rapid eye movement sleep abnormalities in children with pediatric acute-onset neuropsychiatric syndrome (PANS). *J Clin Sleep Med.* 2016;12(7). DOI: https://doi.org/10.5664/jcsm.5942

37. Toufexis MD, Hommer R, Gerardi DM, et al. Disordered eating and food restrictions in children with PANDAS/PANS. *J Child Adolesc Psychopharmacol.* 2015;25(1):48–56.

38. Norris ML SW, Katzman DK. Update on eating disorders: current perspectives on avoidant/restrictive food intake disorder in children and youth.. *Neuropsychiatr Dis Treat* 2016;12:213–8. doi: 10.2147/NDT.S82538

39. Murphy ML PM. Prospective Identification and Treatment of Children With Pediatric Autoimmune Neuropsychiatric Disorder Associated With Group A Streptococcal Infection (PANDAS). *Arch Pediatr Adolesc Med.* 2002;156(4):356–361. doi: 10.1001/archpedi.156.4.356

40. Feinstein AR, Wood HF, Epstein JA, Taranta A, Simpson R, Turksy E. A controlled study of three methods of prophylaxis against streptococcal infection in a population of rheumatic children. II. Results of the first three years of the study, including methods for evaluating the maintenance of oral prophylaxis. *N Engl J Med.* 1969;260(14):697–702.

41. Gerber MA, Baltimore RS, Eaton CB, et al. Prevention of rheumatic fever and diagnosis and treatment of acute streptococcal pharyngitis. A scientific statement from the American Heart Association Rheumatic Fever, Endocarditis, and Kawasaki Disease Committee of the Council on Cardiovascular Disease in the Young, the Interdisciplinary Council on Functional Genomics and Translational Biology, and the Interdisciplinary Council on Quality of Care and Outcomes Research. *Circulation.* 2009;119(11):1541–1551.

42. Sigra S, Hesselmark E, Bejerot S. Treatment of PANDAS and PANS: a systematic review. *Neurosci Biobehav Rev.* 2018;86:51–65.

43. American Academy of Pediatrics, Committee on Infectious Diseases. Recommendations for prevention and control of influenza in children, 2024–2025: Policy statement. *Pediatrics.* 2024;154(4):e2024068507.

44. Spalice A. *Mycoplasma pneumoniae* infection with neurologic complications. *Ital J Pediatr.* 2015;41:A67.

45. Frankovich J, Swedo S, Murphy T, et al; PANS/PANDAS Consortium. Clinical management of pediatric acute-onset neuropsychiatric syndrome: Part II—use of immunomodulatory therapies. *J Child Adolesc Psychopharmacol.* 2017;27(7):574–593.

46. Williams KA SS, Farmer CA, Grantz H, Grant PJ, D'Souza P, Hommer R, Katsovich L, King RA, Leckman JF. Randomized, Controlled Trial of Intravenous Immunoglobulin for Pediatric Autoimmune Neuropsychiatric Disorders Associated With Streptococcal Infections. *J Am Acad Child Adolesc Psychiatry.* 2016;55(10):860–867.e2. doi: 10.1016/j.jaac.2016.06.017

47. American Academy of Pediatrics. *Bright Futures: Family-Centered Care.* American Academy of Pediatrics; 2021. Accessed April 5, 2022. https://brightfutures.aap.org/families/Pages/default.aspx

Perinatal Urinary Tract Dilation: Recommendations on Pre-/Postnatal Imaging, Prophylactic Antibiotics, and Follow-up

- *Clinical Report*
  - *PPI: AAP Partnership for Policy Implementation See Appendix 1 for more information.*

American Academy of Pediatrics
DEDICATED TO THE HEALTH OF ALL CHILDREN®

AAP Partnership for Policy Implementation

CLINICAL REPORT Guidance for the Clinician in Rendering Pediatric Care

American Academy of Pediatrics

DEDICATED TO THE HEALTH OF ALL CHILDREN™

Perinatal Urinary Tract Dilation: Recommendations on Pre-/Postnatal Imaging, Prophylactic Antibiotics, and Follow-up: Clinical Report

C. D. Anthony Herndon, MD, FAAP,[1] Hansel J. Otero, MD, FAAP,[2] David Hains, MD, FAAP,[3] Rebecca M. Sweeney, MD, FAAP,[4] Gina M. Lockwood, MD, MS, FAAP,[5] and the Section on Urology, Section on Nephrology, Section on Radiology, and Section on Hospital Medicine

abstract

Perinatal urinary tract dilation (UTD) occurs in approximately 1% of all pregnancies and represents the second most common congenital anomaly detected prenatally, second only to cardiac defects. Causes of UTD include transient dilation, vesicoureteral reflux (VUR) and genitourinary obstruction. A vast majority of these conditions will never require surgical intervention. However, a subset of patients will be at increased risk of urologic and kidney disease. The purpose of this clinical report will be to review the current imaging modalities used for the evaluation of perinatal UTD and discuss the risk stratification for UTD, the indications for prophylactic antibiotics, and the use of lower tract imaging and renal scintigraphy (RS). Ultimately, the management of these children is individualized and should involve a shared-decision making process between the physician and parent/guardian that is evidence based.

The evaluation and management of more severe forms of bilateral UTD in boys who are at high risk for bladder outlet obstruction is outside of the scope of this document. Any concern for this entity should prompt an immediate consultation with a nephrology/urology specialist.

[1]Department of Urology, Children's Hospital of Richmond at VCU, Richmond, Virginia; [2]Department of Radiology, Children's Hospital of Philadelphia, Philadelphia, Pennsylvania; [3]Division of Pediatric Nephrology and Hypertension, Riley Hospital for Children, Indianapolis, Indiana; [4]Oxford University Hospital NHSFT, Oxford, United Kingdom; and [5]Department of Urology, University of Iowa Health Care, Iowa City, Iowa

CONFLICT OF INTEREST DISCLOSURE: The authors have indicated they have no potential conflicts of interest to disclose.

To cite: Anthony Herndon CD, Otero HJ, Hains D, et al; American Academy of Pediatrics, and the Section on Urology, Section on Nephrology, Section on Radiology, and Section on Hospital Medicine. Perinatal Urinary Tract Dilation: Recommendations on Pre-/Postnatal Imaging, Prophylactic Antibiotics, and Follow-up: Clinical Report. *Pediatrics.* 2025; 156(1):e2025071814

INTRODUCTION

The benefit of the detection of antenatal urinary tract dilation (UTD) continues to evolve as its natural history is better understood. In the 1980s, the properties of fetal ultrasonography (US) afforded the discovery of hydronephrosis in 1% to 3% of pregnancies, which led to a paradigm shift in the diagnosis of conditions such as ureteropelvic junction (UPJ) obstruction and vesicoureteral reflux (VUR). Early discovery of UTD prompted indiscriminate recommendations for prophylactic antibiotics, lower urinary tract imaging, and early surgical intervention in an effort to prevent urinary tract infections (UTIs) or deterioration in kidney function. These recommendations were made with good intentions but were not evidence based. Fortunately, most patients had good outcomes, which has afforded a more pragmatic approach over the last decade.

To this end, great effort has been made to work toward a model of care that maximizes the benefit of detection while minimizing evaluation and treatment that may not be evidenced based. Recent prospective registries have given insight into resolution rates for UTD, identified risk factors for UTI, and better informed the use of antibiotic prophylaxis.[1–4]

This report provides a framework for the pediatrician to better understand and educate parents on UTD in the context of recommendations for surveillance, use of prophylactic antibiotics, use of adjunct genitourinary imaging, and referral to a specialist. It is important to note that generally speaking, this report is aimed at patients with UTD and little to no concern for bladder outlet obstruction from various causes (eg, posterior urethral valves). Cases of bilateral UTD, especially those that are severe in nature and suggestive of bladder outlet obstruction, often associated with bilateral hydroureteronephrosis, bladder and urethral abnormalities, and/or oligohydramnios, are managed using a different paradigm both prenatally and postnatally.

ANTENATAL EVALUATION OF URINARY TRACT DILATION

Fetal Development and Detection of UTD Prenatally

Fetal genitourinary development begins early in the first trimester with urine production occurring around 14 weeks' gestational age, and it continues through the postnatal period.[5] The kidneys and bladder can reliably be detected on antenatal US by the end of the first trimester. US has a high sensitivity for UTD with large studies reporting sensitivities up to 91%.[6] The most severe abnormalities are likely to appear on the first screening US, which in the United States is recommended to be performed between 18 and 22 weeks of gestational age.[7,8] Pathology associated with UTD, thus, can have a significant impact on kidney development and ultimately function. Abnormalities detected on this screening US often prompt referral to a specialized practice able to perform a comprehensive US to confirm the abnormality as well as screen other organ systems.

Etiologies of UTD and Effect on the Kidney and Bladder

Diagnosing the precise etiology of UTD on antenatal imaging can be difficult. Causes of antenatal UTD are diverse and include transient/physiologic dilation, VUR, and any cause of obstructive uropathy (eg, ureteropelvic junction obstruction, posterior urethral valves, ureterocele, ectopic ureter, ureterovesical junction obstruction). The impact of UTD on the renal unit and the patient is also variable, ranging from no effect to increased risk of UTI, renal scarring, and dysplasia of the kidney.

Natural History of Antenatal Urinary Tract Dilation

Many cases of antenatal UTD are transient and spontaneously resolve. Two meta-analyses found spontaneous resolution rates of 64% to 75%.[9,10] More recent observational studies have equally found spontaneous resolution rates of 25% to 55%.[11,12]

Association Between Degree of UTD with Diagnosis and Outcome

Several studies have demonstrated that the less severe the antenatal UTD, the more likely it is to spontaneously resolve,[10–15] whereas the more severe the antenatal UTD, the more likely it was caused by an obstructive uropathy.[9,14,16,17] A meta-analysis by Lee et al found that the greater the degree of antenatal UTD, the greater the risk of specific pathologies including UPJ obstruction and posterior urethral valves.[9] In contrast, VUR is poorly correlated with degree of dilation.[9,18]

Although the number of patients with antenatal UTD who ultimately require postnatal surgery is quite low,[19] several studies show that the more severe the antenatal hydronephrosis, the more likely the patient will require surgical intervention.[11,12,15,17,20] One study found that patients whose UTD worsened between the second and third trimesters were more likely to require surgery.[21]

Goals of Antenatal Detection

The main benefit for detection prenatally is to afford the opportunity for consultation with pediatric specialists. Antenatal discussions should be framed around the differential diagnosis, indications for perinatal intervention; potential need for postnatal imaging, including renal and bladder ultrasonography (RBUS), voiding cystourethrogram (VCUG), and/or functional imaging; and recommendations for prophylactic antibiotics for those thought to be at increased risk of UTI. An algorithm is provided in the Supplemental Files to guide clinical decision making.

Historical Timing of Imaging

In the United States, women with low-risk pregnancies undergo 2 antenatal USs, and those with high-risk pregnancies will undergo more. Historically, when a diagnosis of antenatal UTD is made, there has been lack of consensus regarding the frequency and timing of antenatal and postnatal follow-up imaging. A 2006 meta-analysis by Lee et al[9] found large variability among protocols. Recommendations ranged from vague (eg, "serially as needed") to specific (eg, "once at 32–34 weeks") and from infrequent (eg, "once in the third trimester") to numerous (eg, "once per month"). This guideline strives to delineate the ideal frequency and timing of follow-up based on current evidence.

Technique and Limitations of Antenatal Ultrasonography

Adherence to a standardized technique for antenatal US is recommended to allow accuracy and consistency across studies with a goal that future research might discover correlations between specific antenatal findings and underlying etiologies. **The measurement of the anteroposterior renal pelvis diameter (APD) prenatally should be performed with the fetal spine in the 6 o'clock or 12 o'clock position, and position should remain consistent from US to US.** Specific antenatal values (ie, all 7 UTD parameters) should be communicated to all postnatal providers, including the clinician performing the initial newborn examination and the primary care pediatrician, as these will guide management (Table 1). When feasible, images should be made available to the practitioner for review. Accuracy of antenatal US imaging is not only operator dependent but based on fetal positioning as well.[18] In most instances it should be used as a screening modality that sets the stage for in-depth postnatal evaluation to determine the exact etiology of UTD. Fetal MRI could be useful in certain cases when US fails, such as cases of anhydramnios or oligohydramnios. However, there is not sufficient evidence to support wide adoption, and access is not universal.

ULTRASONOGRAPHIC CLASSIFICATION SYSTEMS FOR ANTENATAL AND POSTNATAL URINARY TRACT DILATION

A diagnosis of antenatal UTD often necessitates postnatal imaging. Historically, several grading systems have been utilized with incomplete, heterogenous adoption[22] to classify and risk-stratify urinary tract dilation on US. A recent focus has been placed on use of a system that can be translated across time and specialties.

Anteroposterior Renal Pelvis Diameter

The measurement of APD has historically been the most commonly used system to measure urinary tract dilation on US. APD is an objective measurement of the renal pelvis at the mid-point of the kidney in the transverse plane. Normative values exist that account for gestational age. The established antenatal normal limits are APD less than 4 mm under 28 weeks and less than 7 mm after 28 weeks. The main advantage of this system is the objective nature of reporting. Disadvantages include that it is operator dependent and does not account for abnormalities of the rest of the collecting system, ureters or bladder. For obstructive lesions, the system demonstrates high specificity for severe dilation, and several studies have identified 15 mm of APD detected in the third trimester as a threshold predictive of UPJ obstruction.[17,23,24]

Society for Fetal Urology Grading System

The Society for Fetal Urology (SFU) grading system is a subjective assessment of kidney dilation and parenchymal integrity[25] (Figure 1). Currently, this is the most common system used postnatally.[26] The SFU system demonstrates high positive predictive value for both kidney function and need for surgical intervention in UPJ obstruction.

TABLE 1. Items Evaluated During Renal and Bladder Ultrasound

US Parameter	Measurement/ Findings	Notes
Anterior posterior renal pelvis diameter (APD)	(mm)	Measured on transverse image at max diameter of renal pelvis; measured with spine in 6 o'clock or 12 o'clock position Normal Ranges by Age • Prenatal <28 weeks: < 4 mm • Prenatal ≥28 weeks: < 7 mm • Postnatal: < 10 mm
Calyceal dilation		
Central (major calyces)	Present/Absent	Subjective assessment
Peripheral (minor calyces)	Present/Absent	Subjective assessment
Parenchymal thickness	Normal/Abnormal	Subjective assessment
Parenchymal appearance	Normal/Abnormal	Evaluation of echogenicity, corticomedullary differentiation, and for cortical cysts
Ureter	Normal/Abnormal	Visualization is considered dilated and abnormal, though intermittent visualization of the ureter is considered normal postnatally.
Bladder	Normal/Abnormal	Evaluation of bladder wall thickness, presence of ureterocele, dilated posterior urethra
Unexplained oligohydramnios	Present/Absent	

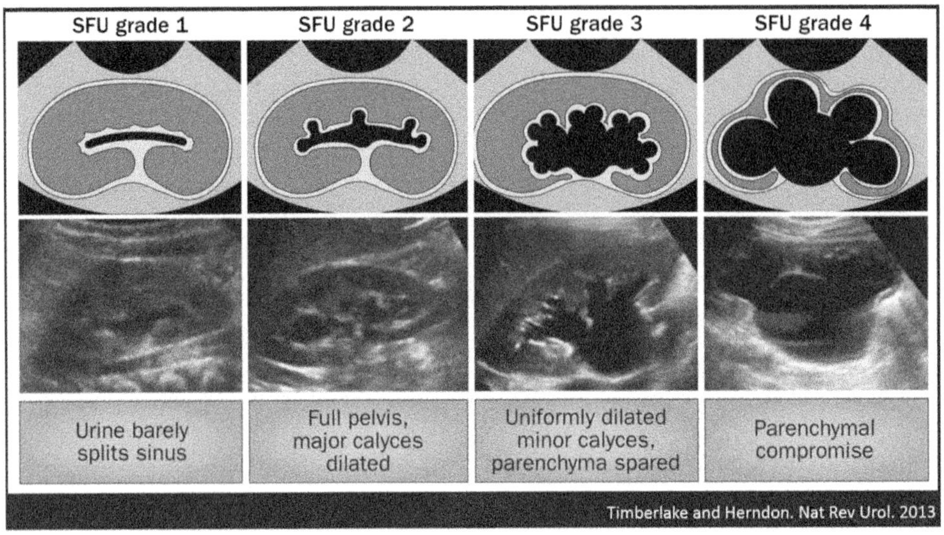

FIGURE 1.
Society for Fetal Urology Grading System.

The advantages are its ease of learning and application. Disadvantages include its limited adoption by other specialists outside of pediatric urology, its subjective nature, as well as the lack of inclusion of the entire collecting system including the ureters and bladder during assessment.

Urinary Tract Dilation (UTD) Grading System

In 2014, a multidisciplinary consensus meeting including representatives from 8 professional societies involved in the diagnosis and management of UTD was held to unify the grading systems and establish a common language among practitioners.[18] The goals were to develop a standard process for imaging and reporting of US results both antenatally and postnatally. Additionally, postnatal normative values that represented physiologic dilation (APD < 10 mm) were agreed upon to curtail low-yield testing and interventions. The term UTD was chosen to describe all degrees of antenatal and postnatal dilation, as opposed to the terms *hydronephrosis, pelviectasis, caliectasis,* and *pelvicaliectasis.* The UTD system is a combination of both the objective and subjective characteristics of the APD and SFU systems and measures variables that include: APD, central calyceal dilation, peripheral calyceal dilation, appearance and thickness of kidney parenchyma, appearance of ureters, appearance of bladder, and unexplained oligohydramnios (Table 1).

ANTENATAL RISK STRATIFICATION/MANAGEMENT

Thresholds for antenatal diagnosis of UTD are based on gestational age at the time of imaging, whether less than or greater than 28 weeks gestation (Figure 2). For both age groups, fetuses are classified into a low-risk group (UTD A1 [denoted A for antenatal]) or an increased risk group (UTD A2-3). In addition to the common parameters between antenatal and postnatal systems, the antenatal system also considers presence or absence of unexplained oligohydramnios. Unlike the postnatal classification, the intermediate and high-risk groups are combined in the antenatal system. This difference relates to the difficulty in accurately differentiating central vs peripheral calyceal dilation in the antenatal US. In both the antenatal and postnatal risk classifications, the most concerning abnormal finding is used to place the patient into a higher risk category (ie, if there is ureteral dilation but the APD is less than 10 mm at greater than 28 weeks gestation, the fetus is still considered UTD A2-3).

The antenatal recommendations are based on the timing of the US and severity of UTD. If UTD is low-risk prior to 28 weeks, then only one US is recommended after 32 weeks' gestation. On the other hand, if the UTD is intermediate/high-risk, then serial US every 4 weeks is recommended. The need/timing for specialty consultation with urology and/or nephrology equally varies by severity of disease (Figure 3).

POSTNATAL EVALUATION OF UTD

Multiple imaging modalities are commonly used to better classify UTD and diagnose its exact cause postnatally. These tests and their uses, as well as risks and benefits are described in Table 2.

Renal and Bladder Ultrasonography

RBUS is the initial imaging study of choice to evaluate children with perinatal UTD. The postnatal degree of dilation of the pelvicalyceal system and ureters helps guide additional

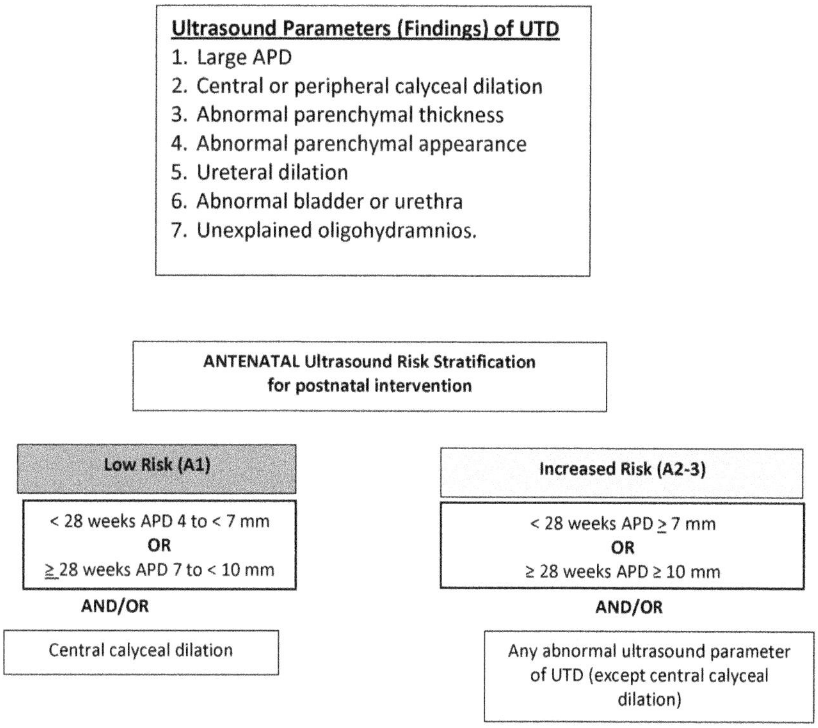

FIGURE 2.
*Prenatal ultrasound risk stratification. **Stratification is based upon the most concerning ultrasound finding**. For example, a fetus with an anterior-posterior renal pelvis diameter (APD) within the UTD A1 range but with peripheral calyceal dilation would be classified as UTD A2-3.

	Follow-Up Ultrasound	Urology/Nephrology Consultation
Low Risk (A1)	Repeat once prenatally at ≥ 32 weeks	Not indicated prenatally
Increased Risk (A2-3)	Repeat every 4 weeks until delivery	Consider prenatal consult

FIGURE 3.
Suggested PRENATAL Management Based Upon US < 32 weeks.

investigations and interventions.[18,27] RBUS advantages include that it is noninvasive, is widely available, is quickly performed, lacks ionizing radiation, and is less costly than other imaging modalities.[28] Additionally, RBUS does not require specific patient positioning, infants can be imaged supine, prone, or while being held in the upright position. However, scanning newborns and infants in the prone position may overestimate the degree of dilation in up to 10% of patients, and this consideration should be taken into account especially in the first postnatal study.[29] For optimal assessment of UTD, RBUS should be performed after 48 hours of life, as studies during the first 48 hours of life might underestimate the degree of dilation due to physiologic neonatal third spacing, which does not fully resolve until day 7 to 10.[30–34]

Adherence to standard technique for postnatal US and reporting of results is paramount to maintain consistency (see Table 1). The first postnatal US serves as a determinant of risk because, in general, higher levels of dilation correspond with higher need for surgery.[20,35,36]

TABLE 2. Risks and Benefits for Postnatal Radiologic Imaging

Features / Imaging Modality	Anatomy versus Function	Anatomy Assessed: Kidneys	Bladder	Ureters	Urethra	Duration (min)	Prep S/H/UC	Ionizing radiation (Yes/No)	Nephrotoxic (Yes/No)	Relative cost
Ultrasound	Anatomy	Yes	Yes	Only if abnormal	Yes	30	None	No	No	$
VCUG	Anatomy	Collecting systems (if reflux)	Yes	Yes (if reflux)	Yes	30	UC	Yes	No	$$
ceVUS	Anatomy	Collecting systems (if reflux)	Yes	Yes (if dilated or reflux)	Yes	30	UC	No	No	$$
MAG 3 diuretic renography	Function	Renal function	No	No	No	90	H/UC	Yes	No	$$$
MR Urography	Anatomy & Function	Anatomy & function	Yes	Yes	Yes	60	S/H/UC	No	No**	$$$$

S/H/UC: Refers to the need of sedation (S), intravenous hydration (H) and urinary catheter (UC) placement for the completion of the study. In general, sedation for any of these imaging tests is only needed in patients older than 6 months and under 5 years of age.
**Gadolinium-based contrast agents used for MR Urography have a small risk of adverse allergy-like reactions and linked to nephrogenic systemic fibrosis (NSF) a rare disease reported in patients that receive gadolinium and have end-stage renal disease.

Voiding Cystourethrography

Fluoroscopic VCUG is the gold standard for diagnosing and grading VUR,[37,38] which occurs in 15% of children with prenatally diagnosed isolated UTD.[39–41] It can also yield information about bladder or urethral abnormalities contributing to UTD. The standards for technique, image acquisition and interpretation have been previously reported by the American Academy of Pediatrics in a joint publication from the sections of urology and radiology.[38] In terms of technique, a VCUG study consists of instilling iodinated contrast material into the bladder via a urinary catheter and imaging with pulsed fluoroscopy. The key images include the bladder at different levels of filling, the urethra during voiding, and the renal fossae immediately after voiding, to document the presence and grade of reflux.[37,38] Imaging during multiple filling cycles of the bladder is helpful in infants who void at low volumes.[37]

A normal postnatal US does not exclude reflux.[42] The risk of VUR in patients with a nondilated or a mildly dilated collecting system may be as high as 25%.[43] Fortunately, VUR associated with prenatally detected UTD has a high incidence of spontaneous resolution.[42,44] Historically, some authors recommended VCUG in all children with prenatally detected UTD, and there was great practice variability.[45] Between 26% and 57% of pediatric urologists will recommend VCUG and antibiotics for patients with UTD P2, and between 85% and 88% will recommend them for patients with UTD P3.[46] Currently, it is largely accepted that UTD in itself should not be considered an indication for VCUG in asymptomatic neonates and infants, and its optimal use is an area of ongoing research.[19]

Contrast-Enhanced Voiding Urosonography

In addition to VCUG, similar information can be extracted from contrast-enhanced voiding urosonography (ceVUS).[47,48] CeVUS has shown to be more sensitive in detecting VUR than VCUG, with a higher grade of reflux in a majority of patients.[49,50] CeVUS is not uniformly available at most institutions, which limits its application.

If ceVUS is chosen as an alternative to VCUG, US instead of fluoroscopy is used for imaging and the iodinated contrast instilled into the bladder is substituted by a US contrast agent (ie, microbubbles). While the images of the kidneys and bladder are acquired in a similar fashion as a regular RBUS, images of the urethra during voiding are necessary and usually obtained via a suprapubic and/or transperineal approach.

Functional Renal Imaging - Renal Scintigraphy

Functional nuclear medicine renal imaging, known under several names including renal scintigraphy (RS), diuretic renography, furosemide renography, radionuclide RS, radioisotope renography, and nuclear medicine renogram, follow the uptake of radiotracers by the kidneys and their excretion through the collecting system. RS imaging captures gamma rays emitted by the patient after intravenous radiotracer administration and follow the biodistribution of radiotracer throughout the body. The most commonly used radiotracer in the evaluation of UTD is ^{99m}Tc-MAG3 (technetium-99m-labeled-mercaptoacetyl triglycine), which reaches the collecting system via tubular secretion[51–54] and offers better overall quality of the images, even in patients with a low glomerular filtration rate, edema, or ascites.[55] Several other radiotracers can be used to calculate kidney function as well, including ^{99m}Tc-DMSA (technetium-99m-labeled-dimercaptosuccinic acid) and ^{99m}Tc-DTPA (technetium-99m-labeled-diethylenetriamine penta-acetic acid). ^{99m}Tc-DMSA undergoes cortical tubular binding while ^{99m}Tc-DTPA measures glomerular filtration.[51–54]

The RS (^{99m}Tc-MAG3) technique requires a well-hydrated patient using intravenous or oral hydration protocols. Before beginning the study, a urinary catheter is placed to create an unobstructed outlet system to reduce the potential negative effect of a distended bladder on radiotracer excretion and the confounding effect from possible high-grade vesicoureteral reflux. With RS, there is concern about the use of radiation. However, the effective radiation dose is low, and more than 95% of the radiotracer is cleared within 3 hours in patients with normal kidney function,[51,56,57] which allows the child to safely go to clinic or home after the study is performed.

In cases of UTD, RS is used to establish a baseline differential kidney function, which indicates the relative contribution of each kidney to the overall kidney function (warranting intervention if functional decline is documented) and to differentiate between dilated collecting systems *with* or *without* obstruction. RS ^{99m}Tc-MAG3 measures 2 important parameters. First, the parenchymal uptake (first pass from the circulation into the kidney), which reflects the split renal function (or differential renal function). Second, clearance is evaluated over 30 minutes to determine the presence and level of obstruction of the collecting system from the UPJ to the ureterovesical junction.[53,54] If there is retained radiotracer in the collecting system after 15 or 20 minutes, a diuretic (furosemide, 1.0 mg/kg; maximum dose of 40 mg) is administered to differentiate dilated systems *with* from those *without* a critical obstruction.[58] A dilated but unobstructed system will respond to diuretics, while a truly obstructed system will retain radiotracer as it is unable to increase the rate of clearance through the critically narrowed segment. This is crucial because only obstructed systems require (and benefit from) surgery. Note that after surgical intervention, a previously dilated and capacious system may not regress back to normal and does not indicate failure of surgery. In normal subjects, ^{99m}Tc-MAG3 split renal function values ranges from 42% to 58%,[58] and thus a threshold of 40% split function is used to identify those in which the obstruction is felt to be compromising kidney function.

Accurate RS results in infants with UTD rely on adequate renal blood flow and kidney development; thus, tests should ideally be deferred until at least 6 to 12 weeks of age. During the first months of life, kidney immaturity results in low uptake of ^{99m}Tc-MAG3 and slower cortical transit times. While there is evidence that RS can be performed at any age, and the decision of timing is based on the specific clinical indication, practitioners often delay for up to 6 to 12 weeks.[59–62] Studies performed before 6 to 12 weeks may over- or underestimate the kidney function and are not generally predictive of outcome.[63,64]

Functional Magnetic Resonance Urography

Magnetic resonance urography (MRU) is a reliable and safe diagnostic tool that can substitute RS for the determination of differential kidney function and provide detailed information about the morphology of the kidney with a dilated collecting system.[65] MRU provides morphologic characterization of the kidney parenchyma and the entire urinary tract, which can be advantageous in the diagnostic and/or presurgical work up of neonatal UTD.[66,67] Similar to RS, MRU aims to differentiate between capacious and obstructed systems, determine the level of the obstruction, and estimate the relative contribution of each kidney to the overall kidney function. Despite advantages related to providing high-quality anatomical and functional data in a single examination that lacks radiation, MRU has ancillary disadvantages including need for sedation or anesthesia for the younger children, higher cost, and relatively limited availability.[28]

As part of the protocol and similar to RS, patients receive hydration and diuretics (furosemide), but hydration is given intravenously and the furosemide is administered prior to image acquisition for better resolution. During the dynamic scan, the enhancement of the aorta, the kidneys, and in most cases the initial drainage flow of the urinary system are obtained and used to calculate quantitative parameters as well as enhancement and excretion curves.[68] The enhancement and excretion curves are a display of the change of signal intensity over time and calculated for the aorta, renal parenchyma, pelvis, and calyces with higher spatial resolution than nuclear medicine studies. The important clinical functional information obtained from analyzing contrast flow dynamics allows differentiation of obstructed from nonobstructed renal collecting systems.[69]

POSTNATAL UTD RISK STRATIFICATION

Under the current UTD classification (Figures 4a, 4b), patients are stratified into 3 tiers postnatally based on their RBUS: low (UTD P1), intermediate (UTD P2), and high (UTD P3) risk.[18] The risk classification helps clinicians decide the need for investigations such as lower urinary tract imaging (eg, VCUG or ceVUS) or functional imaging.

POSTNATAL MANAGEMENT OF UTD

Over the last 2 decades, there has been a focus of research on analysis of outcomes in patients with UTD to better inform providers as to which patients truly benefit from additional evaluation and treatment for UTD. This research has informed creation of both antenatal and postnatal recommendations for patients with UTD regarding US surveillance, subspecialist referral, need for additional imaging studies and need for antibiotic prophylaxis, although there is lack of consensus on some of these topics (Figures 5 and 6).

Consideration of UTI, Renal Scarring, and Antibiotic Prophylaxis in the Management of UTD

Diagnosis and treatment of UTI is outside of the scope of this report. UTIs in this report refer to febrile UTI and, thus, are presumed to be pyelonephritis. Imaging confirmation of pyelonephritis is not always available or necessary for management.

Emerging research has endeavored to determine the frequency of UTI and renal scarring in patients with UTD, the timing of UTI if it does occur, whether certain subpopulations are at higher risk than others for UTI and renal scarring, and whether prophylactic antibiotics decrease any of these risks. This report summarizes the current evidence, acknowledging this is a dynamic area of active research subject to change.

Risk of UTI in Children with UTD and Which Subpopulations Are at Increased Risk

Estimates of UTI rates in patients with prenatally diagnosed UTD range from 8% to 22% with a linear relationship between the degree of dilation and the development of a UTI.[9] Most recently, data from the SFU multicenter prospective hydronephrosis registry evaluated 801 patients over a 12-year interval enrolled prospectively from 2008–2020.[70] In patients with isolated hydronephrosis, the overall UTI rate was 4.2%. When stratified, the UTI rate in patients with high-grade hydronephrosis was 6.0% compared with 3.2% in those with low-grade hydronephrosis. Another report from the same registry identified ureteral dilation ≥7 mm as a significant risk factor for UTI in over 200 patients.[71] These findings are consistent with numerous prior studies, which have demonstrated higher rates of UTI in patients with *high-grade* UTD[3,4,72–78] and/or hydroureteronephrosis.[3,72,76,78,79] In addition to these 2 findings, other risk factors that have been shown to increase risk of UTI in patients with UTD include: female gender,[1,3,15,73,75,80–82] intact foreskin,[1,3,19,72,73,75] and obstructive uropathy[78] (Table 3a). Studies that assessed whether or not patients with both UTD and VUR are at increased risk for UTI (compared to UTD in the absence of VUR) show conflicting results.[1,3,15,72–75,77] Of note, most of the mentioned studies excluded patients with known uropathy at birth (eg, solitary kidney). These frequently excluded patient populations are listed within Table 3b and should also be considered at increased risk.

Knowledge of timing will also affect the clinician and family's management decisions. The incidence of UTI prior to the first postnatal ultrasound is low (1.4%).[83] Regarding longer term data, Zee et al reported prospective data from the multicenter SFU registry on 213 patients with antenatal UTD, showing that 89% of UTIs in this cohort occurred before the first year of life.[4]

UTI and Renal Scarring

The goal of preventing UTIs is to prevent their short-term sequelae, such as bacteremia, and long-term sequelae, such as renal scarring, hypertension, chronic kidney disease, and kidney failure. A more recent study, in which Shaikh et al combined data from the RIVUR and CUTIE studies, found similar results: higher rates of renal scarring in patients with more frequent UTIs. Compared with patients with a history of one UTI, having 2 UTIs increased the odds of renal scarring by a factor of 12 and having 3 UTIs by a factor of 14.[84] The odds of renal scarring were also higher in patients who were toilet-trained or had hydronephrosis, high-grade VUR, or ureteral duplication.[85]

Effectiveness of Continuous Antibiotic Prophylaxis in Children with UTD

Historically, patients with antenatal UTD were empirically prescribed continuous antibiotic prophylaxis to prevent UTI and, ultimately, kidney damage. To date, no studies have addressed the effect of continuous antibiotic prophylaxis (CAP) on renal scarring in patients with UTD. Multiple studies, including some meta-analyses, have assessed the benefits of CAP to prevent scarring in other patient populations (such as VUR). None found a reduction in renal scarring, although they were not powered appropriately to answer this clinical question.[85–93]

Moreover, in recent years, conflicting studies/reports have questioned the efficacy of CAP in patients with UTD, especially in patients with low-risk UTD. A recent 2017 meta-analysis by Easterbrook et al found no significant difference in UTI rates between patients that were (9.9%) or were not (7.5%) given CAP.[73] An older meta-analysis by Braga et al found that CAP prevented UTIs in patients with *high-grade* UTD (NNT = 7) but made no difference in patients with *low-grade* UTD.[74] Notably,

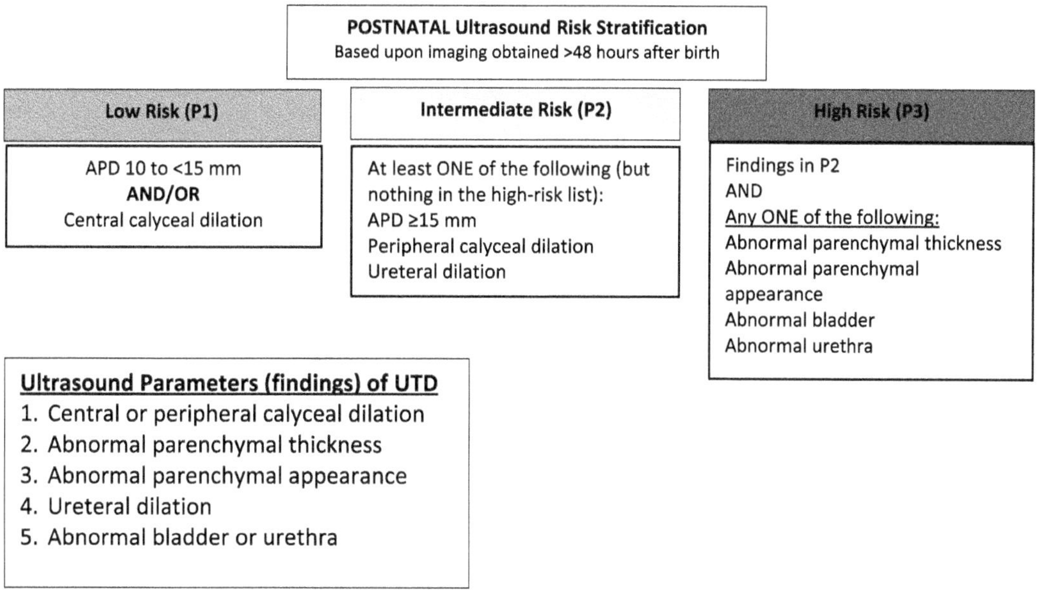

(A)

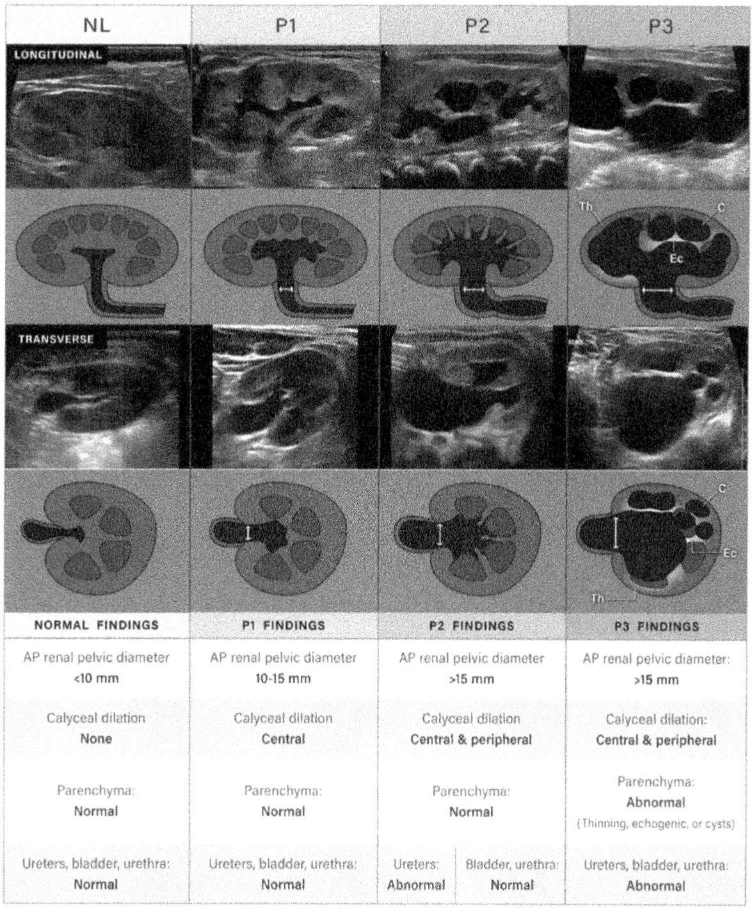

(B)

FIGURE 4.

(A) Postnatal ultrasound risk stratification. **Stratification is based upon the most concerning ultrasound finding**. For example, if the anterior-posterior renal pelvis diameter (APD) is in the UTD P1 range, but there is peripheral calyceal dilation, the classification is UTD P2. Similarly, the presence of parenchymal abnormalities denotes UTD P3 classification, regardless of APD measurement. (B) Postnatal Urinary Tract Dilation Grading System.

UTD Classification	Definition	Initial Postnatal US	Urology/Nephrology Consultation
Incomplete or Unclear Classification		Follow postnatal evaluation similar to UTD A1	Follow postnatal evaluation similar to UTD A1
Resolved at Last Prenatal Ultrasound		If prior US were all A1 --> No postnatal evaluation or surveillance required If any prior US was A2-3 --> Manage according to recommendations for "Increased Risk (A2-3)" below.	
Low Risk (A1)	≥ 28 weeks APD 7 to <10 mm **AND/OR** central calyceal dilation	≥48 hrs to 6 weeks of age Need not delay discharge*	May consider with outpatient follow-up
Increased Risk (A2-3)	≥ 28 weeks APD ≥10 mm **OR** any abnormal parameter (except central calyceal dilation)	Prior to discharge. Ideally after 48 hr of life.	Recommended prior to discharge

The ultrasound should be prioritized and can either be ordered prior to discharge or at the first primary care visit to allow for imaging within 4-6 weeks of life.

FIGURE 5.
Suggested Subsequent POSTNATAL Management Based Upon Antenatal Ultrasound.

UTD Classification	Definition/Circumstance	Follow-Up Ultrasound (2nd Postnatal Ultrasound)	Antibiotic Prophylaxis	VCUG/ceVUS	MAG3/fMRU	Urology/Nephrology Consultation
Resolved		3-9 month of age	Not recommended	Not recommended	Not recommended	Not recommended
Low Risk (P1)	APD 10 to <15 mm **AND/OR** central calyceal dilation	3-6 months of age	Not recommended	Not recommended	Not recommended	Outpatient
Intermediate Risk (P2)	APD ≥15 mm **AND/OR** peripheral calyceal dilation	1-3 months of age	Use shared decision making to determine use	Use shared decision making to determine need	Use shared decision making to obtain at >6 weeks of age	Inpatient consult or expedited outpatient referral
	Ureteral dilation ≥7 mm	1-3 months of age	Recommended	Recommended within 1-3 months of age	Use shared decision making to obtain at >6 weeks of age	Inpatient consult or expedited outpatient referral
High Risk (P3)	Findings in P2 **AND** abnormal parenchymal thickness **or** appearance **or** abnormal bladder	1 month of age	Recommended	Recommended within 1-3 months of age	Recommended at >6 weeks of age.	Inpatient consult or expedited outpatient referral

fMRU indicates functional magnetic resonance urography.

FIGURE 6.
Suggested Subsequent POSTNATAL Management Based Upon Initial Postnatal Ultrasound. fMRU indicates functional magnetic resonance urography. Most studies evaluating risk factors for UTI with UTD and/or VUR have excluded known uropathies. It is recommended that children with these diagnoses be considered high risk, as most are associated with obstructive uropathy or VUR.

TABLE 3A. Children With UTD AND Risk Factors for UTI
Female gender
Intact foreskin (UTD P2/P3)
UTD P3
Distal ureteral dilation ≥7mm
Vesicoureteral reflux
Obstructive uropathy (suggested by bilateral UTD)

TABLE 3B. Children With Known Uropathy at Birth
Ureteropelvic Junction Obstruction
Posterior Urethral Valves
Ectopic ureter
Duplex ureter
Solitary kidney
Multi-cystic dysplastic kidney
Bladder diverticulum
Neurogenic bladder
Bladder exstrophy
Spina bifida
Horseshoe kidney
Crossed-fused ectopia
Cloacal exstrophy

neither meta-analysis included any RCTs. A recent 2021 study by Holzman et al also found that CAP prevented UTIs in patients with *high-risk* UTD with concomitant ureteral dilation ≥7 mm and VUR.[71] However, data from the same year from the SFU Hydronephrosis Registry demonstrated no benefit for CAP for isolated UPJ-like hydronephrosis, even when they adjusted for grade of UTD or other risk factors (eg, female gender).[70] Four systematic reviews and 2 recent observational studies also document conflicting results.[72,80,81,83,94,95]

Some studies have shown circumcision to be an equally preventive alternative to antibiotic prophylaxis for prevention of UTI in boys with UTD. As previously mentioned, most UTIs occur within the first year of life, and rates beyond that age are low. Clinicians should therefore consider stopping antibiotic prophylaxis at 12 months of age, unless the child has VUR or ureteral dilation ≥7 mm.

Numerous studies have evaluated bacterial resistance in children on CAP with diagnoses other than UTD, such as VUR. Two meta-analyses calculated that CAP increased the odds of multidrug-resistant infection by 6.5 to 9 times.[86,96] A Cochrane review found similar, although not statistically significant, results.[97] There is also growing interest in the question of how CAP affects the microbiome.

Amoxicillin is the primary antibiotic prescribed for UTI prophylaxis in the newborn in the United States. It covers some gram-negative rods and *Enterococcus* species. After 2 months of life, the most commonly prescribed antibiotic for prophylaxis is trimethoprim-sulfamethoxazole, which attains high concentrations in the urine and results in less bacterial resistance. Before 2 months' corrected gestational age, trimethoprim-sulfamethoxazole can cause bilirubin displacement leading to kernicterus. Nitrofurantoin is an equally effective prophylaxis and is excreted primarily in the urine and has poor tissue penetration thus decreasing impact on the gut microbiome. If a cephalosporin is chosen, the clinician should strongly consider using a first-generation cephalosporin as bacterial resistance remains low.[98] Local patterns of resistance should be considered using the hospital antibiogram or other sources of community antibiotic sensitivity information.

A shared decision-making model that includes the benefits and risks of CAP should be discussed with the family prior to implementation of therapy. In general, the higher degree of suspicion for obstructive UTD, the more CAP benefits the patient and outweighs the inherent risk of developing an infection with a multidrug-resistant organism.

POSTNATAL DIAGNOSIS OF THE COMMON ETIOLOGIES OF UTD AND NEED FOR ADJUNCT IMAGING

Specific diagnosis of the cause of UTD is made most often postnatally, whether through RBUS alone or with the aid of the aforementioned adjunct imaging studies. The most common causes of prenatally diagnosed UTD are transient/physiologic dilation, UPJ obstruction, and vesicoureteral reflux (Table 4).

TRANSIENT UTD

Transient dilation of the urinary tract is the most common etiology of UTD. Two recent reports from large prospective registries affirm that 90% to 100% of patients with P1 will resolve by 4 years of age.[1,2]

UPJ Obstruction

A majority of patients with UPJ-like UTD will not need surgical correction and can be observed with serial imaging.[81,99] Several studies have reported that the antenatal APD threshold may be predictive of the need for surgery for UPJ obstruction.[17,23,100] More recently, a review of more than 1000 patients identified an APD cutoff of 15 mm to be predictive of the need for intervention and confirmed that postnatal measurements were superior to antenatal

TABLE 4. Causes of Urinary Tract Dilation

Non-Obstructive	Obstructive Uropathies
-Transient/physiologic dilation - VUR	Ureteral Obstruction: - ureteropelvic junction (UPJ) obstruction - Ureterocele - Ectopic ureter - Obstructing megaureter Urethral Obstruction: - Posterior urethral valves - Urethral atresia - Other

measurements.[36] Those patients at increased risk can be evaluated with renal functional imaging. However, practice varies and some advocate for the use of serial US.[46,99,101,102]

Vesicoureteral Reflux

Understanding of vesicoureteral reflux and its effects on kidney function have significantly evolved over the last decade. Screening for VUR has traditionally been recommended in patients with prenatally diagnosed UTD, because VUR has been reported in up to 31% of patients with antenatal UTD.[9,103–105] Antenatal UTD correlates poorly with severity of VUR, however.[9] The utility of screening patients for VUR based on UTD has been challenged, as the clinical relevance of reflux in the absence of UTI with normal bladder function is unclear. Two distinct types of patients have been identified who present with VUR. The most common scenario is the child (usually female) with recurrent febrile urinary tract infections. These children usually have less renal scarring and lower grades of VUR. The less common scenario is the child with high grade VUR commonly detected through antenatal screening with significant renal dysplasia ("reflux nephropathy") without UTI.[103] These latter children have high rates of resolution of VUR and low rates of UTI, especially in the circumcised state, suggesting that screening for VUR may not be beneficial based on antenatal UTD alone, in the absence of UTI.

Until further prospective studies can better determine the value of identifying VUR in patients that present with UTD prenatally, a shared decision-making model should be used with families to discuss the benefit of a VCUG/ceVUS. Risk factors such as gender, circumcision status, and/or ureteral dilation should be offset with the benefit of prophylactic antibiotics at mitigating UTI and/or renal scarring.

CONSIDERATIONS FOR SEVERE BILATERAL URINARY TRACT DILATION/SOLITARY FUNCTIONING KIDNEY WITH URINARY TRACT DILATION

The preceding recommendations in this report are not primarily aimed at cases of severe bilateral UTD. Patients with severe bilateral UTD with dilated ureters, abnormal bladder morphology, and oligohydramnios should be evaluated for underlying causes of bladder outlet obstruction, which include posterior urethral valves, urethral atresia, prune belly syndrome, pelvic masses, and spinal dysraphism. If bladder outlet obstruction is suspected prenatally, parents should receive appropriate counseling regarding differential diagnoses, possible effects on bladder and kidney function, and possible postnatal evaluation and management strategies.

Postnatally, infants with suspected bladder outlet obstruction should undergo prompt urology and nephrology consultation, bladder decompression, appropriate imaging, and initiation of antibiotic prophylaxis, ideally all within 48 hours of life. Assessment of overall kidney function with serum testing is also necessary, but it should be remembered that serum creatinine in the neonate will reflect maternal creatinine in the first few days of life.

KEY RECOMMENDATIONS

1. It is important that newborns with UTD receive needed care after discharge. This may include follow-up imaging and subspecialist follow up. It is important that a care plan is developed among treating clinicians and is implemented through coordination between all members of the care team. Communication and definition of roles among all providers and the patients/families/caregivers are needed to clearly delineate responsibility for follow-up related to UTI risk and diagnosis, ordering and reviewing results, providing follow-up care, and communicating the follow-up care plan with the family. Each family's social and economic needs for follow-up care should be assessed with necessary support arranged prior to discharge to reduce barriers to care.
2. Urinary tract dilation should be classified according to the Urinary Tract Dilation Grading System for antenatal (A1-3) and postnatal (P1-3) scoring.
3. **The measurement of the anteroposterior renal pelvis diameter (APD) on antenatal US should be performed with the fetal spine in the 6 o'clock or 12 o'clock position, and position should remain consistent from US to US.**[18]
4. **For gestations identified as *low-risk* (UTD A1) diagnosed prior to 32 weeks, a repeat antenatal US should be obtained at ≥32 weeks[18] to assess for improvement or progression through pregnancy.** Antenatal UTD may improve, remain stable, or progress throughout pregnancy. Resolution in the antenatal period has been shown to occur in approximately 80% of cases when the APD is between 4 and 8 mm during the second trimester.[106–108] Persistent UTD of any severity should prompt postnatal evaluation.
5. **For gestations identified as *low-risk* (UTD A1) that resolve on US after 32 weeks, no postnatal evaluation or surveillance is required.** While some patients with prenatally resolved UTD will have postnatal UTD, these patients are at very low risk for UTI, kidney function deterioration, or need for surgical intervention.[109] Patients with presumed mild or resolved but incomplete or unclear antenatal classification should undergo postnatal evaluation similar to UTD A1.
6. **For gestations identified as *low-risk* (UTD A1) that persists after 32 weeks, postnatal evaluation should include RBUS between 48 hours of life and 6 weeks of life.** It is important that the US be

deferred to after 48 hours to account for intravascular volume depletion that occurs in the fetus after delivery. This form of third spacing redistributes over the first 24 to 48 hours of life and can cause US performed during that period to underestimate UTD.[110] Discharge from birth hospitalization does not need to be prolonged for these *low-risk* infants if clinically stable. The US should be prioritized and can be ordered either prior to discharge or at the first primary care visit to allow for imaging within 4 to 6 weeks of life.

Certain clinical situations may require postnatal US to be performed sooner than 48 hours. With suspected bladder outlet obstruction (eg, posterior urethral valves), urgent intervention may be needed for urinary tract decompression.

7. **For gestations identified as *increased-risk* (UTD A2-3) diagnosed at any time during pregnancy, repeat antenatal US should be obtained every 4 weeks thereafter prior to delivery for reassessment.** Repeat assessment is recommended given possible progression of UTD and implications on management plan and location of delivery (local vs tertiary care center).
8. **For newborns that were identified as *increased-risk* (UTD A2-3) at any time during pregnancy, an RBUS should be obtained during the birth hospitalization to facilitate possible need for antibiotic prophylaxis and to determine need for further imaging. Ideally, this US should be performed after 48 hours of life.** Birth hospitalization need not be prolonged to obtain this first US unless there is suspicion for bladder outlet obstruction.
9. **For gestations identified as *increased-risk* (UTD A2-3), antenatal consultation with nephrology and/or urology should be obtained.** One significant benefit of antenatal detection of urologic abnormalities is antenatal counseling for families. Especially in instances in which urgent or invasive surgical intervention may be warranted postnatally or in which significant compromise of kidney function is anticipated, a discussion before birth can allow time for families to adequately process information and plan for postnatal care. In-person or telemedicine consultation in conjunction with antenatal providers can allow all caregivers for both mother and baby to develop an organized plan of care for the postnatal period. Generally speaking, conditions that most benefit from antenatal multidisciplinary consultation include patients in the UTD A2-3 risk group and any patient with bilateral UTD. Indications for fetal intervention for UTD are outside of the scope of this report. However, intervention for bladder outlet obstruction is offered at some centers, and a candid discussion regarding known risks and benefits with families may be appropriate in some cases.
10. **Orientation and patient position on postnatal US should be documented.** The APD should be calculated at the midpoint of the kidney in the transverse plane (corresponding to the region of the hilar vessels). The maximal diameter should be obtained within the confines of the renal cortex. Standard terminology of the UTD classification system should be used for reporting. Staff performing postnatal US should use techniques and reporting standardized according to the UTD classification system for maximal consistency across studies.[18]
11. **For those patients with indications for postnatal US, a minimum of 2 postnatal renal US should be obtained prior to discontinuation of UTD surveillance.** If UTD is resolved at initial US, at least 1 additional US should be repeated 3 to 6 months later to ensure continued resolution. One study showed that 21% to 28% of children with antenatal UTD had a normal initial postnatal US, but 45% of those patients had a follow-up US that was again abnormal.[111]
12. **For patients identified as *low-risk* (UTD P1) after their initial postnatal US, repeat US should be obtained in 3 to 6 months. Evaluation with VCUG/ceVUS or renal functional imaging, as well as use of antibiotic prophylaxis, is NOT recommended.** Postnatal surveillance with US should be driven by the likelihood of resolution, which occurs in most UTD P1 patients between 24 and 48 months of age.[3,112] Zee et al reported that 90% of UTD P1 patients reached resolution by 48 months.[1] Braga et al also reported that 90% reached resolution by 4 years.[2]

The degree of UTD is not predictive of the presence or severity of VUR and, thus, should not be the sole factor used to determine the need for postnatal VCUG/ceVUS. The risk of UTI should be the main determinant for the need for a VCUG. Two large patient registries have examined risk factors for UTI and utility of antibiotic prophylaxis in children with UTD, and it is agreed upon that patients in this low risk category (UTD P1) receive the least benefit from early VCUG and antibiotic prophylaxis.[4,112] The risk of significant obstructive uropathy in a low-risk child is less than 1%, and thus renal functional imaging is not warranted unless there is worsening dilation over time.[1,2]

13. **For patients identified as *intermediate-risk* (UTD P2), after their first postnatal US, a repeat US should be obtained in 1 to 3 months. Evaluation with VCUG/ceVUS or renal functional imaging, as well as use of antibiotic prophylaxis, should be considered on the basis of a patient's individualized risk.** There is less robust evidence about the utility of VCUG/ceVUS, prophylactic antibiotics and renal functional imaging in the intermediate risk group in preventing UTI and renal function sequelae. An informed

discussion utilizing a shared decision-making approach should be conducted with the family about risks and benefits of testing and antibiotics, as well as chance of future UTI, rate of detection of VUR, its treatment, and natural history.[4,112]

14. **Ureteral dilation (unilateral or bilateral) ≥7 mm increases the risk of UTI. Antibiotic prophylaxis decreases this risk and is recommended as well as a VCUG/ceVUS in this population.**[71] Other factors that may increase UTI risk include female gender, intact foreskin, and certain specific diagnoses.[3,4] **In follow-up, clinicians should consider stopping antibiotic prophylaxis at 12 months of age, unless the child has VUR or persistent ureteral dilation ≥7 mm.**
15. **For patients identified as *high-risk* (UTD P3), a repeat US should be obtained 1 month after their first postnatal US. VCUG/ceVUS, antibiotic prophylaxis, and renal functional imaging are recommended in this group.** This group is known to be at highest risk for urinary tract infection, deterioration of kidney function and need for surgery.[3,4,112] VCUG/ceVUS can be obtained during the birth hospitalization or at the time of second US if there is no concern for conditions leading to bladder outlet obstruction, like posterior urethral valves. If persistent UTD P3 is visualized, a renal functional imaging is usually obtained at 6 to 12 weeks of age. If vesicoureteral reflux is ruled out on VCUG/ceVUS, duration for use of prophylactic antibiotics depends on suspected diagnosis.
16. **If indicated, renal functional imaging should be deferred until at least 6 to 12 weeks of age to allow for appropriate development of renal blood flow, which optimizes the accuracy of testing.** During the first months of life, kidney immaturity results in low uptake of 99mTc-MAG3 and slower cortical transit times. Renal functional studies performed before 6 to 12 weeks may over- or underestimate the kidney function and are not generally predictive of outcome.[63,64]
17. **Any patient with UTD may be referred postnatally to nephrology and/or urology depending on provider comfort level with surveillance of UTD and counseling parents on implications on overall health and natural history.** Nephrology and/or urology consultation is **recommended** early in children in whom the risk of kidney deterioration or need for surgery is high (UTD P2-3) to allow for early shared decision making. Virtual/telemedicine consultation is appropriate.
18. **Any child with known UTD and a fever should be considered for the evaluation of UTI, especially those that have not undergone lower urinary tract imaging. If a febrile UTI is diagnosed in a patient with known UTD, then a VCUG/ceVUS should be performed to evaluate for VUR.** A catheterized urine specimen is preferred if initial urine analysis is suggestive of UTI to minimize rate of contamination and overtesting and treatment. There is not consensus on the need for urine testing with fever and presence of upper respiratory symptoms/other possible sources of fever; however, it should be stated that a high index of suspicion for concomitant UTI, even in the presence of other symptoms, should be maintained. Clinical suspicion should guide evaluation, and a shared decision-making approach should be used.

LEAD AUTHORS

C. D. Anthony Herndon, MD, FAAP
Hansel J. Otero, MD, FAAP
David Hains, MD, FAAP
Rebecca M. Sweeney, MD, FAAP
Gina M. Lockwood, MD, MS, FAAP

CONSULTANTS

Juan D. Chaparro, MD, MS, FAAP
William G. Adams, MD, FAAP

Reza Daugherty, MD, FAAP
Sarah Sarvis Milla, MD, FAAP, Immediate Past Chairperson

STAFF

Laura Laskosz, MPH

SECTION ON HOSPITAL MEDICINE EXECUTIVE COMMITTEE, 2021–22

Geeta Singhal, MD, MEd, FAAP, *Chair*
Rachel Marek, MD, FAAP, *Chair-Elect*
H. Barrett Fromme, MD, MHPE, FAAP, *Immediate Past Chair*
Jessica (Jessie) Allan, MD, FAAP
Zoey Goore, MD, MPH, FAAP
Laura Nell Hodo, MD, FAAP
Dimple Khona, MD, MBA, ABOIM, IFMCP, FAAP, *Community Hospitalist Member*
Tony Tarchichi, MD, FAAP
Jorge Ganem, MD, FAAP, *Task Force on Diversity and Inclusion Chair*
Eleanor Sharp, MD, *Section on Pediatric Trainees Liaison*

STAFF

Dana Bennett-Tejes, MA, MNM

ACKNOWLEDGMENTS

We would like to show our appreciation for the time and commitment put forth by Juan D. Chaparro, MD, FAAP, and Bill Adams, MD, FAAP, for their help with the creation of this document and participation via the Partnership for Policy Implementation, and to Rakhi Gupta Basuray, MD, FAAP, Allison Markowsky, MD, FAAP, and Arun Gupta, MD, FAAP, for their review and feedback of this document on behalf of the Section on Hospital Medicine.

ABBREVIATIONS

APD: anteroposterior renal pelvis diameter
CAP: continuous antibiotic prophylaxis
ceVUS: contrast-enhanced voiding urosonography
MRU: magnetic resonance urography
RBUS: renal and bladder ultrasonography
RS: renal scintigraphy
SFU: Society for Fetal Urology
UPJ: ureteropelvic junction
US: ultrasonography
UTD: urinary tract dilation
UTI: urinary tract infection
VCUG: voiding cystourethrogram
VUR: vesicoureteral reflux
99mTc-DMSA: technetium-99m-labeled-dimercaptosuccinic acid
99mTc-DTPA: technetium-99m-labeled-diethylenetriamine penta-acetic acid
99mTc-MAG3: technetiumm-99m-labeled mercaptoacetyl triglycine

The guidance in this report does not indicate an exclusive course of treatment or serve as a standard of medical care. Variations, taking into account individual circumstances, may be appropriate.

All clinical reports from the American Academy of Pediatrics automatically expire 5 years after publication unless reaffirmed, revised, or retired at or before that time.

FUNDING: No external funding.

https://doi.org/10.1542/peds.2025-071814

REFERENCES

1. Zee RS, Herndon CDA, Cooper CS, et al. Time to resolution: A prospective evaluation from the Society for Fetal Urology hydronephrosis registry. *J Pediatr Urol.* 2017;13(3):316.e1–316.e5. PubMed doi: 10.1016/j.jpurol.2016.12.012
2. Braga LH, McGrath M, Farrokhyar F, Jegatheeswaran K, Lorenzo AJ. Society for Fetal Urology classification vs urinary tract dilation grading system for prognostication in prenatal hydronephrosis: a time to resolution analysis. *J Urol.* 2017;0(0). PubMed doi: 10.1016/j.juro.2017.11.077
3. Braga LH, Farrokhyar F, D'Cruz J, Pemberton J, Lorenzo AJ. Risk factors for febrile urinary tract infection in children with prenatal hydronephrosis: a prospective study. *J Urol.* 2015;193(5)(suppl):1766–1771. PubMed doi: 10.1016/j.juro.2014.10.091
4. Zee RS, Herbst KW, Kim C, et al. Urinary tract infections in children with prenatal hydronephrosis: A risk assessment from the Society for Fetal Urology Hydronephrosis Registry. *J Pediatr Urol.* 2016;12(4):261.e1–261.e7. PubMed doi: 10.1016/j.jpurol.2016.04.024
5. Park JM. Embryology of the genitourinary tract. In: Partin AW, Dmochowski R, Kavoussi L, Peters C, Wein A, eds. *Cambell-Walsh Urology.* 11th ed. Elsevier; 2016:2823–2848.
6. Gonçalves LF, Jeanty P, Piper JM. The accuracy of prenatal ultrasonography in detecting congenital anomalies. *Am J Obstet*

Gynecol. 1994;171(6):1606–1612. PubMed doi: 10.1016/0002-9378(94)90411-1

7. Committee on Practice Bulletins—Obstetrics and the American Institute of Ultrasound in Medicine. Practice Bulletin No. 175: Ultrasound in pregnancy. *Obstet Gynecol.* 2016;128(6):e241–e256. PubMed doi: 10.1097/AOG.0000000000001815
8. American College of Obstetricians and Gynecologists. ACOG Practice Bulletin No. 101: Ultrasonography in pregnancy. *Obstet Gynecol.* 2009;113(2 Pt 1):451–461. PubMed doi: 10.1097/AOG.0b013e31819930b0
9. Lee RS, Cendron M, Kinnamon DD, Nguyen HT. Antenatal hydronephrosis as a predictor of postnatal outcome: a meta-analysis. *Pediatrics.* 2006;118(2):586–593. PubMed doi: 10.1542/peds.2006-0120
10. Sidhu G, Beyene J, Rosenblum ND. Outcome of isolated antenatal hydronephrosis: a systematic review and meta-analysis. *Pediatr Nephrol.* 2006;21(2):218–224. PubMed doi: 10.1007/s00467-005-2100-9
11. Barbosa JABA, Chow JS, Benson CB, et al. Postnatal longitudinal evaluation of children diagnosed with prenatal hydronephrosis: insights in natural history and referral pattern. *Prenat Diagn.* 2012;32(13):1242–1249. PubMed doi: 10.1002/pd.3989
12. Andrés-Jensen L, Jørgensen FS, Thorup J, et al. The outcome of antenatal ultrasound diagnosed anomalies of the kidney and urinary tract in a large Danish birth cohort. *Arch Dis Child.* 2016;101(9):819–824. PubMed doi: 10.1136/archdischild-2015-309784
13. Madden-Fuentes RJ, McNamara ER, Nseyo U, Wiener JS, Routh JC, Ross SS. Resolution rate of isolated low-grade hydronephrosis diagnosed within the first year of life. *J Pediatr Urol.* 2014;10(4):639–644. PubMed doi: 10.1016/j.jpurol.2014.07.004
14. Duin LK, Willekes C, Koster-Kamphuis L, Offermans J, Nijhuis JG. Fetal hydronephrosis: does adding an extra parameter improve detection of neonatal uropathies? *J Matern Fetal Neonatal Med.* 2012;25(7):920–923. PubMed doi: 10.3109/14767058.2011.600365
15. Coelho GM, Bouzada MCF, Pereira AK, et al. Outcome of isolated antenatal hydronephrosis: a prospective cohort study. *Pediatr Nephrol.* 2007;22(10):1727–1734. PubMed doi: 10.1007/s00467-007-0539-6
16. Psooy K, Pike J. Investigation and management of antenatally detected hydronephrosis. *Can Urol Assoc J.* 2009;3(1):69–72. PubMed doi: 10.5489/cuaj.1027
17. Coplen DE, Austin PF, Yan Y, Blanco VM, Dicke JM. The magnitude of fetal renal pelvic dilatation can identify obstructive postnatal hydronephrosis, and direct postnatal evaluation and management. *J Urol.* 2006;176(2):724–727. PubMed doi: 10.1016/j.juro.2006.03.079
18. Nguyen HT, Benson CB, Bromley B, et al. Multidisciplinary consensus on the classification of prenatal and postnatal urinary tract dilation (UTD classification system). *J Pediatr Urol.* 2014;10(6):982–998. PubMed doi: 10.1016/j.jpurol.2014.10.002
19. Sencan A, Carvas F, Hekimoglu IC, et al. Urinary tract infection and vesicoureteral reflux in children with mild antenatal hydronephrosis. *J Pediatr Urol.* 2014;10(6):1008–1013. PubMed doi: 10.1016/j.jpurol.2014.04.001
20. Dias CS, Silva JMP, Pereira AK, et al. Diagnostic accuracy of renal pelvic dilatation for detecting surgically managed ureteropelvic junction obstruction. *J Urol.* 2013;190(2):661–666. PubMed doi: 10.1016/j.juro.2013.02.014
21. Signorelli M, Cerri V, Taddei F, Groli C, Bianchi UA. Prenatal diagnosis and management of mild fetal pyelectasis: implications for neonatal outcome and follow-up. *Eur J Obstet Gynecol Reprod Biol.* 2005;118(2):154–159. PubMed doi: 10.1016/j.ejogrb.2004.04.023
22. Swenson DW, Darge K, Ziniel SI, Chow JS. Characterizing upper urinary tract dilation on ultrasound: a survey of North American pediatric radiologists' practices. *Pediatr Radiol.* 2015;45(5):686–694. PubMed doi: 10.1007/s00247-014-3221-8
23. Dhillon HK. Prenatally diagnosed hydronephrosis: the Great Ormond Street experience. *Br J Urol.* 1998;81(S2)(suppl 2):39–44. PubMed doi: 10.1046/j.1464-410X.1998.0810s2039.x
24. Hothi DK, Wade AS, Gilbert R, Winyard PJD. Mild fetal renal pelvis dilatation: much ado about nothing? *Clin J Am Soc Nephrol.* 2009;4(1):168–177. PubMed doi: 10.2215/CJN.00810208
25. Fernbach SK, Maizels M, Conway JJ. Ultrasound grading of hydronephrosis: introduction to the system used by the Society for Fetal Urology. *Pediatr Radiol.* 1993;23(6):478–480. PubMed doi: 10.1007/BF02012459
26. Zanetta VC, Rosman BM, Bromley B, et al. Variations in management of mild prenatal hydronephrosis among maternal-fetal medicine obstetricians, and pediatric urologists and radiologists. *J Urol.* 2012;188(5):1935–1939. PubMed doi: 10.1016/j.juro.2012.07.011
27. Ismail A, Elkholy A, Zaghmout O, et al. Postnatal management of antenatally diagnosed ureteropelvic junction obstruction. *J Pediatr Urol.* 2006;2(3):163–168. PubMed doi: 10.1016/j.jpurol.2005.07.005
28. Viteri B, Calle-Toro JS, Furth S, Darge K, Hartung EA, Otero H. State-of-the-art renal imaging in children. *Pediatrics.* 2020;145(2):e20190829. PubMed doi: 10.1542/peds.2019-0829
29. Calle-Toro JS, Maya CL, Gorfu Y, Dunn E, Darge K, Back SJ. Supine versus prone positioning for ultrasound evaluation of postnatal urinary tract dilation in children. *Pediatr Radiol.* 2020;50(3):357–362. PubMed doi: 10.1007/s00247-019-04546-7
30. Djahangirian O, Young I, Dorgalli C, et al. Safe discharge parameters for patients with isolated antenatal hydronephrosis. *J Pediatr Urol.* 2018;14(4):321.e1–321.e5. PubMed doi: 10.1016/j.jpurol.2018.04.016
31. Zhang L, Liu C, Li Y, Sun C, Li X. Determination of the need for surgical intervention in infants diagnosed with fetal hydronephrosis in China. *Med Sci Monit.* 2016;22:4210–4217. PubMed doi: 10.12659/MSM.897665
32. Wiener JS, O'Hara SM. Optimal timing of initial postnatal ultrasonography in newborns with prenatal hydronephrosis. *J Urol.* 2002;168(4 Pt 2):1826–1829. PubMed doi: 10.1016/S0022-5347(05)64423-0
33. Laing FC, Burke VD, Wing VW, Jeffrey RB Jr, Hashimoto B. Postpartum evaluation of fetal hydronephrosis: optimal timing for follow-up sonography. *Radiology.* 1984;152(2):423–424. PubMed doi: 10.1148/radiology.152.2.6539930

34. Dejter SW Jr, Gibbons MD. The fate of infant kidneys with fetal hydronephrosis but initially normal postnatal sonography. *J Urol.* 1989;142(2 Pt 2):661–662. PubMed doi: 10.1016/S0022-5347(17)38846-8

35. Passerotti CC, Kalish LA, Chow J, et al. The predictive value of the first postnatal ultrasound in children with antenatal hydronephrosis. *J Pediatr Urol.* 2011;7(2):128–136. PubMed doi: 10.1016/j.jpurol.2010.09.007

36. Arora S, Yadav P, Kumar M, et al. Predictors for the need of surgery in antenatally detected hydronephrosis due to UPJ obstruction–a prospective multivariate analysis. *J Pediatr Urol.* 2015;11(5):248.e1–248.e5. PubMed doi: 10.1016/j.jpurol.2015.02.008

37. American College of Radiology. ACR Practice Guideline for the Performance of Voiding Cystourethrography in Children. Amended 2006. Accessed March 25, 2025. https://raflibrary.com/wp-content/uploads/2022/08/VCUG-Pedi-Guidelines-VCUG-Pedi-Guidelines.pdf

38. Frimberger D, Mercado-Deane M-G, McKenna PH, et al; SECTION ON UROLOGY; SECTION ON RADIOLOGY. Establishing a standard protocol for the voiding cystourethrography. *Pediatrics.* 2016;138(5):e20162590. PubMed doi: 10.1542/peds.2016-2590

39. Phan V, Traubici J, Hershenfield B, Stephens D, Rosenblum ND, Geary DF. Vesicoureteral reflux in infants with isolated antenatal hydronephrosis. *Pediatr Nephrol.* 2003;18(12):1224–1228. PubMed doi: 10.1007/s00467-003-1287-x

40. Gloor JM, Ramsey PS, Ogburn PL Jr, Danilenko-Dixon DR, DiMarco CS, Ramin KD. The association of isolated mild fetal hydronephrosis with postnatal vesicoureteral reflux. *J Matern Fetal Neonatal Med.* 2002;12(3):196–200. PubMed doi: 10.1080/jmf.12.3.196.200

41. van Eerde AM, Meutgeert MH, de Jong TPVM, Giltay JC. Vesicoureteral reflux in children with prenatally detected hydronephrosis: a systematic review. *Ultrasound Obstet Gynecol.* 2007;29(4):463–469. PubMed doi: 10.1002/uog.3975

42. Brophy MM, Austin PF, Yan Y, Coplen DE. Vesicoureteral reflux and clinical outcomes in infants with prenatally detected hydronephrosis. *J Urol.* 2002;168(4 Pt 2):1716–1719. PubMed doi: 10.1097/00005392-200210020-00014

43. Berrocal T, Pinilla I, Gutiérrez J, Prieto C, de Pablo L, Del Hoyo ML. Mild hydronephrosis in newborns and infants: can ultrasound predict the presence of vesicoureteral reflux. *Pediatr Nephrol.* 2007;22(1):91–96. PubMed doi: 10.1007/s00467-006-0285-1

44. Estrada CR, Peters CA, Retik AB, Nguyen HT. Vesicoureteral reflux and urinary tract infection in children with a history of prenatal hydronephrosis–should voiding cystourethrography be performed in cases of postnatally persistent grade II hydronephrosis? *J Urol.* 2009;181(2):801–806. PubMed doi: 10.1016/j.juro.2008.10.057

45. Vemulakonda VM, Chiang G, Corbett ST. Variability in use of voiding cystourethrogram during initial evaluation of infants with congenital hydronephrosis. *Urology.* 2014;83(5):1135–1138. PubMed doi: 10.1016/j.urology.2013.11.011

46. Jackson JN, Zee RS, Martin AN, Corbett ST, Herndon CDA. A practice pattern assessment of members of the Society of Pediatric Urology for evaluation and treatment of urinary tract dilation. *J Pediatr Urol.* 2017;13(6):602–607. PubMed doi: 10.1016/j.jpurol.2017.03.032

47. Papadopoulou F, Efremidis SC, Oiconomou A, et al. Cyclic voiding cystourethrography: is vesicoureteral reflux missed with standard voiding cystourethrography? *Eur Radiol.* 2002;12(3):666–670. PubMed doi: 10.1007/s003300101108

48. Riccabona M, Vivier PH, Ntoulia A, et al; ESPR Uroradiology Task Force. ESPR uroradiology task force imaging recommendations in paediatric uroradiology, part VII: standardised terminology, impact of existing recommendations, and update on contrast-enhanced ultrasound of the paediatric urogenital tract. *Pediatr Radiol.* 2014;44(11):1478–1484. PubMed doi: 10.1007/s00247-014-3135-5

49. Papadopoulou F, Anthopoulou A, Siomou E, Efremidis S, Tsamboulas C, Darge K. Harmonic voiding urosonography with a second-generation contrast agent for the diagnosis of vesicoureteral reflux. *Pediatr Radiol.* 2009;39(3):239–244. PubMed doi: 10.1007/s00247-008-1080-x

50. Darge K. Voiding urosonography with US contrast agents for the diagnosis of vesicoureteric reflux in children. II. Comparison with radiological examinations. *Pediatr Radiol.* 2008;38(1):54–63. PubMed doi: 10.1007/s00247-007-0528-8

51. Taylor AT. Radionuclides in nephrourology, part 1: Radiopharmaceuticals, quality control, and quantitative indices. *J Nucl Med.* 2014;55(4):608–615. PubMed doi: 10.2967/jnumed.113.133447

52. Taylor A Jr, Nally JV. Clinical applications of renal scintigraphy. *AJR Am J Roentgenol.* 1995;164(1):31–41. PubMed doi: 10.2214/ajr.164.1.7998566

53. Ziessman HA. Genitourinary system. In: Ziessman HA, O'Malley J, Thrall J, eds. *Nuclear Medicine: The Requisites.* 4th ed. Elsevier; 2014:168–203.

54. Mujoomdar M, Russell E, Dionne F, et al. *Optimizing Health System Use of Medical Isotopes and Other Imaging Modalities.* Canadian Agency for Drugs and Technologies in Health; 2012.

55. Piepsz A, Ham H. Measurement of GFR in children: means of radionuclide technique. In: Prigent A, Piepsz A, eds. *Functional Imaging in Nephro-Urology.* Routledge; 2006:11–18, 31–35.

56. Stabin M, Taylor A Jr, Eshima D, Wooter W. Radiation dosimetry for technetium-99m-MAG3, technetium-99m-DTPA, and iodine-131-OIH based on human biodistribution studies. *J Nucl Med.* 1992;33(1):33–40. PubMed

57. Durand E, Chaumet-Riffaud P, Grenier N. Functional renal imaging: new trends in radiology and nuclear medicine. *Semin Nucl Med.* 2011;41(1):61–72. PubMed doi: 10.1053/j.semnuclmed.2010.08.003

58. Esteves FP, Taylor A, Manatunga A, Folks RD, Krishnan M, Garcia EV. 99mTc-MAG3 renography: normal values for MAG3 clearance and curve parameters, excretory parameters, and residual urine volume. *AJR Am J Roentgenol.* 2006;187(6):W610–7. PubMed doi: 10.2214/AJR.05.1550

59. Wong JC, Rossleigh MA, Farnsworth RH. Utility of technetium-99m-MAG3 diuretic renography in the neonatal period. *J Nucl Med.* 1995;36(12):2214–2219. PubMed

60. Bayne CE, Majd M, Rushton HG. Diuresis renography in the evaluation and management of pediatric hydronephrosis: What have we learned? *J Pediatr Urol.* 2019;15(2):128–137. PubMed doi: 10.1016/j.jpurol.2019.01.011

61. Chung S, Majd M, Rushton HG, Belman AB. Diuretic renography in the evaluation of neonatal hydronephrosis: is it reliable? *J Urol.* 1993;150(2 Pt 2):765–768. PubMed doi: 10.1016/S0022-5347(17)35609-4

62. Shulkin BL, Mandell GA, Cooper JA, et al. Procedure guideline for diuretic renography in children 3.0. *J Nucl Med Technol.* 2008; 36(3):162–168. PubMed doi: 10.2967/jnmt.108.056622

63. Treves ST, Baker A, Fahey FH, et al. Nuclear Medicine in the First Year of Life. PubMed doi: 10.2967/jnumed.110.084202

64. Gordon I, Piepsz A, Sixt R; Auspices of Paediatric Committee of European Association of Nuclear Medicine. Guidelines for standard and diuretic renogram in children. *Eur J Nucl Med Mol Imaging.* 2011;38(6):1175–1188. PubMed doi: 10.1007/s00259-011-1811-3

65. Pavicevic PK, Saranovic DZ, Mandic MJ, et al. Efficacy of Magnetic Resonance urography in detecting crossing renal vessels in children with ureteropelvic junction obstruction. *Ann Ital Chir.* 2015; 86(5):443–449. PubMed

66. McMann LP, Kirsch AJ, Scherz HC, et al. Magnetic resonance urography in the evaluation of prenatally diagnosed hydronephrosis and renal dysgenesis. *J Urol.* 2006;176(4 Pt 2):1786–1792. PubMed doi: 10.1016/j.juro.2006.05.025

67. Leppert A, Nadalin S, Schirg E, et al. Impact of magnetic resonance urography on preoperative diagnostic workup in children affected by hydronephrosis: should IVU be replaced? *J Pediatr Surg.* 2002;37(10):1441–1445. PubMed doi: 10.1053/jpsu.2002.35408

68. Khrichenko D, Darge K. Functional analysis in MR urography - made simple. *Pediatr Radiol.* 2010;40(2):182–199. PubMed doi: 10.1007/s00247-009-1458-4

69. Jones RA, Perez-Brayfield MR, Kirsch AJ, Grattan-Smith JD. Renal transit time with MR urography in children. *Radiology.* 2004; 233(1):41–50. PubMed doi: 10.1148/radiol.2331031117

70. Chamberlin JD, Braga LH, Davis-Dao CA, et al. Continuous antibiotic prophylaxis in isolated prenatal hydronephrosis. *J Pediatr Urol.* 2022;18(3):363.e1–363.e7. PubMed doi: 10.1016/j.jpurol.2022.03.027

71. Holzman SA, Braga LH, Zee RS, et al. Risk of urinary tract infection in patients with hydroureter: An analysis from the Society of Fetal Urology Prenatal Hydronephrosis Registry. *J Pediatr Urol.* 2021; 17(6):775–781. PubMed doi: 10.1016/j.jpurol.2021.09.001

72. Silay MS, Undre S, Nambiar AK, et al. Role of antibiotic prophylaxis in antenatal hydronephrosis: A systematic review from the European Association of Urology/European Society for Paediatric Urology Guidelines Panel. *J Pediatr Urol.* 2017;13(3):306–315. PubMed doi: 10.1016/j.jpurol.2017.02.023

73. Easterbrook B, Capolicchio JP, Braga LH. Antibiotic prophylaxis for prevention of urinary tract infections in prenatal hydronephrosis: An updated systematic review. *Can Urol Assoc J.* 2017; 11(1–2Suppl1):S3–S11. PubMed doi: 10.5489/cuaj.4384

74. Braga LH, Mijovic H, Farrokhyar F, Pemberton J, DeMaria J, Lorenzo AJ. Antibiotic prophylaxis for urinary tract infections in antenatal hydronephrosis. *Pediatrics* 2013;131(1):e251–e261. PubMed doi: 10.1542/peds.2012-1870

75. Zareba P, Lorenzo AJ, Braga LH. Risk factors for febrile urinary tract infection in infants with prenatal hydronephrosis: comprehensive single center analysis. *J Urol.* 2014;191(5)(suppl):1614–1618. PubMed doi: 10.1016/j.juro.2013.10.035

76. Herz D, Merguerian P, McQuiston L. Continuous antibiotic prophylaxis reduces the risk of febrile UTI in children with asymptomatic antenatal hydronephrosis with either ureteral dilation, high-grade vesicoureteral reflux, or ureterovesical junction obstruction. *J Pediatr Urol.* 2014;10(4):650–654. PubMed doi: 10.1016/j.jpurol.2014.06.009

77. Szymanski KM, Al-Said AN, Pippi Salle JL, Capolicchio JP. Do infants with mild prenatal hydronephrosis benefit from screening for vesicoureteral reflux? *J Urol.* 2012;188(2):576–581. PubMed doi: 10.1016/j.juro.2012.04.017

78. Lee JH, Choi HS, Kim JK, et al. Nonrefluxing neonatal hydronephrosis and the risk of urinary tract infection. *J Urol.* 2008;179(4): 1524–1528. PubMed doi: 10.1016/j.juro.2007.11.090

79. Braga LH, Pemberton J, Heaman J, DeMaria J, Lorenzo AJ. Pilot randomized, placebo controlled trial to investigate the effect of antibiotic prophylaxis on the rate of urinary tract infection in infants with prenatal hydronephrosis. *J Urol.* 2014;191(5)(suppl):1501–1507. PubMed doi: 10.1016/j.juro.2013.10.033

80. Leigh J, Rickard M, Sanger S, Petropoulos J, Braga LH, Chanchlani R. Antibiotic prophylaxis for prevention of urinary tract infections in the first year of life in children with vesicoureteral reflux diagnosed in the workup of antenatal hydronephrosis: a systematic review. *Pediatr Nephrol.* 2020;35(9):1639–1646. PubMed doi: 10.1007/s00467-020-04568-6

81. Braga LH, McGrath M, Farrokhyar F, Jegatheeswaran K, Lorenzo AJ. Associations of initial Society for Fetal Urology grades and urinary tract dilatation risk groups with clinical outcomes in patients with isolated prenatal hydronephrosis. *J Urol.* 2017;197(3 Pt 2): 831–837. PubMed doi: 10.1016/j.juro.2016.08.099

82. Walsh TJ, Hsieh S, Grady R, Mueller BA. Antenatal hydronephrosis and the risk of pyelonephritis hospitalization during the first year of life. *Urology.* 2007;69(5):970–974. PubMed doi: 10.1016/j.urology.2007.01.062

83. Varda BK, Finkelstein JB, Wang HH, Logvinenko T, Nelson CP. The association between continuous antibiotic prophylaxis and UTI from birth until initial postnatal imaging evaluation among newborns with antenatal hydronephrosis. *J Pediatr Urol.* 2018;14(6): 539.e1–539.e6. PubMed doi: 10.1016/j.jpurol.2018.04.022

84. Shaikh N, Haralam MA, Kurs-Lasky M, Hoberman A. Association of renal scarring with number of febrile urinary tract infections in children. *JAMA Pediatr.* 2019;173(10):949–952. PubMed doi: 10.1001/jamapediatrics.2019.2504

85. Hoberman A, Greenfield SP, Mattoo TK, et al; RIVUR Trial Investigators. Antimicrobial prophylaxis for children with vesicoureteral reflux. *N Engl J Med.* 2014;370(25):2367–2376. PubMed doi: 10.1056/NEJMoa1401811

86. Wang HHS, Gbadegesin RA, Foreman JW, et al. Efficacy of antibiotic prophylaxis in children with vesicoureteral reflux: systematic review and meta-analysis. *J Urol.* 2015;193(3):963–969. PubMed doi: 10.1016/j.juro.2014.08.112

87. Hewitt IK, Pennesi M, Morello W, Ronfani L, Montini G. Antibiotic prophylaxis for urinary tract infection-related renal scarring: a systematic review. *Pediatrics.* 2017;139(5):e20163145. PubMed doi: 10.1542/peds.2016-3145

88. Hari P, Hari S, Sinha A, et al. Antibiotic prophylaxis in the management of vesicoureteric reflux: a randomized double-blind placebo-controlled trial. *Pediatr Nephrol.* 2015;30(3):479–486. PubMed doi: 10.1007/s00467-014-2943-z

89. Mattoo TK, Chesney RW, Greenfield SP, et al; RIVUR Trial Investigators. Renal scarring in the randomized intervention for children with vesicoureteral reflux (RIVUR) trial. *Clin J Am Soc Nephrol.* 2016;11(1):54–61. PubMed doi: 10.2215/CJN.05210515

90. Wang ZT, Wehbi E, Alam Y, Khoury A. A reanalysis of the RIVUR Trial using a risk classification system. *J Urol.* 2018;199(6):1608–1614. PubMed doi: 10.1016/j.juro.2017.11.080

91. Pennesi M, Travan L, Peratoner L, et al; North East Italy Prophylaxis in VUR study group. Is antibiotic prophylaxis in children with vesicoureteral reflux effective in preventing pyelonephritis and renal scars? A randomized, controlled trial. *Pediatrics.* 2008;121(6):e1489–e1494. PubMed doi: 10.1542/peds.2007-2652

92. Montini G, Rigon L, Zucchetta P, et al; IRIS Group. Prophylaxis after first febrile urinary tract infection in children? A multicenter, randomized, controlled, noninferiority trial. *Pediatrics.* 2008;122(5):1064–1071. PubMed doi: 10.1542/peds.2007-3770

93. Garin EH, Olavarria F, Garcia Nieto V, Valenciano B, Campos A, Young L. Clinical significance of primary vesicoureteral reflux and urinary antibiotic prophylaxis after acute pyelonephritis: a multicenter, randomized, controlled study. *Pediatrics.* 2006;117(3):626–632. PubMed doi: 10.1542/peds.2005-1362

94. Faiz S, Zaveri MP, Perry JC, Schuetz TM, Cancarevic I. Role of antibiotic prophylaxis in the management of antenatal hydronephrosis, vesicoureteral reflux, and ureterocele in infants. *Cureus.* 2020;12(7):e9064. PubMed doi: 10.7759/cureus.9064

95. Wong NC, Koyle MA, Braga LH. Continuous antibiotic prophylaxis in the setting of prenatal hydronephrosis and vesicoureteral reflux. *Can Urol Assoc J.* 2017;11(1–2S):20. PubMed doi: 10.5489/cuaj.4387

96. Selekman RE, Shapiro DJ, Boscardin J, et al. Uropathogen resistance and antibiotic prophylaxis: a meta-analysis. *Pediatrics.* 2018;142(1):e20180119. PubMed doi: 10.1542/peds.2018-0119

97. Williams G, Craig JC. Long-term antibiotics for preventing recurrent urinary tract infection in children. *Cochrane Database Syst Rev.* 2019;4(4):CD001534. PubMed doi: 10.1002/14651858.CD001534.pub4

98. Fusco NM, Islam S, Polischuk E. Optimal antibiotics at hospital discharge for children with urinary tract infection. *Hosp Pediatr.* 2020;10(5):438–442. PubMed doi: 10.1542/hpeds.2019-0301

99. Herndon CDA. The role of ultrasound in predicting surgical intervention for prenatal hydronephrosis. *J Urol.* 2012;187(5):1535–1536. PubMed doi: 10.1016/j.juro.2012.02.011

100. Shamshirsaz AA, Ravangard SF, Egan JF, et al. Fetal hydronephrosis as a predictor of neonatal urologic outcomes. *J Ultrasound Med.* 2012;31(6):947–954. PubMed doi: 10.7863/jum.2012.31.6.947

101. Burgu B, Aydogdu O, Soygur T, Baker L, Snodgrass W, Wilcox D. When is it necessary to perform nuclear renogram in patients with a unilateral neonatal hydronephrosis? *World J Urol.* 2012;30(3):347–352. PubMed doi: 10.1007/s00345-011-0744-6

102. Erickson BA, Maizels M, Shore RM, et al. Newborn society of fetal urology grade 3 hydronephrosis is equivalent to preserved percentage differential function. *J Pediatr Urol.* 2007;3(5):382–386. PubMed doi: 10.1016/j.jpurol.2007.01.196

103. Herndon CD, McKenna PH, Kolon TF, Gonzales ET, Baker LA, Docimo SG. A multicenter outcomes analysis of patients with neonatal reflux presenting with prenatal hydronephrosis. *J Urol.* 1999;162(3 Pt 2):1203–1208. PubMed doi: 10.1016/S0022-5347(01)68134-5

104. Nguyen HT, Herndon CDA, Cooper C, et al. The Society for Fetal Urology consensus statement on the evaluation and management of antenatal hydronephrosis. *J Pediatr Urol.* 2010;6(3):212–231. PubMed doi: 10.1016/j.jpurol.2010.02.205

105. Upadhyay J, McLorie GA, Bolduc S, Bägli DJ, Khoury AE, Farhat W. Natural history of neonatal reflux associated with prenatal hydronephrosis: long-term results of a prospective study. *J Urol.* 2003;169(5):1837–1841. PubMed doi: 10.1097/01.ju.0000062440.92454.cf

106. Feldman DM, DeCambre M, Kong E, et al. Evaluation and follow-up of fetal hydronephrosis. *J Ultrasound Med.* 2001;20(10):1065–1069. PubMed doi: 10.7863/jum.2001.20.10.1065

107. Podevin G, Mandelbrot L, Vuillard E, Oury JF, Aigrain Y. Outcome of urological abnormalities prenatally diagnosed by ultrasound. *Fetal Diagn Ther.* 1996;11(3):181–190. PubMed doi: 10.1159/000264300

108. Sairam S, Al-Habib A, Sasson S, Thilaganathan B. Natural history of fetal hydronephrosis diagnosed on mid-trimester ultrasound. *Ultrasound Obstet Gynecol.* 2001;17(3):191–196. PubMed doi: 10.1046/j.1469-0705.2001.00333.x

109. Scarborough PL, Ferrara E, Storm DW. Should prenatal hydronephrosis that resolves before birth be followed postnatally? Analysis and comparison to persistent prenatal hydronephrosis. *Pediatr Nephrol.* 2015;30(9):1485–1491. PubMed doi: 10.1007/s00467-015-3080-z

110. Maclaurin JC. Changes in body water distribution during the first two weeks of life. *Arch Dis Child.* 1966;41(217):286–291. PubMed doi: 10.1136/adc.41.217.286

111. Aksu N, Yavaşcan O, Kangin M, et al. Postnatal management of infants with antenatally detected hydronephrosis. *Pediatr Nephrol.* 2005;20(9):1253–1259. PubMed doi: 10.1007/s00467-005-1989-3

112. Capolicchio J-P, Braga LH, Szymanski KM. Canadian Urological Association/Pediatric Urologists of Canada guideline on the investigation and management of antenatally detected hydronephrosis. *Can Urol Assoc J.* 2018;12(4):85–92. PubMed doi: 10.5489/cuaj.5094

Postnatal Cord Blood Sampling

- *Clinical Report*

CLINICAL REPORT Guidance for the Clinician in Rendering Pediatric Care

American Academy of Pediatrics

DEDICATED TO THE HEALTH OF ALL CHILDREN™

Postnatal Cord Blood Sampling: Clinical Report

David A. Kaufman, MD, FAAP,[1] Ashley M. Lucke, MD, FAAP,[2] James J. Cummings, MD, FAAP,[3] and the Committee on Fetus and Newborn

abstract

Blood contained in the umbilical cord after placental separation originates from the infant and can be used for neonatal blood sampling and testing after birth. The most common indications for phlebotomy after birth include care processes for any infant admitted to the neonatal intensive care unit, early-onset sepsis evaluations, and congenital anomalies. Postnatal umbilical cord blood sampling (PCBS), rather than obtaining blood from the neonate, avoids significant neonatal blood loss at a critical time of extrauterine transition and prevents phlebotomy pain in infants without a catheter for blood drawing. Studies of PCBS in very low birth weight infants have demonstrated additional benefits including stable blood pressure, less need for vasopressors and erythrocyte transfusions in the first week, and a potentially decreased risk for intracranial hemorrhage.

PCBS can be used for any full-term or preterm infant when the need for phlebotomy is known at or shorty after delivery. PCBS can be the first option and reliably used for complete blood cell counts, blood cultures, blood typing and crossmatching, newborn screening and metabolic tests, genetic testing, blood chemistries, and coagulation studies. Additionally, PCBS allows the collection of larger blood volumes for blood culture, thereby improving positivity rate. Finally, PCBS can be performed after delayed cord clamping or cord milking and in conjunction with research studies and/or cord blood banking. This report describes the evidence, safety, and methods for collecting cord blood after delivery.

[1]Department of Pediatrics, Division of Neonatology, University of Virginia School of Medicine, Charlottesville, Virginia; [2]Emeritus Professor of Pediatrics and Bioethics, Albany Medical College, Albany, New York; and [3]Department of Pediatrics, Dell Medical School, The University of Texas at Austin, Pediatrix Medical Group of Austin, Austin, Texas

Address correspondence to: David A. Kaufman, MD, FAAP. kaufman.da@gmail.com

Dr Kaufman drafted the initial manuscript, and critically reviewed and revised the manuscript. Drs Lucke and Cummings critically reviewed and revised the manuscript. All authors approved the final manuscript as submitted and agree to be accountable for all aspects of the work.

CONFLICT OF INTEREST DISCLOSURE: The authors have indicated they have no potential conflicts of interest to disclose.

To cite: Kaufman DA, Lucke AM, Cummings JJ; American Academy of Pediatrics, Committee on Fetus and Newborn. Postnatal Cord Blood Sampling: Clinical Report. *Pediatrics.* 2025;155(6):e2025071811

INTRODUCTION

Blood Losses Attributable to Phlebotomy After Birth

Neonates requiring evaluation for infection or neonatal intensive care unit (NICU) admission frequently undergo phlebotomy within the first hours after birth. For preterm infants, this initial blood draw may remove as much as 10% of an infant's blood volume, which may compromise the infant's blood pressure stability.[1] One study of very low birth weight (VLBW) infants measured 7.5 (±5.2) mL/kg of blood loss attributable to phlebotomy in the first 24 hours after birth.[1] In addition to diminishing the neonatal blood volume, phlebotomy removes neonatal blood stem cells and other important cell lines that aid in the recovery, repair, and possibly replacement of injured cells that may contribute to improved outcomes.[2,3] The initial and subsequent phlebotomies directly from neonates during the first days in the NICU result in lower hematocrits in preterm and term infants and are associated with an increase need for vasopressors, early erythrocyte transfusion(s), and potentially severe intraventricular hemorrhage in VLBW infants.[4–8]

Phlebotomy After Birth May Involve One or More Painful Procedures

For infants who do not have a catheter for blood drawing, phlebotomy involves one or more painful procedures to obtain blood via venipuncture, arterial, or capillary puncture. Decreasing pain is a focus for the care of all newborn infants and pain can have particular adverse effects for those of the youngest gestational ages in the first hours after delivery, for whom vital sign changes and stress factor into intracranial hemorrhage risk.[9]

POSTNATAL CORD BLOOD SAMPLING

Blood within the umbilical cord and in the fetal circuit within the placenta is the infant's blood; hence, it is ideal for the infant's initial blood draw.[10–12] The maternal and fetal circulation are separate. PCBS for initial laboratory testing maintains the infant's blood volume at the critical time immediately following delivery, transition, and admission.[5,6] Studies of VLBW infants demonstrated that PCBS results in an increase in stable blood pressures, a higher hemoglobin at 24 hours and fewer patients required vasopressors and erythrocyte transfusions in the first week.[5] Infant blood loss from phlebotomy in the first 24 hours can be decreased to 1.5 ± 2.3 mL/kg when PCBS is used for the initial blood sample from 7.5 ± 5.2 mL/kg when it is not.[1] Furthermore, in one study, the blood volume loss in the first 7 days decreased by 13 mL/kg in infants who underwent PCBS.[1]

PCBS studies have demonstrated a correlation of cord complete blood cell counts (CBCs) with differential with results from infant phlebotomy, an improvement in blood culture detection with less contamination, and that cord blood is an appropriate source of infant blood for blood typing, crossmatching, direct antiglobulin testing (DAT), and other tests (described in more detail in the laboratory test section).[1,10–12] There is sufficient blood left in the placenta and cord for PCBS after delayed cord clamping (DCC).[13] This and other references to DCC in this report apply also to umbilical cord milking in appropriate infants. One study demonstrated that PCBS can successfully be obtained approximately 95% of the time and that its success rate is unaffected by DCC.[5] PCBS can be performed by phlebotomy of the umbilical cord attached to the placenta or an alternate method is isolating (via clamping alone or clamping and cutting) and drawing from a ~ 30 cm segment of blood-filled umbilical cord (Figure 1). Recognized benefits of PCBS are summarized in Table 1.

Clinical conditions such as placental abruption and severe intrauterine growth restriction may affect blood volume in the placenta after delivery. Therefore, once the cord is clamped, ideally after DCC has occurred, the clamp needs to remain on the cord or be replaced with a disposable clamp until PCBS is performed to ensure optimal blood volume.

Key action statement: For PCBS to produce optimal blood volumes, the umbilical cord must remain clamped after DCC until PCBS is performed.

PCBS can be accomplished when cord blood is also obtained for research studies or cord blood banking. PCBS has significant potential benefits in VLBW infants and should be attempted and performed when feasible in infants of all gestational ages.

Key action statement: If there is a need for admission laboratory testing, PCBS should be used in all infants.

The volume available for cord banking for infants ≥1500 g is not significantly affected by PCBS.[13] Cord blood banking should neither take precedence nor serve as a reason not to perform PCBS (or DCC) in VLBW infants.

Key action statement: PCBS followed by research studies if needed and/or cord blood banking using the same or different phlebotomy sites can all be successful in most cases with discussion and planning prior to the delivery. In VLBW infants, PCBS should be prioritized over cord blood banking in most cases.

NEONATAL LABORATORY TESTS WITH BLOOD OBTAINED BY PCBS

The feasibility and accuracy of the tests listed in Table 2 with blood from PCBS have been demonstrated in multiple studies.[7] The most commonly obtained laboratory tests include blood culture, CBC with differential, blood type, and crossmatch. Genetic evaluation via genomic microarray and/or karyotype or newer tests, such as whole-exome and whole-genome sequencing, are often performed as well when indicated and can be part of prenatal planning with many congenital conditions. At some centers, the state newborn screen and coagulation studies can be performed using blood obtained from PCBS. Several other tests can be performed on cord blood, such as bilirubin, albumin, and various biomarkers.[14–17] There are only a few laboratory tests that are not recommended routinely, including HIV DNA and RNA nucleic acid testing, because of the high

Postnatal Cord Blood Sampling (PCBS)

1	**Effectively clamp cord (A).** Leave cord segment clamped (after delayed cord clamping), replace with disposable clamp (optional), and place in sterile basin *-Prevents blood leakage form cord and placenta*
2	**Determine blood tests and blood volume needed.** *-Maximizes the number of tests that can be sent using cord blood to decrease infant blood loss. PCBS volume is about 5 to 10 mL.*
3	**Prepare work space.**
4	**Prep phlebotomy site.** -Dry site and remove coating first with sterile gauze to enhance antiseptic effectiveness. -Then apply antiseptic for 30 seconds (eg, chlorhexidine, povidone-iodine or isopropyl alcohol) and then let dry (takes ≥60 seconds). *-Creates sterility for blood cultures*
5	**Draw laboratory sample** by puncturing the umbilical vein as 1st choice or a large surface vein as 2nd choice **(B and C).** -Limit venipuncture to 2 sites to decrease risk of contamination and of team member injury. -Bevel-down approach improves success by preventing vessel collapse. *-Prevents contamination and staff injury*

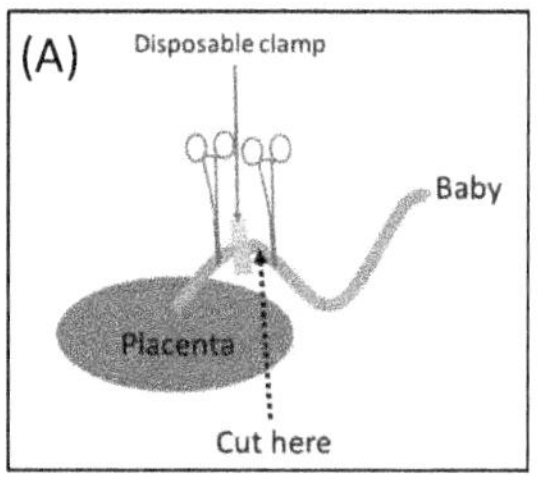

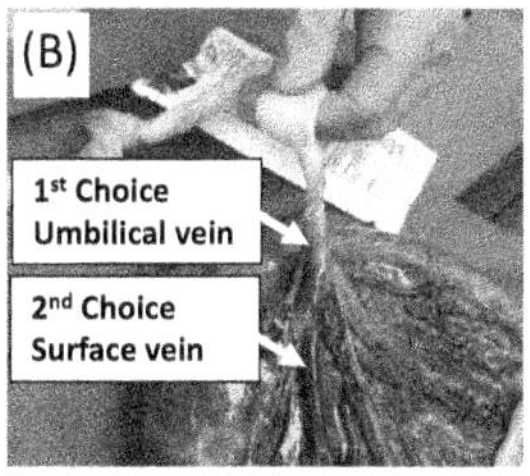

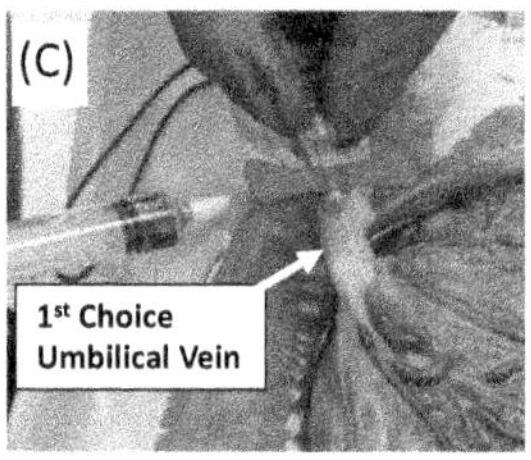

6	**Transfer blood to laboratory tubes.** For blood culture(s), alcohol top of bottle, transfer first with new sterile needle or transfer device. *-Prevents contamination and staff injury*
7	**Return placenta to container.** Do not return to the sterile field. *-Prevents contamination if sterile field present*
8	**Transport blood specimens** to NICU/Nursery. -Label each specimen and the transport bag. -Double bag samples for transport -Print and affix laboratory labels for specimens *-Ensures safe transport and proper assignment of specimens to the correct patient*
9	**Document the procedure.** Include blood culture volume if obtained. Document tests obtained and the disposition of specimens (sent to lab or location stored in some cases—eg, genetics)

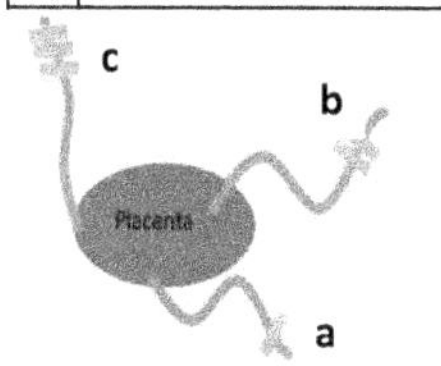

For multiples: 2 clamps for cord of baby "b", 3 clamps on cord of baby "c"

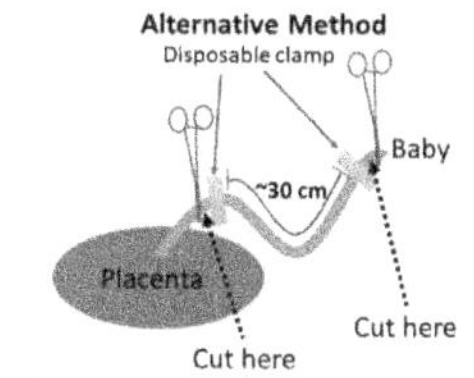

Alternative method: Venipuncture either end of double-clamped blood filled umbilical cord segment (~30 cm)

FIGURE 1.
Postnatal cord blood sampling (PCBS) key steps and rationale.

TABLE 1. Benefits of Postnatal Cord Blood Sampling
Maintains a higher volume of blood cells and plasma in the neonate's circulation at a critical time of neonatal transition
Decreases blood losses attributable to phlebotomy
Prevents hypotension in VLBW infants
Decreases need for vasopressor use in the first 7 d in VLBW infants
Decreases need for early red blood cell transfusions
Decreases risk for intraventricular hemorrhage in VLBW infants
Facilitates improved (larger) blood volume for blood cultures
Easier technique to obtain initial laboratory tests
Potentially reduces one or more procedures associated with unnecessary pain and discomfort and prevents habituation to increased pain response
Abbreviation: VLBW, very low birth weight.

TABLE 2. Studies of Placental Phlebotomy After Delivery for Neonatal Laboratory Tests

Laboratory Test	Number of Studies
Complete blood cell count with differential	11[1,4,5,7,19–24,31]
Blood culture	14[1,4–6,20–23,26–31]
Blood type and crossmatch	4[10–12,34]
Antibody screen	2[4,5]
Genetic studies	1[37]
Coagulation studies	4[1,25,41,42]
Newborn screening tests	2[4,5]

rate of false-positive results and negative results before 14 days after birth are less helpful in excluding HIV infection, though there may be select cases where they may be performed.[18]

CBC With Differential

CBC with differential using blood obtained by PCBS has been validated in several studies. White blood cell count, hemoglobin, and platelet counts may be slightly lower, although not clinically significant, in blood obtained via PCBS when compared with arterial, venous, or capillary blood samples from the neonate.[1,4,5,7,19–24] Some of the differences are attributable to physiologic changes in the first hours of life and are minimized when phlebotomy is timed closest to delivery and within 10 to 30 minutes after delivery.[25] If an isolated double-clamped umbilical cord segment is used, differences are minimized if blood is obtained within 30 minutes after delivery.[25]

Key action statement: PCBS can be used to obtain a reliable CBC with differential.

Blood Cultures

Accuracy and concordance of blood cultures obtained in infants at risk for early-onset sepsis have been examined in several studies.[1,4–6,20–23,26–31] One major advantage of using PCBS is that larger (more optimal) blood volumes of up to 5 mL (for pediatric blood culture bottles) can be obtained, thereby increasing the sensitivity of the blood culture.[30,32] This may also facilitate obtaining anaerobic cultures as part of early-onset infection evaluations.[33,34] Several studies have demonstrated increased detection of early-onset pathogens (eg, *Escherichia coli* and group B streptococci). It is important to remember that the infant, cord, and placenta are delivered through the same environment. Protocols for performing PCBS with appropriate antisepsis of the phlebotomy site, similar to blood culture collection procedures via infant venipuncture or arterial puncture, are critical to obtaining blood cultures without false-positive results or contaminants.[35] Unique to blood culture sampling techniques, the cord phlebotomy site needs to be wiped with sterile gauze to remove coating and dry the site to enhance the effectiveness of the antiseptic applied.[35] Once dry, the antiseptic is applied and allowed to dry, the site kept sterile, blood collected with a sterile needle, followed by changing to a new sterile needle or transfer device before injecting into the blood culture bottle(s). Prior to transfer, the top of blood culture bottles are not sterile and need to be cleaned with alcohol and let dry.

Key action statement: Obtaining PCBS blood cultures, similar to other blood cultures, must be performed as an aseptic procedure.

Blood Type and Crossmatch

Blood typing with antibody and direct antiglobulin testing (DAT) were the first uses of cord blood. Use of PCBS for these tests is a universally accepted standard and newborn practice. PCBS is an appropriate source of infant blood.[1,5,10–12] A recent study of PCBS focused on pretransfusion testing found 100% concordance for ABO and Rh between blood samples obtained by PCBS and infant heel stick.[36] The American Academy of Pediatrics, in the clinical practice guideline on management of hyperbilirubinemia, has recommended that cord blood can be used for blood type, Rh (D) type, and DAT testing.[12]

Key action statement: PCBS can be used to obtain a reliable blood type, DAT testing, and crossmatch.

Genetic Studies

Whole-exome or whole-genome sequencing, chromosomal microarray analysis, and karyotyping are the most common tests to evaluate various neonatal conditions and diseases that may be associated with chromosomal abnormalities.[37,38] PCBS is often used to confirm prenatal genetic diagnoses and to screen for genetic associations or diagnoses for various congenital anomalies. Examples include certain congenital cardiac lesions, nonimmune hydrops fetalis, and congenital diaphragmatic hernia.[39–41] For a perinatal or neonatal death, this may be the only opportunity to obtain important diagnostic information. Depending on the genetic testing needed, significant blood volumes of 2 to 6 mL are often required. Obtaining this volume of blood is more feasible with PCBS than with standard phlebotomy of the neonate after birth.

Other infants worth considering PCBS for genetic (and metabolic) testing include stillborn infants or infants who die in the delivery room or other delivery settings. Cord blood can be collected and then further discussion can occur on which tests to send based on the history and infant findings.

Key action statement: PCBS can be used to obtain genetic studies.

Coagulation Studies

Studies have examined prothrombin time, partial thromboplastin time, fibrinogen, and international normalized ratio and concluded that these tests can be reliably evaluated via PCBS.[1,25,42,43] Because these tests require a large blood volume (minimum of 1.8 mL), PCBS offers a valuable alternative to standard phlebotomy. Optimal timing for blood sampling of coagulation studies is within 30 minutes after delivery.[25]

Key action statement: PCBS can be used to obtain reliable coagulation studies.

Newborn Screening and Metabolic Testing

Blood for newborn screening and metabolic testing may be obtained via PCBS. Because blood products and parenteral nutrition alter newborn screening results and the need for repeat testing, PCBS is ideal as cord blood is unaltered from these interventions. However, obtaining the newborn screen specimen before 24 hours of life (as it would be with PCBS) may result in inaccurate thyroid stimulating hormone, 17-hydroxyprogesterone, and cystic fibrosis (immunoreactive trypsinogen) screens and may necessitate repeat testing. This area is the subject of active research, and further study is needed.[44,45]

Because repeat screening requires additional phlebotomy and in some states additional costs, which sometimes includes the cost of the newborn screening card, each center should discuss the optimal timing of newborn blood screening.

For stillborn infants or infants who die in the delivery room, obtaining blood for the newborn screen could be considered in addition to genetic and other metabolic testing. One can always obtain the cord blood and then discuss further with the team and family.

IMPLEMENTATION

Similar to the institution of any new evidence-based practice, forming a multidisciplinary team with delivery, neonatal, and laboratory personnel that designs and implements PCBS is important for success.[46,47] Evidence continues to emerge supporting the patient benefits presented in this report.[48,49] Baer et al described their implementation and provided a valuable resource as a supplement to their publication.[5] Initial steps include development of a procedural guideline based on key steps outlined in Figure 1 as well as with a detailed procedure guide in the **online appendix**, followed by education of clinicians on the benefits, evidence, and procedure with details on roles and location of supplies. A **fact-sheet** for the delivery team and childbirth providers is included to aid in this education. Establishing a dedicated team to perform PCBS will ensure safety, successful rates of blood collection, sterility for blood cultures, and quality of all blood samples. PCBS does not need to change obstetric practices related to collection of cord blood gases after DCC, just mindfulness to keep the cord clamped to maintain maximal blood volume in the umbilical cord and placenta.[10] When the cord is kept clamped, one will obtain enough blood from the umbilical vein with one phlebotomy in most cases. For team member safety and to decrease risk of contamination, venipuncture should be limited to 2 sites. The need for additional venipuncture usually indicates inadequate blood volume in the cord and placenta and further phlebotomy will not be productive. Some institutions have created carts or packets with supplies located in the delivery areas that can be readily brought to the delivery room or operating suite. Creating carts or packets contributes to the timeliness, organization, and sterility of the procedure.

QUALITY CONTROL

Similar to other process improvement interventions, the implementation of PCBS should include a team champion, a dedicated team to perform PCBS, and a program evaluation using auditing of success frequency and the amount of blood obtained. Programs may develop guidance on the need for confirmatory testing of infants if results report actionable laboratory abnormalities (eg, platelet count $<50\ 000$ μL/mm^3). As with other sources of cultures, microbial growth of a potential contaminant from blood culture may prompt a repeat blood culture immediately in addition to after ≥48 hours of treatment of pathogens to document clearance.

SUMMARY

Blood losses from phlebotomy after birth, and their sequelae, can be minimized by obtaining umbilical cord blood for the initial laboratory tests for term and preterm infants. This benefit is greatest for VLBW infants, improving extrauterine transition and blood pressure and decreasing the need for vasopressors and erythrocyte transfusions in the first week. Blood contained in umbilical cord and placenta after separation originates from the newborn infant. PCBS can be used for CBC, blood culture, blood type and crossmatch, metabolic screen, genetic testing, blood chemistries, and coagulation studies. Compared with phlebotomy, PCBS allows for larger blood culture volumes, which improves the positivity rate. Collection can be performed after DCC and in conjunction with cord blood banking and/or research. PCBS is a safe, accurate, and effective procedure that can be additive to our care benefiting neonates and improving outcomes.

Postnatal Cord Blood Sampling (PCBS) Summary Points:

1. PCBS collects neonatal blood and is a painless procedure that has been well studied and successful 95% of the time in obtaining admission laboratory studies.
2. PCBS can be used to obtain a reliable blood culture, CBC with differential, blood type and crossmatch, genetic and metabolic testing, chemistries, and coagulation studies.
3. If it is determined that blood tests are needed at or shortly after delivery, PCBS should be the first choice for phlebotomy and can be used in newborns of any gestational age in the first hour after birth.
4. PCBS is most commonly performed for infants being admitted to the NICU, early-onset sepsis evaluations, initial and follow-up genetic testing, studies needed for infants with congenital anomalies, and deaths that occur prior to or shortly after delivery.
5. **For PCBS to be successful in obtaining optimal blood volumes** for admission laboratory studies, after delayed cord clamping (or cord milking) **the umbilical cord must remain clamped** (can be quickly changed to a disposable clamp) until PCBS is performed.
6. **PCBS facilitates obtaining larger blood culture volumes** potentially improving early-onset sepsis pathogen detection compared to infant phlebotomy, and similar to obtaining blood cultures from any site, must be performed as an aseptic procedure.
7. **PCBS for admission laboratory tests can be coordinated with research cord studies and cord blood banking.** There may be deliveries where PCBS should be prioritized, for example in VLBW infants, where it prevents hypotension, the need for vasopressors, blood transfusions and potentially intraventricular hemorrhage. PCBS followed by research studies and/or cord blood banking using the same or different phlebotomy sites can all be successful in most cases with discussion and planning prior to the delivery.

LEAD AUTHORS

David A. Kaufman, MD, FAAP
Ashley M. Lucke, MD, FAAP
James J. Cummings, MD, FAAP

COMMITTEE ON FETUS AND NEWBORN, 2024–2025

Eric Eichenwald, MD, FAAP, Chairperson
Namasivayam Ambalavanan, MD, FAAP
Charleta Guillory, MD, FAAP
Mark Hudak, MD, FAAP
David A. Kaufman, MD, FAAP
Camilia Martin, MD, FAAP
Ashley M. Lucke, MD, FAAP
Margaret Parker, MD, FAAP

Arun Pramanik, MD, FAAP
Kelly Wade, MD, FAAP

LIAISONS

Timothy Jancelewicz, MD, FAAP – AAP Section on Surgery
Michael Narvey, MD – Canadian Paediatric Society
Stacy Beck, MD – American College of Obstetricians and Gynecologists
Lisa Grisham, APRN, NNP-BC – National Association of Neonatal Nurses

STAFF

Jim Couto, MA

ACKNOWLEDGMENT

We would like to acknowledge Robert D. Christensen, MD, FAAP, for his contribution as an expert reviewer of this report.

ABBREVIATIONS

CBC: complete blood cell count
DAT: direct antiglobulin testing
DCC: delayed cord clamping
NICU: neonatal intensive care unit
PCBS: postnatal cord blood sampling
VLBW: very low birth weight

FUNDING: No external funding.

https://doi.org/10.1542/peds.2025-071811

REFERENCES

1. Christensen RD, Lambert DK, Baer VL, et al. Postponing or eliminating red blood cell transfusions of very low birth weight neonates by obtaining all baseline laboratory blood tests from otherwise discarded fetal blood in the placenta. *Transfusion.* 2011;51(2):253–258. PubMed doi: 10.1111/j.1537-2995.2010.02827.x
2. Liao Y, Cotten M, Tan S, Kurtzberg J, Cairo MS. Rescuing the neonatal brain from hypoxic injury with autologous cord blood. *Bone Marrow Transplant.* 2013;48(7):890–900. PubMed doi: 10.1038/bmt.2012.169
3. Li J, Yawno T, Sutherland AE, et al. Preterm umbilical cord blood derived mesenchymal stem/stromal cells protect preterm white matter brain development against hypoxia-ischemia. *Exp Neurol.* 2018;308:120–131. PubMed doi: 10.1016/j.expneurol.2018.07.006
4. Christensen RD, Baer VL, Lambert DK, Ilstrup SJ, Eggert LD, Henry E. Association, among very-low-birthweight neonates, between red blood cell transfusions in the week after birth and severe intraventricular hemorrhage. *Transfusion.* 2014;54(1):104–108. PubMed doi: 10.1111/trf.12234
5. Baer VL, Lambert DK, Carroll PD, Gerday E, Christensen RD. Using umbilical cord blood for the initial blood tests of VLBW neonates results in higher hemoglobin and fewer RBC transfusions. *J Perinatol.* 2013;33(5):363–365. PubMed doi: 10.1038/jp.2012.127
6. Moore SP, Newberry DM, Jnah AJ. Use of placental/umbilical blood sampling for neonatal admission blood cultures: benefits, challenges, and strategies for implementation. *Neonatal Netw.* 2017;36(3):152–159. PubMed doi: 10.1891/0730-0832.36.3.152
7. Carroll PD. Umbilical cord blood-an untapped resource: strategies to decrease early red blood cell transfusions and improve neonatal outcomes. *Clin Perinatol.* 2015;42(3):541–556. PubMed doi: 10.1016/j.clp.2015.04.017
8. Backes CH, Huang H, Cua CL, et al. Early versus delayed umbilical cord clamping in infants with congenital heart disease: a pilot, randomized, controlled trial. *J Perinatol.* 2015;35(10):826–831. PubMed doi: 10.1038/jp.2015.89
9. Shiff I, Bucsea O, Pillai Riddell R. Psychosocial and neurobiological vulnerabilities of the hospitalized preterm infant and relevant non-pharmacological pain mitigation strategies. *Front Pediatr.* 2021;9:568755. PubMed doi: 10.3389/fped.2021.568755
10. ACOG Committee on Obstetric Practice. ACOG Committee Opinion No. 348, November 2006: Umbilical cord blood gas and acid-base analysis. *Obstet Gynecol.* 2006;108(5):1319–1322. PubMed doi: 10.1097/00006250-200611000-00058
11. Judd WJ; Scientific Section Coordinating Committee of the AABB. Practice guidelines for prenatal and perinatal immunohematology, revisited. *Transfusion.* 2001;41(11):1445–1452. PubMed doi: 10.1046/j.1537-2995.2001.41111445.x
12. Kemper AR, Newman TB, Slaughter JL, et al. Clinical practice guideline revision: management of hyperbilirubinemia in the newborn infant 35 or more weeks of gestation. *Pediatrics.* 2022;150(3):e2022058859. PubMed doi: 10.1542/peds.2022-058859
13. Carroll PD, Christensen RD. New and underutilized uses of umbilical cord blood in neonatal care. *Matern Health Neonatol Perinatol.* 2015;1(1):16. PubMed doi: 10.1186/s40748-015-0017-2
14. Chakrahari S, Patil M, Bijapure HR. Umbilical cord blood bilirubin, albumin, reticulocyte count, and nucleated red blood cells to predict subsequent hyperbilirubinemia in term neonates: a prospective observational study. *Cureus.* 2023;15(4):e37598. PubMed doi: 10.7759/cureus.37598
15. Şahan H, Gülaşı S, Mert MK, Çekinmez EK. The predictive significance of umbilical cord bilirubin and bilirubin/albumin ratio

for neonatal jaundice in healthy term newborns. *Turk J Med Sci.* 2023;53(2):511–517. PubMed doi: 10.55730/1300-0144.5611

16. Kardum D, Serdarušić I, Biljan B, Šantić K, Živković V, Kos M. Cord blood bilirubin and prediction of neonatal hyperbilirubinemia and perinatal infection in newborns at risk of hemolysis. *J Pediatr (Rio J).* 2021;97(4):440–444. PubMed doi: 10.1016/j.jped.2020.08.009
17. Sharma IK, Kumar D, Singh A, Mahmood T. Ratio of cord blood bilirubin and albumin as predictors of neonatal hyperbilirubinaemia. *Clin Exp Hepatol.* 2020;6(4):384–388. PubMed doi: 10.5114/ceh.2020.102170
18. Chadwick EG, Ezeanolue EE, Hsu KK-C, et al; COMMITTEE ON PEDIATRIC AIDS. Evaluation and management of the infant exposed to HIV in the United States. *Pediatrics.* 2020;146(5):e2020029058. PubMed doi: 10.1542/peds.2020-029058
19. Prakash N, Decristofaro J, Maduekwe ET. One less painful procedure: using umbilical cord blood as alternative source to admission complete blood count. *Am J Perinatol.* 2017;34(12):1178–1184. PubMed doi: 10.1055/s-0037-1601565
20. Greer R, Safarulla A, Koeppel R, Aslam M, Bany-Mohammed FM. Can fetal umbilical venous blood be a reliable source for admission complete blood count and culture in NICU patients? *Neonatology.* 2019;115(1):49–58. PubMed doi: 10.1159/000491993
21. Newberry DM. Comparison of placental and neonatal admission complete blood cell count and blood cultures. *Adv Neonatal Care.* 2018;18(3):215–222. PubMed doi: 10.1097/ANC.0000000000000482
22. Beeram MR, Loughran C, Cipriani C, Govande V. Utilization of umbilical cord blood for the evaluation of group B streptococcal sepsis screening. *Clin Pediatr (Phila).* 2012;51(5):447–453. PubMed doi: 10.1177/0009922811431882
23. Hansen A, Forbes P, Buck R. Potential substitution of cord blood for infant blood in the neonatal sepsis evaluation. *Biol Neonate.* 2005;88(1):12–18. PubMed doi: 10.1159/000083946
24. Carroll PD, Nankervis CA, Iams J, Kelleher K. Umbilical cord blood as a replacement source for admission complete blood count in premature infants. *J Perinatol.* 2012;32(2):97–102. PubMed doi: 10.1038/jp.2011.60
25. Carroll PD, Livingston E, Baer VL, Karkula K, Christensen RD. Evaluating otherwise-discarded umbilical cord blood as a source for a neonate's complete blood cell count at various time points. *Neonatology.* 2018;114(1):82–86. PubMed doi: 10.1159/000488024
26. Kalathia MB, Shingala PA, Parmar PN, Parikh YN, Kalathia IM. Study of umbilical cord blood culture in diagnosis of early-onset sepsis among newborns with high-risk factors. *J Clin Neonatol.* 2013;2(4):169–172. PubMed doi: 10.4103/2249-4847.123092
27. Meena J, Charles MVP, Ali A, Ramakrishnan S, Gosh S, Seetha KS. Utility of cord blood culture in early onset neonatal sepsis. *Australas Med J.* 2015;8(8):263–267. PubMed doi: 10.4066/AMJ.2015.2460
28. Meena R, Meena KK, Athwani V, Gothwal S, Bairwa GS, Sitaraman S. Umbilical cord blood culture in diagnosis of early onset neonatal sepsis. *Indian J Pediatr.* 2020;87(10):793–797. PubMed doi: 10.1007/s12098-020-03345-5
29. Polin JI, Knox I, Baumgart S, Campman E, Mennuti MT, Polin RA. Use of umbilical cord blood culture for detection of neonatal bacteremia. *Obstet Gynecol.* 1981;57(2):233–237. PubMed
30. Herson VC, Block C, McLaughlin JC, Tetreault J, Eisenfeld LI, Krause PJ. Placental blood sampling: an aid to the diagnosis of neonatal sepsis. *J Perinatol.* 1998;18(2):135–137. PubMed
31. Rotshenker-Olshinka K, Shinwell ES, Juster-Reicher A, Rosin I, Flidel-Rimon O. Comparison of hematologic indices and markers of infection in umbilical cord and neonatal blood. *J Matern Fetal Neonatal Med.* 2014;27(6):625–628. PubMed doi: 10.3109/14767058.2013.825597
32. Yaacobi N, Bar-Meir M, Shchors I, Bromiker R. A prospective controlled trial of the optimal volume for neonatal blood cultures. *Pediatr Infect Dis J.* 2015;34(4):351–354. PubMed doi: 10.1097/INF.0000000000000594
33. Mukhopadhyay S, Puopolo KM. Clinical and microbiologic characteristics of early-onset sepsis among very low birth weight infants: opportunities for antibiotic stewardship. *Pediatr Infect Dis J.* 2017;36(5):477–481. PubMed doi: 10.1097/INF.0000000000001473
34. Gottschalk A, Coggins S, Dhudasia MB, et al. Utility of anaerobic blood cultures in neonatal sepsis evaluation. *J Pediatric Infect Dis Soc.* 2024;13(8):406–412. PubMed doi: 10.1093/jpids/piae056
35. Quinones Cardona V, Lowery V, Cooperberg D, Anday EK, Carey AJ. Eliminating contamination in umbilical cord blood culture sampling for early-onset neonatal sepsis. *Front Pediatr.* 2021;9:794710. PubMed doi: 10.3389/fped.2021.794710
36. Alissa R, Williams PD, Baker EL, Hipp JA, Saremian J, Aysola AE. Suitability of placental blood samples of newborns for pre-transfusion testing. *Front Pediatr.* 2021;9:661321. PubMed doi: 10.3389/fped.2021.661321
37. Committee on Genetics and the Society for Maternal-Fetal Medicine. Society for Maternal-Fetal Medicine. Committee Opinion No. 682: Microarrays and next-generation sequencing technology: the use of advanced genetic diagnostic tools in obstetrics and gynecology. *Obstet Gynecol.* 2016;128(6):e262–e268. PubMed doi: 10.1097/AOG.0000000000001817
38. Huang H, Wang Y, Zhang M, et al. Diagnostic accuracy and value of chromosomal microarray analysis for chromosomal abnormalities in prenatal detection: A prospective clinical study. *Medicine (Baltimore).* 2021;100(20):e25999. PubMed doi: 10.1097/MD.0000000000025999
39. Calcagni G, Unolt M, Digilio MC, et al. Congenital heart disease and genetic syndromes: new insights into molecular mechanisms. *Expert Rev Mol Diagn.* 2017;17(9):861–870. PubMed doi: 10.1080/14737159.2017.1360766
40. Mardy AH, Chetty SP, Norton ME, Sparks TN. A system-based approach to the genetic etiologies of non-immune hydrops fetalis. *Prenat Diagn.* 2019;39(9):732–750. PubMed doi: 10.1002/pd.5479
41. Wynn J, Yu L, Chung WK. Genetic causes of congenital diaphragmatic hernia. *Semin Fetal Neonatal Med.* 2014;19(6):324–330. PubMed doi: 10.1016/j.siny.2014.09.003

42. Raffaeli G, Tripodi A, Manzoni F, et al. Is placental blood a reliable source for the evaluation of neonatal hemostasis at birth? *Transfusion*. 2020;60(5):1069–1077. PubMed doi: 10.1111/trf.15785

43. Neary E, McCallion N, Kevane B, et al. Coagulation indices in very preterm infants from cord blood and postnatal samples. *J Thromb Haemost*. 2015;13(11):2021–2030. PubMed doi: 10.1111/jth.13130

44. Mehari A, Challa F, Gebreyesus G, Alemayehu D, Seifu D. Establishment of reference intervals of thyroid function tests from cord blood of neonates in two selected hospitals, Addis Ababa, Ethiopia. *BMC Pediatr*. 2016;16(1):118. PubMed doi: 10.1186/s12887-016-0654-2

45. Held PK, Bird IM, Heather NL. Newborn screening for congenital adrenal hyperplasia: review of factors affecting screening accuracy. *Int J Neonatal Screen*. 2020;6(3):67. PubMed doi: 10.3390/ijns6030067

46. Carroll PD. Cord blood sampling - a review of umbilical cord blood use for admission laboratory tests in the immediate newborn period. *Curr Pediatr Rev*. 2023;19(4):371–375. PubMed doi: 10.2174/1573396319666221125140556

47. Bahr TM, Carroll PD. Cord blood sampling for neonatal admission laboratory testing-An evidence-based blood conservation strategy. *Semin Perinatol*. 2023;47(5):151786. PubMed doi: 10.1016/j.semperi.2023.151786

48. Balasubramanian H, Malpani P, Sindhur M, Kabra NS, Ahmed J, Srinivasan L. Effect of umbilical cord blood sampling versus admission blood sampling on requirement of blood transfusion in extremely preterm infants: a randomized controlled trial. *J Pediatr*. 2019;211:39–45.e2. PubMed doi: 10.1016/j.jpeds.2019.04.033

49. Mu TS, Prescott AC, Haischer-Rollo GD, Aden JK, Shapiro JB. Umbilical cord blood use for admission blood tests of VLBW preterm neonates: a randomized control trial. *Am J Perinatol*. 2023;40(10):1119–1125. PubMed doi: 10.1055/s-0041-1733781

Prescribing Assistive Technology: Focus on Children With Complex Communication Needs

• *Clinical Report*

CLINICAL REPORT Guidance for the Clinician in Rendering Pediatric Care

American Academy of Pediatrics

DEDICATED TO THE HEALTH OF ALL CHILDREN™

Prescribing Assistive Technology: Focus on Children With Complex Communication Needs: Clinical Report

Larry W. Desch, MD, FAAP,[1] Laura J. Hobart-Porter, DO, FAAP, FAAPMR,[2] Amy Houtrow, MD, PhD, MPH, FAAP,[3] and the Council on Children With Disabilities

abstract

The primary care pediatrician and other pediatric physicians play a critical role in the interdisciplinary team effort to provide appropriate augmentative and alternative communication (AAC) technology to children with absent or severely impaired verbal communication, recently recategorized as a complex communication need. This clinical report describes the different types of AAC technology, the device assessment process, and the training required for successful integration into a child's communication. The report further describes the role of the pediatrician in acquisition and appropriate utilization of this technology with a focus on key specialists and funding sources. Decades of research confirm that use of AAC promotes language development; therefore, primary care physicians can reassure families that AAC will likely help their child to learn to communicate more effectively. There is an important need for key resources for AAC to be identified in every community; the majority of relevant professional organizations, including the American Academy of Pediatrics, recognize that these resources are a shared medical, educational, therapeutic, and family responsibility.

[1]Department of Pediatrics, Chicago Medical School, Rosalind Franklin University of Medicine and Science and Advocate Children's Hospital, Oak Lawn, Illinois; [2]Department of Pediatrics, University of Arkansas for Medical Sciences, Arkansas Children's Hospital, Little Rock, Arkansas; and [3]Division of Pediatric Rehabilitation Medicine, Department of Physical Medicine and Rehabilitation, School of Medicine, University of Pittsburgh, Pittsburgh, Pennsylvania

All authors participated in conception, design, drafting, and critical revision of the clinical report and approved the final manuscript as submitted.

FINANCIAL/CONFLICT OF INTEREST DISCLOSURE: The authors have indicated they have no potential conflicts of interest to disclose.

To cite: Desch LW, Hobart-Porter LJ, and Houtrow A; American Academy of Pediatrics, Council on Children With Disabilities. Prescribing Assistive Technology: Focus on Children With Complex Communication Needs: Clinical Report. *Pediatrics*. 2025;156(1):e2025072216

BACKGROUND

Data from the recent 2021–2022 National Survey of Children's Health indicated that nearly 10% of children age 3 to 17 years had speech or other language disorders.[1] Conditions that can cause impairments in communication include cerebral palsy (CP), autism spectrum disorder (ASD), congenital anomalies, deafness, intellectual disabilities, brain injuries, severe speech disorders (eg, dyspraxia, childhood apraxia of speech), and genetic syndromes (such as Down syndrome or Rett syndrome). For these conditions, if speech or verbal language is absent or extremely limited, then a complex communication need (CCN) exists, and the affected child may benefit from augmentative/alternative communication (AAC) systems. If the child has a congenital or early life cause for a CCN, then habilitative treatments are needed. Those with CCN occurring later in life (eg, after a brain injury) will need a more rehabilitative approach to treatment. These treatment methods are often the same or similar. Unfortunately, some insurance companies will only provide payment for rehabilitation services.

Severe limitations in cognition (eg, intellectual developmental disorder) and/or social communication (eg, ASD) can also affect the ability to express oneself. However, since it has been shown that the use of AAC does not prevent or limit acquiring verbal language, it is important for those with severe to profound cognitive and/or social disabilities to be offered some AAC therapeutic interventions as a way to possibly improve functional communication skills.[2,3] There are not prerequisites to the evaluation for and use of appropriate AAC for any child (or adult) who could benefit from AAC, which is in accordance with the American Speech-Language-Hearing Association (ASHA) position statement on access to AAC[4] as well as the "Communication Bill of Rights" from the National Joint Committee for the Communication Needs of Person with Severe Disabilities (NJC).[5]

Children who have severe communication impairments and CCN should be able to anticipate a degree of independence in adult life. AAC can offer the possibility of an occupation that is personally rewarding and results in academical, social, and medical benefits. AAC gives children with CCN the ability to express themselves, allowing them to develop other communication-adjacent skills that can set them up for adulthood with some autonomy. Using AAC may permit increased rates of employment that would otherwise be unavailable; contemporary vocational opportunities are increasingly accessible to adults with physical and communication disabilities. Jobs like editing, writing, and computer applications do not depend on speed of output as much as good judgment and reasoning abilities. Success ultimately depends on quantity and quality of the tools and trainings provided in childhood, such as AAC, and not on prerequisite skills. Even older children with severe functional communication deficits can benefit from AAC intervention that may not have been accessible or needed in their early years, particularly relevant for those children with acquired deficits (eg, brain injuries).

Societal barriers may further limit children with already extant communication impairments. Children who are marginalized by the consequences of racism and poverty have more difficulty accessing care to improve communication.[6] Overall, 24.5% of caregivers of children with a communication impairment report unmet need, but this increases to 29.1% when the children are Black.[6] On the basis of this report by Black et al, children with communication impairment also received inequitable health insurance coverage. Families of children with communication difficulties are less likely to report that their child's health insurance was adequate and also less likely to receive care in a medical home.[6] Even middle class families with incomes between 200% and 299% of the federal poverty level reported difficulty getting access to appropriate devices; 31.3% of children in these families reported unmet needs for their children who require communication aids/devices.[6] The literature on AAC is lacking with regard to children who do not speak English as a primary language but reside in an English language-dominant culture; this may adversely impact access to necessary AAC and trainings. For all children, regardless of primary language or dominant culture, intervention should be culturally responsive. Limited studies in neurotypical children seem to indicate parity between comprehension of Spanish and English on commercially available augmentative communication devices, although this finding cannot reliably be extrapolated to diverse populations.[7] In addition to the issues related to minoritized race, ethnicity, and socioeconomic factors, those children who live in rural areas and who have minimal verbal or nonverbal ASD or other similar disorders also have trouble accessing AAC and related therapy services.[8] For decades, rural school districts have had increasing difficulty recruiting teachers and related staff, including special education teachers and therapists.[8] Poorly resourced rural school districts are often the only programs that are providing help to address a majority of the interventions and referrals needed. In these rural areas, students and families have needs for which they are legally entitled, but in these rural communities there is limited student access to appropriate devices and expertise. As many rural area populations decline, the lack of trained special education teachers and therapists may limit availability of AAC for children with CCN unless access to other interventions (including outpatient services or telehealth) are improved.[9]

Medicine, as a whole, has a long and enduring history of ableism.[10] In the pursuit of wellness and health, there is an inappropriate and dangerous emphasis on normalcy.[11] This emphasis has the effect of marginalizing already vulnerable groups. As Iezzoni states eloquently: Ableism is "rooted in perspectives that characterize disability as 'abnormal' or an individual problem requiring treatment of cure – as opposed to perspectives that acknowledge disability as a normal part of human diversity."[12] Ableism can apply to patients with ASD, CP, and chromosomal disorders, among others. Historically, people with expressive language deficits have been equated with having cognitive or intellectual deficits. Those with cognitive or intellectual deficits often are perceived as less than worthy of attention and care. It is vital that physicians recognize whatever implicit biases they may harbor, acknowledging that diversity is desirable in all its forms. It can feel overwhelming to address these complex issues, but abdicating this duty to others is its own form of ableism we must combat. It is the authors' fervent hope that we may guide the reader to resources that will aid all physicians in the care of patients with CCN.

POPULATIONS OF CCN

CCN spans many clinical groups beyond isolated communication impairments including those with genetic, congenital, and acquired disorders. Sixty percent of children with CP are estimated to have some difficulty in communication[13]; a more recent cohort study revealed 85% of 2-year-olds with CP had significant impairments in speech and language.[14] Children with Down syndrome have also been shown to have significant impairments in expressive language and speech development compared with their peers, even after adjusting for degree of intellectual developmental disorder.[15,16] Approximately 30% of children with ASD who do not have severe intellectual developmental disorder have CCN.[17] Children with a diagnosis of severe intellectual developmental disorder without other developmental disabilities also have a high prevalence of speech and language disabilities.[18]

DEFINITIONS

Assistive technology describes "any item, piece of equipment, or product system, whether acquired commercially off the shelf, modified, or customized, that is used to increase, maintain, or improve functional capabilities of an individual with a disability," as defined by the Individuals with Disability Education Act (IDEA) and the Assistive Technology Act of 2004.[19] Types of assistive technology may include commercial products or accessibility features in products like assistive listening devices (closed captioning software or amplifiers), durable medical equipment including mobility aids (wheelchairs), and speech-generating devices (SGDs) or visual aids (screen-reading software).

The use of an AAC device is another example of assistive technology. While the terms augmentative and alternative are often used interchangeably, they are distinct terms. AAC is augmentative when used to supplement existing speech, and AAC is alternative when used in place of speech that is absent or not functional. For the purposes of this report, the term AAC will refer to any device or system that is used to improve the ability of a child to communicate.

AAC Systems and Devices

AAC is often erroneously thought to refer only to complex electronic devices. Although these advanced devices may be the most appropriate choice for some children, these should be carefully selected on the basis of individual patient needs. Access to powerful technologies has improved for children with complex communication needs, in part because of the widespread availability of mobile technology. The prevalence of said technology has also driven down costs, thus permitting its greater availability for children with limited resources. Other technological advances have also improved access for those with severe motor impairments.

The costs for AAC vary widely depending on the level of complexity and whether or not mass-produced items (like touchscreen tables) are a major component of the device. Although many low-tech and mid-tech AAC solutions are available to assist children with complex communication needs, this report focuses more on high-tech devices, because primary care physicians (PCPs) are sometimes asked to prescribe and approve the use of these more expensive devices.[20] Table 1 describes examples of the variety of AAC currently available. Low-tech strategies describe aids that do not require the use of batteries or electricity. They may include the use of objects, line drawings, and actual photographs or pictures of objects or persons to replace or augment spoken words. Low-tech AAC also includes systems such as lists of words, phrases, or symbols that can be easily understood by others in many environments. Some low-tech options include communication boards, communication books and pragmatic organization dynamic display (PODD). For children with visual impairments, 3-dimensional objects or supports can be substituted for pictures to provide tactile input. Picture Exchange Communication Systems (PECS) is one example of a low-tech intervention program for individuals with ASD and other developmental disabilities that is intended to shape a child's expressive communication abilities using prompting and reinforcement strategies. PECS is a specific approach with specific implementation parameters, based on applied behavior analysis, and consists of 6 progressive instructional phases."[21] Exchanging pictures with a partner to request something (eg, PECS) or using paper communication boards or "flip-books" of familiar images can be quite effective in face-to-face communication. These systems can also be quickly and easily employed in the hospital setting. For children who have visual impairment, 3-dimensional objects that can be felt may be substituted for pictures.[22]

Simple communication boards can be accessed through direct selection or partner-assisted scanning (Figures 1 and 2). In direct selection, the child directly touches or points to the desired target (eg, word, symbol). In partner-assisted scanning, a communication partner goes through showing the available choices until they are stopped by a response from the child (such as an eye blink or signaling device or switch).

Mid-tech devices are typically battery-operated portable voice output storage devices or devices that produce printed text. Devices can store a few recorded or digitized messages, such as "I want to see a movie" or multiple levels of messages. An example of this is the "sequencing

TABLE 1. The Spectrum of Aided Augmentative and Alternative Technology for Communication Impairments[a]

Type of Technology	Characteristics	Examples	Advantages	Disadvantages
Low-tech AAC	Uses paper, plastic, or similar materials Often used as the first-step communication method Also is important as a backup of more complex devices	Simple picture/word boards or cards PECS Eye-gaze picture board Visual scheduler or planner Adapted pens/pencils	Usually low cost Portable Personal Training is quick Readily acceptable to the "listener" Rugged No need for power supply	Very limited speed Very limited vocabulary Unable to use for long-distance communication Requires access to printer and laminator and communication partner to add vocabulary Listening/communication partner needs to have training
Mid-tech AAC	Uses batteries for voice, text, or light output Useful for communication using single words or short phrases Less complex than high-tech devices May also be used as a backup device	Lighted on/off devices "Wrist communicator" (eg, with 2–10 stored vocal outputs) Keyboard with display or printer Scanning light board (eg, with pictures) Sequencing communicators	Low to moderate cost Usually portable Usually personally owned Training is moderate Usually acceptable to listener Occasionally can use for limited long-distance communication Some devices allow for immediate feedback	Limited speed Limited vocabulary Limited distance communication Power supply needed Requires communication partner support for creation of pages and/or recording messages Listening/communication partner needs to have specific training
High-tech AAC	Microcircuits and microcomputer technology Often uses a commercial computer or tablet with dedicated communication software Most commonly used device for those persons needing more complex communication Necessary for persons who have severe movement disorders	Mobile devices: touchscreen tablet programs, adapted laptop computers Visual screen displays Commercially available SGDs: 1) Dynamic displays 2) Touchpads or keyboards Individualized devices (using special inputs, eg, eye blinks, brain waves)	Ease of progressing in skill levels Able to carry out extensive and efficient conversations Usually portable Often can use for long-distance communication (eg, telephone) Able to connect to other devices (eg, for access to computer or for environmental control) Allows for more independence in communication Customizable and adjustable to meet needs as skills improve	Moderate to very high cost Sometimes is not personally owned Need power supply Training is often extensive Listening/communication partner needs to have extensive training Possible security issues if device is connected to a network or the internet

[a] See text for more details on some devices.

communicator" whereby pushing buttons on the AAC device allows a child to have a story read to them as they follow along with a picture book. The stories or messages are typically recorded and changed by the communication partners on the basis of each specific activity. When the desired button is accessed, the recorded message plays. Most mid-tech devices are accessed only through direct selection, using touch, switch access, or a pointer to choose a target.

Low- and mid-tech communication systems have inherent limitations. Vocabulary is limited by what is pictured or stored; therefore, lengthy, novel messages are not feasible. Communication is usually slow and is often more scripted than spontaneous or independent. Mid-tech devices require preprogramming of messages created and managed by a communication partner or caregiver before the activity or may rely on "factory default words" that are already in the device. They may be difficult to use and, thus, inappropriate to use with persons who have fine motor impairments, such as those who have CP or other movement differences.

High-tech AAC devices are electronic devices that have the capacity to store and retrieve messages (Figure 3). Most now have synthesized speech output, allowing the listener to easily receive the message. These are known as SGDs or voice output communication aids (VOCAs). Given the advances in technology, some high-tech AAC devices can be used for more than communication and can now be additionally used with email, word processing or other computer software, or environmental control units. Commercial insurance, however, may not cover high-tech AAC devices that are used for more than communication

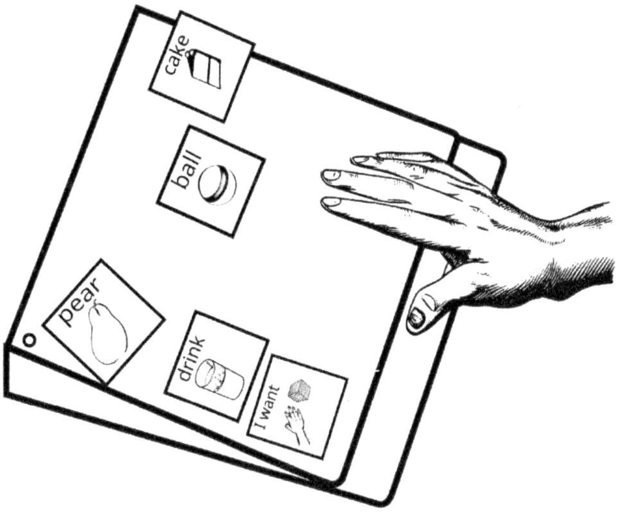

FIGURE 1.
This low-tech communication device allows the user to select one or several images to convey their request.

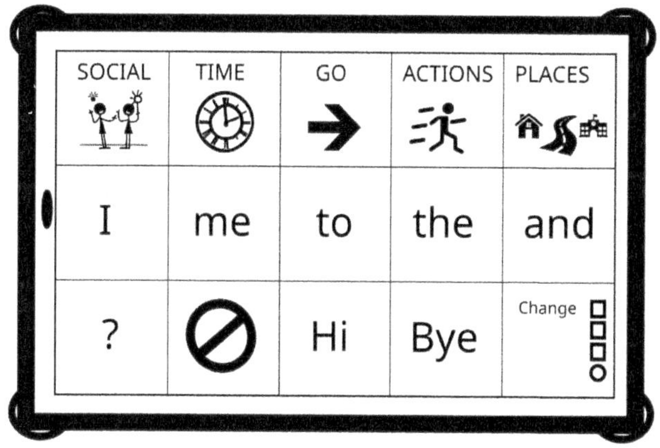

FIGURE 3.
Example of a mid-tech or high-tech spoken word device. If mid-tech, it allows the user to select from a limited set of options. If high-tech, it has a dynamic display and be upgradable to allow for new words to be added and more complex sentences to be constructed. There are several single-use AAC devices and applications for tablets that are commercially available.

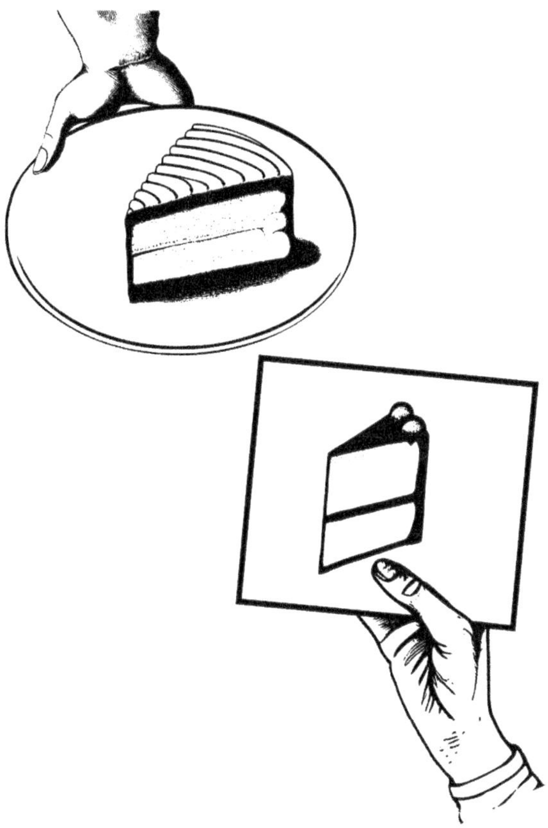

FIGURE 2.
Using a picture of cake selected from the available options in Figure 1, the user can indicate they wish to eat cake by presenting the picture to a communication partner (such as a caregiver).

but may cover AAC software for a privately owned device. SGDs produce voice output by using either digitized recordings of natural speech or the creation of synthesized speech, with the latter allowing for more novel messaging by the user. Unlike mid-tech devices, high-tech devices usually feature a dynamic display that changes with the input so that many levels of symbols, words, or lengthy messages can be stored for quicker retrieval. This improves both the variety of potential vocabulary items and independence in communication. Symbols are displayed on the device in categories such as emotions, objects, actions, people, and concepts. They can be displayed as words, drawings, or photographs, depending on the developmental needs of the child. The needs of the child should dictate the features necessary for system and vocabulary recommendations. With these devices, the user selects a symbol, triggering changes in the set of symbols displayed. This process expands their ability to communicate a novel and often longer message. Symbols are typically placed in a grid with the size and number of the symbols dependent on the child's visual abilities, communication and cognitive skills, and motor control after a comprehensive AAC evaluation.

Over the last decade, there has been an emergence in the use of visual scene displays (VSDs). Rather than using a single symbol to represent an object or person, a VSD can represent a natural life event (eg, a changeable video of a family having a picnic), which can provide a greater context for the child to communicate their message. VSDs can be static or dynamic through the use of preprogrammed videos.[23] VSDs are an additional feature of some vocabulary systems and require programming by a familiar communication partner or professional to support individual needs.

High-tech devices typically have the capability of having multiple access (input) methods ranging from direct selection on a touch screen to various types of scanning, mouse/joystick controllers, or encoding systems. Encoding systems use a simpler set of movements such as a series of eye blinks to represent a longer communication. Some computer-based devices can be accessed via eye gaze. For children who have both severe communication and physical disabilities, these alternative access methods are often needed. Systems that allow direct selection (eg, with a finger) are used with children who have adequate control of movements.

The advantage of high-tech SGDs is their expandability, flexibility, and mobility, especially those that incorporate commercial touchscreen tablets. For children whose communication skills are improving over time, the vocabulary in the SGD can be modified to accommodate the changes to language development and communication needs of the child. Thus, the skills of the child and capability of the device work in tandem and promote communicative proficiency throughout the continuum of care.

As an example, for a child who has ASD but is being limited in communication by using the PECS and low- or mid-tech supports do not meet their expressive communication needs, evaluation for high-tech AAC or SGD is recommended.[24,25] Persons with fine motor impairments may have difficulty accessing hardware connections, and more sophisticated switches may not be able to be used. It is critical that the team include a variety of professionals including occupational therapists (OTs), physical therapists (PTs), assistive technology professionals (ATPs), and speech-language pathologists (SLPs) to identify all the needs of the patient to make the best recommendations for switch access or other access modifications to operate the equipment.

High-tech electronic devices are often constrained by their need for a power source, limiting their usefulness in situations in which battery power gets depleted. A lower-tech solution (such as a word or picture board, a set of pictures or phrases on a ring, or other simple devices) should always be available as a backup for high-tech AAC system users. People who have typical language ability and speech are accustomed to a high rate of expressive speech. Therefore, patience and training are necessary to communicate with an individual who is using an AAC system. Patience and training are particularly important if the child is using a low-tech communication aid, such as a symbol, letter, or word board.

CURRENT RESEARCH AND LIMITATIONS

Prior studies have demonstrated the benefits of early intervention for speech and language disorders, including using augmentative systems, such as pictures or sign language.[26] Furthermore, research has shown that the use of AAC systems does not decrease the use of natural speech and may promote an increase in verbal expression expertise, which should provide reassurance to physicians and families.[27] Multiple systematic reviews and controlled research studies have definitively shown that the use of AAC has not decreased the vocabulary for children with minimal expressive vocabulary; in most cases, AAC use has helped to increase their vocabulary.[28,29] At least one review has also shown evidence of additional improvements in receptive language with the use of AAC.[30] A recent systematic review including studies published in the last decade demonstrated that AAC improves communication (particularly vocabulary) in pediatric AAC users ages 6 to 10 years with various diagnoses.[31] Most of these studies have been conducted with children with ASD and sometimes show improvements in social interactions in addition to increased vocabulary.[32]

AAC use has also been evaluated in children with other disorders and disabilities that cause CCN, including Down syndrome, craniofacial disorders, intellectual developmental disorder, childhood apraxia of speech, severe dysarthria, deafness/hard of hearing or deaf-blindness, and CP and similar motor impairments.[33–38] Some children with ASD develop expressive language through gestalt language processing or scripts, which is a type of language development in which full phrases (scripts) can be memorized and used to communicate ideas before basic units of speech such as individual words or phonemes.[39] Developing competency in AAC can support all children who have unreliable expressive communication skills.

Currently, there is no consensus about the earliest age at which a child can successfully use a more complex AAC device (eg, an SGD), although some have demonstrated successful use of complex devices with children younger than 3 years[40–42] and even children as young as 9 months.[43] Experienced researchers Beukelman and Mirenda have demonstrated the need to study the process by which AAC devices for young children are selected and used.[44] Their research suggested that if a child with severe communication impairment is successfully using an AAC device by first grade, the child will more actively participate in their classroom settings. These findings were reinforced in more recent work in which young children who were skilled and comfortable with their AAC devices communicated more frequently with their typically developing peers.[45] Despite the results of these studies, additional research on early toddler age (12 to 18 months) use of AAC systems is needed to determine whether earlier exposure to communication aids will promote more ease of use and other gains (such as improved social skills and participation).

ASSESSMENT ISSUES

The assessment of a child with a communication disorder and the selection of AAC device(s) is usually performed by an SLP with a team of other trained and experienced professionals (eg, OT, assistive technology). Recently, there has been apparent success with parts or all of this assessment process being conducted virtually, using live 2-way internet access and telehealth, with the child at home or at a different location than the team doing the assessment.[46] Sometimes a child can have limited speech and is having behavior problems possibly attributable to these problems with functional communication skills. In these instances, it is important to determine whether or not the main cause for the misbehaviors is the communication impairments. Evaluations completed in the home can provide critical information that may support decision making but are not required to determine need for AAC supports.

The first and most important step in AAC evaluation is the comprehensive assessment of the person's current functional abilities, environment, and personal preferences (Figure 4). The International Classification of Functioning, Disability and Health (ICF [Figure 5]) for children and youth developed by the World Health Organization can be useful in this process.[47,48] Using this system, one can identify assets and challenges that a person has related to their communication disability. ICF domains include "activities and participation" and subcategories such as "communication" or "mobility." Further information about how the ICF system could possibly be used to address CCN can be obtained by reviewing the recent review by Griffiths et al from England or the tutorial developed by Westby and Washington.[49,50]

A team approach is often needed to properly evaluate both the child and devices and ensure the best match so that the device can be used effectively across environments and communication partners. Depending on the AAC device and the disabilities of the child, this team may include SLPs, OTs, PTs, assistive technology professionals, rehabilitation engineers, PCPs, subspecialists trained in the care of children with disabilities (pediatric physiatrists, developmental and behavioral pediatricians, neurodevelopmentalists, complex care pediatricians, or child neurologists), psychologists, special educators and other school personnel, child care workers, computer specialists, and others in conjunction with the child and family. In most circumstances, the major evaluator is the SLP. Final decisions for the AAC system are made among the family, the SLP and other team members. If a larger interdisciplinary team approach is needed/utilized, it follows that collaborative discussions among team members must occur. For all teams, the team members are expected to have appropriate training regarding evaluation but also provide training to the child and family members. Identified team members are tasked with monitoring the ongoing use of the device and problem-solve with the family if issues arise. The PCP could have an advocacy role to ensure that training and monitoring occur. Abandonment of a device is much less likely to occur when appropriate monitoring and timely assistance are provided.[51]

During the last 15 years, there have been increasing numbers of reports of methods that can improve and standardize the training of communication partners, that is, those persons who will be interacting with the AAC user, including teachers, therapists, parents, and siblings. These methods fall into the category of what has been labeled as "partner augmented input" (most commonly), "modeling" or "communication partner instruction in AAC."[52,53] Evidence-based examples of these teaching methods include SMoRRES, ImPAACT, and an artificial intelligence-assisted automated system that was recently reported.[54–56] Additional research, dissemination, and training of trainers in these methods will likely lead to improvements in how AAC is used and accepted in the "real world" and possibly decrease abandonment of devices.

Children with moderate to severe physical and speech/communicative limitations require an experienced interdisciplinary team, as many of these impairments influence the child's ability to use AAC.[57] Current and future language needs, motor abilities and deficits (including which movements the child can make consistently and whether/how these movements can be used to control a device), cognitive functioning, visual and auditory acuity, anticipated communication partners, environment, and mobility issues must be assessed in detail to determine the features that are necessary for successful AAC implementation. Using this information will help determine the most feasible output method. Output information may vary from a simple laminated card to displays on monitor(s), internet output or synthesized speech. Multiple output types are preferred, especially for those children who have more severe disabilities, as this allows for redundancy should one output fail.

The assessment process for AAC includes consideration of the entire spectrum of AAC (see Figure 4). A patient may need all communication options for all types of communication needs at various times. A dedicated SGD may be recommended, but the child should have access to other communication options during the lengthy waiting period for the prescribed technology. Technology may require repair, charging, or updating or may be unavailable. Low- and mid-tech supports can be included in the plan of care and as part of the comprehensive AAC evaluation.

The basics of the overall assessment process for assistive technology are shown in Figure 4. Steps are ideally repeated periodically as the child's needs change and/or functional changes occur. These steps are outlined in a case example available in Box 1: Identifying the Potential Need, Gathering Information (ie, medical and other history), Capability Profile (Functioning) and Communication Assessment, Feature Match (matching a person's strengths and needs to a device), Trials of Device(s), and Possible Therapies

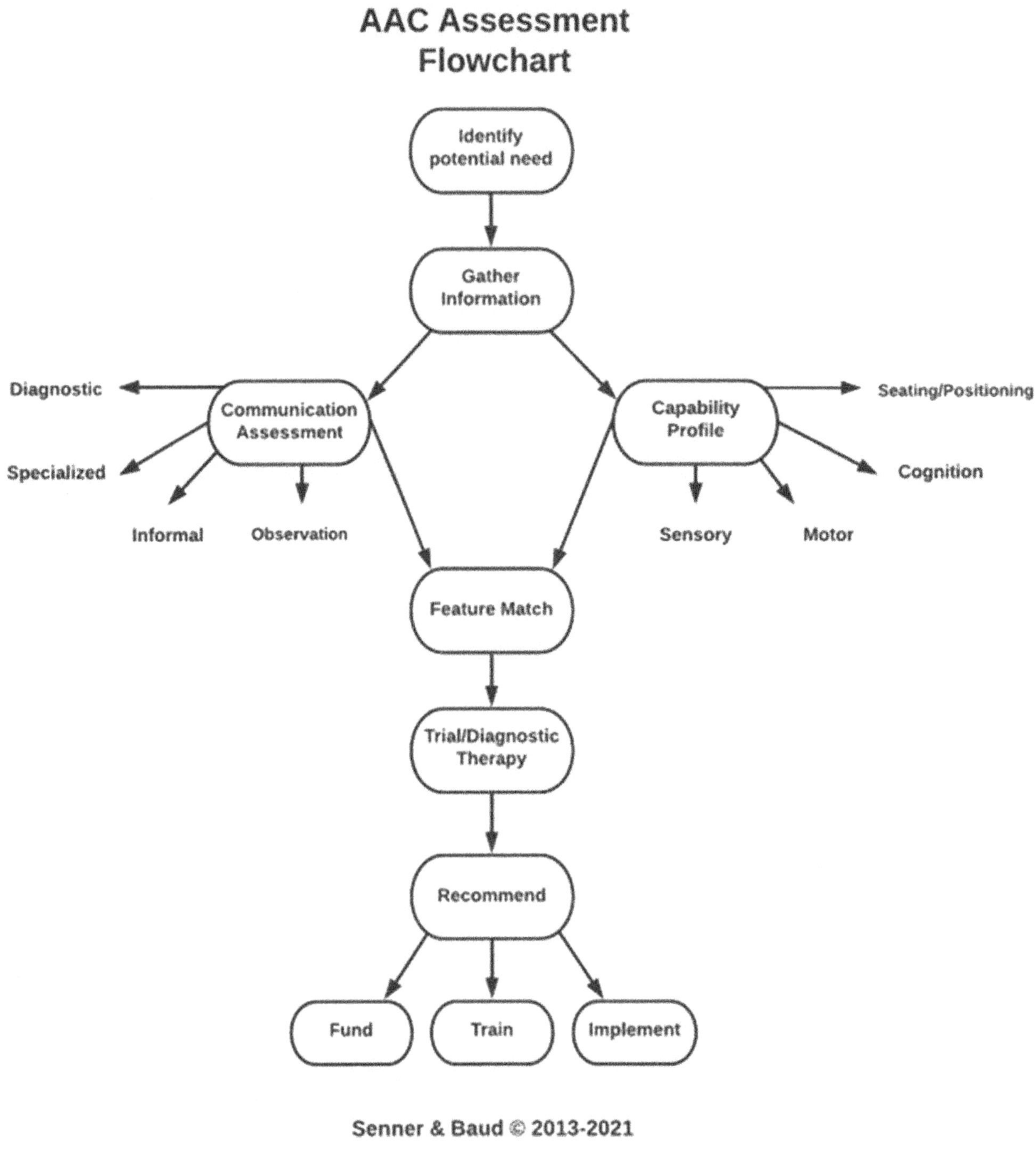

FIGURE 4.
The AAC device assessment cycle. Permission to use granted from Senner & Baud, 2022. From http://talcaac.com.

and Recommending Specific Device. The process culminates with Funding, Training, and Implementation (use) of the device. After implementation, ongoing monitoring, training, and guidance are important for communication and literacy development.

Baseline measurements of function, including cognitive testing, prior to introduction of AAC or assistive technology (AT) and at regular intervals (initially monthly) are essential. The SETT (student, environments, tasks, and tools) system is one framework that uses functional abilities to make assistive technology decisions and recommendations in the classroom environment used to gather this information.[58] This framework is primarily used in schools, and much of this system is available at no cost. Once a baseline is established, ongoing measurements of function can then determine whether progress is being made in distinct

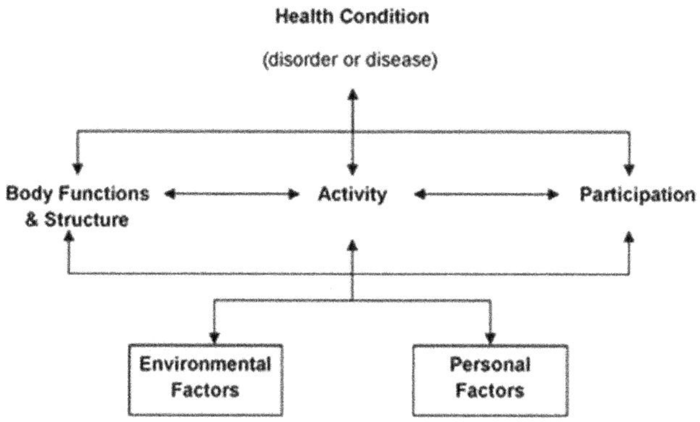

FIGURE 5.
The World Health Organization International Classification of Functioning, Disability and Health. Reproduced from World Health Organization. Towards a common language for functioning, disability and health. In: *International Classification of Functioning, Disability and Health.* Geneva, Switzerland: Copyright © World Health Organization; 2002:9.

domains. Environmental modifications (such as modified wheelchairs, special switches, or other assistive devices) may influence these functional measures and should be accounted for when reporting results. Standardized language-assessment tests could be used to determine progress in communication abilities but may need to be adapted. Caution is advised when children participate in standardized or formal evaluation protocols while using AAC systems, because most standardized evaluations have not been developed with communication supports or devices in mind.[59,60] For school-aged children, the use of any AAC and speech/language services may be covered by a legal document, the individualized education program (IEP).[19] Federal laws governing the IEP require re-evaluations every 3 years or as formally requested by the family or the school. Because of this requirement, if the family or school personnel do not feel that adequate progress using AAC is being made, a re-evaluation can determine actions that lead to improvements. In addition, if the child demonstrates new behavioral issues, it is important to ensure that whatever AAC device (if any) is being used that it is truly meeting the child's current communication needs.

Using the aforementioned steps, the skilled and experienced SLP may select the device(s) that are most likely to meet the child's individual needs on the basis of the child's abilities and communication environments; assistance from other team members may be solicited. Ideally, the child should have a trial period with a rented or loaned unit of the intended device before it is ordered or purchased. A trial period (1- to 2-month) gives the child, family, and educators/caregivers the opportunity to be trained and assess the child's ability to use the device in different settings, identifying the strengths and weaknesses of the system. These steps may reduce purchases of inappropriate devices. Partnering with a reliable technology center (especially at a university program, tertiary care hospital, or nonprofit organization, such as Easter Seals) is often useful, but these may be quite distant or have long waiting lists.[61,62] There may be some families who are uncomfortable with the more complex high-tech AAC devices because of lack of experience or access, and they may require additional instruction and training for the family. This additional family education may prevent abandonment of a device that meets the needs of the child.

Studies have demonstrated that assistive devices may be abandoned shortly after they are obtained in one third of cases; up to 75% of devices are never used successfully[63–65]. Although there has been minimal research done on this issue, this high rate of abandonment may be, at least partially, due to lack of training and support for caregivers, teachers and other therapists in the child's life.[66]

When the child or family's primary language is not English, it may complicate or impair successful uptake of AAC. Low-, mid-, and high-tech devices can usually be easily altered to different languages by labeling and programming of speech, but the paucity of therapists or teachers who are fluent in languages other than English limits their understanding of cultural and linguistic context essential for effective expressive communication. The physician or therapist who prescribes or recommends AAC can help alleviate this with assistance or advocacy for improved initial training for the child or caregiver as well as providing ongoing monitoring of the use of the device. This training is ideally provided in the native language by someone who knows the basics of AAC use, but an interpreter may also be utilized.

During the past 3 decades, methods have been developed to improve the successful matching of assistive devices to users (in adults, "matching person and technology").[67] Similar methods have been used with children and adolescents.[68] In Figure 4, this is the step noted as "Feature Match." If feature matching is well deployed, the best system or device and individualized training can be provided, leading to less chance of system or device abandonment.[50,68,69]

There are many tools and standardized measures available to assist in the process of evaluating the efficacy and performance of assistive devices, including AAC.[70,71] One 10-step framework includes input from caregivers to help professionals obtain assistive technology for young children.[71] These tools are promising but are still in development. In children with motor disabilities such as CP or brain injury or malformation, the types of switches used to access AAC devices are crucial; recent work demonstrates possible pathways to assess these new tools.[72] During the final steps in the assessment process, children needing AAC, no matter the severity, are ideally evaluated, trained, and observed by appropriate professionals using several selected devices, as subtle differences in devices

BOX 1: Case report – Past Medical History of a 5-Year-Old Girl With Speech Impairment
IDENTIFY POTENTIAL NEED – Beatrice (Bee) was born 6 weeks preterm with hyperbilirubinemia (jaundice), requiring a month-long stay in the neonatal intensive care unit. She was discharged with no medications or equipment and a normal newborn hearing screening. She achieved her gross motor milestones within typical age expectations, but her language milestones were significantly delayed. At age 2 years, she whined or grunted while pointing to items of interest, but she did not have any words.
Her physician referred Bee to a state-run early intervention (EI) program, but her parents opted to wait and see how Bee would do for a few more months. When Bee was 32 months of age, her parents had her evaluated by EI therapists because of her lack of progress. Since she was almost 3, she had aged out of EI services and therapies.
GATHERING INFORMATION (assessing communication and physical capabilities) – Based on the EI evaluations, Bee's nonverbal IQ was low average (80). A parent-report instrument indicated that out of 396 possible words, Bee understood 100 words but only said 3 words. An occupational therapist and physical therapist working together found that Bee was not delayed in either fine motor or gross motor skills. She began to work with a private speech-language pathologist (SLP) who introduced her to a picture communication system and encouraged her to speak more words. By 40 months of age, Bee said 15 words but was not using phrases. She remained hard to understand and she consequently became more frustrated and irritable during expressive communication. At 42 months of age, Bee was given a diagnosis of autism spectrum disorder (ASD) by a developmental/behavioral pediatrician.
FEATURE MATCH (What may work best for the child) – Initially, Bee continued with the picture communication system, but her parents were concerned that her worsening temper tantrums might be caused by problems with her not being able to communicate well. Her parents brought this behavior concern to the attention of her pediatrician. Upon re-evaluation, since Bee had no fine motor delays and was used to pointing at pictures and letters on a smartphone, an adapted touchscreen tablet was selected for her. In order to determine Bee's abilities, the SLP selected a system with a dynamic, changeable display, which would allow for more pictures and words being added as her vocabulary increased, adapting with her as she developed.
TRIAL/DIAGNOSTIC TRAINING – The SLP working with Bee and her parents was very experienced with AAC and was fortunate enough to have different tablet-based speech generating systems that she used on a trial basis with Bee. The SLP requested and obtained a loaner copy of a comprehensive but expensive AAC program to try with Bee. After determining the best AAC program to use, the SLP then locked out all the other features of the touchscreen tablet so that Bee could only use the speech-generating program by touching certain pictures. Her parents felt very comfortable with the use of the tablet after training from the SLP.
RECOMMEND/FUNDING – Since the SLP was able to find an AAC system that worked well for Bee and her parents, they prepared a report and recommendations. The SLP assessed funding mechanisms for the recommended AAC system. Bee's physician and SLP sent a letter to the school board describing why AAC is important for children like Bee. Unfortunately, this did not result in the school purchasing a device for her, as Bee's public school early childhood program was poorly resourced and unable to fund her AAC device. Bee's physician and SLP sent a letter of medical necessity and a DME request to the family's insurance company (see Table 3.) Despite 2 appeals over a period of 10 months, the insurance company refused to pay for the tablet-based AAC system, insisting that their policy would only pay for a much more complicated single-use AAC device. The family had a very high-deductible insurance plan and were concerned that they would not be able to pay the deductible. Both the parents and the SLP also felt that Bee would not be able to effectively use such a complex single-use device. Eventually, the family found funding from a philanthropic organization suggested by the company providing the AAC system, and her AAC system was delivered within 2 weeks.
TRAINING/MONITORING – After the AAC system was delivered, the SLP began additional in-person training with Bee, school personnel, and family. Caregivers were taught to how to do minor repairs and updates when needed as well as how to encourage Bee to use it. Bee was quite excited to use the AAC device at school since the other children and her teacher liked to watch her use it. At home, the AAC was rarely used as the parents felt that they could usually understand her when she said 1- or 2-word phrases. Bee's SLP and physician encouraged the parents to work with Bee using the AAC at home to begin putting several words together to make sentences. This "homework" reinforced what was already being done at school and with the private SLP. After a year of using the AAC device, Bee began saying 3-word phrases and sentences using her own voice. She still had trouble being understood most of the time with longer connected speech, although she had hundreds of single words she could say. Using her AAC device, Bee effectively communicated in 6- to 7-word sentences even with unfamiliar communication partners.

may influence its successful uptake. The ultimate goal for using any AAC device is to achieve the highest possible functional communication.

ROLE OF THE PHYSICIAN CARING FOR CHILDREN WITH COMMUNICATION DISORDERS

Identification, Referral, and Care Coordination

Guidance through *Bright Futures: Guidelines for Health Supervision of Infants, Children, and Adolescents* (4th Edition) can equip the PCP to recognize pediatric communication disorders and make appropriate referrals.[73] Children at any age who are nonverbal or have unreliable intelligible speech are potential candidates for AAC. At present, there are many cost- and time-efficient ways to perform screening and surveillance of communication problems, including some clinical guidance from the AAP.[74] Knowing appropriate community resources and professionals for assistive technology is crucial. Children needing AAC systems require services for evaluation, procurement, training, and monitoring of devices and therapy programs. These services are ideally coordinated with existing therapies and educational programs while also being family centered. This integrative process can be confusing and overwhelming for the family, and it is within the role of the pediatric medical home to assist with and make referrals to all available resources.[75] Table 2 lists the 4 major components involved with coordinating care for children with communication disorders. Beyond providing medical home services for individual children, PCPs are also

TABLE 2. The Major Components to Providing Coordinated Care for CCCN

Major Components for Physician in Providing Coordinated Care for Children with Communication Disorders	How the Physician Can Assist	Who and What Can Help the Physician	Justifications for Coordination of Care
Facilitate the assessment process to ensure proper diagnostic and prognostic information	Provide up-to-date diagnoses and information about the current and possible functioning of the child	Pediatric subspecialists (eg, ped neurology, developmental ped); therapists (eg, speech/language, OT)	Without current information about the patient, how to do the assessment and what to look for may be inaccurate.
Guide short- and long-term planning by appropriate professionals, particularly speech-language pathologists (SLPs)	Provide ongoing information if situations change with time, (eg, change in school, discontinuance or startup of new services)	Get 2-way approval from school and therapists to send and receive updated information from all sources	Changes are expected over time. If an AAC device or adaptation is broken or is not being used, the physician may need to order new DME.
Participate in the implementation of the overall plan of use for the AAC in collaboration with the speech-language pathologist, other therapists and educators	Review the initial plan as well as any changes to the plan. This may include assisting family in finding funding sources for the purchase of devices. (See Resources)	If there are questions or concerns about a plan, it is important to discuss these with school and/or therapists.	It is best to discuss the overall plan with all involved individuals, including the family, to ensure agreement. This will lessen the chance for early abandonment.
Work with the family and professional team to evaluate the effectiveness of the efforts being made and to ensure appropriate follow-up	Make appointment for the child and family to be seen in-person (with the AAC) for about 2–4 weeks after delivery. Discuss with family "How's it working?"	Get ongoing reports from the school and/or therapists (especially S/L therapists)	SLPs can often provide objective measures that will help the physician gauge the success or problems with a particular device's implementation.

well poised to advocate on behalf of all of their patients and those children with communication disorders—specifically promoting and advocating that AAC and assistive technology, in general, is a covered service by Medicaid and other payers.

Although others may be involved in the child's care team, the PCP is uniquely positioned to evaluate the child's progress as well as the family's satisfaction or dissatisfaction as the leader of the medical home. For specifics about providing care coordination and care management, the reader is directed to an AAP policy statement that provides additional information and resources.[76]

Prescribing and Funding AAC Technology, Assessments, and Training Technology, including AAC

When pediatric communication disorders are recognized, necessary referrals can be initiated by the child's PCP. Children with communication disorders may be evaluated for AT needs as part of school-based, outpatient, or academic centers. When working with a public school system, the IEP may be utilized. According to the IDEA, AT provided in the school must specifically demonstrate a benefit to the child's participation in the education setting.[77] Unfortunately, equipment purchased by the school is not always sent home with the child for use in the family and community settings. Conversely, a school should not ask for family or insurance funding to purchase educationally necessary AAC (or any other AT). However, if the device is even partially paid for by Medicaid, according to Medicaid rules, it must be made available at home for "educational purposes."[19] The need for the device would be recognized as "medically necessary" and require the support of the medical team. Unless the school itself fully paid for the device, the child and family can keep the device after the child leaves the school or graduates. If a child does have to relinquish the device (for example, during a transition to adult disability or vocational services), there are state vocational/rehabilitation services, insurance changes, and community-based waivers in most states that will often fund purchase of AAC and for trainings.

For infants and toddlers receiving early intervention services through their state, the funding of AAC may be problematic. Early intervention programs are run by the states with some general guidance and requirements provided by federal regulations. These federal regulations, however, do not specifically address the purchase of AAC for children enrolled in early intervention. Therefore, there are historically few state early intervention programs that purchase a high-tech AAC device for a child with CCN. In most states, picture communication systems and some mid-tech devices are frequently used, especially by treating SLPs.[78] Additional information about funding can be found in the Appendix and from the website of the ASHA (asha.org).

For AAC paid for by any type of health insurance, including Medicaid, the PCP may be asked to write a prescription and a letter of medical necessity for AAC. This prescription and letter is written after evaluations by an SLP and other professionals (OT, rehabilitation technology specialist) are completed. A written report from these professionals will be needed to supplement the AAC order. It is important for the physician to have documented the child's communication needs and diagnoses, prescription, letter of medical necessity, and other supporting documentation in the medical record. Many electronic health records permit scanning of outside records to facilitate easier retrieval for the busy clinician.

In rural or other access-limited locations, it may be possible to have one or more evaluations performed by HIPAA-compliant telemedicine.[46,79] Especially since the COVID-19 pandemic, both the availability and the quality of these evaluations have improved greatly. For more information about who might perform these remote evaluations, PCPs or care coordinators may contact major universities in their state who have Departments of Speech/Language (or Communication) or find state-specific information for AAC specialists from the State Technical Assistance Programs (see Appendix). The ASHA (ASHA.org) maintains a list of certified speech-language pathologists (ie, CCC-SLPs). At this time in the United States there is no state or national certification as proof of "expertise" in AAC evaluation and treatment. Since the early 2000s, however, the ASHA certifies speech-language pathologists and verifies competency in AAC. A recent ASHA-certified SLP is, therefore, qualified to provide the necessary evaluation and interventions for AAC without additional state or national certification as proof of "expertise" in AAC. In addition, the American Board of Augmentative and Alternative Communication (see Appendix) is planning to offer additional distinct certification in 2024 for therapists who prefer to have it.

Reports from therapists, particularly from certified SLPs, can greatly assist the PCP in providing an appropriately detailed prescription. Information about the child's current status and expected outcome after using the device may also be requested; this information is often part of the report from the speech-language pathologist. A letter of medical necessity for durable medical equipment is generally needed as part of prescribing an AAC device. A letter of medical necessity provides a detailed summary of evaluation reports and recommendations, concluding that the recommended devices are *medically necessary* for treatment of the child's communication impairment caused by a specific diagnosis (eg, expressive speech impairment secondary to ASD). Insurance companies primarily use the listed *International Classification of Diseases, 10th Revision, Clinical Modification (ICD-10-CM)* codes detailed by the treating PCP as the major justification for the devices or services being requested. An insurance company may have medical necessity policies that define what can be approved on the basis of these codes and/or whether a device is considered rehabilitative or habilitative. Researching relevant insurance policies can assist the PCP in utilizing proper billing codes and diagnoses. If the PCP has access to in-house billing expertise or a care coordinator, these professionals may be helpful in this search process. It may be quite useful for the prescribing PCP to determine ahead of time about these specific policies and the billing codes related to them. Many AAC companies have hired "billing specialists" who can assist the PCP in obtaining this information from insurance companies. However, these "billing specialists" often have significant biases or conflicts of interest regarding what AAC equipment is needed. Table 3 presents a list of commonly necessary points to include in this medical necessity letter.

The AAP has defined medical necessity as "...health care interventions that are evidence-based, evidence-informed, or based on consensus advisory opinion and that are recommended by recognized health care professionals or organizations, such as the AAP, EPSDT services, and *Bright Futures*, to promote optimal growth and development in children and youth and to prevent, detect, diagnose, treat, ameliorate, or palliate the effects of physical, genetic, congenital, developmental, behavioral, or mental conditions, injuries, or disabilities."[80] When justifying medical necessity for any assistive technology (including AAC), the Early and Periodic Screening, Diagnosis and Treatment (EPSDT) benefit standards may provide another authoritative source and help inform medical necessity determinations. The EPSDT's medical necessity standards help ensure care, services, and treatments are commensurate with each child's medical needs, including age-appropriate physical health, mental health, and developmental services across the pediatric continuum.[81] If a health condition is discovered, EPSDT requires the state of a child's residence to provide necessary treatment, although this provision may be neglected by some state agencies. Per EPSDT, states are required to provide all medically necessary services covered by Medicaid, regardless of whether those services are part of the individual state's Medicaid program.[81]

Fortunately, in the last decade, there have been changes in coding and billing that allow the PCP to bill for care coordination activities including developing these prescriptions and letters. For example, chronic care and principal care management Current Procedural Terminology (CPT) services address both physician and clinical staff time spent coordinating and managing multiple or single chronic conditions respectively. Crucial medical home care coordination efforts by pediatricians and PCPs should be paid for by all third-party payers.[76]

Advocacy Information (See Appendix for Resources)

Technology advances quickly, and it is challenging for a physician to stay current with new developments. PCPs often endeavor to serve as informed advocates. Families of children with disabilities can have a variable understanding of AAC, ranging from low knowledge and some hesitancy to extensive knowledge and high expectations. Families may seek answers without support from health care professionals, which can result in inappropriate equipment and failure of AAC acceptance by the child. PCPs have an important advocacy role in this process by advising caregivers, patients, or allied health professionals and providing

TABLE 3. Information and Statements Commonly Needed in a Letter or Certificate of Medical Necessity/Prescription

1. Demographics (Name, Sex, Birth date and Age, Address, Phone and email contacts, Medical and speech/language Diagnoses, and ICD-10CM codes). Patient name: *Beatrice Porter* Patient date of birth: *April 19, 2017* Patient ID: *12345* Diagnoses: *Autism Spectrum Disorder (F84.0), Expressive Communication Disorder (F80.1)*
2. Physician information (Name, Address, Phone/fax, NPI #, Medicaid provider #, Other state-based identification) *Dr. Clarity Speakwell* *1 Children's Lane, Loving, PA* NPI: *123456789* Medicaid Provider: *98765* State License: *PA-61870*
3. Date of face-to-face appointment with the physician and patient when the need for an AAC device was determined. *To Whom it May Concern:* *Beatrice Porter is a patient under my care for autism spectrum disorder and expressive communication disorder. I last evaluated her on October 20, 2022, and determined it is medically necessary that she use the augmentative communication system described below and in supporting speech therapy notes.*
4. Complete list of AAC device and all related components. *She requires a touchscreen tablet with "SuzyTalks" software including the expansion pack.*
5. Statement that the patient has a medical condition which has resulted in a severe expressive language and speech disability such that speaking needs cannot be met by using natural and typical communication methods. *Beatrice has a severe expressive language disability that does not allow for verbal and typical communication methods. She has the cognitive ability for complex communication, but her disability severely impairs this ability.*
6. Statement that the patient has a medically necessary requirement for the AAC device and related components for health reasons (eg, ability to tell others of pain, discomfort, or other medical symptoms). *Beatrice is not able to tell her caregivers verbally if she is in pain without the use of this device and software. This could represent a potentially life-threatening situation if Beatrice is in distress and unable to communicate verbally. She must be able to communicate critical information in her environments at home, at school, and in the community.*
7. A certification or statement that the patient's communication skills will benefit by using the AAC and that other forms of treatment have been tried and were ruled out for being inappropriate or much less effective. *Beatrice has been successful in using a loaner program with "SuzyTalks" software. She has tried several devices with her treating speech-language pathologist, including simple picture exchange systems and more complex speech-generating devices. She has also tried several different software programs and speech-generating applications. She was not able to communicate complex needs with a simple picture exchange system, resulting in complete lack of communication. She was not able to master more complicated speech generating devices, such as the "SUPERMAX TALK 5000" listed in her insurance policy. Beatrice has demonstrated that she can use the "SuzyTalks" in therapeutic, home, and school environments.*
8. Assuming, as is usually the case, that a licensed speech-language pathologist (SLP), or a team led by an SLT, has performed a complete evaluation and produced a report, the physician would review this report. Following this, the physician would include a statement that they agree with the findings of the report and concur that the AAC device and components, as recommended by the SLT, is medically appropriate and necessary. It is important to note that, using internet resources, live video assessments are becoming much more available, even in remote or low=resource locations. The PCP, working with the families' insurance plans, is in a position to help ensure that the best quality evaluations are conducted, even if they are not in-person. (See text.) *I have reviewed the documentation provided by her speech-language pathologist, Rex Theodin, and I agree with both the findings of the report and that the device and software recommended is medically appropriate and necessary.*
9. Finally, a statement such as *"I do hereby attest that the information above is accurate, true, and complete to the best of my knowledge and that any falsifications, omissions, or concealment of any factual materials related to this information may subject me to criminal, civil, or administrative liability and that the signature below is my own."* A legible signature (not a stamp) of the ordering physician is usually needed on the form or letter.

guidance. As such, PCPs can benefit from keeping informed about local resources and professionals who can help provide information about assessments and training.

Several accessible sources of information are described here, and others are in the Appendix. The National Assistive Technology Technical Assistance Partnership oversees the federally mandated but state-funded "assistive tech" projects. These state projects are excellent information hubs and can refer individuals to appropriate service providers. Various organizations for children with disabilities (such as the Council for Exceptional Children and others) have also developed services that can be used to obtain references and abstracts about many facets of disability, especially with regard to school-related services. There are increasing numbers of websites offering resources for using AAC and other AT with children. Clinicians and families should be wary, however, as some are thinly veiled advertisements from companies or groups that may propose "alternative therapies" that are not evidence based and could be harmful (such as the use of vitamins or other supplements at high doses with dubious claims about enhancing language or cognitive development). The ASHA website (www.asha.org) documents communication supports that are not evidence based and not recommended. Physicians, therapists, and families can reach out to ASHA for additional questions.

CONCLUSIONS AND FUTURE DIRECTIONS

Children with communication disabilities can benefit considerably from AAC, as AAC can help maximize their developmental potential. Financial and societal barriers limit the equitable distribution and application of this technology. Much of the recent improvement in AAC devices can be attributed to organizations and companies addressing the principles of "universal design." Universal design is defined as the development of structures or devices that are accessible to both able-bodied persons as well as those persons who have functional limitation, such as touchscreen tablet-based AAC.[82,83] Another example of universal design is the simple wheelchair ramp, which can be used just as effectively by a person able to walk and a user of a wheelchair.

Despite the increasing interest in universal design, some insurance companies and Medicaid/Medicare programs will only pay for "dedicated" (single-use SGDs), which may prevent the option of recommending tablets or laptops as the hardware for AAC devices[84] (see AACfundinghelp.com in the Appendix). This limitation may lead to problems with funding for an AAC device.

Schools are not bound by Medicaid or other health insurance rules, which has led to many AAC devices (especially tablet based) being purchased with school district funds. As mentioned before, schools that pay the entire amount for AAC should be encouraged to provide AAC devices for home use, but they are not legally bound to do so. Encouragement from professionals (including physicians) can help schools understand the importance of using AAC at home and promote acceptance of the device.

Universal design devices are often the ones mainly used for AAC in schools. At this time, the use of AAC in schools is primarily for those children with CCN. School systems also use AAC and other AT to support literacy and written communication needs for children identified with a disability. Only recently has there been any research in the area of AAC use for literacy teaching and improving receptive language skills.[85] For example, many mobile AAC devices use pictures or symbols on the screen that may be selected for voice output of words, phrases, and sentences. Future research is needed to determine how best to teach reading skills to young users of AAC devices. Advocacy for child literacy and communication is essential for all children; this is familiar territory for the PCP.

RECOMMENDATIONS FOR PRIMARY CARE PHYSICIANS

1. In alignment with the principles of the pediatric medical home, the PCP and other pediatric physicians and advanced practice providers should use recommended surveillance and screening methods with their patients to identify children with communication problems and then refer them for appropriate evaluations. The AAP has a clinical report to guide this identification and referral process.[74]
2. If a child may benefit from AAC use, the PCP should ideally make a referral to a an SLP for an AAC assessment. Ideally, the SLP is either qualified in this area or can recommend other SLPs or programs with experience, particularly for patients who have complex needs. Other specialists (such as pediatric physiatrists, neurodevelopmental pediatricians, developmental and behavioral pediatrician, complex care pediatricians, or child neurologists) can assist with identifying SLPs or clinics with expertise if needed. The SLP's AAC assessment report will then support the written durable medical equipment prescription and medical necessity letters.
3. As a part of providing care coordination in the pediatric medical home, the PCP should collaborate with and support the SLP and others in performing appropriate testing for communication disabilities and in communication between the SLP and school personnel. The PCP should evaluate, review, and support the SLP's recommendation for appropriate communication equipment and updating/replacing that equipment as needed. The PCP may write a letter of medical necessity (if needed) or sign off on a letter of medical necessity prepared by the SLP and others, if appropriate. If a subspecialist such as a pediatric physiatrist, a neurodevelopmental pediatrician, a developmental and behavioral pediatrician, a complex care pediatrician, or a child neurologist has assumed the oversight of AT needs, the PCP provides oversight of the medical home neighbors as the leader of the medical home.
4. Primary care pediatricians and other PCP caring for children with CCN can support their patients by having open lines of communication with school personnel and facilitate the SLP's communication with school personnel and outside therapists. Parents and caregivers should feel empowered to discuss in-home use of communication systems or devices with school personnel. AAC use within the home often improves the overall successful use of AAC in educational and community settings.
5. PCPs and other pediatric physicians and advanced practice providers can facilitate guidance, information, training, and support for families of children with CCN to empower families as effective advocates and care coordinators for their children.
6. PCPs and other pediatric physicians and advanced practice providers can have a key role in advocating for the appropriate funding of AAC and related services for children with communication impairments at local, state, and federal levels. There is a critical need for improvements in Medicaid funding of AAC devices and for a more uniform policy and funding stream. Such improvements have already occurred within Medicare Part B; however, Medicaid still has variable state-by-state decision-making processes.
7. PCPs and other pediatric physicians and advanced practice providers can continue to advocate for research to be directed toward new approaches for the assessment of children with CCN, including the study of short- and

long-term effects of using AAC devices (especially SGDs) and evaluating changes in overall learning, social interactions, and participation in recreational and play activities.
8. Further advocacy efforts are needed to simplify and improve the process of determining AAC need and optimizing funding from third-party payers to pay PCPs for activities related to AAC. This would include time spent on care coordination such as making referrals, monitoring of use of and ongoing training for using AAC, and counseling of parents or caregivers.

LEAD AUTHORS

Larry W. Desch, MD, FAAP
Laura Hobart-Porter, DO, FAAP, FAAPMR
Amy Houtrow, MD, PhD, MPH, FAAP

COUNCIL ON CHILDREN WITH DISABILITIES EXECUTIVE COMMITTEE, 2024–2025

Garey Noritz, MD, FAAP, FACP Chairperson
Rishi Agrawal, MD, MPH, FAAP
Deanna S. Bell, MD, FAAP
Jessica E. A. Foster, MD, MPH, FAAP
Ellen Fremion, MD, FAAP, FACP
Sheryl Frierson, MD, MEd, FAAP
Michelle Melicosta, MD, MPH, MSc, FAAP
Barbara S. Saunders, DO, FAAP
Siddharth Srivastava, MD, FAAP
Jilda Vargus-Adams, MD, MSc, FAAP
Katharine E. Zuckerman, MD, MPH, FAAP

PAST COUNCIL ON CHILDREN WITH DISABILITIES EXECUTIVE COMMITTEE MEMBERS

Dennis Z. Kuo, MD, MHS, FAAP, Immediate Past Chairperson

LIAISONS

Jennifer Walton, MD, FAAP – *Section on Developmental and Behavioral Pediatrics*
Matthew Sadof, MD, FAAP – *Section on Home Care*
Allysa Ware, PhD, MSW – *Family Voices*

STAFF

Alexandra Kuznetsov

ABBREVIATIONS

AAC: augmentative/alternative communication
AAP: American Academy of Pediatrics
ASD: autism spectrum disorder
AT: assistive technology
CCN: complex communication needs
CP: cerebral palsy
EPSDT: Early and Periodic Screening, Diagnosis and Treatment
HIPAA: Health Insurance Portability and Accountability Act
ICF: International Classification of Functioning
IDEA: Individuals with Disabilities Education Act
PCP: primary care physician
PECS: Picture Exchange Communication System
SGD: speech-generating device
SLP: speech-language pathologist
VOCA: voice output communication aid
VSD: visual scene display

FUNDING: No external funding.

https://doi.org/10.1542/peds.2025-072216

REFERENCES

1. National Survey of Children's Health. (2021–2022). Accessed July 15, 2024. Available at: https://www.childhealthdata.org/browse/survey/results?q=10474&r=1
2. Müller I, Buchholz M, Ferm U. Text messaging with picture symbols - experiences of seven persons with cognitive and communicative disabilities. *J Assist Technol.* 2010;4(4):11–23. doi: 10.5042/jat.2010.0661.
3. Buchholz M, Müller IM, Ferm U. Text messaging with pictures and speech synthesis for adolescents and adults with cognitive and communicative disabilities – professionals' views about user satisfaction and participation. *Technol Disabil.* 2013;3(14):87–98. doi: 10.3233/TAD-130370.
4. National Joint Committee for the Communication Needs of Persons With Severe Disabilities. Position Statement on Access to Communication Services and Supports: Concerns Regarding the Application of Restrictive "Eligibility" Policies. American School Health Association; 2003. Accessed August 20, 2024. Available at: https://www.asha.org/policy/ps2003-00227
5. Brady NC, Bruce S, Goldman A, et al. Communication services and supports for individuals with severe disabilities: guidance for assessment and intervention. *Am J Intellect Dev*

Disabil. 2016;121(2):121–138. PubMed doi: 10.1352/1944-7558-121.2.121

6. Black LI, Vahratian A, Hoffman HJ. Communication disorders and use of intervention services among children aged 3–17 years: United States, 2012. *NCHS Data Brief.* 2015;(205):1–8. PubMed
7. King MR, Romski M, Sevcik RA. Language differentiation using augmentative and alternative communication: an investigation of Spanish-English bilingual children with and without language impairments. *Am J Speech Lang Pathol.* 2021;30(1):89–104. PubMed doi: 10.1044/2020_ajslp-20-00030
8. Biddle C, Azano AP. Constructing and reconstructing the "rural school problem" a century of rural education research. *Rev Res Educ.* 2016;40(1):298–325. doi: 10.3102/0091732X16667700.
9. Pennington R, Horn C, Berrong A. An evaluation of the differences between big city and small town special education services for low incidence disabilities in Kentucky. *Rural Spec Educ Q.* 2009; 28(4):3–9. doi: 10.1177/875687050902800402.
10. Roy-O'Reilly M, Salles A. Stigma associated with requesting accommodations—the high cost of ableism in medicine. *JAMA Netw Open.* 2023;6(5):e2312131. PubMed doi: 10.1001/jamanetworkopen.2023.12131
11. Christakis DA, Iezzoni LI. Calling on the USPSTF to address ableism and structural ableism. *JAMA.* 2023;330(14):1327–1328. PubMed doi: 10.1001/jama.2023.17092
12. Iezzoni LI. Cancer detection, diagnosis, and treatment for adults with disabilities. *Lancet Oncol.* 2022;23(4):e164–e173. PubMed doi: 10.1016/s1470-2045(22)00018-3
13. Bax M, Tydeman C, Flodmark O. Clinical and MRI correlates of CP: the European CP Study. *JAMA.* 2006;296(13):1602–1608. PubMed doi: 10.1001/jama.296.13.1602
14. Hustad KC, Allison K, McFadd E, Riehle K. Speech and language development in 2-year-old children with cerebral palsy. *Dev Neurorehabil.* 2014;17(3):167–175. PubMed doi: 10.3109/17518423.2012.747009
15. Grieco J, Pulsifer M, Seligsohn K, Skotko B, Schwartz A. Down syndrome: Cognitive and behavioral functioning across the lifespan. *Am J Med Genet C Semin Med Genet.* 2015;169(2):135–149. PubMed doi: 10.1002/ajmg.c.31439
16. Silverman W. Down syndrome: cognitive phenotype. *Ment Retard Dev Disabil Res Rev.* 2007;13(3):228–236. PubMed doi: 10.1002/mrdd.20156
17. Ganz JB. AAC interventions for individuals with autism spectrum disorders: state of the science and future research directions. *Augment Altern Commun.* 2015;31(3):203–214. PubMed doi: 10.3109/07434618.2015.1047532
18. Crowe B, Machalicek W, Wei Q, Drew C, Ganz J. Augmentative and alternative communication for children with intellectual and developmental disability: a mega-review of the literature. *J Dev Phys Disabil.* 2022;34(1):1–42. PubMed doi: 10.1007/s10882-021-09790-0
19. Lin SC, Gold RS. Assistive technology needs, functional difficulties, and services utilization and coordination of children with developmental disabilities in the United States. *Assist Technol.* 2018;30(2):100–106. PubMed doi: 10.1080/10400435.2016.1265023
20. Desch LW. High technology for handicapped children: a pediatrician's viewpoint. *Pediatrics.* 1986;77(1):71–87. PubMed
21. Bondy A, Frost L. The Picture Exchange Communication System. *Behav Modif.* 2001;25(5):725–744. PubMed doi: 10.1177/0145445501255004
22. Gropp M, Johnson E, Bornman J, Koul R. Nurses' perspectives about communication with patients in an intensive care setting using a communication board: A pilot study. *Health SA.* 2019;24:1162. PubMed doi: 10.4102/hsag.v24i0.1162
23. Holyfield C, Drager K, Light J, Caron JG. Typical toddlers' participation in "Just-in-Time" programming of vocabulary for visual scene display augmentative and alternative communication apps on mobile technology: a descriptive study. *Am J Speech Lang Pathol.* 2017;26(3):737–749. PubMed doi: 10.1044/2017_ajslp-15-0197
24. Schepis MM, Reid DH, Behrmann MM, Sutton KA. Increasing communicative interactions of young children with autism using a voice output communication aid and naturalistic teaching. *J Appl Behav Anal.* 1998;31(4):561–578. PubMed doi: 10.1901/jaba.1998.31-561
25. Wendt O, Hsu N, Simon K, Dienhart A, Cain L. Effects of an iPad based speech generating device infused and instruction with the picture exchange communication system for adolescents and young adults with severe autism spectrum disorder. *Behav Modif.* 2019;43(6):898–932. PubMed doi: 10.1177/0145445519870552
26. Leonet O, Orcasitas-Vicandi M, Langarika-Rocafort A, Mondragon NI, Etxebarrieta GR. A systematic review of augmentative and alternative communication interventions for children aged from 0 to 6 years. *Lang Speech Hear Serv Sch.* 2022;53(3):894–920. PubMed doi: 10.1044/2022_lshss-21-00191
27. Berenguer C, Martínez ER, De Stasio S, Baixauli I. Parents' perceptions and experiences with their children's use of augmentative/alternative communication: a systematic review and qualitative meta-synthesis. *Int J Environ Res Public Health.* 2022;19(13):80–91. PubMed doi: 10.3390/ijerph19138091
28. Biggs EE, Carter EW, Gilson CB. Systematic review of interventions involving aided AAC modeling for children with complex communication needs. *Am J Intellect Dev Disabil.* 2018;123(5):443–473. PubMed doi: 10.1352/1944-7558-123.5.443
29. O'Neill T, Light J, Pope L. Effects of interventions that include aided augmentative and alternative communication input on the communication of individuals with complex communication needs: a meta-analysis. *J Speech Lang Hear Res.* 2018;61(7):1743–1765. PubMed doi: 10.1044/2018_jslhr-l-17-0132
30. Dada S, Flores C, Bastable K, Schlosser RW. The effects of augmentative and alternative communication interventions on the receptive language skills of children with developmental disabilities: A scoping review. *Int J Speech Lang Pathol.* 2021;23(3):247–257. PubMed doi: 10.1080/17549507.2020.1797165
31. Langarika-Rocafort A, Mondragon NI, Etxebarrieta GR. A systematic review of research on augmentative and alternative communication interventions for children aged 6–10 in the last decade. *Lang Speech Hear Serv Sch.* 2021;52(3):899–916. PubMed doi: 10.1044/2021_lshss-20-00005
32. Holyfield C, Drager KDR, Kremkow JMD, Light J. Systematic review of AAC intervention research for adolescents and adults with

autism spectrum disorder. *Augment Altern Commun.* 2017;33(4): 201–212. PubMed doi: 10.1080/07434618.2017.1370495

33. Wright CA, Kaiser AP, Reikowsky DI, Roberts MY. Effects of a naturalistic sign intervention on expressive language of toddlers with Down syndrome. *J Speech Lang Hear Res.* 2013;56(3):994–1008. PubMed doi: 10.1044/1092-4388(2012/12-0060)
34. Meinzen-Derr J, Sheldon RM, Henry S, et al. Enhancing language in children who are deaf/hard-of-hearing using augmentative and alternative communication technology strategies. *Int J Pediatr Otorhinolaryngol.* 2019;125:23–31. PubMed doi: 10.1016/j.ijporl.2019.06.015
35. Meinzen-Derr J, Sheldon R, Altaye M, Lane L, Mays L, Wiley S. A technology-assisted language intervention for children who are deaf or hard of hearing: a randomized clinical trial. *Pediatrics.* 2021;147(2):e2020025734. PubMed doi: 10.1542/peds.2020-025734
36. Allen AA, Schlosser RW, Brock KL, Shane HC. The effectiveness of aided augmented input techniques for persons with developmental disabilities: a systematic review. *Augment Altern Commun.* 2017;33(3):149–159. PubMed doi: 10.1080/07434618.2017.1338752
37. Brown MN, Grames LM, Skolnick GB. Augmentative and alternative communication (AAC) use among patients followed by a multidisciplinary cleft and craniofacial team. *Cleft Palate Craniofac J.* 2021;58(3):324–331. PubMed doi: 10.1177/1055665620947606
38. Caynes K, Rose TA, Burmester D, Ware RS, Johnston LM. Reproducibility and validity of the Functional Communication Classification System for young children with cerebral palsy. *Dev Med Child Neurol.* 2021;63(7):866–873. PubMed doi: 10.1111/dmcn.14844
39. Luyster RJ, Zane E, Wisman Weil L. Conventions for unconventional language: Revisiting a framework for spoken language features in autism. *Autism Dev Lang Impair.* 2022;7:23969415221105472. PubMed doi: 10.1177/23969415221105472
40. Cress CJ, Marvin CA. Common questions about AAC services in early intervention. *Augment Altern Commun.* 2003;19(4):254–272. doi: 10.1080/07434610310001598242.
41. Alper S, Raharinirina S. Assistive technology for individuals with disabilities: a review and synthesis of the literature. *J Spec Educ Technol.* 2006;21(2):47–64. doi: 10.1177/016264340602100204.
42. Lorang E, Maltman N, Venker C, Eith A, Sterling A. Speech-language pathologists' practices in augmentative and alternative communication during early intervention. *Augment Altern Commun.* 2022;38(1):41–52. PubMed doi: 10.1080/07434618.2022.2046853
43. Drager K, Light J, McNaughton D. Effects of AAC interventions on communication and language for young children with complex communication needs. *J Pediatr Rehabil Med.* 2010;3(4):303–310. PubMed doi: 10.3233/prm-2010-0141
44. Buekelman DR, Mirenda P. *Augmentative and Alternative Communication: Supporting Children and Adults with Complex Communication Needs.* Paul H. Brookes Co; 2012.
45. Walters C, Sevcik RA, Romski M. Spoken vocabulary outcomes of toddlers with developmental delay after parent-implemented augmented language intervention. *Am J Speech Lang Pathol.* 2021;30(3):1023–1037. PubMed doi: 10.1044/2020_ajslp-20-00093
46. Russell M, Donaldson C, Pleasant J, Roberts K. Using telehealth to adapt service delivery for children during the COVID-19 pandemic. *Dev Disabil Netw J.* 2020;1(2). doi: 10.26077/c6c4-ffdb.
47. World Health Organization. *International Classification of Functioning, Disability and Health- Children and Youth.* World Health Organization; 2001.
48. Nguyen L, Cross A, Rosenbaum P, Gorter JW. Use of the International Classification of Functioning, Disability and Health to support goal-setting practices in pediatric rehabilitation: a rapid review of the literature. *Disabil Rehabil.* 2021;43(6):884–894. PubMed doi: 10.1080/09638288.2019.1643419
49. Griffiths T, Clarke M, Price K. Augmentative and alternative communication for children with speech, language and communication needs. *Paediatr Child Health.* 2022;32(8):277–281. doi: 10.1016/j.paed.2022.05.001.
50. Westby C, Washington KN. Using the International Classification of Functioning, Disability and Health in assessment and intervention of school-aged children with language impairments. *Lang Speech Hear Serv Sch.* 2017;48(3):137–152. PubMed doi: 10.1044/2017_lshss-16-0037
51. Moorcroft A, Scarinci N, Meyer C. Speech pathologist perspectives on the acceptance versus rejection or abandonment of AAC systems for children with complex communication needs. *Augment Altern Commun.* 2019;35(3):193–204. PubMed doi: 10.1080/07434618.2019.1609577
52. Wandin H, Tegler H, Svedberg L, et al. A scoping review of aided AAC modeling for individuals with developmental disabilities and emergent communication. *Curr Dev Disord Rep.* 2023;10(2): 123–131. doi: 10.1007/s40474-023-00275-7.
53. Chazin KT, Ledford JR, Pak NS. A systematic review of augmented input interventions and exploratory analysis of moderators. *Am J Speech Lang Pathol.* 2021;30(3):1210–1223. PubMed doi: 10.1044/2020_ajslp-20-00102
54. Kent-Walsh J, Binger C, Makani MD. Teaching partners to support the communication skills of young children who use AAC: lessons from the ImPAACT program. *Early Child Serv (San Diego Calif).* 2010;4(5):155–170.
55. Senner JE, Post K, Baud MR, et al. Effects of parent instruction in partner-augmented input on parent and child speech generating device use. *Technol Disabil.* 2019;31(1–2):27–38. doi: 10.3233/TAD-190228.
56. Holyfield C, MacNeil S, Caldwell N, et al. Leveraging communication partner speech to automate augmented input for children on the autism spectrum who are minimally verbal: prototype development. *Am J Speech Lang Pathol.* 2024;33(3):1174–1192. PubMed doi: 10.1044/2023_ajslp-23-00224
57. Copley J, Ziviani J. Barriers to the use of assistive technology for children with multiple disabilities. *Occup Ther Int.* 2004;11(4): 229–243. PubMed doi: 10.1002/oti.213
58. Zabala J. SETT Framework. Accessed August 3, 2022. Available at: www.joyzabala.com
59. Ostensjø S, Carlberg EB, Vøllestad NK. The use and impact of assistive devices and other environmental modifications on everyday activities and care in young children with cerebral palsy. *Disabil Rehabil.* 2005; 27(14):849–861. PubMed doi: 10.1080/09638280400018619

60. Rust KL, Smith RO. Assistive technology in the measurement of rehabilitation and health outcomes: a review and analysis of instruments. *Am J Phys Med Rehabil.* 2005;84(10):780–793. PubMed doi: 10.1097/01.phm.0000179520.34844.0e

61. Foster CC, Fuentes MM, Wadlington LA, et al. Caregiver and provider experiences of physical, occupational, and speech therapy for children with medical complexity. *J Pediatr Rehabil Med.* 2021; 14(3):505–516. PubMed doi: 10.3233/prm-190647

62. Graves JM, Mackelprang JL, Moore M, et al. Rural-urban disparities in health care costs and health service utilization following pediatric mild traumatic brain injury. *Health Serv Res.* 2019;54(2): 337–345. PubMed doi: 10.1111/1475-6773.13096

63. Galvin JC, Scherer MJ, eds. *Evaluating, Selecting and Using Appropriate Assistive Technology.* Pro-Ed; 2004.

64. Petrie H, Carmien S, Lewis A. Assistive technology abandonment: research realities and potentials. In: Miesenberger K, Kouroupetroglou G, eds. *Proceedings of the International Conference on Computers Helping People with Special Needs.* Springer; 2018.

65. Waller A. Telling tales: unlocking the potential of AAC technologies. *Int J Lang Commun Disord.* 2019;54(2):159–169. PubMed doi: 10.1111/1460-6984.12449

66. Moorcroft A, Scarinci N, Meyer C. A systematic review of the barriers and facilitators to the provision and use of low-tech and unaided AAC systems for people with complex communication needs and their families. *Disabil Rehabil Assist Technol.* 2019; 14(7):710–731. PubMed doi: 10.1111/1460-6984.12449

67. Scherer MJ. Outcomes of assistive technology use on quality of life. *Disabil Rehabil.* 1996;18(9):439–448. PubMed doi: 10.3109/09638289609165907

68. Zapf SA, Scherer MJ, Baxter MF, H Rintala D. Validating a measure to assess factors that affect assistive technology use by students with disabilities in elementary and secondary education. *Disabil Rehabil Assist Technol.* 2016;11(1):38–49. PubMed doi: 10.3109/17483107.2015.1104559

69. Johnson JM, Inglebret E, Jones C, Ray J. Perspectives of speech language pathologists regarding success versus abandonment of AAC. *Augment Altern Commun.* 2006;22(2):85–99. PubMed doi: 10.1080/07434610500483588

70. Bauer S, Elsaesser LJ. Integrating medical, assistive, and universally designed products and technologies: assistive technology device classification (ATDC). *Disabil Rehabil Assist Technol.* 2012;7(5):350–355. PubMed doi: 10.3109/17483107.2011.653000

71. Long T, Huang L, Woodbridge MM, Woolverton M, Minkel J. Integrating assistive technology into an outcome-driven model of service delivery. *Infants Young Child.* 2003;16:272–284.

72. Nguyen T, Tilbrook A, Sandelance M, Wright FV. The switch access measure: development and evaluation of the reliability and clinical utility of a switching assessment for children with severe and multiple disabilities. *Disabil Rehabil Assist Technol.* 2023;18(5): 673–684. PubMed doi: 10.1080/17483107.2021.1906961

73. Hagan JF, Shaw JS, Duncan PM, eds. *Bright Futures: Guidelines for Health Supervision of Infants, Children, and Adolescents.* 4th ed. American Academy of Pediatrics; 2017.

74. Lipkin PH, Macias MM; COUNCIL ON CHILDREN WITH DISABILITIES, SECTION ON DEVELOPMENTAL AND BEHAVIORAL PEDIATRICS. Promoting optimal development: identifying infants and young children with developmental disorders through developmental surveillance and screening [reaffirmed April 2024]. *Pediatrics.* 2020;145(1):e20193449. PubMed doi: 10.1542/peds.2019-3449

75. Strickland BB, Jones JR, Ghandour RM, Kogan MD, Newacheck PW. The medical home: health care access and impact for children and youth in the United States. *Pediatrics.* 2011;127(4):604–611. PubMed doi: 10.1542/peds.2009-3555

76. Council on Children with Disabilities and Medical Home Implementation Project Advisory Committee. Patient- and family-centered care coordination: a framework for integrating care for children and youth across multiple systems. [reaffirmed April 2023]. *Pediatrics.* 2014;133(5):e1451–e1460. PubMed doi: 10.1542/peds.2014-0318

77. Zirkel PA. Special education law: illustrative basics and nuances of key IDEA components. *Teach Educ Spec Educ.* 2015;38(4):263–275. doi: 10.1177/0888406415575377.

78. Romski M, Sevcik RA. Augmentative communication and early intervention: myths and realities. *Infants Young Child.* 2005;18(3):174–185.

79. Biggs EE, Therrien MCS, Douglas SN, Snodgrass MR. Augmentative and alternative communication telepractice during the COVID-19 pandemic: a national survey of speech-language pathologists. *Am J Speech Lang Pathol.* 2022;31(1):303–321. PubMed doi: 10.1044/2021_ajslp-21-00036

80. Giardino AP, Hudak ML, Sood BG, Pearlman SA; COMMITTEE ON CHILD HEALTH FINANCING. Considerations in the determination of medical necessity in children: application to contractual language. *Pediatrics.* 2022;150(3):e2022058882. PubMed doi: 10.1542/peds.2022-058882

81. Perrin JM. EPSDT (early and periodic screening, diagnosis, and treatment): a primer in time of change. *Ambul Pediatr.* 2006;6 (2):63–64. PubMed doi: 10.1016/j.ambp.2006.02.003

82. Thunberg G, Johnson E, Bornman J, Öhlén J, Nilsson S. Being heard - Supporting person-centred communication in paediatric care using augmentative and alternative communication as universal design: A position paper. *Nurs Inq.* 2022;29(2):e12426. PubMed doi: 10.1111/nin.12426

83. MacKeogh T, Dillenburg K, Donovan J. Applying a universal design approach to empower children with multiple impairments in assistive technology assessment. *Stud Health Technol Inform.* 2018;256:870–880. PubMed

84. Isgett C, Wang S. Challenges regarding assistive technology in special education. 2021 Tenth International Conference of Educational Innovation through Technology; 2021:293–298.

85. Mandak K, Light J, Boyle S. The effects of literacy interventions on single-word reading for individuals who use aided AAC: a systematic review. *Augment Altern Commun.* 2018;34(3):206–218. PubMed doi: 10.1080/07434618.2018.1470668

Promoting Optimal Development: Screening for Mental Health, Emotional, and Behavioral Problems

- *Clinical Report*

CLINICAL REPORT Guidance for the Clinician in Rendering Pediatric Care

American Academy of Pediatrics

DEDICATED TO THE HEALTH OF ALL CHILDREN™

Promoting Optimal Development: Screening for Mental Health, Emotional, and Behavioral Problems: Clinical Report

Carol Weitzman, MD, FAAP,[1] James Guevara, MD, MPH, FAAP,[2] Michelle Curtin, DO, FAAP,[3] Michelle Macias, MD, FAAP,[4] the AAP Section on Developmental and Behavioral Pediatrics; AAP Council on Early Childhood; AAP Committee on Psychosocial Aspects of Child and Family Health; SOCIETY FOR DEVELOPMENTAL AND BEHAVIORAL PEDIATRICS

abstract

Rates of mental health, emotional, and behavioral (MEB) problems in the United States continue to rise, with current estimates of 13% to 20% of children having an MEB disorder and an additional 19% with problems causing impairment or distress that do not meet diagnostic criteria for a specific disorder. This clinical report incorporates and expands on recommendations from the 2019 American Academy of Pediatrics policy statement "Mental Health Competencies for Pediatric Practice" as well as "Recommendations for Preventive Pediatric Health Care." It addresses the rising MEB needs of youth since the previous clinical report, "Promoting Optimal Development: Screening for Behavioral and Emotional Problems," was published in 2015. This report outlines specific guidance for MEB screening, identification, and care of children in pediatric primary care. Screening, as part of regular health supervision visits and surveillance, begins within the first month of life to identify postpartum depression in caregivers. Child-focused screening for MEB problems begins at 6 months of age and continues at 12-, 24-, and 36-month health supervision visits, alternating with recommended developmental and autism spectrum disorder screenings at every visit in the Bright Futures Periodicity schedule and additionally when clinically indicated. After age 3, MEB screening continues annually. This report also 1) reviews updated information on prevalence of MEB problems; 2) articulates the current state of detection of these problems in pediatric primary care; 3) addresses how to manage a positive screen; 4) describes barriers to screening, including special population needs, and potential models

[1]*Department of Pediatrics, Harvard Medical School, Division of Developmental Medicine, Boston Children's Hospital, Boston, Massachusetts;* [2]*Children's Hospital of Philadelphia, Perelman School of Medicine at Penn, Philadelphia, Pennsylvania;* [3]*Department of Pediatrics, Wake Forest University School of Medicine, Winston-Salem, North Carolina; and* [4]*Division of Developmental-Behavioral Pediatrics, Department of Pediatrics, Medical University of South Carolina, Charleston, South Carolina*

Clinical reports from the American Academy of Pediatrics benefit from expertise and resources of liaisons and internal (AAP) and external reviewers. However, clinical reports from the American Academy of Pediatrics may not reflect the views of the liaisons or the organizations or government agencies that they represent.

To cite: Weitzman C, Guevara J, Curtin M, et al; American Academy of Pediatrics, the AAP Section on Developmental and Behavioral Pediatrics; AAP Council on Early Childhood; AAP Committee on Psychosocial Aspects of Child and Family Health; Society for Developmental and Behavioral Pediatrics. Promoting Optimal Development: Screening for Mental Health, Emotional, and Behavioral Problems: Clinical Report. *Pediatrics.* 2025;156(3):e2025073172

to address those barriers; and 5) discusses potential changes at a practice and systems level that facilitate successful MEB screening.

INTRODUCTION

Scope of the Problem

Mental health, emotional, and behavioral problems (collectively referred to as MEB problems[1]) during childhood are common and have reached crisis proportions, yet they often go undetected and untreated despite being responsible for significant morbidity and mortality. By current estimates, approximately 13% to 20% of children in the United States have a behavioral or emotional disorder at any given time,[2,3] including young children ages 2 to 8 years.[4] A substantial number of children have subthreshold MEB problems that cause impairment or distress that do not meet diagnostic criteria for a specific disorder within the *Diagnostic and Statistical Manual of Mental Disorders, Fifth Edition (DSM-5)*.[5,6] MEB problems are among the top 5 chronic pediatric conditions causing functional impairment.[7,8] Between 37% and 39% of children will have an MEB disorder diagnosed by 16 years of age, with the most common diagnoses being disruptive behavior problems, attention-deficit/hyperactivity disorder (ADHD), anxiety, and mood disorders.[2,9,10] Between 23% and 61% of children with an MEB problem diagnosis at one point will have an MEB problem diagnosis in the future, although it is not always the same diagnosis.[2] Children exposed to adversity, including poverty,[11] racism and other forms of discrimination,[12] environmental toxins including lead, and toxic stress[13] (such as exposure to abuse, neglect, parental mental illness, and violence) are more vulnerable to MEB problems. In 2020, suicide became the second leading cause of death in youth 10 to 14 years of age and the third leading cause of death in youth 15 to 24 years of age. This rate increased 41% from 2000 to 2017,[14–16] and individuals with MEB problems have a nearly 8-fold increased risk of death by suicide compared with individuals without MEB problems.[17]

The COVID-19 pandemic exacerbated the prevalence of MEB problems in children. More than 140 000 children lost their primary or secondary caregiver to COVID-19, significantly increasing their psychosocial stress burden.[18] Unprecedented numbers of children presented to emergency departments with serious mental health problems and suicidal ideation. During the winter of 2021, emergency department visits for potential suicide attempts among female youth were 50.6% higher compared with the same period in 2019.[19] These rates remain elevated above prepandemic levels.[20] Data from the Centers for Disease Control and Prevention in 2021 reveal that more than one-third (37%) of high school students reported they experienced poor mental health during the COVID-19 pandemic, and 44% reported that they persistently felt sad or hopeless as compared with 37% in 2019, prior to the start of the pandemic.[21] Some of these symptoms were attributed to traumatic losses, increased psychosocial stressors in the home, disruption of social networks, social isolation, and individual factors including preexisting mental health problems.

The pandemic highlighted inadequacies in existing medical infrastructure including suboptimal detection of MEB problems, an inadequate workforce to treat identified problems, nonexistent or insufficient payment that in many states does not cover costs for screening, a lack of referral sources, and an overall lack of access to care for MEB problems.[22] Approximately 50% of adults with behavioral health problems report that their disorders first manifested in early adolescence.[23,24] Studies have shown that MEB problems detected early in childhood have been shown to have an enduring effect and have a strong association with MEB problems later in adolescence.[25,26] Anxiety disorders and ADHD are the earliest disorders to emerge, often in the preschool and early school-age years, with substance use disorders emerging later. There is an approximately 2- to 4-year period between symptom appearance and the time a child meets diagnostic criteria for an MEB problem, suggesting that there may be opportunities for secondary prevention or early intervention.[27] In 2019, approximately 25% of all children ages 12 to 17 years reported receiving mental health services, reinforcing that MEB problems in children continue to present a substantial public health concern.[28] Although approximately 78% of children with depression received treatment, only 59% of those with anxiety and 53% with behavior problems received treatment, underscoring the need for detection of MEB problems beginning early in childhood so that treatment can be obtained.

Policies in Place

In 2004, the American Academy of Pediatrics (AAP) established the Task Force on Mental Health, which articulated mental health competencies for primary care, developed guidance for addressing systemic and financial barriers to providing mental health care in primary care settings, and provided tools and strategies to assist pediatric primary care clinicians (PPCCs) in applying chronic care principles to children with MEB problems.[29] The task force also provided guidance (through identifying tools and describing strategies) to providers on adapting current practice to include MEB care.[29]

In 2019, the AAP Committee on Psychosocial Aspects of Child and Family Health and Mental Health Leadership Work Group issued "Mental Health Competencies for Pediatric Practice," which was an update of the 2009 policy statement.[30] This updated policy statement outlined mental health competencies needed by PPCCs to promote well-being for children by identifying risks and symptoms of MEB problems, initiating achievable steps within primary care, and collaborating with specialists and community partners to deliver care for children with greater complexity. The authors also developed a process of care algorithm to aid PPCCs in identifying and caring for children who present with mental health problems.

In 2022, the AAP updated the Bright Futures "Recommendations for Preventive Pediatric Health Care," also known as the periodicity schedule.[31] One of the updated topics included changes to recommendations for behavioral/social/emotional screening. The prior recommendation for assessment of psychosocial/behavioral concerns was updated to screening for behavioral/social/emotional problems beginning at the newborn visit to the 21-year-old visit. This update included that the screening should be family centered and may include screening for 1) caregiver emotional and mental health concerns (in addition to already existing recommendations for screening for maternal depression up to 6 months of age); 2) social drivers of health; 3) racism; 4) poverty; 5) relational health; and 6) children's MEB problems. These recommendations were designed to align with existing AAP policy, recommendations of the American College of Obstetricians and Gynecologists Women's Preventive Services Initiative, and guidelines of the American Academy of Child Adolescent Psychiatry.[32,33] This clinical report will focus on the detection of children's MEB problems and describe how they relate to the other concerns included in the list above.

Current State of Detection of MEB Problems and Innovations in Care in Pediatric Settings

In surveys of developmental screening of infants and toddlers, PPCCs increased screening rates from 21% in 2002 to 48% in 2009 and 63% in 2016 (with 98% reporting screening but only 59% reporting using standardized tools in 2019[34]), with a substantial increase in the referral of at-risk patients to early intervention services.[35] Much of this increase is likely attributable to the AAP clinical reports advocating for developmental screening at specified intervals in addition to surveillance.[36] In contrast, there is less research over the same time period on the use of screening tools and routine surveillance for MEB problems. The ability of PPCCs to identify developmental and MEB problems on the basis of clinical judgment alone in the absence of a standardized measure has been shown to have low sensitivity, ranging from 14% to 54%, and a specificity ranging from 69% to 100%.[37]

A number of promising new strategies have been developed since the 2015 clinical report was published to improve the PPCC's ability to screen, identify, and provide care for children with MEB problems, including initiatives such as AAP-sponsored ECHO (Extension for Community Healthcare Outcomes) trainings, learning collaboratives,[38–41] availability of remote psychiatry consultation,[42,43] and integration of mental health providers within pediatric practice.[44,45] Quality improvement learning collaboratives have demonstrated that practices can significantly improve and sustain their screening rates for MEB problems and ability to develop an initial care plan.[38–41]

The failure rate to detect MEB problems ranges from 14% to 40%, moderated by the degree of family distress or known family history risk factors.[46] MEB problems continue to be less likely to be identified by PPCCs in children of color and non–English-speaking children and adolescents related to language and cultural barriers[47,48] or when developmental screening programs are used in isolation, given these screens were not designed to detect MEB problems.[49] Current estimates show that children with identified MEB problems are more likely to receive treatment, suggesting that detection can improve outcome.[22] Surveyed pediatricians overwhelmingly have endorsed that they should be responsible for identifying children with ADHD, eating disorders, depression, substance use disorders, and behavior problems.[50]

Barriers to Early Detection of MEB Problems

Pediatricians have traditionally reported a lack of confidence in their training and ability to identify and successfully manage children's MEB problems; recent interventions such as those described above have improved the skills of PPCCs.[38,39] The most highly reported barriers to adopting new screening practices in pediatrics include lack of time, long waits for children to be seen by mental health providers, and a lack of available mental health providers to whom to refer children.[51] A group of pediatricians were surveyed in 2004 as a part of the AAP periodic survey, and another randomly selected group of AAP members were surveyed in 2013 about barriers to identifying children with MEB problems. Across both surveys, pediatricians reported a lack of training and confidence in the *treatment* of mental health problems. Barriers reported in 2004, including lack of training in *identifying* mental health problems, lack of confidence in diagnosing MEB problems and treating children with medication, inadequate payment, and lack of time were less frequently reported in 2013.[52] Additional screening barriers related to children of different cultures, ethnicities, foster or kinship care placement, developmental status, and language utilization are also noted here, and an in-depth discussion of each unique group warrants further future consideration.

Need for Updates to This Report

Since the publication of the original clinical report in 2015, a series of challenges described earlier have arisen, coupled with continued evidence of a rapidly escalating rise in children with MEB problems. Currently in the United States, there are approximately 755 certified developmental-behavioral pediatricians younger than 70 years currently practicing, 742 adolescent medicine physicians, and 10 500 child and adolescent psychiatrists.[53–55] These numbers equate to fewer than 1 developmental-behavioral pediatrician and only 10 child and adolescent psychiatrists per 100 000 children, despite an estimated need of 47 clinicians per 100 000 children.[56,57] Statistics suggest an aging workforce across fields is worsening the shortage of trained MEB clinicians.[57] This shortage has resulted in an urgent need for PPCCs to identify children with MEB problems within primary care, particularly for those children who do not spontaneously disclose the problem or seek care, so management within the medical home can be initiated early to potentially decrease the need for referrals.

The 2019 AAP policy statement "Mental Health Competencies for Pediatric Practice"[30] outlined a comprehensive approach to mental health identification and treatment within primary care. To complement that statement, this report provides specific guidance to enhance successful MEB surveillance, monitoring, and screening. This updated report offers guidance on: 1) screening intervals at specific time points based on Bright Futures preventive services recommendations and the relationship to ongoing surveillance; 2) the relationship between MEB screens and other recommended screens; 3) managing a positive MEB screen; 4) promoting resilience in children and families; and 5) strategies to organize a pediatric practice for MEB screening, including approaches to developing a workflow and payment.

SCREENING INTERVALS AND TOOLS

Screening Intervals

Screening occurs as one component of the broader landscape of regular health supervision visits and presents an opportunity to use standardized tools to augment clinical practice. Screening builds on consistent surveillance of caregivers' and children's concerns and obtaining input from others familiar with the child, when appropriate, as a part of the continuity of care provided by PPCCs. Screening can be critically important when problems are not readily apparent and issues are not openly disclosed, as clinicians may miss these without formal screening.[47] Screening and surveillance both present an opportunity to initiate conversations with children and families, identify family and child strengths, enhance relationships, and explore findings that may be detected on a screen. Caregivers who have established a trusting, ongoing relationship with their PPCC may be more likely to share personal and confidential information.[58]

Presently, the AAP Bright Futures recommends behavioral/social/emotional screening, which as described earlier includes screening for a number of different concerns and problems starting in the first year of life and continuing at preventive health care visits to 21 years of age. It also recommends depression and suicide risk screening beginning at 12 years of age. The US Preventive Services Task Force (USPSTF) in 2022 recommended annual screening for anxiety in youth aged 8 to 18 years and continues to recommend annual screening for major depressive disorder (MDD)[59] in adolescents 12 to 18 years of age. The AAP and the American Foundation for Suicide Prevention, in partnership with experts from the National Institute of Mental Health, released the "Blueprint for Youth Suicide Prevention" in 2023, recommending annual universal screening for suicide risk in youth 12 years or older and as clinically indicated for children 8 to 11 years of age.[60] The AAP released its "Suicide and Suicide Risk in Adolescents" clinical report in 2024, endorsing the same recommendations.[61] The USPSTF stated that current evidence is insufficient to assess the balance of benefits and harms of screening for suicide risk in children and adolescents.

On the basis of the above stated recommendations, in this clinical report it is recommended that parent-completed MEB screening tools should begin early in the first year of life, beginning with identifying caregiver MEB problems such as perinatal caregiver depression, caregiver-child relational problems, and/or problems with child self-regulation. A recent study in which children were screened yearly for MEB problems beginning at age 2 until age 6 revealed that nearly 34% of children had trajectories over time reflecting elevated levels of severity on the Strengths and Difficulties Questionnaire (SDQ). These findings underscore the need for early screening and detection of young children.[62] There is growing evidence that young children with significant irritability, defined by key features of extreme, unpredictable, and prolonged tantrums; frequent episodes of dysregulation; and problems with anger regulation are more likely to be diagnosed with MEB problems when they reach school age.[63,64] Early identification can trigger exploration of the child's symptoms and functioning to distinguish children with significant irritability from those with age-normative irritability and provide appropriate guidance for caregivers regarding challenging and/or disruptive behavior.

Because of the enduring nature of MEB problems detected early and in accordance with Bright Futures recommendations, it is recommended that MEB screening be conducted at the 6-, 12-, 24-, and 36-month health supervision visits, alternated with the recommended developmental screening at the 9-, 18-, and 30-month and autism spectrum disorder screening at 18- and 24-month health supervision visits. After age 3, screening should occur yearly at routine health supervision visits, as outlined above with surveillance for MEB problems at all visits. At other pediatric visits, including subspeciality, emergency department, and urgent care visits, screening and surveillance should be considered whenever concerns are raised by PPCCs, the caregiver, or the patient. Table 1 summarizes MEB screening recommendations across ages.

Screening Tools

MEB screening tools have advantages and limitations, similar to developmental screening tools. Overall, using standardized screens helps to reduce cognitive and implicit biases that can contribute to misdiagnosis of children. No currently available single screening measure is appropriate for use in children of all ages and for all diagnoses. Tools involve a time commitment for caregivers to complete, staff to score, and PPCCs to interpret and report the results. Several brief tools include a caregiver and child self-report version and versions that can be completed and scored online. Screening tools result in risk categorization (eg, high or low risk) but are not diagnostic. There are global scales that screen for multiple conditions, and there are domain-specific tools that are most useful for screening for a specific problem, such as substance use, ADHD, or adolescent depression and suicidality.

Various screening tools are available and the choice of which to use depends on several considerations. PPCCs should become familiar with the sociodemographic characteristics of the normative population used in screening measure validation studies and choose the screening tool best reflecting the patient population for whom they care. The tool should be culturally relevant and responsive to the PPCC's patient population, although this can be difficult to determine given information in published reports of tools. MEB screening tools that have psychometric validity for children with neurodevelopmental disabilities should be identified with a recognition that there are a limited number available. Although validated screening tools for children with neurodevelopmental disabilities are lacking, this does not mean that screening should be avoided. Tools that have not been specifically tested in this population can still be used with careful interpretation of results. Other important considerations include the availability of the measure in the public domain and the ability to incorporate it into the electronic health record (EHR); the health literacy levels of caregivers, children, and adolescents completing screens; the availability of the screening tool in languages other than English; and whether the person completing the screen will need assistance completing the screen or require the assistance of an interpreter.[65] Although there is no consensus on appropriate values of sensitivity and specificity for MEB screening tools,[66] characteristics to assess a screen's psychometric properties when selecting a screening tool are outlined in Table 2, and commonly used MEB screening tools that are appropriate for use in primary care are described in Supplemental Table 1. The results from a validated screening tool such as those in Supplemental Table 1, combined with findings from regular surveillance, can help determine whether MEB problems are present.

Child and adolescent self-report versions of MEB screening tools provide important information about externalizing conditions, such as ADHD, and internalizing conditions, such as anxiety and depression.[67,68] Some feelings and symptoms are best reported by the individual experiencing them and may not be reliably recognized or observed by caregivers. Self-report tools complement the teacher and caregiver questionnaires and/or rating scales traditionally used to assess various aspects of children's functioning outside the home. Although best practice guidance on when to use self-reports in children is lacking, these can generally be used once children are cognitively able to complete the screen reliably. Most self-report versions provide normative data on children 8 years and older. Cognitive age,

TABLE 1. MEB Screening Interval Recommendations

Age	Interval	Screening recommendations	Screen completer
Birth - 3 y	• 6 mos • 12 mos • 24 mos • 36 mos	• Global MEB screening • Postpartum Depression screening (up to 6 mos)*	• Caregiver
4–7	• Yearly	• Global MEB screening	• Caregiver
8–11	• Yearly	• Global MEB screening • Anxiety screening	• Caregiver • Consider child self-report*
12 y and older	• Yearly	• Global MEB screening • Anxiety Screening • Depression screening** • Suicide screening**	• Caregiver • Adolescent self-report*

* Post-partum Depression screening should begin when the child is 1 month of age until 6 months of age

** Consider child or adolescent cognitive and literacy level

*** This can be initiated by age 8 if clinically indicated based on risk

TABLE 2. Screening Test Properties

- Reliability: ability of a test to produce consistent results.
- Validity: ability of a screening test to discriminate between a child at a determined level of risk for having behavioral or social-emotional problems (ie, high, moderate) from the rest of the population (ie, low risk).
- Sensitivity: accuracy of the test in identifying youth with behavioral or social-emotional problems. Those incorrectly identified as not having behavioral or social-emotional problems developing by the test are *false-negatives.*
- Specificity: accuracy of the test in identifying children who are do not have behavioral or social-emotional problems. Those incorrectly identified as having behavioral or social-emotional problems by the test are *false-positives.*
- Positive predictive value (PPV): the proportion of children with a positive test result who have behavioral or social-emotional disorders; the lower the prevalence or base rate of the disorder, the lower the PPV.
- Negative predictive value (NPV): the proportion of children with negative test results who do not have behavioral or social-emotional disorders; this is also influenced by the prevalence of the disorder.
- Prevalence rate: number of children in population with a disorder, measured at a given time.
- Base rate: rate of a given disorder.
- General screening test: a test that evaluates multiple areas of behavior or social-emotional function.
- Domain-specific screening test: a test that evaluates one area or domain of behavior or social-emotional function.
- Disorder-specific screening test: a test aimed at identifying a specific disorder (eg, ADHD, anxiety, depression).

neurodevelopmental disorders, literacy level of the child, and the language the screen is written in may impact the ability to utilize a self-report tool successfully and accurately. A lack of well-validated self-report tools does not suggest children should not be screened for MEB problems, and the PPCC may need to be more vigilant to detect changes in functioning and MEB signs and symptoms. Youth with disabilities that do not affect their cognitive, literacy, or language abilities should have the option to complete the screening measure using their primary mode of communication (eg, augmentative and alternative communication device or eye gaze technology).

The availability of MEB screening tools in younger children using caregiver-completed screens is more limited than in school-age children, but increasingly reliable, brief tools suitable for use in primary care exist, making it possible to screen all children and adolescents from within the first year of life through 18 years of age.

A list of some of the available MEB screens with acceptable psychometric properties can be found in Supplemental Table 1. This table, although not intended to be exhaustive, includes screens in the public domain as well as those available for a fee. The table also includes limited references to studies, including use in youth with disabilities when available. PPCCs are encouraged to familiarize themselves with different screening tools and choose those that best fit with their patient population and practice needs.

Ideally, PPCCs should complete screening for MEB problems at health supervision visits as recommended in Table 1. However, children may miss well-child visits. Studies have shown an association between increased rates of missed health supervision visits and being publicly insured or uninsured and having a higher level of social drivers of health (SDOH) that are considered barriers, such as financial hardship, housing instability, and lacking social support.[69,70] This association suggests that some of the children most in need of MEB screening and identification of mental health needs may not be accessing routine health supervision visits and subsequently missing opportunities for early detection. Therefore, clinicians should consider MEB screening for children during acute care and/or subspecialty care visits if there are risk factors, such as those discussed above, or the child presents for an urgent visit and MEB problems are suspected.[71–73]

THE RELATIONSHIP BETWEEN MEB SCREENINGS AND OTHER RECOMMENDED SCREENINGS

A child's development, SDOH, family functioning, substance use, and MEB health are often interrelated and impact each other.[11] Therefore, the results of developmental, SDOH, and/or substance use screenings may correlate with findings of MEB screens. Problems identified in any one area should prompt PPCCs to screen in other areas, and identifying all problems is important for treatment planning.

Individuals with developmental and cognitive disorders, including children with intellectual disability, autism spectrum disorder, and physical disabilities, are at a 5-fold higher risk for MEB problems compared with peers without these conditions, and between 40% and 90% will be diagnosed with depression, anxiety disorders, ADHD, suicidality, psychosis, or substance use.[74] It is often MEB problems that most adversely impact functioning and outcomes of children with neurodevelopmental disabilities. If a child is found to be at high risk for developmental delay on screening, then clinicians should consider the need to monitor and screen for MEB problems. Caregivers of children with neurodevelopmental disabilities and MEB problems may experience negative social outcomes because of the increases in caregiving responsibilities as well as the impact on caregiver mental health, career opportunities, and financial resources. Recognizing the intersectionality between youth with disabilities and those facing additional adversities, such as poverty and racism and other forms of discrimination, such as structural ableism, is crucial for addressing the complex interplay of factors that contribute to health disparities.

The presence of MEB problems in children has been demonstrated to be significantly associated with SDOH challenges.[75] Children who experience poverty and racism and other forms of discrimination, such as structural ableism, are more likely to have a range of MEB problems including depression, anxiety, posttraumatic stress disorder, and suicidal ideation. Often this higher rate is attributable to these children experiencing chronic, unremitting toxic stress with possible epigenetic changes to brain development because of a lack of stable, safe nurturing relationships.[13] Recent studies have also suggested that families of color experience significantly more SDOH barriers than white families. Much of this can be attributed to overwhelming structural and social barriers faced by families.[12,76–78] Within a family-centered view of care, caregiver and sibling experiences can impact functioning as well, and some SDOH assessment tools are included in Supplemental Table 1.

Substance use in adolescents, including cannabis, alcohol, and nicotine, has also been found to frequently co-occur with a range of MEB problems, particularly suicidal thoughts and behaviors.[79,80] The AAP recommends a tobacco, alcohol, or drug use assessment yearly after age 11 (Supplemental Table 1). Positive substance use assessments should alert clinicians to screen for MEB problems and vice versa.

ADDRESSING A POSITIVE SCREEN

A positive screen for an MEB problem should prompt the clinician to discuss the findings of the screen to ensure the findings align with child and caregiver perceptions of a problem and to assess the severity and impact of the problem. It is important to make sure that respondents, either patients or caregivers, correctly understood the questions and selected the desired response when assessing a positive screen. When screens are completed by multiple reporters, there may be conflicting findings, and PPCCs will need to review these with the caregivers, child, and other informants to interpret the findings.[81]

An assessment of a child's sleep hygiene, nutrition, exercise, and media exposure should also be ascertained, because problems in any of these areas can mimic or exacerbate MEB problems. As PPCCs assess the type and severity of the problem, they should assess child and family strengths and areas for growth, inquire into potential SDOHs, and observe caregiver-child interactions, building on information obtained during routine clinical care using a trauma-informed approach when appropriate.[13] A physical examination should be completed if indicated, looking for any potential organic or medical causes for the MEB problems or evidence of abuse such as prior injuries, patterned scarring, suspicious bruising, defensive wounds, or evidence of self-harm.

If a positive MEB screen is confirmed, the PPCC needs to determine the severity of the problem to plan next steps. Severity can be assessed by querying the child and family and identifying the extent of impairment or change in functioning in school performance, social interactions, family engagement, and activities of daily living, such as sleep, appetite, and hygiene. Global screening measures often differentiate aspects of an MEB problem and risk stratify based on reported child symptoms and clinical history. For example, in a cross-sectional study of 767 racial and ethnically diverse patients ages 5 to 16 years who underwent behavioral screening in primary care practices, 43% screened positive on the SDQ, a general measure of childhood MEB symptoms.[47] The SDQ allowed for severity classification based on ranges of scores and included subscales for potential types of problems. Of those with a positive screen, the authors reported that 15% scored in the medium severity range and 28% scored in the high severity range. Additionally, of those with a positive screen, 61% reported inattention-hyperactivity symptoms, 50% reported emotional symptoms, 42% reported conduct symptoms, and 30% reported peer relation problems on SDQ subscales. Therefore, in this study, many patients with symptoms in one domain also demonstrated symptoms in at least one other domain, suggesting clustering of symptoms across domains and the need to consider a global approach.

Following the use of a global screen, clinicians can implement a tiered screening approach in which a domain-specific screening measure can be used that identifies specific problems and their severity. For example, the Vanderbilt Rating Scales for ADHD focus on ADHD and its severity.

In addition to the use of standardized screening tools for infants and children, assessment should include an observation of the caregiver-child relationship, with awareness of potential implicit biases. This observation includes an assessment of shared positive engagement and caregiver responsivity and sensitivity to the child's needs.[82] Screening tools for young children may include questions about caregiver stress and mood, and separate tools may be used to assess caregiver functioning. It is important to share observations with families and understand if observations in the clinical setting are reflective of typical interactions, as effective therapeutic interventions exist using a relational approach to foster nurturing caregiver-infant and -young child dyadic relationships.

Children with positive MEB screens who are found to have co-occurring SDOH risks or substance use problems may require interventions that extend beyond focusing solely on the child's MEB problems. This intervention may include addressing caregiver MEB problems, child and caregiver substance use, housing and/or food insecurity, bullying and victimization, and the impact of racism and other forms of discrimination, such as structural ableism.[83,84]

The initial step to addressing any identified MEB problem is building a therapeutic alliance with children and families using a trauma-informed approach when appropriate.[85] The Common Factors approach[86] is a transdiagnostic approach designed to build a therapeutic alliance representing a collaborative bond between a family and clinician. This approach includes therapeutic listening, which allows the child and caregiver to talk about their concerns and worries and delineate concerns.[85] The HEL^{2}P^3 mnemonic (Figure 1) was developed by the AAP Task Force on Mental Health and summarizes components of the Common Factors approach, designed to promote child and family optimism and hope, feelings of well-being, and shared decision making in a culturally relevant way.[30,87] Using the HEL^{2}P^3 approach will aid PPCCs in partnering effectively with children and caregivers to determine best next steps after a positive screen is obtained.

Decisions to involve specialists and referrals to community-based programs for children with a positive MEB screen should be made in collaboration with caregivers and patients. The type of specialist with whom to consult or to whom to refer will depend on the availability of specific types of specialists and programs in the community, the family's readiness to receive that care, and the nature of the problem. For example, a PPCC working at a pediatric practice with an embedded MEB clinician can provide a child with an identified MEB problem a "warm handoff" but may need to refer a child to a community resource, mental health specialist, or developmental-behavioral pediatrician outside the practice if the MEB problem is thought by parents, PPCCs, and/or the embedded MEB clinician to be beyond the scope of the practice—for example, a child with suspected autism spectrum disorder who may require applied behavioral analysis therapy.

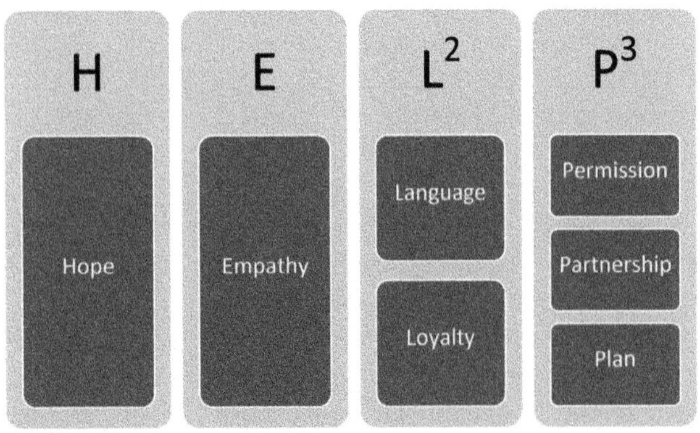

FIGURE 1.
HEL^{2}P.^{3}

For PPCCs with patients whose MEB problem appears complex, a consultation with or referral to a mental health specialist, developmental-behavioral pediatrician, or adolescent medicine physician may be helpful to assess more accurately the nature of the MEB problem following a positive screen. Given the limited availability of specialists, PPCCs should ideally establish referral and consultative relationships with specialists in their community, although it is often difficult to bill for this consultation. Most states and care networks offer telepsychiatry consultative services for local primary care clinicians given the difficulty with in-person mental health referral access.[88] These include well-established programs based on the original Massachusetts Child Psychiatry Access Project and funded through the Pediatric Mental Health Care Access Program.[89] In addition, many states have added PPCC companion guidebooks that address identifying and treating children with MEB problems as well as local resources.

Once a decision on next steps has been reached in partnership with a family, it will be important to ensure an appropriate follow-up plan, which will depend on the nature and severity of the problem, management plan implemented, and patient and family response to the plan.

PROMOTING RESILIENCE AND WELLNESS IN FAMILIES

In addition to screening for MEB problems, families and children benefit from identifying strengths and the promotion of resilience (ie, the ability of individuals to respond to adversity appropriately with a rapid return to homeostasis when the adversity or stressor has remitted).[90] Children with vulnerability in their social-emotional competence, estimated in one study as more than 40% of kindergarten-aged children,[83] can particularly benefit from resilience building. Early childhood may be a time in which prevention and mitigation of harm can be most impactful.[91] The mnemonic "THREADS"[92] (Figure 2), based on the resilience work by Masten,[93] captures key areas in which the PPCC can support children and caregivers. These areas tap into developmental milestones, addressing the changes of childhood growth as well as of parenting skills and intertwining anticipatory guidance with resiliency building. Skill development can be maintained even when children experience significant adversity if these basic adaptational mechanisms are protected.[94]

PPCCs can help strengthen protective factors for children by promoting family strengths within a culturally sensitive framework,[13,95] reducing the effects of adverse childhood experiences through interventions such as positive parenting training,[96] linking children to quality early childhood education, and providing family education on the positive effect of supportive relationships.[97]

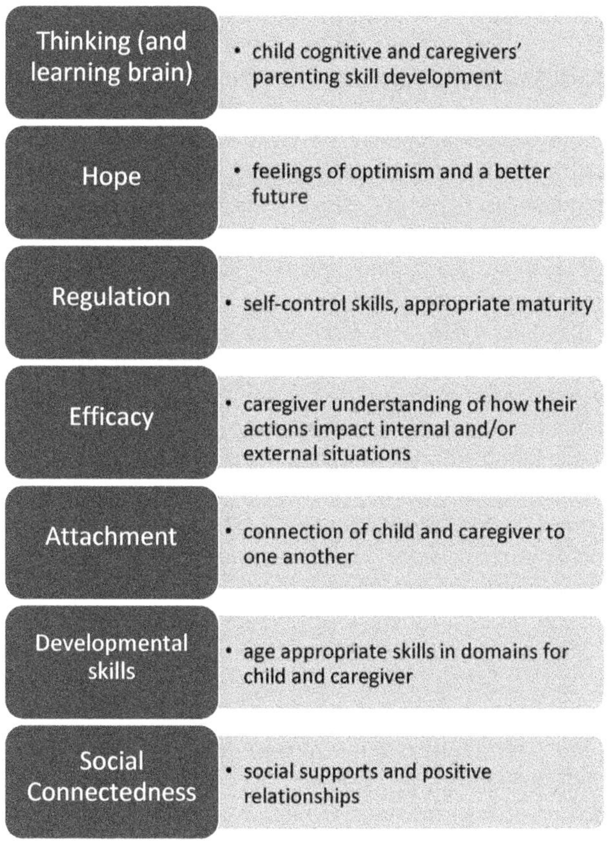

FIGURE 2.
THREADS.

STRATEGIES TO ORGANIZE A PEDIATRIC PRACTICE FOR SCREENING

When implementing MEB screening in practice, whether adding a new measure to an established routine or starting screening for the first time, planning will need to be focused on several key areas. The AAP "Getting Started" worksheet[98] is available for free download and emphasizes key steps in implementing a screening process that includes: 1) identifying current practices around screening; 2) building a practice improvement team around a practice champion; 3) identifying new tools to implement or to replace previous tools that will best serve the practice's patient population; and 4) designing the workflow for the use of new tools. Additional considerations for PPCCs once new or additional screening is in place include: 5) sustaining an established screening system; and 6) appropriate billing and coding for administering, scoring, and reporting screens. The key issues that predict successful screening include ensuring all staff are trained, using shared decision making regarding decisions around screening results, selecting appropriate, culturally relevant screening tools, and combining screening and surveillance to identify children with MEB problems over time. Additionally, "Coding and Valuation," available within AAP practice management resources, maintains updated information around constantly in-flux billing recommendations.

For practices that are part of larger organizations, there may need to be additional advocacy efforts directed at the leadership to promote the value of screening to garner support and integration. Collaboration among pediatricians to share strategies for success will be important for improving widespread adoption.

Identifying Current Practices Around Screening

Currently, many pediatric practices have well-defined processes in place to screen for some disorders such as autism spectrum disorder that typically involve team members across the practice including front desk staff, medical assistants, nurses, PPCCs, and administrators.[99] If a screening process that is currently in place already works well, the team should discuss how adding an additional measure for MEB screening could be successfully incorporated and what modifications to current practice might be needed.

Building a Practice Improvement Team Around a Practice Improvement Champion

Designating a team project champion and a primary practice improvement team who will assume a leadership role in all steps of screening implementation is a critical step to setting up a screening plan or building on an existing structure.

Identifying New Screening Tools or Replacing Previous Ones

Selection of the screening measure, population, and other details are determined in this phase. The entire practice team should be educated on the reason for process change (ie, the need for MEB screening), the chosen measure (eg, scoring, resources related), and the process details to train the team.[100,101] Hands-on opportunities to apply concepts and skills may be more successful than didactics alone.[102]

Designing the Workflow for the Use of New Screening Tools

Steps to determine the practice workflow should include every component of the office sequence, including previsit preparation, patient check-in, rooming, and the examination itself.[99] Data collection on screening may include the number of patients seen; number of patients receiving the screening measure and the number of tools scored; the rates of positive, incomplete, and negative screens; referral rates based on screen results; and management responses to the screens by the team. These data are needed to evaluate successes and areas of suboptimal implementation.[103]

Sustaining an Established Screening System

The framework of the "plan, do, study, act" (PDSA) cycle at the start of a screening initiative should focus on why a particular method was chosen, benefits/limitations, and ongoing process education to promote fidelity.[104–107] A well-delineated system can then be built for sustainability.[108]

Workflow can be enhanced through automation with the EHR platform. The EHR can be designed to alert staff and medical providers of needed screenings based on documentation factors such as patient age or appointment type (eg, sick, well-child, nurse only, etc), and this can be used for previsit preparation. Screening tools can potentially be sent to families prior to the appointment via the EHR patient portal or other secure messaging in the office. Programs are available for purchase in the marketplace to integrate with the EHR to promote screening. The EHR is the key place where documentation should occur.[100] Many EHR systems are equipped to generate a data report to review implementation success.

Data are emerging regarding screening in the setting of telehealth vs in person appointment types. For example, some studies suggest that depression screening may be less likely to happen during telemedicine appointments.[109,110] Telehealth appointments may present additional challenges to initiating a new screening program in a practice but can be used if a similar process to in-person screening is used.[111] Common barriers to virtual screenings can include lack of access to technology and internet connection.[112,113] The *Medicare Claims Processing Manual* from the Centers for Medicare and Medicaid Services states that patients must be present for payment of telehealth services to occur. Coverage and payment guidelines may vary depending on payer policy and payers should be contacted to understand their policies about this.

Billing and Coding of MEB Screenings and Response to Screenings

It is important to document risk and protective factors, screening measure findings, and specific actions or plans discussed with a family. MEB screening tools are billed with the following Current Procedural Terminology (CPT) codes:

- 96127 - Brief emotional/behavioral health screening tools
- 96160 - Assessment of biopsychosocial factors important to physical health and mental health; child completed.
- 96161 codes - Assessment of biopsychosocial factors important to physical health and mental health; Caregiver completed tool for the benefit of the child[114,115]

The appropriate billing code should be selected based on the type of screening performed. These codes include the administration, scoring, and documentation of a standardized measure and should be added to an evaluation and management (E/M) service on the date of service with the time spent administering, scoring, and recording the findings of the measure clearly and separately documented with use of an additional modifier 25.[116,117] Modifier 25 may also be used to bill a separate E/M code when problems are revealed in the context of a well child visit. When billing for multiple units of the same or different tools, modifier 59 may be appropriate.

Payment varies by payors and policies, and claims edits occur within plans regularly. Documentation of the administration of a screening measure must be in its own section of the note, separate from history, physical examination, and medical decision making. For payment purposes, screening and assessment codes are based on the practice expense and professional liability only (eg, cost of furnishing tools, staff time to administer and/or score a measure). The physician's interpretation of the score in the larger clinical context is considered part of the E/M service. When using the Bright Futures recommendation for MEB screening, billing for the screening service is covered as part of the Patient Protection and Affordable Care Act of 2010. For additional information regarding billing and coding, please visit the AAP "Coding and Valuation" section of Practice Management at: https://www.aap.org/en/practice-management/practice-financing/coding-and-valuation/. For more information and advocacy guidance related to access to care and payment in their state, PPCCs are encouraged to contact their AAP state advocacy team at stgov@aap.org.

CLINICAL GUIDANCE FOR MENTAL HEALTH, BEHAVIORAL, AND EMOTIONAL PROBLEM SURVEILLANCE AND SCREENING

This clinical guidance incorporates and builds on the 2014 "Screening for Behavioral and Emotional Problems" clinical report and the 2019 "Mental Health Competencies for Pediatric Practice" policy statement.

For the Medical Home

1. During the first 3 years of life, complete MEB (6-, 12-, 24-, 36-month), developmental (9-, 18-, 30-month), and autism spectrum disorder (18-, 24-month) screenings as a part of a comprehensive, integrated systems approach to pediatric care.
2. Complete MEB screening annually after age 3 for asymptomatic children at preventive health care visits and whenever concerns are raised by the patient, caregiver, or the pediatrician. MEB screening should also be completed at urgent or subspecialty care visits when concerns are raised or there is clinical indication.
3. Beginning at age 8 years, complete global (multiple condition) and domain-specific (single-condition) screens for anxiety, and expand this screening at age 12 years

for depression and suicide if earlier screening is not warranted.

4. Schedule early return visits for continued close surveillance of children whose MEB surveillance raises concerns that are not confirmed by an MEB screening test and/or interview or for those children in whom a positive screen did not lead to additional actions.
5. For patients whose MEB problem appears complex and severe and beyond the scope of the primary care practice, referral for further MEB evaluation and treatment is indicated along with an early return visit to the PPCC to monitor progress, symptom severity, and success of the referral.

For Policy and Advocacy

1. Identify and address barriers to MEB screening in the medical home that include payment for MEB screening and case management, insufficient time to complete screenings and have discussions with families, lack of interprofessional collaboration and discussion of specific children, challenges with telehealth screening, lack of professional and staff knowledge, inflexible EHR systems, and inefficient office workflows to achieve universal screening of all children and adolescents.
2. Reduce disparities in children who are often not adequately screened, including but not exclusive to children of color, children with disabilities, and families with a non-English language preference.
3. Provide appropriate payment for MEB screening, evaluation, and treatment. Payment for these separately identifiable and reportable services should not be bundled into the preventive care visit or any other office visit. Payment for follow-up visits for treatment and to monitor progress and outcomes should also be provided without cost sharing to families.
4. Provide payment for appropriate and necessary ongoing management in the medical home for children identified with an MEB disorder to address the child's ongoing MEB and SDOH needs and to identify and address newly associated conditions and needs.
5. Provide payment for interprofessional collaboration between PPCCs and therapists, specialists, and community programs around the care of children with MEB problems.
6. Advocate for a comprehensive, integrated system within pediatric practices that links to community-based services and supports.
7. Advocate for innovative practice models including collocated services and family navigators and ensure adequate payment for these services.
8. Advocate for training a broader workforce of professionals who can treat children and youth with MEB problems that may include psychologists, psychiatrists, developmental-behavioral pediatricians, and other qualified MEB clinicians.

For Research and Development

1. Encourage ongoing investigation around overall MEB screening and referral rates and for specific MEB disorders. Obstacles and barriers to referral and ongoing management should be identified.
2. Expand the evidence base comparing the effectiveness of MEB surveillance, screening, and their combination in the identification of children with MEB disorders.
3. Identify factors that limit and facilitate PPCCs integration of MEB screening into the medical home.
4. Develop information systems and data-gathering tools to automate and operationalize the surveillance and screening processes recommended within this report. These systems and tools could include integration and documentation into the child's EHR of MEB surveillance and screening of all children as well as chronic condition management of children identified with MEB disorders.
5. Support continued research on the practice of MEB surveillance and screening, including the following:
    a. Examining the efficacy and validity of MEB screening tools in diverse populations (such as non–English-speaking families, refugees,[118,119] etc), at nonscreening health promotion visits and at subspecialty visits;
    b. Assessing the stability of MEB screens over time and trajectories of MEB problems;
    c. Developing MEB screening tools that have psychometric validity for children with neurodevelopmental disabilities, including intellectual disability and autism spectrum disorder;
    d. Expanding the evidence base for the use and effectiveness of optimal ages for recommended MEB screening;
    e. Investigating the short- and long-term benefits of MEB surveillance and screening, given the current limitations of the evidence base; and
    f. Assessing the impact of increased screening on caregivers and youth and their perceptions of the value of screening.

SUMMARY

Promoting optimal child development and well-being includes assessing MEB problems in the context of the family and the community. MEB problems are increasingly common, are persistent, and cause significant functional impairment for many children and adolescents. These problems also have a high likelihood of persisting into adulthood. Pediatricians are ideally situated to prevent, intervene, and ameliorate MEB problems, especially given the 2- to 4-year window that exists between initial presentation of symptoms and the development of a disorder. MEB screening is optimized when it is coupled with regular surveillance. Using reliable and valid MEB screening tools is essential and can be added to a developmental/autism spectrum disorder screening program in the first 3 years of life and annually thereafter; screening should also occur whenever caregivers or children express MEB concerns or behaviors are displayed that suggest an MEB problem. Promising strategies have been developed over the last decade to help organize pediatric practices to improve MEB access and treatment strategies within primary care settings, including learning collaboratives, ECHO trainings, remote subspecialty consultation, and integration of MEB providers within pediatric practice. A strengths-based approach is paramount with promotion of resilience and wellness for children and families. The investments described in this report, financial and otherwise, are critical to ensure a future of thriving and resilient infants, children, and adolescents who will mature into healthy adults.

LEAD AUTHORS

Carol Weitzman, MD, FAAP
James Guevara, MD, MPH, FAAP
Michelle Curtin, DO, FAAP
Michelle Macias, MD, FAAP

AAP SECTION ON DEVELOPMENTAL AND BEHAVIORAL PEDIATRICS EXECUTIVE COMMITTEE, 2024–2025

Jennifer Kinwa Poon, MD, FAAP, Chairperson
Peter J. Joseph Smith, MD, MA, FAAP, Immediate Past Chairperson
Marilyn Christine Augustyn, MD, FAAP
Yi Hui Liu, MD, MPH, FAAP
Adiaha Idara Anopawuia Spinks-Franklin, MD, MPH
Jennifer Marlene Zubler, MD, FAAP
Jennifer Walton, MD, MPH, FAAP

LIAISONS

Jessica E. A. Foster, MD, MPH, FAAP – Council on Children With Disabilities

STAFF

Robyn Wheatley, MPH

AAP COUNCIL ON EARLY CHILDHOOD EXECUTIVE COMMITTEE, 2024–2025

Dipesh Navsaria, MD, MPH, MSLIS, FAAP, Chairperson
Mariana Glusman, MD, FAAP, Chairperson Elect
Chidiogo Uzoatu Anyigbo, MD, MPH, FAAP
Victoria Chen, MD, FAAP
Janis Lynn Gonzales, MD, MPH, FAAP
James P. Guevara, MD, FAAP
Andrew Nobuhide Hashikawa, MD, FAAP
Hilda Marie Loria, MD, MPH, FAAP
Anna Miller-Fitzwater, MD, FAAP
Usha Ramachandran, MD, FAAP
Prachi Edlagan Shah, MD, FAAP

LIAISONS

Rebecca Parlakian – Zero To Three
Jared Boyce – Section on Pediatric Trainees

STAFF

Keisha Wright

AAP COMMITTEE ON PSYCHOSOCIAL ASPECTS OF CHILD AND FAMILY HEALTH, 2024–2025

Arwa Abdulhaq Nasir, MBBS, MSc, MPH, FAAP, Chairperson
Beth Ellen Davis, MD, MPH, FAAP
Pradeep Prem Gidwani, MD, MPH, FAAP
Tiffani Jenae Johnson, MD
Irene P. Mathieu, MD, FAAP
Natasha Kapoor Sriraman, MD, MPH, FABM, FAAP

LIAISONS

Kathleen Hobson Davis – Family Liaison
Elise Michelle Fallucco, MD – American Academy of Child and Adolescent Psychiatry
Heather Fraser – National Association of Social Workers
Elizabeth Hutson – National Association of Pediatric Nurse Practitioners
Terry Stancin, PhD – Society of Pediatric Psychology

STAFF

Robyn Wheatley, MPH

SOCIETY FOR DEVELOPMENTAL AND BEHAVIORAL PEDIATRICS BOARD OF DIRECTORS

Adiaha Spinks-Franklin, MD, President
William J. Barbaresi, MD, President-Elect
Tanya Froehlich, MD, Immediate Past President
Britt Nielsen, PsyD
Jennifer Poon, MD
Jeffrey Yang, MD
Jason Fogler, PhD
Irene Loe, MD
Dinah L. Godwin, MSW
Cy Nadler, PhD
Janice Wilkins
Laura Degnon, CAE

ABBREVIATIONS

AAP: American Academy of Pediatrics
ADHD: attention-deficit/hyperactivity disorder
ECHO: Extension for Community Healthcare Outcomes

EHR: electronic health record
E/M: evaluation and management
CPT: Current Procedural Terminology
MEB: mental health, emotional, and behavioral
MDD: major depressive disorder

PPCCs: pediatric primary care clinicians
SDOH: social drivers of health
SDQ: Strengths and Difficulties Questionnaire
USPSTF: US Preventive Services Task Force

The guidance in this report does not indicate an exclusive course of treatment or serve as a standard of medical care. Variations, taking into account individual circumstances, may be appropriate.

All clinical reports from the American Academy of Pediatrics automatically expire 5 years after publication unless reaffirmed, revised, or retired at or before that time.

All authors contributed equally to the conceptualization, design, drafting, and revision of this clinical report. Each author participated in the literature review, synthesis of evidence, and formulation of recommendations. All authors critically reviewed and approved the final manuscript as submitted and agree to be accountable for all aspects of the work.

CONFLICT OF INTEREST DISCLOSURE: The authors have indicated they have no potential conflicts of interest to disclose.

FUNDING: No external funding.

https://doi.org/10.1542/peds.2025-073172

REFERENCES

1. National Academies of Sciences, Engineering, and Medicine. *Fostering Healthy Mental, Emotional, and Behavioral Development in Children and Youth: A National Agenda.* National Academies Press; 2019.
2. Costello EJ, Mustillo S, Erkanli A, Keeler G, Angold A. Prevalence and development of psychiatric disorders in childhood and adolescence. *Arch Gen Psychiatry.* 2003;60(8):837–844. PubMed doi: 10.1001/archpsyc.60.8.837
3. US Department of Health and Human Services, US Department of Education, US Department of Justice. *Report of the Surgeon General's Conference on Children's Mental Health: A National Action Agenda.* US Department of Health and Human Services; 2000.
4. Cree RA, Bitsko RH, Robinson LR, et al. Health care, family, and community factors associated with mental, behavioral, and developmental disorders and poverty among children aged 2–8 years —United States, 2016. *MMWR Morb Mortal Wkly Rep.* 2018;67(50): 1377–1383. PubMed doi: 10.15585/mmwr.mm6750a1
5. Lewinsohn PM, Shankman SA, Gau JM, Klein DN. The prevalence and co-morbidity of subthreshold psychiatric conditions. *Psychol Med.* 2004;34(4):613–622. PubMed doi: 10.1017/S0033291703001466
6. Johnson JCS, Byrne GJ, Pelecanos AM. The prevalence of subthreshold psychiatric symptoms and associations with alcohol and substance use disorders: from a nationally representative survey of 36,309 adults. *BMC Psychiatry.* 2022;22(1):270. PubMed doi: 10.1186/s12888-022-03834-1
7. Slomski A. Chronic mental health issues in children now loom larger than physical problems. *JAMA.* 2012;308(3):223–225. PubMed doi: 10.1001/jama.2012.6951
8. Halfon N, Houtrow A, Larson K, Newacheck PW. The changing landscape of disability in childhood. *Future Child.* 2012;22(1):13–42. PubMed doi: 10.1353/foc.2012.0004
9. Jaffee SR, Harrington H, Cohen P, Moffitt TE. Cumulative prevalence of psychiatric disorder in youths. *J Am Acad Child Adolesc Psychiatry.* 2005;44(5):406–407. PubMed doi: 10.1097/01.chi.0000155317.38265.61
10. Kim-Cohen J, Caspi A, Moffitt TE, Harrington H, Milne BJ, Poulton R. Prior juvenile diagnoses in adults with mental disorder: developmental follow-back of a prospective-longitudinal cohort. *Arch Gen Psychiatry.* 2003;60(7):709–717. PubMed doi: 10.1001/archpsyc.60.7.709
11. American Academy of Pediatrics, Council on Community Pediatrics. Poverty and child health in the United States [reaffirmed April 2021]. *Pediatrics.* 2016;137(4) doi: https://doi.org/10.1542/peds.2016-0339
12. Trent M, Dooley DG, Dougé J, et al; SECTION ON ADOLESCENT HEALTH; COUNCIL ON COMMUNITY PEDIATRICS; COMMITTEE ON ADOLESCENCE. The impact of racism on child and adolescent health. *Pediatrics.* 2019;144(2):e20191765. PubMed doi: 10.1542/peds.2019-1765
13. Garner A, Yogman M; COMMITTEE ON PSYCHOSOCIAL ASPECTS OF CHILD AND FAMILY HEALTH, SECTION ON DEVELOPMENTAL AND BEHAVIORAL PEDIATRICS, COUNCIL ON EARLY CHILDHOOD. Preventing childhood toxic stress: partnering with families and communities to promote relational health. *Pediatrics.* 2021; 148(2):e2021052582. PubMed doi: 10.1542/peds.2021-052582
14. QuickStats. Death rates for motor vehicle traffic injury, suicide, and homicide among children and adolescents aged 10–14 years—United States, 1999–2014. *MMWR Morb Mortal Wkly Rep.* 2016;65(43):1203. PubMed doi: 10.15585/mmwr.mm6543a8

15. Centers for Disease Control and Prevention, National Center for Injury Prevention and Control. Web-based Injury Statistics Query and Reporting System (WISQARS) [database]. Accessed June 14, 2023. https://www.cdc.gov/injury/wisqars

16. Curtin SC, Heron M. Death rates due to suicide and homicide among persons aged 10–24: United States, 2000–2017. *NCHS Data Brief.* 2019;(352):1–8. PubMed

17. Too LS, Spittal MJ, Bugeja L, Reifels L, Butterworth P, Pirkis J. The association between mental disorders and suicide: A systematic review and meta-analysis of record linkage studies. *J Affect Disord.* 2019;259:302–313. PubMed doi: 10.1016/j.jad.2019.08.054

18. Hillis SD, Blenkinsop A, Villaveces A, et al. COVID-19–associated orphanhood and caregiver death in the United States. *Pediatrics.* 2021;148(6):e2021053760. PubMed doi: 10.1542/peds.2021-053760

19. Leeb RT, Bitsko RH, Radhakrishnan L, Martinez P, Njai R, Holland KM. Mental health–related emergency department visits among children aged <18 years during the COVID-19 pandemic—United States, January 1–October 17, 2020. *MMWR Morb Mortal Wkly Rep.* 2020;69(45):1675–1680. PubMed doi: 10.15585/mmwr.mm6945a3

20. Anderson KN, Johns D, Holland KM, et al. Emergency department visits involving mental health conditions, suicide-related behaviors, and drug overdoses among adolescents—United States, January 2019–February 2023. *MMWR Morb Mortal Wkly Rep.* 2023;72(19):502–512. PubMed doi: 10.15585/mmwr.mm7219a1

21. Jones SE, Ethier KA, Hertz M, et al. Mental health, suicidality, and connectedness among high school students during the COVID-19 pandemic—Adolescent Behaviors and Experiences Survey, United States, January–June 2021. *MMWR Suppl.* 2022;71(3):16–21. PubMed doi: 10.15585/mmwr.su7103a3

22. Ghandour RM, Sherman LJ, Vladutiu CJ, et al. Prevalence and treatment of depression, anxiety, and conduct problems in US children. *J Pediatr.* 2019;206:256–267.e3. PubMed doi: 10.1016/j.jpeds.2018.09.021

23. Kessler RC, Berglund P, Demler O, Jin R, Merikangas KR, Walters EE. Lifetime prevalence and age-of-onset distributions of DSM-IV disorders in the National Comorbidity Survey Replication. *Arch Gen Psychiatry.* 2005;62(6):593–602. PubMed doi: 10.1001/archpsyc.62.6.593

24. Copeland WE, Shanahan L, Costello EJ, Angold A. Childhood and adolescent psychiatric disorders as predictors of young adult disorders. *Arch Gen Psychiatry.* 2009;66(7):764–772. PubMed doi: 10.1001/archgenpsychiatry.2009.85

25. Thomson KC, Richardson CG, Gadermann AM, Emerson SD, Shoveller J, Guhn M. Association of childhood social-emotional functioning profiles at school entry with early-onset mental health conditions. *JAMA Netw Open.* 2019;2(1):e186694. PubMed doi: 10.1001/jamanetworkopen.2018.6694

26. Caspi A, Houts RM, Ambler A, et al. Longitudinal assessment of mental health disorders and comorbidities across 4 decades among participants in the Dunedin Birth Cohort Study. *JAMA Netw Open.* 2020;3(4):e203221. PubMed doi: 10.1001/jamanetwork open.2020.3221

27. National Research Council. Institute of Medicine, Committee on the Prevention of Mental Disorders and Substance Abuse Among Children, Youth and Young Adults: Research Advances and Promising Interventions. O'Connell ME, Boat T, Warner KE, eds. *Preventing Mental, Emotional, and Behavioral Disorders Among Young People: Progress and Possibilities.* National Academies Press; 2009.

28. Bitsko RH, Claussen AH, Lichstein J, et al; Contributor. Mental health surveillance among children—United States, 2013–2019. *MMWR Suppl.* 2022;71(2):1–42. PubMed doi: 10.15585/mmwr.su7102a1

29. Foy JM; American Academy of Pediatrics Task Force on Mental Health. Enhancing pediatric mental health care: report from the American Academy of Pediatrics Task Force on Mental Health. Introduction. *Pediatrics.* 2010;125(suppl 3):S69–S74. PubMed doi: 10.1542/peds.2010-0788C

30. Foy JM, Green CM, Earls MF, et al; COMMITTEE ON PSYCHOSOCIAL ASPECTS OF CHILD AND FAMILY HEALTH, MENTAL HEALTH LEADERSHIP WORK GROUP. Mental health competencies for pediatric practice. *Pediatrics.* 2019;144(5):e20192757. PubMed doi: 10.1542/peds.2019-2757

31. Hackell JM, Almendarez YM, Cantrell PE, et al; COMMITTEE ON PRACTICE & AMBULATORY MEDICINE. 2024 Recommendations for preventive pediatric health care: policy statement. *Pediatrics.* 2024;154(1):e2024067201. PubMed doi: 10.1542/peds.2024-067201

32. Gregory KD, Chelmow D, Nelson HD, et al; Women's Preventive Services Initiative. Screening for anxiety in adolescent and adult women: a recommendation from the Women's Preventive Services Initiative. *Ann Intern Med.* 2020;173(1):48–56. PubMed doi: 10.7326/M20-0580

33. Walter HJ, Bukstein OG, Abright AR, et al. Clinical practice guideline for the assessment and treatment of children and adolescents with anxiety disorders. *J Am Acad Child Adolesc Psychiatry.* 2020;59(10):1107–1124. PubMed doi: 10.1016/j.jaac.2020.05.005

34. Coker TR, Gottschlich EA, Burr WH, Lipkin PH. Early childhood screening practices and barriers: a national survey of primary care pediatricians. *Pediatrics.* 2024;154(2):e2023065552. PubMed doi: 10.1542/peds.2023-065552

35. Lipkin PH, Macias MM, Baer Chen B, et al. Trends in pediatricians' developmental screening: 2002–2016. *Pediatrics.* 2020;145(4):e20190851. PubMed doi: 10.1542/peds.2019-0851

36. Lipkin PH, Macias MM, Norwood KW Jr, et al; COUNCIL ON CHILDREN WITH DISABILITIES, SECTION ON DEVELOPMENTAL AND BEHAVIORAL PEDIATRICS. Promoting optimal development: identifying infants and young children with developmental disorders through developmental surveillance and screening. *Pediatrics.* 2020;145(1):e20193449. PubMed doi: 10.1542/peds.2019-3449

37. Sheldrick RC, Merchant S, Perrin EC. Identification of developmental-behavioral problems in primary care: a systematic review. *Pediatrics.* 2011;128(2):356–363. PubMed doi: 10.1542/peds.2010-3261

38. Walter HJ, Vernacchio L, Trudell EK, et al. Five-year outcomes of behavioral health integration in pediatric primary care.

Pediatrics. 2019;144(1):e20183243. PubMed doi: 10.1542/peds.2018-3243

39. Beers LS, Godoy L, John T, et al. Mental health screening quality improvement learning collaborative in pediatric primary care. *Pediatrics.* 2017;140(6):e20162966. PubMed doi: 10.1542/peds.2016-2966
40. Beck KE, Snyder D, Toth C, et al. Improving primary care adolescent depression screening and initial management: a quality improvement study. *Pediatr Qual Saf.* 2022;7(2):e549. PubMed doi: 10.1097/pq9.0000000000000549
41. Harder VS, Barry SE, French S, Consigli AB, Frankowski BL. Improving adolescent depression screening in pediatric primary care. *Acad Pediatr.* 2019;19(8):925–933. PubMed doi: 10.1016/j.acap.2019.02.014
42. Cama S, Knee A, Sarvet B. Impact of child psychiatry access programs on mental health care in pediatric primary care: measuring the parent experience. *Psychiatr Serv.* 2020;71(1):43–48. PubMed doi: 10.1176/appi.ps.201800324
43. Van Cleave J, Holifield C, Perrin JM. Primary care providers' use of a child psychiatry telephone support program. *Acad Pediatr.* 2018;18(3):266–272. PubMed doi: 10.1016/j.acap.2017.11.007
44. Njoroge WF, Hostutler CA, Schwartz BS, Mautone JA. Integrated behavioral health in pediatric primary care. *Curr Psychiatry Rep.* 2016;18(12):106. PubMed doi: 10.1007/s11920-016-0745-7
45. Mathews TL, Klepper CN, Roberts HJ, Paff ML, Mullarkey JP, Jordan P. Screening for pediatric behavioral health in primary care in rural and urban clinics. *Fam Syst Health.* 2023;41(1):44–53. PubMed doi: 10.1037/fsh0000707
46. Dulcan MK, Costello EJ, Costello AJ, Edelbrock C, Brent D, Janiszewski S. The pediatrician as gatekeeper to mental health care for children: do parents' concerns open the gate? *J Am Acad Child Adolesc Psychiatry.* 1990;29(3):453–458. PubMed doi: 10.1097/00004583-199005000-00018
47. Brown JD, Wissow LS. Screening to identify mental health problems in pediatric primary care: considerations for practice. *Int J Psychiatry Med.* 2010;40(1):1–19. PubMed doi: 10.2190/PM.40.1.a
48. Guevara JP, Mandell DS, Rostain AL, Zhao H, Hadley TR. Disparities in the reporting and treatment of health conditions in children: an analysis of the Medical Expenditure Panel Survey. *Health Serv Res.* 2006;41(2):532–549. PubMed doi: 10.1111/j.1475-6773.2005.00484.x
49. Williams ME, Zamora I, Akinsilo O, Chen AH, Poulsen MK. Broad developmental screening misses young children with social-emotional needs. *Clin Pediatr (Phila).* 2018;57(7):844–849. PubMed doi: 10.1177/0009922817733700
50. Stein REK, Horwitz SM, Storfer-Isser A, Heneghan A, Olson L, Hoagwood KE. Do pediatricians think they are responsible for identification and management of child mental health problems? Results of the AAP periodic survey. *Ambul Pediatr.* 2008;8(1):11–17. PubMed doi: 10.1016/j.ambp.2007.10.006
51. O'Brien D, Harvey K, Howse J, Reardon T, Creswell C. Barriers to managing child and adolescent mental health problems: a systematic review of primary care practitioners' perceptions. *Br J Gen Pract.* 2016;66(651):e693–e707. PubMed doi: 10.3399/bjgp16X687061
52. Horwitz SM, Storfer-Isser A, Kerker BD, et al. Barriers to the identification and management of psychosocial problems: changes from 2004 to 2013. *Acad Pediatr.* 2015;15(6):613–620. PubMed doi: 10.1016/j.acap.2015.08.006
53. Weitzman CC, Baum RA, Fussell J, et al. Defining developmental-behavioral pediatrics. *Pediatrics.* 2022;149(4):e2021054771. PubMed doi: 10.1542/peds.2021-054771
54. American Academy of Child and Adolescent Psychiatry. Severe Shortage of Child and Adolescent Psychiatrists Illustrated in AACAP Workforce Maps. Published May 4, 2022. Accessed June 16, 2023. https://www.aacap.org/aacap/zLatest_News/Severe_Shortage_Child_Adolescent_Psychiatrists_Illustrated_AACAP_Workforce_Maps.aspx
55. American Board of Pediatrics. Pediatric Subspecialty US State and County Maps. Last updated August 21, 2024. Accessed June 15, 2023. https://www.abp.org/dashboards/pediatric-subspecialty-us-state-and-county-maps
56. Lim L, Stamm K. *The Child and Adolescent Psychologist Workforce.* University of Michigan Behavioral Health Workforce Research Center; 2020.
57. Bridgemohan C, Bauer NS, Nielsen BA, et al. A workforce survey on developmental-behavioral pediatrics. *Pediatrics.* 2018;141(3):e20172164. PubMed doi: 10.1542/peds.2017-2164
58. Wissow LS, Larson SM, Roter D, et al; SAFE Home Project. Longitudinal care improves disclosure of psychosocial information. *Arch Pediatr Adolesc Med.* 2003;157(5):419–424. PubMed doi: 10.1001/archpedi.157.5.419
59. US Preventive Services Task Force. Depression and Suicide Risk in Children and Adolescents: Screening. Published October 11, 2022. Accessed June 13, 2023. https://www.uspreventiveservicestaskforce.org/uspstf/recommendation/screening-depression-suicide-risk-children-adolescents
60. American Academy of Pediatrics, American Foundation for Suicide Prevention, National Institute of Mental Health. Suicide: Blueprint for Youth Suicide Prevention. Accessed June 13, 2023. https://www.aap.org/en/patient-care/blueprint-for-youth-suicide-prevention
61. Hua LL, Lee J, Rahmandar MH, Sigel EJ; COMMITTEE ON ADOLESCENCE; COUNCIL ON INJURY, VIOLENCE, AND POISON PREVENTION. Council on Injury, Violence, and Poison Prevention. Suicide and suicide risk in adolescents: clinical report. *Pediatrics.* 2024;153(1):e2023064800. PubMed doi: 10.1542/peds.2023-064800
62. Ammerman RT, Mara CA, Anyigbo C, et al. Behavior problems in low-income young children screened in pediatric primary care. *JAMA Pediatr.* 2023;177(12):1306–1313. PubMed doi: 10.1001/jamapediatrics.2023.4229
63. Wakschlag LS, Estabrook R, Petitclerc A, et al. Clinical implications of a dimensional approach: the normal:abnormal spectrum of early irritability. *J Am Acad Child Adolesc Psychiatry.* 2015;54(8):626–634. PubMed doi: 10.1016/j.jaac.2015.05.016

64. Wiggins JL, Briggs-Gowan MJ, Estabrook R, et al. Identifying clinically significant irritability in early childhood. *J Am Acad Child Adolesc Psychiatry.* 2018;57(3):191–199.e2. PubMed doi: 10.1016/j.jaac.2017.12.008

65. Trevethan R. Sensitivity, specificity, and predictive values: foundations, pliabilities, and pitfalls in research and practice. *Front Public Health.* 2017;5:307. PubMed doi: 10.3389/fpubh.2017.00307

66. Sheldrick RC, Garfinkel D. Is a positive developmental-behavioral screening score sufficient to justify referral? A review of evidence and theory. *Acad Pediatr.* 2017;17(5):464–470. PubMed doi: 10.1016/j.acap.2017.01.016

67. Vugteveen J, de Bildt A, Theunissen M, Reijneveld SA, Timmerman M. Validity Aspects of the Strengths and Difficulties Questionnaire (SDQ) Adolescent Self-Report and Parent-Report Versions Among Dutch Adolescents. *Assessment.* 2021;28(2):601–616. PubMed doi: 10.1177/1073191119858416

68. Etkin RG, Shimshoni Y, Lebowitz ER, Silverman WK. Using evaluative criteria to review youth anxiety measures, part I: self-report. *J Clin Child Adolesc Psychol.* 2021;50(1):58–76. PubMed doi: 10.1080/15374416.2020.1802736

69. Wolf ER, Hochheimer CJ, Sabo RT, et al. Gaps in well-child care attendance among primary care clinics serving low-income families. *Pediatrics.* 2018;142(5):e20174019. PubMed doi: 10.1542/peds.2017-4019

70. Roberts W, Kim EJ, Martinez J, Uwemedimo OT. Associations of adverse social determinants of health with missed well-child visits and the role of caregiver social support. *J Adv Pediatr Child Health.* 2021;4:067–072. doi: https://doi.org/10.29328/journal.japch.1001036

71. Cocozza V, Sickbert L, Kenny T, et al. Increasing mental health screening in pediatric subspecialty clinics: an improvement project at Brooke Army Medical Center. *Mil Med.* 2024;189(3–4):e789–e794. PubMed doi: 10.1093/milmed/usad373

72. Iturralde E, Adams RN, Barley RC, et al. Implementation of depression screening and global health assessment in pediatric subspecialty clinics. *J Adolesc Health.* 2017;61(5):591–598. PubMed doi: 10.1016/j.jadohealth.2017.05.030

73. Esposito J. Suicide screening and behavioral health assessment in the emergency department. *Clin Pediatr Emerg Med.* 2019;20(1):63–70. doi: 10.1016/j.cpem.2019.02.002

74. Eapen V. Developmental and mental health disorders: two sides of the same coin. *Asian J Psychiatr.* 2014;8:7–11. PubMed doi: 10.1016/j.ajp.2013.10.007

75. Prokosch C, Fertig AR, Ojebuoboh AR, et al. Exploring associations between social determinants of health and mental health outcomes in families from socioeconomically and racially and ethnically diverse households. *Prev Med.* 2022;161:107150. PubMed doi: 10.1016/j.ypmed.2022.107150

76. Brody GH, Yu T, Chen E, Miller GE, Kogan SM, Beach SR. Is resilience only skin deep?: rural African Americans' socioeconomic status-related risk and competence in preadolescence and psychological adjustment and allostatic load at age 19. *Psychol Sci.* 2013;24(7):1285–1293. PubMed doi: 10.1177/0956797612471954

77. Chen E, Miller GE, Brody GH, Lei M. Neighborhood poverty, college attendance, and diverging profiles of substance use and allostatic load in rural African American youth. *Clin Psychol Sci.* 2015;3(5):675–685. PubMed doi: 10.1177/2167702614546639

78. Hatsu IE, Eiterman L, Stern M, et al. Household food insecurity is associated with symptoms of emotional dysregulation in children with attention deficit hyperactivity disorder: The MADDY Study. *Nutrients.* 2022;14(6):1306. PubMed doi: 10.3390/nu14061306

79. Quimby EG, Brogan L, Atte T, Diamond G, Fein JA. Evaluating adolescent substance use and suicide in the pediatric emergency department. *Pediatr Emerg Care.* 2022;38(2):e595–e599. PubMed doi: 10.1097/PEC.0000000000002453

80. Tervo-Clemmens B, Gilman JM, Evins AE, et al. Substance use, suicidal thoughts, and psychiatric comorbidities among high school students. *JAMA Pediatr.* 2024;178(3):310–313. PubMed doi: 10.1001/jamapediatrics.2023.6263

81. Forkey H, Szilagyi M, Kelly ET, et al; COUNCIL ON FOSTER CARE, ADOPTION, AND KINSHIP CARE, COUNCIL ON COMMUNITY PEDIATRICS, COUNCIL ON CHILD ABUSE AND NEGLECT, COMMITTEE ON PSYCHOSOCIAL ASPECTS OF CHILD AND FAMILY HEALTH. Trauma-Informed Care. *Pediatrics.* 2021;148(2):e2021052580. PubMed doi: 10.1542/peds.2021-052580

82. Loop L, Mouton B, Brassart E, Roskam I. The observation of child behavior during parent-child interaction: the psychometric properties of the Crowell procedure. *J Child Fam Stud.* 2017;26(4):1040–1050. doi: 10.1007/s10826-016-0625-0

83. Thomson KC, Guhn M, Richardson CG, Ark TK, Shoveller J. Profiles of children's social-emotional health at school entry and associated income, gender and language inequalities: a cross-sectional population-based study in British Columbia, Canada. *BMJ Open.* 2017;7(7):e015353. PubMed doi: 10.1136/bmjopen-2016-015353

84. Peltz A, Rogers S, Garg A. An equity lens for identifying and addressing social needs within pediatric value-based care. *Pediatrics.* 2020;146(4):e20200320. PubMed doi: 10.1542/peds.2020-0320

85. Wissow L, Anthony B, Brown J, et al. A common factors approach to improving the mental health capacity of pediatric primary care. *Adm Policy Ment Health.* 2008;35(4):305–318. PubMed doi: 10.1007/s10488-008-0178-7

86. American Academy of Pediatrics. What is the common factors approach? In: Forman SG, Shahidullah JD, Hostutler CA, Green CM, Baum RA, eds. *Mental Health Strategies for Pediatric Care.* American Academy of Pediatrics; 2022:21–42.

87. American Academy of Pediatrics. Practice Tools. Common Factors Approach: HEL^{2}P^3 to Build a Better Alliance. Accessed August 20, 2024. https://downloads.aap.org/AAP/PDF/mhtk2e_commonfactorsapproach.pdf

88. National Network of Child Psychiatry Access Programs. Child Psychiatry Access Programs in the United States. Accessed August 20, 2024. https://www.nncpap.org/map

89. Sarvet B, Gold J, Bostic JQ, et al. Improving access to mental health care for children: the Massachusetts Child Psychiatry Access Project. *Pediatrics.* 2010;126(6):1191–1200. PubMed doi: 10.1542/peds.2009-1340

90. Southwick SM, Bonanno GA, Masten AS, Panter-Brick C, Yehuda R. Resilience definitions, theory, and challenges: interdisciplinary perspectives. *Eur J Psychotraumatol.* 2014;5(1):25338. PubMed doi: 10.3402/ejpt.v5.25338

91. Harvard University, Center on the Developing Child. Excessive Stress Disrupts the Architecture of the Developing Brain: Working Paper No. 3. Updated Edition. 2005/2014. Accessed January 27, 2025. https://developingchild.harvard.edu/resources/working-paper/wp3/

92. Svendsen S, Griffin J, Forkey H. Using the attachment relationship and positive parenting principles to build childhood resilience. *Adv Pediatr.* 2020;67:15–28. PubMed doi: 10.1016/j.yapd.2020.04.004

93. Masten AS. Ordinary magic. Resilience processes in development. *Am Psychol.* 2001;56(3):227–238. PubMed doi: 10.1037/0003-066X.56.3.227

94. Gupta RC, Randell KA, Dowd MD. Addressing parental adverse childhood experiences in the pediatric setting. *Adv Pediatr.* 2021;68:71–88. PubMed doi: 10.1016/j.yapd.2021.05.003

95. Sege RD, Harper Browne C. Responding to ACEs with HOPE: health outcomes from positive experiences. *Acad Pediatr.* 2017;17(7S): S79–S85. PubMed doi: 10.1016/j.acap.2017.03.007

96. Yamaoka Y, Bard DE. Positive parenting matters in the face of early adversity. *Am J Prev Med.* 2019;56(4):530–539. PubMed doi: 10.1016/j.amepre.2018.11.018

97. Gilgoff R, Schwartz T, Owen M, Bhushan D, Burke Harris N. Opportunities to treat toxic stress. *Pediatrics.* 2023;151(1): e2021055591. PubMed doi: 10.1542/peds.2021-055591

98. American Academy of Pediatrics. Getting Started: Implementing a Screening Process. Accessed August 21, 2023. https://www.aap.org/en/patient-care/screening-technical-assistance-and-resource-center/surveillancemonitoring-and-screening/

99. Meurer J, Rohloff R, Rein L, et al. Improving child development screening: implications for professional practice and patient equity. *J Prim Care Community Health.* 2022;13:21501319211062676. PubMed doi: 10.1177/21501319211062676

100. Talmi A, Bunik M, Asherin R, et al. Improving developmental screening documentation and referral completion. *Pediatrics.* 2014;134(4):e1181–e1188. PubMed doi: 10.1542/peds.2012-1151

101. Pinto-Martin JA, Dunkle M, Earls M, Fliedner D, Landes C. Developmental stages of developmental screening: steps to implementation of a successful program. *Am J Public Health.* 2005;95(11):1928–1932. PubMed doi: 10.2105/AJPH.2004.052167

102. Davis MV, Vincus A, Eggers M, et al. Effectiveness of public health quality improvement training approaches: application, application, application. *J Public Health Manag Pract.* 2012;18(1):E1–E7. PubMed doi: 10.1097/PHH.0b013e3182249505

103. Berry AD, Garzon DL, Mack P, Kanwischer KZ, Beck DG. Implementing an early childhood developmental screening and surveillance program in primary care settings: lessons learned from a project in Illinois. *J Pediatr Health Care.* 2014;28(6): 516–525. PubMed doi: 10.1016/j.pedhc.2014.04.008

104. Nicolay CR, Purkayastha S, Greenhalgh A, et al. Systematic review of the application of quality improvement methodologies from the manufacturing industry to surgical healthcare. *Br J Surg.* 2012;99(3):324–335. PubMed doi: 10.1002/bjs.7803

105. Christoff P. Running PDSA cycles. *Curr Probl Pediatr Adolesc Health Care.* 2018;48(8):198–201. PubMed https://doi.org/10.1016/j.cppeds.2018.08.006

106. Taylor MJ, McNicholas C, Nicolay C, Darzi A, Bell D, Reed JE. Systematic review of the application of the plan-do-study-act method to improve quality in healthcare. *BMJ Qual Saf.* 2014;23(4):290–298. PubMed doi: 10.1136/bmjqs-2013-001862

107. McNicholas C, Lennox L, Woodcock T, Bell D, Reed JE. Evolving quality improvement support strategies to improve Plan-Do-Study-Act cycle fidelity: a retrospective mixed-methods study. *BMJ Qual Saf.* 2019;28(5):356–365. PubMed doi: 10.1136/bmjqs-2017-007605

108. First 5 LA, University of Southern California, University Center for Excellence in Developmental Disabilities. Early Screening, Better Outcomes: Developmental Screening & Referral Toolkit for Pediatric Medical Clinics. Accessed June 15, 2023. http://publichealth.lacounty.gov/mch/HelpMeGrow/docs/EarlyScreeningBetterOutcomes.pdf

109. Curfman A, Hackell JM, Herendeen NE, et al. Telehealth: opportunities to improve access, quality, and cost in pediatric care. *Pediatrics.* 2022;149(3):e2021056035. PubMed doi: 10.1542/peds.2021-056035

110. Blackstone SR, Sebring AN, Allen C, Tan JS, Compton R. Improving depression screening in primary care: a quality improvement initiative. *J Community Health.* 2022;47(3):400–407. PubMed doi: 10.1007/s10900-022-01068-6

111. American Academy of Pediatrics. Screening Technical Assistance and Resource (STAR) Center. Accessed June 21, 2023. https://www.aap.org/en/patient-care/screening-technical-assistance-and-resource-center/

112. Ftouni R, AlJardali B, Hamdanieh M, Ftouni L, Salem N. Challenges of telemedicine during the COVID-19 pandemic: a systematic review. *BMC Med Inform Decis Mak. 3* 2022;22(1):207. doi: https://doi.org/10.1186/s12911-022-01952-0

113. Family Voices. Nuts and Bolts of Telemedicine: Essentials for a Family-Centered Experience. Accessed June 15, 2023. https://familyvoices.org/telehealth/curriculum/

114. American Academy of Family Practice. Four screening codes you should be using. Accessed June 15, 2023. https://www.aafp.org/pubs/fpm/blogs/inpractice/entry/screening_codes.html

115. Wang K. CPT Screening Codes. *AACAP News.* May/June 2018: 121–122. Accessed January 27, 2025. https://www.aacap.org/App_Themes/AACAP/Docs/member_resources/aacap_news/2018/AACAP-News-May-June-2018-CPT-Screening-Codes.pdf

116. Hughes C. Getting paid for screening and assessment services. *Fam Pract Manag.* 2017;24(6):25–29. PubMed

117. American Academy of Pediatrics. Coding and Valuation. Accessed June 15, 2023. https://www.aap.org/en/practice-management/practice-financing/coding-and-valuation/

118. Caballero TM, DeCamp LR, Platt RE, et al. Addressing the mental health needs of Latino children in immigrant families. *Clin Pediatr (Phila)*. 2017;56(7):648–658. PubMed doi: 10.1177/0009922816679509

119. Knuti Rodrigues K, Hambidge SJ, Dickinson M, Richardson DB, Davidson AJ. Developmental screening disparities for languages other than English and Spanish. *Acad Pediatr*. 2016;16(7):653–659. PubMed doi: 10.1016/j.acap.2015.12.007

Recognition and Management of Iatrogenically Induced Opioid Dependence and Withdrawal in Children

- *Clinical Report*

CLINICAL REPORT Guidance for the Clinician in Rendering Pediatric Care

American Academy of Pediatrics

DEDICATED TO THE HEALTH OF ALL CHILDREN™

Recognition and Management of Iatrogenically Induced Opioid Dependence and Withdrawal in Children: Clinical Report

Adam C. Adler, MD, MS, FAAP, FASE,[1] Linda B. Siegel, MD, FAAP, FAAHPM,[2] Robert T. Wilder, MD, PhD, FAAP,[3] Julie Good, MD, FAAP,[4] and the Committee on Drugs, Section on Critical Care, and Section on Anesthesiology and Pain Medicine

Opioids are often prescribed to children for pain relief related to procedures, acute injuries, and chronic conditions. Around-the-clock dosing of opioids can produce physiologic opioid dependence within 5 days. According to a 2001 consensus paper from the American Academy of Pain Medicine, American Pain Society, and American Society of Addiction Medicine, dependence is defined as "a state of adaptation that is manifested by a drug class specific withdrawal syndrome that can be produced by abrupt cessation, rapid dose reduction, decreasing blood level of the drug, or administration of an antagonist." The experience of children undergoing iatrogenic withdrawal symptoms is variable and may be mild and go unreported or can be severe and even life threatening. Guidance on opioid withdrawal is available only for adults and primarily for adults with substance use disorders. This report will summarize existing literature and provide readers with information on how to screen for symptoms of iatrogenic opioid withdrawal as well as mechanisms for opioid withdrawal prevention.

abstract

[1]*Department of Anesthesiology, Perioperative and Pain Medicine, Texas Children's Hospital, Baylor College of Medicine, Houston, Texas;* [2]*Northwell, New Hyde Park, New York; Department of Pediatrics, Division of Critical Care, Zucker School of Medicine, Cohen Children's Medical Center, Queens, New York;* [3]*Department of Anesthesiology and Perioperative Medicine, Mayo Clinic, Rochester, Minnesota; and* [4]*Department of Anesthesiology, Perioperative and Pain Medicine, Stanford University School of Medicine, Stanford Medicine Children's Health, Stanford, California*

Drs Adler, Siegel, Wilder, and Good all contributed to the writing and editing of this statement and have approved the final submission.

FINANCIAL/CONFLICT OF INTEREST DISCLOSURE: The authors have indicated they have no potential conflicts of interest to disclose.

FUNDING: No external funding.

To cite: Adler AC, Siegel LB, Wilder RT, et al; American Academy of Pediatrics, Committee on Drugs; Section on Critical Care; and Section on Anesthesiology and Pain Medicine. Recognition and Management of Iatrogenically Induced Opioid Dependence and Withdrawal in Children: Clinical Report. *Pediatrics.* 2025;156(3):e2025073169

INTRODUCTION

Opioids are commonly used for analgesia and sedation for children of all ages.[1] Primarily, opioids are used in short duration for analgesia required after a major procedure or an acute injury. Opioids have also been used in children requiring analgesia and sedation in the intensive care unit (ICU). Although the utilization of opioids in these circumstances is widely accepted, it is important to realize that children prescribed opioids regularly for as few as 5 days can develop physiologic opioid dependence and exhibit drug-specific withdrawal symptoms on abrupt discontinuation or tapering of these medications.[2,3]

Children in the ICU are especially prone to these issues, because they are often exposed to opioids at high doses and for longer periods of time, as they have ongoing pain or require long-term sedation/analgesia as part of their care. Children in the ICU require pain management for a variety of different reasons. Some of the etiologies of pain in children in the ICU include trauma, surgery, cancer, and pain and discomfort associated with an endotracheal tubes or other invasive devices. Children who are intubated in the pediatric intensive care unit (PICU) require pain control and sedation in order to tolerate noxious devices and avoid harming themselves by pulling out indwelling tubes or lines.[4] In the past, sedation was used along with pain management, but sedation with benzodiazepines has been found to be associated with the development of delirium and other adverse outcomes.[4–7] Therefore, reliance on opioids for analgesia and sedation, along with dexmedetomidine for additional sedation, is now more common and may lead to more opioid withdrawal symptoms in the PICU population. Additionally, opioids are frequently prescribed on an outpatient basis for pediatric patients following acute injuries and surgical or dental procedures. This type of outpatient prescribing is a source of medically prescribed opioids in children.

To understand the consequences of opioid use for sedation purposes, it is important to define physiologic withdrawal and tolerance. The most accepted definitions for these terms are based on the *Diagnostic and Statistical Manual of Mental Disorders, 5th Edition (DSM-5)*.[8] The definitions are as follows:

- Withdrawal is a syndrome that occurs when blood or tissue concentrations of a substance decline in an individual who had maintained prolonged heavy use of the substance.
- Tolerance is signaled by requiring a markedly increased dose of the substance to achieve the desired effect or a markedly reduced effect when the usual dose is consumed.

It is important not to conflate addiction, also known as an opioid use disorder, with physiologic dependence or tolerance, because patients appropriately treated with prolonged opioid therapy may develop physiological dependence and sometimes tolerance.[8,9] Although the physiology of opioid dependence may be similar between patients with iatrogenic opioid dependence and those with opioid use disorder, the psychology and approach between these two groups is quite different.

The experience of many children undergoing iatrogenically induced withdrawal is variable; it may be mild or go unreported, or it can be severe and potentially life threatening. Guidance for neonates and infants including those exposed in utero is available from the American Academy of Pediatrics.[10] Until recently, guidance was derived from literature concerning adults with substance use disorders. However, work with the Sophia Observation Scale (SOS) and the Withdrawal Symptoms Scale, Version 1 (WAT-1) has provided a lot of directed evidence for pediatric patients experiencing iatrogenic withdrawal. This clinical report serves as an update to the prior 2014 statement and summarizes the existing literature on iatrogenically induced opioid withdrawal and serves to update assessment tools and strategies for weaning opioids in this pediatric population.[11] The scope of this document is limited to children who received opioid medications exclusive of those being treated for neonatal abstinence syndrome (withdrawal from prenatal drug exposure).

Infants are a distinct patient population that merits brief mention, because they can live with withdrawal symptoms related to maternal opioid use (called neonatal abstinence syndrome [NAS] or neonatal opioid withdrawal syndrome [NOWS]), as well as from iatrogenic withdrawal, which occurs after postnatal exposure to opioids. This current report specifically addresses care for those infants affected by iatrogenic withdrawal syndrome (IWS) as these infants are cared for in both the neonatal ICU and PICU settings. The diagnosis and treatment of neonates with IWS is the same as for older children.[12,13] The WAT-1 and the SOS have both been validated in neonates and are commonly used to diagnose IWS in neonates.

BEHAVIORAL AND PHYSIOLOGIC CHARACTERISTICS OF OPIOID DEPENDENCE AND WITHDRAWAL

In most situations, opioid dependence does not manifest any symptoms until opioid administration is abruptly decreased or discontinued, resulting in symptoms of withdrawal. Care should be taken during opioid transitions, such as when converting from intravenous to oral opioids or when changing from one type of opioid to another (eg, fentanyl to morphine) because of reduced analgesic effect or presence of side effects, because the expected blood concentration of opioid may be less than expected and withdrawal symptoms can occur. Additionally, standardly applied medication doses may be ineffective for some patients or result in harm in others.[14,15] These differences in effect have been well described for medications such as codeine and tramadol, with increasing evidence for other opioid medications.[14,16] Individual differences can lead to pharmacogenomic differences (ie, differences in the metabolism and processing of the drug), resulting in an unpredictable bioavailability and, thus, an unpredictable effect between patients. Although "standard" opioid doses are effective in most patients, individual patient differences in pharmacogenomics may result in less predictable effects for the patient, which may be observed as either over effective (eg, excessive sedation) or not effective enough (eg, reduced analgesia, signs of opioid withdrawal).[13,17]

The signs and symptoms associated with withdrawal in the pediatric population can vary somewhat by age but are relatively consistent overall.[18,19] Neuropsychiatric symptoms are often the primary manifestation of withdrawal and include anxiety, agitation, insomnia, and tremulousness (or tremors). In addition to behavioral symptoms, physiologic changes commonly seen in withdrawal include increased muscle tone, nausea, vomiting, diarrhea, decreased appetite, tachypnea, tachycardia, fever, sweating, and hypertension. Care *must* be taken to rule out other causes of these symptoms, such as infection and sepsis. These symptoms can also be masked in patients taking other medications (eg, alpha-2 agonists, beta blockers, antipyretics, antihypertensives).

Many of these symptoms are assessed in tools used to monitor children undergoing potential opioid withdrawal.[18] Specific scales for children include the SOS and WAT-1, both of which have been validated in ICU patients.[20–22] These scales rely on patient observations related to vital signs, autonomic or gastrointestinal dysfunction, and central nervous system changes to assess for the occurrence and severity of withdrawal and are comparable in terms of accuracy and ease of use.[13] Providers should familiarize themselves with the foundation of these scales so they may be aware of potentially developing symptoms and signs of withdrawal when prescribing or assessing patients who have been prescribed opioids. Unfortunately, because of the overlap in symptoms, these scales are not able to differentiate between withdrawal from opioids or benzodiazepines. Amirnovin et al provide a stratified weaning protocol to address weaning in patients habituated on opioids and benzodiazepines, although weaning one class of medications at a time is generally preferred.[23] Lastly, these scales are not recommended for assessing patients experiencing withdrawal from illicit substance use (ie, not iatrogenic withdrawal) as these scales have not be validated for assessing patients with opioid use disorders. Consistently using and becoming familiar with either of these scales will allow a clinician a means of detecting early signs of withdrawal so a treatment strategy can be implemented. Clinicians should interpret results from the use of these scales within the clinical context of each individual patient, because there may be reasons other than opioid withdrawal that could explain certain behaviors or vital sign changes being scored (eg, a patient may be experiencing tachycardia and tachypnea attributable to sepsis and not opioid withdrawal).

MANAGEMENT STRATEGIES FOR APPROPRIATE WEANING OF OPIOIDS AND TREATMENT OF WITHDRAWAL SYMPTOMS

Withdrawal symptoms can be experienced with regular opioid administration of ≥5 days.[4,19,24] As such, if prescribing opioids for a duration of ≥5 days, providers should consider preemptively tapering the opioids over time rather than abruptly discontinuing the medication.[4] Unfortunately, evidence supporting the efficacy of tapering is of low quality.[4,25,26]

When planning to taper and/or discontinue an opioid, the first steps are to 1) decide whether the patient is at risk for opioid withdrawal; and 2) assess any continued analgesic need. Most patients who have received an opioid for fewer than 5 days do not live with withdrawal and can have their opioids prescribed on the basis of their current analgesic requirements. Patients who have been exposed to an opioid for longer than 5 days should taper their dose of opioids and should be assessed regularly for withdrawal symptoms. Patients taking higher doses of opioids or those taking opioids for prolonged durations (eg, weeks to months) are more likely to experience withdrawal symptoms.[27] A patient should not have ongoing painful stimuli or a condition that requires continuation or escalation of opioid dose to adequately manage pain before weaning. For the patient who needs to be continued on an opioid to adequately manage pain, the focus is to match the opioid analgesic requirement while assessing for and preventing withdrawal. Lastly, the patient should be clinically stable such that other signs (eg, hypertension, hypotension, sepsis) are not mistaken for withdrawal symptoms.

When it is determined that a patient should be weaned off an opioid, a protocol such as a weaning/tapering schedule should be used that generally considers both the length of opioid exposure and the total daily opioid dose. The use of a weaning/tapering protocol is advised to reduce the frequency of IWS and to decrease the total duration of opioid exposure.[28–32] However, no universally accepted protocol has been developed. Monitoring the individual patient's response to tapering is generally more important than following a rigid schedule. Once the patient is stabilized on a starting dose schedule, opioid weaning is typically accomplished by reducing the original doses in 10% to 20% decrements every 24 to 48 hours, depending on the half-life of the opioid chosen, although such advice is anecdotal and may be influenced by pharmacokinetic variables.[33,34] For example, drugs with longer half-lives such as methadone should be tapered more slowly. A wide range of opioid tapering doses are reported, and slower weans should be considered in patients at increased risk for IWS. Patients <6 years of age, especially those <6 months of age, and those with preexisting cognitive impairment may be at increased risk for experiencing withdrawal symptoms that go unrecognized.[4,26] A rescue opioid dose (single, as-needed dose) should be administered to patients determined to be in withdrawal (eg, ≥3 for WAT-1). The WAT-1 scale may also be used for patients who are nonverbal, as it relies on observer signs and symptoms that are irrespective of patient communication.

Adjunct medications (eg, dexmedetomidine), although not approved for the treatment of withdrawal in children, have been used, although there is little information at present to support their use in children for the treatment of opioid withdrawal. Dexmedetomidine has been shown both to be neuroprotective and to reduce inflammation, although more research is needed.[35] The role of adjunctive medications to prevent or manage iatrogenic opioid withdrawal symptoms needs further study. A common clinical scenario in patients with opioid dependence is concomitant benzodiazepine and/or alpha-2 agonist dependence, so one needs to anticipate the need for weaning from several classes of medication simultaneously. There are no accepted evidenced-based guidelines for the concurrent weaning of benzodiazepines, alpha-2 agonists, and opioids. Although multidrug weaning is out of the scope of this clinical report, one option may be to wean one class of medication at a time rather than attempt to wean from several simultaneously. Using this strategy, signs of withdrawal can be more clearly attributed to a particular class of medication.

For patients receiving prolonged opioid therapy (more than 5 days), it is best to develop a plan to taper the opioid therapy while minimizing withdrawal symptoms. The plan should include patient's support structure (eg, family member, prescribing physician, and other care team members [physical therapists]) and ideally be guided by the patient's primary care physician, particularly in the outpatient setting. Given the success of multidisciplinary pain management interventions, behavioral therapy may be a useful part of any weaning program to help with sleep hygiene, anxiety/mood symptoms, and gastrointestinal and pain-related symptoms that may occur during the tapering period. Behavioral management (eg, eat, sleep, console) has been used to treat infants with withdrawal symptoms from maternal opioid exposure; however, limited evidence exists to support application of these strategies to iatrogenic withdrawal in children.[36,37] Child life specialists can be helpful in providing developmentally appropriate support during tapering. Nonopioid analgesics such as acetaminophen, dexmedetomidine, ketamine, nonsteroidal anti-inflammatory drugs, and modulators such as gabapentin and local anesthetics can be particularly beneficial for patients with ongoing analgesia needs and can be used to reduce opioid requirements. Regional or neuraxial anesthesia techniques can be used when there is a nidus for pain (eg, postoperatively) and can be performed as a single, one-time block or as continuous therapy. Physical or occupational therapy aimed at improving function and mobility should be a mainstay in the treatment plan.

The most common pitfalls in tapering opioids are using a weaning schedule that is too rapid, failure to reassess and individualize a patient's tapering schedule, or inadequately accounting for analgesic needs of a patient during the process should pain occur. Lastly, nonrecognition of withdrawal symptoms or attribution of symptoms unrelated to withdrawal can complicate weaning.

CONCLUSIONS

Prescription opioid use is prevalent in both pediatric inpatient and outpatient settings. Abrupt discontinuation of opioids can lead to drug-specific withdrawal symptoms. For patients receiving prolonged opioid therapy (more than 5 days), it is best to develop a plan to taper the opioid therapy while minimizing withdrawal symptoms. The plan should include patient's support structure, eg, family member, prescribing physician, primary care pediatrician, and other care team members such as physical and emotional therapists. Use of an opioid-tapering strategy should be employed alongside a validated score for assessing withdrawal symptoms. Nonopioid adjuncts should be used for analgesia, when possible, to minimize opioid exposure.

LEAD AUTHORS

Adam C. Adler, MD, MS, FAAP, FASE
Linda B. Siegel, MD, FAAP, FAAHPM
Robert T. Wilder, MD, PhD, FAAP
Julie Good, MD, FAAP

Linda Siegel, MD, FAAP, FAAHPM
Vijay Srinivasan, MD, FAAP

LIAISONS

Nicholas Ettinger, MD, PhD, CPPS, FAAP – AAP Committee on Hospital Care
Steve Bondi, MD, JD, FAAP – AAP Committee on Medical Liability and Risk Management
Toni Gross, MD, MPH, FAAP – AAP Committee on Pediatric Emergency Medicine
Matthew Harting, MD, MS, FACS – AAP Section on Surgery
Tessie October, MD, MPH, FAAP – National Institute of Child Health and Human Development
Robert Francis Tamburro, Jr, MD, FAAP – Society of Critical Care Medicine
Mark Hall, MD, FCCM – World Federation of Pediatric Intensive & Critical Care Societies

STAFF

Sue Tellez

SECTION ON ANESTHESIOLOGY AND PAIN MEDICINE EXECUTIVE COMMITTEE, 2023-2024

Debnath Chatterjee, MD, FAAP, Chairperson
Christina Diaz, MD, FAAP, Chairperson-Elect
Elizabeth T. Drum, MD, FAAP
Justin B. Long, MD, MS, FAAP
Lena S. Sun, MD, FAAP
Brittany L. Willer, MD, FAAP
Mary Landrigan-Ossar, MD, FAAP, Immediate Past Chairperson

LIAISONS

James J. Fehr, MD, FAAP – Society for Pediatric Anesthesia
Yuan-Chi Lin, MD, FAAP – Society for Pediatric Pain Medicine
Debnath Chatterjee, MD, FAAP – American Society of Anesthesiologists Committee on Pediatric Anesthesia
Adam C. Adler, MD, MS, FAAP, FASE – AAP Committee on Drugs

STAFF

Jennifer Riefe, MEd
Address correspondence to lead authors:

- Adam C. Adler MD, MS, FAAP adamcadler@gmail.com
- Linda Siegal Lsiegs64@gmail.com
- Julie Wood jjkaleba@yahoo.com
- Robert Wilder wilder.robert@me.com

ABBREVIATIONS

IWS: iatrogenic withdrawal symptoms
PICU: pediatric intensive care unit
SOS: Sophia Observation Scale
WAT-1: Withdrawal Symptoms Scale, Version 1.

The guidance in this report does not indicate an exclusive course of treatment or serve as a standard of medical care. Variations, taking into account individual circumstances, may be appropriate.

All clinical reports from the American Academy of Pediatrics automatically expire 5 years after publication unless reaffirmed, revised, or retired at or before that time.

https://doi.org/10.1542/peds.2025-073169

REFERENCES

1. Volkow ND, McLellan TA, Cotto JH, Karithanom M, Weiss SR. Characteristics of opioid prescriptions in 2009. *JAMA*. 2011;305(13):1299–1301. PubMed doi: 10.1001/jama.2011.401
2. Arnold JH, Truog RD, Orav EJ, Scavone JM, Hershenson MB. Tolerance and dependence in neonates sedated with fentanyl during extracorporeal membrane oxygenation. *Anesthesiology*. 1990;73(6):1136–1140. PubMed doi: 10.1097/00000542-199012000-00011
3. Harris J, Ramelet AS, van Dijk M, et al. Clinical recommendations for pain, sedation, withdrawal and delirium assessment in critically ill infants and children: an ESPNIC position statement for healthcare professionals. *Intensive Care Med*. 2016;42(6):972–986. PubMed doi: 10.1007/s00134-016-4344-1
4. Smith HAB, Besunder JB, Betters KA, et al. 2022 Society of Critical Care Medicine Clinical Practice Guidelines on Prevention and Management of Pain, Agitation, Neuromuscular Blockade, and Delirium in Critically Ill Pediatric Patients With Consideration of the ICU Environment and Early Mobility. *Pediatr Crit Care Med*. 2022;23(2):e74–e110. PubMed doi: 10.1097/PCC.0000000000002873
5. Smith HAB, Gangopadhyay M, Goben CM, et al. Delirium and Benzodiazepines Associated With Prolonged ICU Stay in

Critically Ill Infants and Young Children. *Crit Care Med.* 2017;45(9): 1427–1435. PubMed doi: 10.1097/CCM.0000000000002515

6. Dervan LA, Di Gennaro JL, Farris RWD, Watson RS. Delirium in a Tertiary PICU: Risk Factors and Outcomes. *Pediatr Crit Care Med.* 2020;21(1):21–32. PubMed doi: 10.1097/PCC.0000000000002126
7. Mody K, Kaur S, Mauer EA, et al. Benzodiazepines and Development of Delirium in Critically Ill Children: Estimating the Causal Effect. *Crit Care Med.* 2018;46(9):1486–1491. PubMed doi: 10.1097/CCM.0000000000003194
8. Association AP. *Diagnostic and Statistical Manual of Mental Disorders.* 5th Ed. ed. American Psychiatric Publishing; 2013:992.
9. Zieli ski J, Morawska-Kochman M, Dudek K, Czapla M, Zato ski T. The Effect of Pre-Emptive Analgesia on the Postoperative Pain in Pediatric Otolaryngology: A Randomized, Controlled Trial. *J Clin Med.* 2022;11(10):2713. PubMed doi: 10.3390/jcm11102713
10. Patrick SW, Barfield WD, Poindexter BB, et al; COMMITTEE ON FETUS AND NEWBORN, COMMITTEE ON SUBSTANCE USE AND PREVENTION. Neonatal Opioid Withdrawal Syndrome. *Pediatrics.* 2020;146(5): e2020029074. PubMed doi: 10.1542/peds.2020-029074
11. Galinkin J, Koh JL, Frattarelli DAC, et al; Committee on Drugs; Section On Anesthesiology and Pain Medicine; American Academy of Pediatrics. Recognition and management of iatrogenically induced opioid dependence and withdrawal in children. *Pediatrics.* 2014;133(1):152–155. PubMed doi: 10.1542/peds.2013-3398
12. Isaac L, van den Hoogen NJ, Habib S, Trang T. Maternal and iatrogenic neonatal opioid withdrawal syndrome: Differences and similarities in recognition, management, and consequences. *J Neurosci Res.* 2022;100(1):373–395. PubMed doi: 10.1002/jnr.24811
13. Achuff BJ, Lemming K, Causey JC, et al. Opioid Weaning Protocol Using Morphine Compared With Nonprotocolized Methadone Associated With Decreased Dose and Duration of Opioid After Norwood Procedure. *Pediatr Crit Care Med.* 2022;23(5):361–370. PubMed doi: 10.1097/PCC.0000000000002885
14. Wong AK, Somogyi AA, Rubio J, Philip J. The Role of Pharmacogenomics in Opioid Prescribing. *Curr Treat Options Oncol.* 2022;23(10):1353–1369. PubMed doi: 10.1007/s11864-022-01010-x
15. Allegaert K, Rochette A, Veyckemans F. Developmental pharmacology of tramadol during infancy: ontogeny, pharmacogenetics and elimination clearance. *Paediatr Anaesth.* 2011;21(3):266–273. PubMed doi: 10.1111/j.1460-9592.2010.03389.x
16. Williams DG, Patel A, Howard RF. Pharmacogenetics of codeine metabolism in an urban population of children and its implications for analgesic reliability. *Br J Anaesth.* 2002;89(6):839–845. PubMed doi: 10.1093/bja/aef284
17. Wilson SH, Hellman KM, James D, Adler AC, Chandrakantan A. Mechanisms, diagnosis, prevention and management of perioperative opioid-induced hyperalgesia. *Pain Manag.* 2021;11(4):405–417. PubMed doi: 10.2217/pmt-2020-0105
18. Ista E, van Dijk M, Gamel C, Tibboel D, de Hoog M. Withdrawal symptoms in critically ill children after long-term administration of sedatives and/or analgesics: a first evaluation. *Crit Care Med.* 2008;36(8):2427–2432. PubMed doi: 10.1097/CCM.0b013e318181600d
19. Anand KJ, Willson DF, Berger J, et al; Eunice Kennedy Shriver National Institute of Child Health and Human Development Collaborative Pediatric Critical Care Research Network. Tolerance and withdrawal from prolonged opioid use in critically ill children. *Pediatrics.* 2010;125(5):e1208–e1225. PubMed doi: 10.1542/peds.2009-0489
20. Ista E, de Hoog M, Tibboel D, Duivenvoorden HJ, van Dijk M. Psychometric evaluation of the Sophia Observation withdrawal symptoms scale in critically ill children. *Pediatr Crit Care Med.* 2013;14(8):761–769. PubMed doi: 10.1097/PCC.0b013e31829f5be1
21. Franck LS, Harris SK, Soetenga DJ, Amling JK, Curley MA. The Withdrawal Assessment Tool-1 (WAT-1): an assessment instrument for monitoring opioid and benzodiazepine withdrawal symptoms in pediatric patients. *Pediatr Crit Care Med.* 2008;9(6):573–580. PubMed doi: 10.1097/PCC.0b013e31818c8328
22. Franck LS, Scoppettuolo LA, Wypij D, Curley MAQ. Validity and generalizability of the Withdrawal Assessment Tool-1 (WAT-1) for monitoring iatrogenic withdrawal syndrome in pediatric patients. *Pain.* 2012;153(1):142–148. PubMed doi: 10.1016/j.pain.2011.10.003
23. Amirnovin R, Sanchez-Pinto LN, Okuhara C, et al. Implementation of a Risk-Stratified Opioid and Benzodiazepine Weaning Protocol in a Pediatric Cardiac ICU. *Pediatr Crit Care Med.* 2018;19(11):1024–1032. PubMed doi: 10.1097/PCC.0000000000001719
24. Mondardini MC, Sperotto F, Daverio M, Amigoni A. Analgesia and sedation in critically ill pediatric patients: an update from the recent guidelines and point of view. *Eur J Pediatr.* 2023;182(5): 2013–2026. PubMed doi: 10.1007/s00431-023-04905-5
25. Sneyers B, Duceppe MA, Frenette AJ, et al. Strategies for the Prevention and Treatment of Iatrogenic Withdrawal from Opioids and Benzodiazepines in Critically Ill Neonates, Children and Adults: A Systematic Review of Clinical Studies. *Drugs.* 2020;80(12):1211–1233. PubMed doi: 10.1007/s40265-020-01338-4
26. Klein K, Pereira JS, Curtinaz K, Jantsch LB, Souza NS, Carvalho PRA. Strategies for the management and prevention of withdrawal syndrome in critically ill pediatric patients: a systematic review. *Rev Bras Ter Intensiva.* Oct-Dec 2022;34(4):507–518. Estrategias para manejo e prevencao da sindrome de abstinencia em pacientes pediatricos criticos: revisao sistematica. doi: 10.5935/0103-507X.20220145-pt
27. Best KM, Boullata JI, Curley MA. Risk factors associated with iatrogenic opioid and benzodiazepine withdrawal in critically ill pediatric patients: a systematic review and conceptual model. *Pediatr Crit Care Med.* 2015;16(2):175–183. PubMed doi: 10.1097/PCC.0000000000000306
28. Dokken M, Rustøen T, Diep LM, et al. Implementation of an algorithm for tapering analgosedation reduces iatrogenic withdrawal syndrome in pediatric intensive care. *Acta Anaesthesiol Scand.* 2023;67(9):1229–1238. PubMed doi: 10.1111/aas.14288

29. Dokken M, Rustøen T, Diep LM, et al. Iatrogenic withdrawal syndrome frequently occurs in paediatric intensive care without algorithm for tapering of analgosedation. *Acta Anaesthesiol Scand.* 2021;65(7):928–935. PubMed doi: 10.1111/aas.13818

30. Wilson AK, Ragsdale CE, Sehgal I, et al. Exposure-Based Methadone and Lorazepam Weaning Protocol Reduces Wean Length in Children. *J Pediatr Pharmacol Ther.* 2021;26(1):42–49. PubMed doi: 10.5863/1551-6776-26.1.42

31. Vyas D, Quinones Cardona V, Carroll A, Markel C, Young M, Fleishman R. Standardized Scoring Tool and Weaning Guideline to Reduce Opioids in Critically Ill Neonates. *Pediatr Qual Saf.* 2022;7(3):e562. PubMed doi: 10.1097/pq9.0000000000000562

32. Ford J, Harthan A, McGarvey J, Mischler M. Implementation of an Opioid Weaning Protocol at a Tertiary Care Children's Hospital. *Hosp Pediatr.* 2022;12(11):945–953. PubMed doi: 10.1542/hpeds.2021-006306

33. Morales Castro D, Dresser L, Granton J, Fan E. Pharmacokinetic Alterations Associated with Critical Illness. *Clin Pharmacokinet.* 2023;62(2):209–220. PubMed doi: 10.1007/s40262-023-01213-x

34. Tobias JD. Methadone: applications in pediatric anesthesiology and critical care medicine. *J Anesth.* 2021;35(1):130–141. PubMed doi: 10.1007/s00540-020-02887-4

35. Liaquat Z, Xu X, Zilundu PLM, Fu R, Zhou L. The Current Role of Dexmedetomidine as Neuroprotective Agent: An Updated Review. *Brain Sci.* 2021;11(7):846. PubMed doi: 10.3390/brainsci11070846

36. Barfield WD. Hush Little Baby - Promise of the Eat, Sleep, Console Approach. *N Engl J Med.* 2023;388(25):2391–2392. PubMed doi: 10.1056/NEJMe2304989

37. Young LW, Ounpraseuth ST, Merhar SL, et al; ACT NOW Collaborative. Eat, Sleep, Console Approach or Usual Care for Neonatal Opioid Withdrawal. *N Engl J Med.* 2023;388(25):2326–2337. PubMed doi: 10.1056/NEJMoa2214470

Recommendations for COVID-19 Vaccines in Infants, Children, and Adolescents

- *Policy Statement*

POLICY STATEMENT Organizational Principles to Guide and Define the Child Health System and/or Improve the Health of All Children

American Academy of Pediatrics

DEDICATED TO THE HEALTH OF ALL CHILDREN™

Recommendations for COVID-19 Vaccines in Infants, Children, and Adolescents: Policy Statement

Committee on Infectious Diseases

INTRODUCTION

This policy statement updates the recommendations of the American Academy of Pediatrics (AAP)[1] for the use of coronavirus disease 2019 (COVID-19) vaccines in the prevention of severe COVID-19 in children. These COVID-19 vaccine recommendations may change in future seasons or as additional variants emerge.

COVID-19 continues to be a cause of hospitalization[2,3] and death[4] in the pediatric population. COVID-19 vaccines are safe[5–12] and effective[13] in protecting individuals and populations against serious outcomes associated with severe acute respiratory syndrome coronavirus 2 (SARS-CoV-2) infection, including post-acute sequelae of SARS-CoV-2 infection (PASC)[14] and multisystem inflammatory syndrome in children (MIS-C).[15]

RECOMMENDATIONS

- Infants and children 6 through 23 months of age are at high risk for severe COVID-19.[2–4] The AAP recommends all infants and children in this age group who do not have contraindications* receive 2025–2026 COVID-19 vaccine, as follows:
  - Those who are previously unvaccinated should receive an initial vaccine series.
  - Those who are previously vaccinated but did not complete their initial vaccine series should complete their initial vaccine series.
  - Those who are previously vaccinated and completed their initial series should receive a single dose. This dose should be administered at least 8 weeks after the last dose was received.
  - Those with a previous asymptomatic infection or symptomatic disease caused by SARS-CoV-2 should also receive COVID-19 vaccination.
- Children 6 months through 18 years of age who are moderately or severely immunocompromised require 2 or more doses of age-appropriate 2025–2026 COVID-19 vaccine depending on previous

*COVID-19 vaccine contraindication includes a history of severe allergic reaction (eg, anaphylaxis) after a previous dose or to a component of the COVID-19 vaccine.

CONFLICT OF INTEREST DISCLOSURE: Sean O'Leary, MD, MPH, FAAP, has no potential conflicts of interest to disclose. José Romero, MD, FAAP, has disclosed a financial relationship with Pfizer in an advisory role regarding COVID-19 vaccination for adults. Robert W. Frenck Jr, MD, FAAP, disclosed relationships with Pfizer and Moderna. Neither Dr. Romero nor Dr Frenck participated in making recommendations or development of this statement. Other disclosures of committee members were reviewed and determined not relevant to the work related to the statement.

FUNDING: No external funding.

https://doi.org/10.1542/peds.2025-073924

To cite: American Academy of Pediatrics, Committee on Infectious Diseases. Recommendations for COVID-19 Vaccines in Infants, Children, and Adolescents: Policy Statement. *Pediatrics*. 2025;156(5):e2025073924

TABLE 1. Populations Recommended for Vaccination Including Those at High Risk for Severe COVID-19 Among Children Aged 6 Months Through 18 Years[a]

Population Characteristics	
Infants and children 6 through 23 mos of age	
Residents of long-term care facilities or other congregate settings[b]	
Children who have never been vaccinated against COVID-19	
Infants and children with household contacts who are at high risk for severe COVID-19[2,7]	
Underlying condition or treatment with common examples[c]	
Chronic pulmonary disease	Asthma/reactive airway disease Chronic lung disease of prematurity Compromised respiratory function (eg, abnormality of airway, tracheostomy, or ventilator dependent)
Cardiovascular disease	Congenital heart disease
Gastrointestinal disorders	Feeding tube dependent Inflammatory bowel disease
Hepatic disease	Chronic liver disease
Hematologic disease	Sickle cell disease
Metabolic disorders	Diabetes mellitus
Obesity	BMI ≥ the 95th percentile in children
Neurologic and neurodevelopmental conditions	Cerebral palsy Epilepsy Intellectual developmental disorder Compromised mobility (eg, wheelchair dependent)
Immunosuppressive conditions[d]	Receipt of immunosuppressive therapy Primary immunodeficiency HIV infection Receipt of hematopoietic cell transplant or solid organ transplant
Rheumatologic, autoimmune disease	Systemic lupus erythematosus Juvenile idiopathic arthritis

Abbreviation: BMI, body mass index.

[a] Adapted from Free RJ, Patel K, Taylor CA, et al. Hospitalization for COVID-19 and risk factors for severe disease among children: 2022–2024. *Pediatrics*. Published online July 3, 2025. doi: 10.1542/peds.2025-072788.[2]

[b] Congregate care settings refer to places where individuals live together in structured environments outside of their home, including residential treatment facilities, group homes, emergency shelters, juvenile detention centers, etc.

[c] List of examples is not exhaustive.

[d] Children who are **moderately or severely immunocompromised require 2 or more doses** of COVID-19 vaccine. Additional doses may be administered at ≥2-month intervals, informed by the clinical judgment of a health care provider and personal preference and circumstances.[16] Refer to AAP Recommended Child and Adolescent Immunization Schedule for dosing guidance at AAP.org/ImmunizationSchedule.

vaccination status.[16] Refer to the AAP Recommended Child and Adolescent Immunization Schedule for dosing recommendations at AAP.org/ImmunizationSchedule.

- The AAP recommends a single dose of age-appropriate 2025–2026 COVID-19 vaccine for all children and adolescents 2 through 18 years of age in the following risk groups (as described in Table 1) regardless of prior COVID-19 vaccination status:
    - Persons at high risk of severe COVID-19[2]
    - Residents of long-term care facilities or other congregate settings
    - Persons who have never been vaccinated against COVID-19
    - Persons whose household contacts are at high risk for severe COVID-19[2,17]
- Children 2 through 18 years of age not included in the risk groups above whose parent or guardian desires their protection from COVID-19 should be offered a single dose of age-appropriate 2025–2026 COVID-19 vaccine.[18] This dose should be administered at least 8 weeks after the last dose was received.
- Any available COVID-19 vaccine appropriate by age and health status that is approved by the US Food and Drug Administration through a biologics license application can be used. The most updated version of the COVID-19 vaccine that is available should be used.

For additional clinical guidance on COVID-19, refer to the *Red Book: 2024 Report of the Committee on Infectious Diseases* (https://publications.aap.org/redbook). For more information on the dosing and administration of COVID-19 vaccines, storage and handling, reporting, and patient education, visit https://www.aap.org/en/patient-care/covid-19/.

COMMITTEE ON INFECTIOUS DISEASES, 2025–2026

Sean T. O'Leary, MD, MPH, FAAP, Chairperson
James D. Campbell, MD, MS, FAAP, Vice Chairperson
Monica I. Ardura, DO, MSCS, FAAP
Kristina A. Bryant, MD, FAAP, *Red Book Online* Team Lead
Roberta L. DeBiasi, MD, MS, FAAP
Claudia Espinosa, MD, MSc, FAAP
Robert W. Frenck, Jr, MD, FAAP
C. Mary Healy, MD
Betsy C. Herold, MD, FAAP
Chandy C. John, MD, MS, FAAP
Aaron M. Milstone, MD, MHS, FAAP
Angela L. Myers MD, MPH, FAAP
Pia S. Pannaraj, MD, MPH, FAAP
Adam J. Ratner, MD, MPH, FAAP, *Red Book* Associate Editor
José R. Romero, MD, FAAP
Matthew Zahn, MD, FAAP

EX-OFFICIO

David W. Kimberlin, MD, FAAP, *Red Book* Editor
Ritu Banerjee, MD, PhD, FAAP, *Red Book* Associate Editor
Elizabeth D. Barnett, MD, FAAP, *Red Book* Associate Editor
Ruth Lynfield, MD, FAAP, *Red Book* Associate Editor

LIAISONS

Amina Ahmed, MD, FAAP, American Thoracic Society

Michelle Barton, MD, Canadian Paediatric Society
Carolyn Cleary, MD, FAAP, AAP Committee on Practice and Ambulatory Medicine
Denee J. Moore, MD, American Academy of Family Physicians
Jennifer L. Thompson, MD, American College of Obstetricians and Gynecologists
Juan P. Torres, MD, PhD, Sociedad Latinoamericana de Infectología Pediátrica
Charles R. Woods, Jr., MD, MS, FAAP, Pediatric Infectious Diseases Society

STAFF

Gillian Gibbs, MPH
Sunnah Kim

ACKNOWLEDGMENTS

The Committee on Infectious Diseases gratefully acknowledges Sean O'Leary, MD, MPH, FAAP, for his leadership in drafting the policy statement.

REFERENCES

1. COMMITTEE ON INFECTIOUS DISEASES. COVID-19 vaccines in infants, children, and adolescents. *Pediatrics*. 2022;150(3):e2022058700. PubMed doi: 10.1542/peds.2022-058700
2. Free RJ, Patel K, Taylor CA, et al. Hospitalization for COVID-19 and risk factors for severe disease among children: 2022–2024. *Pediatrics*. 2025;e2025072788. Published online July 3, 2025 PubMed doi: 10.1542/peds.2025-072788
3. Centers for Disease Control and Prevention. COVID-19 Hospitalization Surveillance Network (COVID-NET). Accessed August 7, 2025. https://www.cdc.gov/covid/php/covid-net/index.html
4. Centers for Disease Control and Prevention, National Center for Health Statistics. Provisional Mortality Statistics. CDC WONDER [database]. Accessed July 29, 2025. https://wonder.cdc.gov/mcd-icd10-provisional.html
5. Hause AM, Shay DK, Klein NP, et al. Safety of COVID-19 vaccination in United States children ages 5 to 11 years. *Pediatrics*. 2022;150(2):e2022057313. PubMed doi: 10.1542/peds.2022-057313
6. Hause AM, Marquez P, Zhang B, et al. Safety monitoring of mRNA COVID-19 vaccine third doses among children aged 6 months–5 years—United States, June 17, 2022–May 7, 2023. *MMWR Morb Mortal Wkly Rep*. 2023;72(23):621–626. PubMed doi: 10.15585/mmwr.mm7223a2
7. Hesse EM, Hause A, Myers T, et al; MIS-C REVIEW GROUP. COVID-19 vaccine safety first year findings in adolescents. *Pediatrics*. 2023;151(5):e2022060295. PubMed doi: 10.1542/peds.2022-060295
8. Hause AM, Marquez P, Zhang B, et al. Safety monitoring of bivalent COVID-19 mRNA vaccine booster doses among children aged 5–11 years—United States, October 12–January 1, 2023. *MMWR Morb Mortal Wkly Rep*. 2023;72(2):39–43. PubMed doi: 10.15585/mmwr.mm7202a5
9. Hause AM, Marquez P, Zhang B, et al. COVID-19 mRNA vaccine safety among children aged 6 months–5 years—United States, June 18, 2022–August 21, 2022. *MMWR Morb Mortal Wkly Rep*. 2022;71(35):1115–1120. PubMed doi: 10.15585/mmwr.mm7135a3
10. Goddard K, Donahue JG, Lewis N, et al. Safety of COVID-19 mRNA vaccination among young children in the Vaccine Safety Datalink. *Pediatrics*. 2023;152(1):e2023061894. PubMed doi: 10.1542/peds.2023-061894
11. Cortese MM, Taylor AW, Akinbami LJ, et al. Surveillance for multisystem inflammatory syndrome in US children aged 5–11 years who received Pfizer-BioNTech COVID-19 vaccine, November 2021 through March 2022. *J Infect Dis*. 2023;228(2):143–148. PubMed doi: 10.1093/infdis/jiad051
12. Yousaf AR, Cortese MM, Taylor AW, et al; MIS-C Investigation Authorship Group. Reported cases of multisystem inflammatory syndrome in children aged 12–20 years in the USA who received a COVID-19 vaccine, December, 2020, through August, 2021: a surveillance investigation. *Lancet Child Adolesc Health*. 2022;6(5):303–312. PubMed doi: 10.1016/S2352-4642(22)00028-1
13. Link-Gelles R, Ciesla AA, Rowley EAK, et al. Effectiveness of monovalent and bivalent mRNA vaccines in preventing COVID-19–associated emergency department and urgent care encounters among children aged 6 months–5 years — VISION Network, United States, July 2022–June 2023. *MMWR Morb Mortal Wkly Rep*. 2023;72(33):886–892. PubMed doi: 10.15585/mmwr.mm7233a2
14. Yousaf AR, Mak J, Gwynn L, et al. COVID-19 vaccination and odds of post–COVID-19 condition symptoms in children aged 5 to 17 years. *JAMA Netw Open*. 2025;8(2):e2459672. PubMed doi: 10.1001/jamanetworkopen.2024.59672
15. Hamad Saied M, van der Griend L, van Straalen JW, Wulffraat NM, Vastert S, Jansen MHA. The protective effect of COVID-19 vaccines on developing multisystem inflammatory syndrome in children (MIS-C): a systematic literature review and meta-analysis. *Pediatr Rheumatol Online J*. 2023;21(1):80. PubMed doi: 10.1186/s12969-023-00848-1
16. Roper LE, Godfrey M, Link-Gelles R, et al. Use of additional doses of 2024–2025 COVID-19 vaccine for adults aged ≥65 years and persons aged ≥6 months with moderate or severe immunocompromise: recommendations of the Advisory Committee on Immunization Practices—United States, 2024. *MMWR Morb Mortal Wkly Rep*. 2024;73(49):1118–1123. doi: 10.15585/mmwr.mm7349a2
17. Yek C, Warner S, Wiltz JL, et al. Risk factors for severe COVID-19 outcomes among persons aged ≥18 years who completed a primary COVID-19 vaccination series—465 health care facilities, United States, December 2020–October 2021. *MMWR Morb Mortal Wkly Rep*. 2022;71(1):19–25. PubMed doi: 10.15585/mmwr.mm7101a4
18. National Center for Immunization and Respiratory Diseases, US Centers for Disease Control and Prevention. Use of 2025-2026 COVID-19 Vaccines: Work Group Considerations. Accessed August 7, 2025. https://www.cdc.gov/acip/downloads/slides-2025-04-15-16/05-Panagiotakopoulos-COVID-508.pdf

Recommendations for Prevention and Control of Influenza in Children, 2025–2026

- *Policy Statement*
  - *PPI: AAP Partnership for Policy Implementation See Appendix 1 for more information.*

American Academy of Pediatrics
DEDICATED TO THE HEALTH OF ALL CHILDREN®

AAP Partnership for Policy Implementation

POLICY STATEMENT Organizational Principles to Guide and Define the Child Health Care System and/or Improve the Health of All Children

American Academy of Pediatrics

DEDICATED TO THE HEALTH OF ALL CHILDREN™

Recommendations for Prevention and Control of Influenza in Children, 2025–2026: Policy Statement

Committee on Infectious Diseases

abstract

This statement updates the recommendations of the American Academy of Pediatrics (AAP) for the use of influenza vaccines and antiviral medications in the prevention and treatment of influenza in children during the 2025–2026 influenza season. A review of the evidence supporting these recommendations is in the accompanying technical report (https://doi.org/10.1542/peds.2025-073622).

The AAP recommends annual influenza vaccination of all children without medical contraindications starting at 6 months of age. Influenza vaccination is an important strategy for protecting children and the broader community as well as reducing the overall burden of respiratory illnesses when other viruses are cocirculating. Any licensed influenza vaccine appropriate for age and health status can be administered, as soon as possible in the season, without preference for one product or formulation.

Antiviral treatment of influenza is recommended for children with suspected or confirmed influenza who are hospitalized or have severe or progressive disease or have underlying conditions that increase their risk of complications of influenza. In this situation, antiviral treatment should be started as soon as possible regardless of duration of illness. Antiviral treatment is an option in the outpatient setting for other children with suspected or confirmed influenza in some circumstances.

Antiviral chemoprophylaxis is an option in certain individuals, especially exposed children who are asymptomatic and are at high risk for influenza complications but have not yet been immunized or those who are not expected to mount an effective immune response.

Address correspondence to: Kristina A. Bryant, MD, FAAP. k0brya01@louisville.edu

CONFLICT OF INTEREST DISCLOSURE: Dr Bryant has no disclosed conflicts related to the content of this statement. Dr Bryant has disclosed completed or ongoing research relationships with Gilead, Pfizer, Sanofi, and Enanta that were reviewed and determined not relevant to influenza. Dr Bryant receives honoraria from WebMed, a stipend from the American Society of Nephrology, and royalties from Oxford University Press. Committee on Infectious Diseases members who disclosed relevant conflicts did not participate in the development of this statement.

FUNDING: No external funding.

To cite: American Academy of Pediatrics, Committee on Infectious Diseases. Recommendations for Prevention and Control of Influenza in Children, 2025–2026: Policy Statement. *Pediatrics.* 2025;156(6):e2025073620

INTRODUCTION

Children, especially those younger than 5 years and those with certain underlying medical conditions, can experience substantial morbidity, including severe or fatal complications, from influenza virus infection.[1–3] Children also play a pivotal role in the transmission of influenza virus infection to household and other close contacts.[4–6]

Influenza vaccination of children can reduce disease burden directly and among household members, close contacts, and community members of all ages.[7,8] By reducing the burden of respiratory illnesses, influenza vaccination helps to preserve health care capacity, especially when other viruses are cocirculating. The American Academy of Pediatrics (AAP) recommends routine influenza vaccination of children ≥6 months of age for the prevention of influenza. Despite this recommendation, influenza vaccination coverage decreased again during the 2024–2025 influenza season. Through April 26, 2025, only 49.2% of children 6 months through 17 years had been vaccinated, 14.5 percentage points lower than at the end of 2020 (https://www.cdc.gov/fluvaxview/interactive/general-population-coverage.html). Differences in vaccination rates were noted by age, race, and ethnicity; poverty status; urbanicity; and maternal immunization status.[9] Continued efforts to increase influenza vaccination, including strategies to decrease disparities in vaccine access and delivery and to counter vaccine hesitancy, are urgently needed.

This policy statement summarizes updates and recommendations for the 2025–2026 influenza season. An accompanying technical report provides further detail.[10]

UPDATES FOR THE 2025–2026 INFLUENZA SEASON

1. All licensed vaccines available in the United States this season are trivalent.
2. The compositions of influenza vaccines for the 2025–2026 season have been updated (Table 1).
3. Recommendations for influenza treatment and prophylaxis have been simplified.
4. Live attenuated influenza vaccine (LAIV) is available for administration in the home by a caregiver for eligible children ≥2 years of age.
5. Recombinant baculovirus-expressed hemagglutinin (HA) influenza vaccine (RIV3) is now licensed for individuals as young as 9 years of age.[11]

HIGH-RISK GROUPS IN PEDIATRICS

Children younger than 5 years, especially those younger than 2 years, and children with certain underlying medical conditions are at increased risk of hospitalization and complications attributable to influenza (Table 2).[10] Although influenza vaccination is recommended for everyone starting at 6 months of age, emphasis should be placed on ensuring that high-risk children, medically vulnerable children, and children with medical complexity, as well as their parents/guardians, other household contacts, and caregivers, receive annual influenza vaccine (Table 3). Additionally, increased efforts are needed to eliminate barriers to vaccination in all persons experiencing higher rates of adverse outcomes from influenza. Racial and ethnic disparities exist in severe outcomes from influenza, with some group experiencing higher rates of severe outcomes.[12] In 1 cross-sectional study spanning 10 influenza seasons, Black, Hispanic, and American Indian/Alaska Native people had higher rates of influenza-associated hospitalizations and intensive care unit admissions, and disparities were highest in children ≤4 years of age.[12] Influenza-associated in-hospital deaths were three- to 4-fold higher in Black, Hispanic, and Asian/Pacific Islander children compared with white children.[12] Inequities in health care system access and other social drivers of health contribute to severe outcomes and increased mortality in these groups.

TABLE 1. Trivalent Influenza Vaccine Composition for the 2025–2026 Season

	Specific Strain
Influenza A	
H1N1	A/Victoria/4897/2022 (H1N1)pdm09-like virus (egg-based)[a]
	A/Wisconsin/67/2022 (H1N1)pdm09-like virus (cell culture-based or recombinant)[a]
H3N2	A/Croatia/10136RV/2023 (H3N2)-like virus (egg-based)[b]
	A/District of Columbia/27/2023 (H3N2)-like virus (cell culture-based or recombinant)[b]
Influenza B	
Victoria	B/Austria/1359417/2021-like virus (B/Victoria lineage)[a]

Quadrivalent vaccines are still available outside the United States.
[a] Unchanged this season.
[b] New this season.

SEASONAL INFLUENZA VACCINES

The seasonal influenza vaccines licensed for children for the 2025–2026 season are described in Table 4. As in the 2024–2025 season, all 2025–2026 seasonal influenza vaccines available in the United States are trivalent and contain hemagglutinin derived from the same influenza strains as recommended by the World Health Organization (WHO) and the US Food and Drug Administration (FDA) for the Northern Hemisphere (Table 1).[13,14] The influenza A (H3N2) vaccine component for the 2025–2026 season has been updated. The influenza A (H1N1) and influenza B Victoria lineage are unchanged.

INFLUENZA VACCINE RECOMMENDATIONS

General Recommendations

1. The AAP recommends influenza vaccination of everyone 6 months and older during the 2025–2026 influenza season.

TABLE 2. High-Risk Groups for Influenza Complications

Category	Description
Demographic Characteristics	Children <5 y, especially those <2 y[a]
	Children born preterm or early term[b]
	Residents of a chronic care facility or nursing home
Underlying Condition or Treatment with Common Examples[c]	
Chronic pulmonary disease	Asthma[21]
	Cystic fibrosis Bronchopulmonary dysplasia[21]
	Compromised respiratory function (eg, requiring mechanical ventilation, tracheostomy)
Cardiovascular disease	Hemodynamically significant conditions (excluding hypertension alone)
Kidney disease	Chronic kidney disease, including end-stage kidney disease Dialysis
Hepatic disease	Chronic liver disease Cirrhosis[22,23]
Hematologic disease	Sickle cell disease
	Other hemoglobinopathies
Metabolic disorders	Diabetes mellitus
Neurologic and neurodevelopmental conditions	Cerebral palsy
	Epilepsy
	Stroke
	Intellectual developmental disorder
	Moderate to severe developmental delay
	Neuromuscular disorders, including muscular dystrophy
	Spinal cord injury
Extreme obesity	BMI ≥40 for adults; BMI ≥the 95th percentile in children[d]
Immunosuppression	Receipt of immunocompromising medications
	Receipt of hematopoietic cell transplant or solid organ transplant
	Congenital or acquired immune deficiency, including HIV
	Asplenia
Receiving treatment with aspirin or salicylate-containing therapies[e]	
Pregnancy and up to 2 weeks postpartum	

Abbreviation: BMI, body mass index.
[a] Regardless of the presence of underlying medical conditions.
[b] Higher risk of influenza hospitalization in the first 5 years of life.
[c] List of examples is not exhaustive.
[d] BMI associated with increased risk not well-defined in children but could consider BMI at or above the 95th percentile for children and adolescents of the same age and sex.[24,25]
[e] Applies to children and adolescents <19 years who may be at increased risk of Reye syndrome.
Grohskopf LA, Ferdinands JM, Blanton LH, Broder KR, Loehr J. Prevention and control of seasonal influenza with vaccines: recommendations of the Advisory Committee on Immunization Practices–United States, 2024–25 influenza season. *MMWR Recomm Rep.* 2024;73(RR-5):1–25.

TABLE 3. Strategies for Increasing Childhood Influenza Vaccination

Clinician/Care Team
• Offer strong, presumptive influenza vaccine recommendation • Bundle recommendation for influenza vaccine with recommendations for other needed vaccines • Use consistent messaging across care team members • Identify influenza vaccine champion(s)
Practice/Health System
• Review influenza vaccination status at all visits • Bundle influenza vaccine with other needed vaccines • Vaccinate at all visit types (eg, well child, acute care visits) • Vaccinate in all health care settings (eg, hospital, emergency department, subspecialty practice) • Increase access to influenza vaccine (eg, expanded hours, vaccine-only clinic) • Provide evidence-based information to patients and families (eg, office-based educational handout) • Offer scripting for staff and messaging for patients and families to address common questions, including frequent misconceptions and relevant contraindications and precautions, including allergies • Consider an early or expedited allergy referral for patients with a potential flu vaccine allergy to ensure timely vaccination when appropriate • Send influenza vaccine reminder/recall messages • Use electronic health record (EHR)-based tools to identify and classify high-risk patients for targeted outreach • Utilize standing orders for influenza vaccine • Implement influenza vaccine prompts/clinical decision support • Perform audits and share feedback reports
Community/Public Health
• Integrate electronic health record with regional or state immunization information system (IIS) and automate reconciliation of electronically received influenza vaccine administration data • Partner with stakeholders to support vaccine initiatives within the community, including school-based programs and pharmacies • Engage with communities affected by health disparities to develop tailored strategies that promote trust, encourage dialogue, and increase access to preventive services

2. The AAP recommends any licensed influenza vaccine product appropriate for age and health status and does not prefer one product over another, including inactivated (non-live) influenza vaccine (IIV) or recombinant influenza vaccine (RIV) and LAIV. RIV is now an option for persons ≥9 years of age.[11] Influenza vaccination should not be delayed to obtain a specific product, including a thimerosal-free product. The safety of thimerosal-containing vaccines is discussed in the technical report in the section "Safety of IIV and RIV" (https://doi.org/10.1542/peds.2025-073622).
3. LAIV should not be used for immunocompromised persons and persons with certain chronic medical conditions (Table 5).
4. The number of influenza vaccine doses recommended for children remains unchanged in the 2025–2026 influenza season and depends on the child's age at first

TABLE 4. Recommended Seasonal Influenza Vaccines for Children and Adolescents: United States, 2025–2026 Influenza Season

Vaccine	Trade Name (Manufacturer)	Age Group	Presentation and Hemagglutinin Antigen Content (IIVs and RIV3) or Virus Count (LAIV3) per Dose for Each Antigen	Recommended Dose	Thimerosal Mercury Content[a] (mcg Hg/0.5-mL dose)
Trivalent Standard Dose – Egg-Based Vaccines					
IIV3	Afluria *(Seqirus)*[b]	≥36 mo	0.5-mL prefilled syringe (15 mcg/0.5 mL)	0.5 mL	0 0
IIV3	Fluarix *(GlaxoSmithKline)*	≥6 mo	0.5-mL prefilled syringe (15 mcg/0.5 mL)	0.5 mL	0
IIV3	FluLaval *(GlaxoSmithKline)*	≥6 mo	0.5-mL prefilled syringe (15 mcg/0.5 mL)	0.5 mL	0
IIV3	Fluzone *(Sanofi Pasteur)*	≥6 mo 6 through 35 mo ≥36 mo	0.5-mL prefilled syringe (15 mcg/0.5 mL) 5-mL multidose vial[c,d] (15 mcg/0.5 mL) 5-mL multidose vial[c] (15 mcg/0.5 mL)	0.5 mL 0.25 or 0.5 mL 0.5 mL	0 25 25
Trivalent Standard Dose – Cell Culture-Based Vaccines					
ccIIV3	Flucelvax *(Seqirus)*	≥6 mo	0.5-mL prefilled syringe (15 mcg/0.5 mL)	0.5 mL	0
Recombinant Vaccine					
RIV3	Flublok *(Sanofi Pasteur)*	≥9 y	0.5-mL prefilled syringe (45 mcg/0.5 mL)	0.5 mL	0
Live Attenuated Vaccine-Egg Based Vaccine					
LAIV3	FluMist *(AstraZeneca)*	2–49 y	0.2-mL prefilled intranasal sprayer (Virus dose: $10^{6.5–7.5}$ FFU/0.2 mL)	0.2 mL (0.1 mL per nostril)	0

Abbreviations: IIV3, trivalent adjuvanted inactivated (non-live) influenza vaccine; ccIIV3, trivalent cell culture-based inactivated (non-live) influenza vaccine; FFU, fluorescent focus unit; LAIV3, trivalent live attenuated influenza vaccine; RIV3, trivalent recombinant influenza vaccine.

[a] See section on Thimerosal-Containing Vaccines.

[b] For children through 35 months, the dose of Afluria is 0.25 mL, but the manufacturer reports that neither 0.25 mL pre-filled syringes or multidose vials will be available during the 2025-2026 season.

[c] For vaccines that include a multidose vial presentation, the maximum number of doses withdrawn should not exceed the number specified in the package insert (eg, 10 doses for Fluzone). Residual product should be discarded.

[d] A total of 0.25 mL drawn from a multidose vial is an acceptable dose for children 6 to 35 months of age.

Implementation guidance on supply, pricing, payment, billing, coding, and liability issues can be found at aap.org/influenza.

dose administration and influenza vaccination history (Figure 1). Doses given up to 4 days prior to the minimum suggested interval are acceptable.

5. When a child is recommended to receive 2 doses of vaccine in a given season, the doses do not need to be the same brand or formulation. A child may receive a combination of IIV, RIV, and LAIV if appropriate for age and health status.
6. Influenza vaccine should be offered to children as soon as it becomes available, especially to those recommended to receive 2 doses. The recommended dose(s) ideally should be received by the end of October for optimal protection before the influenza season.
7. For children with malignant neoplasms receiving chemotherapy, IIV or RIV should be administered ≥2 weeks before cytotoxic chemotherapy, when clinically possible.
8. For children who will be starting anti-B cell therapies (eg, rituximab, alemtuzumab), IIV or RIV should optimally be provided at least 2 to 4 weeks before starting these therapies. For children who have received anti-B cell therapies, IIV should be deferred for 6 months after last dose, and ideally once there is evidence of B cell recovery.
9. Non-live vaccines should be considered ≥6 months after CD19-targeted chimeric antigen receptor (CAR)-T–cell infusion in patients who are in remission and do not require additional chemotherapy or hematopoietic cell transplantation.
10. For hematopoietic cell transplant (HCT) recipients, IIV or RIV can be given starting 4 to 6 months after transplantation.
11. Although high-dose IIV is not approved for use in children, clinicians could consider administering 2 doses of high-dose trivalent inactivated (non-live) influenza vaccine (IIV3) 28 to 42 days apart in pediatric HCT recipients 3 to 17 years of age.[15,16]
12. For solid organ transplant (SOT) recipients, IIV or RIV can be given starting 3 months after receipt of an SOT, although it may be considered ≥1 month after SOT during the influenza season.
13. Household contacts of immunocompromised individuals should receive influenza vaccine annually.

Additional Recommendations for Pregnant and Breastfeeding Persons

14. Pediatricians who interact with pregnant individuals should recommend influenza vaccination, emphasizing the benefits of vaccination for them and their infants.

TABLE 5. Influenza Vaccine Contraindications and Precautions

Vaccine	Contraindication	Precaution	Clinician Discretion	Not Contraindication or Precaution
Egg-based inactivated (non-live) influenza vaccine (IIV)[a]	• Anaphylaxis or severe allergic reaction to any previous influenza vaccination or to any vaccine component	• Moderate to severe acute illness with or without fever, including COVID-19 • History of Guillain-Barré syndrome (GBS) within 6 weeks of prior influenza vaccination		• Mild illness, with or without fever • Egg allergy
Cell culture-based inactivated (non-live) influenza vaccine (ccIIV)[a]	• Anaphylaxis or severe allergic reaction to previous dose of ccIIV or any component of ccIIV3	• Moderate to severe acute illness with or without fever, including COVID-19 • History of GBS within 6 weeks of prior influenza vaccination • Anaphylaxis or severe allergic reaction to any other influenza vaccine (ie, any egg-based IIV, LAIV, or RIV)		• Mild illness, with or without fever • Egg allergy
Live attenuated influenza vaccine (LAIV)[a]	• Anaphylaxis or severe allergic reaction to any previous influenza vaccination or to any vaccine component, including gelatin • Age 2–4 y with diagnosis of asthma or history of wheezing in last 12 mos • Cochlear implants • Active cerebrospinal fluid leaks • Immunosuppression due to any cause, including: ◦ Primary or acquired immunodeficiency, including HIV ◦ Immunosuppressive or immunomodulatory therapy ◦ Anatomic or functional asplenia • Close contacts or caregivers of severely immunocompromised individuals • Taking aspirin or salicylate-containing medications • Receiving or recently received influenza antiviral medication[b] • Currently pregnant[c]	• Moderate to severe acute illness with or without fever, including COVID-19 • History of GBS within 6 weeks of prior influenza vaccination • Diagnosis of asthma and age ≥5 y • Certain underlying chronic conditions that might predispose to complications after influenza (eg, chronic pulmonary disease, cardiovascular disease, renal, hepatic, neurologic, hematologic, or metabolic disorders)	• Defer to resolution of symptoms or use IIV if a patient has nasal congestion that could impede vaccine delivery	• Mild illness, with or without fever • Egg allergy
Recombinant HA vaccine (RIV3)[a]	• Anaphylaxis or severe allergic reaction to previous dose of RIV3 or any component of RIV3	• Moderate to severe illness, with or without fever, including COVID-19 • History of GBS within 6 weeks of prior influenza vaccination • Anaphylaxis or severe allergic reaction to any other influenza vaccine (ie, any egg-based IIV, LAIV, or ccIIV)		• Mild illness, with or without fever • Egg allergy

[a] Egg-based IIVs for children include Afluria, Fluarix, FluLaval, and Fluzone. Cell-culture based IIV includes Flucelvax. RIV includes Flublok. LAIV includes FluMist.
[b] Within 48 hours (oseltamivir, zanamivir), 5 days (peramivir), or 17 days (baloxavir) of stopping influenza antiviral therapy.
[c] Pregnancy is not a labeled contraindication for LAIV. The prescribing information for FluMist Quadrivalent, 2023–2024 formula indicated that FluMist is not absorbed systemically following intranasal administration and use during pregnancy is not expected to result in fetal exposure to the drug.

15. Pregnant individuals may receive IIV or RIV at any time during pregnancy to protect themselves and their infants. Those who do not receive it during pregnancy should receive influenza vaccine before hospital discharge. Those who decline the vaccine during hospitalization should be encouraged to discuss influenza vaccination with their obstetrician, family physician, nurse midwife, or other trusted clinician.
16. Influenza vaccination of a breastfeeding parent provides protection to both the parent and the infant and is recommended and safe.

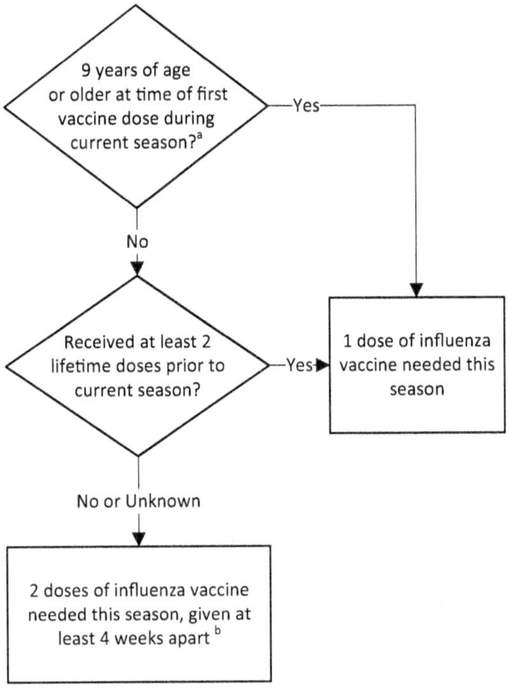

FIGURE 1.
Number of 2025–2026 seasonal influenza vaccine doses recommended for children based on age and prior vaccination history.
[a]Must be at least 6 months of age to be eligible for influenza vaccine.
[b]Second dose still required for children who turn 9 between first and second dose.

Additional Recommendations for Travelers

17. Individuals traveling to the tropics, on cruise ships, or to the Southern hemisphere during April to September should consider seasonal influenza vaccination ≥2 weeks before departure if not vaccinated during the preceding fall or winter and if vaccine is available (see section "Timing of Influenza Vaccination and Duration of Protection" in the technical report [https://doi.org/10.1542/peds.2025-073622]).[10]

Additional Recommendations for Health Care Personnel

18. The AAP supports influenza vaccination of health care personnel as a condition of employment as a crucial strategy for reducing health care-associated influenza virus infections.

Influenza Vaccine Implementation

19. Efforts should be made to promote influenza vaccination of all children, especially children younger than 5 years and those in high-risk groups (Table 2) and their contacts, unless contraindicated (Table 5), using evidence-based strategies (Table 3). To promote influenza vaccination in communities affected by health disparities, it is important to include community members in the development of culturally relevant strategies.
20. Strategies for communicating with families about vaccines and promoting vaccine confidence are available at https://www.aap.org/vaccinecommunication.
21. Increasing access and reducing barriers to vaccination through schools, pharmacies, hospitals, and other nontraditional settings may improve vaccination rates. However, vaccination in the medical home is the preferred option for young children to facilitate other necessary services, including well care, preventive screening, anticipatory guidance, and other important childhood vaccinations. For patients and families for whom resource constraints would present an obstacle to receiving the vaccine in the medical home, at-home administration of LAIV is an alternative for some eligible individuals 2 through 49 years of age. Practical considerations for LAIV administered in the home setting are presented in the technical report (https://doi.org/10.1542/peds.2025-073622).[10]
22. When influenza vaccination takes place in a nontraditional setting, appropriate documentation should be provided to patients and the medical home and submitted to the state or regional immunization information systems (IISs).
23. Practices serving children and adolescents may consider offering influenza vaccine to family members and close contacts.[17]

Influenza Vaccine Advocacy

24. All participants in immunization efforts should work to eliminate disparities in influenza vaccine supply between privately insured patients and those eligible for vaccination through the Vaccines for Children (VFC) program.
25. Information about influenza vaccine and influenza vaccine clinics should be provided to eligible children and their families in their preferred language, especially those who may experience barriers to preventive care.
26. Public and private payers should offer adequate payment for influenza vaccine supply and administration to pediatric populations, update payments for influenza vaccine so that physicians and other clinicians who care for children are paid for administering doses in July and August and eliminate remaining "patient responsibility" cost barriers to influenza vaccination where they still exist.

INFLUENZA VACCINE CONTRAINDICATIONS AND PRECAUTIONS

Contraindications and precautions for the use of influenza vaccines are described in Table 5, and further details are provided in the technical report.[10] Key points include:

1. Product-specific contraindications must be considered when selecting the type of influenza vaccine to administer.[18]
2. Although a history of severe allergic reaction (eg, anaphylaxis) to any influenza vaccine is generally a contraindication to future receipt of influenza vaccines, children who have had a severe allergic reaction after influenza vaccination should be evaluated by an allergist to help identify the vaccine component responsible for the reaction and to determine whether future vaccine receipt is appropriate. Children who are allergic to gelatin (very rare) should receive IIV (or RIV if age appropriate) instead of LAIV. Overlap between gelatin and alpha-gal allergy has been reported.[19]
3. Children with egg allergy can receive any influenza vaccine without any additional precautions beyond those recommended for all vaccines.
4. Children with acute moderate or severe illness may receive influenza vaccine as soon as their acute illness has improved; strategies to promote timely receipt once recovered from illness should be employed (ie, schedule return visit; send reminder message; if hospitalized, administer prior to discharge from hospital setting); children with mild illness, including a low-grade fever, should still be vaccinated.

INFLUENZA TESTING

Influenza Testing Recommendations Are Informed by Setting and Anticipated Impact on Clinical Management

1. Influenza testing should be performed in children with signs and symptoms of influenza when test results are anticipated to impact clinical management (eg, to inform the decision to initiate antiviral or avoid antibiotic therapy, pursue other diagnostic testing, initiate infection prevention and control measures, or distinguish from other respiratory viruses with similar symptoms). Testing for avian influenza or other novel strains should be performed at the direction of public health authorities.[20] Clinicians should consider asking about exposures to sick or dead animals, particularly wild birds, poultry, or dairy cows, to inform the need for testing for avian influenza.
2. When influenza is circulating in the community, hospitalized patients with signs and symptoms of influenza should be tested with a nucleic acid amplification test with high sensitivity and specificity (eg, reverse transcriptase-polymerase chain reaction [RT-PCR]).
3. At-home tests are available for children as young as 2 years of age (https://www.fda.gov/medical-devices/in-vitro-diagnostics/influenza-diagnostic-tests), but data on the use of these tests in pediatric patients is limited. The use of at-home test results to inform treatment decisions should be informed by the sensitivity and specificity of the test, the prevalence of influenza in the community, the presence and duration of compatible signs and symptoms, and individual risk factors and comorbidities.

INFLUENZA TREATMENT

Antiviral medications (Table 6) are an important adjunct in the control of influenza but are not a substitute for influenza vaccination. The role of antivirals for the prevention and treatment of influenza in children depends on illness severity and risk considerations (Table 7). Options for antiviral medications along with potential benefits and harms of antiviral treatment are summarized in the technical report [https://doi.org/10.1542/peds.2025-073622]; see section "Rationale for Influenza Treatment in Children").[10] Although best results are observed when the child is treated within 48 hours of symptom onset, antiviral therapy should still be considered beyond 48 hours in certain cases.

1. Physicians and other clinicians who care for children should promptly identify patients suspected of having influenza for timely initiation of antiviral treatment, when indicated, to reduce morbidity and mortality. Treatment of children who are not at high risk for influenza complications in the outpatient setting should be based on shared decision making between the clinician and child's parent/guardian.
2. Provision of antiviral therapy does not require a positive test for influenza when influenza is circulating in the community. Initiation of antiviral therapy should be based on signs and symptoms consistent with influenza infection, patient risk factors, and epidemiologic factors (eg, influenza circulating in the community, known exposure, etc).
3. The AAP considers oseltamivir the preferred antiviral medication for patients with influenza A and B because of the cumulative experience of this drug in children, relative cost, and ease of administration. Clinicians should refer to the CDC (https://www.cdc.gov/flu/hcp/antivirals/summary-clinicians.html#cdc_generic_section_9-influenza-antiviral-resistance-considerations; recommendations for the use of oseltamivir differ from FDA-approved labeling) for the most up-to-date information on antiviral susceptibilities.

Recommendations for Treatment and Chemoprophylaxis of Specific Populations

4. Antiviral treatment should be offered as early as possible to the following individuals, regardless of influenza vaccination status and duration of symptoms[1]:
   - Any child hospitalized with suspected or confirmed influenza disease.
   - Any child with severe, complicated, or progressive influenza disease, regardless of health care setting (ie, inpatient or outpatient).

TABLE 6. Recommended Dosage and Schedule of Influenza Antiviral Medications for Treatment and Chemoprophylaxis in Children for the 2025–2026 Influenza Season: United States

Medication	Treatment		Chemoprophylaxis		Common Adverse Events[a]
	Dosage	Duration	Dosage	Duration After Last Exposure	
Oseltamivir[b,c]					
Adults	75 mg, twice daily, orally or by feeding tube	5 d	75 mg, once daily	7 d	
Children ≥12 mo					
≤15 kg	30 mg, twice daily, orally or by feeding tube	5 d	30 mg, once daily	7 d	Nausea Vomiting Headache
>15 kg–23 kg	45 mg, twice daily, orally or by feeding tube	5 d	45 mg, once daily	7 d	
>23 kg–40 kg	60 mg, twice daily, orally or by feeding tube	5 d	60 mg, once daily	7 d	
>40 kg	75 mg, twice daily, orally or by feeding tube	5 d	75 mg, once daily	7 d	
Infants 9–11 mo[d]	3.5 mg/kg per dose, twice daily, orally or by feeding tube	5 d	3.5 mg/kg per dose, once daily	7 d	Skin reactions Diarrhea (children <1 y of age)
Term infants 0–8 mo[d]	3 mg/kg per dose, twice daily, orally or by feeding tube	5 d	3–8 mo: 3 mg/kg per dose, once daily	7 d	
Preterm infants[e]					
<38 weeks' PMA	1 mg/kg per dose, twice daily, orally or by feeding tube	5 d	See footnote		
38–40 weeks' PMA	1.5 mg/kg per dose, twice daily, orally or by feeding tube	5 d			
>40 weeks' PMA	3 mg/kg per dose, twice daily, orally or by feeding tube	5 d			
Zanamivir[c,f]					
Adults	10 mg (two 5-mg inhalations), twice daily	5 d	10 mg (two 5-mg inhalations), once daily	7 d[c]	Bronchospasm Skin reactions Sinusitis Dizziness
Children	≥7 y: 10 mg (two 5-mg inhalations), twice daily	5 d	≥5 y: 10 mg (two 5-mg inhalations), once daily	7 d[b]	
Peramivir[g]					
Adults	One 600-mg dose via intravenous infusion, given over 15–30 min	N/A	Not recommended		Diarrhea Skin reactions
Children 6 mos–12 y	One 12-mg/kg dose (600 mg maximum) via intravenous infusion over 15–30 min	N/A	Not recommended		
13–17 y	One 600-mg dose, via intravenous infusion over 15–30 min	N/A	Not recommended		
Baloxavir[h]					
Individuals ≥5 y					
<20 kg	One 2-mg/kg dose, orally or by feeding tube	N/A	2 mg/kg as single dose, orally	N/A	Adverse events reported in clinical trials, including nausea, vomiting, and diarrhea, similar to placebo
20 kg–<80 kg	One 40-mg dose, orally or by feeding tube	N/A	One 40-mg dose	N/A	
≥80 kg	One 80-mg dose, orally or by feeding tube	N/A	One 80-mg dose, orally	N/A	

[a] Although only common adverse events are listed in this table, hypersensitivity reactions, including anaphylaxis, have been reported postmarketing with oseltamivir and baloxavir. Hypersensitivity reactions have also been reported with peramivir and zanamivir.

[b] Oseltamivir is administered orally or by feeding tube without regard to meals, although administration with meals may improve gastrointestinal tolerability. Oseltamivir is available as a generic drug or as Tamiflu in 30-mg, 45-mg, and 75-mg capsules and as a powder for oral suspension that is reconstituted to provide a final concentration of 6 mg/mL. For the 6-mg/mL suspension, a 30-mg dose is given with 5 mL of oral suspension, a 45-mg dose is given with 7.5 mL oral suspension, a 60-mg dose is given with 10 mL oral suspension, and a 75-mg dose is given with 12.5 mL oral suspension. If the commercially manufactured oral suspension is not available, a suspension can be compounded by retail pharmacies (final concentration also 6 mg/mL), based on instructions contained in the package label. For infants younger than 1 year, an appropriate measuring device such as a 3-mL or 5-mL oral syringe should be used to measure the dose instead of the syringe supplied.

In patients with renal insufficiency, the dose should be adjusted on the basis of creatinine clearance. Renal dosing of oseltamivir is not available in the package insert for pediatric patients. However, the package insert instructions may useful for children who qualify for adult doses based on weight >40 kg. For treatment of patients with creatinine clearance 10–30 mL/min: 75 mg, once daily, for 5 days. For chemoprophylaxis of patients with creatinine clearance 10–30 mL/min: 30 mg, once daily, for 10 days after exposure or 75 mg, once every other day, for 10 days after exposure (5 doses).

(Continued on next page)

TABLE 6. Recommended Dosage and Schedule of Influenza Antiviral Medications for Treatment and Chemoprophylaxis in Children for the 2025–2026 Influenza Season: United States (Continued)

[c] The Centers for Disease Control and Prevention (CDC) recommends routine chemoprophylaxis with oseltamivir or zanamivir for 7 days after last known exposure; minimum of 14 days and continuing for 7 days after last known exposure if part of institutional outbreak (https://www.cdc.gov/flu/hcp/antivirals/summary-clinicians.html). This differs from the package insert for zanamivir, which recommends prophylaxis for 10 days in community settings and 28 days in community outbreaks (https://www.accessdata.fda.gov/drugsatfda_docs/label/2010/021036s025lbl.pdf).

[d] Approved by the US Food and Drug Administration (FDA) for treatment of children as young as 2 weeks of age. Given preliminary pharmacokinetic data and limited safety data, oseltamivir can be used to treat influenza in both term and preterm infants from birth because benefits of therapy are likely to outweigh possible risks of treatment. Oseltamivir is not FDA-approved for postexposure prophylaxis (PEP) in children younger than 1 year. Oseltamivir is not recommended by the American Academy of Pediatrics (AAP) or CDC for chemoprophylaxis of infants <3 months because of limited safety and efficacy data in this age group. Of note, the dose recommended by the AAP for treatment of infants 9 to 11 months of age is higher than the FDA approved dose of 3.0 mg/kg, twice daily and is based on data that indicated that the higher dose was needed to achieve the protocol-defined targeted exposure for infants in this age group as defined in the National Institute of Allergy and Infectious Diseases Collaborative Antiviral Study Group 114 study.[27] The CDC recommends a dose of 3.0 mg/kg, twice daily, for all infants <12 months; the IDSA guidelines[26] include both AAP and CDC recommendations.

[e] Oseltamivir dosing for preterm infants. The weight-based dosing recommendation for preterm infants is lower than for term infants.[28–30] Preterm infants may have lower clearance of oseltamivir because of immature renal function, and doses recommended for full-term infants may lead to very high drug concentrations in this age group. Limited data from the National Institute of Allergy and Infectious Diseases Collaborative Antiviral Study Group provide the basis for dosing preterm infants using their postmenstrual age (PMA) (gestational age + chronologic age). For extremely preterm infants (<28 weeks), please consult a pediatric infectious disease physician. PEP is not generally recommended for preterm infants because of limited data on use in these infants unless PEP is determined to be essential for outbreak control based on clinician judgment. Optimal dosing has not been defined in this circumstance.

[f] Zanamivir is administered by inhalation using a proprietary "Diskhaler" device distributed together with the medication. Zanamivir is a dry powder, not an aerosol, and should not be administered using nebulizers, ventilators, or other devices typically used for administering medications in aerosolized solutions. Zanamivir is not recommended for people with chronic respiratory diseases, such as asthma or chronic obstructive pulmonary disease, which increase the risk of bronchospasm.

[g] Peramivir requires dose adjustment in patients with renal insufficiency. For treatment of pediatric patients 6 months to 12 years of age: 2 mg/kg if creatinine clearance is 10–29 mL/min; 4 mg/kg if creatinine clearance is 30 to 49 mL/min. For treatment of adolescents 13 years and older, 100 mg if creatinine is clearance 10–29 mL/min; 200 mg if creatinine clearance is 30 to 49 mL/min (https://www.accessdata.fda.gov/drugsatfda_docs/label/2017/206426s004lbl.pdf).

[h] Oral baloxavir marboxil is approved by the FDA for treatment of acute uncomplicated influenza within 2 days of illness onset. It should not be administered with dairy products, calcium-fortified beverages, polyvalent cation-containing laxatives, antacids, or oral supplements (eg, calcium, iron, magnesium, selenium, or zinc). Baloxavir marboxil is not recommended as monotherapy for treatment of influenza in individuals who are severely immunocompromised. It is not recommended for persons who are pregnant or breastfeeding.

Sources: IDSA[26] and https://www.cdc.gov/flu/hcp/antivirals/summary-clinicians.html?CDC_AAref_Val=https://www.cdc.gov/flu/professionals/antivirals/summary-clinicians.htm.

- Any child with suspected or confirmed influenza disease of any severity if they are younger than 5 years or they belong to other high-risk groups for influenza complications, regardless of health care setting (ie, inpatient or outpatient) (Table 2).

5. Treatment is an option for the following individuals in the outpatient setting:
   - Any child with suspected or confirmed influenza disease who is not at high risk for influenza complications, if treatment can be initiated within 48 hours of illness onset.
   - Any child with suspected or confirmed influenza disease whose siblings or household contacts are either younger than 6 months or at high risk for influenza complications (Table 2).

INFLUENZA CHEMOPROPHYLAXIS RECOMMENDATIONS

1. Chemoprophylaxis is not a substitute for vaccination, and among some high-risk people, both vaccination with IIV or RIV and antiviral chemoprophylaxis is an option.
2. The AAP considers oseltamivir to be the preferred postexposure chemoprophylaxis for influenza A and/or B.
3. Postexposure chemoprophylaxis should only be used when antiviral agents can be initiated within 48 hours of exposure.
4. Postexposure chemoprophylaxis should not be used for routine or widespread prophylaxis outside of institutional outbreaks. Postexposure chemoprophylaxis is recommended for unvaccinated staff and unvaccinated children in a closed institutional setting with children at high risk for influenza complications (eg, extended-care facilities) to control influenza outbreaks.
5. Postexposure chemoprophylaxis can be considered after known or suspected influenza exposure for children in the following situations:
   - Any child at high risk for influenza complications if:
     - They cannot receive the influenza vaccine.
     - They have not yet been administered influenza vaccination this season.
     - They received influenza vaccine in the past 2 weeks or may not have mounted a sufficient response because of immunosuppression (ie, suboptimal immunity).
     - Influenza virus strains circulating in the community are not well-matched with those of the seasonal influenza vaccine.
   - Any unvaccinated child with a family member or close contact who is at high risk for influenza complications and is unable to be otherwise effectively protected from influenza.
6. Postexposure chemoprophylaxis can be considered for known or suspected influenza exposed family members or close contacts of children at high risk for influenza complication in the following situations:
   - Unvaccinated family members and close contacts who are likely to have ongoing, close exposure to unvaccinated children at high risk for influenza complications or unvaccinated children who are younger than 24 months.

TABLE 7. Summary of Antiviral Treatment and Chemoprophylaxis Recommendations

Applicable Subpopulation	Who Would Receive Antiviral Medications	Time Since Symptoms or Exposure	Medication Plan
Hospitalized children	Child with symptoms and known or suspected infection[a]	No time limit on starting although treatment should ideally be started as soon as possible after symptom onset	Recommend treatment
Children with severe illness	Child with symptoms and known or suspected infection[a]	No time limit on starting	Recommend treatment
Children with complicated illness	Child with symptoms and known or suspected infection[a]	No time limit on starting	Recommend treatment
Children with progressive illness	Child with symptoms and known or suspected infection[a]	No time limit on starting	Recommend treatment
Children at higher risk for complications (<5 y of age or with underlying condition [Table 2])	Child with symptoms and known or suspected infection[a]	No time limit on starting	Recommend treatment
Children with household contacts at high risk	Child with symptoms and known or suspected infection[a]	No time limit on starting	Consider treatment
Children with household contacts under age 6 mos	Child with symptoms and known or suspected infection[a]	No time limit on starting	Consider treatment
Other children with flu-like symptoms	Child with symptoms and known or suspected infection[a]	Within 48 h of symptoms starting	Consider treatment
Unvaccinated or incompletely vaccinated children at high risk of complications	Asymptomatic child with known or suspected exposure	Within 48 h of exposure	Consider chemoprophylaxis
Vaccinated children at high risk of complications who may have not mounted an immune response	Asymptomatic child with known or suspected exposure	Within 48 h of exposure	Consider chemoprophylaxis
Vaccinated children at high risk of complications when vaccination strain does not match or is ineffective against circulating strains	Asymptomatic child with known or suspected exposure	Within 48 h of exposure	Consider chemoprophylaxis
Unvaccinated children with a family member or close contact who is at high risk for influenza complications and is unable to be otherwise effectively protected from influenza	Asymptomatic child with known or suspected exposure	Within 48 h of exposure	Consider chemoprophylaxis
Unvaccinated family members and close contacts of unvaccinated children at high risk of complications or unvaccinated children under 24 mos old	Asymptomatic close contact with known or suspected exposure	Within 48 h of exposure	Consider chemoprophylaxis
Family members and close contacts of children at high risk of complications when vaccination strain does not match or is ineffective against circulating strains	Asymptomatic close contact with known or suspected exposure	Within 48 h of exposure	Consider chemoprophylaxis

[a] Once testing results are available, treatment could be tailored accordingly.

- Influenza virus strains circulating in the community are not well matched with those of the seasonal influenza vaccine, per the CDC.

COMMITTEE ON INFECTIOUS DISEASES, 2024–2025

Sean T. O'Leary, MD, MPH, FAAP, Chairperson
James D. Campbell, MD, MS, FAAP, Vice Chairperson
Monica I. Ardura, DO, MSCS, FAAP
Kristina A. Bryant, MD, FAAP, *Red Book Online* Team Lead
Mary T. Caserta, MD, FAAP
Claudia Espinosa, MD, MSc, FAAP
Robert W. Frenck, Jr, MD, FAAP
C. Mary Healy, MD
Chandy C. John, MD, MS, FAAP
Aaron M. Milstone, MD, MHS, FAAP
Angela L. Myers, MD, MPH, FAAP
Pia Pannaraj, MD, MPH, FAAP
Adam J. Ratner, MD, MPH, FAAP, *Red Book* Associate Editor
José R. Romero, MD, FAAP
Matthew Zahn, MD, FAAP

CONTRIBUTORS

Kristina A. Bryant, MD, FAAP
Annika M. Hofstetter, MD, PhD, MPH, FAAP

PARTNERSHIP FOR POLICY IMPLEMENTATION

Juan D. Chaparro, MD, MS, FAAP
Jeremy J. Michel, MD, MHS, FAAP

EX OFFICIO

David W. Kimberlin, MD, FAAP, *Red Book* Editor
Ritu Banerjee, MD, PhD, FAAP, *Red Book* Associate Editor
Elizabeth D. Barnett MD, FAAP, *Red Book* Associate Editor
Ruth Lynfield, MD, FAAP, *Red Book* Associate Editor

LIAISONS

Amina Ahmed, MD, FAAP, American Thoracic Society
Michelle Barton, MD, Canadian Paediatric Society
Lisa M. Kafer, MD, FAAP, AAP Committee on Practice and Ambulatory Medicine
Denee J. Moore, MD, American Academy of Family Physicians
Jennifer L. Thompson, MD, American College of Obstetricians and Gynecologists
Juan P. Torres, MD, PhD, Sociedad Latinoamericana de Infectología Pediátrica
Charles R. Woods, Jr, MD, MS, FAAP, Pediatric Infectious Diseases Society

STAFF

Gillian Gibbs, MPH

ACKNOWLEDGMENTS

The Committee on Infectious Diseases gratefully acknowledges Kristina A. Bryant, MD, FAAP, and Annika M. Hofstetter, MD, PhD, MPH, FAAP, for their leadership in drafting the policy statement and technical report, and Juan D. Chaparro, MD, MS, FAAP, and Jeremy J. Michel, MD, MHS, FAAP, for their significant contributions in providing input on the initial drafts on behalf of the AAP Partnership for Policy Implementation.

ABBREVIATIONS

AAP: American Academy of Pediatrics
FDA: US Food and Drug Administration
ccIIV: cell culture-based inactivated (non-live) influenza vaccine
ccIIV3: trivalent cell culture-based inactivated (non-live) influenza vaccine
IIV: inactivated (non-live) influenza vaccine
IIV3: trivalent inactivated (non-live) influenza vaccine
LAIV: live attenuated influenza vaccine
LAIV3: trivalent live attenuated influenza vaccine
RIV: recombinant influenza vaccine
RIV3: trivalent recombinant influenza vaccine
WHO: World Health Organization

All policy statements from the American Academy of Pediatrics automatically expire 5 years after publication unless reaffirmed, revised, or retired at or before that time.

Embedded links to cdc.gov and fda.gov sites were active and reviewed by AAP subject matter experts as of July 5, 2025.

https://doi.org/10.1542/peds.2025-073620

COMPANION PAPER: A companion to this article can be found online at www.pediatrics.org/cgi/doi/10.1542/peds.2025-073622.

REFERENCES

1. Grohskopf LA, Ferdinands JM, Blanton LH, Broder KR, Loehr J. Prevention and control of seasonal influenza with vaccines: recommendations of the Advisory Committee on Immunization Practices–United States, 2024–25 influenza season. *MMWR Recomm Rep.* 2024;73(RR-5):1–25. doi: 10.15585/mmwr.rr7305a1
2. White EB, O'Halloran A, Sundaresan D, et al. High influenza incidence and disease severity among children and adolescents aged <18 years—United States, 2022–23 season. *MMWR Morb Mortal Wkly Rep.* 2023;72(41):1108–1114. PubMed doi: 10.15585/mmwr.mm7241a2
3. Hauge SH, de Blasio BF, Håberg SE, Oakley L. Influenza hospitalizations during childhood in children born preterm. *Influenza Other Respir Viruses.* 2022;16(2):247–254. PubMed doi: 10.1111/irv.12908
4. Neuzil KM, Hohlbein C, Zhu Y. Illness among schoolchildren during influenza season: effect on school absenteeism, parental absenteeism from work, and secondary illness in families. *Arch Pediatr Adolesc Med.* 2002;156(10):986–991. PubMed doi: 10.1001/archpedi.156.10.986
5. Shope TR, Walker BH, Aird LD, Southward L, McCown JS, Martin JM. Pandemic influenza preparedness among child care center

directors in 2008 and 2016. *Pediatrics.* 2017;139(6):e20163690. PubMed doi: 10.1542/peds.2016-3690

6. Petrie JG, Ohmit SE, Cowling BJ, et al. Influenza transmission in a cohort of households with children: 2010–2011. *PLoS One.* 2013; 8(9):e75339. PubMed doi: 10.1371/journal.pone.0075339
7. Loeb M, Russell ML, Moss L, et al. Effect of influenza vaccination of children on infection rates in Hutterite communities: a randomized trial. *JAMA.* 2010;303(10):943–950. PubMed doi: 10.1001/jama.2010.250
8. Pannaraj PS, Wang HL, Rivas H, et al. School-located influenza vaccination decreases laboratory-confirmed influenza and improves school attendance. *Clin Infect Dis.* 2014;59(3):325–332. PubMed doi: 10.1093/cid/ciu340
9. Centers for Disease Control and Prevention. Weekly Flu Vaccination Dashboard: Influenza Vaccination Coverage, Children 6 months through 17 years, United States. Accessed August 3, 2025. https://www.cdc.gov/fluvaxview/dashboard/children-vaccination-coverage.html
10. American Academy of Pediatrics, Committee on Infectious Diseases. Recommendations for prevention and control of influenza in children, 2025–2026: Technical report. *Pediatrics.* 2025; 156(4):e2025073622. doi: 10.1542/peds.2025-073622
11. US Food and Drug Administration. Flublok package insert. Accessed March 25, 2025. https://www.fda.gov/media/179778/download
12. O'Halloran AC, Holstein R, Cummings C, et al. Rates of influenza-associated hospitalization, intensive care unit admission, and in-hospital death by race and ethnicity in the United States from 2009 to 2019. *JAMA Netw Open.* 2021;4(8):e2121880. PubMed doi: 10.1001/jamanetworkopen.2021.21880
13. World Health Organization. Recommendations announced for influenza vaccine composition for the 2025–2026 northern hemisphere influenza season. Accessed March 25, 2025. https://www.who.int/news/item/28-02-2025-recommendations-announced-for-influenza-vaccine-composition-for-the-2025-2026-northern-hemisphere-influenza-season
14. US Food and Drug Administration. Influenza Vaccine Composition for the 2025–2026 U.S. Influenza Season. Accessed March 25, 2025. https://www.fda.gov/vaccines-blood-biologics/influenza-vaccine-composition-2025-2026-us-influenza-season
15. Schuster JE, Hamdan L, Dulek DE, et al; Pediatric HCT Flu Study Group. Influenza vaccine in pediatric recipients of hematopoietic-cell transplants. *N Engl J Med.* 2023;388(4):374–376. PubMed doi: 10.1056/NEJMc2210825
16. Schuster JE, Hamdan L, Dulek DE, et al; Pediatric HCT Flu Study. Pediatric HCT Flu Study. The durability of antibody responses of two doses of high-dose relative to two doses of standard-dose inactivated influenza vaccine in pediatric hematopoietic cell transplant recipients: a multi-center randomized controlled trial. *Clin Infect Dis.* 2024;78(1):217–226. PubMed doi: 10.1093/cid/ciad534
17. Lessin HR, Edwards KM; American Academy of Pediatrics, Committee on Practice and Ambulatory Medicine, Committee on Infectious Diseases. Immunizing parents and other close family contacts in the pediatric office setting. *Pediatrics.* 2012; 129(1):e247–e253. PubMed doi: 10.1542/peds.2011-2937
18. US Food and Drug Administration. Vaccines licensed for use in the United States. Accessed May 25, 2025. https://www.fda.gov/vaccines-blood-biologics/vaccines/vaccines-licensed-use-united-states
19. Moschese V, Montin D, Ottaviano G, et al; within the Italian Society of Pediatric Allergology and Immunology (SIAIP) Vaccine Committee. Vaccines and allergy: Back to the right places. *Pediatr Allergy Immunol.* 2024;35(9):e14236. PubMed doi: 10.1111/pai.14236
20. Centers for Disease Control and Prevention. Avian Influenza (Bird Flu). Laboratory and Testing Information for Novel Influenza A Viruses. Accessed May 25, 2025. https://www.cdc.gov/bird-flu/php/severe-potential/index.html
21. Homaira N, Briggs N, Oei JL, et al. Impact of influenza on hospitalization rates in children with a range of chronic lung diseases. *Influenza Other Respir Viruses.* 2019;13(3):233–239. PubMed doi: 10.1111/irv.12633
22. Schütte A, Ciesek S, Wedemeyer H, Lange CM. Influenza virus infection as precipitating event of acute-on-chronic liver failure. *J Hepatol.* 2019;70(4):797–799. PubMed doi: 10.1016/j.jhep.2018.11.015
23. Premkumar M, Devurgowda D, Dudha S, et al. A/H1N1/09 influenza is associated with high mortality in liver cirrhosis. *J Clin Exp Hepatol.* 2019;9(2):162–170. PubMed doi: 10.1016/j.jceh.2018.04.006
24. Hampl SE, Hassink SG, Skinner AC, et al. Clinical practice guideline for the evaluation and treatment of children and adolescents with obesity. *Pediatrics.* 2023;151(2):e2022060640. PubMed doi: 10.1542/peds.2022-060640
25. Vitoratou D-I, Milas G-P, Korovessi P, Kostaridou S, Koletsi P. Obesity as a risk factor for severe influenza infection in children and adolescents: a systematic review and meta-analysis. *Eur J Pediatr.* 2023;182(1):363–374. PubMed doi: 10.1007/s00431-022-04689-0
26. Uyeki TM, Bernstein HH, Bradley JS, et al. Clinical practice guidelines by the Infectious Diseases Society of America (IDSA): 2018 Update diagnosis, treatment, chemoprophylaxis and institutional outbreak management of seasonal influenza. *Clin Infect Dis.* 2019; 68(6):e1–e47. PubMed doi: 10.1093/cid/ciy866
27. Kimberlin DW, Acosta EP, Prichard MN, et al; National Institute of Allergy and Infectious Diseases Collaborative Antiviral Study Group. Oseltamivir pharmacokinetics, dosing, and resistance among children aged <2 years with influenza. *J Infect Dis.* 2013;207(5):709–720. PubMed doi: 10.1093/infdis/jis765
28. Pannaraj PS, Tam B, Akan D. Oseltamivir treatment and prophylaxis in a neonatal intensive care unit during a 2009 H1N1 influenza outbreak. *J Perinatol.* 2011;31(7):487–493. PubMed doi: 10.1038/jp.2010.159
29. Acosta EP, Jester P, Gal P, et al; National Institute of Allergy and Infectious Diseases Collaborative Antiviral Study Group. Oseltamivir dosing for influenza infection in premature neonates. *J Infect Dis.* 2010;202(4):563–566. PubMed doi: 10.1086/654930
30. McPherson C, Warner B, Hunstad DA, Elward A, Acosta EP. Oseltamivir dosing in premature infants. *J Infect Dis.* 2012; 206(6):847–850. PubMed doi: 10.1093/infdis/jis471

Recommendations for Prevention and Control of Influenza in Children, 2025–2026 (Technical Report)

- *Technical Report*
  - *PPI: AAP Partnership for Policy Implementation See Appendix 1 for more information.*

American Academy of Pediatrics
DEDICATED TO THE HEALTH OF ALL CHILDREN®

AAP Partnership for Policy Implementation

TECHNICAL REPORT

American Academy of Pediatrics

DEDICATED TO THE HEALTH OF ALL CHILDREN™

Recommendations for Prevention and Control of Influenza in Children, 2025–2026: Technical Report

Committee on Infectious Diseases

abstract

This technical report accompanies the recommendations of the American Academy of Pediatrics for the routine use of influenza vaccine and antiviral medications in the prevention and treatment of influenza in children during the 2025–2026 influenza season. The rationale for the American Academy of Pediatrics recommendation for annual influenza vaccination of all children without medical contraindications starting at 6 months of age is provided. Influenza vaccination is an important strategy for protecting children and the broader community against influenza. This technical report summarizes recent influenza seasons, morbidity and mortality in children, vaccine effectiveness, and vaccination coverage and provides detailed guidance on vaccine storage, administration, and implementation. The report also provides a brief background on inactivated (non-live) and live attenuated influenza vaccines, available vaccines for the 2025–2026 influenza season, vaccination during pregnancy and breastfeeding, diagnostic testing for influenza, and antiviral medications for treatment and chemoprophylaxis. Strategies to promote vaccine uptake are emphasized.

CONFLICT OF INTEREST DISCLOSURE: Dr Bryant has no disclosed conflicts related to the content of this statement. Dr Bryant has disclosed completed or ongoing research relationships with Gilead, Pfizer, Sanofi, and Enanta that were reviewed and determined not relevant to influenza. Dr Bryant receives honoraria from WebMed, a stipend from the American Society of Nephrology, and royalties from Oxford University Press. Committee on Infectious Diseases members who disclosed relevant conflicts did not participate in the development of this statement.

FUNDING: No external funding.

To cite: American Academy of Pediatrics, Committee on Infectious Diseases. Recommendations for Prevention and Control of Influenza in Children, 2025–2026: Technical Report. *Pediatrics*. 2025;156(6):e2025073622

INTRODUCTION

This technical report accompanies the recommendations of the American Academy of Pediatrics (AAP) for the routine use of influenza vaccine and antiviral medications in the prevention and treatment of influenza in children during the 2025–2026 season.[1]

SUMMARY OF RECENT INFLUENZA ACTIVITY IN THE UNITED STATES

Recent influenza seasons in the US have varied by severity, duration, and impact on children's health (Table 1). Influenza vaccine effectiveness has

TABLE 1. Summary of Recent Influenza Seasons

	2020–2021	2021–2022	2022–2023[a]	2023–2024[b]
Severity	Low	Low	Moderate with high severity in children	Moderately severe
Duration	—	—	—	—
Predominant Viruses	Influenza A(H3N2) Influenza B (Victoria)	Influenza A(H3N2)	Influenza A(H3N2)	A(H1N1)pdm09
Vaccination Coverage in Children	58.2%	57.8%	55.1%	53.8
Hospitalization Rate	0.8/100 000 overall rate	32.1/100 000 (0–4 y) 14.1/100 000 (5–17 y)	112/100 000 (0–4 y) 42.1/100 000 (5–17 y)	86.1/100 000 (0–4 y) 34.3/100 000 (5–17 y)
Characteristics of Hospitalized Children	• Not available because of low case numbers	54.1% had ≥1 underlying condition[c] • Asthma 28.% • Neurologic disorder 16.9% • Obesity 13.3%	51.9% had ≥1 underlying condition[c] • Asthma 27.6% • Neurologic disorder 15.7% • Obesity 14.4%	54.6% had ≥1 underlying condition[c] • Asthma 24.5% • Neurologic disorder 18.7% • Obesity 16.1%
Pediatric Deaths[d]	1	49 • 39.1% without underlying condition • Bacterial co-infection in 53.8%	187 • 53.4% without underlying condition • Bacterial coinfection in 51.4%	207 • 51% without underlying condition • Bacterial co-infection in 48% • 17.2% of vaccine-eligible children fully vaccinated[e]
Notable Findings	• Low severity season likely because of COVID-19 mitigation measures reducing spread of all respiratory illnesses • 1 reported case of novel influenza A(H1N2) in the US	• Influenza activity began to increase in November, declined in January 2022, increased again in March 2022 and remained elevated until mid-June 2022 • Higher number of hospitalizations in the second wave • 13 human infections with novel influenza A virus identified, including 1 case of avian influenza A(H5) virus (first in a human in the US)	• Influenza activity began in October (earlier than prior seasons)[f] • Low proportion of children vaccinated at onset of season • High pediatric hospitalization rates, especially in the southeast • Co-circulation of SARS-CoV2 and RSV	• Influenza activity began to increase in early November and peaked in late December 2023, similar to pre-pandemic pattern of circulation • A(H3N2) and B/Victoria virus activity increased at end of season 21 novel influenza A virus infections identified, including 14 avian influenza A(H5) virus (all cases in adults) and 7 variant viruses (3 in children <18 y)

—, not reported.

[a] Centers for Disease Control and Prevention. Preliminary estimated influenza illnesses, medical visits, hospitalizations, and deaths in the United States—2022–2023 Influenza Season. Accessed June 1, 2025. Available at: https://www.cdc.gov/flu-burden/php/data-vis/2022-2023.html

[b] Centers for Disease Control and Prevention. Influenza Activity in the United States during the 2023–2024 Season and Composition of the 2024–2025 Influenza Vaccine. Accessed March 30, 2025. https://www.cdc.gov/flu/whats-new/flu-summary-2023-2024.html

[c] Data abstracted from: https://www.cdc.gov/flu-burden/php/data-vis/2022-2023.html; Accessed June 1, 2025.

[d] Data abstracted from: https://gis.cdc.gov/GRASP/Fluview/PedFluDeath.html. Accessed June 1, 2025.

[e] Based on interim analysis of 197 deaths and 157 children and adolescents eligible for influenza vaccination (age ≥6 months at date of illness onset) and for whom vaccination status was known.

[f] White EB, O'Halloran A, Sundaresan D, et al. High influenza incidence and disease severity among children and adolescents aged <18 years—United States, 2022–23 season. *MMWR Morb Mortal Wkly Rep.* 2023;72(41):1108–1114.

likewise varied by year, influenza type and influenza A virus subtype, and age group of the child immunized (Figure 1 and https://www.cdc.gov/flu-vaccines-work/php/effectiveness-studies/index.html).

2024–2025 Influenza Season

According to the Centers for Disease Control and Prevention (CDC), the 2024–2025 influenza season was a high-severity season for persons of all ages, including children, in terms of outpatient medical visits, hospitalizations, and death.[2] This was the first high-severity season since 2017–2018. Nationally, between October 1, 2024, and May 17, 2025, the CDC estimated the burden of influenza in individuals of all ages to include 47 to 82 million illnesses, 21 to 37 million influenza-related medical visits, and 610 000 to 1 300 000 influenza-and influenza-related hospitalizations (https://www.cdc.gov/flu-burden/php/data-vis/2024-2025.html). The proportion of outpatient visits for influenza-like illness was highest in children 0 to 4 years of age, peaking at 18% in February 2025. Through August 2, 2025, hospitalization rates in children were highest among those <1 year of age (149.4/100 000), similar to rates in persons 50 to 64 years of age (https://gis.cdc.gov/GRASP/Fluview/FluHospRates.html). Cumulative hospitalization rates for influenza among children were higher than observed in the 2023–2024 season (100.8/100 000 vs 84.3/100 000 in patients 0 to 4 years of age; rates were similar in children 5–17 years of age (39.3/100 000 vs 39.9/100 000). In a sample of hospitalized children reported to the Influenza Hospital Surveillance Network (FluSurv-NET), 54% had at least 1 underlying medical condition. As in prior years, the most common underlying condition observed in hospitalized children was asthma (26.2%; https://gis.cdc.gov/grasp/fluview/FluHospChars.html. Other common underlying conditions in hospitalized children included neurologic disease (17.5%) and obesity (13.2%).

Through July 5, 2025, 260-related pediatric deaths were reported by the CDC[2] (Figure 2). Of these, 43.6% occurred in children without a high-risk medical condition. Among children who were eligible for influenza vaccination and with known vaccine status, 90% of reported pediatric deaths have occurred in children who were not fully vaccinated against influenza.

Through June 21, 2025, more than 89% of the influenza viruses identified were influenza A, with similar proportions of H1N1pdm09 (52.8% of isolates with subtyping performed) and H3N2 (47.1%). In an interim analysis posted by the CDC on May 23, 2025, of the subset of virus characterized, most influenza A(H1N1)pdm09 viruses (99.5%) and influenza B/Victoria viruses (96.2%) were antigenically similar to viruses contained in seasonal influenza

Influenza Type/ Age Group	2019–2020 B/Victoria and A(H1N1)pdm09 VE% (95% CI)	2021–2022 A(H3N2) VE% (95% CI)	2022–2023 A(H3N2) VE% (95% CI)	2023–2024 A(H3N2)[c] VE% (95% CI)
Influenza A and B				
Overall all ages	39 (32, 44)	36 (21, 48)[†]	49 (36, 60)[†]	67 (48, 80)
6 mo–8 y	34 (19, 46)	Not reported	Not reported	
9–17 y	40 (22, 53)	Not reported	Not reported	
Influenza A(H1N1)pdm09				
Overall all ages	30 (21, 39)	Not reported	56 (28, 72)	61 (26, 81)
6 mo–8 y	23 (-3, 42)	Not reported		
9–17 y	29 (-7, 52)	Not reported		
Influenza A(H3N2)				
Overall all ages	Not reported	36 (20, 49)	45 (29, 58)	Not reported
6 mo–8 y	Not reported	51 (19, 70)		
9–17 y	Not reported	34 (-7, 59)		
Influenza B Victoria				
Overall all ages	45 (37, 52)	Not reported	Not reported	Not reported
6 mo–8 y	39 (20, 54)	Not reported	Not reported	89 (70, 97)
9–17 y	43 (23, 58)	Not reported	Not reported	Not reported

FIGURE 1.

Adjusted Vaccine Effectiveness (VE)[a] in Children in the United States, by Season, as Reported by the Centers for Disease Control and Prevention (CDC), US Influenza Vaccine Effectiveness Network.[b]

[a]VE is estimated as 100% x (1 – odds ratio [ratio of odds of being vaccinated among outpatients with CDC's real-time RT-PCR influenza-positive test results to the odds of being vaccinated among outpatients with influenza-negative test results]); odds ratios were estimated using logistic regression. Adjusted for study site, age group, sex, race/ethnicity, self-rated general health, number of days from illness onset to enrollment, and month of illness using logistic regression.**VE 0–30 %** **>30%–50%** **>50%**

[b]VE could not be assessed for 2020–2021 season because of low virus circulation. However, the A(H1N1)pdm09, A(H3N2), and B/Victoria strains that were genetically characterized were similar to the strains included in the vaccine.

[c] Interim VE estimates.[268]

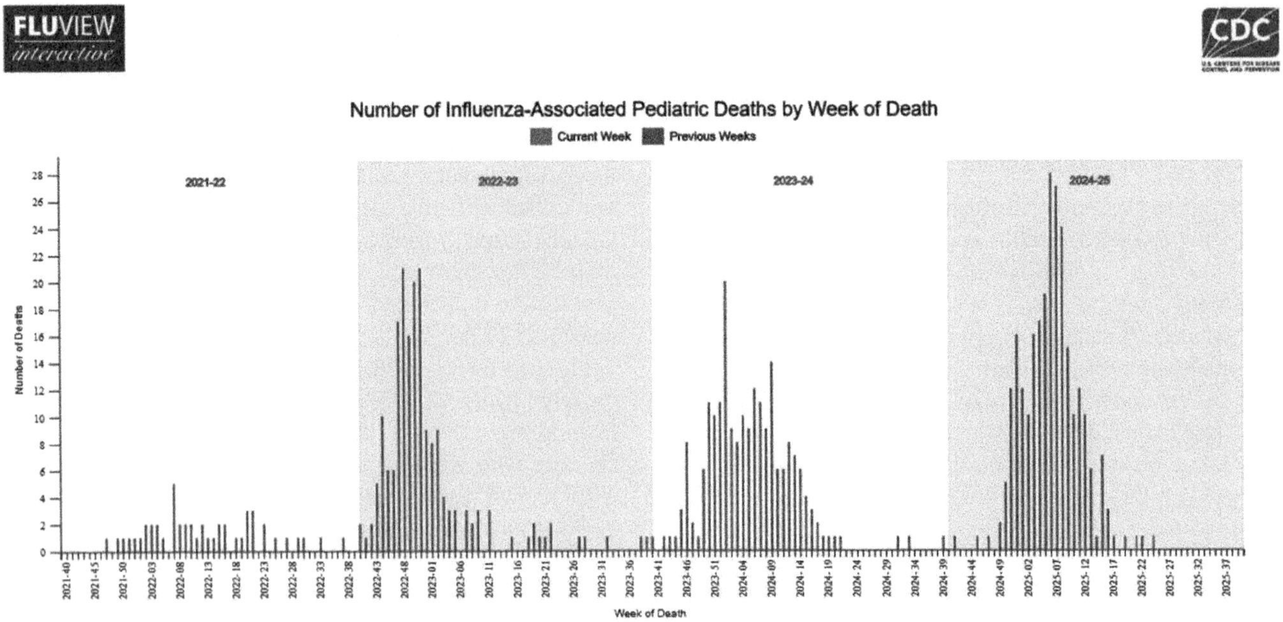

Seasons	Total Deaths	Deaths reported During the Week Ending 05 Jul 2025
2021-22	49	0
2022-23	187	0
2023-24	207	0
2024-25	260	4

FIGURE 2.
Influenza-Associated Pediatric Deaths by Season. From: https://gis.cdc.gov/GRASP/Fluview/PedFluDeath.html. Accessed July 16, 2025.

vaccines compared with 58.6% of influenza A(H3N2) viruses (https://www.cdc.gov/fluview/surveillance/2025-week-20.html). In an interim analysis of vaccine effectiveness (VE) during the 2024–2025 season, VE against any influenza-associated acute respiratory tract infection for children 6 months through 17 years of age ranged from 32% to 60% in outpatient settings; VE was 63% to 78% against influenza-associated hospitalization.[3] Effectiveness against influenza A varied by subtype and surveillance network. In the New Vaccine Surveillance Network (NVSN), VE in outpatient settings was 72% against influenza A(H1N1)pdm09 and 42% against H3N2. In the US Influenza Vaccine Effectiveness Network, VE in outpatient settings was 53% against influenza A(H1N1)pdm09 but was not statistically significant against H3N2 (16%; 95% CI −34% to 49%). VE against influenza hospitalization measured in the NVSN was 63% against influenza A(H1N1)pdm09 and 55% against H3N2.

Highly pathogenic avian influenza (HPAI) A(H5N1) continues to circulate among wild birds in the US, with sporadic outbreaks in poultry, backyard flocks, and dairy cattle. Sporadic cases occur in mammals, including cats. Human cases remain rare. As July 1, 2025, 70 human cases had been reported in the US, and most were in adults with exposure to dairy cattle (n = 41) or poultry farms and culling operations (n = 24). In November 2024, the first reported case of H5N1 infection in a child in the US was reported in California; the child experienced mild illness and recovered.[4] A second infected child in California was reported in January of 2025 and was unrelated to the first. The child had fever and conjunctivitis and recovered.[5] The source of infection has not been determined for either child. A severe case of H5N1 was identified in an adolescent with underlying medical conditions in British Columbia, Canada.[6] The adolescent required mechanical ventilation and extracorporeal membrane oxygenation support but ultimately recovered. The virus recovered from the patient was closely related to viruses detected in wild birds in the region. Fatal pediatric cases have also been reported in 2025 from Mexico, Cambodia, and India; Vietnam reported a severe H5N1 avian flu infection in an 8-year-old girl diagnosed with encephalitis.[7] The CDC provides H5N1 situation updates at https://www.cdc.gov/bird-flu/situation-summary/index.html.

Information about influenza surveillance is available through the CDC Voice Information System (1-800-232-4636) and is posted weekly on the CDC website (www.cdc.gov/flu/index.htm).

INFLUENZA MORBIDITY AND MORTALITY IN CHILDREN

In a typical influenza season, the disease burden among children is substantial. Each year, an estimated 8% to 10% of US children develop symptomatic influenza virus infection, although even higher proportions are observed in some seasons.[8,9] Children infected with influenza virus are more likely to exhibit symptoms than adults. In 2 community-based prospective cohort studies conducted in Managua, Nicaragua, influenza was asymptomatic in just 6.6% of infected children ≤14 years of age, although the asymptomatic fraction increased with age (1.7%, 3.5%, and 9.1% for ages 0–1, 2–4, and 5–14 years, respectively; $P < .001$).[10]

Common clinical syndromes associated with seasonal influenza virus infection include a nonspecific febrile illness with or without upper respiratory symptoms, bronchiolitis, croup, or a pertussis-like illness. Gastrointestinal symptoms, including vomiting, diarrhea, and abdominal pain, are frequently seen in young children.[11] Ocular manifestations, including conjunctivitis, occur uncommonly.[12]

A variety of complications have been reported with influenza virus infection, including myocarditis, pericarditis, myositis, and rhabdomyolysis.[13] Neurologic complications of influenza include febrile seizures, nonfebrile seizures, ataxia, encephalitis, and encephalopathy. In a cohort of children <5 years of age enrolled in 1 state Medicaid program, neurologic complications were uncommon but higher in children younger than 2 years and those with underlying neurologic conditions.[14] Approximately 8% to 11% of children hospitalized with influenza experience neurologic complications, and these are more frequent in children with underlying neurologic conditions and children who are unimmunized.[15,16]

In January 2025, the CDC received anecdotal reports of critical illness and death in children with acute necrotizing encephalopathy (ANE).[17] ANE is a severe form of influenza-associated encephalopathy or encephalitis (IAE) characterized by rapid neurologic deterioration and bilateral symmetric lesions usually affecting the thalami; lesions can also be seen in periventricular white matter, internal capsules, putamina, temporal lobes, upper brainstem tegmentum, or cerebellum.[18] In response to these reports, the Influenza-Associated Pediatric Mortality Surveillance System was queried to assess the frequency of IAE. Of the 1840 pediatric influenza-associated deaths reported by state health departments to CDC using this system during the 2010–2011 through 2024–2025 influenza seasons, 166 (9%) had IAE, ranging from 0% (2020–21 season) to 14% (2011–12 season). IAE prevalence was highest among children aged 2 to 4 years (34 [10%] of 334 total fatal cases), and more than half (89; 54%) had no underlying medical condition. Through February 8, 2025, of the 2024–2025 influenza season, 9 pediatric influenza-associated deaths in children with IAE were reported to the CDC, 4 cases of which were ANE. Case ascertainment is ongoing. Because no dedicated national surveillance for IAE or ANE exists, it is unknown whether the numbers of cases this season vary from expected numbers.

Bacterial complications of influenza virus infection include otitis media, pneumonia, sinusitis, and bloodstream infections. Among children <16 years of age hospitalized with laboratory-confirmed influenza at 12 Canadian hospitals, bloodstream infections occurred in 0.9% and were associated with intensive care unit admission, need for mechanical ventilation, and longer lengths of stay.[19] *Staphylococcus aureus* and *Streptococcus pneumoniae* were the most common pathogens. Viral infections, including influenza, have previously been identified as risk factors for invasive bacterial infections, including invasive group A streptococcal infections.[20,21] According to the CDC, from 2016 to 2022, increases in invasive group A streptococcal infections coincided with seasonal peaks in respiratory syncytial virus (RSV) and influenza hospitalization rates during most years except 2021.

As many as 10% of all pediatric hospitalizations during the winter are attributable to influenza.[22,23] Hospitalization rates of children with influenza are highest in those younger than 5 years; rates are typically the highest among infants <6 months of age and decrease with increasing age.[8,24] Over 12 influenza seasons in the US following the 2009 H1N1 pandemic, laboratory-confirmed influenza-associated hospitalization rates in children 0 to 4 years ranged from 16 (2011–2012; 95% CI [14.2–17.9]) to 91.4 (2019–2020; 95% CI [86.9–96.0]) per 100 000 children.[25] Influenza-associated hospitalization rates in children 5 to 17 years ranged from 4 (2011–2012; 95%CI [3.5–4.6]) to 30.3 (2022–2023; 95% CI [28.7–31.8]) per 100 000 children. Hospitalization rates were not reported for 2020–2021, a year in which there was not substantial circulation of influenza viruses.

The highest influenza-associated hospitalization rates are caused by influenza A virus infection. Some data suggest that influenza subtype influences disease severity and the risk of hospitalization. Across seasons, the greatest proportion of influenza-associated hospitalizations in children are attributable to influenza A(H3N2).[25] However, in 1 large, prospective, multicenter study conducted between 2015 and 2020 in children who were hospitalized or seen in the emergency department, children with influenza A (H1N1)pdm09 had more severe disease, with increased incidence of hospitalization, compared to those with influenza A(H3N2) and B.[26]

Morbidity in children hospitalized with influenza is substantial, as demonstrated by population-based surveillance for influenza-associated hospitalizations conducted by the Influenza Hospitalization Surveillance Network (FluSurv-NET).[27] In the 2017–2018 through 2019–2020 seasons, 6774 children 0 through 17 years of age were hospitalized with influenza; 17.8% had pneumonia, 21.6% required admission to the intensive care unit (ICU), and 5.3% were mechanically ventilated.

Children hospitalized with influenza are commonly treated with antibiotics for suspected bacterial infections, and many children receive antibiotics inappropriately.[28] In 1 active surveillance study of pediatric influenza hospitalizations in Canada over 11 seasons, 71.6% (6424/8971) received an antibiotic, including 53% of those without an appropriate indication.

Postdischarge respiratory sequelae occur in children hospitalized with critical respiratory illness attributable to influenza. In 1 study (n = 165), 78% of children with preexisting asthma experienced asthma symptoms in the 90 days after discharge, and 13% required readmission to the hospital.[29] Among patients without preexisting asthma, 11.1% had asthma newly diagnosed (n = 10).

During 12 of 13 recent influenza seasons, influenza-associated deaths in children have ranged from 37 in the 2011–2012 season to 207 in the 2023–2024 season (a single pediatric death was reported during the 2020–2021 season, coincident with very low circulation of seasonal influenza viruses) (https://gis.cdc.gov/GRASP/Fluview/PedFluDeath.html).[30,31] According to the CDC, pediatric influenza deaths are likely underreported, as not all children whose death was related to influenza virus infection may have had viral testing.[32] Statistical models predict that during the 2023–2024 influenza season, for example, as many as 724 children could have died from the flu compared with the 207 reported (https://www.cdc.gov/flu/whats-new/flu-summary-addendum-2023-2024.html).

HIGH-RISK GROUPS IN PEDIATRICS

Children younger than 5 years (especially those younger than 2 years) and children of any age with certain underlying medical conditions have a high risk of complications from influenza (see Table 2 in the policy statement [https://doi.org/10.1542/peds.2025-073620]). These medical conditions include obesity, a condition that affects more than 14 million children and adolescents in the US.[33] In a recent systematic review and meta-analysis, obesity increased the odds of hospitalization in children with influenza, although the definition of obesity varied among included studies.[34] Additionally, in children hospitalized for influenza, obesity was associated with a worse prognosis, including ICU admission and death.

Influenza vaccination is particularly important in these high-risk groups (see Table 2 in the policy statement) and populations disproportionately affected by severe influenza outcomes. Health disparities are apparent in both

TABLE 2. Adjusted Influenza Vaccine Effectiveness (VE) Against Influenza Hospitalization[a]

Author/Setting	Seasons Included	Population Studied	N	Adjusted VE Partially Vaccinated[b] (95% CI)	Adjusted VE Fully Vaccinated (95% CI)
Feldstein/US New Vaccine Surveillance Network	2015–2016	6 mo to 17 y	1653	18% (−44, 54)	56% (34, 71)
Israel/Segaloff	2015–2016 2016–2017 2017–2018	6 mo to 8 y	3147	25.6% (−3.0, 47.0)	53.9% (38.6, 68.3)
Australia/Blyth	2018	≤16 y	458	NR	86.1% (76.3, 91.9)
United Kingdom/Pebody	2018–2019	2 to 17 y	986	NR	53.0% (33.3, 66.8) • A(H1N1): 63.5% (34.4, 79.7) • A(H3N2): 31.1% (53.9, 69.2)
Systematic Review/Kalligeros	2005–2019	6 mo to 17 y	NR	33.91(21.12, 46.69)	61.79 (54.45, 69.13)
Japan/Shinjoh	2018–2019	6 mo to 15 y	205	NR	56% (16, 77)[c]
Atlanta, Georgia/Yildirim	2012–2013 2013–2014 2014–2015 2016–2016 2016–2017	6 mo to 17 y	980	46.8% (23.8, 62.8)	55.3% (31.7, 70.7)
Hong Kong/Cowling	2023	9 mo to 17 y	1671	NR	69.6% (49.3%, 81.7%)

Abbreviation: NR, not reported.
[a] Laboratory-confirmed influenza hospitalization.
[b] Included only patients 6 months to 8 years.
[c] Included patients with full and partial vaccination.

influenza diagnosis as well as influenza morbidity and mortality.[35]

In 1 test-negative case-control study conducted in an urban population of children <14 years of age, public or self-pay insurance was associated with increased risk of an influenza diagnosis.[36] In a retrospective cohort study using the National Inpatient Sample from January 1, 2008, to December 31, 2017, Hispanic (adjusted odds ratio [aOR], 1.25; 95% CI, 1.17 to 1.33), non-Hispanic-Black (aOR, 1.21; 95% CI, 1.17 to 1.33) and non-Hispanic other children (aOR, 1.11; 95% CI, 1.04 to 1.19) were more likely to be hospitalized with an influenza diagnosis than non-Hispanic white children, although mortality was similar.[37] In a cross-sectional study that included 10 influenza seasons, higher rates of severe influenza disease were reported in Black, Hispanic, American Indian/Alaska Native, and Asian/Pacific Islander people compared with white people, and differences were pronounced in children ≤4 years of age.[38] In this age group, hospitalization rates were higher in Black children (relative risk [RR], 2.21; 95% CI, 2.10 to 2.33), Hispanic children (RR, 1.87; 95% CI, 1.77 to 1.97), American Indian/Alaska Native children (RR, 3.00; 95% CI, 2.55 to 3.53), and Asian/Pacific Islander children (RR, 1.26; 95% CI, 1.16 to 1.38) compared with white children. Rates of ICU admission were also higher (Black children: RR, 2.74; 95% CI, 2.43 to 3.09; Hispanic children: RR, 1.96; 95% CI, 1.73 to 2.23; American Indian/Alaska Native children: RR, 3.51; 95% CI, 2.45 to 5.05). The rate of in-hospital death was 3-fold to 4-fold higher in Black, Hispanic, and Asian/Pacific Islander children compared with white children.

Disparities have also been noted in subpopulations of children with high-risk medical conditions. In pediatric solid organ transplant recipients, for example, the risk of an influenza-associated hospital encounter was higher in non-Hispanic Black patients (adjusted subdistribution hazard ratio [aSHR], 1.63; 95% CI, 1.28 to 2.07; $P < .001$) and Hispanic patients (aSHR, 1.57; 95% CI, 1.27 to 1.94; $P < .001$) compared with non-Hispanic white patients.[39] Importantly, factors associated with disparities observed with other respiratory viruses (eg, SARS-CoV-2 and RSV),[40,41] including lack of access to quality health care, crowded living conditions, and social vulnerability, were not evaluated in these studies.

Additional research is needed to understand how social drivers of health impact influenza-associated hospitalization, but 1 study that utilized hospitalization data collected by FluSERV-NET during the 2010–2011 and 2011–2012 seasons found increasing rates of influenza-related hospitalization with increasing census tract poverty.[42] This association was found in all ages and racial/ethnic groups. Additional strategies are needed to understand and address disparities in influenza-associated morbidity, including social needs screening/assessment to identify high-risk populations and increase their access to quality health care.

Although protecting all children against influenza through timely vaccination remains critically important, increased efforts are needed to eliminate barriers to immunization in all people experiencing higher rates of complications from infection with influenza viruses.

EFFECTIVENESS OF INFLUENZA VACCINATION ON MORTALITY, HOSPITALIZATION, LABORATORY-CONFIRMED INFLUENZA ILLNESS IN AMBULATORY CHILDREN, AND ANTIBIOTIC USE

Although influenza vaccination does not prevent all cases of influenza, it does offer substantial health benefits, including protection against severe and life-threatening disease and reduced health resources utilization.[43]

Mortality

Historically, up to 80% of influenza-associated pediatric deaths have occurred in unvaccinated or incompletely vaccinated children.[44] Influenza vaccination is associated with reduced risk of laboratory-confirmed influenza-related pediatric death.[45] In 1 case-cohort analysis of laboratory-confirmed influenza-associated pediatric deaths in the US from 2010 to 2014, overall VE against influenza-associated death in all children was 65% (95% CI, 54% to 74%) and 51% (95% CI, 31% to 67%) in children with underlying conditions.[45] Similarly, in a case-control study conducted over 2 influenza seasons (2010 to 2012), influenza vaccination was associated with a three-quarters reduction in the risk of life-threatening influenza illness in children.[46] During the 2023–2024 season, influenza vaccination prevented an estimated 266 deaths in children 6 months through 17 years of age (https://www.cdc.gov/flu-burden/php/data-vis-vac/2023-2024-prevented.html).[47]

Hospitalization

A robust body of evidence supports the effectiveness of influenza vaccination in preventing hospitalization in children, even during seasons in which overall VE is lower (Table 2).[48–60] According to a systematic review, VE is the highest in children younger than 5 years.[52] During the 2023–2024 season, the CDC estimates that influenza vaccination prevented 19 946 hospitalizations in children 6 months through 17 years of age (https://www.cdc.gov/flu-burden/php/data-vis-vac/2023-2024-prevented.html).[47]

Laboratory-Confirmed Influenza Illness and Medically Attended Influenza Illness in Ambulatory Settings

In an analysis of US Influenza Vaccine Effectiveness Network data that included 9 seasons (from 2011–2012 through 2019–2020), pooled VE against outpatient influenza illness was 46% (95% CI, 43 to 50).[61] VE was lowest against influenza A(H3N2)-associated illness (33%

[95% CI, 27 to 39]), and estimates were similar for influenza B (54% [95% CI, 49 to 59]) and influenza A(H1N1)pdm09 (57% [95% CI: 51 to 62]). VE was highest for children 6 through 59 months of age compared with older children. During the 2023–2024 season, the CDC estimates that influenza vaccination prevented 3 098 105 symptomatic flu-related illnesses and 1 611 014 medical visits in children 5 through 17 years of age, a group in whom adjusted VE was 52% (95% CI, 51.8 to 52.2) (https://www.cdc.gov/flu-burden/php/data-vis-vac/2023-2024-prevented.html). In children 6 months through 4 years of age, adjusted VE was higher (65% [95% CI, 64.7 to 65.3]), resulting in an estimated 1 422 807 symptomatic flu-related illnesses and 953 281 medical visits prevented.

Antibiotic Use in Ambulatory Children

Antibiotics are prescribed for an estimated 11% to 43% of patients of all ages in whom influenza is diagnosed,[62–64] and not all prescribing is appropriate. Patients are prescribed antibiotics with and without recognized bacterial complications of influenza, including pneumonia, otitis media, and sinusitis.[65] In 1 population-based retrospective cohort study spanning 2012 to 2017, the antibiotic prescription rate in ambulatory children declined by 3/1000 person-months for each 1% increase in influenza vaccination coverage.[66]

Household and Community Transmission

Influenza vaccination of children may reduce influenza virus transmission in the home and in the community. In a prospective case-ascertained household transmission cohort study that enrolled patients over 3 consecutive influenza seasons (2017 to 2020), influenza VE for preventing secondary infections among household contacts was 21% (95% CI, 1.4% to 36.7%) and varied by influenza type.[67]

Increasing vaccination rates in schools may protect unvaccinated students. In 1 prospective cohort study that evaluated school-located vaccination programs on laboratory-confirmed influenza and absenteeism, vaccination of nearly 50% of a school's enrollees conferred 54% indirect protection to unvaccinated children.[68]

SEASONAL INFLUENZA VACCINES

The seasonal influenza vaccines licensed for children and adolescents for the 2025–2026 season are described in Table 4 of the policy statement. All 2025–2026 seasonal influenza vaccines for use in the US are trivalent and contain hemagglutinin derived from the same influenza strains as recommended by the World Health Organization (WHO) and the US Food and Drug Administration (FDA) for the Northern Hemisphere (see Table 1 in the policy statement [https://doi.org/10.1542/peds.2025-073620]).[69,70] The influenza A(H3N2) component is different this season compared with last season, whereas the influenza A (H1N) and influenza B Victoria lineage components are unchanged. Different but antigenically related influenza A strains are included in this season's egg-based and cell-based or recombinant vaccines. However, they are still matched to the strains expected to circulate in the 2025–2026 season.

Inactivated Influenza Vaccine (IIV)

For the 2025–2026 season, among inactivated influenza vaccines available for children, 4 are egg-based (seed strains grown in eggs), and 1 is cell culture-based (seed strains grown in Madin-Darby canine kidney cells) (see Table 4 in policy statement [https://doi.org/10.1542/peds.2025-073620]). All inactivated egg-based vaccines (Afluria, Fluarix, FluLaval, and Fluzone) and 1 cell culture-based based vaccine (Flucelvax) are licensed for children 6 months and older, and all are available in single-dose, thimerosal-free, prefilled syringes.[71]

A trivalent recombinant baculovirus-expressed hemagglutinin (HA) influenza vaccine (RIV3 [Flublok]) was originally licensed only for people 18 years and older, but on March 31, 2025, the FDA approved the use of use of this vaccine in individuals as young as 9 years of age.[72] In 1 randomized controlled trial that enrolled 159 children 9 to 17 years of age, the safety and immunogenicity of RIV4 was similar to the comparator IIV.[73]

A trivalent high-dose inactivated (non-live) influenza vaccine (HD-IIV3 [Fluzone High Dose) and a trivalent MF-59 adjuvanted inactivated vaccine (aIIV3 [Fluad]) are licensed for people 65 years and older. Adjuvanted seasonal influenza vaccines are not licensed for children in the US; however, studies of adjuvanted vaccines in children have been performed, and evaluation is ongoing.[74–77]

Children 6 months and older can receive any licensed, age-appropriate inactivated (non-live) influenza vaccine (IIV). Trivalent egg-based and cell culture-based IIVs contain 15 μg HA from each strain in 0.5-mL. The recommended dose volume (and, therefore, the recommended antigen content) for younger children varies by product. The dose of Fluarix, FluLaval, and Flucelvax is 0.5-mL for all children 6 months and older.[78] Children 6 through 35 months of age can receive a 0.25-mL or 0.5-mL dose of Fluzone from a multidose vial; 0.5-mL prefilled syringes are also available.[79] These 2 doses demonstrated comparable safety and immunogenicity in a single, randomized multicenter study.[80] Children 3 years and older should receive 0.5 mL. Afluria is supplied in 0.5-mL single-dose syringes. The dose of Afluria is 0.5 mL for children 3 years and older and 0.25 mL for children 6 through 35 months of age.[81]

The dose of RIV3 for children 9 years and older is also 0.5 mL. Each dose is 135 μg HA per 0.5 mL (45 μg HA from each influenza virus strain) and is available in prefilled syringes.

IIV Storage

The CDC has published best practice guidelines (https://www.cdc.gov/vaccines/hcp/imz-best-practices/ and https://www.cdc.gov/vaccines/hcp/storage-handling/) for vaccine storage and administration. Additionally, the AAP offers guidance on the components of a written disaster plan, including a comprehensive vaccine management protocol to keep the vaccine storage temperature constant during a power failure or other disaster (see the AAP Pediatric Preparedness Resource Kit at https://downloads.aap.org/AAP/PDF/PedPreparednessKit.pdf).

IIVs for intramuscular injection are shipped and stored at 2 °C to 8 °C (36 °F to 46 °F); vaccines that are inadvertently frozen should not be used.

IIV Administration

Vaccines are administered intramuscularly into the anterolateral thigh of infants and young children and into the deltoid muscle of older children and adults. Given that various IIV formulations are available, careful attention should be paid to ensure that each product is used according to its approved age indication, dosing, and volume of administration (see Table 4 in policy statement [https://doi.org/10.1542/peds.2025-073620]).

For vaccines that include a multidose vial option, the maximum number of doses drawn from a multidose vial is specified in the package insert and should not be exceeded; residual product must be discarded regardless of the remaining volume in the vial. A 0.5-mL prefilled syringe of any IIV should not be split into 2 separate 0.25-mL doses. If a prefilled syringe of Fluzone is used for a child younger than 36 months, the dose volume will be 0.5 mL per dose. If a child is inadvertently vaccinated with a formulation only approved for older children or adults, the dose is counted as valid. If a lower dose than recommended is inadvertently administered to a child 36 months or older (eg, 0.25 mL), an additional 0.25-mL dose is to be administered to provide a full dose of 0.5 mL as soon as possible.

COADMINISTRATION OF INACTIVATED INFLUENZA VACCINE AND OTHER IMMUNIZATIONS

In general, all vaccines indicated on a given day can be administered. Influenza vaccine can also be administered concomitantly or any time before or after currently available COVID-19 vaccines.[82–85] Overall, the benefits of timely vaccination with same-day administration of IIV and other recommended vaccines outweigh the risk of potential reactogenicity in children. Influenza vaccine can also be administered to children concomitantly or at any time before or after administration of nirsevimab or clesrovimab.

Neither the CDC nor AAP define the maximum volumes that can be injected into each muscle group in different age groups (https://www.aap.org/en/patient-care/respiratory-syncytial-virus-rsv-prevention/nirsevimab-frequently-asked-questions/). Separating injection sites by 1 inch or more, if possible, is a recommended practice.

Safety of IIV and RIV

IIVs are well tolerated in children and can be used in healthy children as well as those with underlying chronic medical conditions. The most common injection site adverse reactions following administration of IIV in children are pain (17%–67%), redness (13%–37%), and swelling (10%–25%). The most commonly reported systemic adverse events are drowsiness (13%–38%), irritability (14%–54%), abnormal crying (33%–41%), loss of appetite (11%–32%), fatigue (10%–20%), muscle aches (10%–39%), headache (10%–23%), arthralgia (10%–13%), and gastrointestinal tract symptoms (10%–20%). Fever can occur, especially in children 6 through 35 months of age, but is uncommon. RIV is also well-tolerated. In 1 clinical trial enrolling children 9 through 17 years of age, the most common solicited injection-site adverse reaction was pain (34.4%). The most common solicited systemic adverse reaction was myalgia (19.3%), followed by headache (18.5%) and malaise (16.1).[72] Package inserts for US-licensed vaccines are available on the FDA website.[78]

The AAP continues to support the current WHO recommendations for use of thimerosal as a preservative in multiuse vials in the global vaccine supply.[86] Thimerosal-containing vaccines are not associated with an increased risk of autism spectrum disorder in children.[87,88] Thimerosal from vaccines has not been linked to any neurologic condition. Despite the lack of evidence of harm, some states have legislation restricting the use of vaccines that contain even trace amounts of thimerosal and in June 2025, the Advisory Committee on Immunization Practices (ACIP) recommended that children and adults only receive influenza vaccine in single-dose formulations that are free of thimerosal as a preservative.[89] The benefits of protecting children against the known risks of influenza are clear. Therefore, to the extent permitted by state law, children should receive any available formulation of IIV rather than delaying vaccination while waiting for reduced-thimerosal content or thimerosal-free vaccines. IIV formulations that are free of even trace amounts of thimerosal are widely available, as described in the policy statement. Additional information to assist clinicians in responding to parental concerns about thimerosal is available from the Children's Hospital of Philadelphia Vaccine Education Center (https://www.chop.edu/sites/default/files/vaccine-education-center-thimerosal.pdf).

Vaccination in the Setting of Immunosuppression

Non-live vaccines, including IIVs, are safe in persons with altered immune competence, but immunogenicity may be diminished. Decreases in immunogenicity vary by

TABLE 3. Value Sets for Underlying Conditions of High-Risk Groups for Influenza Complications

Category	Description	Established Value Sets	Object Identifier (OID)	Code System	Steward
Underlying Condition or Treatment with Common Examples[a]					
Chronic Pulmonary Disease	Asthma	Asthma Diagnosis ICD-10 Asthma Diagnosis Grouping	2.16.840.1.113762.1.4.1047.308 2.16.840.1.113762.1.4.1047.309	ICD10CM ICD10CM ICD9CM SNOMEDCT	American Academy of Allergy Asthma and Immunology American Academy of Allergy Asthma and Immunology
	Cystic fibrosis	Cystic Fibrosis Cystic Fibrosis Lung Disease	2.16.840.1.113883.3.464.1003.102.12.1002 2.16.840.1.113762.1.4.1219.15	ICD10CM ICD9CM SNOMEDCT ICD10CM SNOMEDCT	National Committee for Quality Assurance CMS Documentation Requirement Lookup Service
	Compromised respiratory function (eg, requiring mechanical ventilation, tracheostomy or baseline oxygen requirement)	Mechanical Ventilation	2.16.840.1.113762.1.4.1248.107	ICD10PCS SNOMEDCT	American Institutes for Research
Cardiovascular Disease	Hemodynamically significant conditions (excluding hypertension alone)	No Existing Value Set			
Kidney Disease	Dialysis Chronic kidney disease, including end-stage kidney disease	Dialysis Services	2.16.840.1.113883.3.464.1003.109.11.1026	CPT	National Committee for Quality Assurance
Hepatic Disease	Chronic liver disease Cirrhosis	Chronic Liver Disease Cirrhosis	2.16.840.1.113883.3.464.1003.199.12.1035 2.16.840.1.113762.1.4.1248.149	ICD10CM ICD9CM SNOMEDCT ICD10CM SNOMEDCT	National Committee for Quality Assurance American Institutes for Research
Hematologic Disease	Sickle cell disease	Sickle Cell Anemia and HB S Disease	2.16.840.1.113762.1.4.1235.222	ICD10CM SNOMEDCT	B.well Connected Health
	Other hemoglobinopathies	No Existing Value Set			
Metabolic Disorders	Diabetes mellitus	Diabetes	2.16.840.1.113883.3.464.1003.103.12.1001	ICD10CM SNOMEDCT	National Committee for Quality Assurance
Neurologic and Neurodevelopmental Conditions	Cerebral palsy	Congenital or Infantile Cerebral Palsy Group	2.16.840.1.113883.3.666.5.1580	ICD10CM ICD9CM SNOMEDCT	Lantana
	Epilepsy	Epilepsy Seizure Disorder	2.16.840.1.113762.1.4.1034.51 2.16.840.1.113883.3.464.1003.105.12.1206	ICD10CM ICD9CM SNOMEDCT ICD10CM ICD9CM SNOMEDCT	American Academy of Neurology National Committee for Quality Assurance
	Stroke	Stroke	2.16.840.1.113762.1.4.1248.176	ICD10CM	American Institutes for Research
	Intellectual developmental disorder	No Existing Value Set			

(Continued on next page)

TABLE 3. Value Sets for Underlying Conditions of High-Risk Groups for Influenza Complications (Continued)

Category	Description	Established Value Sets	Object Identifier (OID)	Code System	Steward
	Moderate to severe developmental delay	No Existing Value Set			
	Muscular dystrophy	No Existing Value Set			
	Spinal cord injury	Spinal Cord Injury	2.16.840.1.113883.3.7587.3.1009	ICD10CM ICD9CM SNOMEDCT	American Academy of Physical Medicine and Rehabilitation
Extreme Obesity	BMI ≥40 for adults[b]	No Existing Value Set			
Immunosuppression	Receipt of immunocompromising medications	No Existing Value Set			
	Congenital or acquired immune deficiency, including HIV	Immunodeficiency Syndromes HIV	2.16.840.1.113762.1.4.1200.189 2.16.840.1.113883.3.464.1003.120.12.1003	ICD10CM ICD10CM ICD9CM SNOMEDCT	Cliniwiz National Committee for Quality Assurance
	Asplenia	Anatomic or Functional Asplenia_HD_CN_Grouping	2.16.840.1.113762.1.4.1235.219	ICD10CM ICD9CM SNOMEDCT	B.well Connected Health
Receiving Treatment with Aspirin or Salicylate-Containing Therapies[c]		No Existing Value Set			
Pregnancy and Up to 2 Weeks Postpartum		No Existing Value Set			

The sets provided are previously published value sets available at the Value Set Authority Center (a service of the National Library of Medicine) and can be accessed at https://vsac.nlm.nih.org. These sets are provided by the relevant steward listed and are not endorsed by the AAP but may serve as a starting point for organizations creating electronic clinical decision support systems.

[a] List of examples is not exhaustive.

[b] Not well-defined in children but could consider BMI ≥95% for age.

[c] Applies to children and adolescents <19 years who may be at increased risk of Reye syndrome.

Source: Grohskopf LA, Ferdinands JM, Blanton LH, Broder KR, Loehr J. Prevention and control of seasonal influenza with vaccines: recommendations of the Advisory Committee on Immunization Practices—United States, 2024–25 influenza season. *MMWR Recomm Rep*. 2024;73(RR-5):1–25.

TABLE 4. Comparison of Types of Influenza Diagnostic Tests

Testing Category[a]	Method	Influenza Viruses Detected	Distinguishes Influenza A Virus Subtypes	Typical Time to Results	Performance
Rapid molecular assay	Nucleic acid amplification	Influenza A or B viral RNA	No	15–30 min	High sensitivity; high specificity
Rapid influenza diagnostic test	Antigen detection	Influenza A or B virus antigens	No	10–15 min	Moderate sensitivity (higher with analyzer reader device; high specificity
Direct and indirect immunofluorescence assays	Antigen detection	Influenza A or B virus antigens	No	2–4 h	Moderate sensitivity; high specificity
Molecular assays (including RT-PCR)	Nucleic acid amplification	Influenza A or B viral RNA	Yes, if subtype primers are used	1–8 h	Very high sensitivity; very high specificity
Multiplex molecular assays	Nucleic acid amplification	Influenza A or B viral RNA, other viral or bacterial targets (RNA or DNA)	Yes, if subtype primers are used	1–2 h	High sensitivity; high specificity
Rapid cell culture (shell vial and cell mixtures)	Virus isolation	Influenza A or B virus	Yes	1–3 d	High sensitivity; high specificity
Viral culture (tissue cell culture)	Virus isolation	Influenza A or B virus	Yes	3–10 d	High sensitivity; high specificity

[a] Negative results may not rule out influenza. Respiratory tract specimens should be collected as close to illness onset as possible for testing. Clinicians should consult the manufacturer's package insert for the specific test for the approved respiratory specimen(s). Specificities are generally high (>90%) for all tests compared with reverse transcriptase-polymerase chain reaction (RT-PCR). Sensitivities of rapid influenza diagnostic tests vary by test and are lower compared with RT-PCR and viral culture. The typical sensitivity of a rapid test performed in a physician's office is 50% to 70%, and clinicians may wish to confirm negative test results with molecular assays, especially during peak community influenza activity. Some FDA-cleared rapid influenza diagnostic tests are CLIA-waived; most FDA-cleared rapid influenza molecular assays are CLIA-waived, depending on the complexity.

Sources: Uyeki[209] and https://www.cdc.gov/flu/php/laboratories/table-testing-methods.html.

underlying condition. Guidelines for the immunization of immunocompromised children and adults have been published by the Infectious Diseases Society of America and the CDC.[90,91] Guidelines for the immunization of solid organ transplant recipients have been published by the American Society of Transplantation.[92] The CDC has published additional recommendations for influenza immunization of adult solid organ transplant recipients.[71] In June 2024, the CDC ACIP recommended high-dose inactivated (HD-IIV3) and adjuvanted inactivated (aIIV3) influenza vaccines as acceptable options for influenza vaccination of solid organ transplant recipients aged 18 through 64 years who are on immunosuppressive medication regimens, without a preference over other age-appropriate IIV3s or RIV3. Studies in pediatric solid organ transplant recipients are ongoing.

Live Attenuated (Intranasal) Influenza Vaccine

Overview

The history of live attenuated influenza vaccine (LAIV) use in the US, along with a detailed discussion of VE over serial seasons, is available in the 2021 technical report.[93] For the 2025–2026 season, trivalent live attenuated influenza vaccine (LAIV3) has replaced quadrivalent live attenuated influenza vaccine (LAIV4).

Storage and Administration

The cold-adapted, temperature-sensitive LAIV3 formulation is shipped and stored at 2 °C to 8 °C (36 °F to 46 °F). LAIV3 is administered intranasally in a prefilled, single-use sprayer containing 0.2-mL of vaccine. A removable dose-divider clip is attached to the sprayer to facilitate administration of 0.1-mL separately into each nostril. If the child sneezes immediately after administration, the dose should not be repeated. Administration of LAIV intranasally is not an aerosol-generating procedure; however, vaccine administrators are advised to wear gloves when administering LAIV given the potential for contact with respiratory secretions.

Coadministration of LAIV and Other Vaccines

LAIV may be administered simultaneously with other inactivated or live vaccines. If not administered simultaneously, it is recommended that administration of injectable live vaccines is separated by a 4-week interval from LAIV vaccination. Oral typhoid vaccine can be administered simultaneously with or at any interval before or after LAIV.[94]

In addition to LAIV administration in traditional settings, in September 2024, the FDA approved an application from Astra Zeneca to allow eligible adult patients to self-administer LAIV; caregivers will be allowed to administer the vaccine to eligible children 2 years and older.[95] To access LAIV for home administration, the guardian completes an online application for each eligible household member. A health care professional at a centralized pharmacy reviews the application for eligibility; if approved, LAIV is mailed to the patient's home with detailed directions for storage and administration with a phone number to call for any questions. Caregivers attest electronically that vaccine has been administered, and the dispensing pharmacy will submit the administration to state immunization registries.

In a small pilot feasibility study that enrolled 27 parents/caregivers and 41 children (age range 2.6 to 17.9 years of age; mean 10.5 years), LAIV was successfully administered in the home setting by all participants.[96] Participating parents/caregivers voiced a preference for administration of home administration of LAIV. Additional practical considerations for home LAIV are presented in Box 1.

Because administration cannot be verified, LAIV home administration is not recommended in situations in which influenza vaccine is mandated. This includes children required to have an influenza vaccine for child care attendance or health care personnel (HCP) who have influenza vaccination as a condition of employment.

Box 1. Considerations for Use of LAIV in the Home Setting

Logistical Considerations

Caregiver/patient must initiate the process to receive LAIV at home

- Prescription by patient's physician not required; after eligibility is determined, a prescription is generated through an online pharmacy service.
- Modest shipping and processing fee charged at time of order.
- Shipped to patient home using validated and approved cold-chain procedures and packaging.
- Detailed instructions for use provided in updated package insert[95] and videos available via product website portal.
- Updated package insert instructs vaccine recipient or caregiver to seek immediate medical attention if the vaccine recipient experiences any symptoms of an acute allergic reaction.
- Pharmacist documents in IIS based on caregiver attestation that vaccine administered.
- Used sprayer is mailed to medical waste company in a pre-labeled, prepaid envelope for disposal.

Administration of Partial Dose

Caregiver contacts pharmacist at online pharmacy service to determine next steps (if an additional dose is to be sent or recommendation to seek vaccination through a retail or clinic setting).

Financial Considerations

- Not covered as part of Vaccines for Children in the 2025–2026 influenza season.
- Privately insured patients will pay a modest shipping and processing fee.

Safety of LAIV

The most common solicited adverse reactions after LAIV administration in clinical trials included runny nose or nasal congestion (recipients 2 years through 49 years), fever >100 °F (children ages 2 years through 6 years), and sore throat (adults ages 18 years through 49 years).[97]

LAIV and Immunocompromised Hosts

IIV (or RIV, if age-eligible) is the vaccine of choice for severely immunocompromised patients and anyone in close contact with a subset of severely immunocompromised people (ie, those requiring a protected environment). This preference is based on the theoretical risk of infection attributable to an LAIV strain in an immunocompromised contact of an LAIV-immunized person. HCP immunized with LAIV may continue to work in most units of a hospital, including the neonatal intensive care unit and general oncology ward, using standard infection control techniques. As a precautionary measure, people recently vaccinated with LAIV should restrict contact with severely immunocompromised patients (eg, those requiring a protective environment) for 7 days after vaccination, although there have been no reports of LAIV transmission from an LAIV-vaccinated person to an immunocompromised person.[98] In the theoretical scenario in which an immunocompromised host develops a symptomatic LAIV infection, the LAIV strains are susceptible to antiviral medications.

LAIV and Asthma/Wheezing

The AAP and ACIP currently consider asthma in persons ≥5 years of age to be a precaution for LAIV. The LAIV package insert states, "Children younger than 5 years of age with recurrent wheezing and persons of any age with asthma may be at increased risk of wheezing following administration of FluMist." Although LAIV administration is currently contraindicated in children 2 through 4 years of age with asthma or a history of recurrent wheezing,[1,71] 1 systematic literature review of 14 studies over 20 years[99] demonstrated that LAIV was well tolerated in children and adults 2 through 49 years of age with mild to moderate asthma or recurrent wheeze, with no safety concerns or increased risk identified for any of the respiratory outcomes measured when comparing LAIV-AA with injectable influenza vaccines or nonvaccine controls. In a more recent systematic literature review, Bandell et al found no difference in the number or severity of asthma exacerbations among 5- to 17-year-olds with asthma and no increase in medically significant wheezing among 2- to 17-year-olds with asthma or recurrent wheeze following LAIV vs IIV administration.[100] One cited study observed a higher incidence of rhinitis after LAIV administration in patients aged 6 to 17 years with asthma. They also found no difference in medical resource utilization and a similar or lower incidence of emergency department (ED) visits or hospitalizations after LAIV vs

IIV administration. Based on these data, several countries, including Canada, have issued more permissive guidelines regarding LAIV use in children with asthma and/or recurrent wheeze.[101] The use of LAIV in children with asthma and wheezing deserves additional review. As of July 5, 2025, the ACIP recommendations are unchanged while data continue to accumulate and are reviewed by expert groups.

TIMING OF INFLUENZA VACCINATION AND DURATION OF PROTECTION

Although peak influenza activity in the US typically occurs from January through March, influenza viruses can begin to circulate in early fall (October), as occurred in the 2022–2023 season. Circulation can continue to late spring (May or later), with 1 or more disease peaks, as was the case in the 2021–2022 season. The typical pattern of circulation was substantially altered during the COVID-19 pandemic, although prepandemic patterns have been observed in recent seasons. Still, predicting the onset and duration or the severity of the influenza season with accuracy is impossible. Timely influenza vaccination is important to ensure that individuals are optimally protected before influenza viruses are circulating in the community. Thus, the AAP and CDC recommend children, especially those who need 2 doses, should be immunized as soon as vaccine becomes available and complete influenza vaccination by the end of October. Because the duration of the influenza season is unpredictable, vaccination should continue as long as influenza viruses are circulating and unexpired vaccine is available (no influenza vaccines in the US are labeled with an expiration date past June 30 of the prior influenza season[102]).

Immunity after influenza vaccination can wane over time.[103] Studies in adults suggest that very early vaccination (July or August) might be associated with suboptimal immunity before the end of the influenza season, and the CDC now discourages influenza vaccination in the summer months for most adults.[71] There is less evidence of waning immunity in children.[104–106] In some studies in children, VE decreased within a single influenza season, and this decrease correlated with increasing time after vaccination. However, this decay in VE was not consistent across different age groups and varied by season and virus types and influenza A virus subtypes.[103,107–114] Waning VE was more evident among older adults and younger children[108–110] and with influenza A(H3N2) viruses more than influenza A(H1N1) or B viruses.[104,109,113] Most recently, waning immunity after influenza vaccination was studied over 9 influenza seasons in Ontario, Canada.[115] In a cohort of individuals ≥6 months vaccinated during the 2011–2012 to the 2018–2019 seasons, the odds of laboratory-confirmed influenza increased 1.09 times every 28 days since vaccination, but waning immunity varied by season, influenza subtype and age group. Unlike older persons, individuals <18 years had lower odds of influenza at subsequent intervals and waning protection was not observed. A systematic review and meta-analysis that included 3 studies of influenza-vaccinated children found that antibody levels waned over time but remained elevated compared with prevaccination levels for 6 months after vaccination.[116] Adjuvanted vaccines, which are not currently available for children, elicited higher antibody responses than standard vaccines. In a cohort of influenza vaccine-naive patients 6 to <24 months of age in Nicaragua who received a single dose of vaccine, VE against laboratory-confirmed influenza illness declined 9% per month in the first 4 months following immunization and then plateaued.[117] Waning of immunity after 2 doses of vaccine, as is recommended in the US, was not studied. Collectively, these studies support the current recommendation to immunize children as soon as possible after vaccine becomes available. An early onset of the influenza season, as occurred for the 2022–2023 season, is a concern when considering delaying vaccination, and delays increase the likelihood of missing influenza vaccination altogether.[71]

Although influenza activity in the US is typically low during the summer, influenza cases and outbreaks can occur, particularly among international travelers, who may be exposed to influenza year-round, depending on destination. Influenza can occur throughout the year in the tropics. The CDC has recommended that individuals who did not receive the current seasonal influenza vaccine during the Northern Hemisphere fall/winter season and who are traveling to parts of the world where influenza activity is ongoing should consider seasonal influenza vaccination ≥2 weeks before departure, if available.[118] This includes persons traveling to the tropics, to destinations in the Southern Hemisphere during the Southern Hemisphere influenza season (April to September), or on cruise ships or with organized tourist groups during an influenza season.[71]

INFLUENZA VACCINE CONSIDERATIONS FOR SUBPOPULATIONS, INCLUDING CONTRAINDICATIONS AND PRECAUTIONS

Contraindications and precautions to available influenza vaccines are detailed in Table 5 in the policy statement[1] (https://doi.org/10.1542/peds.2025-073620). A precaution for vaccination is a condition that might increase the risk or seriousness of a vaccine-related adverse reaction, might compromise the ability of the host to develop immunity after vaccination, or might cause diagnostic confusion.[119] Vaccination may be recommended in the presence of a precaution if the benefit of protection from the vaccine outweighs the potential risks.

Previous Allergic Reaction: Contraindication

Although a severe allergic reaction (eg, anaphylaxis) to a previous dose of any influenza vaccine is generally a contraindication to future receipt of influenza vaccines, the AAP recommends that children who have had an allergic reaction after a previous dose of any influenza vaccine be evaluated by an allergist to determine whether future receipt of the vaccine is appropriate. Children who are allergic to gelatin (very rare) should receive IIV3 instead of LAIV3. RIV3 is an option for patients with gelatin allergy who are ≥9 years of age.

Moderate or Severe Illness, Including COVID-19: Delay Is Recommended

Mild illnesses, with or without fever, are neither precautions nor contraindications to the use of influenza vaccines, including among children with mild upper respiratory infection symptoms or allergic rhinitis. In children judged by the clinician to have a moderate to severe illness, vaccination should be deferred until resolution of the illness. Children with an amount of nasal congestion that would notably impede vaccine delivery into the nasopharyngeal mucosa may receive IIV or should have LAIV deferred until symptom resolution.

Guillain-Barré Syndrome: Precaution

History of Guillain-Barré syndrome (GBS) following influenza vaccine is considered a precaution for the administration of influenza vaccines. GBS is rare, especially in children, and there is a lack of evidence on the risk of GBS following influenza vaccination in children. Nonetheless, regardless of age, a history of GBS less than 6 weeks after a previous dose of influenza vaccine is a precaution for administration of influenza vaccine. GBS may occur after influenza virus infection. The benefits of influenza vaccination might outweigh the risks for certain people who have a history of GBS (particularly if not temporally occurring after prior influenza vaccination) and who also are at high risk for severe complications from influenza.

Influenza Vaccines and Egg Allergy: Not a Contraindication or Precaution

There is strong evidence that individuals with egg allergy can safely receive influenza vaccine without any additional precautions beyond those recommended for any vaccine.[120,121] The presence of egg allergy in an individual is not a contraindication to receive IIV or LAIV. Vaccine recipients with egg allergy are at no greater risk for a systemic allergic reaction than those without egg allergy. Therefore, precautions such as choice of a particular vaccine, special observation periods, or restriction of administration to particular medical settings are not warranted and constitute an unnecessary barrier to vaccination. It is not necessary to inquire about egg allergy prior to the administration of any influenza vaccine, including on screening forms. Routine prevaccination questions regarding anaphylaxis after receipt of any vaccine are appropriate. Standard vaccination practice for all vaccines in children should include the ability to respond to rare acute hypersensitivity reactions.

Pregnancy: IIV Recommended, Not a Contraindication or Precaution

Influenza vaccination is recommended by the ACIP, the American College of Obstetricians and Gynecologists (ACOG), and the American Academy of Family Physicians (AAFP) for all pregnant individuals, during any trimester of gestation, to protect against influenza and its complications.[71,122] Influenza vaccination prevents laboratory-confirmed influenza disease and its complications in pregnant individuals and protects their infants in the first months of life (up to 6 months) through transplacental passage of antibodies.[122–132] Two recently published studies reinforce the benefits of influenza vaccination during pregnancy to infants. Over 9 influenza seasons in Ontario, Canada, vaccination during any trimester was associated with reduced risk of laboratory-confirmed influenza (VE 64% [95% CI, 50% to 74%]) and influenza hospitalization (VE 67% [95% CI, 50% to 78%]) during the first 6 months of life.[133] In a prospective, test-negative case-control study that analyzed data from the NVSN (2016–2017 to 2019–2020), VE in infants younger than 6 months was 39% against influenza-associated hospitalization (95% CI, 12% to 58%) and 19% against influenza-associated ED visits (95% CI, −24% to 48%).[134] Effectiveness was highest among infants <3 months (53% [95% CI, 30% to 68%]) and infants whose birthing parent was vaccinated during the third trimester (52% [95% CI, 30% to 68%]).

Any licensed, recommended, and age-appropriate IIV or RIV may be administered to pregnant individuals during any trimester of gestation and postpartum. The AAP and ACIP consider LAIV to be contraindicated during pregnancy. This differs from the prescribing information for FluMist 2024–2025 Formula, which indicates that FluMist is not absorbed systemically following intranasal administration and use during pregnancy is not expected to result in fetal exposure to the drug.[95] Influenza vaccine may be administered during the same visit as other recommended vaccines, including RSV, COVID-19, and Tdap vaccines. Data on the safety of influenza vaccination at any time during pregnancy continues to support the safety of influenza immunization during pregnancy.[122,124–135] Most studies demonstrate that vaccination during pregnancy, including during the first trimester, is not associated with a risk of spontaneous abortion[136–139] or with the overall risk of major congenital malformations,[140–143] autism spectrum disorder, or other neurodevelopmental disorders.[144,145] Assessments of any association with influenza vaccination and preterm birth and small-for-gestational-age infants have yielded inconsistent results, with most studies reporting a protective effect or no association with these outcomes.[146–149]

Despite clear evidence of benefit to pregnant individuals and their infants, influenza vaccination in this population is suboptimal. During the 2024–2025 influenza season, 38% of pregnant individuals were vaccinated through March 29, 2025.[150] Vaccination coverage was highest among non-Hispanic Asian pregnant persons (53.1%) and lowest among non-Hispanic Black pregnant persons (26.4%).

Racial disparities in uptake of influenza vaccine during pregnancy have been identified previously, with Black women consistently having the lowest rates.[134,151] Black women report a lower rate of being offered or recommended to receive influenza vaccine, despite evidence that a provider recommendation is associated with vaccine acceptance.[151] Lower influenza vaccination coverage also has been reported in Medicaid-insured pregnant women compared with privately insured women and in women residing in rural areas compared with those residing in urban areas.[152,153] A comprehensive intervention that coupled a strong provider recommendation for influenza immunization with patient education and point-of-care availability of vaccine improved immunization rates in pregnant persons attending 1 urban prenatal clinic in Canada.[154]

Breastfeeding: Recommended, Not a Contraindication or Precaution

Influenza vaccination with IIV, RIV, or LAIV during breastfeeding is safe for lactating individuals and their infants, and vaccination is recommended for individuals not already vaccinated during the current season. Breastfeeding is strongly recommended to protect infants against influenza viruses by activating innate antiviral mechanisms, specifically type-1 interferons. Human milk from pregnant individuals vaccinated during the third trimester also contains higher levels of influenza-specific immunoglobulin A.[155] Greater exclusivity of breastfeeding in the first 6 months of life decreases the episodes of respiratory illness with fever in infants of vaccinated lactating parents. For infants whose birthing parent has confirmed influenza illness at delivery, breastfeeding is encouraged, and guidance on breastfeeding practices is available on the CDC website (https://www.cdc.gov/breastfeeding-special-circumstances/hcp/illnesses-conditions/flu.html and https://www.cdc.gov/flu/hcp/infection-control/peri-post-settings.html). Birthing parents may pump and feed expressed breast milk if they or their infants are too ill to breastfeed.

INFLUENZA VACCINATION COVERAGE

Influenza vaccination coverage of children decreased coincident with the COVID-19 pandemic, mirroring the declines in other routine pediatric vaccines during the pandemic, and has not returned to prepandemic levels.[156–159] During the 2024–2025 season, influenza vaccination coverage decreased for the fifth year in a row, remaining well below the Healthy People 2030 target of 70% (Figure 3).[160,161] Through April 26, 2025, only 49.2% of children 6 months through 17 years had been vaccinated, 14.5 percentage points lower than in at the end of the 2019–2020 (https://www.cdc.gov/fluvaxview/interactive/general-population-coverage.html). Historically, the lowest influenza immunization rates have been observed in non-Hispanic Black children. This season, non-Hispanic white children had the lowest influenza vaccine coverage (46.2%) compared with several groups with higher coverage, including non-Hispanic Black children (47.8%), Hispanic children (53.1%), and children identified as other/non-Hispanic (55.3%). Coverage levels were also lower among children residing in rural areas (36.5%) compared with suburban (49%) or urban (56.2%) areas. Coverage rates also varied by poverty level, with the lowest coverage among children classified as "above poverty, income < $75,000" (42.4%). Higher rates were reported in children classified as "poverty status unknown" (44.6%), "below poverty" (49.4%) and "above poverty, income ≥$75,000" (53.3%).

Disparities by insurance type have previously been reported. In a cross-sectional study using the Massachusetts All Payer Claims Database (2014–2018), privately insured children with asthma were significantly more likely to receive an influenza vaccination than Medicaid-insured children with asthma,[162] although vaccination coverage in both groups was low (51.3% vs 45.1%). Because National Immunization Survey-Flu data may overestimate vaccination rates in some populations, actual immunization rates may be lower.[163]

Factors contributing to declining influenza vaccination coverage in the early years of the pandemic included logistical barriers, including lack of transportation and altered school and work schedules, which may reduce access to routine medical care.[164] Some of these barriers persist. A recent analysis of data from the National Immunization Survey-Child found that estimated coverage with most of the routinely recommended childhood vaccines by age 24 months, including influenza vaccine, was lower among children born in 2020 and 2021 compared with coverage among those born in 2018 and 2019.[165] Vaccination coverage was lower among Black, Hispanic, and AI/AN children, those insured by Medicaid or other nonprivate insurance, uninsured children, children living in more rural areas, and children in families with incomes below the federal poverty level. These data suggest the need to reduce financial obstacles and improve access to vaccination services.

Parental vaccine hesitancy may also contribute to suboptimal influenza immunization rates.[166] Data collected by the CDC through National Immunization Survey-Flu in 2019 found that 1 in 5 US children had a parent who was vaccine hesitant, and hesitancy was negatively associated with childhood influenza vaccination.[166] Between 2019 and 2022, parental vaccine hesitancy toward routine childhood

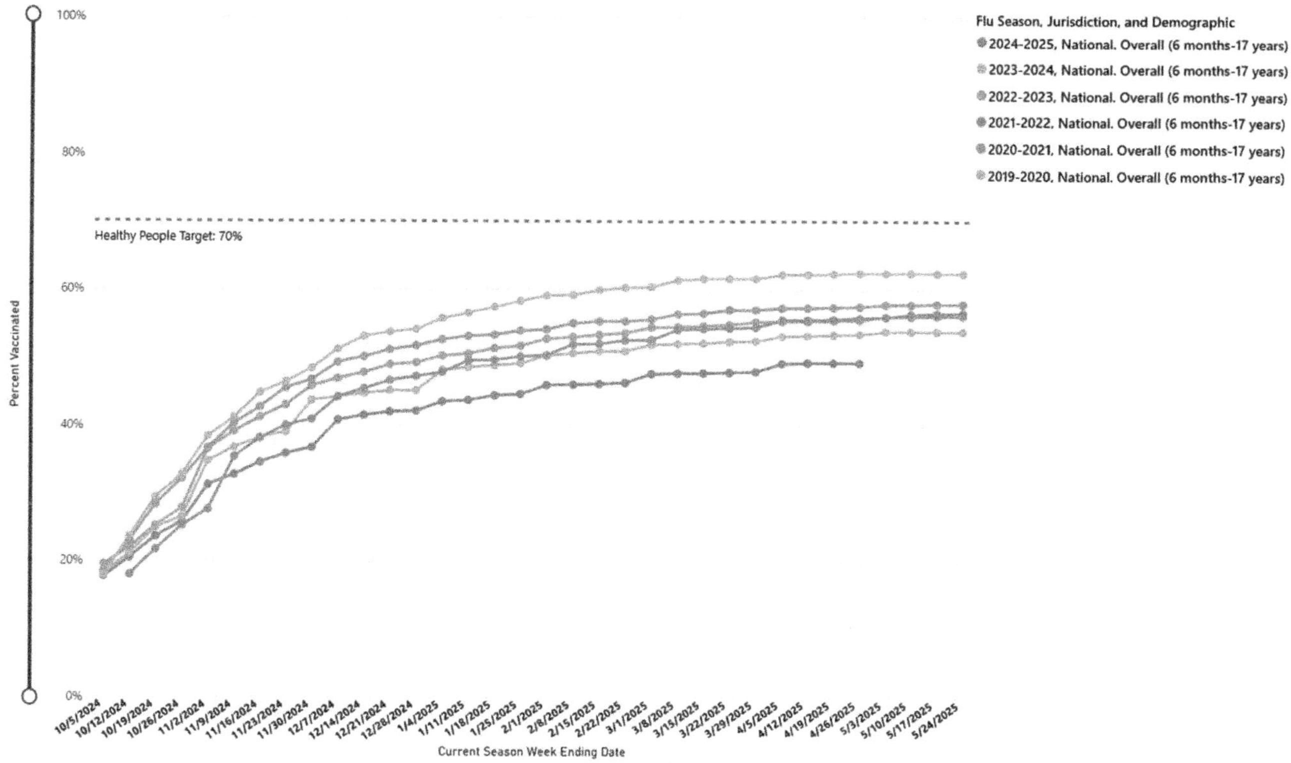

FIGURE 3.
Influenza Vaccination Coverage in Children 6 Months to 17 Years of Age in the United States, 2019–2020 to 2024–2025. Influenza vaccination coverage in children 6 months to 17 years of age in the US, 2019–2020 to 2024–2025 From Centers for Disease Control and Prevention. Influenza Vaccination Coverage, Children 6 months through 17 years, United States. Data source: NIS-Flu. Available at: https://www.cdc.gov/fluvaxview/dashboard/children-vaccination-coverage.html. Accessed July 6, 2025.

vaccines remained stable at ~ 19%.[167] A higher percentage of parents voice hesitancy about influenza vaccine compared to routine childhood vaccines, although that percentage has remained relatively stable (33.8% in 2020 vs 30.9% on 2022–2023).[166] Parental surveys collected through the National Immunization Survey-Child COVID-19 Module October 2022 through April 2023 found the highest rates of parental vaccine hesitancy among parents of Black children (39.8%) and children of other or multiple races (35.3%) compared with parents of white (30.2%), Asian (20.3%), and Hispanic (27.9%) children.

Rates of influenza vaccine hesitancy by race and ethnicity have been previously reported and suggest the need for tailored interventions. For example, in 1 small mixed-methods study of parents and legal guardians presenting with their children to a pediatric emergency department (ED) during the 2021–2022 influenza season, Black caregivers expressed more hesitancy to vaccinate their children for influenza than did white caregivers (42% vs 21%; $P = .01$).[168] Hispanic caregivers also expressed more hesitancy than white caregivers (37%), but this difference was not statistically significant. Barriers to influenza vaccination voiced by Black and Hispanic caregivers included perceived vaccine side effects, lack of necessity, inadequate data, and distrust of the science, health care system, and government. Vaccine hesitancy in Black communities is rooted in part in historical trauma, including unethical medical trials, and has persisted because of ongoing experiences of discrimination, racism, mistreatment, and other health disparities.[169,170] Black caregivers highlighted the importance of health care personnel communicating about vaccines in a transparent, nonjudgmental way. Facilitators of vaccination emphasized by Black and Hispanic caregivers included desire to protect others, employer facilitation of vaccination, and personal stories from others. The use of trusted messengers in their communities, such as faith-based leaders, to promote vaccination is also paramount.[169]

Vaccination interventions must balance the considerable diversity that exists within racial and ethnic groups. For example, within a study enrolling 309 economically marginalized Hispanic mothers of children younger than 5 years of age in the US, there were notable differences in intent to vaccinate, mistrust of influenza vaccine and access to vaccine, suggesting the need for person-centered strategies.[171]

Influenza immunization rates in groups of children with health conditions that increase the risk for severe influenza[172–175] trend higher than rates in children without these health conditions, but opportunities for improvement persist. Tailored interventions may also be needed for these populations. For example, adolescent patients with rheumatic disease receiving immunosuppression (n = 81) and their parents (n = 145) were surveyed about their knowledge of influenza and barriers to influenza vaccination.[172] Commonly cited reasons for not receiving the influenza vaccine included worry about disease flare (25.6%), concern the vaccine will cause influenza (25.6%), and lack of vaccine effectiveness (20.5%).

Achieving high influenza vaccination coverage of infants, children, and adolescents remains a priority to protect them against influenza disease and its complications. Multifaceted strategies are needed to increase influenza vaccination coverage, especially in vulnerable, high-risk populations.

INFLUENZA VACCINE DELIVERY AND IMPLEMENTATION STRATEGIES

Timely annual distribution of influenza vaccine to health care facilities serving children and adolescents, especially primary medical homes, may help avoid missed opportunities. Placing initial vaccine orders early and creating systems for tracking and reordering when necessary throughout the season may optimize supply. Such efforts may be particularly important when there are disruptions in vaccine delivery because of supply chain issues, inclement weather, or other unforeseen circumstances, along with prioritizing delivery to primary care settings, especially when supply is limited or delayed. The AAP has developed guidance for addressing influenza vaccine supply, payment, coding, and liability issues (https://www.aap.org/influenza).

The AAP and CDC recommend influenza vaccination at any visit to the medical home during influenza season. Influenza vaccination in the medical home is ideal, especially for the youngest children. Administering influenza vaccine in diverse locations, such as subspecialty practices, perioperative clinics, urgent care clinics, EDs, schools, and pharmacies, may help augment these efforts.[176–178] This may be particularly useful for children at high risk for influenza-related complications and children who do not have or cannot readily access their medical home, including those residing in rural areas where coverage levels are markedly lower than in suburban or urban areas. EDs are an underutilized resource. In 1 tertiary care ED and 3 affiliated sites, a standardized influenza vaccination program consisting of nursing education, standing orders, and a best practice advisory in the electronic health record (EHR) significantly increased the number of influenza vaccines administered.[179] Children vaccinated during the intervention period were more likely to be of Black race (8.4% vs 7.2%) or multiple/other race (26.0% vs 19.8%), Hispanic ethnicity (46.0% vs 34.7%), and with public insurance (64.3% vs 56.0%), suggesting a standardized ED influenza vaccination program could be an effective way to increase immunization rates among minority and government-insured children. In a recent national survey completed by 142 pediatric emergency medicine physicians representing 61 EDs, only 26 of 61 (44%) administer any influenza vaccine and 17 of 61 (28%) administered <50 vaccines annually.[180] Investigators projected that up to 18 750 additional patients could receive influenza vaccine annually if nonvaccinating EDs offered influenza vaccine to children and achieved a 10% acceptance rate.

Expanding pharmacy-based influenza vaccine administration is another strategy with the potential to increase vaccine access, as an estimated 93% of the population lives within 5 miles of a pharmacy.[181,182] The number of children immunized by pharmacists has been increasing but still remains relatively low. In 1 retrospective cohort study that utilized a claims data warehouse of commercially insured persons to analyze influenza vaccines administered to children between July 1, 2016, and June 30, 2017, only 5.2% of vaccines were administered by pharmacists.[182] State-specific restrictions on the minimum age for pharmacist-administered vaccinations vary and may limit the number of children who can be immunized in this setting.[181]

Hospitalized patients should be vaccinated before discharge, unless medically contraindicated. Historically, a substantial proportion of children hospitalized for influenza have been hospitalized previously during the same season; failure to offer vaccine to hospitalized children is a missed opportunity.[183] An automated, hospital-based influenza vaccination screening program integrated into the hospital medical record may increase vaccination of eligible patients.[184]

A system for reporting influenza vaccine administrations is crucial to ensure adequate communication and maintain accurate patient records across settings. Integration of immunization information systems (IISs) with EHR systems can enhance data accuracy and up-to-date vaccination status.[185]

For patients with a fragmented medical home or in communities where patients often receive vaccines in diverse settings, querying the IIS prior to administration of vaccination may prevent unnecessary vaccine administration. Use of patient portals for parents to self-report vaccination is one strategy for health systems looking to calculate influenza vaccination coverage of their patient population and to decrease unnecessary communications to patients who received vaccinations outside the medical home.

Practices should prepare in advance for their influenza vaccine campaign and leverage a range of evidence-based strategies[186,187] throughout the season to increase vaccination rates in their patient population (see Table 3 in the policy statement[1] [https://doi.org/10.1542/peds.2025-073620]). The AAP has created tools to help practices in this work (https://www.aap.org/influenza). Some practices expand their hours of operation (ie, evenings, weekends) or schedule vaccine-only clinics to increase patient access to influenza vaccine early in the season and during peak periods. Sending reminder/recall messages using a modality (ie, telephone, text, letter, email, messaging via the patient portal) that is feasible for their practice and aligns with the preferences of their patient population may improve immunization rates.[188–190] A Cochrane Review from 2018 concluded that reminder/recall improves childhood influenza vaccination with moderate certainty of evidence (RR, 1.51; 95% CI, 1.14 to 1.99).[191] Effective messages notify families of influenza vaccine availability and provide other key information such as the child's vaccination status and where, when, and why the child should receive the vaccine. This information is beneficial early in the campaign as well as throughout the season. For example, 1 clinical trial[192] found that sending text message reminders to parents of children who remain unvaccinated in the late fall increased influenza vaccine uptake. Another trial[193] demonstrated the effectiveness of using text message reminders for children requiring 2 doses in a season, particularly when the messages embedded information regarding the need for a timely second dose. Not all studies have shown an impact, including a recent study of text vs patient portal messaging,[194] neither of which improved overall immunization rates. Other strategies may be needed, such as those addressing vaccine hesitancy.

Effective influenza vaccine communication with patients and families is crucial. Messaging should be consistent across all members of the care team, including front office staff, medical assistants, nurses, physicians and advanced practice providers (including those specializing in primary care and subspecialty care). Practices should educate their staff, physicians, and other clinicians about influenza and influenza vaccine-related topics, including the importance of annual vaccination, vaccine effectiveness and safety, the 2-dose requirement for certain children, vaccine contraindications, and common parental concerns. Making vaccine-related information readily available (ie, via a practice website, social media platform, or educational handout)[195,196] and tailoring this information for their patients and families (ie, materials in preferred language) have been effective. Resources are available from the AAP at https://www.aap.org/en/patient-care/influenza/social-media-toolkit-influenza/.

Digital storytelling, featuring compelling accounts of lived experience, is a promising behavioral intervention that could be leveraged to improve influenza immunization rates.[197]

Care team members should use evidence-based communication strategies in their conversations with patients and families. These include offering a strong, presumptive influenza vaccine recommendation, bundling their recommendation for influenza vaccine with recommendations for other needed vaccines, and pursuing their initial recommendation when families initially decline the vaccine.[198–201] Moreover, communication should be tailored to address the specific vaccine-related concerns of patients and families. Resources regarding effective vaccine communication techniques are available on the AAP website at https://aap.org/vaccinecommunication.

Practices, staff, physicians, and other clinicians should consider expanding their conversations and messaging campaigns about influenza to include other preventable respiratory illnesses (ie, RSV, COVID-19). Messaging examples from the AAP are available at https://www.healthychildren.org/English/tips-tools/ask-the-pediatrician/Pages/can-children-get-COVID-19.aspx. Exact language is particularly important in their discussions and messaging to patients and families. While acknowledging that influenza can sometime cause gastrointestinal symptoms, especially in young children, referring to all viral gastrointestinal illnesses as "stomach flu," creates unnecessary confusion. In Spanish, the term "gripe" is commonly used to refer to viral influenza but is a nonprecise term referring to respiratory illnesses. Using this term may cause confusion about the actual illness prevented by influenza vaccine and result in decreased confidence about vaccine effectiveness. "Influenza" rather than "la gripe" is preferred when discussing influenza and influenza vaccine with Spanish-speaking patients and families.

Strategies to reduce missed opportunities during patient visits include standardization of practice workflow to screen all patients for influenza vaccine eligibility and administer the vaccine to any patient who is due for the vaccine. This workflow could be utilized at all visit types, including preventive care, acute care, and mental/behavioral health visits. Influenza vaccination can be administered when patients present for other needed vaccines as well. Practices may identify influenza vaccine champion(s) within their practice to spearhead these efforts. Informatic tools can also facilitate influenza vaccination. For example, studies have shown that standing vaccine orders and vaccine prompts in the EHR increase influenza vaccine uptake in both inpatient and outpatient settings.[202,203] Audits and performance feedback for providers have also been shown to be effective as part of multimodal interventions.[187] Additionally, these tools can be used to identify patients who have a precaution or contraindication to a particular formulation or who need repeat vaccinations and support future dose scheduling. Practices should attempt to schedule a timely return visit for any patient identified as needing a future dose (eg, vaccine dose deferred because of concomitant moderate or severe illness or second dose indicated because of age). Additionally, health systems looking to identify patients at high risk for severe influenza illness can leverage information from the EHR to identify patients at risk and provide targeted communications. Sample value sets for use in creating electronic clinical decision support tools are presented in Table 3. Implementation can be challenging, but some institutions have used these sources. Local adaptation may be needed.

For practices that choose to offer influenza vaccine to family members and other close contacts of children and adolescent patients, the AAP technical report, "Immunizing Parents and Other Close Family Contacts in the Pediatric Office Setting,"[204] provides medical liability risk management guidance on documenting in a separate record screening, informed consent, and National Vaccine Injury Compensations Program (VICP)-required immunization administration data. Guidance is provided on ascertaining whether immunizing adults is covered by customary pediatric medical liability insurance policies for any adverse events not covered by the VICP; logistical and financial barriers are also addressed. Practices that participate in value-based care contracts with insurance companies should understand the plan-specific implications of immunizing parents. In some cases, immunizing a parent or adult caregiver could result in that individual being attributed to the pediatrician's roster and result in negative financial consequences. Additional resources are available at https://aap.org/immunization.

Partnership with community entities, including early childhood learning centers, schools, school-based health centers, public health agencies, pharmacies, and other organizations, can optimize influenza vaccine distribution, communication, and administration. These partnerships may be particularly important for reaching patients with limited access to care, including those residing in rural areas. For example, practices could help with outreach initiatives such as influenza vaccine fairs or mobile vaccine vans. Partnering with faith-based organizations may be an effective intervention to increase immunization rates in communities in which mistrust and vaccine hesitancy are high.[205] Collectively, practices and partners can educate families and community members on the importance of influenza vaccination and address common concerns. The AAP has created communication resources to convey key messages and to help the public understand influenza vaccination recommendations on the AAP website at https://www.aap.org/en/news-room/campaigns-and-toolkits/flu-campaign-toolkit.

The AAP supports influenza vaccination as a condition of employment for HCP in all settings, including outpatient locations. Optimal prevention of influenza in these settings requires that at least 90% of HCP are vaccinated. Estimated influenza vaccination coverage of HCP was 75.4% during the 2023–2024 season, similar to coverage of 75.9% in 2022–2023, but decreased from 80.6% during the 2021–2022 season.[206] Coverage levels continued to be the highest among HCP who reported an employer requirement for influenza vaccination (97.5%). Coverage levels were also higher among HCP working in hospitals (89.1%) compared with those working in ambulatory settings (74.6%) or long-term care and home health care settings (65.2%). Influenza vaccination programs for HCP benefit the health of employees, their patients, and members of the community, especially because HCP frequently come into contact with high-risk patients in their clinical settings. The programs reduce HCP absenteeism and may reduce disruptions in care delivery associated with personnel shortages.[207] Influenza vaccination as a condition of employment for HCPs is considered ethical, just, and necessary to improve patient safety. For the prevention and control of influenza, HCP must prioritize the health and safety of their patients, honor the requirement of causing no harm, and act as role models for both their patients and colleagues by receiving influenza vaccination annually.

INFLUENZA TREATMENT AND CHEMOPROPHYLAXIS

Antiviral Therapy

The AAP, CDC,[208] Infectious Diseases Society of America,[209] and Pediatric Infectious Diseases Society recommend antiviral treatment for children with serious, complicated, or progressive disease presumptively or definitively caused by influenza, irrespective of influenza vaccination status (the circulating strains may not be well matched with vaccine strains) or whether illness began >48 hours before presentation. Earlier treatment provides better clinical responses, but treatment after 48 hours of symptoms in adults and children with moderate to severe disease or with progressive disease has been shown to provide some benefit and should be offered.[210–212] Additionally, the AAP recommends treatment of children at risk for severe complications of influenza, regardless of duration of symptoms. Otherwise healthy children who have suspected or confirmed influenza with an uncomplicated presentation should be considered for antiviral medication, particularly if they are in contact with other children who either are younger than 6 months (as they are not able to receive influenza vaccine) or have high-risk conditions (including age <5 years) that predispose them to complications of influenza, when influenza viruses are known to be circulating in the community. Antiviral treatment should be started as soon as possible after illness onset and should not be delayed while waiting for a definitive influenza test result, because early therapy provides the best outcomes. Algorithms for interpreting positive and negative influenza tests are available (https://www.cdc.gov/flu/hcp/testing-methods/algorithm-results-circulating.html).

The balance between benefits and harms should be considered when making decisions about the use of antiviral agents for either treatment or chemoprophylaxis of influenza. The cost of antiviral therapy may be a barrier to treatment for some families. When there are shortages of antiviral agents, antivirals are prioritized for patients at greatest risk of influenza-related complications and those who are hospitalized.[213]

Antiviral agents available for both influenza treatment and chemoprophylaxis in children of all ages can be found in Table 6 in the policy statement[11] (https://doi.org/10.1542/peds.2025-073620) (including doses for preterm infants that have not been evaluated by the FDA) and on the CDC website.[208] These include the neuraminidase inhibitors (NAIs [oseltamivir, zanamivir, peramivir]) and a selective inhibitor of influenza cap-dependent endonuclease (baloxavir), all of which have activity against influenza A and B viruses.[209]

The AAP considers oseltamivir (Tamiflu), administered orally or by feeding tube, to be the antiviral drug of choice for the management of illness caused by influenza virus infections. This is the only drug recommended by the AAP for treatment of hospitalized children (AAP recommendations for use of oseltamivir differ from FDA-approved labeling). Oseltamivir is preferred because of the cumulative experience of this drug in children, relative cost, and ease of administration. The FDA has approved oseltamivir for treatment of children as young as 2 weeks of age. Given preliminary pharmacokinetic data and limited safety data, the CDC and AAP support the use of oseltamivir to treat influenza in both term and preterm infants from birth, because benefits of therapy for neonatal influenza are likely to outweigh possible risks of treatment. If the breastfeeding parent requires antivirals, treatment with oral oseltamivir is preferred.

Other Antivirals for the Treatment of Influenza

Although more difficult to administer, inhaled zanamivir (Relenza) is an acceptable alternative for patients 7 years and older who do not have chronic respiratory disease. In 1 nationwide, population-based cohort study that included ambulatory children and adults who were treated with antiviral medications within 48 hours of a clinical diagnosis of influenza, inhaled zanamivir was not inferior to oral oseltamivir in preventing influenza-related hospitalization or death, but an exploratory subgroup analysis favored oseltamivir in children 5 through 17 years of age. This may reflect the ability of children to correctly use a zanamivir inhaler.

A single dose of intravenous peramivir (Rapivab) is approved for the treatment of acute uncomplicated influenza in ambulatory children 6 months and older who have been symptomatic for no more than 2 days. The efficacy of peramivir in patients with serious influenza requiring hospitalization has not been established.[209] In a retrospective cohort study of children 0 to 5 years of age hospitalized with influenza in China, oral oseltamivir and IV peramivir were associated with similar clinical outcomes when used for the treatment of influenza B.[214] In children with influenza A, oseltamivir treatment was associated with improved recovery and shorter hospital stays (5 vs 6 days; $P = 0.02$). In another retrospective cohort study of 97 children 29 days to 18 years of age hospitalized with influenza and treated with peramivir, duration of fever and influenza nucleic acid amplification test positivity were shorter in children infected with influenza A H3N2 compared with children with influenza B; other outcomes were similar.[215]

Baloxavir marboxil (Xofluza) is approved for treatment of acute uncomplicated influenza in healthy individuals as young as 5 years of age and all individuals 12 years and older, including those at high risk of developing influenza-related complications.[216] It is also approved by the FDA for postexposure prophylaxis of influenza for persons ≥5 years of age within 48 hours of contact with an individual with influenza. At present, the CDC does not recommend use of baloxavir for outpatients with complicated or progressive illness, severely immunosuppressed people, hospitalized patients or during pregnancy or breastfeeding because of the lack of information on use of baloxavir in these groups (https://www.cdc.gov/flu/treatment/baloxavir-marboxil.html). There are no available data regarding the presence of baloxavir in human milk, the effects on the breastfed infant, or the effects on milk production.

Baloxavir is administered as a single dose and could be considered as an alternative to oseltamivir for eligible patients when compliance is a concern or there is poor tolerance of an antiviral regimen requiring multiple medication doses.

Outcomes in patients treated with baloxavir are generally similar to those for NAIs.[217,218] In a randomized controlled trial (RCT) that enrolled adolescents and adults, baloxavir had better efficacy than oseltamivir in the treatment of influenza B.[219] Some observational studies suggest more rapid resolution of fever in children treated with baloxavir compared with oseltamivir.[220,221] In an observational study conducted at 10 outpatient clinics across 9 prefectures in Japan during the 2012–2013 and 2019–2020 influenza seasons, baloxavir compared with oseltamivir significantly reduced the median duration of fever in children with influenza B (20.3 hours [95% CI, 9.4 to 31.3] vs 35.0 hours [95% CI, 21.3 to 59.0]).[222] Median duration of fever was similar in children with influenza A(H1N1)pdm09 or A(H3N2). A post hoc analysis of an RCT demonstrated similar durations of fever in children 5 to 11 years of age treated with baloxavir or oseltamivir.[223] In a post hoc analysis of 2 open label studies of baloxavir in children 1 to <12 years of age in Japan, symptom recurrence after day 4 was noted in 54.5% of treated children <6 years of age, while fever recurrence was noted in 50%.[224] In some patients, fever and symptom recurrence occurred during or after increases in virus titer, although titer increases were transient and all patients with symptom recurrence recovered without the need for additional antiviral treatment. In 2 studies, baloxavir treatment reduced the duration of viral shedding compared with oseltamivir treatment in patients infected with influenza.[223,225]

The oral suspension formulation of baloxavir was not available in the US for the 2024–2025 influenza season, limiting use in children who were old enough to receive the drug but weigh less than 20 kg.[226] Availability of this formulation for the 2025–2026 influenza season is unknown at this time.

Rationale for Influenza Treatment in Children

The rationale for influenza treatment recommendations are 3-fold: 1) reduce the duration of symptoms; 2) reduce complication of influenza, including hospitalization and death; and 3) potentially reduce transmission. RCTs to evaluate the efficacy of influenza antiviral medications among outpatients with uncomplicated influenza have found that timely treatment (optimally ≤2 days from symptom onset) can reduce the duration of influenza symptoms and fever in pediatric and adult populations.[227–231] Observational studies in pediatric and adult populations suggest that antivirals are safe and could reduce the risk of certain influenza complications, including hospitalization and death.[232–236]

A Cochrane review of 6 RCTs involving treatment of 2356 children with clinically diagnosed influenza, of whom 1255 had laboratory-confirmed influenza, showed that in children with laboratory-confirmed influenza, oral oseltamivir and inhaled zanamivir reduced median duration of illness by 36 hours (26%; $P<.001$) and 1.3 days (24%, $P<.001$), respectively.[231] Among the studies reviewed, 1 trial of oseltamivir in children with asthma who had laboratory-confirmed influenza showed a nonsignificant reduction in illness duration (10.4 hours; 8%; $P=.542$). Another Cochrane review of RCTs in adults and children, which included 20 oseltamivir (9623 participants) and 26 zanamivir trials (14 628 participants)[228] found no effect of oseltamivir in reducing the duration of illness in asthmatic children, but in otherwise healthy children, there was a reduction by a mean difference of 29 hours (95% CI, 12 hours to 47 hours; $P=.001$). No significant effect was observed with zanamivir. This review did not find a significant effect of NAIs on reducing hospitalizations, pneumonia, bronchitis, otitis media, or sinusitis in children.[228] More recently, a meta-analysis of 5 new RCTs that included 1598 children with laboratory-confirmed influenza showed that treatment with oseltamivir significantly reduced the duration of illness in this population by 17.6 hours (95% CI, −34.7 hours to −0.62 hours).[229] When children with asthma were excluded, this difference was larger (−29.9 hours; 95% CI, −53.9 hours to −5.8 hours). The risk of otitis media was 34% lower in this group as well. Similarly, a meta-analysis conducted by Tejada et al showed a statistically significant reduction in the risk of acute otitis media occurrence among treated children over placebo recipients (odds ratio [OR]: 0.48; 95% CI, 0.30 to 0.77).[236] Overall, efficacy outcomes are best demonstrated in patients with laboratory-confirmed influenza.

There are no prospective, fully enrolled, completed RCTs of antivirals vs placebo for treatment of influenza in hospitalized children or pediatric patients with comorbidities, and prospectively collected data to determine the role of antiviral agents in treating severe influenza are limited. One RCT of oseltamivir treatment of influenza in hospitalized children in El Salvador and Panama suggested clinical benefit, but no statistically significant findings were reported, because only 21% of the target sample size was enrolled, and therefore, the study was substantially underpowered.[237] Nevertheless, on the basis of information obtained from retrospective observational studies and meta-analyses conducted to date in both adults and children, most experts support the use of antiviral medications as soon as possible to treat pediatric patients with severe influenza, including hospitalized patients.[229–234,237]

In a retrospective study of 784 pediatric intensive care unit admissions from 2009 to 2012, the estimated risk of death was reduced in 653 NAI-treated individuals (OR, 0.36; 95% CI, 0.16 to 0.83).[210] In a retrospective analysis of data from the US Influenza Hospitalization Surveillance Network, administration of antiviral agents ≤2 days after illness onset was associated with shorter lengths of stay in children admitted to the intensive care unit (adjusted hazard ratio: 1.46; $P=.007$) and in children with underlying medical conditions not admitted to the ICU (adjusted hazard ratio: 1.37; $P=.02$). In the relatively small number of patients studied, antiviral treatment ≥3 days after illness onset had no significant effect in either cohort.[238] Similarly, early antiviral treatment of children with tracheostomy hospitalized with influenza reduced length of stay by 1 day (6.4 vs 7.5 days; $P=0.01$).[239] In a multicenter, retrospective cohort study involving 55 799 children hospitalized with influenza between 2007 and 2020, oseltamivir use on hospital day 0 or 1 was associated with shorter hospital stays and lower odds of readmission within 7 days, transfer to the ICU and the composite outcome use of extracorporeal membrane oxygenation and in-hospital mortality.[240]

Several studies also suggest that treatment of index patients with influenza reduces transmission to household contacts to some extent, but the magnitude of the effect is inconsistent across published reports.[241]

Potential limitations of the trials conducted to date in children include the study size (the number of events might not be sufficient to assess specific outcomes in small studies), variations in the case definition of influenza illness (clinically diagnosed vs laboratory confirmed), time of treatment administration in relation to the onset of illness, and inclusion of children of varying ages and underlying health conditions. Observational studies using administrative data may be biased by misclassification of both influenza infection status and oseltamivir exposure.[242]

Nevertheless, the totality of available evidence supports the treatment of children with influenza.

No additional benefit exists for double-dose NAI therapy on reduction of mortality or viral clearance, compared with standard-dose therapy, on the basis of a recent systematic review and meta-analysis of 10 published studies[243] (4 RCTs and 6 observational studies) involving 20 947 adult and pediatric patients. In a randomized, parallel-group, double-blind, placebo-controlled, superiority trial, combining baloxavir with NAIs did not result in superior clinical outcomes compared with NAIs alone in patients 12 years and older hospitalized with laboratory-confirmed influenza.[244]

Oseltamivir Adverse Effects

In adverse event data collected systematically in prospective trials, vomiting was the only adverse effect reported more often with oseltamivir compared with placebo when studied in children 1 through 12 years of age (ie, 15% of treated children vs 9% receiving placebo). Diarrhea was reported in clinical trials of oseltamivir in 7% of treated children <1 year of age. Following reports from Japan of possible oseltamivir-attributable neuropsychiatric adverse effects, a review of controlled clinical trial data and ongoing surveillance has failed to establish a link between this drug and neurologic or psychiatric events.[245,246] Neurologic and neuropsychiatric complications including abnormal behavior occur in children with influenza in the absence of exposure to oseltamivir.[247] In a retrospective cohort study of children 5 through 17 years of age in Tennessee, the incidence rate of neuropsychiatric events was 51 per 100 000 person-weeks of influenza, and rates were higher among adolescents and those with risk factors for influenza complications.[248] The study did not support an association between oseltamivir and neuropsychiatric events, but was unable to characterize the dose, duration, or timing of oseltamivir administration in relation to the onset of neuropsychiatric events.

Adherence to Antiviral Treatment Guidance

Despite the body of evidence supporting antiviral treatment of children hospitalized with confirmed or suspected influenza and longstanding guidance recommending antiviral use in children at high risk for complications, antiviral prescribing is suboptimal.[249–253]

A multicenter, prospective surveillance cohort study conducted from 1 December 2016 to 31 March 2020 at 7 pediatric medical centers as a part of the NVSN confirmed that children hospitalized with laboratory-confirmed influenza frequently do not receive antiviral treatment.[254] Of 1213 children with laboratory-confirmed influenza, 652 children (53.8%) received an antiviral. A hematologic disorder (aOR = 1.76; 95% CI, 1.03 to 3.02), an oncologic or immunocompromising disorder (aOR = 2.41; 95% CI, 1.13 to 5.11), receipt of antivirals for current illness prior to hospitalization (aOR 2.34; 95% CI, 1.49 to 3.67), and ICU admission at presentation (aOR 1.53; 95% CI, 1.02 to 2.29) were associated with receipt of an antiviral medication. Rates of antiviral therapy differed 5-fold across sites.

Data from the NSVN and FluSurv-NET indicate that antiviral treatment of children and adolescents hospitalized with influenza declined during the pandemic and has not returned to prepandemic levels.[255] The overall percentage of hospitalized patients aged <18 years with laboratory-confirmed influenza who were treated with antiviral medications during the 2017–2018 season was 70% in NVSN and 86% in FluSurv-NET. During the 2023–2024 season, only 52% (NVSN) and 59% (FluSurv-NET) of children and adolescents hospitalized with influenza received antiviral treatment. A higher proportion of children aged <6 months received antiviral treatment (68% [NVSN]; 73% [FluSurv-NET]) compared with older children. Antiviral treatment was also more prevalent among children admitted to an ICU (84% [NVSN]; 82% [FluSurv-NET]) or who received noninvasive or invasive ventilation (89%–94% [NVSN]; 82% [FluSurv-NET]).

In the ambulatory setting, only 31% of children and adolescents recommended to receive antiviral treatment were prescribed antivirals. The percentage of prescriptions was highest among children aged <6 months (49%), a group known to be a high-risk for complications of influenza.

Additional studies are needed to explore barriers to treatment of children with influenza and test multifactorial interventions to increase the number of children with influenza who are treated in accordance with recommendations.

INFLUENZA CHEMOPROPHYLAXIS

Antiviral medications are important adjuncts to influenza vaccination for control and prevention of influenza disease in children who are at least 3 months of age. Randomized placebo-controlled studies showed that oral oseltamivir and inhaled zanamivir were efficacious when administered as chemoprophylaxis to household contacts after a family member had laboratory-confirmed influenza.[209] The efficacy of baloxavir was demonstrated in a randomized, placebo-controlled trial in Japan conducted during the 2018–2019 influenza season. Among household members ≥5 years of age treated with a single dose of baloxavir within 48 hours of exposure to a symptomatic household contact with influenza, 2% developed influenza compared with 13% in the placebo group (aRR, 0.14).[256] For additional context, 73% started baloxavir within 24 hours of the index case's symptom onset, an exercise that would be difficult to replicate in practice in the US. There are no data on intravenous peramivir for chemoprophylaxis.

Decisions on whether to administer antiviral chemoprophylaxis should include consideration of the exposed person's risk of influenza complications, vaccination status, type and duration of contact, time since exposure, recommendations from local or public health authorities, and clinical judgment. Optimally, postexposure chemoprophylaxis should only be used when antiviral agents can be started within 48 hours of exposure; the lower once-daily dosing for chemoprophylaxis with oral oseltamivir or inhaled zanamivir should not be used for treatment of children symptomatic with influenza.[209] Early, full treatment dosing (rather than once-daily chemoprophylaxis dosing) should be used in high-risk symptomatic patients without waiting for laboratory confirmation.

Toxicities may be associated with antiviral agents, and indiscriminate use might limit availability. Pediatricians should inform recipients of antiviral chemoprophylaxis that risk of influenza is lowered, but not eliminated, while taking the medication, and susceptibility to influenza returns when medication is discontinued. Chemoprophylaxis is not a substitute for vaccination and among some high-risk people, both vaccination with IIV and antiviral chemoprophylaxis may be considered.[209] The effectiveness of LAIV but not IIV or RIV will be decreased for children receiving oseltamivir or other influenza antivirals.[209] Updates will be available at www.aapredbook.org and www.cdc.gov/flu/professionals/antivirals/index.htm.

ANTIVIRAL RESISTANCE

Resistance to any antiviral drug can emerge, necessitating continuous population-based assessment. In 2023, global surveillance of influenza virus isolates available in the Global Initiative on Sharing All Influenza Data identified an increase in the number of influenza A(H1N1)pdm09 viruses with mutations conferring decreased susceptibility to neuraminidase inhibitors.[257] Fortunately, for nearly all influenza A isolates in the 2024–2025 season to date, antiviral resistance was rarely detected.[258] One influenza A(H1N1)pdm09 isolate (<0.1% of all viruses tested) exhibited reduced inhibition by oseltamivir; 5 influenza A(H1N1)pdm09 isolates exhibited highly reduced inhibition by oseltamivir and peramivir (0.2% of all viruses tested).

Influenza viruses with reduced baloxavir susceptibility have been identified coincident with treatment in children. In an analysis of 4 pediatric trials, the incidence of subjects with treatment-emergent resistance substitutions after baloxavir use was highest in subjects <5 years of age with a clear peak of resistance in subjects 2 to 4 years of age (https://www.fda.gov/media/162113/download). Resistance was substantially higher in subjects infected with influenza A(H3N2). Knowledge of the circulating influenza strain may influence the decision to use baloxavir. Surveillance in the US during the 2024–2025 season did not detect significant resistance to baloxavir. One influenza A(H1N1)pdm09 virus (<0.1%) and 1 influenza A H3N2 virus (0.1%) exhibited decreased susceptibility to baloxavir.

Influenza B Victoria viruses represented a small proportion of infections in the US during the 2024–2025 influenza season. No influenza B Victoria viruses exhibited reduced susceptibility to antiviral agents (https://www.cdc.gov/fluview/surveillance/2025-week-16.html).

High levels of resistance to amantadine and rimantadine persist among the seasonal influenza A viruses currently circulating; neither drug is effective against influenza B viruses. Adamantane medications are not currently recommended for use against seasonal influenza.[209]

To date, most novel influenza A virus, including avian influenza A(H5N1) have been susceptible to antivirals recommended for treatment of seasonal influenza, including oseltamivir, peramivir, zanamivir, and baloxavir.[259] Oseltamivir resistance has been reported in a case of influenza A H5N1 infection associated with a fatal outcome.[260]

If a newly emergent antiviral-resistant virus is a concern, recommendations for alternative treatment will be available from the AAP and CDC. Resistance characteristics can change for an individual patient over the duration of a treatment course, especially in those who are severely immunocompromised. Information on current recommendations and therapeutic options can be found on the AAP website (www.aap.org or www.aapredbook.org), through state-specific AAP chapter websites, or on the CDC website (https://www.cdc.gov/flu/hcp/antivirals/summary-clinicians.html).

DIAGNOSTIC TESTS FOR INFLUENZA

Diagnostic testing for influenza may be beneficial when results will be used to inform clinical management or infection prevention measures and to distinguish from other respiratory viruses with similar symptoms. Performance characteristics of tests vary and are impacted by duration of illness in the person being tested and proper specimen collection and handling. Test results must be interpreted in the context of community influenza activity (Table 4); false-positive test results may occur during periods of low influenza activity.

Molecular assays include rapid molecular tests, reverse-transcriptase polymerase chain reaction (RT-PCR) test, and other nucleic acid amplification tests. Multiplex assays that allow for the simultaneous detection of influenza viruses plus SARS-CoV-2 and RSV are available. These assays can be particularly useful when these viruses are cocirculating, because signs and symptoms of these viruses may be similar, clinical differentiation is difficult, and different treatment strategies are recommended. A list of FDA-cleared and FDA-authorized tests is available at https://www.fda.gov/medical-devices/in-vitro-diagnostics/influenza-diagnostic-tests.

Antigen detection tests include rapid influenza diagnostic tests (RIDTs) and immunofluorescence assays. Some available RIDTs detect SARS-CoV-2 as well as influenza A and B. An updated list of RIDTs is available at https://www.cdc.gov/flu/professionals/diagnosis/table-ridt.html.

Rapid molecular assays are highly sensitive and are preferred over RIDTs in ambulatory children in whom testing is performed. During periods of high community influenza activity, clinicians should consider confirming negative RIDTs with a molecular test. When influenza is circulating in the community, hospitalized patients with signs and symptoms of influenza should be tested with a molecular assay with high sensitivity and specificity.

Most influenza tests ordered in clinical settings do not distinguish avian influenza A(H5) viruses from seasonal influenza A viruses.[261] In January 2025, amid the ongoing avian influenza A(H5) virus animal outbreak in the US and an increasing number of sporadic human cases, the CDC recommended expedited subtyping of influenza A specimens recovered from hospitalized patients, particularly those in intensive care units. When isolates test positive for influenza A but negative for seasonal influenza A virus subtypes (ie, A[H1] and A[H3]), further testing at public health laboratories is indicated as soon as possible and within 24 hours of obtaining results to evaluate for influenza A(H5).

Over-the-counter at-home tests are available under FDA emergency use authorization to diagnose both influenza A and B and SARS-CoV-2 in symptomatic individuals as young as 2 years. There are multiplex antigen tests that detect SARS-CoV-2 and influenza A/B viruses in upper respiratory tract specimens, and 1 multiplex molecular assay that detects SARS-CoV-2 and influenza A/B (https://www.fda.gov/medical-devices/in-vitro-diagnostics/influenza-diagnostic-tests). At a minimum, parents, especially those of children at high risk for complications of influenza, will benefit from counseling about timely communication with the medical home about the results of home tests and education that a negative test result cannot completely exclude influenza.

FUTURE DIRECTIONS

Safety and Effectiveness of Available Influenza Vaccines

Continued evaluation of the safety, immunogenicity, and effectiveness of influenza vaccines, especially for at-risk and diverse populations, is important. The safety of LAIV in children with asthma/recurrent wheeze deserves additional review. If guidelines for administration are revised, safety should be monitored using existing systems, including the Vaccine Adverse Event Reporting System (VAERS), the Clinical Immunization Safety Assessment Project, and the Vaccine Safety Datalink.

The duration of protection, potential role of previous influenza vaccination on overall VE, and VE by vaccine formulation, virus strain, timing of vaccination, and subject age and health status in preventing outpatient medical visits, hospitalizations, and deaths continue to be evaluated. Additional controlled data are needed to inform the timing, schedule, and type of influenza vaccine for optimal vaccine immunogenicity among immunocompromised children, but use of high-dose IIV in selected populations is a promising strategy. In a phase 2, multicenter, double-blind, randomized, controlled trial comparing immunogenicity and safety of high-dose trivalent influenza vaccine (HD-TIV) and standard-dose quadrivalent influenza vaccine (SD-QIV) in children and adolescents 3 through 17 years of age who had received an allogeneic hematopoietic cell transplant 3 to 35 months earlier, 2 doses of HD-TIV were more immunogenic than 2 doses of SD-QIV.[262] Two doses of either vaccine were more immunogenic than a single dose. The greatest benefit of HD-TIV relative to SD-QIV was in individuals receiving their first influenza immunization 6 months or more after receiving a hematopoietic cell transplant.[263] The safety profile of vaccines was similar, although mild to moderate injection site reactions were slightly higher after the second dose of HD-TIV.[262,263] In a subcohort of 65 patients re-enrolled and vaccinated in a second season, a single dose of HD-TIV or SD-QIV was more immunogenic in year 2 than 2 doses of the same formulation in year 1.[264] Injection site and systemic reactions were similar.

Influenza Vaccines in Development

Development efforts continue for universal influenza vaccines that induce broader protection and eliminate the need for annual vaccination. The success of mRNA and other novel technologies used in the development of COVID-19 vaccines may accelerate the prospects of broad influenza vaccines. Ongoing federal support of National Institutes of Health (NIH)-sponsored research related to vaccine development is crucial. Understanding the establishment of immunity against influenza in early life and developing a safe, immunogenic vaccine for infants younger than 6 months are essential. Studies on the effectiveness and safety of influenza vaccines containing adjuvants that enhance immune responses to influenza vaccines or that use novel routes of administration are needed in children. Efforts to improve the vaccine development process to allow for a shorter interval between identification of vaccine strains and vaccine production continue.

Promoting Vaccine Confidence and Increasing Vaccination Coverage

Systematic health services research is needed to examine influenza vaccination coverage, factors associated with undervaccination, and interventions to increase uptake in diverse populations. Prospective assessment of the impact of at-home administration of LAIV on immunization rates is warranted, as well as logistical challenges such as accurate and timely reporting of doses.

National data from 2019 found that 25.8% of parents were hesitant about influenza vaccine.[265] Children of parents who were hesitant about childhood vaccines had 25.6% lower influenza vaccination coverage in the influenza 2018–2019 season compared with children of parents not reporting hesitancy.[266] Vaccine hesitancy remains a major public health threat. Future studies, including those funded by the NIH, should aim to improve our understanding of influenza vaccine hesitancy and identify effective strategies to respond to parental concerns, address misinformation/disinformation, foster greater vaccine confidence, and increase influenza vaccine acceptance.[200] Although social media may be a source of misinformation about influenza vaccine, it has also been used as tool to increase acceptance of vaccines.[267] The AAP has created a resource to help pediatricians respond to vaccine misinformation on social media (https://www.aap.org/vaccinecommunication). Additional research is needed to understand the impact of social media messaging on influenza vaccination rates.

Engagement of key stakeholder groups in addressing vaccine hesitancy is crucial, including patients and families, health care professionals, practices as well as health systems, public health officials, and community leaders. Enhanced collaboration may facilitate more equitable influenza vaccine supply and delivery and more effective community outreach, particularly to vulnerable populations. Novel approaches for reducing barriers to accessing preventive care services may also help to reduce disparities in influenza vaccination coverage. Ongoing efforts should include broader implementation and evaluation of mandatory HCP vaccination programs in both inpatient and outpatient settings.

Antiviral Treatment

New antiviral drugs are in various development phases, given the need to improve options for the treatment and chemoprophylaxis of influenza. Additionally, with limited data on the use of antivirals in hospitalized children and in children with underlying medical conditions, prospective clinical trials to inform optimal timing and efficacy of antiviral treatment in these populations are warranted, particularly as new antivirals or new indications for existing antivirals become available. Barriers to timely treatment of children at high risk for complications, especially hospitalized patients, must be explored.

ADDITIONAL RESOURCES

Pediatricians can remain informed of advances and other updates during the influenza season by following the CDC Influenza page (www.cdc.gov/flu) and the AAP Red Book Online Respiratory Illness Season News and Resources Page (https://publications.aap.org/redbook/resources/15189).

COMMITTEE ON INFECTIOUS DISEASES, 2024–2025

Sean T. O'Leary, MD, MPH, FAAP, Chairperson
James D. Campbell, MD, MS, FAAP, Vice Chairperson
Monica I. Ardura, DO, MSCS, FAAP
Kristina A. Bryant, MD, FAAP, *Red Book Online* Team Lead
Mary T. Caserta, MD, FAAP
Claudia Espinosa, MD, MSc, FAAP
Robert W. Frenck, Jr, MD, FAAP
C. Mary Healy, MD
Chandy C. John, MD, MS, FAAP
Aaron M. Milstone, MD, MHS, FAAP
Angela L. Myers, MD, MPH, FAAP
Pia Pannaraj, MD, MPH, FAAP
Adam J. Ratner, MD, MPH, FAAP, *Red Book* Associate Editor
José R. Romero, MD, FAAP
Matthew Zahn, MD, FAAP

CONTRIBUTORS

Kristina A. Bryant, MD, FAAP
Annika M. Hofstetter, MD, PhD, MPH, FAAP

PARTNERSHIP FOR POLICY IMPLEMENTATION

Juan D. Chaparro, MD, MS, FAAP
Jeremy J. Michel, MD, MHS, FAAP

EX OFFICIO

David W. Kimberlin, MD, FAAP – *Red Book* Editor
Ritu Banerjee, MD, PhD, FAAP – *Red Book* Associate Editor
Elizabeth D. Barnett MD, FAAP– *Red Book* Associate Editor
Ruth Lynfield, MD, FAAP - *Red Book* Associate Editor

LIAISONS

Amina Ahmed, MD, FAAP, American Thoracic Society
Michelle Barton, MD, Canadian Paediatric Society
Lisa M. Kafer, MD, FAAP, AAP Committee on Practice and Ambulatory Medicine
Denee J. Moore, MD, American Academy of Family Physicians
Jennifer L. Thompson, MD, American College of Obstetricians and Gynecologists
Juan P. Torres, MD, PhD, Sociedad Latinoamericana de Infectología Pediátrica
Charles R. Woods, Jr, MD, MS, FAAP, Pediatric Infectious Diseases Society

STAFF

Gillian Gibbs, MPH

ACKNOWLEDGMENTS

The Committee on Infectious Diseases gratefully acknowledges Kristina A. Bryant, MD, FAAP, and Annika M. Hofstetter, MD, PhD, MPH, FAAP, for their leadership in drafting the policy statement and technical report; and Juan D. Chaparro, MD, MS, FAAP, and Jeremy J. Michel, MD, MHS, FAAP, for their significant contributions in providing input on the initial drafts on behalf of the AAP Partnership for Policy Implementation.

ABBREVIATIONS

AAP: American Academy of Pediatrics
ACIP: Advisory Committee on Immunization Practices
ANE: acute necrotizing encephalopathy
aOR: adjusted odds ratio
ccIIV: cell culture-based inactivated (non-live) influenza vaccine
ccIIV3: trivalent cell culture-based inactivated (non-live) influenza vaccine
CDC: Centers for Disease Control and Prevention
ED: emergency department
EHR: electronic health record
FDA: US Food and Drug Administration
GBS: Guillain-Barré syndrome
HA: hemagglutinin
HCP: health care personnel
HD-TIV: high-dose trivalent influenza vaccine
IAE: influenza-associated encephalopathy or encephalitis
ICU: intensive care unit
IIV: inactivated (non-live) influenza vaccine
IIV3: trivalent inactivated (non-live) influenza vaccine
IIV3: trivalent inactivated (non-live) influenza vaccine
LAIV: live attenuated influenza vaccine
LAIV3: trivalent live attenuated influenza vaccine
NAI: neuraminidase inhibitor
NIH: National Institutes of Health
NVSN: New Vaccine Surveillance Network
RCT: randomized controlled trial
RIDT: rapid influenza diagnostic tests
RIV: recombinant influenza vaccine
RIV3: trivalent recombinant influenza vaccine
RSV: respiratory syncytial virus
SD-QIV: standard-dose quadrivalent influenza vaccine
VE: vaccine effectiveness
WHO: World Health Organization

Embedded links to cdc.gov and fda.gov sites were active and reviewed by AAP subject matter experts as of July 5, 2025.

https://doi.org/10.1542/peds.2025-073622

COMPANION PAPER: A companion to this article can be found online at www.pediatrics.org/cgi/doi/10.1542/peds.2025-073620.

ADDITIONAL RESOURCES

Lessin HR, Edwards KM; Committee On Practice And Ambulatory Medicine; Committee On Infectious Diseases. Immunizing parents and other close family contacts in the pediatric office setting. *Pediatrics.* 2012;129(1):e247–e253. PubMed doi: 10.1542/peds.2011-2937

American Academy of Pediatrics, Committee on Infectious Diseases. Policy statement: Influenza immunization for all health care personnel: keep it mandatory. *Pediatrics.* 2015;136(4):809–818. Reaffirmed March 2020.

American Academy of Pediatrics, Committee on Pediatric Emergency Medicine. Preparation for emergencies in the offices of pediatricians and pediatric primary care providers. *Pediatrics.* 2007;120(1):200–212. Reaffirmed November 2018.

American Academy of Pediatrics, Committee on Practice and Ambulatory Medicine, Committee on Infectious Diseases, Committee on State Government Affairs, Council on School Health. Medical versus nonmedical immunization exemptions for child care and school attendance: Policy statement. *Pediatrics.* 2025;156(2):e2025072714.

O'Leary ST, Opel DJ, Cataldi JR, et al; Committee on Infectious Diseases; Committee on Practice and Ambulatory Medicine; Committee on Bioethics. Strategies for Improving Vaccine Communication and Uptake. *Pediatrics.* 2024;153(3):e2023065483. PubMed doi: 10.1542/peds.2023-065483

American Academy of Pediatrics. Influenza. In: Kimberlin DW, Banerjee R, Barnett ED, Lynfield R, Sawyer MH, eds. *Red Book: 2024 Report of the Committee on Infectious Diseases.* 33rd ed. American Academy of Pediatrics; 2024:511–522. Available at: http://aapredbook.org

Hackell JM, Palevsky SL, Resnick M; Committee on Practice and Ambulatory Medicine, Council on Clinical Information Technology, Section on Early Career Physicians. Immunization Information Systems. *Pediatrics.* 2022;150(4):e2022059281. PubMed doi: 10.1542/peds.2022-059281

REFERENCES

1. American Academy of Pediatrics, Committee on Infectious Diseases. Recommendations for prevention and control of influenza in children, 2025–2026: Policy statement. *Pediatrics.* 2025; 156(4):e2025073620. doi: 10.1542/peds.2025-073620
2. Centers for Disease Control and Prevention. Weekly US Influenza Surveillance Report: Key Updates for Week 14, ending April 5, 2025. Accessed April 18, 2025. https://www.cdc.gov/fluview/surveillance/2025-week-14.html
3. Frutos AM, Cleary S, Reeves EL, et al; CDC Influenza Vaccine Effectiveness Collaborators. Interim estimates of 2024-2025 seasonal influenza vaccine effectiveness—four vaccine effectiveness networks, United States, October 2024–February 2025. *MMWR Morb Mortal Wkly Rep.* 2025;74(6):83–90. PubMed doi: 10.15585/mmwr.mm7406a2
4. Centers for Disease Control and Prevention. CDC confirms H5N1 Bird Flu Infection in a Child in California. Accessed May 25, 2025. https://www.cdc.gov/media/releases/2024/p1122-h5n1-bird-flu.html
5. San Francisco Department of Public Health. Presumptive Bird Flu Case Identified in San Francisco Resident. Accessed May 25, 2025. https://www.sf.gov/news–presumptive-bird-flu-case-identified-san-francisco-resident
6. Jassem AN, Roberts A, Tyson J, et al. Critical illness in an adolescent with influenza A(H5N1) virus infection. *N Engl J Med.* 2025; 392(9):927–929. PubMed doi: 10.1056/NEJMc2415890
7. World Health Organization. Influenza at the human-animal interface Summary and risk assessment, from 20 March to 22 April 2025. https://cdn.who.int/media/docs/default-source/influenza/human-animal-interface-risk-assessments/influenza-at-the-human-animal-interface-summary-and-assessment–from-20-march-to-22-april-2025.pdf. Accessed June 1, 2025.
8. Tokars JI, Olsen SJ, Reed C. Seasonal incidence of symptomatic influenza in the United States. *Clin Infect Dis.* 2018;66(10):1511–1518. PubMed doi: 10.1093/cid/cix1060
9. Centers for Disease Control and Prevention. Influenza (Flu). Accessed June 1, 2025. https://www.cdc.gov/flu/about/index.html
10. Hoy G, Kuan G, López R, et al. The spectrum of influenza in children. *Clin Infect Dis.* 2023;76(3):e1012–e1020. PubMed doi: 10.1093/cid/ciac734
11. Uyeki TM, Hui DS, Zambon M, Wentworth DE, Monto AS. Influenza. *Lancet.* 2022;400(10353):693–706. PubMed doi: 10.1016/S0140-6736(22)00982-5
12. Belser JA, Lash RR, Garg S, Tumpey TM, Maines TR. The eyes have it: influenza virus infection beyond the respiratory tract. *Lancet Infect Dis.* 2018;18(7):e220–e227. PubMed doi: 10.1016/S1473-3099(18)30102-6
13. Ghebrehewet S, MacPherson P, Ho A. Influenza. *BMJ.* 2016;355: i6258. PubMed doi: 10.1136/bmj.i6258
14. Quertermous BP, Williams DJ, Bruce J, et al. Serious neurologic events with seasonal influenza in young children. *Acad Pediatr.* 2025;25(4):102801. PubMed doi: 10.1016/j.acap.2025.102801
15. Antoon JW, Hall M, Herndon A, et al. Prevalence, risk factors, and outcomes of influenza-associated neurologic complications in children. *J Pediatr.* 2021;239:32–38.e5. PubMed doi: 10.1016/j.jpeds.2021.06.075
16. Frankl S, Coffin SE, Harrison JB, Swami SK, McGuire JL. Influenza-associated neurologic complications in hospitalized children. *J Pediatr.* 2021;239:24–31.e1. PubMed doi: 10.1016/j.jpeds.2021.07.039
17. Fazal A, Reinhart K, Huang S, et al. Reports of encephalopathy among children with influenza-associated mortality—United States, 2010–11 through 2024–25 influenza seasons. *MMWR Morb Mortal Wkly Rep.* 2025;74(6):91–95. PubMed doi: 10.15585/mmwr.mm7406a3
18. Sakuma H, Thomas T, Debinski C, et al. International consensus definitions for infection-triggered encephalopathy syndromes. *Dev Med Child Neurol.* 2025;67(2):195–207. PubMed doi: 10.1111/dmcn.16067
19. Modler J, Morris SK, Bettinger JA, et al; Canadian Immunization Monitoring Program Active (IMPACT) Investigators. Bloodstream infections in children hospitalized for influenza, the Canadian Immunization Monitoring Program Active (IMPACT). *Pediatr Infect Dis J.* 2023; advance online publication. PubMed
20. Herrera AL, Huber VC, Chaussee MS. The association between invasive group A streptococcal diseases and viral respiratory tract infections. *Front Microbiol.* 2016;7:342. PubMed doi: 10.3389/fmicb.2016.00342
21. Barnes M, Youngkin E, Zipprich J, et al. Notes from the field: increase in pediatric invasive group A Streptococcus infections—Colorado and Minnesota, October–December 2022. *MMWR Morb Mortal Wkly Rep.* 2023;72(10):265–267. PubMed doi: 10.15585/mmwr.mm7210a4
22. Rolfes MA, Foppa IM, Garg S, et al. Annual estimates of the burden of seasonal influenza in the United States: A tool for strengthening influenza surveillance and preparedness. *Influenza Other Respir Viruses.* 2018;12(1):132–137. PubMed doi: 10.1111/irv.12486
23. Wolf RM, Antoon JW. Influenza in children and adolescents: epidemiology, management, and prevention. *Pediatr Rev.* 2023; 44(11):605–617. PubMed doi: 10.1542/pir.2023-005962
24. Kamidani S, Garg S, Rolfes MA, et al. Epidemiology, clinical characteristics, and outcomes of influenza-associated hospitalizations in U.S. children over 9 seasons following the 2009 H1N1 pandemic. *Clin Infect Dis.* 2022;75(11):1930–1939. PubMed doi: 10.1093/cid/ciac296
25. Naquin A, O'Halloran A, Ujamaa D, et al. Laboratory-confirmed influenza-associated hospitalizations among children and adults—Influenza Hospitalization Surveillance Network, United States, 2010–2023. *MMWR Surveill Summ.* 2024;73(6):1–18. PubMed doi: 10.15585/mmwr.ss7706a1
26. Grioni HM, Sullivan E, Strelitz B, et al. Pediatric clinical influenza disease by type and subtype 2015-2020: a multicenter, prospective study. *J Pediatric Infect Dis Soc.* 2025;14(1):piae108. PubMed doi: 10.1093/jpids/piae108
27. Delahoy MJ, Ujamaa D, Taylor CA, et al. Comparison of influenza and coronavirus disease 2019-associated hospitalizations among children younger than 18 years old in the United States: FluSurv-NET (October–April 2017–2021) and COVID-NET

(October 2020–September 2021). *Clin Infect Dis.* 2023;76(3):e450–e459. PubMed doi: 10.1093/cid/ciac388

28. Schober T, Morris SK, Bettinger JA, et al; Canadian Immunization Monitoring Program Active (IMPACT) Investigators. Antibiotic use in children hospitalised for influenza, 2010-2021: the Canadian Immunization Monitoring Program Active (IMPACT). *Infection.* 2024;52(3):865–875. PubMed doi: 10.1007/s15010-023-02124-6
29. Maddux AB, Grunwell JR, Newhams MM, et al; PALISI Pediatric Intensive Care Influenza Network Investigators. Association of asthma with treatments and outcomes in children with critical influenza. *J Allergy Clin Immunol Pract.* 2023;11(3):836–843.e3. PubMed doi: 10.1016/j.jaip.2022.10.045
30. Centers for Disease Control and Prevention. 2020-2021 Flu Season. Accessed May 25, 2025. https://www.cdc.gov/flu/season/2020-2021.html
31. Centers for Disease Control and Prevention. Flu Deaths in Children Last Season Reach 199, Matching Record. Accessed June 1, 2025. https://www.cdc.gov/flu/whats-new/2023-2024-flu-deaths-children.html
32. Centers for Disease Control and Prevention. 2023-2024 Influenza Season Summary: Influenza Severity Assessment, Burden and Burden Prevented Accessed May 25, 2025 https://www.cdc.gov/flu/whats-new/flu-summary-addendum-2023-2024.html
33. Centers for Disease Control and Prevention. Childhood Obesity Facts. Accessed May 25, 2025. https://www.cdc.gov/obesity/childhood-obesity-facts/childhood-obesity-facts.html
34. Vitoratou D-I, Milas G-P, Korovessi P, Kostaridou S, Koletsi P. Obesity as a risk factor for severe influenza infection in children and adolescents: a systematic review and meta-analysis. *Eur J Pediatr.* 2023;182(1):363–374. PubMed doi: 10.1007/s00431-022-04689-0
35. Centers for Disease Control and Prevention. Flu and Healthy Lives for All. Accessed June 2, 2025. Available at: https://www.cdc.gov/flu/healthy-living
36. Feiler MO, Yucel R, Liu Z, et al. Trends and non-clinical predictors of respiratory syncytial virus (RSV) and influenza diagnosis in an urban pediatric population. *Int J Pediatr Res.* 2023;9(1):112. PubMed
37. O'Bryant SC, Dongarwar D, Salihu HM, Gillespie S. Racial and ethnic differences of influenza-associated pediatric hospitalizations and deaths, 2008-2017. *Pediatr Allergy Immunol Pulmonol.* 2022;35(2):102–108. PubMed doi: 10.1089/ped.2021.0199
38. O'Halloran AC, Holstein R, Cummings C, et al. Rates of influenza-associated hospitalization, intensive care unit admission, and in-hospital death by race and ethnicity in the United States From 2009 to 2019. *JAMA Netw Open.* 2021;4(8):e2121880. PubMed doi: 10.1001/jamanetworkopen.2021.21880
39. Haddadin Z, Spieker AJ, Amarin JZ, et al. Incidence of and risk factors for influenza-associated hospital encounters in pediatric solid organ transplant recipients. *Am J Transplant.* 2023;23(5):659–665. PubMed doi: 10.1016/j.ajt.2023.01.024
40. Mackey K, Ayers CK, Kondo KK, et al. Racial and ethnic disparities in COVID-19-related infections, hospitalizations, and deaths: a systematic review. *Ann Intern Med.* 2021;174(3):362–373. PubMed doi: 10.7326/M20-6306
41. Fitzpatrick T, McNally JD, Stukel TA, et al. Family and Child Risk Factors for Early-Life RSV Illness. *Pediatrics.* 2021;147(4):e2020029090. PubMed doi: 10.1542/peds.2020-029090
42. Hadler JL, Yousey-Hindes K, Pérez A, et al. Influenza-related hospitalizations and poverty levels—United States, 2010–2012. *MMWR Morb Mortal Wkly Rep.* 2016;65(5):101–105. PubMed doi: 10.15585/mmwr.mm6505a1
43. Sumner KM, Sahni LC, Boom JA, et al; New Vaccine Surveillance Network Collaborators. Estimated vaccine effectiveness for pediatric patients with severe influenza, 2015-2020. *JAMA Netw Open.* 2024;7(12):e2452512. PubMed doi: 10.1001/jamanetworkopen.2024.52512
44. Shang M, Blanton L, Brammer L, Olsen SJ, Fry AM. Influenza-associated pediatric deaths in the United States, 2010-2016. *Pediatrics.* 2018;141(4):e20172918. PubMed doi: 10.1542/peds.2017-2918
45. Flannery B, Reynolds SB, Blanton L, et al. Influenza vaccine effectiveness against pediatric deaths: 2010-2014. *Pediatrics.* 2017;139(5):e20164244. PubMed doi: 10.1542/peds.2016-4244
46. Ferdinands JM, Olsho LE, Agan AA, et al; Pediatric Acute Lung Injury and Sepsis Investigators (PALISI) Network. Effectiveness of influenza vaccine against life-threatening RT-PCR-confirmed influenza illness in US children, 2010-2012. *J Infect Dis.* 2014;210(5):674–683. PubMed doi: 10.1093/infdis/jiu185
47. Centers for Disease Control and Prevention. Flu Burden Prevented by Vaccination 2023-2024 Flu Season. Accessed May 25, 2025. https://www.cdc.gov/flu-burden/php/data-vis-vac/2023-2024-prevented.html
48. Olson SM, Newhams MM, Halasa NB, et al; Pediatric Intensive Care Influenza Investigators. Vaccine effectiveness against life-threatening influenza illness in US children. *Clin Infect Dis.* 2022;75(2):230–238. PubMed doi: 10.1093/cid/ciab931
49. Feldstein LR, Ogokeh C, Rha B, et al. Vaccine effectiveness against influenza hospitalization among children in the United States, 2015-2016. *J Pediatric Infect Dis Soc.* 2021;10(2):75–82. PubMed doi: 10.1093/jpids/piaa017
50. Segaloff HE, Leventer-Roberts M, Riesel D, et al. Influenza vaccine effectiveness against hospitalization in fully and partially vaccinated children in Israel: 2015-2016, 2016-2017, and 2017-2018. *Clin Infect Dis.* 2019;69(12):2153-2161. PubMed doi: 10.1093/cid/ciz125
51. Blyth CC, Cheng AC, Crawford NW, et al; Paediatric Active Enhanced Disease Surveillance (PAEDS), Influenza Complications Alert Network (FluCAN) Collaboration. The impact of new universal child influenza programs in Australia: Vaccine coverage, effectiveness and disease epidemiology in hospitalised children in 2018. *Vaccine.* 2020;38(13):2779–2787. PubMed doi: 10.1016/j.vaccine.2020.02.031
52. Kalligeros M, Shehadeh F, Mylona EK, et al. Influenza vaccine effectiveness against influenza-associated hospitalization in children: A systematic review and meta-analysis. *Vaccine.* 2020;38(14):2893–2903. PubMed doi: 10.1016/j.vaccine.2020.02.049
53. Pebody RG, Zhao H, Whitaker HJ, et al. Effectiveness of influenza vaccine in children in preventing influenza associated

hospitalisation, 2018/19, England. *Vaccine.* 2020;38(2):158–164. PubMed doi: 10.1016/j.vaccine.2019.10.035

54. Shinjoh M, Sugaya N, Yamaguchi Y, et al. Influenza vaccine effectiveness against influenza A in children based on the results of various rapid influenza tests in the 2018/19 season. *PLoS One.* 2021;16(3):e0249005. PubMed doi: 10.1371/journal.pone.0249005
55. Yildirim I, Kao CM, Tippett A, et al. A retrospective test-negative case-control study to evaluate influenza vaccine effectiveness in preventing hospitalizations in children. *Clin Infect Dis.* 2021;73(10):1759–1767. PubMed doi: 10.1093/cid/ciab709
56. Tran D, Vaudry W, Moore D, et al; members of the Canadian Immunization Monitoring Program Active. Hospitalization for Influenza A Versus B. *Pediatrics.* 2016;138(3):e20154643. PubMed doi: 10.1542/peds.2015-4643
57. Campbell AP, Ogokeh C, Weinberg GA, et al; New Vaccine Surveillance Network (NVSN). Effect of vaccination on preventing influenza-associated hospitalizations among children during a severe season associated with B/Victoria viruses, 2019-2020. *Clin Infect Dis.* 2021;73(4):e947–e954. PubMed doi: 10.1093/cid/ciab060
58. Chung JR, Rolfes MA, Flannery B, et al; US Influenza Vaccine Effectiveness Network, the Influenza Hospitalization Surveillance Network, and the Assessment Branch, Immunization Services Division, Centers for Disease Control and Prevention. Effects of influenza vaccination in the United States during the 2018–2019 influenza season. *Clin Infect Dis.* 2020;71(8):e368–e376. PubMed doi: 10.1093/cid/ciz1244
59. Cowling BJ, Kwan MYW, Murphy C, et al. Influenza vaccine effectiveness against influenza-associated hospitalization in Hong Kong children aged 9 months to 17 years, March–June 2023. *J Pediatric Infect Dis Soc.* 2023;12(11):586–589. PubMed doi: 10.1093/jpids/piad083
60. Adams K, Weber ZA, Yang D-H, et al. Vaccine effectiveness against pediatric influenza-A-associated urgent care, emergency department, and hospital encounters during the 2022–2023 season: VISION Network. *Clin Infect Dis.* 2023; advance online publication. PubMed
61. Hood N, Flannery B, Gaglani M, et al. Influenza vaccine effectiveness among children: 2011-2020. *Pediatrics.* 2023;151(4):e2022059922. PubMed doi: 10.1542/peds.2022-059922
62. Cadieux G, Tamblyn R, Dauphinee D, Libman M. Predictors of inappropriate antibiotic prescribing among primary care physicians. *CMAJ.* 2007;177(8):877–883. PubMed doi: 10.1503/cmaj.070151
63. Ciesla G, Leader S, Stoddard J. Antibiotic prescribing rates in the US ambulatory care setting for patients diagnosed with influenza, 1997-2001. *Respir Med.* 2004;98(11):1093–1101. PubMed doi: 10.1016/j.rmed.2004.03.021
64. Wang EE, Einarson TR, Kellner JD, Conly JM. Antibiotic prescribing for Canadian preschool children: evidence of overprescribing for viral respiratory infections. *Clin Infect Dis.* 1999;29(1):155–160. PubMed doi: 10.1086/520145
65. Smith ER, Fry AM, Hicks LA, et al. Reducing antibiotic use in ambulatory care through influenza vaccination. *Clin Infect Dis.* 2020;71(11):e726–e734. PubMed doi: 10.1093/cid/ciaa464
66. Younas M, Royer J, Winders HR, et al. Temporal association between influenza vaccination coverage and ambulatory antibiotic use in children. *Pediatr Infect Dis J.* 2022;41(7):600–602. PubMed doi: 10.1097/INF.0000000000003533
67. Grijalva CG, Nguyen HQ, Zhu Y, et al. Estimated effectiveness of influenza vaccines in preventing secondary infections in households. *JAMA Netw Open.* 2024;7(11):e2446814. PubMed doi: 10.1001/jamanetworkopen.2024.46814
68. Pannaraj PS, Wang HL, Rivas H, et al. School-located influenza vaccination decreases laboratory-confirmed influenza and improves school attendance. *Clin Infect Dis.* 2014;59(3):325–332. PubMed doi: 10.1093/cid/ciu340
69. World Health Organization. Recommendations announced for influenza vaccine composition for the 2025–2026 northern hemisphere influenza season. Accessed March 25, 2025. https://www.who.int/news/item/28-02-2025-recommendations-announced-for-influenza-vaccine-composition-for-the-2025-2026-northern-hemisphere-influenza-season
70. US Food and Drug Administration. Influenza Vaccine Composition for the 2025-2026 U.S. Influenza Season. Accessed March 25, 2025. https://www.fda.gov/vaccines-blood-biologics/lot-release/use-trivalent-influenza-vaccines-2024-2025-us-influenza-season
71. Grohskopf LA, Ferdinands JM, Blanton LH, Broder KR,Loehr J. Prevention and control of seasonal influenza with vaccines: recommendations of the Advisory Committee on Immunization Practices-United States, 2024–25 influenza season. *MMWR Recomm Rep.* 2024;73(RR-5):1–25. doi: 10.15585/mmwr.rr7305a1
72. US Food and Drug Administration. Flublok package insert. Accessed May 25, 2025. https://www.fda.gov/media/179778/download
73. Dunkle LM, Izikson R, Patriarca PA, Goldenthal KL, Cox M, Treanor JJ. Safety and immunogenicity of a recombinant influenza vaccine: a randomized trial. *Pediatrics.* 2018;141(5):e20173021. PubMed doi: 10.1542/peds.2017-3021
74. Kim JH, Drame M, Puthanakit T, et al. Immunogenicity and safety of AS03-adjuvanted H5N1 influenza vaccine in children 6–35 months of age. *Pediatr Infect Dis J.* 2021;40(9):e333–e339. PubMed doi: 10.1097/INF.0000000000003247
75. Vesikari T, Kirstein J, Devota Go G, et al. Efficacy, immunogenicity, and safety evaluation of an MF59-adjuvanted quadrivalent influenza virus vaccine compared with non-adjuvanted influenza vaccine in children: a multicentre, randomised controlled, observer-blinded, phase 3 trial. *Lancet Respir Med.* 2018;6(5):345–356. PubMed doi: 10.1016/S2213-2600(18)30108-5
76. Palladino G, Ferrari A, Music N, Settembre EC, Wen Y. Improved immunologic responses to heterologous influenza strains in children with low preexisting antibody response vaccinated with MF59-adjuvanted influenza vaccine. *Vaccine.* 2021;39(38):5351–5357. PubMed doi: 10.1016/j.vaccine.2021.08.021
77. Chanthavanich P, Versage E, Van Twuijver E, Hohenboken M. Antibody responses against heterologous A/H5N1 strains for an

MF59-adjuvanted cell culture-derived A/H5N1 (aH5N1c) influenza vaccine in healthy pediatric subjects. *Vaccine.* 2021;39(47):6930–6935. PubMed doi: 10.1016/j.vaccine.2021.10.010

78. US Food and Drug Administration. Vaccines Licensed for Use in the United States. Accessed June 3, 2024. https://www.fda.gov/vaccines-blood-biologics/vaccines/vaccines-licensed-use-united-states.
79. US Food and Drug Administration. Fluzone quadrivalent, fluzone high-dose quadrivalent, fluzone, intradermal quadrivalent, fluzone quadrivalent southern hemisphere. Accessed May 2, 2022. https://www.fda.gov/vaccines-blood-biologics/vaccines/fluzone-quadrivalent
80. Robertson CA, Mercer M, Selmani A, Klein NP, Jeanfreau R, Greenberg DP. Safety and immunogenicity of a full-dose, split-virion, inactivated, quadrivalent influenza vaccine in healthy children 6–35 months of age: a randomized controlled clinical trial. *Pediatr Infect Dis J.* 2019;38(3):323–328. PubMed doi: 10.1097/INF.0000000000002227
81. US Food and Drug Administration. Afluria Quadrivalent. July 13, 2018. Accessed June 24, 2019. https://www.fda.gov/vaccines-blood-biologics/vaccines/afluria-quadrivalent
82. Janssen C, Mosnier A, Gavazzi G, et al. Coadministration of seasonal influenza and COVID-19 vaccines: A systematic review of clinical studies. *Hum Vaccin Immunother.* 2022;18(6):2131166. PubMed doi: 10.1080/21645515.2022.2131166
83. Moro PL, Zhang B, Ennulat C, et al. Safety of co-administration of mRNA COVID-19 and seasonal inactivated influenza vaccines in the vaccine adverse event reporting system (VAERS) during July 1, 2021-June 30, 2022. *Vaccine.* 2023;41(11):1859–1863. PubMed doi: 10.1016/j.vaccine.2022.12.069
84. Hause AM, Zhang B, Yue X, et al. Reactogenicity of simultaneous COVID-19 mRNA booster and influenza vaccination in the US. *JAMA Netw Open.* 2022;5(7):e2222241. PubMed doi: 10.1001/jamanetworkopen.2022.22241
85.. Centers for Disease Control and Prevention. Interim Clinical Considerations for Use of COVID-19 Vaccines Currently Authorized in the United States. Available at: https://www.cdc.gov/vaccines/covid-19/clinical-considerations/covid-19-vaccines-us.html. Accessed July 14, 2024.
86. World Health Organization, Global Advisory Committee on Vaccine Safety. Thimerosal in Vaccines. *Wkly Epidemiol Rec.* 2012;87:277–288.
87. Verstraeten T, Davis RL, DeStefano F, et al; Vaccine Safety Datalink Team. Safety of thimerosal-containing vaccines: a two-phased study of computerized health maintenance organization databases. *Pediatrics.* 2003;112(5):1039–1048. PubMed doi: 10.1542/peds.112.5.1039
88. Stehr-Green P, Tull P, Stellfeld M, Mortenson PB, Simpson D. Autism and thimerosal-containing vaccines: lack of consistent evidence for an association. *Am J Prev Med.* 2003;25(2):101–106. PubMed doi: 10.1016/S0749-3797(03)00113-2
89. Jenco M. CDC vaccine advisers call for flu vaccines without thimerosal; discussion based on misinformation. *AAP News.* June 26, 2025. Accessed July 5, 2025. https://publications.aap.org/aapnews/news/32530/CDC-vaccine-advisers-call-for-flu-vaccines-without?autologincheck=redirected
90. Rubin LG, Levin MJ, Ljungman P, et al; Infectious Diseases Society of America. 2013 IDSA clinical practice guideline for vaccination of the immunocompromised host. *Clin Infect Dis.* 2014;58(3):309–318. PubMed doi: 10.1093/cid/cit816
91. Centers for Disease Control and Prevention. Altered Immunocompetence. Accessed May 25, 2025. https://www.cdc.gov/vaccines/hcp/imz-best-practices/altered-immunocompetence.html
92. Danziger-Isakov L, Kumar D; AST ID Community of Practice. Vaccination of solid organ transplant candidates and recipients: Guidelines from the American society of transplantation infectious diseases community of practice. *Clin Transplant.* 2019;33(9):e13563. PubMed doi: 10.1111/ctr.13563
93. Maldonado YA, O'Leary ST, Ardura MI, et al; COMMITTEE ON INFECTIOUS DISEASES. Technical report. Recommendations for prevention and control of influenza in children, 2021–2022. *Pediatrics.* 2021;148(4):e2021053745. PubMed doi: 10.1542/peds.2021-053745
94. Centers for Disease Control and Prevention. General recommendations on immunization. Recommendations of the Advisory Committee on Immunization Practices (ACIP). *MMWR Recomm Rep.* 1994;43(RR-1):1–38. PubMed
95. US Food and Drug Administration. FluMist. Accessed May 25, 2025. https://www.fda.gov/media/180697/download?attachment
96. Jhaveri R, Allyne K. A feasibility trial of home administration of intranasal vaccine by parents to eligible children. *Clin Ther.* 2017;39(1):204-211.e4. PubMed doi: 10.1016/j.clinthera.2016.11.018
97. US Food and Drug Administration. FluMist package insert. Accessed June 6, 2023. https://www.fda.gov/media/160349/download
98. Centers for Disease Control and Prevention. General Best Practice Guidelines for Immunization. Altered Immunocompetence. Accessed May 31, 2025. https://www.cdc.gov/vaccines/hcp/imz-best-practices/altered-immunocompetence.html
99. Bandell A, Ambrose CS, Maniaci J, Wojtczak H. Safety of live attenuated influenza vaccine (LAIV) in children and adults with asthma: a systematic literature review and narrative synthesis. *Expert Rev Vaccines.* 2021;20(6):717–728. PubMed doi: 10.1080/14760584.2021.1925113
100. Bandell A, Giles L, Cervelo Bouzo P, et al. Safety of LAIV vaccination in asthma or wheeze: a systematic review and GRADE assessment. *Pediatrics.* 2025;155(5):e2024068459. PubMed doi: 10.1542/peds.2024-068459
101. Public Health Agency of Canada. Contraindications and precautions: Canadian Immunization Guide. Accessed May 25, 2025. https://www.canada.ca/en/public-health/services/publications/healthy-living/canadian-immunization-guide-part-2-vaccine-safety/page-3-contraindications-precautions-concerns.html
102. Weir JP, Gruber MF. An overview of the regulation of influenza vaccines in the United States. *Influenza Other Respir Viruses.* 2016;10(5):354–360. PubMed doi: 10.1111/irv.12383

103. Petrie JG, Ohmit SE, Truscon R, et al. Modest waning of influenza vaccine efficacy and antibody titers during the 2007-2008 influenza season. *J Infect Dis.* 2016;214(8):1142–1149. PubMed doi: 10.1093/infdis/jiw105

104. Radin JM, Hawksworth AW, Myers CA, Ricketts MN, Hansen EA, Brice GT. Influenza vaccine effectiveness: Maintained protection throughout the duration of influenza seasons 2010-2011 through 2013-2014. *Vaccine.* 2016;34(33):3907–3912. PubMed doi: 10.1016/j.vaccine.2016.05.034

105. Powell LN, Bégué RE. Influenza vaccine effectiveness among children for the 2017-2018 season. *J Pediatric Infect Dis Soc.* 2020; 9(4):468–473. PubMed doi: 10.1093/jpids/piz077

106. Sahni LC, Naioti EA, Olson SM, et al. Sustained within-season vaccine effectiveness against influenza-associated hospitalization in children: evidence from the New Vaccine Surveillance Network, 2015-2016 through 2019-2020. *Clin Infect Dis.* 2022; online ahead of print. PubMed

107. Ferdinands JM, Fry AM, Reynolds S, et al. Intraseason waning of influenza vaccine protection: Evidence from the US Influenza Vaccine Effectiveness Network, 2011-12 through 2014-15. *Clin Infect Dis.* 2017;64(5):544–550. PubMed doi: 10.1093/cid/ciw816

108. Castilla J, Martínez-Baz I, Martínez-Artola V, et al; Primary Health Care Sentinel Network; Network for Influenza Surveillance in Hospitals of Navarre. Decline in influenza vaccine effectiveness with time after vaccination, Navarre, Spain, season 2011/12. *Euro Surveill.* 2013;18(5):20388. PubMed doi: 10.2807/ese.18.05.20388-en

109. Kissling E, Valenciano M, Larrauri A, et al. Low and decreasing vaccine effectiveness against influenza A(H3) in 2011/12 among vaccination target groups in Europe: results from the I-MOVE multicentre case-control study. *Euro Surveill.* 2013;18(5):20390. PubMed doi: 10.2807/ese.18.05.20390-en

110. Belongia EA, Sundaram ME, McClure DL, Meece JK, Ferdinands J, VanWormer JJ. Waning vaccine protection against influenza A (H3N2) illness in children and older adults during a single season. *Vaccine.* 2015;33(1):246–251. PubMed doi: 10.1016/j.vaccine.2014.06.052

111. Puig-Barberà J, Mira-Iglesias A, Tortajada-Girbés M, et al; Valencia Hospital Network for the Study of Influenza and other Respiratory Viruses (VAHNSI, Spain). Waning protection of influenza vaccination during four influenza seasons, 2011/2012 to 2014/2015. *Vaccine.* 2017;35(43):5799–5807. PubMed doi: 10.1016/j.vaccine.2017.09.035

112. Ray GT, Lewis N, Klein NP, et al. Intraseason waning of influenza vaccine effectiveness. *Clin Infect Dis.* 2019;68(10):1623–1630. PubMed doi: 10.1093/cid/ciy770

113. Kissling E, Nunes B, Robertson C, et al; I-MOVE case–control study team. I-MOVE multicentre case-control study 2010/11 to 2014/15: Is there within-season waning of influenza type/subtype vaccine effectiveness with increasing time since vaccination? *Euro Surveill.* 2016;21(16). PubMed doi: 10.2807/1560-7917.ES.2016.21.16.30201

114. Pebody R, Andrews N, McMenamin J, et al. Vaccine effectiveness of 2011/12 trivalent seasonal influenza vaccine in preventing laboratory-confirmed influenza in primary care in the United Kingdom: evidence of waning intra-seasonal protection. *Euro Surveill.* 2013;18(5):20389. PubMed doi: 10.2807/ese.18.05.20389-en

115. Chung H, Campitelli MA, Buchan SA, et al; Canadian Immunization Research Network (CIRN) Provincial Collaborative Network (PCN) Investigators. Measuring waning protection from seasonal influenza vaccination during nine influenza seasons, Ontario, Canada, 2010/11 to 2018/19. *Euro Surveill.* 2024;29(8):2300239. PubMed doi: 10.2807/1560-7917.ES.2024.29.8.2300239

116. Doyon-Plourde P, Przepiorkowski J, Young K, Zhao L, Sinilaite A. Intraseasonal waning immunity of seasonal influenza vaccine - A systematic review and meta-analysis. *Vaccine.* 2023;41(31): 4462–4471. PubMed doi: 10.1016/j.vaccine.2023.06.038

117. Wagner AL, Sanchez N, Kubale J, et al. Single-dose vaccination among infants and toddlers provides modest protection against influenza illness, which wanes after 5 months. *J Infect Dis.* 2022; 227(1):87–91. PubMed doi: 10.1093/infdis/jiac288

118. Centers for Disease Control and Prevention. *CDC Yellow Book: Health Information for International Travel.* Atlanta, GA: Centers for Disease Control and Prevention; 2024. Accessed June 4, 2024. https://wwwnc.cdc.gov/travel/page/yellowbook-home

119. Centers for Disease Control and Prevention. General Best Practices for Immunization. Accessed May 25, 2025. https://www.cdc.gov/vaccines/hcp/imz-best-practices

120. Kelso JM, Greenhawt MJ, Li JT; Joint Task Force on Practice Parameters (JTFPP). Update on influenza vaccination of egg allergic patients. *Ann Allergy Asthma Immunol.* 2013;111(4):301–302. PubMed doi: 10.1016/j.anai.2013.07.030

121. Greenhawt M, Turner PJ, Kelso JM. Administration of influenza vaccines to egg allergic recipients: A practice parameter update 2017. *Ann Allergy Asthma Immunol.* 2018;120(1):49–52. PubMed doi: 10.1016/j.anai.2017.10.020

122. American College of Obstetricians and Gynecologists. ACOG Committee Opinion No. 732: Influenza vaccination during pregnancy. *Obstet Gynecol.* 2018;131(4):e109–e114. PubMed doi: 10.1097/AOG.0000000000002588

123. Robison SG, Osborn AW. The concordance of parent and child immunization. *Pediatrics.* 2017;139(5):e20162883. PubMed doi: 10.1542/peds.2016-2883

124. Zaman K, Roy E, Arifeen SE, et al. Effectiveness of maternal influenza immunization in mothers and infants. *N Engl J Med.* 2008; 359(15):1555–1564. PubMed doi: 10.1056/NEJMoa0708630

125. Tapia MD, Sow SO, Tamboura B, et al. Maternal immunisation with trivalent inactivated influenza vaccine for prevention of influenza in infants in Mali: a prospective, active-controlled, observer-blind, randomised phase 4 trial. *Lancet Infect Dis.* 2016;16(9):1026–1035. PubMed doi: 10.1016/S1473-3099(16)30054-8

126. Madhi SA, Cutland CL, Kuwanda L, et al; Maternal Flu Trial (Matflu) Team. Influenza vaccination of pregnant women and protection of their infants. *N Engl J Med.* 2014;371(10):918–931. PubMed doi: 10.1056/NEJMoa1401480

127. Steinhoff MC, Katz J, Englund JA, et al. Year-round influenza immunisation during pregnancy in Nepal: a phase 4, randomised,

placebo-controlled trial. *Lancet Infect Dis.* 2017;17(9):981–989. PubMed doi: 10.1016/S1473-3099(17)30252-9

128. Shakib JH, Korgenski K, Presson AP, et al. Influenza in infants born to women vaccinated during pregnancy. *Pediatrics.* 2016;137(6): e20152360. PubMed doi: 10.1542/peds.2015-2360

129. Nunes MC, Madhi SA. Influenza vaccination during pregnancy for prevention of influenza confirmed illness in the infants: A systematic review and meta-analysis. *Hum Vaccin Immunother.* 2018; 14(3):758–766. PubMed doi: 10.1080/21645515.2017.1345385

130. Thompson MG, Kwong JC, Regan AK, et al; PREVENT Workgroup. Influenza vaccine effectiveness in preventing influenza-associated hospitalizations during pregnancy: a multi-country retrospective test negative design study, 2010-2016. *Clin Infect Dis.* 2019;68(9): 1444–1453. PubMed doi: 10.1093/cid/ciy737

131. Nunes MC, Madhi SA. Prevention of influenza-related illness in young infants by maternal vaccination during pregnancy. *F1000 Res.* 2018;7:122. PubMed doi: 10.12688/f1000research.12473.1

132. Omer SB, Clark DR, Aqil AR, et al; for BMGF Supported Maternal Influenza Immunization Trials Investigators Group. Maternal influenza immunization and prevention of severe clinical pneumonia in young infants: analysis of randomized controlled trials conducted in Nepal, Mali and South Africa. *Pediatr Infect Dis J.* 2018;37(5):436–440. PubMed doi: 10.1097/INF.0000000000001914

133. Fell DB, Russell M, Fung SG, et al. Effectiveness of maternal influenza vaccination during pregnancy against laboratory-confirmed seasonal influenza among infants under 6 months of age in Ontario, Canada. *J Infect Dis.* 2024;230(1):e80–e92. PubMed doi: 10.1093/infdis/jiad539

134. Sahni LC, Olson SM, Halasa NB, et al; New Vaccine Surveillance Network Collaborators. Maternal Vaccine Effectiveness Against Influenza-Associated Hospitalizations and Emergency Department Visits in Infants. *JAMA Pediatr.* 2024;178(2):176–184. PubMed doi: 10.1001/jamapediatrics.2023.5639

135. Munoz FM, Jackson LA, Swamy GK, et al. Safety and immunogenicity of seasonal trivalent inactivated influenza vaccines in pregnant women. *Vaccine.* 2018;36(52):8054–8061. PubMed doi: 10.1016/j.vaccine.2018.10.088

136. Chambers CD, Johnson DL, Xu R, et al; OTIS Collaborative Research Group. Safety of the 2010-11, 2011-12, 2012-13, and 2013-14 seasonal influenza vaccines in pregnancy: Birth defects, spontaneous abortion, preterm delivery, and small for gestational age infants, a study from the cohort arm of VAMPSS. *Vaccine.* 2016;34(37): 4443–4449. PubMed doi: 10.1016/j.vaccine.2016.06.054

137. Donahue JG, Kieke BA, King JP, et al. Association of spontaneous abortion with receipt of inactivated influenza vaccine containing H1N1pdm09 in 2010-11 and 2011-12. *Vaccine.* 2017;35(40):5314–5322. PubMed doi: 10.1016/j.vaccine.2017.06.069

138. Donahue JG, Kieke BA, King JP, et al. Inactivated influenza vaccine and spontaneous abortion in the Vaccine Safety Datalink in 2012-13, 2013-14, and 2014-15. *Vaccine.* 2019;37(44):6673–6681. PubMed doi: 10.1016/j.vaccine.2019.09.035

139. Regan AK, Sullivan SG, Arah OA. Maternal influenza vaccination and associated risk of fetal loss: a claims-based prospective cohort study. *Vaccine.* 2024;42(26):126256. doi: 10.1016/j.vaccine.2024.126256

140. Sheffield JS, Greer LG, Rogers VL, et al. Effect of influenza vaccination in the first trimester of pregnancy. *Obstet Gynecol.* 2012; 120(3):532–537. PubMed doi: 10.1097/AOG.0b013e318263a278

141. Polyzos KA, Konstantelias AA, Pitsa CE, Falagas ME. Maternal influenza vaccination and risk for congenital malformations: a systematic review and meta-analysis. *Obstet Gynecol.* 2015;126(5): 1075–1084. PubMed doi: 10.1097/AOG.0000000000001068

142. Peppa M, Thomas SL, Minassian C, et al. Seasonal influenza vaccination during pregnancy and the risk of major congenital malformations in live-born infants: a 2010-2016 historical cohort study. *Clin Infect Dis.* 2021;73(11):e4296–e4304. PubMed doi: 10.1093/cid/ciaa845

143. Palmsten K, Suhl J, Conway KM, et al; National Birth Defects Prevention Study. Influenza vaccination during pregnancy and risk of selected major structural congenital heart defects, National Birth Defects Prevention Study 2006-2011. *Birth Defects Res.* 2023;115(1):88–95. PubMed doi: 10.1002/bdr2.2114

144. Becerra-Culqui TA, Getahun D, Chiu V, Sy LS, Tseng HF. Prenatal influenza vaccination or influenza infection and autism spectrum disorder in offspring. *Clin Infect Dis.* 2022;75(7):1140–1148. PubMed doi: 10.1093/cid/ciac101

145. Foo D, Sarna M, Pereira G, Moore HC, Regan AK. Association between maternal influenza vaccination and neurodevelopmental disorders in childhood: a longitudinal, population-based linked cohort study. *Arch Dis Child.* 2023;108(8):647–653. PubMed doi: 10.1136/archdischild-2022-324269

146. Chambers CD, Johnson D, Xu R, et al; OTIS Collaborative Research Group. Risks and safety of pandemic H1N1 influenza vaccine in pregnancy: birth defects, spontaneous abortion, preterm delivery, and small for gestational age infants. *Vaccine.* 2013;31(44): 5026–5032. PubMed doi: 10.1016/j.vaccine.2013.08.097

147. Nordin JD, Kharbanda EO, Vazquez Benitez G, Lipkind H, Vellozzi C, Destefano F; Vaccine Safety Datalink. Maternal influenza vaccine and risks for preterm or small for gestational age birth. *J Pediatr.* 2014;164(5):1051–1057.e2. PubMed doi: 10.1016/j.jpeds.2014.01.037

148. Robinson C, Oberye J, van Boxmeer J, et al. A prospective cohort study on pregnancy outcomes of persons immunized with a seasonal quadrivalent inactivated influenza vaccine during pregnancy. *Vaccines (Basel).* 2022;10(10):1577. PubMed doi: 10.3390/vaccines10101577

149. Duque J, Howe AS, Azziz-Baumgartner E, Petousis-Harris H. Multi-decade national cohort identifies adverse pregnancy and birth outcomes associated with acute respiratory illness hospitalisations during the influenza season. *Influenza Other Respir Viruses.* 2023;17(1):e13063. PubMed doi: 10.1111/irv.13063

150. Centers for Disease Control and Prevention. Influenza Vaccination Coverage, Pregnant Women, United States. Accessed May 25, 2025. https://www.cdc.gov/fluvaxview/dashboard/pregnant-women-coverage.html

151. Callahan AG, Coleman-Cowger VH, Schulkin J, Power ML. Racial disparities in influenza immunization during pregnancy in the

United States: A narrative review of the evidence for disparities and potential interventions. *Vaccine.* 2021;39(35):4938–4948. PubMed doi: 10.1016/j.vaccine.2021.07.028

152. Moll K, Wong HL, Fingar K, et al. Vaccine exposure during pregnancy among privately and publicly insured women in the United States, 2016-2018. *Vaccine.* 2021;39(41):6095–6103. PubMed doi: 10.1016/j.vaccine.2021.08.091

153. Kaur R, Callaghan T, Regan AK. Disparities in maternal influenza immunization among women in rural and urban areas of the United States. *Prev Med.* 2021;147:106531. PubMed doi: 10.1016/j.ypmed.2021.106531

154. Manji S, Idarraga Reyes L, McDonald S, et al. Improving influenza vaccine uptake during pregnancy through vaccination at point of care: a before-and-after study. *J Obstet Gynaecol Can.* 2024;46(11):102656. PubMed doi: 10.1016/j.jogc.2024.102656

155. Schlaudecker EP, Steinhoff MC, Omer SB, et al. IgA and neutralizing antibodies to influenza a virus in human milk: a randomized trial of antenatal influenza immunization. *PLoS One.* 2013;8(8):e70867. PubMed doi: 10.1371/journal.pone.0070867

156. Ackerson BK, Sy LS, Glenn SC, et al. Pediatric vaccination during the COVID-19 pandemic. *Pediatrics.* 2021;148(1):e2020047092. PubMed doi: 10.1542/peds.2020-047092

157. Bramer CA, Kimmins LM, Swanson R, et al. Decline in child vaccination coverage during the COVID-19 pandemic – Michigan Care Improvement Registry, May 2016-May 2020. *MMWR Morb Mortal Wkly Rep.* 2020;69(20):630–631. PubMed doi: 10.15585/mmwr.mm6920e1

158. O'Leary ST, Trefren L, Roth H, Moss A, Severson R, Kempe A. Number of childhood and adolescent vaccinations administered before and after the COVID-19 outbreak in Colorado. *JAMA Pediatr.* 2021;175(3):305–307. PubMed doi: 10.1001/jamapediatrics.2020.4733

159. Santoli JM, Lindley MC, DeSilva MB, et al. Effects of the COVID-19 pandemic on routine pediatric vaccine ordering and administration—United States, 2020. *MMWR Morb Mortal Wkly Rep.* 2020;69(19):591–593. PubMed doi: 10.15585/mmwr.mm6919e2

160. US Department of Health and Human Services, Office of Disease Prevention and Health Promotion. Healthy People 2030. Vaccination. Accessed June 4, 2024. https://health.gov/healthypeople/objectives-and-data/browse-objectives/vaccination

161. Centers for Disease Control and Prevention. Influenza Vaccination Coverage, Children 6 months through 17 years, United States. Accessed July 5, 2025. https://www.cdc.gov/fluvaxview/dashboard/children-vaccination-coverage.html

162. Geissler KH, Shieh M-S, Evans V, et al. Influenza vaccinations among privately and publicly insured children with asthma. *Acad Pediatr.* 2023;23(7):1368–1375. PubMed doi: 10.1016/j.acap.2023.02.010

163. Gates DM, Cohen SA, Orr K, Caffrey AR. Pediatric influenza vaccination rates lower than previous estimates in the United States. *Vaccine.* 2022;40(44):6337–6343. PubMed doi: 10.1016/j.vaccine.2022.09.053

164. Fogel B, Schaefer EW, Hicks SD. Early influenza vaccination rates decline in children during the COVID-19 pandemic. *Vaccine.* 2021;39(31):4291–4295. PubMed doi: 10.1016/j.vaccine.2021.06.041

165. Hill HA, Yankey D, Elam-Evans LD, et al. Decline in vaccination coverage by age 24 months and vaccination inequities among children born in 2020 and 2021—National Immunization Survey-Child, United States, 2021–2023. *MMWR Morb Mortal Wkly Rep.* 2024;73(38):844–853. PubMed doi: 10.15585/mmwr.mm7338a3

166. Santibanez TA, Nguyen KH, Greby SM, et al. Parental vaccine hesitancy and childhood influenza vaccination. *Pediatrics.* 2020;146(6):e2020007609. PubMed doi: 10.1542/peds.2020-007609

167. Vashist K, Yankey D, Elam-Evans LD, et al. Changes in vaccine hesitancy among parents of children aged 6 months - 17 Years, National Immunization Surveys, 2019-2022. *Vaccine.* 2024;42(20):125989. PubMed doi: 10.1016/j.vaccine.2024.05.037

168. Baumer-Mouradian SH, Hart RJ, Visotcky A, et al. Understanding influenza and SARS-CoV-2 vaccine hesitancy in racial and ethnic minority caregivers. *Vaccines (Basel).* 2022;10(11):1968. PubMed doi: 10.3390/vaccines10111968

169. Savoia E, Masterson E, Olander DR, Anderson E, Mohamed Farah A, Pirrotta L. Determinants of vaccine hesitancy among African American and Black individuals in the United States of America: a systematic literature review. *Vaccines (Basel).* 2024;12(3):277. PubMed doi: 10.3390/vaccines12030277

170. Freimuth VS, Jamison AM, An J, Hancock GR, Quinn SC. Determinants of trust in the flu vaccine for African Americans and Whites. *Soc Sci Med.* 2017;193:70–79. PubMed doi: 10.1016/j.socscimed.2017.10.001

171. Park YW, Bragard E, Madhivanan P, Fisher CB. A latent profile analysis of COVID-19 and influenza vaccine hesitancy among economically marginalized Hispanic mothers of children under five years of age in the US. *J Racial Ethn Health Disparities.* 2025;12(3):1824–1835. PubMed doi: 10.1007/s40615-024-02012-1

172. Harris JG, Favier L, Jones JT, et al. Influenza knowledge and barriers to vaccination in immunosuppressed patients in the pediatric rheumatology clinic. *Pediatr Rheumatol Online J.* 2024;22(1):104. PubMed doi: 10.1186/s12969-024-01048-1

173. Graham RJ, Enriquez LF, Elmi AF, et al. Influenza and COVID-19 vaccination rates among children receiving long-term ventilation. *JAMA Netw Open.* 2024;7(8):e2430989. PubMed doi: 10.1001/jamanetworkopen.2024.30989

174. Walden J, Stanek JR, Young J, Griffith MM, Nahata L, Creary SE. Influenza vaccine uptake among youth with sickle cell disease who are seen in clinic before and after the COVID-19 pandemic. *Vaccine.* 2024;42(22):126212. PubMed doi: 10.1016/j.vaccine.2024.126212

175. Yarnall JN, Mertens A, Yee M, Orenstein E, Lai KW, Wasilewski-Masker K. Influenza vaccination receipt in pediatric patients with cancer or sickle cell disease. *J Pediatr Hematol Oncol.* 2023;45(2):e228–e235. PubMed doi: 10.1097/MPH.0000000000002559

176. Hofstetter AM, Schaffer S. Childhood and adolescent vaccination in alternative settings. *Acad Pediatr.* 2021;21(4S):S50–S56. PubMed doi: 10.1016/j.acap.2021.02.001

177. Hart RJ, Paul RI, Levine A, Sikes K, Bryant K, Stevenson MD. Parent intent and willingness to immunize children against influenza in the pediatric emergency department. *Pediatr Emerg Care.* 2019;35(7):493–497. PubMed doi: 10.1097/PEC.0000000000001869

178. Meyer AJ, Smith JR, Wright TL, Engler LJ, Bigham MT, Bhalla T. Pediatric influenza vaccination in the perioperative setting: A quality improvement project. *Paediatr Anaesth.* 2024;34(2):167–174. PubMed doi: 10.1111/pan.14790

179. Alayari A, Ziniel SI, Hawkins E, Mackenzie J, Rao S. Evaluation of an influenza vaccination program in the pediatric emergency department. *J Pediatr.* 2025;282:114541. PubMed doi: 10.1016/j.jpeds.2025.114541

180. Hart R, Feygin Y, Kluthe T, Quinn KG, Rao S, Baumer-Mouradian SH. Emergency departments: An underutilized resource to address pediatric influenza vaccine coverage. *Vaccine.* 2023;41(47):7026–7032. PubMed doi: 10.1016/j.vaccine.2023.10.039

181. Westrick SC, Patterson BJ, Kader MS, Rashid S, Buck PO, Rothholz MC. National survey of pharmacy-based immunization services. *Vaccine.* 2018;36(37):5657–5664. PubMed doi: 10.1016/j.vaccine.2018.07.027

182. Gates DM, Cohen SA, Orr K, Caffrey AR. Demographic and clinical predictors of pharmacist-administered pediatric influenza immunization. *J Pharm Pract.* 2024;37(3):612–624. PubMed doi: 10.1177/08971900231155223

183. Zerr DM, Englund JA, Robertson AS, Marcuse EK, Garrison MM, Christakis DA. Hospital-based influenza vaccination of children: an opportunity to prevent subsequent hospitalization. *Pediatrics.* 2008;121(2):345–348. PubMed doi: 10.1542/peds.2007-2812

184. Pollack AH, Kronman MP, Zhou C, Zerr DM. Automated screening of hospitalized children for influenza vaccination. *J Pediatric Infect Dis Soc.* 2014;3(1):7–14. PubMed doi: 10.1093/jpids/pit044

185. Stockwell MS, Natarajan K, Ramakrishnan R, et al. Immunization data exchange with electronic health records. *Pediatrics.* 2016;137(6):e20154335. PubMed doi: 10.1542/peds.2015-4335

186. Stokley S, Kempe A, Stockwell MS, Szilagyi PG. Improving pediatric vaccination coverage in the United States. *Acad Pediatr.* 2021;21(4S):S1–S2. PubMed doi: 10.1016/j.acap.2021.03.004

187. Cataldi JR, Kerns ME, O'Leary ST. Evidence-based strategies to increase vaccination uptake: a review. *Curr Opin Pediatr.* 2020;32(1):151–159. PubMed doi: 10.1097/MOP.0000000000000843

188. Clark SJ, Butchart A, Kennedy A, Dombkowski KJ. Parents' experiences with and preferences for immunization reminder/recall technologies. *Pediatrics.* 2011;128(5):e1100–e1105. PubMed doi: 10.1542/peds.2011-0270

189. Daley MF, Barrow J, Pearson K, et al. Identification and recall of children with chronic medical conditions for influenza vaccination. *Pediatrics.* 2004;113(1 Pt 1):e26–e33. PubMed doi: 10.1542/peds.113.1.e26

190. Tuckerman J, Harper K, Sullivan TR, et al. Short message service reminder nudge for parents and influenza vaccination uptake in children and adolescents with special risk medical conditions: The Flutext-4U randomized clinical trial. *JAMA Pediatr.* 2023;177(4):337–344. PubMed doi: 10.1001/jamapediatrics.2022.6145

191. Jacobson Vann JC, Jacobson RM, Coyne-Beasley T, Asafu-Adjei JK, Szilagyi PG. Patient reminder and recall interventions to improve immunization rates. *Cochrane Database Syst Rev.* 2018;1(1):CD003941. PubMed doi: 10.1002/14651858.CD003941.pub3

192. Hofstetter AM, Vargas CY, Camargo S, et al. Impacting delayed pediatric influenza vaccination: a randomized controlled trial of text message reminders. *Am J Prev Med.* 2015;48(4):392–401. PubMed doi: 10.1016/j.amepre.2014.10.023

193. Stockwell MS, Hofstetter AM, DuRivage N, et al. Text message reminders for second dose of influenza vaccine: a randomized controlled trial. *Pediatrics.* 2015;135(1):e83–e91. PubMed doi: 10.1542/peds.2014-2475

194. Szilagyi PG, Duru OK, Casillas A, et al. Text vs patient portal messaging to improve influenza vaccination coverage: a health system-wide randomized clinical trial. *JAMA Intern Med.* 2024;184(5):519–527. PubMed doi: 10.1001/jamainternmed.2024.0001

195. Scott VP, Opel DJ, Reifler J, et al. Office-based educational handout for influenza vaccination: a randomized controlled trial. *Pediatrics.* 2019;144(2):e20182580. PubMed doi: 10.1542/peds.2018-2580

196. Daley MF, Narwaney KJ, Shoup JA, Wagner NM, Glanz JM. Addressing parents' vaccine concerns: a randomized trial of a social media intervention. *Am J Prev Med.* 2018;55(1):44–54. PubMed doi: 10.1016/j.amepre.2018.04.010

197. Williams JTB, Johnson D, Weinshenker D, O'Leary ST. Co-creation of pediatric influenza digital stories via rapid community translation. *Vaccine.* 2025;51:126866. PubMed doi: 10.1016/j.vaccine.2025.126866

198. Hofstetter AM, Robinson JD, Lepere K, Cunningham M, Etsekson N, Opel DJ. Clinician-parent discussions about influenza vaccination of children and their association with vaccine acceptance. *Vaccine.* 2017;35(20):2709–2715. PubMed doi: 10.1016/j.vaccine.2017.03.077

199. Limaye RJ, Opel DJ, Dempsey A, et al. Communicating with vaccine-hesitant parents: a narrative review. *Acad Pediatr.* 2021;21(4S):S24–S29. PubMed doi: 10.1016/j.acap.2021.01.018

200. Stephens AB, Hofstetter AM, Stockwell MS. Influenza vaccine hesitancy: scope, influencing factors, and strategic interventions. *Pediatr Clin North Am.* 2023;70(2):227–241. PubMed doi: 10.1016/j.pcl.2022.11.003

201. O'Leary ST, Opel DJ, Cataldi JR, et al; COMMITTEE ON INFECTIOUS DISEASES; COMMITTEE ON PRACTICE AND AMBULATORY MEDICINE; COMMITTEE ON BIOETHICS. Strategies for improving vaccine communication and uptake. *Pediatrics.* 2024;153(3):e2023065483. PubMed doi: 10.1542/peds.2023-065483

202. Rao S, Ziniel SI, Khan I, Dempsey A. Be inFLUential: Evaluation of a multifaceted intervention to increase influenza vaccination rates among pediatric inpatients. *Vaccine.* 2020;38(6):1370–1377. PubMed doi: 10.1016/j.vaccine.2019.12.010

203. Stockwell MS, Catallozzi M, Camargo S, et al. Registry-linked electronic influenza vaccine provider reminders: a cluster-crossover trial. *Pediatrics.* 2015;135(1):e75–e82. PubMed doi: 10.1542/peds.2014-2616

204. Lessin HR, Edwards KM; American Academy of Pediatrics, Committee on Practice and Ambulatory Medicine, Committee on Infectious Diseases. Immunizing parents and other close family contacts in the pediatric office setting. *Pediatrics.* 2012;129(1): e247–e253. Reaffirmed August 2016.

205. Corley AMS, Gomes SM, Crosby LE, et al. Partnering with faith-based organizations to offer flu vaccination and other preventive services. *Pediatrics.* 2022;150(3):e2022056193. PubMed doi: 10.1542/peds.2022-056193

206. Centers for Disease Control and Prevention. Influenza and COVID-19 Vaccination Coverage Among Health Care Personnel – United States, 2023-24 Influenza Season. Accessed May 25, 2025. https://www.cdc.gov/fluvaxview/coverage-by-season/health-care-personnel-coverage-2023-24.html

207. Frederick J, Brown AC, Cummings DA, et al. Protecting healthcare personnel in outpatient settings: the influences of mandatory versus nonmandatory influenza vaccination policies on workplace absenteeism during multiple respiratory virus seasons. *Infect Control Hosp Epidemiol.* 2018;39(4):452–461. PubMed doi: 10.1017/ice.2018.9

208. Centers for Disease Control and Prevention. Influenza Antiviral Medications. Accessed April 14, 2022. https://www.cdc.gov/flu/hcp/antivirals/summary-clinicians.html#Table1

209. Uyeki TM, Bernstein HH, Bradley JS, et al. Clinical practice guidelines by the Infectious Diseases Society of America (IDSA): 2018 Update diagnosis, treatment, chemoprophylaxis and institutional outbreak management of seasonal influenza. *Clin Infect Dis.* 2019; 68(6):e1–e47. PubMed doi: 10.1093/cid/ciy866

210. Louie JK, Yang S, Samuel MC, Uyeki TM, Schechter R. Neuraminidase inhibitors for critically ill children with influenza. *Pediatrics.* 2013;132(6):e1539–e1545. PubMed doi: 10.1542/peds.2013-2149

211. Katzen J, Kohn R, Houk JL, Ison MG. Early oseltamivir after hospital admission is associated with shortened hospitalization: a 5-year analysis of oseltamivir timing and clinical outcomes. *Clin Infect Dis.* 2019;69(1):52–58. PubMed doi: 10.1093/cid/ciy860

212. Ramirez J, Peyrani P, Wiemken T, Chaves SS, Fry AM. A randomized study evaluating the effectiveness of oseltamivir initiated at the time of hospital admission in adults hospitalized with influenza-associated lower respiratory tract infections. *Clin Infect Dis.* 2018;67(5):736–742. PubMed doi: 10.1093/cid/ciy163

213. Centers for Disease Control and Prevention, Health Alert Network. Interim Guidance for Clinicians to Prioritize Antiviral Treatment of Influenza in the Setting of Reduced Availability of Oseltamivir. Accessed April 11, 2023. https://emergency.cdc.gov/han/2022/han00482.asp

214. Xu M, Cai T, Yue T, et al. Comparative effectiveness of oseltamivir versus peramivir for hospitalized children (aged 0-5 years) with influenza infection. *Int J Infect Dis.* 2023;128:157–165. PubMed doi: 10.1016/j.ijid.2022.12.043

215. Wang J, Chen H, Zhuo L, et al. Effectiveness of intravenous peramivir for the treatment of influenza A/H3N2 and influenza B/Victoria in hospitalized children. *J Infect Chemother.* 2023;29(9): 843–848. PubMed doi: 10.1016/j.jiac.2023.05.004

216. US Food and Drug Administration. Approval package for XOFLUZA. Accessed May 29, 2022. https://www.accessdata.fda.gov/drugsatfda_docs/nda/2019/210854Orig1s001.pdf

217. Baker J, Block SL, Matharu B, et al. Baloxavir marboxil single-dose treatment in influenza-infected children: a randomized, double-blind, active controlled phase 3 safety and efficacy trial (miniSTONE-2). *Pediatr Infect Dis J.* 2020;39(8):700–705. PubMed doi: 10.1097/INF.0000000000002747

218. Taieb V, Ikeoka H, Wojciechowski P, et al. Efficacy and safety of baloxavir marboxil versus neuraminidase inhibitors in the treatment of influenza virus infection in high-risk and uncomplicated patients - a Bayesian network meta-analysis. *Curr Med Res Opin.* 2021;37(2):225–244. PubMed doi: 10.1080/03007995.2020.1839400

219. Ison MG, Portsmouth S, Yoshida Y, et al. Early treatment with baloxavir marboxil in high-risk adolescent and adult outpatients with uncomplicated influenza (CAPSTONE-2): a randomised, placebo-controlled, phase 3 trial. *Lancet Infect Dis.* 2020;20(10): 1204–1214. PubMed doi: 10.1016/S1473-3099(20)30004-9

220. Kakuya F, Haga S, Okubo H, Fujiyasu H, Kinebuchi T. Effectiveness of baloxavir marboxil against influenza in children. *Pediatr Int.* 2019; 61(6):616–618. PubMed doi: 10.1111/ped.13855

221. Nezu K, Hayashida S, Nagano N, Udagawa S, Morioka I. Early fever resolution in early childhood influenza treated with baloxavir marboxil: a retrospective study compared to those with oseltamivir. *Medicina (Kaunas).* 2023;59(9):1543. PubMed doi: 10.3390/medicina59091543

222. Sun Y, Wagatsuma K, Saito R, et al. Duration of fever in children infected with influenza A(H1N1)pdm09, A(H3N2) or B virus and treated with baloxavir marboxil, oseltamivir, laninamivir, or zanamivir in Japan during the 2012-2013 and 2019-2020 influenza seasons. *Antiviral Res.* 2024;228:105938. PubMed doi: 10.1016/j.antiviral.2024.105938

223. Baker JB, Block SL, Cagas SE, et al. Safety and efficacy of baloxavir marboxil in influenza-infected children 5-11 years of age: a post hoc analysis of a phase 3 study. *Pediatr Infect Dis J.* 2023;42(11): 983–989. PubMed doi: 10.1097/INF.0000000000004062

224. Hirotsu N, Sakaguchi H, Fukao K, et al. Baloxavir safety and clinical and virologic outcomes in influenza virus-infected pediatric patients by age group: age-based pooled analysis of two pediatric studies conducted in Japan. *BMC Pediatr.* 2023;23(1):35. PubMed doi: 10.1186/s12887-023-03841-5

225. Ison MG, Portsmouth S, Yoshida Y, Shishido T, Hayden F, Uehara T. LB16. Phase 3 trial of baloxavir marboxil in high-risk influenza patients (CAPSTONE-2 Study). *Open Forum Infect Dis.* 2018; 5(suppl 1):S764–S765. doi: 10.1093/ofid/ofy229.2190

226. US Food and Drug Administration. 2024-2025 Influenza Season: Availability of Antiviral Medications (Updated 3/13/25). Available at: https://www.fda.gov/media/120654/download. Accessed March 30, 2025.

227. Dobson J, Whitley RJ, Pocock S, Monto AS. Oseltamivir treatment for influenza in adults: a meta-analysis of randomised controlled trials. *Lancet.* 2015;385(9979):1729–1737. PubMed doi: 10.1016/S0140-6736(14)62449-1

228. Jefferson T, Jones MA, Doshi P, et al. Neuraminidase inhibitors for preventing and treating influenza in healthy adults and children. *Cochrane Database Syst Rev.* 2012;1(4):CD008965. PubMed

229. Malosh RE, Martin ET, Heikkinen T, Brooks WA, Whitley RJ, Monto AS. Efficacy and safety of oseltamivir in children: systematic review and individual patient data meta-analysis of randomized controlled trials. *Clin Infect Dis.* 2018;66(10):1492–1500. PubMed doi: 10.1093/cid/cix1040

230. Uyeki TM. Oseltamivir treatment of influenza in children. *Clin Infect Dis.* 2018;66(10):1501–1503. PubMed doi: 10.1093/cid/cix1150

231. Wang K, Shun-Shin M, Gill P, Perera R, Harnden A. Neuraminidase inhibitors for preventing and treating influenza in children (published trials only) [Review]. *Cochrane Database Syst Rev.* 2012; 2012(4):CD002744. PubMed doi: 10.1002/14651858.CD002744.pub4

232. Domínguez A, Romero-Tamarit A, Soldevila N, et al; Surveillance of Hospitalized Cases of Severe Influenza in Catalonia Working Group. Effectiveness of antiviral treatment in preventing death in severe hospitalised influenza cases over six seasons. *Epidemiol Infect.* 2018;146(7):799–808. PubMed doi: 10.1017/S0950268818000663

233. Hsu J, Santesso N, Mustafa R, et al. Antivirals for treatment of influenza: a systematic review and meta-analysis of observational studies. *Ann Intern Med.* 2012;156(7):512–524. PubMed doi: 10.7326/0003-4819-156-7-201204030-00411

234. Muthuri SG, Venkatesan S, Myles PR, et al; PRIDE Consortium Investigators. Effectiveness of neuraminidase inhibitors in reducing mortality in patients admitted to hospital with influenza A H1N1pdm09 virus infection: a meta-analysis of individual participant data. *Lancet Respir Med.* 2014;2(5):395–404. PubMed doi: 10.1016/S2213-2600(14)70041-4

235. Venkatesan S, Myles PR, Leonardi-Bee J, et al. Impact of outpatient neuraminidase inhibitor treatment in patients infected with influenza A(/H1N1)pdm09 at high risk of hospitalization: an individual participant data metaanalysis. *Clin Infect Dis.* 2017;64(10):1328–1334. PubMed doi: 10.1093/cid/cix127

236. Tejada S, Tejo AM, Peña-López Y, Forero CG, Corbella X, Rello J. Neuraminidase inhibitors and single dose baloxavir are effective and safe in uncomplicated influenza: a meta-analysis of randomized controlled trials. *Expert Rev Clin Pharmacol.* 2021;14(7):901–918. PubMed doi: 10.1080/17512433.2021.1917378

237. Dawood FS, Jara J, Gonzalez R, et al. A randomized, double-blind, placebo-controlled trial evaluating the safety of early oseltamivir treatment among children 0-9 years of age hospitalized with influenza in El Salvador and Panama. *Antiviral Res.* 2016;133:85–94. PubMed doi: 10.1016/j.antiviral.2016.07.007

238. Campbell AP, Tokars JI, Reynolds S, et al. Influenza antiviral treatment and length of stay. *Pediatrics.* 2021;148(4):e2021050417. PubMed doi: 10.1542/peds.2021-050417

239. Miyakawa R, Barreto NB, Kato RM, Neely MN, Russell CJ. Early use of anti-influenza medications in hospitalized children with tracheostomy. *Pediatrics.* 2019;143(3):e20182608. PubMed doi: 10.1542/peds.2018-2608

240. Walsh PS, Schnadower D, Zhang Y, Ramgopal S, Shah SS, Wilson PM. Association of early oseltamivir with improved outcomes in hospitalized children with influenza, 2007-2020. *JAMA Pediatr.* 2022; 176(11):e223261. PubMed doi: 10.1001/jamapediatrics.2022.3261

241. Hayden FG, Asher J, Cowling BJ, et al. Reducing influenza virus transmission: the potential value of antiviral treatment. *Clin Infect Dis.* 2022;74(3):532–540. PubMed doi: 10.1093/cid/ciab625

242. Bassett HK, Coon ER, Mansbach JM, Snow K, Wheeler M, Schroeder AR. Misclassification of both influenza infection and oseltamivir exposure status in administrative data. *JAMA Pediatr.* 2024; 178(2):201–203. PubMed doi: 10.1001/jamapediatrics.2023.5731

243. Li L, Liu J, Qin K. Comparison of double-dose vs standard-dose oseltamivir in the treatment of influenza: A systematic review and meta-analysis. *J Clin Pharm Ther.* 2020;45(5):918–926. Published online June 4, 2020 PubMed doi: 10.1111/jcpt.13203

244. Kumar D, Ison MG, Mira JP, et al. Combining baloxavir marboxil with standard-of-care neuraminidase inhibitor in patients hospitalised with severe influenza (FLAGSTONE): a randomised, parallel-group, double-blind, placebo-controlled, superiority trial. *Lancet Infect Dis.* 2022;22(5):718–730. PubMed doi: 10.1016/S1473-3099(21)00469-2

245. Howard A, Uyeki TM, Fergie J. Influenza-associated acute necrotizing encephalopathy in siblings. *J Pediatric Infect Dis Soc.* 2018; 7(3):e172–e177. PubMed doi: 10.1093/jpids/piy033

246. Takeuchi S, Tetsuhashi M, Sato D. Oseltamivir phosphate-Lifting the restriction on its use to treat teenagers with influenza in Japan [commentary]. *Pharmacoepidemiol Drug Saf.* 2019;28(4): 434–436. PubMed doi: 10.1002/pds.4721

247. Toovey S, Prinssen EP, Rayner CR, et al. Post-marketing assessment of neuropsychiatric adverse events in influenza patients treated with oseltamivir: an updated review. *Adv Ther.* 2012; 29(10):826–848. PubMed doi: 10.1007/s12325-012-0050-8

248. Antoon JW, Williams DJ, Bruce J, et al. Population-based incidence of influenza-associated serious neuropsychiatric events in children and adolescents. *JAMA Pediatr.* 2023;177(9):967–969. PubMed doi: 10.1001/jamapediatrics.2023.2304

249. Antoon JW, Sarker J, Abdelaziz A, et al. Trends in outpatient influenza antiviral use among children and adolescents in the United States. *Pediatrics.* 2023;152(6):e2023061960. PubMed doi: 10.1542/peds.2023-061960

250. Antoon JW, Hall M, Feinstein JA, et al. Guideline-concordant antiviral treatment in children at high risk for influenza complications. *Clin Infect Dis.* 2023;76(3):e1040–e1046. PubMed doi: 10.1093/cid/ciac606

251. Hamdan L, Probst V, Haddadin Z, et al. Influenza clinical testing and oseltamivir treatment in hospitalized children with acute respiratory illness, 2015-2016. *Influenza Other Respir Viruses.* 2022; 16(2):289–297. PubMed doi: 10.1111/irv.12927

252. Mehta K, Morris SK, Bettinger JA, et al; Canadian Immunization Monitoring Program Active (IMPACT) Investigators. Antiviral use in Canadian children hospitalized for influenza. *Pediatrics.* 2021;148(4):e2020049672. PubMed doi: 10.1542/peds.2020-049672

253. Walsh PS, Schnadower D, Zhang Y, Ramgopal S, Shah SS, Wilson PM. Assessment of temporal patterns and patient factors associated with oseltamivir administration in children hospitalized

with influenza, 2007-2020. *JAMA Netw Open.* 2022;5(9):e2233027. PubMed doi: 10.1001/jamanetworkopen.2022.33027

254. Antoon JW, Amarin JZ, Hamdan O, et al. Antiviral use among children hospitalized with laboratory-confirmed influenza illness: a prospective, multicenter surveillance study. *Clin Infect Dis.* 2024;ciae573. PubMed doi: 10.1093/cid/ciae573

255. Frutos AM, Ahmad HM, Ujamaa D, et al. Underutilization of influenza antiviral treatment among children and adolescents at higher risk for influenza-associated complications—United States, 2023–2024. *MMWR Morb Mortal Wkly Rep.* 2024;73(45): 1022–1029. PubMed doi: 10.15585/mmwr.mm7345a2

256. Ikematsu H, Hayden FG, Kawaguchi K, et al. Baloxavir marboxil for prophylaxis against influenza in household contacts. *N Engl J Med.* 2020;383(4):309–320. PubMed doi: 10.1056/NEJMoa1915341

257. Leung RC, Ip JD, Chen LL, Chan WM, To KK. Global emergence of neuraminidase inhibitor-resistant influenza A(H1N1)pdm09 viruses with I223V and S247N mutations: implications for antiviral resistance monitoring. *Lancet Microbe.* 2024;5(7):627–628. PubMed doi: 10.1016/S2666-5247(24)00037-5

258. Centers for Disease Control and Prevention. Weekly US Influenza Surveillance Report: Key Updates for Week 11, ending March 15, 2025. Accessed May 25, 2025. https://www.cdc.gov/fluview/surveillance/2025-week-11.html

259. Centers for Disease Control and Prevention. Interim guidance on the use of antiviral medications for treatment of human infections with novel influenza A viruses associated with severe human disease. Accessed April 16, 2025. https://www.cdc.gov/bird-flu/hcp/novel-av-treatment-guidance/index.html

260. de Jong MD, Tran TT, Truong HK, et al. Oseltamivir resistance during treatment of influenza A (H5N1) infection. *N Engl J Med.* 2005; 353(25):2667–2672. PubMed doi: 10.1056/NEJMoa054512

261. Centers for Disease Control and Prevention Health Alert Network. Accelerated Subtyping of Influenza A in Hospitalized Patients. Accessed March 29, 2025. https://www.cdc.gov/han/2025/han00520.html

262. Schuster JE, Hamdan L, Dulek DE, et al; Pediatric HCT Flu Study Group. Influenza vaccine in pediatric recipients of hematopoietic-cell transplants. *N Engl J Med.* 2023;388(4):374–376. PubMed doi: 10.1056/NEJMc2210825

263. Schuster JE, Hamdan L, Dulek DE, et al; Pediatric HCT Flu Study. The durability of antibody responses of two doses of high-dose relative to two doses of standard-dose inactivated influenza vaccine in pediatric hematopoietic cell transplant recipients: a multi-center randomized controlled trial. *Clin Infect Dis.* 2024;78(1):217–226. PubMed doi: 10.1093/cid/ciad534

264. Bahakel H, Spieker AJ, Hayek H, et al; Pediatric HCT Flu Study. Immunogenicity and reactogenicity of high- or standard-dose influenza vaccine in a second consecutive influenza season. *J Infect Dis.* 2025;231(1):e123–e131. PubMed doi: 10.1093/infdis/jiae454

265. Kempe A, Saville AW, Albertin C, et al. Parental hesitancy about routine childhood and influenza vaccinations: a national survey. *Pediatrics.* 2020;146(1):e20193852. PubMed doi: 10.1542/peds.2019-3852

266. Santibanez TA, Black CL, Zhou T, Srivastav A, Singleton JA. Parental hesitancy about COVID-19, influenza, HPV, and other childhood vaccines. *Vaccine.* 2024;42(25):126139. doi: 10.1016/j.vaccine.2024.07.040

267. Glanz JM, Wagner NM, Narwaney KJ, et al. Web-based social media intervention to increase vaccine acceptance: a randomized controlled trial. *Pediatrics.* 2017;140(6):e20171117. PubMed doi: 10.1542/peds.2017-1117

268. Frutos AM, Price AM, Harker E, et al; CDC Influenza Vaccine Effectiveness Collaborators. Interim estimates of 2023–24 seasonal influenza vaccine effectiveness—United States. *MMWR Morb Mortal Wkly Rep.* 2024;73(8):168–174. PubMed doi: 10.15585/mmwr.mm7308a3

Recommendations for the Prevention of RSV Disease in Infants and Children

- *Policy Statement*

POLICY STATEMENT Organizational Principles to Guide and Define the Child Health System and/or Improve the Health of All Children

American Academy of Pediatrics

DEDICATED TO THE HEALTH OF ALL CHILDREN™

Recommendations for the Prevention of RSV Disease in Infants and Children: Policy Statement

Committee on Infectious Diseases

RECOMMENDED POPULATIONS

The American Academy of Pediatrics (AAP) recommends respiratory syncytial virus (RSV) immunization[1] for:

- infants <8 months of age born during or entering their first RSV season if:
  - pregnant parent did not receive RSVpreF vaccine during this pregnancy,
  - pregnant parent's RSVpreF vaccination status is unknown, or
  - infant was born <14 days after the pregnant parent's RSVpreF vaccination
- infants and children 8 through 19 months of age at high risk of severe RSV disease and entering their second RSV season, regardless of the RSV vaccination status of the pregnant parent or the child's prior receipt of nirsevimab or clesrovimab when <8 months of age in their first RSV season. High-risk criteria include the following:
  - Children with chronic lung disease of prematurity who required medical support (chronic corticosteroid therapy, diuretic therapy, or supplemental oxygen) at any time during the 6-month period before the start of the second RSV season
  - Children with severe immunocompromise
  - Children with cystic fibrosis who have either:
    - manifestations of severe lung disease (previous hospitalization for pulmonary exacerbation in the first year of life or abnormalities on chest imaging that persist when stable), or
    - weight-for-length that is less than the 10th percentile
  - American Indian or Alaska Native children

Note that all ages refer to chronologic age, not corrected age.

EQUITY CONSIDERATIONS

American Indian and Alaska Native Children are included in the high-risk category, because they experience significantly higher rates of severe RSV

CONFLICT OF INTEREST DISCLOSURE: Sean O'Leary, MD, MPH, FAAP, has no potential conflicts of interest to disclose. Claudia Espinosa, MD, MSc, FAAP, has disclosed a direct to institution financial relationship with Merck and Sanofi as a research site Principal Investigator. Dr Espinosa did not participate in making recommendations or development of this statement. Other disclosures of committee members were reviewed and determined not relevant to the work related to the statement.

FUNDING: No external funding.

Policy statements from the American Academy of Pediatrics benefit from expertise and resources of liaisons and internal (AAP) and external reviewers. However, policy statements from the American Academy of Pediatrics may not reflect the views of the liaisons or the organizations or government agencies that they represent.

The guidance in this statement does not indicate an exclusive course of treatment or serve as a standard of medical care. Variations, taking into account individual circumstances, may be appropriate.

All policy statements from the American Academy of Pediatrics automatically expire 5 years after publication unless reaffirmed, revised, or retired at or before that time.

https://doi.org/10.1542/peds.2025-073923

To cite: American Academy of Pediatrics, Committee on Infectious Diseases. Recommendations for the Prevention of RSV Disease in Infants and Children: Policy Statement. *Pediatrics*. 2025;156(5):e2025073923

disease and hospitalization, with children living in rural and reservation communities most impacted. Evidence supports that this increased risk is associated with social drivers of health, with specific attention to running water access, transportation difficulties, household crowding, and indoor air quality.[2]

APPROVED PRODUCTS

Nirsevimab and Clesrovimab

Nirsevimab and clesrovimab[3,4] are considered the first-line recommended immunization products for administration to infants to protect against medically attended RSV disease. They are long-acting monoclonal antibody products administered as a single dose for administration during an infant's first RSV season. The AAP recommends any licensed RSV immunization product appropriate for age and health status and does not prefer one product over another.

- Only children 8 through 19 months who meet high-risk criteria should receive RSV immunization in their second RSV season. Nirsevimab is approved for this indication; clesrovimab is not.
- While the timing of the onset and duration of RSV season may vary, RSV immunization may be administered from October through the end of March in most of the continental United States. The timing of the onset, peak, and decline of RSV activity vary geographically, and providers may adjust timing of administration based on guidance from public health authorities (eg, Centers for Disease Control and Prevention [CDC], local health departments) or regional medical centers.
- Infants born during the RSV season should receive RSV immunization within 1 week of birth, ideally during their birth hospitalization. However, administration can occur during any visit to a health care setting, including well-child visits.
- Eligible infants with prolonged birth hospitalizations because of prematurity or other causes, who are discharged during RSV season, should receive RSV immunization shortly before or promptly after discharge from the hospital.
- Eligible infants who are <8 months of age and born outside of RSV season should receive RSV immunization shortly before or during the RSV season. Administration can occur during any visit to a health care setting, including well-child visits.
- In accordance with AAP's general best practices for immunizations, (https://publications.aap.org/redbook) simultaneous administration of RSV immunization with age-appropriate vaccines is recommended. In clinical trials, when RSV immunization was administered concomitantly with routine childhood vaccines, the safety and reactogenicity profile of the concomitantly administered regimen was similar to that of the childhood vaccines administered alone. When concomitantly administered, RSV immunization is not expected to interfere with the immune response to other vaccines.
- Immunization is not needed for most infants <8 months of age whose pregnant parent received RSVpreF vaccine during the pregnancy and ≥14 days before giving birth. RSV immunization may be considered for infants born to a vaccinated pregnant parent in rare circumstances when, based on the clinical judgment of the health care provider, the potential incremental benefit of administration is warranted. These situations include, but are not limited to:
  - Infants born to pregnant people who may not mount an adequate immune response to RSV vaccination (eg, pregnant people with immunocompromising conditions)
  - Infants born to pregnant people who have medical conditions associated with reduced transplacental antibody transfer (eg, pregnant people living with HIV infection)
  - Infants who have undergone cardiopulmonary bypass (see nirsevimab FDA package insert and clesrovimab FDA package insert) or extracorporeal membrane oxygenation (ECMO), leading to loss of maternal antibodies
  - Infants with substantial increased risk for severe RSV disease (eg, hemodynamically significant congenital heart disease, intensive care admission with a requirement of oxygen at discharge)

Palivizumab

Palivizumab is a short-acting monoclonal antibody product that is administered in monthly doses during the RSV season. Palivizumab is no longer routinely recommended for use and will be discontinued as of December 31, 2025.

Additional Information

- RSV Immunization Administration Visual Guide (AAP.org/rsv)
- RSV Immunization Frequently Asked Questions (AAP.org/rsv)
- *Red Book* Chapter on Respiratory Syncytial Virus (https://publications.aap.org/redbook)
- RSV Immunization Information Statement (https://www.immunize.org/vaccines/vis/iis-rsv/)

COMMITTEE ON INFECTIOUS DISEASES, 2025–2026

Sean T. O'Leary, MD, MPH, FAAP, Chairperson
James D. Campbell, MD, MS, FAAP, Vice Chairperson
Monica I. Ardura, DO, MSCS, FAAP
Kristina A. Bryant, MD, FAAP, *Red Book Online* Team Lead
Roberta L. DeBiasi, MD, MS, FAAP
Claudia Espinosa, MD, MSc, FAAP

Robert W. Frenck, Jr, MD, FAAP
C. Mary Healy, MD
Betsy C. Herold, MD, FAAP
Chandy C. John, MD, MS, FAAP
Aaron M. Milstone, MD, MHS, FAAP
Angela L. Myers MD, MPH, FAAP
Pia S. Pannaraj, MD, MPH, FAAP
Adam J. Ratner, MD, MPH, FAAP, *Red Book* Associate Editor
José R. Romero, MD, FAAP
Matthew Zahn, MD, FAAP

EX-OFFICIO

David W. Kimberlin, MD, FAAP, *Red Book* Editor
Ritu Banerjee, MD, PhD, FAAP, *Red Book* Associate Editor
Elizabeth D. Barnett, MD, FAAP, *Red Book* Associate Editor
Ruth Lynfield, MD, FAAP, *Red Book* Associate Editor

LIAISONS

Amina Ahmed, MD, FAAP, American Thoracic Society
Michelle Barton, MD, Canadian Paediatric Society
Carolyn Cleary, MD, FAAP, AAP Committee on Practice and Ambulatory Medicine
Denee J. Moore, MD, American Academy of Family Physicians
Jennifer L. Thompson, MD, American College of Obstetricians and Gynecologists
Juan P. Torres, MD, PhD, Sociedad Latinoamericana de Infectología Pediátrica
Charles R. Woods, Jr., MD, MS, FAAP, Pediatric Infectious Diseases Society

STAFF

Sunnah Kim; Gillian Gibbs, MPH

ACKNOWLEDGMENTS

The Committee on Infectious Diseases gratefully acknowledges Sean O'Leary, MD, MPH, FAAP, for his leadership in drafting the policy statement.

REFERENCES

1. American Academy of Pediatrics. Respiratory syncytial virus. In: Kimberlin DW, Banerjee R, Barnett ED, Lynfield R, Sawyer MH, eds. *Red Book: 2024 Report of the Committee on Infectious Diseases*. 33rd ed. American Academy of Pediatrics; 2024:713–721.
2. Atwell JE, Hartman RM, Parker D, et al. RSV among American Indian and Alaska Native children: 2019 to 2020. *Pediatrics*. 2023;152(2):e2022060435. PubMed doi: 10.1542/peds.2022-060435
3. Zar HJ, Simoes E, Madhi S, et al. 166. A phase 2b/3 study to evaluate the efficacy and safety of an investigational respiratory syncytial virus (RSV) antibody, clesrovimab, in healthy preterm and full-term infants [abstr]. *Open Forum Infect Dis*. 2025;12(Suppl 1):ofae631.003. doi: https://doi.org/10.1093/ofid/ofae631.003
4. Moulia D; Maternal/Pediatric RSV Work Group. Centers for Disease Control and Prevention. Evidence to Recommendations Framework: Clesrovimab. Accessed August 8, 2025. https://www.cdc.gov/acip/downloads/slides-2025-04-15-16/02-Moulia-maternal-peds-RSV-508.pdf

Recommended Childhood and Adolescent Immunization Schedule: United States, 2026

- *Policy Statement*

POLICY STATEMENT Organizational Principles to Guide and Define the Child Health Care System and/or Improve the Health of All Children

American Academy of Pediatrics

DEDICATED TO THE HEALTH OF ALL CHILDREN™

Recommended Childhood and Adolescent Immunization Schedule: United States, 2026: Policy Statement

Sean T. O'Leary, MD, MPH, FAAP and the Committee on Infectious Diseases

The 2026 recommended childhood and adolescent immunization schedule has been published by the American Academy of Pediatrics (AAP). The schedule is revised annually to reflect current recommendations for the use of vaccines licensed by the US Food and Drug Administration. At this time, the AAP no longer endorses the recommended childhood and adolescent immunization schedule from the Centers for Disease Control and Prevention.

Members of the AAP Committee on Infectious Diseases participated in the immunization work groups of the Advisory Committee on Immunization Practices through May of 2025. The Evidence to Recommendations framework was used by the work groups and informed the 2026 pediatric recommendations.[1]

The **cover page** includes a table with an alphabetical listing of vaccines and other immunizing agents, approved abbreviations for each agent, and trade names.

Table 1 contains the recommended immunization schedule from birth to 18 years of age.

Table 2 is the catch-up immunization schedule for persons 4 months to 18 years of age who start late or who are more than 1 month behind the recommended age for vaccine administration.

Table 3 lists the immunizations that may be indicated for children and adolescents 18 years of age or younger on the basis of medical conditions.

The **Notes** provide additional information and are presented in alphabetical order of the vaccine or other immunizing agent.

The **Appendix** provides conditions when vaccines and other immunizing agents are contraindicated or not recommended or when precautions should be considered.

The **Addendum** summarizes new and updated AAP recommendations that occur after the 2026 immunization schedule is published.

The **Endorsements** list the logos of the medical and health organizations endorsing the AAP schedule.

All authors contributed substantially to the conception and design; review and interpretation of relevant literature; drafting and revisions; and final approval of the published version.

All authors have filed conflict of interest statements with the American Academy of Pediatrics. Any conflicts have been resolved through a process approved by the Board of Directors. Author disclosures are provided at the end of this article. The American Academy of Pediatrics has neither solicited nor accepted any commercial involvement in the development of the content of this publication.

Policy statements from the American Academy of Pediatrics benefit from expertise and resources of liaisons and internal (AAP) and external reviewers. However, policy statements from the American Academy of Pediatrics may not reflect the views of the liaisons or the organizations or government agencies that they represent.

To cite: O'Leary ST; American Academy of Pediatrics, Committee on Infectious Diseases. Recommended Childhood and Adolescent Immunization Schedule: United States, 2026: Policy Statement. *Pediatrics.* 2026;157(3):e2025075754

The following changes have been made since the publication of the original 2025 schedule in November 2024:

OVERALL SCHEDULE

- Where relevant, webpage resources were changed from federal websites to trusted webpage resources from AAP and partners. Where federal webpage resources are listed, "Accessed on" dates were added.

COVER PAGE

- In the table listing immunization names and abbreviations, Enflonsia, Penmenvy and Flublok were added.
- Other information was updated on the page, including:
  - Added information on 12 medical and health organizations endorsing the AAP schedule.
  - Added information on how to report clinically significant adverse events for RSV-mAb products to MedWatch, a reporting system that supports the Food and Drug Administration (FDA)'s postmarketing safety surveillance for drugs and therapeutic biologics.
  - Changed Questions or comments contact to an AAP submission form.
  - Updated link for the current Vaccine Information Statements.
  - Updated QR code and immunization schedule landing page.

TABLE 1

Recommended Child and Adolescent Immunization Schedule by Age

- **Legend** colors and text were updated as follows:
  - Blue: Range of recommended ages for all children.
  - Purple: Range of recommended ages for catch-up vaccination.
  - Orange: Range of recommended ages for certain high-risk groups or populations.
  - Blue with dots: A new legend was added for recommended vaccination for those who desire protection.
  - Blue with diagonal lines: Recommended vaccination based on shared clinical decision-making.
  - Legends for recommended vaccination can begin in this age group and no guidance/not applicable were removed.
- **Respiratory syncytial virus (RSV) monoclonal antibody (mAb):** Added clesrovimab[2] to RSV immunizations. To provide additional clarity, the overlying text for birth through 7 months for all children was changed to "1 dose during RSV season depending on maternal RSV vaccination status (See Notes)" and for 8 months through 19 months for high risk groups was changed to "1 dose nirsevimab during RSV season (See Notes)."
- **Influenza:** Combined rows for IIV3, ccIIV3 and LAIV3 into one row for simplicity.
- **Human papillomavirus (HPV):** Changed HPV age range for recommendation to 9–12 years, to align with AAP policy.[3]
- **COVID-19:** Updated COVID recommendations to align with updated AAP policy.[4]
  - Universal recommendation for all children 6–23 months of age.
  - Risk-based recommendation for children 2–17 years of age.
  - Recommendation for those 2–17 years of age who desire protection.
  - See notes for full details.
- **RSV vaccine:** Added "if not previously vaccinated" to overlying text for clarity.

TABLE 2

Recommended Catch-up Immunization Schedule for Persons 4 Months to 18 Years of Age

- No updates were made to Table 2.

TABLE 3

Recommended Schedule by Medical Indication

- **Legend** colors and text were updated as follows:
  - Blue: Recommended for all age-eligible children who lack documentation of a complete immunization series.
  - Orange: Not recommended for all children, but recommended for some children based on increased risk for severe outcomes from disease.
  - Purple: Recommended for all age-eligible children, and additional doses may be necessary based on medical condition or other indications.
  - Pink with diagonal red lines: Precaution: Might be indicated if benefit of protection outweighs risk of adverse reaction.
  - Gray legend for No Guidance/Not Applicable was removed, and table is blank where no guidance is provided.
- **RSV-mAb:** Added clesrovimab to immunizing agents. For clarification, added a blue legend with overlying text "1 dose clesrovimab or nirsevimab during 1st RSV season depending on maternal RSV vaccination status (See Notes)." Added "nirsevimab" in purple legend to clarify only nirsevimab is recommended for 2nd RSV season for high risk individuals.

- **COVID-19:** Added an asterisk for pregnancy with a link to the American College of Obstetricians & Gynecologists (ACOG) practice advisory that states: *For more information, refer to https://www.acog.org/clinical/clinical-guidance/practice-advisory/articles/2020/12/covid-19-vaccination-considerations-for-obstetric-gynecologic-care.

NOTES

- **COVID-19:**
  - This section has been updated with new recommendations per AAP policy[4] and to reflect the change in FDA approval of Pfizer-BioNTech Comirnaty from children 6 months of age and older to children 5 years of age and older and addition of Moderna mNEXSPIKE for age 12 + years.
  - The AAP's COVID-19 Vaccine Dosing Guide was added for reference. Dosing guidance was updated for 6–23-month old who has previously received 1 dose prior formulation of Pfizer-BioNTech vaccine and for age 6 months–4 years moderately or severely immunocompromised who has previously received 1 dose prior formulation of Pfizer-BioNTech vaccine.
  - New references were added for revaccination guidance for children with hematologic malignancy post-hematopoietic cell transplant or CAR T-cell therapy.
- **Dengue:** Added a note that dengue vaccine distribution in the US was discontinued September 2025 (with a shelf life up to September 2026).[5]
- **Hepatitis B:** Removed recommendations for PreHevbrio since it was discontinued.[6]
- **HPV:** Updated language to align with AAP policy.[3]
- **Influenza:** Updated dates to reflect 2025–2026 season and added a link to AAP influenza vaccine recommendations.[7]
- **Measles, mumps, and rubella (MMR):** Updated note to align with AAP policy[8] that the AAP expresses no preference between MMR plus monovalent varicella vaccine or MMRV for toddlers receiving their first immunization of this kind.
- **Meningococcal serogroup A, C, W, Y Vaccination:**
  - Moved recommendations on MenACWY-TT/MenB-FHb and MenACWY-CRM/MenB-4C to new notes section on Meningococcal serogroup A, B, C, W, Y.
  - Clarified language for military recruits and first-year college students who live in residential housing.
  - Added product Penmenvy to note about Penbraya as an alternative to separate administration of MenACWY and MenB when both vaccines would be given on the same clinic day.
  - Added chronic GVHD as an additional example of functional asplenia.
- **Meningococcal serogroup B:** Moved recommendations on MenACWY-TT/MenB-FHb and MenACWY-CRM/MenB-4C to new notes section on Meningococcal serogroup A, B, C, W, Y and added chronic GVHD as an additional example of functional asplenia.
- **Meningococcal serogroup A, B, C, W, Y:** Added a new notes section with recommendations on the use of MenACWY-TT/MenB-FHb and MenACWY-CRM/MenB-4C.
- **RSV Immunization:** Added clesrovimab as an available product for infants <8 months[2] and updated notes to align with AAP policy,[9] including the removal of guidance on palivizumab.
- **RSV Vaccination:** Added clesrovimab under Routine vaccination to "Either maternal RSV vaccination with Abrysvo or infant immunization with nirsevimab or clesrovimab is recommended to prevent severe RSV disease in infants," and under Subsequent pregnancies, "Infants born to pregnant women who received RSV vaccine during a previous pregnancy should receive nirsevimab or clesrovimab."
- **Varicella:** Updated note to align with AAP policy[7] that the AAP expresses no preference between MMR plus monovalent varicella vaccine or MMRV combination vaccine for toddlers receiving their first immunization of this kind.

APPENDIX (CONTRAINDICATIONS AND PRECAUTIONS)

- **Meningococcal ABCWY:** Added Penmenvy product and added contraindications for MenACWY-CRM/MenB-4C and MenACWY-TT/MenB-FHbp.

The AAP's 2026 version of Tables 1 through 3, notes, appendix, and addendum are available on the American Academy of Pediatrics website (https://aap.org/ImmunizationSchedule). A parent-friendly vaccine schedule for children and adolescents is available at http://www.healthychildren.org/immunizationschedules. Clinically significant adverse events that follow vaccines should be reported to the Vaccine Adverse Event Reporting System (VAERS). Guidance about how to obtain and complete a Vaccine Adverse Event Reporting System form can be obtained at http://www.vaers.hhs.gov or by calling 800-822-7967. For RSV-mAb products, clinically significant adverse events should be reported to MedWatch Adverse Event Reporting program at www.accessdata.fda.gov/scripts/medwatch/index.cfm. If RSV-mAb is co-administered with other products, then report to VAERS.

Additional information can be found in the *Red Book* and at *Red Book Online* (https://publications.aap.org/redbook). Information on new vaccine releases, vaccine supplies, and interim recommendations resulting from vaccine shortages and statements on specific vaccines can be found at https://publications.aap.org/redbook.

COMMITTEE ON INFECTIOUS DISEASES 2025–2026

Sean T. O'Leary, MD, MPH, FAAP, Chairperson
James D. Campbell, MD, MS, FAAP, Vice Chairperson
Monica I. Ardura, DO, MSCS, FAAP
Kristina A. Bryant, MD, FAAP, *Red Book Online* Team Lead
Roberta L. DeBiasi, MD, MS, FAAP
Claudia Espinosa, MD, MSc, FAAP
Robert W. Frenck, Jr., MD, FAAP
C. Mary Healy, MD
Betsy C. Herold, MD, FAAP
Chandy C. John, MD, MS, FAAP
Aaron M. Milstone, MD, MHS, FAAP
Angela L. Myers MD, MPH, FAAP
Pia S. Pannaraj, MD, MPH, FAAP
Adam J. Ratner, MD, MPH, FAAP, *Red Book* Associate Editor
José R. Romero, MD, FAAP
Matthew Zahn, MD, FAAP

EX-OFFICIO

David W. Kimberlin, MD, FAAP, *Red Book* Editor
Ritu Banerjee, MD, PhD, FAAP, *Red Book* Associate Editor
Elizabeth D. Barnett, MD, FAAP, *Red Book* Associate Editor
Ruth Lynfield, MD, FAAP, *Red Book* Associate Editor

LIAISONS

Amina Ahmed, MD, FAAP, American Thoracic Society
Michelle Barton, MD, Canadian Paediatric Society
Carolyn Cleary, MD, FAAP, AAP Committee on Practice and Ambulatory Medicine
Denee J. Moore, MD, American Academy of Family Physicians
Jennifer L. Thompson, MD, American College of Obstetricians and Gynecologists
Juan P. Torres, MD, PhD, Sociedad Latinoamericana de Infectología Pediátrica
Charles R. Woods, Jr., MD, MS, FAAP, Pediatric Infectious Diseases Society

STAFF

Gillian Gibbs, MPH

ABBREVIATIONS

AAP: American Academy of Pediatrics
ACIP: Advisory Committee on Immunization Practices
aIIV3: adjuvanted inactivated influenza vaccine, trivalent
ccIIV3: cell-culture inactivated influenza vaccine, trivalent
CDC: Centers for Disease Control and Prevention
DTaP: diphtheria and tetanus toxoids and acellular pertussis vaccine
HD-IIV3: high-dose inactivated influenza vaccine, trivalent
Hib: *Haemophilus influenzae* type b vaccine
IPV: inactivated poliovirus vaccine
MenB: meningococcal serogroup B vaccine
MMR: measles, mumps, and rubella vaccine
MMRV: measles, mumps, rubella, and varicella vaccine
PCV: pneumococcal conjugate vaccine
PPSV23: pneumococcal polysaccharide vaccine, 23-valent
RSV: respiratory syncytial virus
RSV-mAb: respiratory syncytial virus monoclonal antibody
Td: tetanus toxoid, reduced diphtheria toxoid

The guidance in this statement does not indicate an exclusive course of treatment or serve as a standard of medical care. Variations, taking into account individual circumstances, may be appropriate.

All policy statements, clinical reports, and technical reports from the American Academy of Pediatrics automatically expire 5 years after publication unless reaffirmed, revised, or retired at or before that time.

FINANCIAL/CONFLICT OF INTEREST DISCLOSURES: The author had no disclosures.

Disclosures are reviewed and mitigated through a conflict-of-interest process that consists of reviewing pertinent information which is then used to decide what action is required to maintain content integrity. Disclosures may include salary, wages or other remuneration of any kind (including but not limited to consulting or advising fees, speaking fees, research funding, ownership interests, honoraria, participation in pension or benefit plans or programs or other perquisites, and reimbursement for travel, lodging, and meals) given for services rendered or other activities for which remuneration is received or expected, whether that compensation or other remuneration is paid directly to the individual or to the individual's employer or another third party. A disclosure does not necessarily imply a real or perceived conflict of interest.

Members of the Committee on Infectious Diseases assisted in the development of this policy statement. AAP requires committee members to mitigate any perceived or actual conflict of interest which may include recusal from participating in policy development.

FUNDING: No external funding.

https://doi.org/10.1542/peds.2025-075754

REFERENCES

1. Lee G, Carr W, Reingold A, et al; ACIP Evidence-Based Recommendations Work Group; ACIP Evidence Based Recommendations Work Group. Updated Framework for Development of Evidence-Based Recommendations by the Advisory Committee on Immunization Practices. *MMWR Morb Mortal Wkly Rep.* 2018;67(45):1271–1272. PubMed doi: 10.15585/mmwr.mm6745a4
2. Moulia DL, Link-Gelles R, Chu HY, et al. Use of clesrovimab for prevention of severe respiratory syncytial virus–associated lower respiratory tract infections in infants: recommendations of the Advisory Committee on Immunization Practices—United States, 2025. *MMWR Morb Mortal Wkly Rep.* 2025;74(32):508–514. PubMed doi: 10.15585/mmwr.mm7432a3
3. American Academy of Pediatrics. Human papillomaviruses. In: Kimberlin DW, Banerjee R, Barnett ED, Lynfield R, Sawyer MH, eds. *Red Book: 2024 Report of the Committee on Infectious Diseases.* American Academy of Pediatrics; 2024:503–511. doi: https://doi.org/10.1542/9781610027373-S3_008_018
4. O'Leary ST, Campbell JD, Ardura MI, et al; Committee on Infectious Diseases. Recommendations for COVID-19 vaccines in infants, children, and adolescents: Policy statement. *Pediatrics.* 2025;156(5):e2025073924. PubMed doi: 10.1542/peds.2025-073924
5. Department of Health and Human Services. Food and Drug Administration, Center for Biologics Evaluation and Research. Memorandum. Dengvaxia (Dengue Tetravalent Vaccine, Live). April 29–30, 2025. Accessed December 11, 2025. https://www.fda.gov/media/187189/download?attachment
6. VBI Vaccines Inc. VBI Vaccines Issues Voluntary Nationwide Recall of All PreHevbrio® Vaccine Within Expiry Due to Discontinuation of Co Operations. Accessed December 11, 2025. https://www.prehevbrio.com/
7. O'Leary ST, Campbell JD, Ardura MI, et al; Committee on Infectious Diseases. Recommendations for prevention and control of influenza in children, 2025–2026: Policy statement. *Pediatrics.* 2025;156(6):e2025073620. PubMed doi: 10.1542/peds.2025-073620
8. American Academy of Pediatrics. Measles. In: Kimberlin DW, Banerjee R, Barnett ED, Lynfield R, Sawyer MH, eds. *Red Book: 2024 Report of the Committee on Infectious Diseases.* American Academy of Pediatrics; 2024:570–585. doi: https://doi.org/10.1542/9781610027373-S3_012_002
9. O'Leary ST, Campbell JD, Ardura MI, et al; Committee on Infectious Diseases. Recommendations for the prevention of RSV disease in infants and children: Policy statement. *Pediatrics.* 2025;156(5):e2025073923. PubMed doi: 10.1542/peds.2025-073923

Systems-Based Care of the Injured Child

- *Policy Statement*

POLICY STATEMENT Organizational Principles to Guide and Define the Child Health Care System and/or Improve the Health of All Children

American Academy of Pediatrics

DEDICATED TO THE HEALTH OF ALL CHILDREN™

Systems-Based Care of the Injured Child: Policy Statement

Katherine T. Flynn-O'Brien, MD, MPH, FAAP, FACS,[1] Vijay Srinivasan, MBBS, MD, FCCM, FAAP,[2] Mary E. Fallat, MD, FAAP, FACS,[3] Committee on Pediatric Emergency Medicine; Council on Injury, Violence, and Poison Prevention; Section on Critical Care; Section on Surgery; Section on Transport Medicine; PEDIATRIC TRAUMA SOCIETY; SOCIETY OF TRAUMA NURSES; Pediatric Committee

abstract

Injury is the leading cause of death and a frequent cause of disability in children and negatively affects physical health, mental health, and quality of life in both the short- and long-term. The goal of a pediatric trauma system is to optimize the care for children within a state or region encompassing the entire continuum of care regardless of where children live or where traumatic events occur. This continuum includes injury prevention, prehospital care, emergency department care, interfacility transport, acute and critical inpatient care, inpatient and outpatient rehabilitation, and reintegration into the community and primary care medical home. A systems-based approach requires distinct elements of structure and function to perform together in an interrelated and cohesive manner to improve care quality. In this case, it represents a sequential practice of evidence-based evaluation and management along the continuum of care. To improve outcomes after injury, a cohesive system must effectively provide optimal care for the "right child, at the right place, at the right time" across this continuum.

[1]Division of Pediatric Surgery, Department of Surgery, Children's Wisconsin and Medical College of Wisconsin, Milwaukee, Wisconsin; [2]Children's Healthcare of Atlanta, Department of Pediatrics, Emory University, Atlanta, Georgia; and [3]Division of Pediatric Surgery, Department of Surgery, Norton Children's and University of Louisville, Louisville, Kentucky

Drs Fallat and Flynn-O'Brien conceptualized and organized the policy statement, coordinated and supervised the manuscript drafting, drafted sections of the initial manuscript, edited the initial manuscript as a whole and critically reviewed and revised the manuscript. Dr Srinivasan drafted sections of the initial manuscript, edited the initial manuscript as a whole and critically reviewed and revised the manuscript. All authors approved the final manuscript as submitted and agree to be accountable for all aspects of the work.

CONFLICT OF INTEREST DISCLOSURE: The authors have indicated they have no potential conflicts of interest to disclose.

FUNDING: No external funding.

To cite: Flynn-O'Brien KT, Srinivasan V, Fallat ME; American Academy of Pediatrics, Committee on Pediatric Emergency Medicine; Council on Injury, Violence, and Poison Prevention; Section on Critical Care; Section on Surgery; Section on Transport Medicine; PEDIATRIC TRAUMA SOCIETY; SOCIETY OF TRAUMA NURSES; Pediatric Committee. Systems-Based Care of the Injured Child: Policy Statement. *Pediatrics.* 2025;156(3): e2025072720

INTRODUCTION

Injury has been the leading cause of death in children in the United States for decades.[1,2] Injury leads to more years of potential life lost than cancer, congenital anomalies, and perinatal health issues combined.[1,3] Survivors of childhood injury frequently suffer mental and behavioral health sequelae and physical disabilities.[4,5] Improving outcomes requires an approach that recognizes childhood injury as a significant public health problem. The continuum of care model for trauma system development and planning provides a framework to integrate care and optimize outcomes.[6] This continuum includes injury prevention, prehospital care, interfacility transport, acute and critical inpatient care, inpatient and outpatient rehabilitation, and reintegration into the community and primary care medical home. A systems-based approach requires distinct elements of structure and function to perform seamlessly together to improve care quality.[7,8] Current pediatric trauma care lacks cohesion and has notable gaps in pediatric readiness across the nation, leading to preventable deaths and inferior outcomes. Furthermore, recent data have highlighted disparities in care and outcomes after pediatric injury, lack of equitable access to resources, and the relationship between injury and poor mental health outcomes and quality of life.[9–13] The goal of a comprehensive and cohesive national pediatric trauma system is to provide equitable and optimal access to care for all injured children.

TRAUMA SYSTEMS

Optimally, trauma systems are inclusive of prehospital care, hospital-based care, and rehabilitation/reintegration, to deliver coordinated care for the injured child throughout the care continuum. Timely access to care is critical; however, access to pediatric trauma centers varies by state and/or region.[14] Pediatric trauma systems optimally define age ranges and injury severity criteria for field triage of pediatric patients on the basis of specific hospital and trauma team resource availability. The American College of Surgeons (ACS) Committee on Trauma and the Centers for Disease Control and Prevention provide regular updates and recommendations for field triage criteria that can be used by emergency medical services (EMS) and hospital systems to coordinate care for children.[15–17] State trauma program managers, emergency medical services for children (EMSC) managers, and Pediatric Emergency Care Coordinators are key partners to facilitate how all hospitals with emergency departments (EDs) can safely evaluate and initiate resuscitation of injured children with processes to streamline coordinated care after initial stabilization.[18] Regional medical operations coordinating centers can coordinate care across EMS agencies, hospitals, and public health and emergency management leadership, particularly in the circumstance of a disaster. They can effectively load-balance a trauma system ensuring each child receives the optimal care at the appropriate facility.[19] Coordination of state operations with pediatric trauma system development and embedded continuous improvement should be part of an all-hazards approach to care that includes state, regional, and national partners with a vested interest in children along the care continuum.

INTEGRATION OF PEDIATRIC CARE

Injury Prevention

Injury prevention is the cornerstone of pediatric trauma care. The field of injury prevention employs scientific principles to identify areas for intervention and best practices. The Haddon matrix is a foundational systematic and scientific approach to injury prevention. This matrix analyzes injuries by considering how the host (ie, child) is susceptible to or injured by an agent (eg, motor vehicle, firearm) in a specific environment (eg, physical, social, economic) and in 3 different temporal phases: preinjury, during the injury event, and postinjury.[20,21] Overall, a multipronged approach to injury prevention is essential and may include legislation, advancing safety technology, improving the built environment, anticipatory guidance, and education of caregivers.[20]

Data from the local community, institutional trauma registries, or regional and national databases and trauma registries may be used to identify high-risk injury-prevention needs at the local level and beyond. Ideally, a wide range of medical and non-medical community members and organizations will collaborate to develop and implement injury-prevention programs and education. Physicians and nonphysician clinicians (eg, nurses, nurse practitioners, or physician assistants) are encouraged to emphasize age-appropriate safety topics during well-child visits and other health care encounters to educate families on injury prevention using available resources from the American Academy of Pediatrics (AAP) and other organizations.[22,23]

Prehospital Care and Pediatric Readiness

Prehospital care of children should follow best practices aligned with current evidence.[24] As an example, up-to-date EMS field triage guidelines and protocols that involve children are important resources to proactively have in place to guide prehospital teams.[17] Regular assessment of knowledge, iterative training on how to use essential equipment in children, pediatric-specific skill retention, and continuous evaluation of performance are crucial for EMS clinicians.[25] Pediatric readiness checklists and toolkits for both the prehospital and the ED settings are publicly available from the EMSC Innovation and Improvement Center website.[26] The national EMSC program uses performance measures to gauge state progress at integration of children into the emergency care network, including 3 prehospital EMS systems-based measures and 6 hospital-based measures.[27] The ACS Committee on Trauma is a partner in pediatric readiness and has outlined a blueprint along with recommendations for incorporating pediatric readiness into trauma system development.[28]

Community Care and Interfacility Transport

Key to a cohesive pediatric trauma system is timely and effective care concordant with a child's needs and seamless provision of care across the care continuum. Although critically injured children may need to be transferred to a higher level of pediatric trauma care, many children can be effectively and safely cared for in the community and/or at facilities that are not pediatric trauma centers (PTCs). Irrespective of care location, it is important that the

necessary equipment and supplies to adequately care for children are available. The National Pediatric Readiness Project
provides resources for pediatric injury care, including standardized guidelines, weight-based pediatric drug dosing, and checklists.[29] Prehospital and ED pediatric readiness across the country are essential component of pediatric trauma systems,[28,30] and have been associated with reduced mortality and improved outcomes.[31–33] To the extent possible, pediatric care at all locations should align with national or multi-institutional guidelines (eg, Image Gently using "as low as reasonably achievable" principles, and the American Pediatric Surgery Association solid organ injury guidelines). The Pediatric Trauma Society (PTS) Hub provides updated and vetted guidelines for the acute management of injuries by body system and is readily accessible to the public on the PTS website.[34] Transfer decisions and destination must be guided by the needs of the child. As soon as it is recognized that a child will likely need transfer to a higher level of care, further diagnostic tests beyond basic laboratory tests can be limited to those that will inform the need for intervention prior to transfer or those that dictate the need for transfer after consultation with pediatric trauma center personnel. Only necessary imaging studies should be completed to minimize radiation and to avoid the need for repeat imaging after transfer.[35]

Interfacility transfers can be best informed by official transfer guidelines, policies, and procedures that are reviewed and updated at regular intervals. Efficient and effective systems can facilitate transfer with multidisciplinary team involvement using centralized "transfer centers" allowing hospitals that initially treat children to initiate transfer to higher levels of care with a single call. These calls facilitate guidance on when and how children should be transferred based on their physiology and injuries, including recommendations for diagnostic and therapeutic interventions prior to transfer and preferred transport method (eg, ground vs aeromedical, one-way vs two-way with a specialized team, advanced vs basic life support). Templates for pediatric transfer protocols and guidelines are available online from the EMSC Innovation and Improvement Center (EIIC) website.[26] Readily available communication systems and image sharing technology across regional and state trauma systems facilitates consultation for, and coordination of, pediatric trauma care.

The Role of the Pediatric Trauma Center

Trauma centers are described by their ability to provide trauma-specific care, with level I being the highest, most comprehensive, level of care. [14] Trauma centers can be self-described, state-designated, and/or ACS-verified, and trauma systems may include as many as 4 or 5 levels. The ACS verifies level I and level II PTCs through a process that involves 4 components: adherence to standards, comprehensive infrastructure, rigorous data to guide quality improvement, and external peer review.[36] Regional PTCs have the necessary capacity to care for all life- and limb-threatening injuries in an expeditious manner to optimize outcomes. PTCs may have pediatric-trained physicians, nonphysician clinicians, specialists and subspecialists, therapists, physiatrists (rehabilitation medicine physicians), pharmacists, and other staff with pediatric expertise. The PTC in the regional trauma system plays an essential role in care provision and education. The PTC is generally readily available for consultation regarding care recommendations and/or transfer guidance, highlighting the importance of interhospital coordination and collaboration across the continuum of care. Expanding telehealth and remote consultation may be an opportunity to expand reach and improve care.[37]

Continuing pediatric-specific trauma education is important and can be accomplished by courses that provide training in key components of pediatric care. The highest-level trauma centers (pediatric and/or combined adult and pediatric) in each regional system generally provide education and outreach to local and regional community centers and state agencies to improve care for children. Trauma centers often involve EMS clinicians in their trauma quality improvement committees and activities, recognizing them as an essential part of the team.

SPECIAL CONSIDERATIONS

Child Abuse

A unique aspect of pediatric trauma care is the need for awareness and recognition of signs of child abuse and neglect, best accomplished by implementation of a standardized screening tool[38] and training of health care team members in nonbiased screening for, and identification of, child abuse.[39] Institutional resources to facilitate early and timely reporting to child protective services and law enforcement are important, with some caveats. Significant race- and ethnicity-based disparities in abusive head trauma evaluation and reporting have been highlighted in the past by several authors.[40] Possible biases on the part of mandated reporters may contribute to selective reporting that affects minority populations disproportionately. Training on implicit and explicit bias, utilizing diverse multidisciplinary teams and objective screening tools, and consultation with child abuse specialists are possible strategies to mitigate disparities.[40] Across the pediatric trauma system, capturing data on abuse screening and diagnosis for benchmarking and quality improvement has the potential to better understand and mitigate disparities.[38,39]

Injury Trends (Firearm Violence)

Historically, the leading cause of injury-related death in children, adolescents, and young adults 1 to 19 years of age was motor vehicle collisions; however, in 2019 firearm injury became the leading cause of death in this population.[2] Both the ACS and the AAP have published resources for health care workers, patients, and families regarding firearm injury prevention and safe storage.[23,41] The ACS, AAP, and American College of Emergency Physicians have all published position statements, policy statements, and/or technical reports on firearm safety and firearm-related injury prevention as part of their individual advocacy strategies.[42–44]

Disparities in Care

Inequity and disparities in pediatric trauma care are recognized as increasingly important considerations and key determinants of short- and long-term outcomes.[12,45,46] Disproportionate numbers of injuries and outcomes variation are seen in certain groups of minoritized children and adolescents. For example, minoritized children are at higher risk for injuries by firearms, have less access to pediatric trauma facilities and have fewer resources for rehabilitation and they may return to communities where there is additional exposure to violence. Because disparities occur along the continuum of the pediatric trauma care, equity-based efforts to address these disparities must also span the continuum of care. Next steps at the ACS level involve including an equity-focused framework into quality data reporting systems such as the Trauma Quality Improvement Program and beginning to study patient reported outcomes, which may provide more insight into disparities in care.[47,48] Pediatric trauma systems must work to provide equitable care to all injured children throughout the care continuum.

Recovery From Injury

The goal of a comprehensive pediatric trauma system is to return children to full, age-appropriate function with the ability to reach maximum adult potential. Care provided should be trauma informed, which takes into account the child's life experiences and social drivers of health to optimize patient care, child and family engagement, and health outcomes.[49,50] This care includes reintegration into the family, community, school/educational environment, and primary care medical home. Mental health sequalae, such as posttraumatic stress disorder and depression, are common after pediatric injury. Postinjury mental health screening designed to identify children in need of early intervention and/or referral is an important aspect of trauma care.[51] For children with extensive mental and/or physical needs after injury, the availability of rehabilitation resources specifically for children is a scarce yet vital component of trauma care. Physical, occupational, cognitive, speech, and appropriate trauma informed psychological and social supports are essential elements of a comprehensive rehabilitation effort for the injured child and family, and the importance of early rehabilitation during the inpatient phase of care cannot be overemphasized.

Research and Advocacy

Individuals and organizations at every level across the care continuum can participate in research and advocacy efforts to prevent injury, and, also to help improve the lives of children after injury. Institutional, state, and federal financial support of these initiatives is important to discover, improve, and support the best care for children. Systematic and transparent data collection and data sharing at the local, regional, and national levels is imperative to support these efforts.

SUMMARY/CONCLUSIONS

Injury is the leading cause of death for children in the United States. Using a systems-based approach along the continuum of care for trauma system development and planning provides a framework to integrate care and optimize outcomes. The ideal pediatric trauma system is comprehensive and cohesive providing optimal and equitable care for the "right child, at the right place, at the right time" across the care continuum. National trauma and EMS organizations should include children's unique needs and interests in their programs to ensure that children receive timely and appropriate care no matter where they are injured. State and federal financial support for research, advocacy, education, and trauma system development and maintenance are important.

RECOMMENDATIONS

1. The unique needs of injured children and their families should be integrated into trauma systems and disaster planning at the local, state, regional, and national levels.
2. An integrated public health approach to pediatric injury should address the needs of children *across* the continuum of care, including injury prevention, prehospital care, emergency and acute hospital care, rehabilitation, and long-term follow-up, to optimize successful reintegration into the community.
3. Evaluation and management of the injured child begins with EMS clinicians in the field and clinicians in urgent care centers and emergency departments who have education, competency, and proficiency in pediatric readiness at the point of trauma care.
4. Emergency departments throughout the United States should refer to pediatric readiness guidelines to facilitate appropriate care for all children.
5. Specialized pediatric trauma centers are essential components of trauma systems and should provide support and guidance to non-pediatric and non-trauma centers as part of their outreach mission.

6. All members of the health care team across the care continuum must be aware of potential abuse when evaluating injured children including equitable reporting of concerns to the appropriate authorities.
7. Optimal recovery after injury requires a trauma-informed approach, and the mental health needs of injured children and their families should be supported through screening and the provision of appropriate resources tailored to their needs after injury.
8. National organizations with a special interest in pediatric trauma should work together to ensure pediatric trauma care is multidisciplinary and collaborative to provide the highest quality of care.
9. Pediatric trauma care teams should actively work to provide equitable care to all injured children.
10. Systematic and transparent data collection and data sharing must occur at local, regional and national levels to inform all aspects of trauma care, from injury prevention to research and advocacy.

ACTION AND IMPLEMENTATION STRATEGIES

1. State and federal institutions should financially support pediatric trauma system development and maintenance, disaster planning, data collection and sharing, research, and education.
2. Every state or region should identify specialized trauma centers with the resources to care for injured children and establish systems to triage injured children appropriately based on their needs.
3. Health care systems should actively participate in and cultivate injury-prevention programming to reduce the rate of pediatric injuries.
4. Prehospital and hospital clinicians should make every effort to stay current in the management of injured children, including the ability to evaluate, stabilize, and transfer acutely injured children. Direct feedback from trauma centers can assist with continued process improvement for prehospital teams and agencies.
5. Interfacility transfer guidelines and protocols should be in place to facilitate rapid transport of critically injured children to trauma centers that can provide an appropriate level of care. EMS professionals and transport teams with pediatric expertise should be used in the interfacility transport of critically injured children.
6. Evidence-based protocols for the management of the injured child should be developed for essential aspects of care *across* the continuum of care. These should be continuously revised to reflect current evidence, with the goal to improve outcomes after injury.
7. Evidence-based mental health screening tools should be developed for use in the acute setting and in follow-up to aid in the early detection of children at risk for development of posttraumatic stress disorder. Those at risk should be provided resources and/or referral for early intervention by mental health professionals trained in trauma-informed care.
8. Established performance improvement and quality improvement programs should be established at all centers caring for injured children. Closed loop communication in the form of direct, constructive feedback should be provided by, and to, pediatric trauma centers to allow for continued education and improved pediatric care.

LEAD AUTHORS

Katherine T. Flynn-O'Brien, MD, MPH, FAAP, FACS
Vijay Srinivasan, MBBS, MD, FCCM, FAAP
Mary E. Fallat, MD, FAAP, FACS

AMERICAN ACADEMY OF PEDIATRICS

Committee on Pediatric Emergency Medicine, 2024-2025

Toni K. Gross MD, MPH, FAAP, FAEMS, Chairperson
Kerry S. Caperell, MD, FAAP
Jennifer A. Hoffmann, MD, MS, FAAP
Jennifer E. McCain, MD, FAAP
Sylvia Owusu-Ansah, MD, MPH, FAAP
Christian D. Pulcini, MD, MEd, MPH, FAAP
Mohsen Saidinejad, MD, MS, MBA, FAAP
David Schnadower, MD, MPH, FAAP
Caleb E. Ward, MB, BChir, MPH, FAAP
Muhammad Waseem, MD, FAAP

FORMER COMMITTEE MEMBER CONTRIBUTORS, 2021-2024

Gregory P. Conners, MD, MPH, MBA, FAAP, Chairperson 2020-2024
Benson S. Hsu, MD, MBA, FAAP, FCCM
Deborah C.W. Hsu, MD, MEd, FAAP
Lois K. Lee, MD, MPH, FAAP
Suzan S. Mazor, MD
Ronald I. Paul, MD, FAAP

LIAISONS

Christopher S. Amato, MD, FAAP, FACEP – *American College of Emergency Physicians*
Mary E. Fallat, MD, FAAP, FACS – *American College of Surgeons/AAP Section on Surgery*
Kathryn Kothari, MD – *National Association of EMS Physicians*
Cynthiana Lightfoot – *AAP FamilY Partnerships Network*
Katherine E. Remick, MD, FAAP, FACEP, FAEMS – *National Association of Emergency Medical Technicians*
Sam Shahid, MBBS, MPH – *American College of Emergency Physicians*
Elizabeth L. Stone, RN, PhD, CEN – *Emergency Nurses Association*
Cynthia J. Wright-Johnson, MSN, RN – *National Association of State EMS Officials*

STAFF

Susan Tellez

COUNCIL ON INJURY, VIOLENCE, AND POISON PREVENTION EXECUTIVE COMMITTEE, 2024-2025

Lois K. Lee, MD, MPH, FAAP, Chairperson
Alison Culyba, MD, MPH, PhD, FAAP
James Dodington, MD, FAAP
Katherine T. Flynn-O'Brien, MD, MPH, FAAP
Aimee Grace, MD, FAAP
Maya Haasz, MD, FAAP
Sadiqa A. I. Kendi, MD, MPH, FAAP
Andrew Waititu Kiragu, MD, FAAP
Terri D. McFadden, MD, MPH, FAAP
Kevin C. Osterhoudt, MD, MS, FAAP
Benjamin D. Hoffman, MD, FAAP, Immediate Past Chairperson

FORMER COMMITTEE MEMBER CONTRIBUTORS, 2021-2014

Brian D. Johnston, MD, MPH, FAAP
Milton Tenenbein, MD, FAAP

LIAISONS

Suzanne M. Beno, MD – *Canadian Paediatric Society*

STAFF

Bonnie Kozial

SECTION ON CRITICAL CARE EXECUTIVE COMMITTEE, 2024-2025

Vijay Srinivasan, MBBS, MD, FCCM, FAAP, Chairperson
Benson S. Hsu, MD, MBA, FCCM, FAAP, Immediate Past Chairperson
Wendy G. Hasson, MD, FAAP
Jimmy W. Huh, MD, FAAP
Jason (Jake) M. Kane, MD, MS, FAAP, FCCM
Lia H. Lowrie, MD, FAAP
Simon-Noel Ndely, MD, FAAP
Margaret A. Satchell, MD, FAAP

LIAISONS

Michael S.D. Agus, MD, FAAP – *Pediatric Critical Care Chiefs Network, Pediatric Intermediate Care Network*
Rajit K. Basu, MD, MS, FCCM – *Society of Critical Care Medicine*
Mary Lihinie deAlmeida, MD – *World Federation of Pediatric Intensive and Critical Care Societies*

FORMER COMMITTEE MEMBER CONTRIBUTORS, 2021-2024

Scottie B. Day, MD
Nicholas A. Ettinger, MD, PhD, CPPS, FAAP
Steven Loscalzo, MD
Elizabeth Mack, MD, MS, FAAP, Chairperson 2018-2021
Linda B. Siegel, FAAP, FAAHPM

STAFF

Susan Tellez

SECTION ON SURGERY EXECUTIVE COMMITTEE, 2024-2025

Marybeth Browne, MD, MS, FAAP, Chairperson
Elizabeth Beierle, MD, FAAP
Barbara Anne Gaines, MD, FAAP
Saleem Islam, MD, MPH, FAAP, Immediate Past Chair
Marc P. Michalsky, MD, MBA, FAAP
Mehul V. Raval, MD, MS, FAAP
Danielle Saunders Walsh, MD, FAAP

FORMER COMMITTEE MEMBER CONTRIBUTORS, 2021-2024

Andrew Davidoff, MD, FAAP
Cynthia Downard, MD, FAAP
Kenneth Gow, MD, MHA, FAAP

LIAISONS

Mary E. Fallat, MD, FAAP, FACS – *American College of Surgeons/AAP Section on Surgery*

STAFF

Vivian Thorne

SECTION ON TRANSPORT MEDICINE EXECUTIVE COMMITTEE, 2024-2025

Michael Stroud, MD, FAAP, Chairperson
Archana Dhar, MD, FAAP
Matthew Harris, MD, FAAP
Rudy Kink, MD, FAAP
Emily Krennerich, MD, FAAP
Franscesca Miquel Verges, MD, FAAP
Holly Engelstad, MD, FAAP

LIAISONS

Michael Bigham, MD, FAAP – *Air Medical Physician Association (AMPA)*
Beth Diehl, DNP, NNP-BC CCRN, LNCC – *National Association of Neonatal Nurses (NANN)*
Robert Holcomb, Jr, MD, FAAP – *Commission on Accreditation of Medical Transport Systems*
Corina Noje, MD, FAAP – *Ground Air Medical qUality Transport Quality Improvement Collaborative (GAMUT)*
Tammy Rush, MSN, RN, C-NPT, EMT – *National Association of Neonatal Nurses*
Hamilton Schwartz, MD, FAAP – *National Association of EMS Physicians (NAEMSP)*

AFFILIATES TRANSPORT MEDICINE SPECIALISTS

Tammy Rush, MSN, RN, C-NPT, EMT, Chairperson
Lisa Pruitt, BSN, RN, C-NPT, Vice Chairperson
Timothy Farmer, MSc, RRT-NPS
Laura Westley, RN
Jessica Wright, BSN, RNC, NPT
Richard Zimmerman, RRT-NPS, C-NPT, FP-C
Webra Price Douglas, CRNP, PhD
Beth C. Diehl, DNP, NNP-BC, CCRN, LNCC

STAFF

Dana Bennett-Tejes, MA, MNM

ABBREVIATIONS

ACS: American College of Surgeons
ED: emergency department
EMS: emergency medical services
EMSC: emergency medical services for children
PTC: pediatric trauma center

Policy statements from the American Academy of Pediatrics benefit from expertise and resources of liaisons and internal (AAP) and external reviewers. However, policy statements from the American Academy of Pediatrics may not reflect the views of the liaisons or the organizations or government agencies that they represent.

The guidance in this statement does not indicate an exclusive course of treatment or serve as a standard of medical care. Variations, taking into account individual circumstances, may be appropriate.

All policy statements from the American Academy of Pediatrics automatically expire 5 years after publication unless reaffirmed, revised, or retired at or before that time.

https://doi.org/10.1542/peds.2025-072720

COMPANION PAPER: A companion to this article can be found online at www.pediatrics.org/cgi/doi/10.1542/peds.2025-072721.

REFERENCES

1. Centers for Disease Control and Prevention, National Center for Injury Prevention and Control. *Web-based Injury Statistics Query and Reporting System*. WISQARS; 2023. [online]. Accessed April 1, 2023 www.cdc.gov/injury/wisqars
2. Goldstick JE, Cunningham RM, Carter PM. Current Causes of Death in Children and Adolescents in the United States. *N Engl J Med*. 2022;386(20):1955–1956. PubMed doi: 10.1056/NEJMc2201761
3. Cunningham RM, Walton MA, Carter PM. The Major Causes of Death in Children and Adolescents in the United States. *N Engl J Med*. 2018;379(25):2468–2475. PubMed doi: 10.1056/NEJMsr1804754
4. Oddo ER, Maldonado L, Hink AB, Simpson AN, Andrews AL. Increase in Mental Health Diagnoses Among Youth With Nonfatal Firearm Injuries. *Acad Pediatr*. 2021;21(7):1203–1208. PubMed doi: 10.1016/j.acap.2021.06.003
5. Burd RS, Jensen AR, VanBuren JM, et al; Eunice Kennedy Shriver National Institute of Child Health and Human Development Collaborative Pediatric Critical Care Research Network Assessment of Functional Outcomes and Health-Related Quality of Life after Pediatric Trauma Investigators. Long-Term Outcomes after Pediatric Injury: Results of the Assessment of Functional Outcomes and Health-Related Quality of Life after Pediatric Trauma Study. *J Am Coll Surg*. 2021;233(6):666–675.e2. PubMed doi: 10.1016/j.jamcollsurg.2021.08.693
6. Sacco WJ, Long WB, Copes WS, et al. Continuum of care trauma outcome evaluation. *Socioecon Plann Sci*. 1993;27(3):219–232. doi: 10.1016/0038-0121(93)90006-5
7. Kaplan G, Bo-Linn G, Carayon P, et al. *Bringing a Systems Approach to Health*. Discussion Paper. Institute of Medicine and National Academy of Engineering; 2013
8. US Department of Health and Human Services. Systems-Based Approach to Helathcare Incident Managment. *Public Health Emergency* 2023; https://www.phe.gov/Preparedness/planning/mscc/healthcarecoalition/chapter1/Pages/systemsbasedapproach.aspx. Accessed April 6, 2023.
9. Ranney M, Karb R, Ehrlich P, Bromwich K, Cunningham R, Beidas RS; FACTS Consortium. What are the long-term consequences of youth exposure to firearm injury, and how do we prevent them? A scoping review. *J Behav Med*. 2019;42(4):724–740. PubMed doi: 10.1007/s10865-019-00035-2
10. Burdick KJ, Lee LK, Mannix R, Monuteaux MC, Hirsh MP, Fleegler EW. Racial and ethnic disparities in access to pediatric trauma centers in the United States: a geographic information systems analysis. *Ann Emerg Med*. 2023;81:325–333. doi: 10.1016/j.annemergmed.2022.08.454
11. Jimenez N, Quistberg A, Vavilala MS, Jaffe KM, Rivara FP. Utilization of Mental Health Services After Mild Pediatric Traumatic Brain Injury. *Pediatrics*. 2017;139(3):e20162462. PubMed doi: 10.1542/peds.2016-2462

12. LaPlant MB, Hess DJ. A review of racial/ethnic disparities in pediatric trauma care, treatment, and outcomes. *J Trauma Acute Care Surg.* 2019;86(3):540–550. PubMed doi: 10.1097/TA.0000000000002160

13. Yue JK, Upadhyayula PS, Avalos LN, Cage TA. Pediatric Traumatic Brain Injury in the United States: Rural-Urban Disparities and Considerations. *Brain Sci.* 2020;10(3):135. PubMed doi: 10.3390/brainsci10030135

14. United States Government Accountability Office. Pediatric Trauma Centers: Availabilty, Outcomes, and Federal Support Related to Pediatric Trauma Care. 2017; https://www.gao.gov/products/gao-17-334. Accessed November 28, 2022.

15. Fischer PE, Gestring ML, Sagraves SG, et al. The national trauma triage protocol: how EMS perspective can inform the guideline revision. *Trauma Surg Acute Care Open.* 2022;7(1):e000879. PubMed doi: 10.1136/tsaco-2021-000879

16. Lupton JR, Davis-O'Reilly C, Jungbauer RM, et al. Under-Triage and Over-Triage Using the Field Triage Guidelines for Injured Patients: A Systematic Review. *Prehosp Emerg Care.* 2023;27(1):38–45. PubMed

17. Newgard CD, Fischer PE, Gestring M, et al; Writing Group for the 2021 National Expert Panel on Field Triage. National guideline for the field triage of injured patients: Recommendations of the National Expert Panel on Field Triage, 2021. *J Trauma Acute Care Surg.* 2022;93(2):e49–e60. PubMed doi: 10.1097/TA.0000000000003627

18. Brown KM, Ackerman AD, Ruttan TK, et al; COMMITTEE ON PEDIATRIC EMERGENCY MEDICINE; AMERICAN COLLEGE OF EMERGENCY PHYSICIANS, PEDIATRIC EMERGENCY MEDICINE COMMITTEE; EMERGENCY NURSES ASSOCIATION, PEDIATRIC COMMITTEE, 2018–2019. Access to Optimal Emergency Care for Children. *Pediatrics.* 2021;147(5):e2021050787. PubMed doi: 10.1542/peds.2021-050787

19. Administration for Strategic Preparedness and Response, TRACIE. Medical Operations Coordination Centers (MOCC): Patient Load-Balancing- Summary of Lessons Learned during COVID-19. 2022. Accessed February 1, 2024. https://files.asprtracie.hhs.gov/documents/mocc-patient-load-balancing-summary-of-lessons-learned-during-covid-19.pdf

20. Dorney K, Dodington JM, Rees CA, et al; Injury Free Coalition for Kids®. Preventing injuries must be a priority to prevent disease in the twenty-first century. *Pediatr Res.* 2020;87(2):282–292. PubMed doi: 10.1038/s41390-019-0549-7

21. Haddon W Jr. A logical framework for categorizing highway safety phenomena and activity. *J Trauma.* 1972;12(3):193–207. PubMed doi: 10.1097/00005373-197203000-00002

22. TIPP (The Injury Prevention Program). https://publications.aap.org/patiented/pages/c_tipp?autologincheck=redirected. Accessed May 30, 2022.

23. Safer: Storing Firearms Prevents Harm. https://shop.aap.org/safer-storing-firearms-prevents-harm/. Accessed December 10, 2022.

24. EMSC Innovation and Improvement Center. Prehospital Pediatric Readiness. https://emscimprovement.center/domains/prehospital-care/prehospital-pediatric-readiness/. Accessed July 7, 2022.

25. Lammers RL, Willoughby-Byrwa MJ, Vos DG, Fales WD. Comparison of Four Methods of Paramedic Continuing Education in the Management of Pediatric Emergencies. *Prehosp Emerg Care.* 2022;26(4):463–475. PubMed doi: 10.1080/10903127.2021.1916140

26. EMSC Innovation and Improvement Center. ED Checklist and Toolkit. https://emscimprovement.center/domains/pediatric-readiness-project/readiness-toolkit/#:~:text=The%20NPRP%20Toolkit%20is%20a,contribution%20of%20numerous%20national%20experts. Accessed April 4, 2023.

27. Emergency Medical Services for Children Program. Performance Measures Manual. Department of Health and Human Services, Health Resources and Services Administration, Emergency Medical Services for Children Program; 2023

28. Ross SW, Campion E, Jensen AR, et al. Prehospital and emergency department pediatric readiness for injured children: A statement from the American College of Surgeons Committee on Trauma Emergency Medical Services Committee. *J Trauma Acute Care Surg.* 2023;95(2):e6–e10. PubMed doi: 10.1097/TA.0000000000003997

29. EMSC Innovation and Improvement Center. National Pediatric Readiness Project. https://emscimprovement.center/domains/pediatric-readiness-project/. Accessed March 30, 2024.

30. Remick K, Gausche-Hill M, Joseph MM, Brown K, Snow SK, Wright JL; AMERICAN ACADEMY OF PEDIATRICS Committee on Pediatric Emergency Medicine and Section on Surgery; AMERICAN COLLEGE OF EMERGENCY PHYSICIANS Pediatric Emergency Medicine Committee; EMERGENCY NURSES ASSOCIATION Pediatric Committee. Pediatric Readiness in the Emergency Department. *Pediatrics.* 2018;142(5):e20182459. PubMed doi: 10.1542/peds.2018-2459

31. Newgard CD, Lin A, Olson LM, et al; Pediatric Readiness Study Group. Evaluation of Emergency Department Pediatric Readiness and Outcomes Among US Trauma Centers. *JAMA Pediatr.* 2021;175(9):947–956. PubMed doi: 10.1001/jamapediatrics.2021.1319

32. Melhado C, Remick K, Miskovic A, et al. The Association between Pediatric Readiness and Mortality for Injured Children Treated at US Trauma Centers. *Ann Surg.* 2024;280(6):e26–e33. PubMed

33. Newgard CD, Lin A, Malveau S, et al; Pediatric Readiness Study Group. Emergency Department Pediatric Readiness and Short-term and Long-term Mortality Among Children Receiving Emergency Care. *JAMA Netw Open.* 2023;6(1):e2250941. PubMed doi: 10.1001/jamanetworkopen.2022.50941

34. Pediatric Trauma Society. PTS Guidelines HUB. 2023; https://pediatrictraumasociety.org/resources/guidelines/. Accessed April 9, 2023

35. Brinkman AS, Gill KG, Leys CM, Gosain A. Computed tomography-related radiation exposure in children transferred to a Level I pediatric trauma center. *J Trauma Acute Care Surg.* 2015;78(6):1134–1137. PubMed doi: 10.1097/TA.0000000000000645

36. American College of Surgeons. *Resources for Optimal Care of the Injured Patient.* American College of Surgeons; 2022

37. Kohler JE, Falcone RA Jr, Fallat ME. Rural health, telemedicine and access for pediatric surgery. *Curr Opin Pediatr.* 2019;31(3):391–398. PubMed doi: 10.1097/MOP.0000000000000763

38. Escobar MA Jr, Wallenstein KG, Christison-Lagay ER, Naiditch JA, Petty JK. Child abuse and the pediatric surgeon: A position statement from the Trauma Committee, the Board of Governors and the Membership of the American Pediatric Surgical Association. *J Pediatr Surg.* 2019;54(7):1277–1285. PubMed doi: 10.1016/j.jpedsurg.2019.03.009

39. American College of Surgeons Trauma Quality Programs. *Best Practices Guidelines for Trauma Center Recognition of Child Abuse, Elder Abuse, and Intimate Partner Violence.* American College of Surgeons; 2019

40. Palusci VJ, Botash AS. Race and Bias in Child Maltreatment Diagnosis and Reporting. *Pediatrics.* 2021;148(1):e2020049625. PubMed doi: 10.1542/peds.2020-049625

41. American College of Surgeons Committee on Trauma. Firearm Injury Prevention Activities. 2023; https://www.facs.org/quality-programs/trauma/advocacy-and-injury-prevention/firearm-injury-prevention-activities/. Accessed April 9, 2023.

42. American College of Emergency Physicians. Firearm Safety and Injury Prevention. *Ann Emerg Med.* 2020;76(4):e99–e100. PubMed doi: 10.1016/j.annemergmed.2020.08.001

43. Lee LK, Fleegler EW, Goyal MK, et al. Policy Statement: Firearm-Related Injuries and Deaths in Children and Youth: Injury Prevention and Harm Reduction. *Pediatrics.* 2022;150(6):e2022060070. doi: 10.1542/peds.2022-060070

44. American College of Surgeons. Statement on Firearm Injuries. 2013; https://www.facs.org/about-acs/statements/firearm-injuries/. Accessed April 9, 2023.

45. Mitchell HK, Reddy A, Perry MA, Gathers C-A, Fowler JC, Yehya N. Racial, ethnic, and socioeconomic disparities in paediatric critical care in the USA. *Lancet Child Adolesc Health.* 2021;5(10):739–750. PubMed doi: 10.1016/S2352-4642(21)00161-9

46. Kendi S, Macy ML. The Injury Equity Framework - Establishing a Unified Approach for Addressing Inequities. *N Engl J Med.* 2023;388(9):774–776. PubMed doi: 10.1056/NEJMp2212378

47. Herrera-Escobar JP, Osman SY, Das S, et al; National Trauma Research Action Plan (NTRAP) Investigators Group. Long-term patient-reported outcomes and patient-reported outcome measures after injury: the National Trauma Research Action Plan (NTRAP) scoping review. *J Trauma Acute Care Surg.* 2021;90(5):891–900. PubMed doi: 10.1097/TA.0000000000003108

48. Trauma Quality Improvement Programs. https://www.facs.org/quality-programs/trauma/quality/trauma-quality-improvement-program/. Accessed February 1, 2024.

49. Menschner C, Maul A. Key Ingredients for Successful Trauma-Informed Care Implementation. *Brief.* Center for Health Care Strategies; April 2016. Accessed April 3, 2024. www.chcs.org/resource/key-ingredients-for-successful-trauma-informed-care-implementation/

50. Forkey H, Szilagyi M, Kelly ET, et al; COUNCIL ON FOSTER CARE, ADOPTION, AND KINSHIP CARE, COUNCIL ON COMMUNITY PEDIATRICS, COUNCIL ON CHILD ABUSE AND NEGLECT, COMMITTEE ON PSYCHOSOCIAL ASPECTS OF CHILD AND FAMILY HEALTH. Trauma-Informed Care. *Pediatrics.* 2021;148(2):e2021052580. PubMed doi: 10.1542/peds.2021-052580

51. American College of Surgeons Trauma Quality Programs. *Best Practice Guidelines: Screening and Intervention for Mental Health Disorders and Substance Use and Misuse in the Acute Trauma Patient.* American College of Surgeons; 2022.

Systems-Based Care of the Injured Child (Technical Report)

- *Technical Report*

TECHNICAL REPORT

American Academy of Pediatrics

DEDICATED TO THE HEALTH OF ALL CHILDREN™

Systems-Based Care of the Injured Child: Technical Report

Katherine T. Flynn-O'Brien, MD, MPH, FAAP, FACS,[1] Vijay Srinivasan, MBBS, MD, FCCM, FAAP,[2] Mary E. Fallat, MD, FAAP, FACS,[3] Committee on Pediatric Emergency Medicine; Council on Injury, Violence, and Poison Prevention; Section on Critical Care; Section on Surgery; Section on Transport Medicine; Pediatric Trauma Society; Society of Trauma Nurses; Pediatric Committee

abstract

Injury is the leading cause of death and a cause of disability in children and negatively affects physical health, mental health, and quality of life in both the short- and long-term. The goal of a pediatric trauma system is to optimize the care for children within a state, regional, or national trauma system across the entire continuum of care regardless of where they live or where the traumatic event occurs. This continuum includes injury prevention, prehospital care, interfacility transport between hospitals providing different levels of care, acute and critical inpatient care, inpatient and outpatient rehabilitation, and reintegration into the community and primary care medical home. A systems-based approach, one that requires distinct elements of structure and function to perform together in an interrelated and cohesive manner to improve care quality, is essential. To improve outcomes after injury, a cohesive system must effectively provide optimal care for the "right child, at the right place, at the right time" across this continuum.

[1]Division of Pediatric Surgery, Department of Surgery, Children's Wisconsin and Medical College of Wisconsin, Milwaukee, Wisconsin; [2]Departments of Anesthesiology, Critical Care and Pediatrics, Children's Hospital of Atlanta, Atlanta, Georgia; and [3]Division of Pediatric Surgery, Department of Surgery, Norton Children's and University of Louisville, Louisville, Kentucky

Drs Fallat and Flynn-O'Brien conceptualized and organized the technical report, coordinated and supervised the manuscript drafting, drafted sections of the initial manuscript, edited the initial manuscript as a whole, and critically reviewed and revised the manuscript. Dr Srinivasan drafted sections of the initial manuscript, edited the initial manuscript as a whole, and critically reviewed and revised the manuscript. All authors approved the final manuscript as submitted and agree to be accountable for all aspects of the work.

CONFLICT OF INTEREST DISCLOSURE: The authors have indicated they have no potential conflicts of interest to disclose.

FUNDING: No external funding.

Policy statements from the American Academy of Pediatrics benefit from expertise and resources of liaisons and internal (AAP) and external reviewers. (Continued)

To cite: Flynn-O'Brien KT, Srinivasan V, Fallat ME; American Academy of Pediatrics, Committee on Pediatric Emergency Medicine; Council on Injury, Violence, and Poison Prevention; Section on Critical Care; Section on Surgery; Section on Transport Medicine; Pediatric Trauma Society; Society of Trauma Nurses; Pediatric Committee. Systems-Based Care of the Injured Child: Technical Report. *Pediatrics.* 2025;156(3): e2025072721

INTRODUCTION

Injury has been the leading cause of death and a cause of disability in children in the United States for decades.[1,2] Injury leads to more years of potential life lost than cancer, congenital anomalies, and perinatal health issues combined.[1,3] Survivors of childhood injury frequently suffer mental and behavioral health sequelae and physical disabilities, sometimes with long-term consequences.[4,5] Improving outcomes requires an approach that recognizes childhood injury as a significant public health problem. Using the continuum of care model for trauma system development and planning provides a framework to integrate care and optimize outcomes.[6] This continuum of care includes injury prevention, prehospital care, emergency department (ED) care, interfacility transport, acute and critical inpatient care, inpatient and outpatient rehabilitation, and reintegration into the community and primary care

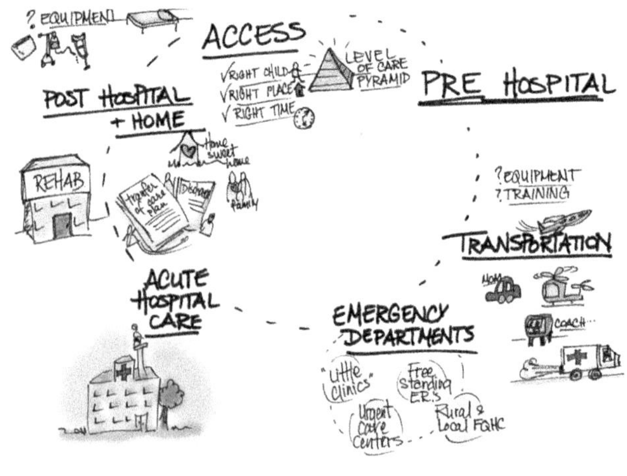

FIGURE 1.
Trauma system continuum of care.[7]
Figure developed by Tanya Gerber, graphic recorder. Reprinted with permission.

medical home (Figure 1).[7] A systems-based approach requires distinct elements of structure and function to perform together in an interrelated and cohesive manner.[8,9] A functional trauma system is represented by a sequential practice of evidence-based evaluation and management along the continuum of care and needs to be team-based, cohesive, and seamless to improve care quality in an efficient and effective manner.

Current pediatric trauma care lacks cohesion and has notable gaps in pediatric readiness across the nation, leading to preventable death and inferior outcomes.[10] Recent data have highlighted disparities in care and outcomes after pediatric injury, lack of equitable access to resources, and the importance of the relationship between injury and poor mental health outcomes and quality of life.[5,10–17] Systems-based approaches to pediatric trauma readiness, child abuse, head injury, and imaging practices have also been developed and/or updated.[18–22]

TRAUMA SYSTEMS

Children are injured in a variety of geographic locations, and involvement of emergency medical services (EMS) and both local and regional hospital systems is paramount to optimizing care. Pediatric trauma care refers to the care received in any setting by a child who has suffered a traumatic injury, and a trauma center is a hospital-based setting specifically designated or verified to provide trauma care.[23,24] Trauma care is provided in a variety of settings including in the field, at non-trauma hospitals or centers, and at adult and/or pediatric trauma centers (PTCs). Additionally, in addition to the ED, minor trauma care may be provided at urgent care and private practice clinics.

Ideally, a *comprehensive* pediatric trauma system incorporates prehospital and hospital-based care capable of initial stabilization of children of any age and their transfer, when needed, to centers providing advanced pediatric trauma care. A *cohesive* system allows for prompt communication and coordination, with tiered care concordant with patient needs. A trauma system focuses not only on survival but survivorship,[25] following the patient through discharge to a rehabilitation or home environment. Integration of disaster response systems at the local, state, regional, and national levels is an essential component of any functional trauma system.[26] Coordination of trauma system development generally includes physicians and nonphysician clinicians (eg, nurses, nurse practitioners, or physician assistants) and their professional organizations; hospital, state, and regional emergency management teams; the Administration for Strategic Preparedness and Response Hospital Preparedness Program; state hospital associations; local and state departments of health; state and regional trauma advisory councils; state legislatures; and local community leaders, among others (Table 1).

Effectiveness of state or regional pediatric trauma systems across the country has not traditionally been assessed. However, a state-based scoring system was created in 2022, called the Pediatric Trauma System Assessment Score (PTSAS), to measure each state's pediatric trauma capacity within the context of their trauma system (Figure 2). Through a Delphi process, 6 domains were chosen (injury prevention and recognition, access to care, quality improvement and trauma registry, disaster, legislation, and funding), each of which included 3 to 5 seminal parameters reflecting a state's pediatric trauma capabilities. A PTSAS summary score ranging from 0 to 100 was computed based on the weighted averages of each domain (with a score of 100 being the highest capabilities). The PTSAS score has been associated with both out-of-hospital and in-hospital deaths, and every 1-point increase in PTSAS has been associated with a decrease in overall state-based mortality of 0.12 (95% confidence interval [CI]: −0.22, −0.02) deaths per 100 000 children (Figure 3).

Because of regional geography and the limited number of PTCs, timely access to pediatric trauma care varies significantly across the nation.[24,27,28] A 2017 US Government Accountability Office report found that only 57% of children in the United States lived within 30 miles of an American College of Surgeons (ACS)- and/or state-designated PTC, defined as centers able to treat children of all ages and all injuries regardless of severity.[24] Considerable variation existed by state, with 15 states having less than a quarter of children living within 30 miles of a PTC.[24] In 2023, Burdick et al reported that the percentage of US children younger than 15 years who could not reach a level I, II, or III PTC within an hour of injury was 45.5% by ground and 25.9% by air transport.[15] Non-PTCs within the trauma system, including adult trauma centers (ATCs), community hospitals, rural or critical access hospitals, and adult regional hospitals, among others, are relied on to safely

TABLE 1. Partnering Organizations Important for the Optimal Care of the Injured Child[a,b]

Organization	Acronym	Contact/website
Administration for Strategic Preparedness and Response Hospital Preparedness Program	ASPR/HPP	https://aspr.hhs.gov/HealthCareReadiness/HPP
American Academy of Child and Adolescent Psychiatry	AACAP	https://www.aacap.org/
American Academy of Pediatrics	AAP	https://www.aap.org/
American Association of Neurological Surgeons	AANS/CNS	https://www.aans.org/en/Membership/AANSCNS-Sections
American Association of Nurse Anesthesiology	AANA	https://www.aana.com
American College of Emergency Physicians	ACEP	https://www.acep.org/
American College of Radiology	ACR	https://www.acr.org/
American College of Surgeons Committee on Trauma	ACS/COT	https://www.facs.org/quality-programs/trauma/
American Congress of Rehabilitation Medicine - Pediatric Rehabilitation Networking Group	ACRM	https://acrm.org/acrm-communities/pediatrics/
American Pediatric Surgical Association	APSA	https://apsapedsurg.org/
American Society of Anesthesiologists	ASA	https://www.asahq.org/
American Society of Pediatric Neurosurgeons	ASPN	https://www.aspn.org/
Association of Child Life Professionals	ACLP	https://www.childlife.org/
Eastern Association for the Surgery of Trauma	EAST	https://www.east.org/
Emergency Nurses Association	ENA	https://www.ena.org/
Health Resources and Services Administration	HRSA	https://www.hrsa.gov/
National Association of Emergency Medical Technicians	NAEMT	https://naemt.org/
National Association of EMS Educators	NAEMSE	https://naemse.org/
National Association of EMS Physicians	NAEMSP	https://naemsp.org/
National Association of Pediatric Nurse Practitioners	NAPNAP	https://www.napnap.org/
National Association of Social Workers	NASW	https://www.socialworkers.org/
National Association of State EMS Officials	NASEMSO	https://nasemso.org/
National EMS Management Association	NEMSMA	https://www.nemsma.org/
Pediatric Orthopaedic Society of North America	POSNA	https://posna.org/
Pediatric Trauma Society	PTS	https://pediatrictraumasociety.org/
Society for Pediatric Anesthesia	SPA	https://pedsanesthesia.org/
Society of Pediatric Psychology	SPP	https://pedpsych.org/
Society of Trauma Nurses	STN	https://www.traumanurses.org/
The American Association for the Surgery of Trauma	AAST	https://www.aast.org/Default.aspx
The Society for Pediatric Radiology	SPR	https://www.spr.org/
Urgent Care Association	UCA	https://urgentcareassociation.org/
Western Trauma Association	WTA	https://www.westerntrauma.org

[a] Other subspecialty societies including but not limited to Hospital Medicine, Urology, Otolaryngology, Vascular Surgery, Ophthalmology, Plastic surgery, and Oral and Maxillofacial Surgery, among others.
[b] Independent public health organizations and agencies associated with families and child health are also important partners.

provide stabilization and initial management of an injured child. This phenomenon is particularly true in rural and underserved areas of the country (Figure 4). Hence, it is essential that any hospital, health care center, or urgent care site that may treat injured children have the necessary training and resources to provide pediatric-specific care (see section on Pediatric Readiness). Collaborative efforts are important, as are novel approaches to improve care for children without immediate access to a trauma center (eg, teleconsultation/telemedicine).[29]

INJURY PREVENTION

Injury prevention is the cornerstone of pediatric trauma care. The field of injury prevention employs scientific principles to identify areas for intervention and best practices. The Haddon matrix is a popular systematic approach to injury prevention, analyzing injuries by considering how the host (ie, child) is susceptible to or injured by an agent (eg, motor vehicle, firearm) in a specific environment (eg, physical, social, economic) and in 3 different temporal phases: preinjury, during the injury event, and

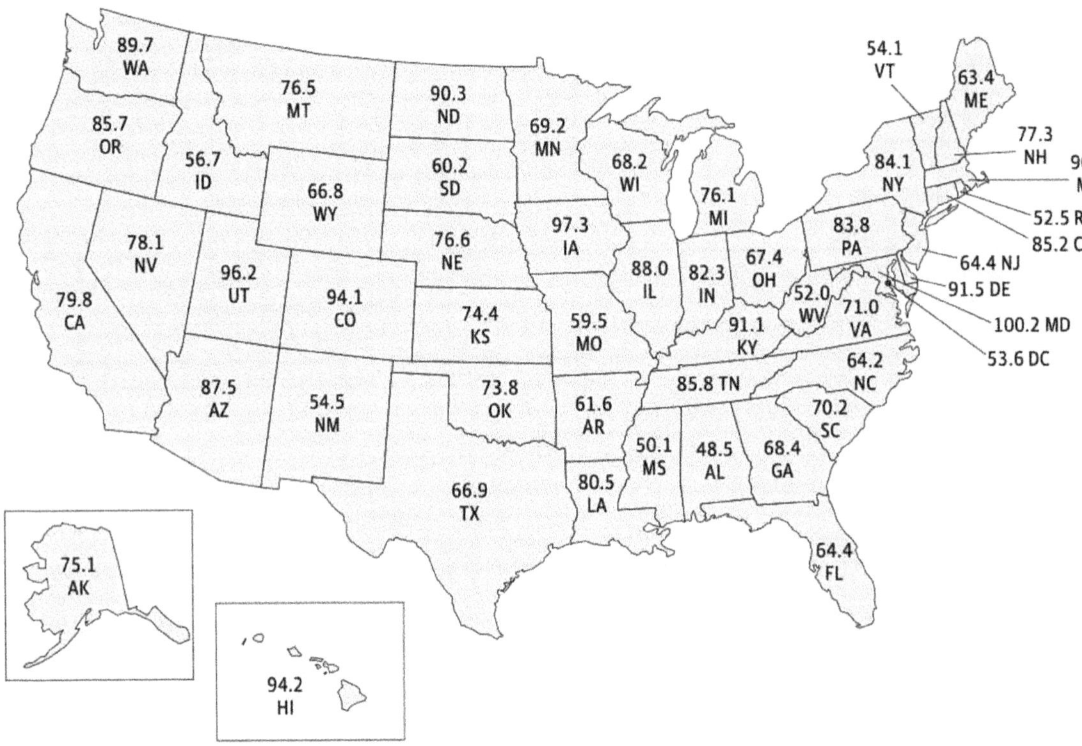

FIGURE 2.
Summary Pediatric Trauma System Assessment scores by state.
Source: Fallat ME, Treager C, Humphrey S, et al. *JAMA Surg.* 2022;157(11):1042–1049.

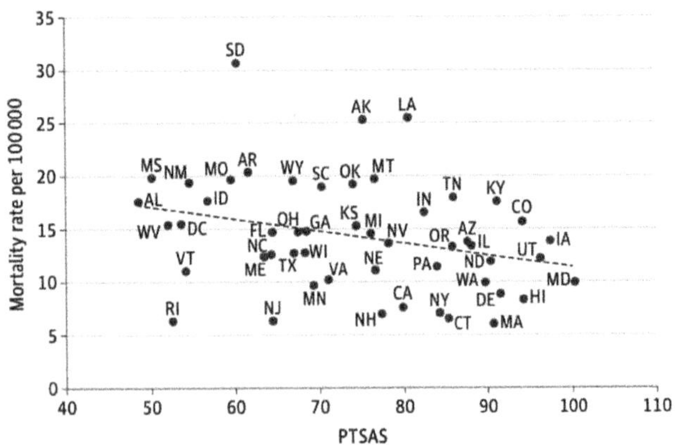

FIGURE 3.
Mortality rate by state and Pediatric Trauma System Assessment score.
Source: Fallat ME, Treager C, Humphrey S, et al. *JAMA Surg.* 2022;157 (11):1042–1049.

postinjury.[29,30] Building on the Haddon matrix, an injury equity framework was recently designed to "provide clinicians, researchers, public health professionals, and policymakers a theoretical basis for identifying and analyzing factors that influence who is injured, the severity of the injury, and the injury outcome using an equity lens."[31] The framework highlights the intersectionality between historical and current societal factors and community, family, and individual factors within the Haddon matrix structure. Overall, a multipronged approach to injury prevention is essential and may include legislation, advancing safety technology, improving the built environment (eg, parks, roadways), address risk factors related to a child's environment (eg, home, school), anticipatory guidance, and education of caregivers.[29] Furthermore, interventions should be evidence based and equity focused.[31]

Mechanism- and community-specific injury prevention initiatives have a long history of success, including the traffic safety, safe storage of firearms, window falls, and car seat programs, to name a few.[29,32–35] More than 20 years ago, Dr Maureen Durkin and colleagues studied the incidence of severe traffic injuries before and after a community-based intervention involving the creation of safe and accessible play areas, traffic safety education, and supervised activities for school-aged children.[34] During the intervention period, a 36% unadjusted reduction in the incidence of traffic injuries to school-aged children was observed (rate ratio [RR]: 0.64; 95% CI: 0.58, 0.72). Comparable reductions in traffic-related injuries were not identified in younger children (ages 0–4 years) or school-aged children who were not targeted by the program or for traffic fatalities involving school-aged residents in other communities in the city.[34] Policy-based injury prevention efforts that were legislated to become state or federal statutes have proven some of the

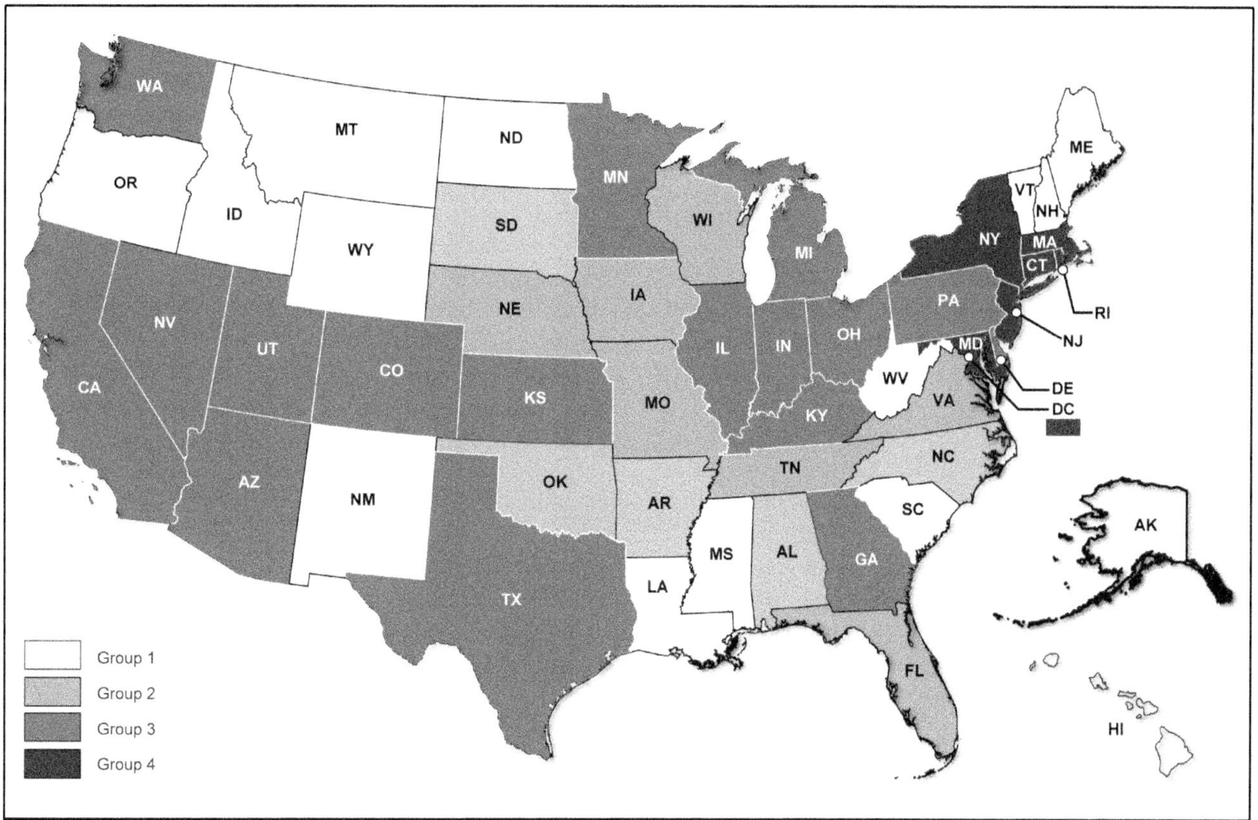

Group 1 0-24.9% of state's children lived within 30 miles of a high-level pediatric trauma center	Group 2 25-49.9% of state's children lived within 30 miles of a high-level pediatric trauma center	Group 3 50-74.9% of state's children lived within 30 miles of a high-level pediatric trauma center	Group 4 75-100% of state's children lived within 30 miles of a high-level pediatric trauma center
● 15 states ● 393,628 children within 30 miles ● 8 states with no children within 30 miles	● 12 states ● 6.7 million children within 30 miles	● 17 states ● 26.1 million children within 30 miles	● 7 states ● 8.8 million children within 30 miles ● 4 states with 90% or more children within 30 miles

Sources: GAO analysis of American Trauma Society and U.S. Census Bureau data (data); Map Resources (map). | GAO-17-334

FIGURE 4.
Estimated percentage of children who lived within 30 miles of a high-level pediatric trauma center, by state, 2011–2015.
Source: GAO analysis of American Trauma Society and US Census Bureau data (data): Map Resources. GAO 17-17-334. US Government Accountability Office. Pediatric Trauma Centers: Availability, Outcomes and Federal Support Related to Pediatric Trauma Care. Published March 27, 2017. Accessed September 12, 2023. https://www.gao.gov/products/gao-17-334

most effective, including seat belt and child passenger safety legislation.[29,36]

Often, a combination of approaches is essential. Dr Barbara Barlow was instrumental in identifying, describing, and promoting regulatory changes related to window falls by children in New York City.[32] After Dr Barlow's work in Washington Heights led to a 1979 ordinance requiring landlords to install window guards, the number of injuries children sustained from falling out of windows decreased in the neighborhood by 96%.[37] Effective public health messaging through the "Children Don't Fly" campaign helped solidify and disseminate her pivotal work.

More recently, Dr Lois Lee and colleagues summarized the evidence regarding firearm injury prevention and harm reduction, describing safe firearm storage, anticipatory guidance, lethal means counseling, and legislation through an American Academy of Pediatrics (AAP) policy statement.[35] Policy statements endorsed by national organizations like the AAP have wide distribution, and often guide advocacy efforts nationwide. The AAP has published a number of policy statements, clinical reports, technical reports, and other resources related to injury prevention in childhood. These include drowning prevention, pedestrian safety, child passenger safety, helmet use, and more.[38–42] More resources can be found on the AAP website at https://www.aap.org/en/policy/ and for families at healthchildren.org. The AAP also designed The Injury Prevention Program (TIPP), which helps pediatricians provide injury-related anticipatory guidance using a developmentally based schedule and supports pediatricians by providing a standardized resource about injury prevention for parents and caregivers. TIPP has recently been shown in a cluster randomized controlled trial to result in a reduction of parent-reported injuries in children.[43] This highlights the important role of pediatric physicians and nonphysician clinicians (eg, nurses, nurse practitioners, or physician assistants) in injury prevention, and supports emphasize of age-appropriate safety topics during well-child visits and other health care encounters to educate families on injury prevention using available resources from the AAP and other organizations.[44,45]

The Consumer Product Safety Commission (CPSC) has been instrumental in industry-specific injury prevention initiatives, including but not limited to baby walker-related injuries, furniture safety, and more. Federal agencies like the Centers for Disease Control and Prevention (CDC) have routinely contributed to injury prevention efforts. One example is sports-related injury prevention with resources, education, and guidance for health care staff, coaches, and parents regarding concussions and protective equipment.[46] The CDC also provides research and resources related to child abuse and neglect.[47] The Health Resources and Services Administration (HRSA)'s National Fetal, Infant, and Child Death Review Program and local child death review programs have traditionally helped with outreach messaging. There are now child death review teams in all 50 states and most US territories, which generally incorporate multidisciplinary approaches to the community's death review process.[48,49]

Finally, nonprofit organizations have, and continue to, contribute to injury prevention. Safe Kids, Prevent Child Injury, Charlie's House, Prevent Child Abuse America, and the Injury Free Coalition for Kids have addressed injury risks related to drowning, television and furniture tip overs, child abuse, and all-terrain vehicle use, to name a few. Many of these organizations promote risk reduction behaviors such as bike helmet use and safe teen driving. Both Safe Kids and the Injury Free Coalition for Kids have been instrumental in research, education, and advocacy for childhood injury prevention nationwide, and Prevent Child Injury provides multimedia toolkits on injury prevention topics, including information for families and providers, reports and data, and social media materials for outreach.[50–54]

Despite incredible efforts in the injury prevention space, it is important to note that many causes of injury to children have not changed over the past decade.[55] Aside from deaths due to motor vehicle collisions and pedestrian injuries, which have declined substantially, many injury-related causes of deaths have not changed for 20 years.[2,40] This highlights the importance of continued focus on injury prevention initiatives at local, regional, and national levels.

PEDIATRIC READINESS

The 2006 Institute of Medicine report evaluating the US emergency care system described care for children as uneven and found that many of the country's EDs lacked the necessary equipment, drugs, and supplies to care for children adequately.[56] The National Pediatric Readiness Project works to address these gaps with strategies to improve children's care including standardized guidelines and checklists. This includes the recommendation that there be a Pediatric Emergency Care Coordinator (PECC) position established in every ED in the nation. The PECC is tasked with providing education and training, ensuring maintenance of equipment and supplies, and completing quality improvement related to all types of pediatric trauma care and has been associated with improved ED pediatric readiness.[57] The HRSA-funded Emergency Medical Services for Children (EMSC) Program has incorporated the National Pediatric Readiness Project performance measures for assessment of state-based programs (Table 2).[58]

Prehospital and ED pediatric readiness across the country is an essential component of pediatric trauma systems.[59] New studies have validated the effectiveness of pediatric readiness in reducing in-hospital mortality after injury and critical illness.[18,60,61] ED pediatric readiness is also independently associated with long-term survival among injured children.[61,62] This makes pediatric readiness of all EDs across the country an essential component of health care safety and quality.[18,63–65] Because of its success, the program has also been extended to the prehospital care environment.[66,67] The ACS Committee on Trauma is a partner in pediatric readiness and has outlined a blueprint along with recommendations for incorporating pediatric readiness into trauma system development.[59]

PREHOSPITAL AND INTERFACILITY PEDIATRIC TRAUMA CARE

Prehospital Care

Prehospital care may be provided by a variety of emergency health care clinicians, including emergency medical technicians, advanced emergency medical technicians, emergency medical responders, and paramedics.[68] Police and/or fire departments, private or third-party ambulance services, and public agencies all play a role in parts of the country. Aside from specialty units associated with large children's hospitals, individual prehospital nonphysician clinicians infrequently care for critically ill or injured children, particularly those who volunteer or work in rural or underserved areas. Limited knowledge and experience with pediatric trauma patients are addressed by continuing education efforts through established courses supported by the AAP, American College of Emergency Physicians, American Heart Association, National Association of Emergency Medical Technicians, National Association of

TABLE 2. Emergency Medical Services for Children Performance Measures
Adapted from "Emergency Medical Services for Children Performance Measures: 2023 Implementation Manual for State Partnership Grantees"[58]

Performance Measure	Measurement Details
Objective 1: Expand uptake of pediatric readiness in EDs	
Hospital Emergency Department Pediatric Readiness Recognition Program (EMSC 04)	States/jurisdictions have a standardized pediatric readiness recognition program for EDs
Hospital Emergency Department Pediatric Emergency Care Coordinator	Hospital EDs have a designated pediatric emergency care coordinator
Hospital Emergency Department Weigh and Record Children's Weight in Kilograms	Hospital EDs weigh and record children's weight in kilograms
Hospital Emergency Department Disaster Plan	Hospital EDs have disaster plans that address the needs of children
Objective 2: Improve pediatric readiness in EMS systems	
Prehospital Emergency Medical Services Pediatric Readiness Recognition Program	States/jurisdictions have a standardized pediatric readiness recognition program for prehospital EMS agencies
Prehospital Emergency Medical Services Pediatric Emergency Care Coordinator (EMSC 02)	Prehospital EMS agencies have a designated pediatric emergency care coordinator
Prehospital Emergency Medical Services Use of Pediatric-Specific Equipment (EMSC 03)	Prehospital EMS agencies have a process for conducting a pediatric skills-check on the use of pediatric equipment
Prehospital Emergency Medical Services Disaster Plan	Prehospital EMS agencies have disaster plans that address the needs of children
Objective 3: Prioritize and advance family partnership and leadership in efforts to improve EMSC systems of care	
Family Representation on the State EMSC Advisory Committee	States/jurisdictions have a family representative on their State EMSC Advisory Committee who represents the emergency needs of children in their community
Program performance evaluation	
Established Permanence of EMSC (EMSC 08)	Degree to which the state has established permanence of EMSC in the state EMS system
Established Permanence of EMSC by Integrating EMSC Priorities Into Statutes/Regulations (EMSC 09)	Degree to which the state has established permanence of EMSC in the state EMS system by integrating EMSC priorities into statutes or regulations

EMS Educators, and National Association of EMS Physicians, among others. Local and regional EMS-based pediatric-specific educational initiatives and practical experience at children's hospitals have been utilized to optimize competency and comfort with care of the injured child. Additional methods for skill maintenance include simulation and online and remote training.[69–72] Simulation-based training for prehospital personnel in the management of pediatric emergencies is associated with improvement in some skills (ie, choosing the correct airway equipment and use of Broselow tape), and data suggest low-fidelity simulation training is more effective than high-fidelity simulation at improving pediatric resuscitation skills.[71] However, limited exposure of any training (whether simulation-based, lecture, or online self-study) may not be sufficient to substantially improve skills,[71] highlighting the need for iterative and varied approaches to capacity building and skill maintenance. The EMSC Program has introduced pediatric readiness to EMS systems, using collaborative approaches and promoting a PECC for each EMS service. The PECC is responsible for pediatric quality improvement to make sure pediatric equipment is up to date and working, that all emergency health care clinicians know how to use the equipment, and to use periodic simulation to refresh skills.

Individual states have the responsibility of regulating their own EMS system. In some states, EMS agencies are required to submit practice guidelines and protocols to the state medical director for approval and other states require a standardized state protocol. Evidence-based and standardized pediatric-specific protocols for prehospital care are an essential component. In all states, licensure of EMS agencies requires an approved number of education hours and/or experience dependent on the level of service provided, although these hours may or may not include pediatric education.

Direct feedback from trauma centers can assist with continued process improvement for EMS teams and agencies. Feedback can be provided in real-time by including EMS teams in trauma quality improvement meetings, in case reviews, and/or in written or oral feedback through direct communication after a child's injury-related encounter is complete. Examples of follow-up guidelines and communications are included in the EMSC Inter-facility Toolkit.[73]

Although evidence guiding prehospital care is limited, there are increasing data regarding best practices for pediatric resuscitation in out-of-hospital traumatic cardiac arrest; fluid, drug, and product administration; cervical spine stabilization; and airway management.[74–77] Field triage criteria are updated regularly by the ACS Committee on

Trauma and the CDC.[78–80] These criteria include anatomic and physiologic parameters that indicate whether transport to the highest level trauma center available within the geographic constraints of a regional trauma system is indicated. Additional parameters, including mechanism of injury and other considerations (including young age and concerns for child abuse) suggest transfer to a trauma center, although not necessarily the highest level.[79] In general, trauma systems have a goal of under-triaging no more than 5% and over-triaging between 25% and 35%. Iterative review of field criteria is essential and guides updates to national field triage guidelines.[81,82]

Community Care and Interfacility Transport

More than 27% of injury- and poison-related ED visits in the United States in 2020 were for children younger than 18 years.[83] Because of specific hospital characteristics, local triage patterns, and regional geography, many children are treated at community and/or adult-focused hospitals, including urgent care centers and EDs, with or without pediatric-specific protocols and programs. Although young and/or critically injured children may need transfer to a higher level of pediatric trauma care, many children are effectively and safely cared for at facilities that are not PTCs. For centers that evaluate and transfer injured children, there are national or multi-institutional guidelines that can guide pediatric care (eg, Image Gently using "as low as reasonably achievable" [ALARA] principles).[65,84,85] Nearly 25% of EDs do not have reduced-dose radiation protocols for computed tomography and radiographic imaging.[86] Partnering with trauma centers that care for children for advice on appropriate workup before transfer is ideal. For centers that routinely care for and admit children, other guidelines are accessible through national organizations. For example, the Pediatric Trauma Society (PTS) Hub provides updated and vetted guidelines for the acute management of injuries by body system and is readily accessible to the public on the PTS website.[87] The EMSC Inter-facility Toolkit provides guidance on specific components associated with interfacility transfer, including templates and examples of guidelines and agreements for public use, summaries of standards and regulations, and family considerations.[73]

Interhospital transfer guidelines, policies, and procedures facilitate patient transfer, often through multidisciplinary centralized "transfer centers." Transfer centers allow hospitals that initially treat children to efficiently initiate transfer to higher levels of care with a single call. These calls can facilitate guidance on when and how a child should be transferred on the basis of their physiology and injuries, what diagnostic and therapeutic interventions are indicated prior to transfer, and what method of transport is most appropriate (eg, ground vs aeromedical, one-way vs two-way with a specialized team, advanced life support vs basic life support). Pediatric transport teams may be the best resource for severely injured children because of their specific expertise in pediatric resuscitation and trauma care.[88–90] Generally, as soon as it is recognized that a child will likely need transfer to a higher level of care, further diagnostic tests beyond basic laboratory tests can be limited to those that will inform the need for intervention prior to transfer or those that dictate the need for transfer after consultation with pediatric trauma center personnel. Only necessary imaging studies should be completed to minimize radiation and to avoid the need for repeat imaging after transfer.[91,92]

Transport decisions are a collaborative effort between referring and accepting physicians to determine mode (air vs ground), the appropriate level of expertise of transport team members, and the necessary equipment to ensure a safe transport to optimize patient care, all while considering the cost and time for the mobilization of each transport type and the respective travel times.[90] Although the patient's health is the utmost priority to guide interfacility transport decisions, recognizing of the impact of transport on the child and family (eg, separation of child and parent) are important.

Telemedicine and Teleradiology

The use of technology to support clinical care decision making has increased over the past decade. Telehealth services have the potential to enhance the reach of tertiary trauma care for children in rural and underserved areas where pediatric specialty care is not readily available.[93] Services can include education, protocol sharing, ALARA-based guidelines, and administrative oversight.[93] As a consequence of the COVID-19 pandemic, teleradiology has been progressively utilized around the nation. Data suggest that efficient cloud-based imaging may lead to decreased repeat imaging, lower costs, and fewer delays in care for pediatric trauma patients.[94] With the growth of telehealth opportunities to improve care, appropriate and commensurate payment models must be developed to support telehealth services.

TRAUMA CENTERS

In 2006, the National Study on Costs and Outcomes of Trauma found that trauma center care was associated with decreased mortality, particularly for the most critically injured patients.[95] In general, trauma centers are described by their ability to provide trauma-specific care, with level I being the highest, most comprehensive level of care (Table 3).[24] Trauma centers can be self-described, state-designated, and/or ACS-verified. They can be classified as PTCs, ATCs, or combined adult/pediatric trauma centers. The ACS verifies ATCs as Level I, II, and III, and pediatric centers as Level I or II, with Level I as the highest level. Verification by the ACS is a process that is integrated into

TABLE 3. General Criteria for Trauma Centers
Adapted from the American College of Surgeons' "Resources for the Optimal Care of the Injured Patient, 2022 Standards"

Level I	Level I trauma centers must be capable of providing system leadership and comprehensive trauma care for all injuries. In its central role, a level I trauma center must have adequate depth of resources and personnel. Most level I trauma centers are university-based teaching hospitals because of the resources required for patient care, education, and research. In addition to providing acute trauma care, these centers have an important role in local trauma system development, regional disaster planning, increasing capacity, and advancing trauma care through research.
Level II	Level II trauma centers are expected to provide initial definitive trauma care for a wide range of injuries and injury severity and may take on additional responsibilities in the region related to education, system leadership, and disaster planning.
Level III	Level III trauma centers typically serve communities that may not have timely access to a level I or II trauma center and fulfill a critical role in much of the United States by serving more remote and/or rural populations. Level III trauma centers provide definitive care to patients with mild to moderate injuries, allowing patients to be cared for closer to home. These centers also have processes in place for the prompt evaluation, initial management, and transfer of patients whose needs might exceed the resources available.

their quality programs and involves 4 components: adherence to standards, comprehensive infrastructure, rigorous data to guide quality improvement, and external peer review. State criteria for trauma level designation may differ from or be identical to ACS verification criteria and may include as many as 4 or 5 levels. ACS verification criteria are reviewed and updated at regular intervals and published as "Resources for the Optimal Care of the Injured Patient," which provides a comprehensive description of the necessary resources to provide optimal care for injured adults and children.[23] A 2022 standard for ACS verification at all levels of trauma centers addresses the pediatric readiness of the hospital ED: "In all trauma centers, the emergency department must evaluate its pediatric readiness and have a plan to address any deficiencies."[23] This standard aims to raise awareness of the importance of pediatric readiness, include the trauma surgeon as part of the team, and begin to optimize resources for pediatric care in all settings.

Injured children, including adolescents, may have improved outcomes at PTCs, although the data are mixed.[24,96–100] For example, a 2019 analysis of Healthcare Cost and Utilization Project data for injured children 16 years and younger demonstrated improved mortality for children who were treated at a level 1 PTC compared with a level 1 trauma centers with no pediatric verification (adjusted odds: 0.6; 95% CI: 0.4, 0.9).[96] Similarly, a 2024 Trauma Quality Improvement Program analysis of injured children 15 years and younger with severe injury found treatment at a level 1 or level II PTC was associated with decreased mortality (adjusted odds: 0.72; 95% CI: 0.61, 0.85) compared to centers without pediatric verification. In firearm-specific injury data from the 2010–2016 National Trauma Databank files in children 13 to 16 years of age, odds of mortality were 2.88 times higher at ATCs compared with PTCs (95% CI: 1.55, 5.36; $P < .001$). However, using a 1:1 propensity score matching model, no difference in mortality was found by trauma center type.[98] Perhaps most importantly, recent data suggests risk-adjusted benchmarking in adults is not a reliable surrogate for pediatric outcomes.[101] Hence, it is imperative pediatric-specific metrics are measured and targeted for quality improvement.[102]

PTCs are generally capable of providing a broad range of pediatric services delivered by pediatric-focused staff, including physicians and nonphysician clinicians trained in pediatric emergency medicine, nurses with demonstrated competency in the care of injured children, pediatric anesthesia providers, and pediatric medical subspecialists and surgical specialists. Resources at PTCs required by the ACS include readily available/on-site interventional radiology, pediatric anesthesiology, pediatric surgery, pediatric orthopedic and neurosurgical care, and pediatric critical care, among others. A protocol for screening patients at high risk for psychological sequelae from their injury is also required, along with a process for referral to a mental health clinician trained in trauma informed care.[23] For the appropriately trained clinician, examples of evidence based therapies may include Trauma-Focused Cognitive Behavioral Therapy (TF-CBT) and Alternatives for Families: A Cognitive Behavioral Therapy (AF-CBT). To help guide trauma centers, the ACS Committee on Trauma has published best practice guidelines to guide screening and intervention for mental health disorders in the acute trauma patient, including pediatric-specific resources.[103] PTCs also often have certified child life specialists, and the 2023 standard for ACS verification requires all PTCs to have a child life program. In addition, PTCs often have child abuse physicians; pediatric registered dietitians and pharmacists; pediatric physiatrists; pediatric occupational, physical, and speech therapists; pediatric pain medicine specialists; and pediatric palliative care services. Many of these specialized services can be offered through consultation, and in some cases, telemedicine.

Emergency Department at the Trauma Center

Once a child arrives at the ED of the PTC, care continues by initiating or continuing resuscitation and identification of injuries, regardless of whether the child arrives from the field or is transferred from a referral center. Transferred patients meeting triage criteria are evaluated in the same manner as patients who have not been evaluated elsewhere.

The ACS requires all trauma centers to have clearly defined tiered activation criteria to efficiently and expeditiously mobilize the appropriate staff and resources as a team.[23] These criteria are used to ensure the resources and personnel are available that are commensurate with the needs of the patient. The ACS defines patient criteria and trauma surgeons response times for the highest level of activation.[23] Some critically injured patients may need to transition directly to the operating room or interventional radiology suite. Protocols for massive transfusion, management of noncompressible hemorrhage, replants, vascular injuries/critical limb ischemia, spine and neurological trauma, and others are critical to provide prompt limb and lifesaving care.[104–107] Special consideration should be taken to formalize systems for optimal and efficient care for injuries that may require coordination with an adult center (ie, vascular injury/compromise, replants, complex pelvic trauma). Additionally, guidelines for body region-specific imaging are critical to limit radiation and the need for repeat studies.[84,85,108–111]

Critical Care, Acute Care, and Operative Resources at the Trauma Center

A well-equipped and staffed pediatric intensive care unit (PICU) is essential for optimal care of the injured child,[112] and the availability of PICU beds within a region may improve survival in pediatric trauma.[113] PICUs offer a setting with necessary equipment and advanced technology to support physiologically unstable or intubated patients who need advanced monitoring. PICUs are staffed by physicians and nonphysician clinicians with pediatric critical care training or expertise. PICU resources are essential for the management of severe traumatic brain injury and advanced burn resuscitation.[19,114] In the PICU, attention is paid not only to physiologic stability but also to minimizing secondary harm (eg, preventable delirium, decubitus ulcers, hospital acquired infections). The ACS recommends that surgeons be the primary physicians and/or involved on all patients admitted with traumatic injuries; however, notable variability exists in the structure and care processes in place for critically injured children.[115] Critically injured children likely benefit from collaborative care by both the trauma and PICU services. Likewise, co-management with medical teams on acute care floors is often beneficial and/or essential depending on hospital-specific resources and processes (ie, which teams are in house, relative expertise, etc) and patient age and comorbid diagnoses (ie, uncontrolled diabetes, prematurity, psychosis, complex care needs, etc).

The acute care hospitalization at a PTC frequently incorporates a multidisciplinary team, including physical therapists, occupational therapists, speech therapists, and mental and behavioral health specialists (among others) concordant with each child's needs. Readily available access to the operating room at all times is critical, and the ACS requires an operating room to be staffed and available within 15 minutes of notification for level I and II centers for cases that are considered to be emergencies.[23] Urgent cases include the timely fixation of orthopedic fractures, and level I and II trauma centers must have a dedicated operating room prioritized for fracture care in nonemergent orthopedic trauma.[23]

SPECIAL CONSIDERATIONS

Issues unique to management of children, irrespective of where they receive definitive care, include reducing diagnostic radiation exposure; addressing pain during invasive procedures; weight-based fluid, drug, and electrolyte management and blood transfusions; family-centered care; and child life specialty care, among others. Careful consideration of the extent of diagnostic radiation for trauma evaluation is important because of the risk of radiation-related malignancies over the lifetime of a child.[21,22,116] Patterns of injury and pathology in children are different than those of adult patients, and much of the imaging protocols in adult trauma patients do not apply to pediatric trauma patient.[22] Knowledge of incidental findings and normal variations of pediatric anatomy may mitigate false-positive diagnoses. The ability to provide a full range of safe but effective pain management strategies for children is important, including nonpharmacologic techniques.[117,118] A child- and family-centered environment facilitates family presence during care that may range from wound debridement, suturing and dressings, fracture reduction, or post-arrest resuscitations, and optimizes communication and education between the treatment team and family.[119] The presence of child life specialists before, during, and/or after invasive procedures has been associated with improved care-experiences.[120] Family presence during trauma resuscitations requires a designated team member to be with the family at all times, when possible, to support the family and help them understand and process the events. Overall, trauma-informed care from the time of injury and throughout the care continuum, including rehabilitation, is critical.[121]

Child Abuse

A unique aspect of pediatric trauma care is the need for awareness and recognition of signs of child abuse and neglect. Various historical factors, examination findings, and diagnostic testing results are associated with child physical abuse.[122–124] A combination of these findings are often included in institution-specific screening tools. It is important to note that multiple reports have identified disparities in child abuse reporting, with children from historically marginalized racial or ethnic groups disproportionately identified as potential victims of abuse and more likely to be investigated, to be subject to unnecessary tests, and to have a change of caregiver at discharge.[125–132] Minimizing disparities in reporting (and unnecessary tests) requires a multipronged approach, including clinical pathways/guidelines and staff education on bias reduction.

Multidisciplinary teams that care for children with suspected child abuse often include social work and pediatricians with expertise in child abuse recognition and management, if available.[132] The use of telemedicine or remote consultation may help expand the reach of trained child abuse pediatricians and their expertise. The ACS, EMSC Innovation and Improvement Center, and American Pediatric Surgical Association have all published resources and/or guidelines for assessment of child abuse. For children with suspected physical abuse, the ACS recommends consultation with a surgical trauma service, in addition to a child abuse physician and social worker.[20,133,134] Diagnostic studies beyond what would typically be pursued for the injury of presentation may be required, including imaging to detect previous occult injuries and specific laboratory studies.[22] Commonly used clinical decision rules (eg, Pediatric Emergency Care and Research Network [PECARN] tools for traumatic brain injury and intra-abdominal injury) do not apply in child abuse.[135–138] Although there is variability in state statutes, all health care workers in all states are mandated by law to report concern for child maltreatment.[139]

The AAP Council on Child Abuse and Neglect has resources, including clinical reports, policy statements, technical reports, and educational offerings for physicians, patients, and families[140] pertaining to child abuse and neglect, including special populations and situations (eg, children with disabilities, sex trafficking, abusive head trauma, child abuse fatalities, and long-term sequelae and management of abuse).[140–147]

Injury Trends

Historically, the leading cause of injury-related death in children, adolescents, and young adults 1 to 19 years of age was motor vehicle collisions. In 2019, firearm injury became the leading cause of death in this population.[2] Both the ACS and the AAP have published resources for health care workers, patients, and families regarding firearm injury prevention and safe storage.[45,148] The ACS, AAP, and American College of Emergency Physicians have all published position statements, policy statements, and/or technical reports on firearm safety and firearm-related injury prevention.[33,35,149–151] There has also been an increase in suicide among adolescents and young adults in recent decades, highlighting the need for evidence-based suicide prevention strategies and suicide screening.[152–155] The AAP Blueprint on Youth Suicide Prevention is a free online education resource to support pediatric health clinicians "identify equitable youth suicide prevention strategies" (https://www.aap.org/suicideprevention).[154] Overall, since 2010, trauma-related ED visits have been increasing, although with fewer hospitalizations.[156] The COVID-19 pandemic was associated with further shifts in injury epidemiology among children and adolescents.[122,157–168]

REHABILITATION AND REINTEGRATION INTO THE COMMUNITY

Injury during childhood has been associated with poor educational outcomes, functional status and quality of life.[5,169–173] The trauma community has more recently emphasized survivorship and recovery given the potential long-term physical and mental health effects of trauma on the child, family, and community.[174] To this end, postinjury trauma-informed care, along with recovery and resiliency programs, are becoming more common.[175–178] The goal of a trauma system is to return children to full, age-appropriate function with the ability to reach maximum adult potential. This process includes reintegration into the community, school or educational environment, and primary care medical home. The primary care pediatrician is an essential navigator in this post injury phase of care, supporting children and adolescents with short- and long-term sequelae, in addition to assisting in the transition to adult trauma-informed care clinicians. Crisis intervention and ongoing support can be offered through hospital-based violence intervention programs to youth who are injured through interpersonal violence and are at risk of reinjury and psychosocial trauma.[179–181] For injured children with extensive care needs after the acute injury, the availability of both inpatient and outpatient rehabilitation resources specifically for children is a scarce yet vital component of trauma care. Physical, occupational, cognitive, speech, and play therapy, along with psychological and social support, are essential elements of a comprehensive rehabilitation effort for the injured child and family. The ability to begin early rehabilitation during the acute hospitalization, particularly for children with traumatic brain injury and cognitive challenges or with fractures and mobility requirements, is inherent to recovery and reintegration.[182–184] There are many areas of the country with no inpatient pediatric rehabilitation resources and limited outpatient resources that are barriers to optimal or expeditious recovery. Novel approaches to care, such as telehealth and mobile or wearable health technologies, may help increase access to pediatric-specific care to meet the needs of all children, despite where they live, grow, and play.

Mental Health

The impact of injury on a child goes well beyond the initial hospital encounter. Mental health sequalae, such as posttraumatic stress disorder (PTSD) and depression, are common after pediatric injury. An estimated 20% of children report posttraumatic stress symptoms after injury, and previous injury is also associated with anxiety and depressive symptoms.[16,103,185] In a managed Medicaid population (using the MarketScan database), an estimated 25%

of children 0 to 17 years of age with nonfatal firearm injury were diagnosed with a new mental health condition.[4] In another MarketScan study, documented mental health diagnoses increased by 63% in the 12 months after unintentional injury, from 95.9/1000 person-years preinjury to 156.7/1000 person-years postinjury (RR: 1.63; 95% CI: 1.39, 1.92). The rate of psychotropic prescriptions also increased from 121.7/1000 person-years preinjury to 310.9/1000 person-years postinjury (RR: 2.55; 95% CI: 2.26, 2.89).[186] Similar trends have been identified in injury-specific pediatric populations, particularly among children and youth with firearm injuries.[4,187] Estimates do vary, as yet another MarketScan study looking at and evaluating children 6 to 17 years of age admitted for traumatic injury found only 3.3% developed a subsequent mental health diagnosis (ie, PTSD, depression, anxiety, or adjustment disorder), and only 1.6% developed PTSD, presumably because of suboptimal recognition of these symptoms.[17] Despite variability in estimates, there is widespread understanding that injury is intricately related to mental health and quality of life after injury and also affects families, parents, and caregivers.[5,185,188] Resources including screening tools for children and adolescents can be found in the ACS "Best Practice Guidelines: Screening and Intervention for Mental Health Disorders and Substance Use and Misuse in the Acute Trauma Patient."[103]

PERFORMANCE IMPROVEMENT, EDUCATION, AND OUTREACH

Effective clinical performance and quality improvement are integral components of trauma programs and indirectly for trauma systems as a whole. Performance improvement efforts often focus on patient safety and harm prevention, reporting of delays in diagnosis or care, near misses, trends in morbidity across service lines, mortality review to recognize opportunities for improvement, and/or communication issues. Review of trauma care provided to children is facilitated by comprehensive chart review. Collaborative reviews between transferring and receiving institutions and transport teams are important for children transferred for additional care. Each dedicated trauma center has an institutional trauma registry, which exports data to state and (often) national databases so that outcomes can be risk-adjusted and benchmarked to allow for evaluation of care quality across institutions and inform opportunities for improvement. Quality review generally adopts the Donabedian framework of structure, process, and outcomes, with selection of performance improvement initiatives based on performance indicators that fall below a specific threshold based on benchmarking.[189,190] Quality indicators should be remeasured after implementation, with reassessment of outcomes. Outcomes are compared through programs like the ACS Pediatric Trauma Quality Improvement Program (TQIP), the Cardiac Arrest Registry to Enhance Survival (CARES), and the National EMS Information System (NEMSIS). Data systems, however, continue to be disjointed and lack the ability to link across data sets to fully understand the continuum of care and the connection between processes and outcomes. One consideration is to create a National Unique Identifier for each trauma patient that starts from the initial encounter (eg, EMS, urgent care, or other) and is added to all centers (and their data set), at which the patient is treated. This identifier would follow a child from initial evaluation through acute treatment, rehabilitation, and post-discharge follow-up. This is an important step to obtain comprehensive understanding of the impact of a pediatric trauma system on long-term outcomes.

At all institutions that treat injured children, systematic child mortality and morbidity review processes help identify variations in standard of care, trends in outcomes, and systematic risk factors for which interventions can be developed, evaluated, and improved. The implementation of technologies such as video review of trauma activations aids in ongoing improvement of team dynamics, improvement of trauma and emergency resuscitation quality, and multidisciplinary team education.[23,191]

Capacity-building, education, and training at all health care centers that treat injured children is important. The highest-level trauma centers often provide education and outreach to local and regional community centers and state agencies to improve care for children. National trauma and EMS organizations work jointly to include children's unique needs and interests in their programs to ensure that children receive timely and appropriate care no matter where they are injured. Continuing trauma education for physicians, nurses, and prehospital professionals can be accomplished by courses such as the Advanced Trauma Care for Nurses (ATCN), Trauma Nursing Core Course (TNCC), PTS/STN Pediatric Trauma Across the Care Continuum nursing course, PALS Plus: Trauma, NAEMT's PHTLS and EPC courses for prehospital providers, and the Advanced Trauma Life Support (ATLS) courses, all of which includes key components for children. The Emergency Nursing Pediatric Course has injury-specific modules as well.

PEDIATRIC DISASTER PREPAREDNESS AND SURGE

Disaster preparedness for adults and children in the United States has improved significantly since Hurricane Katrina in 2005. Hospital accreditation programs including The Joint Commission have strengthened their disaster preparedness requirements for institutions. There is considerable federal support through the Administration for Strategic Preparedness and Response Hospital Preparedness Program and the HRSA Regional Pediatric Pandemic Network (PPN) to improve pediatric disaster care nationally.[192–195] As of 2022, there were 10 children's hospitals partnering with professional associations, nonprofit organizations, government agencies, and others through the PPN to improve the pediatric readiness of health care systems and ensure high-quality, equitable pediatric care in emergencies, disasters, and pandemics.

Children have unique needs for health care in mass casualty incidents involving trauma and burns.[26] Along with physiologic considerations unique to the trauma management of children, additional issues of triage, identification, decontamination, tracking, and reunification are considered. Support services including child life, social work, child and adolescent psychologists, and bereavement counselors, among others, are important to recovery.[196] Children and youth with special health care needs (CYSHCN) are a vulnerable population during disasters because of mobility challenges, language impairment, executive functioning and sensory difficulties, medical conditions with and without technology dependence, and other trauma exposure.[195] Even with disaster planning, households with individuals with disabilities are less likely to be prepared, and very few studies have examined the optimal methods of disaster communication tailored for families of CYSHCN.[197,198] The AAP has resources available for patients, families, and physicians related to CYSHCN to prepare before, help during, and recover after disasters.[199,200]

A process for recruiting pediatric health care professionals when a surge response is needed is a mainstay of institutional disaster plans. Although the needs of children in disasters can be anticipated, the capability of a trauma system to meet these needs requires frequent simulation practice and mock disaster drills, including multi-institutional, state, and regional planning.[201] State, regional, and federal agencies manage the legal, operational, and information systems to provide effective pediatric mass casualty care through the following: (1) pre-disaster/mass casualty planning, management, and assessment with input from child health professionals; (2) close cooperation, agreements, public-private partnerships, and unique delivery systems; and (3) use of existing public health data to assess pediatric populations at risk and to model graded response plans on the basis of increasing patient volume and acuity.[202] Regional Medical Operations Coordinating Centers (MOCCs) can coordinate care across EMS agencies, hospitals, public health, and emergency management leadership.[203] They can effectively load-balance a trauma system ensuring each child receives optimal care at the appropriate facility.[204] Pediatric trauma systems may play a role in supporting adult centers during crisis, such as occurred during the COVID-19 pandemic, during which surgeons boarded in trauma and critical care provided intensive care services for adults.[205]

HEALTH EQUITY AND DISPARITIES IN CARE

Inequity and disparities in pediatric injury prevalence, trauma care, and outcomes are recognized as increasingly important considerations and key determinants of short- and long-term outcomes.[13,31,206,207] Although the extensive use of protocol-guided management during trauma care might be presumed to mitigate treatment disparities, the evidence suggests otherwise.[13] Disparities in injury incidence, treatment, and outcomes frequently result from racial, economic, and geographic drivers of health and may be attributable to individual or systemic bias or a combination of these.[31,208–212]

The burden of injury falls disproportionately on minoritized children and those who are economically or geographically disadvantaged.[159,207,213,214] Studies examining the impact of socioeconomic status on injury outcomes often use insurance coverage and median household income as proxies, as they are readily available data elements that may reflect financial and educational resources available to children and their families for primary, secondary, and tertiary injury prevention and trauma care.[215] Recent literature explores composite scores of deprivation (or disadvantage or vulnerability), based on different geographic areas of residence (ie, census tract, census block, zip code, or county), and have consistently identified an association between increased "deprivation" and incidence of injury and specific injury types.[207] Additionally, disparities exist related to treatment experiences in the ED, such as pain control and sedation during fracture management, radiographic evaluations, child abuse screening, transfer to PTCs, and discharge to inpatient rehabilitation.[126,216–218]

Many studies have examined the association of race or ethnicity and/or insurance status with mortality. Black and Hispanic children who require operative intervention following major abdominopelvic trauma have a higher risk of postoperative mortality compared with white children.[219] In other studies, lack of insurance and disparities in socioeconomic status were associated with mortality after pediatric injury.[220–222] There are limited data on racial and ethnic disparities in pediatric trauma morbidities such as disability, quality of life, and mental health; however, studies suggest Black children have worse functional outcomes after traumatic brain injury.[223,224] These differences are not due to a biologic difference, but reflect complex underlying disparities.

Community violence exposure is also a prominent determinant of negative physical and mental health outcomes. Community violence exposure is linked to numerous negative psychological outcomes in children, such as PTSD, externalizing behavior, and internalizing symptoms as well as obesity, asthma, and health-risk behaviors. All pediatricians, pediatric subspecialists, and pediatric trauma care clinicians and partners can address community violence exposure and related health disparities by developing trauma-informed systems that routinely screen for community violence exposure, provide basic support for affected families, and link those in need to trauma-focused interventions through the mechanisms of trauma-informed care.[225]

Next steps at the ACS level involve including an equity-focused quality framework into data systems such as the Trauma Quality Improvement Program (TQIP) and beginning to study patient-reported outcomes, which may provide more insight into disparities in care.[226,227] The Center for Disease Control and Prevention's Division of Adolescent and School Health has defined action steps to address health disparities and include focused programmatic efforts, raising awareness, building partnerships, and documenting impact.[228] Additionally, the US Department of Health and Human Services and the Office of Disease Prevention and Health Promotion's Healthy People 2030 focuses on 'eliminating health disparities and creating equitable opportunities for people to live healthy lives.' More information on Health Equity in Healthy People 2030, including goals, objectives and tools for action, can be found online (http://odphp.health.gov/).[228] Altogether, disparities occur along the continuum of the pediatric trauma care and equity-based efforts to address these disparities must also span the continuum of care.

RESEARCH

State and federal financial support for research, advocacy, education, and trauma system development and maintenance provides integration of pediatric and adult care in all phases of planning and implementation of trauma systems. Regional, state, and national organizations advocate for the comprehensive support of pediatric trauma-related research. Current examples of organizations that fund or perform at least some pediatric trauma research include certain federally funded HRSA programs (eg, the EMSC Program, EMSC Innovation and Improvement Center, Pediatric Emergency Care and Research Network, and PPN), the Pediatric Emergency Research Network, the Injury Free Coalition for Kids, Safe Kids, the Childress Institute for Pediatric Trauma, the PTS, the American Pediatric Surgical Association, the CDC, and the National Institutes for Health, among others. Research efforts to address disparities in pediatric injury are essential.[229]

The National Academies of Sciences, Engineering, and Medicine (NASEM) called for a National Trauma Research Action Plan (NTRAP) in 2016, and the Department of Defense Combat Casualty Care Research Program funded its development in 2018. The NTRAP brings the "research and medical community of trauma systems across the United States together around a prioritized, comprehensive research agenda, develops the best assessment tools for long-term functional outcomes for injured patients, and identifies regulatory barriers to conducting trauma research and develops recommendations for best practices."[230] Since its inception, the NTRAP has used Delphi methodology to develop priorities of research regarding long-term outcomes, pediatrics, and injury prevention, among others.[226,231,232]

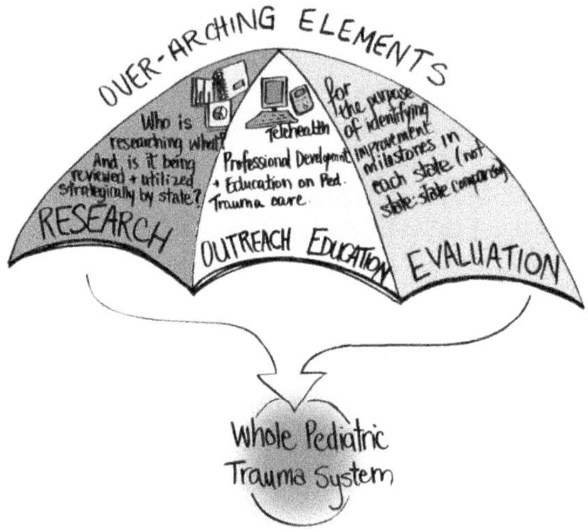

FIGURE 5.
Graphic depicting trauma system involvement above and beyond patient care.[7]
Figure developed by Tanya Gerber, graphic recorder. Reprinted with permission.

ADVOCACY

Advocating for the health and wellness of children and youth is integral to preventing death and disability from trauma and can lead to improved funding and resources to optimize both prevention initiatives and health care provided. The AAP is one of many organizations active in advocacy for child health and injury prevention at the national and state levels. Organizations including the ACS and the AAP offer advocacy-focused conferences for members and they partner with many other organizations, including SafeKids, to promote issues such as injury prevention and firearm safety.[45,50,148]

SUMMARY/CONCLUSIONS

Injury is the leading cause of death and a cause of disability in children in the United States. Using a systems-based approach along the continuum of care for trauma system development and planning along with integration of research, outreach, and iterative evaluation (Figure 5) provides a framework to integrate care and optimize outcomes. The ideal pediatric trauma system is comprehensive and cohesive but seamlessly integrated with the adult trauma system of care to provide optimal and equitable care for the "right child, at the right place, and at the right time" across this continuum.

LEAD AUTHORS

Katherine T. Flynn-O'Brien, MD, MPH, FAAP, FACS
Vijay Srinivasan, MBBS, MD, FCCM, FAAP
Mary E. Fallat, MD, FAAP, FACS

AMERICAN ACADEMY OF PEDIATRICS

Committee on Pediatric Emergency Medicine, 2024–2025

Toni K. Gross MD, MPH, FAAP, FAEMS, Chairperson
Kerry S. Caperell, MD, FAAP
Jennifer A. Hoffmann, MD, MS, FAAP
Jennifer E. McCain, MD, FAAP
Sylvia Owusu-Ansah, MD, MPH, FAAP
Christian D. Pulcini, MD, MEd, MPH, FAAP
Mohsen Saidinejad, MD, MS, MBA, FAAP
David Schnadower, MD, MPH, FAAP
Caleb E. Ward, MB, BChir, MPH, FAAP
Muhammad Waseem, MD, FAAP

Former Committee Member Contributors, 2021–2024

Gregory P. Conners, MD, MPH, MBA, FAAP, Chairperson 2020–2024
Benson S. Hsu, MD, MBA, FAAP, FCCM
Deborah C.W. Hsu, MD, MEd, FAAP
Lois K. Lee, MD, MPH, FAAP
Suzan S. Mazor, MD
Ronald I. Paul, MD, FAAP

Liaisons

Christopher S. Amato, MD, FAAP, FACEP - *American College of Emergency Physicians*
Mary E. Fallat, MD, FAAP, FACS - *American College of Surgeons/AAP Section on Surgery*
Kathryn Kothari, MD - *National Association of EMS Physicians*
Cynthiana Lightfoot - *AAP FamilY Partnerships Network*
Katherine E. Remick, MD, FAAP, FACEP, FAEMS - *National Association of Emergency Medical Technicians*
Sam Shahid, MBBS, MPH - *American College of Emergency Physicians*
Elizabeth L. Stone, RN, PhD, CEN - *Emergency Nurses Association*
Cynthia J. Wright-Johnson, MSN, RN - *National Association of State EMS Officials*

Staff

Susan Tellez

Council on Injury, Violence, and Poison Prevention Executive Committee, 2024–2025

Lois K. Lee, MD, MPH, FAAP, Chairperson
Alison Culyba, MD, MPH, PhD, FAAP
James Dodington, MD, FAAP
Katherine T. Flynn-O'Brien, MD, MPH, FAAP
Aimee Grace, MD, FAAP
Maya Haasz, MD, FAAP
Sadiqa A. I. Kendi, MD, MPH, FAAP
Andrew Waititu Kiragu, MD, FAAP
Terri D. McFadden, MD, MPH, FAAP
Kevin C. Osterhoudt, MD, MS, FAAP
Benjamin D. Hoffman, MD, FAAP, Immediate Past Chairperson

Former Committee Member Contributors, 2021–2014

Brian D. Johnston, MD, MPH, FAAP
Milton Tenenbein, MD, FAAP

Liaisons

Suzanne M. Beno, MD - *Canadian Paediatric Society*

Staff

Bonnie Kozial

Section on Critical Care Executive Committee, 2024–2025

Vijay Srinivasan, MBBS, MD, FCCM, FAAP, Chairperson
Benson S. Hsu, MD, MBA, FCCM, FAAP, Immediate Past Chairperson
Wendy G. Hasson, MD, FAAP
Jimmy W. Huh, MD, FAAP
Jason (Jake) M. Kane, MD, MS, FAAP, FCCM
Lia H. Lowrie, MD, FAAP
Simon-Noel Ndely, MD, FAAP
Margaret A. Satchell, MD, FAAP

Liaisons

Michael S.D. Agus, MD, FAAP - *Pediatric Critical Care Chiefs Network, Pediatric Intermediate Care Network*
Rajit K. Basu, MD, MS, FCCM - *Society of Critical Care Medicine*
Mary Lihinie deAlmeida, MD - *World Federation of Pediatric Intensive and Critical Care Societies*

Former Committee Member Contributors, 2021–2024

Scottie B. Day, MD
Nicholas A. Ettinger, MD, PhD, CPPS, FAAP
Steven Loscalzo, MD
Elizabeth Mack, MD, MS, FAAP, Chairperson 2018-2021
Linda B. Siegel, FAAP, FAAHPM

Staff

Susan Tellez

Section on Surgery Executive Committee, 2024–2025

Marybeth Browne, MD, MS, FAAP, Chairperson
Elizabeth Beierle, MD, FAAP
Barbara Anne Gaines, MD, FAAP
Saleem Islam, MD, MPH, FAAP, Immediate Past Chair
Marc P. Michalsky, MD, MBA, FAAP
Mehul V. Raval, MD, MS, FAAP
Danielle Saunders Walsh, MD, FAAP

Former Committee Member Contributors, 2021–2024

Andrew Davidoff, MD, FAAP
Cynthia Downard, MD, FAAP
Kenneth Gow, MD, MHA, FAAP

Liaisons

Mary E. Fallat, MD, FAAP, FACS - *American College of Surgeons/AAP Section on Surgery*

Staff

Vivian Thorne

Section on Transport Medicine Executive Committee, 2024–2025

Michael Stroud, MD, FAAP, Chairperson
Archana Dhar, MD, FAAP
Matthew Harris, MD, FAAP
Rudy Kink, MD, FAAP
Emily Krennerich, MD, FAAP
Franscesca Miquel Verges, MD, FAAP
Holly Engelstad, MD, FAAP

Liaisons

Michael Bigham, MD, FAAP - *Air Medical Physician Association (AMPA)*
Beth Diehl, DNP, NNP-BC CCRN, LNCC - *National Association of Neonatal Nurses (NANN)*
Robert Holcomb, Jr, MD, FAAP - *Commission on Accreditation of Medical Transport Systems*
Corina Noje, MD, FAAP - *Ground Air Medical qUality Transport Quality Improvement Collaborative (GAMUT)*
Tammy Rush, MSN, RN, C-NPT, EMT - *National Association of Neonatal Nurses*
Hamilton Schwartz, MD, FAAP - *National Association of EMS Physicians (NAEMSP)*

Affiliates Transport Medicine Specialists

Tammy Rush, MSN, RN, C-NPT, EMT, Chairperson
Lisa Pruitt, BSN, RN, C-NPT, Vice Chairperson
Timothy Farmer, MSc, RRT-NPS
Laura Westley, RN
Jessica Wright, BSN, RNC, NPT
Richard Zimmerman, RRT-NPS, C-NPT, FP-C
Webra Price Douglas, CRNP, PhD
Beth C. Diehl, DNP, NNP-BC, CCRN, LNCC

Staff

Dana Bennett-Tejes, MA, MNM

ABBREVIATIONS

AAP: American Academy of Pediatrics
ACS: American College of Surgeons
ATC: adult trauma center
CDC: Centers for Disease Control and Prevention
CYSHCN: children and youth with special health care needs
COT: Committee on Trauma
ED: emergency department
EMS: emergency medical services
EMSC: Emergency Medical Services for Children
HRSA: Health Resources and Services Administration
NTRAP: National Trauma Research Action Plan
PICU: pediatric intensive care unit
PPN: pediatric pandemic network
PTC: pediatric trauma center
PTS: Pediatric Trauma Society
PTSAS: Pediatric Trauma System Assessment Score

However, policy statements from the American Academy of Pediatrics may not reflect the views of the liaisons or the organizations or government agencies that they represent.

The guidance in this statement does not indicate an exclusive course of treatment or serve as a standard of medical care. Variations, taking into account individual circumstances, may be appropriate.

All policy statements from the American Academy of Pediatrics automatically expire 5 years after publication unless reaffirmed, revised, or retired at or before that time.

https://doi.org/10.1542/peds.2025-072721

COMPANION PAPER: A companion to this article can be found online at www.pediatrics.org/cgi/doi/10.1542/peds.2025-072720.

REFERENCES

1. Centers for Disease Control and Prevention, National Center for Injury Prevention and Control. Web-based Injury Statistics Query and Reporting System (WISQARS) [online]. 2023; https://wisqars.cdc.gov/. Accessed April 1, 2023.
2. Goldstick JE, Cunningham RM, Carter PM. Current Causes of Death in Children and Adolescents in the United States. *N Engl J Med.* 2022;386(20):1955–1956. PubMed doi: 10.1056/NEJMc2201761
3. Cunningham RM, Walton MA, Carter PM. The Major Causes of Death in Children and Adolescents in the United States. *N Engl J Med.* 2018;379(25):2468–2475. PubMed doi: 10.1056/NEJMsr1804754
4. Oddo ER, Maldonado L, Hink AB, Simpson AN, Andrews AL. Increase in Mental Health Diagnoses Among Youth With Nonfatal Firearm Injuries. *Acad Pediatr.* 2021;21(7):1203–1208. PubMed doi: 10.1016/j.acap.2021.06.003
5. Burd RS, Jensen AR, VanBuren JM, et al; Eunice Kennedy Shriver National Institute of Child Health and Human Development Collaborative Pediatric Critical Care Research Network Assessment of Functional Outcomes and Health-Related Quality of Life after Pediatric Trauma Investigators. Long-Term Outcomes after Pediatric Injury: Results of the Assessment of Functional Outcomes and Health-Related Quality of Life after Pediatric Trauma Study. *J Am Coll Surg.* 2021;233(6):666–675.e2. PubMed doi: 10.1016/j.jamcollsurg.2021.08.693
6. Sacco WJ, Long WB, Copes WS, et al. Continuum of care trauma outcome evaluation. *Socioecon Plann Sci.* 1993;27(3):219–232. doi: 10.1016/0038-0121(93)90006-5
7. Fallat ME, Gaines BA, Haley K, Meredith JW, Mooney DP, Upperman JS. Proceedings of the second Childress Summit on pediatric trauma. *J Trauma Acute Care Surg.* 2016;81(4):795–801. doi: 10.1097/TA.0000000000001197
8. Kaplan G, Bo-Linn G, Carayon P, Pronovost P, Rouse W, Reid P, Saunders R. *Bringing a Systems Approach to Health.* Discussion Paper. Institute of Medicine and National Academy of Engineering; 2013. Accessed July 11, 2025. http://nam.edu/wp-content/uploads/2015/06/systemsapproaches.
9. US Department of Health and Human Services. Systems-Based Approach to Helathcare Incident Managment. *Public Health Emergency* 2023; https://www.phe.gov/Preparedness/planning/mscc/healthcarecoalition/chapter1/Pages/systemsbasedapproach.aspx. Accessed April 6, 2023.
10. Fallat ME, Treager C, Humphrey S, et al. A Novel Approach to Assessment of US Pediatric Trauma System Development. *JAMA Surg.* 2022;157(11):1042–1049. PubMed doi: 10.1001/jamasurg.2022.4303
11. Ranney M, Karb R, Ehrlich P, Bromwich K, Cunningham R, Beidas RS; FACTS Consortium. What are the long-term consequences of youth exposure to firearm injury, and how do we prevent them? A scoping review. *J Behav Med.* 2019;42(4):724–740. PubMed doi: 10.1007/s10865-019-00035-2
12. Jimenez N, Quistberg A, Vavilala MS, Jaffe KM, Rivara FP. Utilization of Mental Health Services After Mild Pediatric Traumatic Brain Injury. *Pediatrics.* 2017;139(3):e20162462. PubMed doi: 10.1542/peds.2016-2462
13. LaPlant MB, Hess DJ. A review of racial/ethnic disparities in pediatric trauma care, treatment, and outcomes. *J Trauma Acute Care Surg.* 2019;86(3):540–550. PubMed doi: 10.1097/TA.0000000000002160
14. Yue JK, Upadhyayula PS, Avalos LN, Cage TA. Pediatric Traumatic Brain Injury in the United States: Rural-Urban Disparities and Considerations. *Brain Sci.* 2020;10(3):135. PubMed doi: 10.3390/brainsci10030135
15. Burdick KJ, Lee LK, Mannix R, Monuteaux MC, Hirsh MP, Fleegler EW. Racial and Ethnic Disparities in Access to Pediatric Trauma Centers in the United States: A Geographic Information Systems Analysis. *Ann Emerg Med.* 2023;81(3):325–333. PubMed doi: 10.1016/j.annemergmed.2022.08.454
16. Jenness JL, Witt CE, Quistberg DA, et al. Association of physical injury and mental health: Results from the national comorbidity survey- adolescent supplement. *J Psychiatr Res.* 2017;92:101–107. PubMed doi: 10.1016/j.jpsychires.2017.03.022
17. Chandler JM, Chan KS, Han R, Chao SD. Mental health outcomes in pediatric trauma patients: A 10 year real world analysis using a large database approach. *J Pediatr Surg.* 2022;57(2):291–296. PubMed doi: 10.1016/j.jpedsurg.2021.09.049
18. Newgard CD, Lin A, Olson LM, et al; Pediatric Readiness Study Group. Evaluation of Emergency Department Pediatric Readiness and Outcomes Among US Trauma Centers. *JAMA Pediatr.* 2021;175(9):947–956. PubMed doi: 10.1001/jamapediatrics.2021.1319
19. Kochanek PM, Tasker RC, Carney N, et al. Guidelines for the Management of Pediatric Severe Traumatic Brain Injury, Third Edition: Update of the Brain Trauma Foundation Guidelines. *Pediatr Crit Care Med.* 2019;20(3S Suppl 1):S1–S82.
20. American College of Surgeons Trauma Quality Programs. *Best Practices Guidelines for Trauma Center Recognition of Child Abuse, Elder Abuse, and Intimate Partner Violence.* American College of Surgeons; 2019
21. The Image Gently Aliance. Accessed May 26, 2022. http://imagegently.org/.
22. American College of Surgeons Trauma Quality Programs. *ACS TQIP Best Practices Guidelines in Imaging.* American College of Surgeons; 2018
23. American College of Surgeons. *Resources for Optimal Care of the Injured Patient.* American College of Surgeons; 2022
24. United States Government Accountability Office. Pediatric Trauma Centers: Availability, Outcomes, and Federal Support Related to Pediatric Trauma Care. 2017; https://www.gao.gov/products/gao-17-334. Accessed November 28, 2022.
25. Livingston DH. Survivorship. *J Trauma Acute Care Surg.* 2023;94(1):1–7. PubMed doi: 10.1097/TA.0000000000003806

26. Disaster Preparedness Advisory CDISASTER PREPAREDNESS ADVISORY COUNCIL; COMMITTEE ON PEDIATRIC EMERGENCY MEDICINE. Ensuring the Health of Children in Disasters. *Pediatrics.* 2015;136(5):e1407–e1417. PubMed doi: 10.1542/peds. 2015-3112

27. Carr BG, Nance ML. Access to pediatric trauma care: alignment of providers and health systems. *Curr Opin Pediatr.* 2010;22(3):326–331. PubMed doi: 10.1097/MOP.0b013e3283392a48

28. Burdick KJ, Lee LK, Mannix R, Monuteaux MC, Hirsh MP, Fleegler EW. Racial and ethnic disparities in access to pediatric trauma centers in the United States: a geographic information systems analysis. *Ann Emerg Med.* 2023;81(3):325–333. doi: 10.1016/j. annemergmed.2022.08.454

29. Dorney K, Dodington JM, Rees CA, et al; and the Injury Free Coalition for Kids®. Preventing injuries must be a priority to prevent disease in the twenty-first century. *Pediatr Res.* 2020;87(2): 282–292. PubMed doi: 10.1038/s41390-019-0549-7

30. Haddon W Jr. A logical framework for categorizing highway safety phenomena and activity. *J Trauma.* 1972;12(3):193–207. PubMed doi: 10.1097/00005373-197203000-00002

31. Kendi S, Macy ML. The Injury Equity Framework - Establishing a Unified Approach for Addressing Inequities. *N Engl J Med.* 2023; 388(9):774–776. PubMed doi: 10.1056/NEJMp2212378

32. Pressley JC, Barlow B. Child and adolescent injury as a result of falls from buildings and structures. *Inj Prev.* 2005;11(5):267–273. PubMed doi: 10.1136/ip.2004.007724

33. Lee LK, Fleegler EW, Goyal MK, et al. Techical report: Firearm-Related Injuries and Deaths in Children and Youth. *Pediatrics.* 2022;150(6).

34. Durkin MS, Laraque D, Lubman I, Barlow B. Epidemiology and prevention of traffic injuries to urban children and adolescents. *Pediatrics.* 1999;103(6):e74. PubMed doi: 10.1542/peds.103.6.e74

35. Lee LK, Fleegler EW, Goyal MK, et al. Policy statement: Firearm-Related Injuries and Deaths in Children and Youth: Injury Prevention and Harm Reduction. *Pediatrics.* 2022;150(6).

36. Durbin DR, Hoffman BD, Agran PF, et al; Council On Injury, Violence, and Poison Prevention. Child Passenger Safety. *Pediatrics.* 2018; 142(5):e20182460. doi: 10.1542/peds.2018-2460

37. Dr. Barbara Barlow. *Changing the Face of Medicine* 2015; https:// cfmedicine.nlm.nih.gov/physicians/biography_22.html. Accessed September 1, 2023.

38. Denny SA, Quan L, Gilchrist J, et al; COUNCIL ON INJURY, VIOLENCE, AND POISON PREVENTION. Prevention of Drowning. *Pediatrics.* 2019;143(5):e20190850. PubMed doi: 10.1542/peds.2019-0850

39. Kendi S, Johnston BD; Council On Injury, Violence, and Poison Prevention. Child Pedestrian Safety. *Pediatrics.* 2023;152(1)

40. Kendi S, Johnston BD, Hoffman B, et al. Council On Injury V, Poison P. Epidemiology and Prevention of Child Pedestrian Injury. *Pediatrics.* 2023;152(1):e2023062508. doi: 10.1542/peds.2023-062508

41. Lee LK, Flaherty MR, Blanchard AM, Agarwal M; Council On Injury, Violence, and Poison Prevention. Helmet Use in Preventing Head Injuries in Bicycling, Snow Sports, and Other Recreational Activities and Sports. *Pediatrics.* 2022;150(3):e2022058878. doi: 10.1542/peds.2022-058878

42. Melhado C, Remick K, Miskovic A, et al. The Association between Pediatric Readiness and Mortality for Injured Children Treated at US Trauma Centers. *Ann Surg.* 2023. PubMed

43. Perrin EM, Skinner AC, Sanders LM, et al. The Injury Prevention Program to Reduce Early Childhood Injuries: A Cluster Randomized Trial. *Pediatrics.* 2024;153(5):e2023062966. PubMed doi: 10.1542/peds.2023-062966

44. TIPP (The Injury Prevention Program). https://publications.aap.org/patiented/pages/c_tipp?autologincheck=redirected. Accessed May 30, 2022.

45. Safer: Storing Firearms Prevents Harm. https://shop.aap.org/safer-storing-firearms-prevents-harm/. Accessed December 10, 2022.

46. Centers for Disease Control and Prevention. CDC HeadsUp. Safe Brain. Safe Future. 2023; https://www.cdc.gov/headsup/index.html. Accessed April 14, 2023.

47. Centers for Disease Control and Prevention. Child Abuse and Neglect. 2023; https://www.cdc.gov/violence-prevention/. Accessed April 14, 2023.

48. American Academy of Pediatrics. AAP Message from the Section on Child Death Review and Prevention Chair. Accessed January 26, 2024. https://www.aap.org/en/community/aap-sections/child-death-review-and-prevention/about-socdrp/message-from-the-socdrp-chair/

49. Batra EK, Quinlan K, Palusci VJ, et al; AAP SECTION ON CHILD DEATH REVIEW AND PREVENTION; COUNCIL ON INJURY, VIOLENCE, AND POISON PREVENTION; COUNCIL ON CHILD ABUSE AND NEGLECT. Child Fatality Review. *Pediatrics.* 2024;153(3):e2023065481. PubMed doi: 10.1542/peds.2023-065481

50. Safe Kids Worldwide. https://www.safekids.org/. Accessed May 30, 2022.

51. Injury Free Coalition for Kids. https://www.injuryfree.org/. Accessed May 30, 2022.

52. Prevent Child Injury. https://www.preventchildinjury.org/. Accessed September 1, 2023.

53. Prevent Child Abuse America. https://preventchildabuse.org/. Accessed January 21, 2014.

54. Charlie's House. https://www.charlieshouse.org/. Accessed Janurary 21, 2024.

55. Tomas C, Kallies K, Levas M, deRoon-Cassini T, Cassidy L, Flynn-O'Brien K. Mechanisms of paediatric injury: an 11-year review of injury trends from the National Trauma Data Bank. *Inj Prev.* 2025;31(2):107–113. PubMed doi: 10.1136/ip-2024-045440

56. Institute of Medicine. *Emergency Care for Children: Growing Pains.* The National Academies Press; 2007.

57. Gausche-Hill M, Ely M, Schmuhl P, et al. A national assessment of pediatric readiness of emergency departments. *JAMA Pediatr.* 2015;169(6):527–534. PubMed doi: 10.1001/jamapediatrics.2015.138

58. Department of Health and Human Services, Health Resources and Services Administration, Emergency Medical Services for Children Program. Performance Measures Manual. Health Resources and Services Administration; 2023

59. Ross SW, Campion E, Jensen AR, et al. Prehospital and emergency department pediatric readiness for injured children: A statement from the American College of Surgeons Committee on Trauma Emergency Medical Services Committee. *J Trauma Acute Care Surg.* 2023;95(2):e6–e10. PubMed doi: 10.1097/TA.0000000000003997

60. Ames SG, Davis BS, Marin JR, et al. Emergency Department Pediatric Readiness and Mortality in Critically Ill Children. *Pediatrics.* 2019;144(3):e20190568. PubMed doi: 10.1542/peds.2019-0568

61. Newgard CD, Lin A, Malveau S, et al; Pediatric Readiness Study Group. Emergency Department Pediatric Readiness and Short-term and Long-term Mortality Among Children Receiving Emergency Care. *JAMA Netw Open.* 2023;6(1):e2250941. PubMed doi: 10.1001/jamanetworkopen.2022.50941

62. Newgard CD, Lin A, Goldhaber-Fiebert JD, et al; Pediatric Readiness Study Group. Association of Emergency Department Pediatric Readiness With Mortality to 1 Year Among Injured Children Treated at Trauma Centers. *JAMA Surg.* 2022;157(4):e217419. PubMed doi: 10.1001/jamasurg.2021.7419

63. American Academy of PediatricsCommittee on Pediatric Emergency MedicineAmerican College of Emergency PhysiciansPediatric CommitteeEmergency Nurses Association Pediatric Committee. Joint policy statement–guidelines for care of children in the emergency department. *Pediatrics.* 2009;124(4):1233–1243. PubMed doi: 10.1542/peds.2009-1807

64. Brown KM, Ackerman AD, Ruttan TK, et al; COMMITTEE ON PEDIATRIC EMERGENCY MEDICINE; AMERICAN COLLEGE OF EMERGENCY PHYSICIANS, PEDIATRIC EMERGENCY MEDICINE COMMITTEE; EMERGENCY NURSES ASSOCIATION, PEDIATRIC COMMITTEE, 2018–2019. Access to Optimal Emergency Care for Children. *Pediatrics.* 2021;147(5):e2021050787. PubMed doi: 10.1542/peds.2021-050787

65. Remick K, Gausche-Hill M, Joseph MM, Brown K, Snow SK, Wright JL; AMERICAN ACADEMY OF PEDIATRICS Committee on Pediatric Emergency Medicine and Section on Surgery; AMERICAN COLLEGE OF EMERGENCY PHYSICIANS Pediatric Emergency Medicine Committee; EMERGENCY NURSES ASSOCIATION Pediatric Committee. Pediatric Readiness in the Emergency Department. *Pediatrics.* 2018;142(5):e20182459. PubMed doi: 10.1542/peds.2018-2459

66. Moore B, Shah MI, Owusu-Ansah S, et al; AMERICAN ACADEMY OF PEDIATRICS COMMITTEE ON PEDIATRIC EMERGENCY MEDICINE AND SECTION ON EMERGENCY MEDICINE EMS SUBCOMMITTEE; AMERICAN COLLEGE OF EMERGENCY PHYSICIANS EMERGENCY MEDICAL SERVICES COMMITTEE; EMERGENCY NURSES ASSOCIATION PEDIATRIC COMMITTEE; NATIONAL ASSOCIATION OF EMERGENCY MEDICAL SERVICES PHYSICIANS STANDARDS AND CLINICAL PRACTICE COMMITTEE; NATIONAL ASSOCIATION OF EMERGENCY MEDICAL TECHNICIANS EMERGENCY PEDIATRIC CARE COMMITTEE. Pediatric Readiness in Emergency Medical Services Systems. *Pediatrics.* 2020;145(1):e20193307. PubMed doi: 10.1542/peds.2019-3307

67. Owusu-Ansah S, Moore B, Shah MI, et al; COMMITTEE ON PEDIATRIC EMERGENCY MEDICINE, SECTION ON EMERGENCY MEDICINE; EMS SUBCOMMITTEE, SECTION ON SURGERY. Pediatric Readiness in Emergency Medical Services Systems. *Pediatrics.* 2020;145(1):e20193308. PubMed doi: 10.1542/peds.2019-3308

68. National Association of Emergency Medical System Physicians. About EMS: Who Provides EMS? https://www.naemt.org/about-ems/EMS-overview. Accessed July 7, 2022.

69. Eppich WJ, Nypaver MM, Mahajan P, et al. The role of high-fidelity simulation in training pediatric emergency medicine fellows in the United States and Canada. *Pediatr Emerg Care.* 2013;29(1):1–7. PubMed doi: 10.1097/PEC.0b013e31827b20d0

70. Warren L, Sapien R, Fullerton-Gleason L. Is online pediatric continuing education effective in a rural state? *Prehosp Emerg Care.* 2008;12(4):498–502. PubMed doi: 10.1080/10903120802096753

71. Lammers RL, Willoughby-Byrwa MJ, Vos DG, Fales WD. Comparison of Four Methods of Paramedic Continuing Education in the Management of Pediatric Emergencies. *Prehosp Emerg Care.* 2022;26(4):463–475. PubMed doi: 10.1080/10903127.2021.1916140

72. Farrell C, Dorney K, Mathews B, et al. A Statewide Collaboration to Deliver and Evaluate a Pediatric Critical Care Simulation Curriculum for Emergency Medical Services. *Front Pediatr.* 2022;10:903950. PubMed doi: 10.3389/fped.2022.903950

73. Emergency Medical Services for Children. *Inter Facility Transfer Tool Kit for the Pediatric Patient.* EMSC Innovation and Improvement Center; 2018.

74. Fischer PE, Perina DG, Delbridge TR, et al. Spinal Motion Restriction in the Trauma Patient - A Joint Position Statement. *Prehosp Emerg Care.* 2018;22(6):659–661. PubMed doi: 10.1080/10903127.2018.1481476

75. Fallat ME; American College of Surgeons Committee on Trauma; American College of Emergency Physicians Pediatric Emergency Medicine Committee; National Association of EMS Physicians; American Academy of Pediatrics Committee on Pediatric Emergency Medicine. Withholding or termination of resuscitation in pediatric out-of-hospital traumatic cardiopulmonary arrest. *Ann Emerg Med.* 2014;63(4):504–515. PubMed doi: 10.1016/j.annemergmed.2014.01.013

76. Bosson N, Hansen M, Gausche-Hill M, et al. Design of a novel clinical trial of prehospital pediatric airway management. *Clin Trials.* 2022;19(1):62–70. PubMed doi: 10.1177/17407745211059855

77. Polites SF, Moody S, Williams RF, et al. Timing and volume of crystalloid and blood products in pediatric trauma: An Eastern Association for the Surgery of Trauma multicenter prospective observational study. *J Trauma Acute Care Surg.* 2020;89(1):36–42. PubMed doi: 10.1097/TA.0000000000002702

78. McCoy CE, Chakravarthy B, Lotfipour S. Guidelines for Field Triage of Injured Patients: In conjunction with the Morbidity and Mortality Weekly Report published by the Center for Disease Control and Prevention. *West J Emerg Med.* 2013;14(1):69–76. PubMed doi: 10.5811/westjem.2013.1.15981

79. American College of Surgeons. National Guideline for the Field Triage of Injured Patients Patients. American College of Surgeons; 2022

80. Newgard CD, Fischer PE, Gestring M, et al; Writing Group for the 2021 National Expert Panel on Field Triage. National guideline for the field triage of injured patients: Recommendations of the National Expert Panel on Field Triage, 2021. *J Trauma Acute*

Care Surg. 2022;93(2):e49–e60. PubMed doi: 10.1097/TA.0000000000003627

81. Lupton JR, Davis-O'Reilly C, Jungbauer RM, et al. Mechanism of injury and special considerations as predictive of serious injury: A systematic review. *Acad Emerg Med.* 2022;29(9):1106–1117. PubMed doi: 10.1111/acem.14489
82. Lupton JR, Davis-O'Reilly C, Jungbauer RM, et al. Under-Triage and Over-Triage Using the Field Triage Guidelines for Injured Patients: A Systematic Review. *Prehosp Emerg Care.* 2022;27(1):1–8. PubMed
83. National Center for Health Statistics. *Emergency Department Visits in the United States, 2016–2020.* Accessed January 10, 2023. https://www.cdc.gov/nchs/dhcs/ed-visits/index.htm
84. Marin JR, Lyons TW, Claudius I, et al; AMERICAN ACADEMY OF PEDIATRICS Committee on Pediatric Emergency Medicine, Section on Radiology; AMERICAN COLLEGE OF RADIOLOGY; AMERICAN COLLEGE OF EMERGENCY PHYSICIANS Pediatric Emergency Medicine Committee. Optimizing Advanced Imaging of the Pediatric Patient in the Emergency Department: Technical Report. *Pediatrics.* 2024;154(1):e2024066855. PubMed doi: 10.1542/peds.2024-066855
85. Marin JR, Lyons TW, Claudius I, et al; AMERICAN ACADEMY OF PEDIATRICS Committee on Pediatric Emergency Medicine, Section on Radiology; AMERICAN COLLEGE OF RADIOLOGY; AMERICAN COLLEGE OF EMERGENCY PHYSICIANS Pediatric Emergency Medicine Committee. Optimizing Advanced Imaging of the Pediatric Patient in the Emergency Department: Policy Statement. *Pediatrics.* 2024;154(1):e2024066854. PubMed doi: 10.1542/peds.2024-066854
86. Remick KE, Hewes HA, Ely M, et al. National Assessment of Pediatric Readiness of US Emergency Departments During the COVID-19 Pandemic. *JAMA Netw Open.* 2023;6(7):e2321707. PubMed doi: 10.1001/jamanetworkopen.2023.21707
87. Pediatric Trauma Society. PTS Guidelines HUB. 2023; https://pediatrictraumasociety.org/resources/guidelines/. Accessed April 9, 2023.
88. Orr RA, Felmet KA, Han Y, et al. Pediatric specialized transport teams are associated with improved outcomes. *Pediatrics.* 2009;124(1):40–48. PubMed doi: 10.1542/peds.2008-0515
89. Calhoun A, Keller M, Shi J, et al. Do Pediatric Teams Affect Outcomes of Injured Children Requiring Inter-hospital Transport? *Prehosp Emerg Care.* 2017;21(2):192–200. PubMed doi: 10.1080/10903127.2016.1218983
90. Stroud MH, Trautman MS, Meyer K, et al. Pediatric and neonatal interfacility transport: results from a national consensus conference. *Pediatrics.* 2013;132(2):359–366. PubMed doi: 10.1542/peds.2013-0529
91. Brinkman AS, Gill KG, Leys CM, Gosain A. Computed tomography-related radiation exposure in children transferred to a Level I pediatric trauma center. *J Trauma Acute Care Surg.* 2015;78(6):1134–1137. PubMed doi: 10.1097/TA.0000000000000645
92. Chwals WJ, Robinson AV, Sivit CJ, Alaedeen D, Fitzenrider E, Cizmar L. Computed tomography before transfer to a level I pediatric trauma center risks duplication with associated increased radiation exposure. *J Pediatr Surg.* 2008;43(12):2268–2272. PubMed doi: 10.1016/j.jpedsurg.2008.08.061
93. Kohler JE, Falcone RA Jr, Fallat ME. Rural health, telemedicine and access for pediatric surgery. *Curr Opin Pediatr.* 2019;31(3):391–398. PubMed doi: 10.1097/MOP.0000000000000763
94. Puckett Y, To A. Pediatric Trauma Transfer Imaging Inefficiencies-Opportunities for Improvement with Cloud Technology. *AIMS Public Health.* 2016;3(1):49–53. PubMed doi: 10.3934/publichealth.2016.1.49
95. MacKenzie EJ, Rivara FP, Jurkovich GJ, et al. A national evaluation of the effect of trauma-center care on mortality. *N Engl J Med.* 2006;354(4):366–378. PubMed doi: 10.1056/NEJMsa052049
96. Myers SR, Branas CC, French B, Nance ML, Carr BG. A National Analysis of Pediatric Trauma Care Utilization and Outcomes in the United States. *Pediatr Emerg Care.* 2019;35(1):1–7. PubMed doi: 10.1097/PEC.0000000000000902
97. Dreyfus J, Flood A, Cutler G, Ortega H, Kreykes N, Kharbanda A. Comparison of pediatric motor vehicle collision injury outcomes at Level I trauma centers. *J Pediatr Surg.* 2016;51(10):1693–1699. PubMed doi: 10.1016/j.jpedsurg.2016.04.005
98. Swendiman RA, Luks VL, Hatchimonji JS, et al. Mortality After Adolescent Firearm Injury: Effect of Trauma Center Designation. *J Adolesc Health.* 2021;68(5):978–984. PubMed doi: 10.1016/j.jadohealth.2020.09.004
99. Walther AE, Falcone RA, Pritts TA, Hanseman DJ, Robinson BR. Pediatric and adult trauma centers differ in evaluation, treatment, and outcomes for severely injured adolescents. *J Pediatr Surg.* 2016;51(8):1346–1350. PubMed doi: 10.1016/j.jpedsurg.2016.03.016
100. Ramsey WA, Huerta CT, O'Neil CF, et al. Admission to a Verified Pediatric Trauma Center is Associated With Improved Outcomes in Severely Injured Children. *J Pediatr Surg.* 2024;59(3):488–493. PubMed doi: 10.1016/j.jpedsurg.2023.10.064
101. Melhado C, Evans LL, Miskovic A, et al. Benchmarking Pediatric Trauma Care in Mixed Trauma Centers: Adult Risk-Adjusted Mortality Is Not a Reliable Indicator of Pediatric Outcomes. *J Am Coll Surg.* 2024;238(3):243–251. PubMed doi: 10.1097/XCS.0000000000000919
102. Fallat ME. Invited Commentary: A Common-Sense Approach to Improving Pediatric Trauma Care in Mixed Trauma Centers. *J Am Coll Surg.* 2024;238(3):251–253. PubMed doi: 10.1097/XCS.0000000000000903
103. American College of Surgeons Trauma Quality Programs. *Best Practice Guidelines: Screening and Intervention for Mental Health Disorders and Substance Use and Misuse in the Acute Trauma Patient.* American College of Surgeons; 2022
104. Evangelista ME, Gaffley M, Neff LP. Massive Transfusion Protocols for Pediatric Patients: Current Perspectives. *J Blood Med.* 2020;11:163–172. PubMed doi: 10.2147/JBM.S205132
105. Neff LP, Beckwith MA, Russell RT, Cannon JW, Spinella PC. Massive Transfusion in Pediatric Patients. *Clin Lab Med.* 2021;41(1):35–49. PubMed doi: 10.1016/j.cll.2020.10.003

106. Martin MJ, Brasel KJ, Brown CVR, et al. Pediatric emergency resuscitative thoracotomy: A Western Trauma Association, Pediatric Trauma Society, and Eastern Association for the Surgery of Trauma collaborative critical decisions algorithm. *J Trauma Acute Care Surg.* 2023;95(4):583–591. PubMed doi: 10.1097/TA.0000000000004055

107. Selesner L, Yorkgitis B, Martin M, et al. Emergency department thoracotomy in children: A Pediatric Trauma Society, Western Trauma Association, and Eastern Association for the Surgery of Trauma systematic review and practice management guideline. *J Trauma Acute Care Surg.* 2023;95(3):432–441. PubMed doi: 10.1097/TA.0000000000003879

108. Letica-Kriegel AS, Kaplan A, Orlas C, Masiakos PT. Variability of Pediatric Cervical Spine Clearance Protocols: A Systematic Review. *Ann Surg.* 2022;276(6):989–994. PubMed doi: 10.1097/SLA.0000000000005453

109. Ozcan A, Ahn T, Akay B, Menoch M. Imaging for Pediatric Blunt Abdominal Trauma With Different Prediction Rules: Is the Outcome the Same? *Pediatr Emerg Care.* 2022;38(2):e654–e658. PubMed doi: 10.1097/PEC.0000000000002346

110. Stephens CQ, Boulos MC, Connelly CR, Gee A, Jafri M, Krishnaswami S. Limiting thoracic CT: a rule for use during initial pediatric trauma evaluation. *J Pediatr Surg.* 2017;52(12):2031–2037. PubMed doi: 10.1016/j.jpedsurg.2017.08.039

111. Babl FE, Borland ML, Phillips N, et al; Paediatric Research in Emergency Departments International Collaborative (PREDICT). Accuracy of PECARN, CATCH, and CHALICE head injury decision rules in children: a prospective cohort study. *Lancet.* 2017;389(10087):2393–2402. PubMed doi: 10.1016/S0140-6736(17)30555-X

112. Hsu BS, Hill V, Frankel LR, et al. Executive Summary: Criteria for Critical Care of Infants and Children: PICU Admission, Discharge, and Triage Practice Statement and Levels of Care Guidance. *Pediatrics.* 2019;144(4):2019–2433. PubMed doi: 10.1542/peds.2019-2433

113. Odetola FO, Miller WC, Davis MM, Bratton SL. The relationship between the location of pediatric intensive care unit facilities and child death from trauma: a county-level ecologic study. *J Pediatr.* 2005;147(1):74–77. PubMed doi: 10.1016/j.jpeds.2005.02.012

114. Advanced Burn Life Support Course, Provider Manual 2023 update. American Burn Association; 2023

115. Flynn-O'Brien KT, Thompson LL, Gall CM, Fallat ME, Rice TB, Rivara FP. Variability in the structure and care processes for critically injured children: A multicenter survey of trauma bay and intensive care units. *J Pediatr Surg.* 2016;51(3):490–498. PubMed doi: 10.1016/j.jpedsurg.2015.09.006

116. Brody AS, Frush DP, Huda W, Brent RL; American Academy of Pediatrics Section on Radiology. Radiation risk to children from computed tomography. *Pediatrics.* 2007;120(3):677–682. PubMed doi: 10.1542/peds.2007-1910

117. Chou R, Gordon DB, de Leon-Casasola OA, et al. Management of Postoperative Pain: A Clinical Practice Guideline From the American Pain Society, the American Society of Regional Anesthesia and Pain Medicine, and the American Society of Anesthesiologists' Committee on Regional Anesthesia, Executive Committee, and Administrative Council. *J Pain.* 2016;17(2):131–157. PubMed doi: 10.1016/j.jpain.2015.12.008

118. Smith HAB, Besunder JB, Betters KA, et al. 2022 Society of Critical Care Medicine Clinical Practice Guidelines on Prevention and Management of Pain, Agitation, Neuromuscular Blockade, and Delirium in Critically Ill Pediatric Patients With Consideration of the ICU Environment and Early Mobility. *Pediatr Crit Care Med.* 2022;23(2):e74–e110. PubMed doi: 10.1097/PCC.0000000000002873

119. Leske JS, McAndrew NS, Brasel KJ, Feetham S. Family Presence During Resuscitation After Trauma. *J Trauma Nurs.* 2017;24(2):85–96. PubMed doi: 10.1097/JTN.0000000000000271

120. Hall JE, Patel DP, Thomas JW, Richards CA, Rogers PE, Pruitt CM. Certified Child Life Specialists Lessen Emotional Distress of Children Undergoing Laceration Repair in the Emergency Department. *Pediatr Emerg Care.* 2018;34(9):603–606. PubMed doi: 10.1097/PEC.0000000000001559

121. Forkey H, Szilagyi M, Kelly ET, et al; COUNCIL ON FOSTER CARE, ADOPTION, AND KINSHIP CARE, COUNCIL ON COMMUNITY PEDIATRICS, COUNCIL ON CHILD ABUSE AND NEGLECT, COMMITTEE ON PSYCHOSOCIAL ASPECTS OF CHILD AND FAMILY HEALTH. Trauma-Informed Care. *Pediatrics.* 2021;148(2):e2021052580. PubMed doi: 10.1542/peds.2021-052580

122. Escobar MA Jr, Flynn-O'Brien KT, Auerbach M, et al. The association of nonaccidental trauma with historical factors, examination findings, and diagnostic testing during the initial trauma evaluation. *J Trauma Acute Care Surg.* 2017;82(6):1147–1157. PubMed doi: 10.1097/TA.0000000000001441

123. Christian CW; Committee on Child Abuse and Neglect, American Academy of Pediatrics. The evaluation of suspected child physical abuse. *Pediatrics.* 2015;135(5):e1337–e1354. PubMed doi: 10.1542/peds.2015-0356

124. Pierce MC, Kaczor K, Lorenz DJ, et al. Validation of a Clinical Decision Rule to Predict Abuse in Young Children Based on Bruising Characteristics. *JAMA Netw Open.* 2021;4(4):e215832. PubMed doi: 10.1001/jamanetworkopen.2021.5832

125. Joseph B, Sakran JV, Obaid O, et al. Nationwide Management of Trauma in Child Abuse: Exploring the Racial, Ethnic, and Socioeconomic Disparities. *Ann Surg.* 2022;276(3):500–510. PubMed doi: 10.1097/SLA.0000000000005548

126. Diyaolu M, Ye C, Huang Z, et al. Disparities in detection of suspected child abuse. *J Pediatr Surg.* 2022. PubMed

127. Edwards F, Wakefield S, Healy K, Wildeman C. Contact with Child Protective Services is pervasive but unequally distributed by race and ethnicity in large US counties. *Proc Natl Acad Sci U S A.* 2021;118(30):e2106272118. PubMed doi: 10.1073/pnas.2106272118

128. Lane WG, Rubin DM, Monteith R, Christian CW. Racial differences in the evaluation of pediatric fractures for physical abuse. *JAMA.* 2002;288(13):1603–1609. PubMed doi: 10.1001/jama.288.13.1603

129. Palusci VJ, Botash AS. Race and Bias in Child Maltreatment Diagnosis and Reporting. *Pediatrics.* 2021;148(1):e2020049625. PubMed doi: 10.1542/peds.2020-049625

130. Raz M. Unintended Consequences of Expanded Mandatory Reporting Laws. *Pediatrics.* 2017;139(4):e20163511. PubMed doi: 10.1542/peds.2016-3511

131. Raz M, Dettlaff A, Edwards F. The Perils of Child "Protection" for Children of Color: Lessons From History. *Pediatrics*. 2021; 148(1):e2021050237. PubMed doi: 10.1542/peds.2021-050237

132. Raz M, Gupta-Kagan J, Asnes AG; Using Child Abuse Specialists to Reduce Unnecessary Child Protective Services Reports and Investigations. Using Child Abuse Specialists to Reduce Unnecessary Child Protective Services Reports and Investigations. *JAMA Pediatr.* 2023;177(12):1249–1250. PubMed doi: 10.1001/jamapediatrics.2023.3676

133. Escobar MA Jr, Wallenstein KG, Christison-Lagay ER, Naiditch JA, Petty JK. Child abuse and the pediatric surgeon: A position statement from the Trauma Committee, the Board of Governors and the Membership of the American Pediatric Surgical Association. *J Pediatr Surg.* 2019;54(7):1277–1285. PubMed doi: 10.1016/j.jpedsurg.2019.03.009

134. EMSC Innovation and Improvement Center. Pediatric Education and Advocacy Kit (PEAK): Child Abuse. https://emscimprovement.center/education-and-resources/peak/child-abuse/. Accessed January 27, 2024.

135. Magana JN, Kuppermann N. The PECARN TBI Rules Do Not Apply to Abusive Head Trauma. *Acad Emerg Med.* 2017;24(3):382–384. PubMed doi: 10.1111/acem.13155

136. Ide K, Uematsu S, Tetsuhara K, Yoshimura S, Kato T, Kobayashi T. External Validation of the PECARN Head Trauma Prediction Rules in Japan. *Acad Emerg Med.* 2017;24(3):308–314. PubMed doi: 10.1111/acem.13129

137. Holmes JF, Lillis K, Monroe D, et al; Pediatric Emergency Care Applied Research Network (PECARN). Identifying children at very low risk of clinically important blunt abdominal injuries. *Ann Emerg Med.* 2013;62(2):107–116.e2. PubMed doi: 10.1016/j.annemergmed.2012.11.009

138. Springer E, Frazier SB, Arnold DH, Vukovic AA. External validation of a clinical prediction rule for very low risk pediatric blunt abdominal trauma. *Am J Emerg Med.* 2019;37(9):1643–1648. PubMed doi: 10.1016/j.ajem.2018.11.031

139. Child Welfare Information Gateway. *Mandatory Reporters of Child Abuse and Neglect.* US Department of Health and HumanServices, Administration for Children and Families, Children's Bureau; 2019. Accessed July 11, 2025. https://www.childwelfare.gov/topics/systemwide/laws-policies/statutes/manda/

140. American Academy of Pediatrics. Child Abuse and Neglect. 2023; https://www.aap.org/en/patient-care/child-abuse-and-neglect/#:~:text=The%20Federal%20Child%20Abuse%20Prevention,younger%20than%2018%20years%20of. Accessed April 9, 2023.

141. Flaherty E, Legano L, Idzerda S, et al; COUNCIL ON CHILD ABUSE AND NEGLECT. Ongoing Pediatric Health Care for the Child Who Has Been Maltreated. *Pediatrics.* 2019;143(4):e20190284. PubMed doi: 10.1542/peds.2019-0284

142. Greenbaum J, Bodrick NCOMMITTEE ON CHILD ABUSE AND NEGLECT; SECTION ON INTERNATIONAL CHILD HEALTH. Global Human Trafficking and Child Victimization. *Pediatrics.* 2017;140(6):e20173138. PubMed doi: 10.1542/peds.2017-3138

143. Legano LA, Desch LW, Messner SA, et al; COUNCIL ON CHILD ABUSE AND NEGLECT; COUNCIL ON CHILDREN WITH DISABILITIES. Maltreatment of Children With Disabilities. *Pediatrics.* 2021; 147(5):e2021050920. PubMed doi: 10.1542/peds.2021-050920

144. Sege RD, Amaya-Jackson L, Flaherty EG, et al; AMERICAN ACADEMY OF PEDIATRICS Committee on Child Abuse and Neglect, Council on Foster Care, Adoption, and Kinship Care; AMERICAN ACADEMY OF CHILD AND ADOLESCENT PSYCHIATRY Committee on Child Maltreatment and Violence; NATIONAL CENTER FOR CHILD TRAUMATIC STRESS. Clinical Considerations Related to the Behavioral Manifestations of Child Maltreatment. *Pediatrics.* 2017;139(4):e20170100. PubMed doi: 10.1542/peds.2017-0100

145. Palusci VJ, Kay AJ, Batra E, et al; Council on Child Abuse and Neglect; Section on Child Death Review and Prevention; Task Force on Sudden Infant Death Syndrome; NATIONAL ASSOCIATION OF MEDICAL EXAMINERS. Identifying Child Abuse Fatalities During Infancy. *Pediatrics.* 2019;144(3):e20192076. PubMed doi: 10.1542/peds.2019-2076

146. Keeshin B, Forkey HC, Fouras G, et al; AMERICAN ACADEMY OF PEDIATRICS, COUNCIL ON CHILD ABUSE AND NEGLECT, COUNCIL ON FOSTER CARE, ADOPTION, AND KINSHIP CARE, AMERICAN ACADEMY OF CHILD AND ADOLESCENT PSYCHIATRY, COMMITTEE ON CHILD MALTREATMENT AND VIOLENCE, COMMITTEE ON ADOPTION AND FOSTER CARE. Children Exposed to Maltreatment: Assessment and the Role of Psychotropic Medication. *Pediatrics.* 2020;145(2):e20193751. PubMed doi: 10.1542/peds.2019-3751

147. Narang SK, Fingarson A, Lukefahr J, et al; COUNCIL ON CHILD ABUSE AND NEGLECT. Abusive Head Trauma in Infants and Children. *Pediatrics.* 2020;145(4):e20200203. PubMed doi: 10.1542/peds.2020-0203

148. American College of Surgeons Committee on Trauma. Firearm Injury Prevention Activities. 2023; https://www.facs.org/quality-programs/trauma/advocacy-and-injury-prevention/firearm-injury-prevention-activities/. Accessed April 9, 2023.

149. American College of Emergency Physicians. Firearm Safety and Injury Prevention. *Ann Emerg Med.* 2020;76(4):e99–e100. PubMed doi: 10.1016/j.annemergmed.2020.08.001

150. Petty JK, Henry MCW, Nance ML, Ford HR; APSA Board of Governors. Firearm Injuries and Children: Position Statement of the American Pediatric Surgical Association. *Pediatrics.* 2019;144(1):e20183058. PubMed doi: 10.1542/peds.2018-3058

151. American College of Surgeons. Statement on Firearm Injuries. 2013; https://www.facs.org/about-acs/statements/firearm-injuries/. Accessed April 9, 2023.

152. Ramchand R, Gordon JA, Pearson JL. Trends in Suicide Rates by Race and Ethnicity in the United States. *JAMA Netw Open.* 2021; 4(5):e2111563. PubMed doi: 10.1001/jamanetworkopen.2021.11563

153. Mann JJ, Michel CA, Auerbach RP. Improving Suicide Prevention Through Evidence-Based Strategies: A Systematic Review. *Am J Psychiatry.* 2021;178(7):611–624. PubMed doi: 10.1176/appi.ajp.2020.20060864

154. American Academy of Pediatrics. Screening for Suicide in Clinical Practice *Suicide: Blueprint for Youth Suicide Prevention* 2023; https://www.aap.org/en/patient-care/blueprint-for-youth-suicide-prevention/strategies-for-clinical-settings-for-youth-suicide-

prevention/screening-for-suicide-risk-in-clinical-practice/. Accessed August 15, 2023.

155. Theodorou CM, Yamashiro KJ, Stokes SC, Salcedo ES, Hirose S, Beres AL. Pediatric suicide by violent means: a cry for help and a call for action. *Inj Epidemiol.* 2022;9(1):13. PubMed doi: 10.1186/s40621-022-00378-6

156. Lee LK, Porter JJ, Mannix R, et al. Pediatric Traumatic Injury Emergency Department Visits and Management in US Children's Hospitals From 2010 to 2019. *Ann Emerg Med.* 2022;79(3):279–287. PubMed doi: 10.1016/j.annemergmed.2021.10.008

157. Collings AT, Farazi M, Van Arendonk KJ, et al; Midwest Pediatric Surgery Consortium. The COVID-19 pandemic and associated rise in pediatric firearm injuries: A multi-institutional study. *J Pediatr Surg.* 2022;57(7):1370–1376. PubMed doi: 10.1016/j.jpedsurg.2022.03.034

158. Collings AT, Farazi M, Van Arendonk K, et al; Midwest Pediatric Surgery Consortium. Impact of "Stay-at-Home" orders on non-accidental trauma: A multi-institutional study. *J Pediatr Surg.* 2022;57(6):1062–1066. PubMed doi: 10.1016/j.jpedsurg.2022.01.056

159. Flynn-O'Brien KT, Collings AT, Farazi M, et al; Midwest Pediatric Surgery Consortium. Pediatric injury trends and relationships with social vulnerability during the COVID-19 pandemic: A multi-institutional analysis. *J Trauma Acute Care Surg.* 2023;94(1):133–140. PubMed doi: 10.1097/TA.0000000000003687

160. Georgeades CM, Collings AT, Farazi M, et al. A multi-institutional study evaluating pediatric burn injuries during the COVID-19 pandemic. *J Burn Care Res.* 2023;44(2):399–407. PubMed doi: 10.1093/jbcr/irac118

161. Bell TM, Robbins C, Gosain A. The Influence of the COVID-19 Pandemic on Pediatric Firearm Injuries. *Pediatrics.* 2021;148(1):e2020049746. PubMed doi: 10.1542/peds.2020-049746

162. Bessoff KE, Han RW, Cho M, et al. Epidemiology of pediatric trauma during the COVID-19 pandemic shelter in place. *Surg Open Sci.* 2021;6:5–9. PubMed doi: 10.1016/j.sopen.2021.06.001

163. Bullinger LR, Boy A, Messner S, Self-Brown S. Pediatric emergency department visits due to child abuse and neglect following COVID-19 public health emergency declaration in the Southeastern United States. *BMC Pediatr.* 2021;21(1):401. PubMed doi: 10.1186/s12887-021-02870-2

164. Cappa C, Jijon I. COVID-19 and violence against children: A review of early studies. *Child Abuse Negl.* 2021;116(Pt 2):105053. PubMed doi: 10.1016/j.chiabu.2021.105053

165. DeLaroche AM, Rodean J, Aronson PL, et al. Pediatric Emergency Department Visits at US Children's Hospitals During the COVID-19 Pandemic. *Pediatrics.* 2021;147(4):e2020039628. PubMed doi: 10.1542/peds.2020-039628

166. Gastineau KAB, Williams DJ, Hall M, et al. Pediatric Firearm-Related Hospital Encounters During the SARS-CoV-2 Pandemic. *Pediatrics.* 2021;148(2):e2021050223. PubMed doi: 10.1542/peds.2021-050223

167. Pelletier JH, Rakkar J, Au AK, Fuhrman D, Clark RSB, Horvat CM. Trends in US Pediatric Hospital Admissions in 2020 Compared With the Decade Before the COVID-19 Pandemic. *JAMA Netw Open.* 2021;4(2):e2037227. PubMed doi: 10.1001/jamanetworkopen.2020.37227

168. Sheridan GA, Nagle M, Russell S, et al. Pediatric Trauma and the COVID-19 Pandemic: A 12-Year Comparison in a Level-1 Trauma Center. *HSS J.* 2020;16:(suppl 1):92–96. PubMed doi: 10.1007/s11420-020-09807-y

169. Visnick MJ, Pell JP, Mackay DF, Clark D, King A, Fleming M. Educational and employment outcomes associated with childhood traumatic brain injury in Scotland: A population-based record-linkage cohort study. *PLoS Med.* 2023;20(3):e1004204. PubMed doi: 10.1371/journal.pmed.1004204

170. Evans A, Dunstan F, Fone DL, et al. The role of health and social factors in education outcome: A record-linked electronic birth cohort analysis. *PLoS One.* 2019;14(8):e0220771. PubMed doi: 10.1371/journal.pone.0220771

171. Vassel-Hitier J, Verdier V, Rasquier S, Chalard A, Laurent-Vannier A, Chevignard M. Language, intellectual and educational outcomes after moderate-to-severe traumatic brain injury sustained before the age of 18 months. *Brain Inj.* 2019;33(8):1105–1115. PubMed doi: 10.1080/02699052.2019.1623420

172. Pruente J, Heinemann AW, Zebracki K, Mukherjee S, Gaebler-Spira D. Adult outcomes for children who sustained firearm-related spinal cord injuries. *J Spinal Cord Med.* 2023;46(1):68–74. PubMed doi: 10.1080/10790268.2021.1943250

173. Burd RS, Jensen AR, VanBuren JM, et al; Eunice Kennedy Shriver National Institute of Child Health and Human Development Collaborative Pediatric Critical Care Research Network Assessment of Health-Related Quality of Life and Functional Outcomes After Pediatric Trauma Investigators. Factors Associated With Functional Impairment After Pediatric Injury. *JAMA Surg.* 2021;156(8):e212058. PubMed doi: 10.1001/jamasurg.2021.2058

174. Herrera-Escobar JP, Schneider JC. From Survival to Survivorship - Framing Traumatic Injury as a Chronic Condition. *N Engl J Med.* 2022;387(7):581–583. PubMed doi: 10.1056/NEJMp2205162

175. Ridings LE, Anton MT, Winkelmann J, et al. Trauma Resilience and Recovery Program: Addressing Mental Health in Pediatric Trauma Centers. *J Pediatr Psychol.* 2019;44(9):1046–1056. PubMed doi: 10.1093/jpepsy/jsz053

176. Livingston DH, La Bagnara S, Sieck D, et al. The Center for Trauma Survivorship: Addressing the great unmet need for posttrauma center care. *J Trauma Acute Care Surg.* 2020;89(5):940–946. PubMed doi: 10.1097/TA.0000000000002775

177. Dicker RA, Thomas A, Bulger EM, et al; ISAVE Workgroup; Members of the ISAVE Workgroup. Strategies for Trauma Centers to Address the Root Causes of Violence: Recommendations from the Improving Social Determinants to Attenuate Violence (ISAVE) Workgroup of the American College of Surgeons Committee on Trauma. *J Am Coll Surg.* 2021;233(3):471–478.e1. PubMed doi: 10.1016/j.jamcollsurg.2021.06.016

178. Marsac ML, Kassam-Adams N, Hildenbrand AK, et al. Implementing a Trauma-Informed Approach in Pediatric Health Care Networks. *JAMA Pediatr.* 2016;170(1):70–77. PubMed doi: 10.1001/jamapediatrics.2015.2206

179. The Health Alliance for Violence Intervention. https://www.thehavi.org/. Accessed May 30, 2022.

180. National Network for Hospital-based Violence Intervention Programs. *NNHVIP Policy White Paper, Hospital-based Violence Intervention: Practices and Policies to End the Cycle of Violence*. National Network for Hospital-based Violence Intervention Programs; 2019

181. Bonne S, Hink A, Violano P, et al. Understanding the makeup of a growing field: A committee on trauma survey of the national network of hospital-based violence intervention programs. *Am J Surg*. 2022;223(1):137–145. PubMed doi: 10.1016/j.amjsurg.2021.07.032

182. Fink EL, Beers SR, Houtrow AJ, et al; PICU-Rehabilitation Study Group. Early Protocolized Versus Usual Care Rehabilitation for Pediatric Neurocritical Care Patients: A Randomized Controlled Trial. *Pediatr Crit Care Med*. 2019;20(6):540–550. PubMed doi: 10.1097/PCC.0000000000001881

183. Wieczorek B, Burke C, Al-Harbi A, Kudchadkar SR. Early Mobilization in the Pediatric Intensive Care Unit- A Systematic Review. *J Pediatr Intensive Care*. 2015;4:212–217. doi: 10.1055/s-0035-1563386

184. Niedzwecki CM, Rogers AT, Fallat ME. Using Rehabilitation along the Pediatric Trauma Continuum as a Strategy to Define Outcomes in Traumatic Brain Injury. *Clin Pediatr Emerg Med*. 2018;19(3):260–271. doi: 10.1016/j.cpem.2018.08.005

185. Kassam-Adams N, Marsac ML, Hildenbrand A, Winston F. Posttraumatic stress following pediatric injury: update on diagnosis, risk factors, and intervention. *JAMA Pediatr*. 2013;167(12):1158–1165. PubMed doi: 10.1001/jamapediatrics.2013.2741

186. Bushroe KM, Hade EM, McCarthy TA, Bridge JA, Leonard JC. Mental Health after Unintentional Injury in a Pediatric Managed-Medicaid Population. *J Pediatr*. 2018;199:29–34.e16. PubMed doi: 10.1016/j.jpeds.2018.03.039

187. Ehrlich PF, Pulcini CD, De Souza HG, et al. Mental Health Care Following Firearm and Motor Vehicle-related Injuries: Differences Impacting Our Treatment Strategies. *Ann Surg*. 2022;276(3):463–471. PubMed doi: 10.1097/SLA.0000000000005557

188. Herrera-Escobar JP, de Jager E, McCarty JC, et al. Patient-reported Outcomes at 6 to 12 Months Among Survivors of Firearm Injury in the United States. *Ann Surg*. 2021;274(6):e1247–e1251. PubMed doi: 10.1097/SLA.0000000000003797

189. Moore L, Lavoie A, Bourgeois G, Lapointe J. Donabedian's structure-process-outcome quality of care model: Validation in an integrated trauma system. *J Trauma Acute Care Surg*. 2015;78(6):1168–1175. PubMed doi: 10.1097/TA.0000000000000663

190. Donabedian A. *An Introduction to Quality Assurance in Health Care*. Oxford University Press; 2003.

191. Quirion A, Nikouline A, Jung J, Nolan B. Contemporary uses of trauma video review: a scoping review. *CJEM*. 2021;23(6):787–796. PubMed doi: 10.1007/s43678-021-00178-9

192. U.S. Department of Health & Human Services. Hospital Preparedness Program (HPP). https://www.phe.gov/Preparedness/planning/hpp/Pages/default.aspx. Accessed May 30, 2022.

193. US Department of Health and Human Services. *Emergency Preparedness Grant Coordination*. Accessed May 30, 2022. https://www.fema.gov/sites/default/files/2020-09/fema_emergency-preparedness-grant-coordination_02-09-2016.pdf

194. U.S. Department of Health and Human Services. Pediatric Pandemic Network. https://pedspandemicnetwork.org/. Accessed April 4, 2023.

195. US Department of Health and Human Services, Administration for Strategic Preparedness and Response. *HHS Child and Adolescent Health EmergencyPlanning Toolkit: Guidance for Addressing the Needs of Children and Youth with Special Health Care Needs*. US Department of Health and Human Services; January 2023. Accessed April 4, 2023. https://aspr.hhs.gov/at-risk/Pages/CYSHCN-planning-toolkit.aspx

196. Schonfeld DJ, Demaria T. Disaster Preparedness Advisory Committee; DISASTER PREPAREDNESS ADVISORY COUNCIL AND COMMITTEE ON PSYCHOSOCIAL ASPECTS OF CHILD AND FAMILY HEALTH. Providing Psychosocial Support to Children and Families in the Aftermath of Disasters and Crises. *Pediatrics*. 2015;136(4):e1120–e1130. PubMed doi: 10.1542/peds.2015-2861

197. Stough LM, Ducy EM, Kang D. Addressing the Needs of Children With Disabilities Experiencing Disaster or Terrorism. *Curr Psychiatry Rep*. 2017;19(4):24. PubMed doi: 10.1007/s11920-017-0776-8

198. Mann M, McMillan JE, Silver EJ, Stein REK. Children and Adolescents with Disabilities and Exposure to Disasters, Terrorism, and the COVID-19 Pandemic: a Scoping Review. *Curr Psychiatry Rep*. 2021;23(12):80. PubMed doi: 10.1007/s11920-021-01295-z

199. American Academy of Pediatrics. Disaster Preparedness for Children and Youth with Special Health Care Needs. 2023; https://www.aap.org/en/patient-care/disasters-and-children/professional-resources-for-disaster-preparedness/preparedness-for-children-and-youth-with-special-health-care-needs/. Accessed April 8, 2023.

200. Callahan JM, Baldwin S, Bodnar C, et al; COMMITTEE ON PEDIATRIC EMERGENCY MEDICINE; COUNCIL ON CLINICAL INFORMATION TECHNOLOGY; COUNCIL ON CHILDREN AND DISASTERS; AMERICAN COLLEGE OF EMERGENCY PHYSICIANS, PEDIATRIC EMERGENCY MEDICINE COMMITTEE. Access to Critical Health Information for Children During Emergencies: Emergency Information Forms and Beyond. *Pediatrics*. 2023;151(3):e2022060970. PubMed doi: 10.1542/peds.2022-060970

201. National Commission on Children and Disasters. *2010 Report to the President and Congress*. AHRQ Publication No. 10-M037. Agency for Healthcare Research and Quality; October 2010

202. Barfield WD, Krug SE, Kanter RK, et al; Task Force for Pediatric Emergency Mass Critical Care. Neonatal and pediatric regionalized systems in pediatric emergency mass critical care. *Pediatr Crit Care Med*. 2011;12(6)(suppl):S128–S134. PubMed doi: 10.1097/PCC.0b013e318234a723

203. Administration for Strategic Preparedness and Response Technical Resources, Assistance Center, and Information Exchange (TRACIE). Medical Operations Coordination Cells: Toolkit Second Edition 2021. Accessed July 11, 2025. https://files.asprtracie.hhs.gov/documents/fema-mocc-toolkit.pdf

204. Administration for Strategic Preparedness and Response Technical Resources, Assistance Center, and Information Exchange (TRACIE). Medical Operations Coordination Centers (MOCC): Patient Load-Balancing- Summary of Lessons Learned during COVID. 2022. Accessed February 1, 2024. https://files.asprtracie.hhs.gov/documents/mocc-patient-load-balancing-summary-of-lessons-learned-during-covid-19.pdf

205. Children's Hospital Association. Coordinating Hospital Care for Children to Increase Capacity for the Surge in COVID-19 Patients [press release]. Children's Hospital Association. April 3, 2020

206. Mitchell HK, Reddy A, Perry MA, Gathers C-A, Fowler JC, Yehya N. Racial, ethnic, and socioeconomic disparities in paediatric critical care in the USA. *Lancet Child Adolesc Health.* 2021;5(10):739–750. PubMed doi: 10.1016/S2352-4642(21)00161-9

207. Trinidad S, Kotagal M. Social determinants of health as drivers of inequities in pediatric injury. *Semin Pediatr Surg.* 2022;31(5):151221. PubMed doi: 10.1016/j.sempedsurg.2022.151221

208. Graves JM, Mackelprang JL, Moore M, et al. Rural-urban disparities in health care costs and health service utilization following pediatric mild traumatic brain injury. *Health Serv Res.* 2019;54(2):337–345. PubMed doi: 10.1111/1475-6773.13096

209. Mokdad AA, Wolf LL, Pandya S, Ryan M, Qureshi FG. Road Traffic Accidents and Disparities in Child Mortality. *Pediatrics.* 2020;146(5):e20193009. PubMed doi: 10.1542/peds.2019-3009

210. Sakran JV, Nance M, Riall T, Asmar S, Chehab M, Joseph B. Pediatric Firearm Injuries and Fatalities: Do Racial Disparities Exist? *Ann Surg.* 2020;272(4):556–561. PubMed doi: 10.1097/SLA.0000000000004390

211. Hughes BD, Cummins CB, Shan Y, Mehta HB, Radhakrishnan RS, Bowen-Jallow KA. Pediatric firearm injuries: Racial disparities and predictors of healthcare outcomes. *J Pediatr Surg.* 2020;55(8):1596–1603. PubMed doi: 10.1016/j.jpedsurg.2020.02.021

212. Alber DA, Dalton MK, Uribe-Leitz T, et al. A Multistate Study of Race and Ethnic Disparities in Access to Trauma Care. *J Surg Res.* 2021;257:486–492. PubMed doi: 10.1016/j.jss.2020.08.031

213. Trinidad S, Brokamp C, Sahay R, et al. Children from disadvantaged neighborhoods experience disproportionate injury from interpersonal violence. *J Pediatr Surg.* 2023;58(3):545–551. PubMed doi: 10.1016/j.jpedsurg.2022.05.023

214. Kayton ML, Staab V, Stahl B, et al. Health Inequities in Pediatric Trauma. *Children (Basel).* 2023;10(2):343. PubMed doi: 10.3390/children10020343

215. Dickens H, Rao U, Sarver D, et al. Racial, Gender, and Neighborhood-Level Disparities in Pediatric Trauma Care. *J Racial Ethn Health Disparities.* 2022. PubMed

216. Kulaylat AN, Hollenbeak CS, Armen SB, Cilley RE, Engbrecht BW. The Association of Race, Sex, and Insurance With Transfer From Adult to Pediatric Trauma Centers. *Pediatr Emerg Care.* 2021;37(12):e1623–e1630. PubMed doi: 10.1097/PEC.0000000000002137

217. Macy ML, Zonfrillo MR, Cook LJ, et al. Patient- and Community-Level Sociodemographic Characteristics Associated with Emergency Department Visits for Childhood Injury. *J Pediatr.* 2015;167(3):711–718 e711-714.

218. Goyal MK, Johnson TJ, Chamberlain JM, et al; PEDIATRIC EMERGENCY CARE APPLIED RESEARCH NETWORK (PECARN). Racial and Ethnic Differences in Emergency Department Pain Management of Children With Fractures. *Pediatrics.* 2020;145(5):e20193370. PubMed doi: 10.1542/peds.2019-3370

219. Willer BL, Mpody C, Thakkar RK, Tobias JD, Nafiu OO. Association of Race With Postoperative Mortality Following Major Abdominopelvic Trauma in Children. *J Surg Res.* 2022;269:178–188. PubMed doi: 10.1016/j.jss.2021.07.034

220. Rangel EL, Burd RS, Falcone RA Jr, Multicenter Child Abuse Disparity G; Multicenter Child Abuse Disparity Group. Socioeconomic disparities in infant mortality after nonaccidental trauma: a multicenter study. *J Trauma.* 2010;69(1):20–25. PubMed doi: 10.1097/TA.0b013e3181bbd7c3

221. Reed CR, Hamill ME, Safford SD. Insurance status, mortality, and hospital use among pediatric trauma patients over three decades. *J Pediatr Surg.* 2017;52(11):1822–1826. PubMed doi: 10.1016/j.jpedsurg.2017.03.041

222. Rosen H, Saleh F, Lipsitz SR, Meara JG, Rogers SO Jr. Lack of insurance negatively affects trauma mortality in US children. *J Pediatr Surg.* 2009;44(10):1952–1957. PubMed doi: 10.1016/j.jpedsurg.2008.12.026

223. Haider AH, Efron DT, Haut ER, DiRusso SM, Sullivan T, Cornwell EE III. Black children experience worse clinical and functional outcomes after traumatic brain injury: an analysis of the National Pediatric Trauma Registry. *J Trauma.* 2007;62(5):1259–1262. PubMed doi: 10.1097/TA.0b013e31803c760e

224. Kelly KA, Patel PD, Salwi S, Iii HNL, Naftel R. Socioeconomic health disparities in pediatric traumatic brain injury on a national level. *J Neurosurg Pediatr.* 2021;29(3):335–341. PubMed doi: 10.3171/2021.7.PEDS20820

225. Stolbach BC, Anam S. Racial and Ethnic Health Disparities and Trauma-Informed Care for Children Exposed to Community Violence. *Pediatr Ann.* 2017;46(10):e377–e381. PubMed doi: 10.3928/19382359-20170920-01

226. Herrera-Escobar JP, Osman SY, Das S, et al; National Trauma Research Action Plan (NTRAP) Investigators Group. Long-term patient-reported outcomes and patient-reported outcome measures after injury: the National Trauma Research Action Plan (NTRAP) scoping review. *J Trauma Acute Care Surg.* 2021;90(5):891–900. PubMed doi: 10.1097/TA.0000000000003108

227. Trauma Quality Improvement Programs. https://www.facs.org/quality-programs/trauma/quality/trauma-quality-improvement-program/. Accessed February 1, 2024.

228. Centers for Disease Control and Prevention, Division of Adolescent and School Health. Action Steps for Disparities. 2024. https://www.cdc.gov/healthy-youth/.

229. Roldos MI, Farhat T, Moehlman T. NIH Portfolio of Unintentional Injury Research Among Racial and Ethnic Minority Children: Current Landscape and Future Opportunities. *J Racial Ethn*

Health Disparities. 2021;8(3):596–606. PubMed doi: 10.1007/s40615-020-00818-3

230. Coalition for National Trauma Research. The National Trauma Reserach Action Plan 2023; https://www.nattrauma.org/research/research-policies-templates-guidelines/national-trauma-research-action-plan-ntrap/. Accessed April 9, 2023.

231. Cooper Z, Herrera-Escobar JP, Phuong J, et al; NTRAP Injury Prevention Panel. Developing a National Trauma Research Action Plan: Results from the injury prevention research gap Delphi survey. *J Trauma Acute Care Surg.* 2022;93(3):367–375. PubMed doi: 10.1097/TA.0000000000003665

232. Groner JI, Phuong J, Price MA, et al. Developing a National Trauma Research Action Plan: Results from the Pediatric Research Gap Delphi Survey. *J Trauma Acute Care Surg.* 2022;93(3):360–366. PubMed doi: 10.1097/TA.0000000000003610

Use of Chaperones for the Pediatric and Adolescent Encounter

- *Policy Statement*

POLICY STATEMENT Organizational Principles to Guide and Define the Child Health Care System and/or Improve the Health of All Children

American Academy of Pediatrics

DEDICATED TO THE HEALTH OF ALL CHILDREN™

Use of Chaperones for the Pediatric and Adolescent Encounter: Policy Statement

Abeba Berhane, MD, FAAP,[1] Jesse M. Hackell, MD, FAAP,[2] Stephenie Wallace, MD, FAAP,[3] the Committee on Practice and Ambulatory Medicine; and the Committee on Adolescence

abstract

Pediatric inpatient and outpatient encounters often include examinations that may be perceived as intrusive or uncomfortable by patients because of examination of sensitive body areas. The presence of a chaperone during these examinations can serve to optimize the patient's sense of comfort and safety, as well as protecting the physician. Chaperones should usually be clinical staff members, although providing adequate staffing may not be feasible for many small practices. Thus, the decision to use a chaperone and the specific choice of chaperone should be made jointly by the patient, parent and clinician providing care, considering the wishes of all parties to the encounter. Certain situations, including telemedicine encounters, unaccompanied minors, patients with intellectual disability, those suffering from abuse, exploitation or trafficking and those who are otherwise unable to assent to care or participate in shared decision making require special consideration for sensitive examinations, with attention paid to principles of trauma-informed care. All outpatient practices and inpatient services should develop policies addressing the situations which might prompt the need for a chaperone, and address their ability to provide one, and be prepared to involve the patient and family in the decision-making process.

[1]Corewell Health West, Helen DeVos Children's Hospital; Department of Pediatrics, Michigan State College of Medicine, Grand Rapids, Michigan; [2]Department of Pediatrics, New York Medical College, Valhalla, New York; and [3]Department of Pediatrics, UAB Heersink School of Medicine, Birmingham, Alabama

All authors were directly involved in determining the need for this statement and in its research, writing, and editing. All authors responded to comments during peer review, and have approved the final version.

CONFLICT OF INTEREST DISCLOSURE: The authors have indicated they have no potential conflicts of interest to disclose.

FUNDING: No external funding.

https://doi.org/10.1542/peds.2025-071810

To cite: Berhane A, Hackell JM, and Wallace S; American Academy of Pediatrics, Committee on Practice and Ambulatory Medicine; Committee on Adolescence. Use of Chaperones for the Pediatric and Adolescent Encounter: Policy Statement. *Pediatrics.* 2025;155(6):e2025071810

INTRODUCTION

An appropriate physical examination is a critical component of any health care encounter for an infant, child, adolescent, or young adult and represents comprehensive, sensitive, and effective health care. The clinical visit or inpatient admission may, at times, include examinations that may be perceived by the patient as intrusive or uncomfortable, such as inspection or palpation of anorectal or genital areas and/or breasts.[1] This part of the examination has the potential to cause distress or discomfort to the patient or create a misunderstanding or concern about appropriate conduct, and pediatricians should approach a sensitive examination/procedure with particular care and attention to any discomfort shown by the patient or caregiver. Although this statement will highlight areas of concern unique to the pediatric and adolescent population, it cannot comprehensively review all possible care scenarios. It is intended to prompt discussion and development of policies, inclusive of inpatient and outpatient care, for all practitioners and institutions that are in the best interests of both clinicians and patients.

The authors recognize that, given the disparity in resources available to pediatric clinicians in practices of different sizes and settings, it would be difficult and unrealistic to make recommendations that can be implemented in every setting and for every encounter. The goal of this policy statement, therefore, will be to discuss the issues surrounding the use of a chaperone, the contexts in which such decisions will be made, and the aspirational best practices in an ideal setting, whether inpatient or outpatient. The authors recognize that implementation of any recommendations may be prohibitive for some clinicians and therefore seek to, at a minimum, increase awareness of the factors that should guide their decisions on the use of chaperones in various settings.

REASONS FOR USE OF A CHAPERONE

The primary purpose for considering the use of a chaperone during a clinical encounter is to optimize the patient's feelings of safety and comfort. This begins with appropriate communication with the patient to help the patient and the parent/guardian/caregiver understand the reasons for the proposed sensitive examination. Open discussion can help engender confidence in patients, caregivers, and clinicians regarding the appropriateness of the examination and/or procedure.

Pediatricians can clearly communicate the suggestion for a chaperone to the patient and caregiver and agree on the inclusion of an appropriate chaperone through shared decision making, especially with adolescents. This discussion would include an explanation of the reasons for the presence of a chaperone ("your comfort is important to me"), the role of the chaperone ("to provide someone to focus on your comfort"), and the option of the patient to decline a chaperone ("the choice is yours") as well as the right of the patient to change their mind at any point. Clinical team members, including primary care clinicians (physicians, physician assistants, nurse practitioners), nurses, or medical assistants, are considered appropriate chaperones. Utilizing nonclinical staff members as chaperones is generally not recommended, although training of nonclinical staff about the role of a chaperone can make it easier for small offices with limited number of staff to safely conduct sensitive examinations. The use of students and residents as chaperones will generally follow institutional guidelines. As with other clinical staff members, the ability of these team members to serve in the role of chaperone depends upon preserving their autonomy and freedom to report possible infractions by clinicians of any status.

ROLE OF THE CHAPERONE

The American Academy of Pediatrics (AAP) recommendation that a chaperone be present for potentially distressing examinations and inspections of certain body areas of children and adolescents[1] is consistent with guidelines and policies from other national organizations of physicians, including the American College of Obstetricians and Gynecologists[2] and the American Medical Association,[3] as well as those issued in other countries, such as the General Medical Council[4] in the United Kingdom.

Ideally, an appropriate member of the health care team will be selected for the role of chaperone, as recommended by the American Medical Association.[3] With their training or professional experience, clinical team members understand the examinations and are familiar with both professional codes of ethics and procedures and can reassure the patient and caregiver of the appropriateness of the examination and be alert for any potential concerns during the encounter. The chaperone should be present during the examination, communicating with the patient and clinician and observing the examination, if necessary. Health care team members assisting with a procedure can also serve in the role of chaperone during these procedures.

When a clinical staff member is unavailable to serve as chaperone, it may be necessary to utilize a nonclinical staff member. However, clinicians should be aware of the risks involved with using nonclinical staff (or a family member) as a chaperone. These risks include missed opportunities to have a person familiar with the examination present to address any potential misunderstanding and ensure the appropriateness of the examination. A policy discussing the limitations of available staff and planning for their response to such scenarios can help when these situations do occur. The presence of a chaperone (name and credentials) should be documented in the encounter note, in addition to any pertinent discussion, especially if the patient declines a chaperone or a nonpreferred person serves in that role.

DECIDING ON A CHAPERONE

There is a paucity of evidence in the literature to guide the decisions regarding the use of a chaperone or the choice of the most appropriate person to fill that role. However, when surveyed in a variety of clinical settings, few adolescents or parents preferred a medical chaperone, generally preferring the presence of a parent over a clinical staff member. Male patients sometimes preferred to be alone or with either parent, regardless of the gender of the practitioner, and female patients generally preferred the presence of a same-sex parent for sensitive examinations, especially when performed by a male clinician.[5]

The role of the chaperone can be explained to the patient and parent/caregiver during the discussions regarding the medical evaluation. When discussing examinations of potentially sensitive areas, the conversation can include who will be in the room during the examination, such as the medical assistant or chaperone, and their role in the care for the patient. The chaperone is generally not needed when the history of the illness is being obtained or after the examination during the discussion and explanation of the findings.

Framing the use of a chaperone as an "opt-out" choice (eg, "For this part of this exam, I will have a chaperone present, as this is our clinic/hospital's best practice. Let me know if you have concerns") can avoid placing the burden of requesting a chaperone on the patient but can also address the patient's desire for a chaperone even if not initially offered.

Discussion about the gender of the chaperone can be included in this discussion. There is no specific evidence in pediatric patients that gender of the chaperone has an impact either on the decision to utilize a chaperone or the patient and clinician satisfaction with the visit,[6] although individual patients may have specific gender, cultural, or other preferences that should be considered. The decision to utilize a chaperone should not be affected by the gender of the patient, clinician, or the available chaperone candidates, and shared decision making may help to increase the patient's comfort with the ultimate choice. The patient's preference for the location and field of view of the chaperone should also be respected to provide an appropriate level of privacy when possible.

For infants and younger children, routine observation and palpation in the anogenital area will generally not require a chaperone; however, more invasive procedures may prompt consideration of the use of a chaperone, as should more than routine observation of sensitive areas in older children and adolescents. The adolescent patient may prefer a parent or caregiver to be present[6] during a sensitive examination or procedure, and these requests can be respected in most circumstances, as they can provide comfort to an anxious child or adolescent. In addition to the family member's presence, especially for patients who have started puberty, clinicians may consider including a chaperone who is a member of the health care team.

Some patients may be uncomfortable with having an unfamiliar person as a chaperone, even a health care team member, and all patients can be encouraged to express these concerns. These conversations should be grounded by cultural awareness and trauma-informed practices, as recommended by the AAP.[7] If the suggestion of a chaperone is declined, the pediatric practitioner can share any concerns about conducting the evaluation without having a chaperone present, including clinic or hospital policy or the practitioner's personal manner of practice. This discussion and opportunity for shared decision making can help to reach a compromise satisfactory to all parties. If the inclusion of a chaperone is declined, the clinician can determine whether the examination or procedure can still be completed without a chaperone; this decision will depend on the nature and urgency of the examination, the ongoing clinician-patient relationship, and other factors. If the examination cannot proceed satisfactorily due to lack of agreement, the practitioner should discuss and document any potential adverse outcomes, such as a delay of care, inaccurate diagnoses, and improper treatments, and use their best clinical judgment to evaluate the illness with the information given, and assist in transferring the patient's care to another clinician, if needed or requested.

SPECIFIC SITUATIONS

Certain clinical situations may require consideration of other factors beyond shared discussion in the decision regarding a chaperone.

Telehealth Visits

Many outpatient encounters relating to sensitive issues or examinations are not appropriate for a telehealth encounter and are more appropriate for in-person visits in which there is access to a chaperone and confidentiality can be preserved. However, there may be times when this is not possible for logistical reasons or when the nature of a telehealth encounter may change to become sensitive during the visit. In this situation, the physicians may determine that patient comfort would be improved with an appropriate chaperone.

As discussed in the AAP policy statement on telehealth,[7] any telehealth visits should be conducted via a HIPAA-compliant platform, which will provide secure transmission of any clinical data. Although a telehealth encounter does not present the same issues regarding inappropriate physical contact, like all encounters, these visits can involve examinations or discussions of a sensitive nature, which should be handled with the same degree of privacy as an in-person visit.[8] The ability of the patient during a telehealth encounter to be able to maintain privacy cannot be determined when the physician's ability to observe the entire surroundings of the patient are limited. A chaperone might be offered in 3 different manners during a telehealth visit. If appropriate based on the nature of the problem, and acceptable to the patient, a parent or guardian might be brought into the visit on the patient's end. This differs from the previous guidance that family members generally do not serve as a chaperone, because in a telehealth visit, there is less need for the chaperone to understand the nature of an examination or procedure. Additionally, an appropriate office staff member could be used as a chaperone on the physician's end of the visit or via a split-screen setup. Finally, in the absence of either of these options, the encounter may be recorded on most platforms. Although this last option may not impact the encounter in real time, it can provide a record of the encounter if either party has concerns about the appropriateness after the encounter. In any case, the pediatrician can support confidentiality on both sides of the telehealth encounter and attempt to provide an appropriate chaperone if desired.

Children in Foster Care or Legal Custody

Children and adolescents in foster care or legal custody may have restricted freedom to participate in shared decision making, yet they may also have a higher incidence of sexual abuse or other trauma and, therefore, be in greater need of care involving sensitive examinations.[9] Like other patients, they may have strong preferences either for or against the presence of a chaperone for these examinations, and these preferences should be taken into account. The default choice for examining an adolescent can be for the presence of a chaperone. Furthermore, if the pediatrician is uncomfortable, has legal or safety concerns, or believes that the adolescent has impaired decision-making capability, the clinician may choose not to perform an examination without a chaperone, while explaining their reasons and the risks of such course to the patient and family. Otherwise, participation of the adolescent in the decision can help increase their comfort level in an already stressful situation and help increase the access to care for a population that often lives with inequities in access.

History of Child Abuse, Sexual Abuse, Exploitation or Other Similar Trauma

As noted earlier, children and adolescents with a history of abuse, exploitation, or other trauma, are often under stresses unrelated to the examination being performed; every effort to reduce that stress should be attempted. When appropriate, depending on the age of the child and the nature of the medical condition being addressed, a child with a history of abuse may be given the option to defer a sensitive examination during a time of extreme stress. A chaperone may serve, in addition to providing protection for both the child and the examiner, to reduce the fears of the child and make the examination less stressful and more productive. Generally, the choice of others in the room should not include anyone who may have been a party to the prior trauma. These issues are discussed further in the AAP policy statement on trauma-informed care.[9]

Patients With Gender Dysphoria/Diversity

Patients with gender dysphoria or gender diversity may have experienced traumatic examinations in the past and should be treated in accordance with the recommendations in the AAP policy statement on trauma-informed care, including but not limited to the use of chaperones for sensitive examinations. Shared decision making is important in this setting.

Patients Unable to Assent to Care or Participate in Shared Decision-Making

This category includes children and adolescents with intellectual and developmental disabilities (IDD) or mental illness as well as those whose cognitive or decision-making capabilities are impaired by alcohol, drugs, or other agents at the time of the sensitive examination/procedure. Because verbal consent and shared decision making cannot always be utilized in patients with IDD, use of a chaperone is strongly recommended. Examination of patients who are unconscious or impaired by substance ingestion should never be performed until those conditions resolve, unless a direct threat to life or health exists at the time. For examinations of children and adolescents who are under anesthesia, other staff members will generally be present, and one staff member can be designated as a chaperone during these procedures.

Unaccompanied Adolescents

The unique nature of the visit with an unaccompanied adolescent can require an extra effort to provide a comfortable environment for the patient. Chaperones should be discussed for all such examinations. If the use of a chaperone cannot be agreed to, pediatric practitioners may use their best clinical judgement to address the concern by using alternative assessments and explaining the limitations in this approach.

BARRIERS TO IMPLEMENTATION

Chaperone use is recommended for a relatively large number of situations and examinations, and this recommendation is equally applicable to both inpatient and outpatient encounters. Especially in smaller clinical settings, this guidance can have a significant impact on both staffing and workflow. Hiring additional staff may not be financially feasible, yet having a chaperone readily available when needed is important, and the appropriate use of chaperones should be recognized as both a patient support and a necessary risk-reduction action for the practice, with potential benefits for both. In addition, the time required for extensive discussion and shared decision-making is generally uncompensated during non-time-based visits (eg, well visits) which places an additional burden on pediatric offices, serving as a further barrier to implementation of these recommendations.

These barriers can be addressed in several ways. In larger clinical settings, it is more likely that there will be adequate staff available to serve as chaperones. The presence of a chaperone in the examination room can be limited to the actual time required for the sensitive parts of the examination, rather than the entire visit. Designation of a single staff member at the start of each clinic session to serve as chaperone when needed can help to preemptively address the availability of a chaperone when needed. Incentives to provide chaperones should be created by medical liability insurers and payers to encourage the appropriate utilization; without these incentives, implementation of these recommended best practices may not occur. Finally, when no other options exist, the use of a specifically trained, nonmedical staff member or a family member, if specifically requested by the patient, as a chaperone may be acceptable, even though it may not be ideal.

RECOMMENDATIONS

1. All clinical practice settings are strongly encouraged to develop chaperone policies to provide a safe and comfortable environment for pediatric patients as well as to help provide liability protection for the clinicians. Policies should be clear on specific age groups (eg, infant/child, prepuberty, adolescent) and examinations (eg, inspection, palpitation, instrumentation) that should prompt consideration and discussion of the use of a chaperone.
2. Keeping in mind patient safety and comfort, as well as facility and staff size, each clinical setting should assess its ability to provide chaperones when determining policies, because workflow and staffing considerations will impact individual practice decisions.
3. Clinical staff members are the preferred choice for chaperones. Any staff members asked to serve as a chaperone should understand their role as the chaperone, including the need to observe the examination or procedure. Trainees may be considered for the role of chaperone, but particular care is needed to assure their autonomy when chaperoning examinations performed by their supervisors and instructors. If a family member is chosen as a chaperone at the request of the patient, patient comfort may be enhanced, but this should be balanced against the possibility of reduced liability protection for the pediatric practitioner.
4. In discussions regarding medical examinations, pediatric clinicians should preferably include the roles of the chaperone using an opt-out approach to avoid any issues of imbalance of power or control. Shared decision making with the patient and/or caregiver will determine how to proceed, and this discussion should be documented.
5. Although telemedicine offers benefits in increasing access to care, encounters related to sensitive physical examinations will in many cases require conversion to in-person visits.
6. The safety and comfort of certain pediatric patients, such as those in foster care/legal system, those who have experienced abuse or trauma, or patients with developmental delays/special needs, should be given extra consideration and protection. Therefore, a chaperone is strongly recommended for potentially sensitive examinations in these situations.

LEAD AUTHORS

Abeba Berhane, MD, FAAP
Jesse M. Hackell, MD, FAAP
Stephenie Wallace, MD, FAAP

COMMITTEE ON PRACTICE AND AMBULATORY MEDICINE, 2023–2024

Jesse M. Hackell, MD, FAAP, Chairperson
Yvette M. Almendarez, MD, FAAP
Patricia E. Cantrell, MD, FAAP
Carolyn Cleary, MD, FAAP
Elizabeth Hawse, MD, FAAP
Lisa M. Kafer, MD, FAAP
Tomitra Latimer, MD, FAAP
Robert H. Wiskind, MD, FAAP

LIAISONS

Seth D. Kaplan, MD, FAAP, Section on Administration and Practice Management
Alisa Skatrud, MPA, Family Partnerships Network

STAFF

Mackenzie Magnus MBA, MPH

COMMITTEE ON ADOLESCENCE, 2023–2024

Elizabeth M. Alderman, MD, FSAHM, FAAP, Chairperson
Elise Berlan, MD, FAAP
Richard J. Chung, MD, FAAP
Michael Colburn, MD, MEd, FAAP
Janet Lee, MD, FAAP
Maria C. Monge, MD, FAAP
Taraneh Shafii, MD, FAAP

LIAISONS

Nancy Sokkary, MD – American College of Obstetricians and Gynecologists
Laura K. Grubb, MD, MPH, FAAP – Society for Adolescent Health and Medicine
Liwei L. Hua, MD, PhD – American Academy of Child and Adolescent Psychiatry
Seema Menon, MD – North American Society of Pediatric and Adolescent Gynecology
Maria Rahmandar, MD, FAAP – Section on Adolescent Health
Ellie Vyver, MD – Canadian Pediatric Society

Lauren B. Zapata, PhD, MSPH – Centers for Disease Control and Prevention

STAFF

Karen Smith

REFERENCES

1. Curry ES; Committee on Practice and Ambulatory Medicine. Use of chaperones during the physical examination of the pediatric patient [reaffirmed June 2022]. *Pediatrics.* 2011;127(5):991–993. PubMed doi: 10.1542/peds.2011-0322
2. American College of Obstetricians and Gynecologists. FAQs. Making the Most of Your Health Care Visit. Frequently Asked Questions. Accessed April 30, 2024. https://www.acog.org/womens-health/faqs/making-the-most-of-your-health-care-visit
3. American Medical Association. Code of Medical Ethics. Use of Chaperones. Opinion 1.2.4. Accessed April 30, 2024. https://code-medical-ethics.ama-assn.org/sites/default/files/2022-08/1.2.4%20Use%20of%20chaperones%20–%20background%20reports_0.pdf
4. United Kingdom General Medical Council. Professional Standards. Intimate Examinations and Chaperones. Updated January 30, 2024. Accessed April 30, 2024. https://www.gmc-uk.org/ethical-guidance/ethical-guidance-for-doctors/intimate-examinations-and-chaperones/endnotes
5. Wilson M, Patel SM, Langhan ML. The use of medical chaperones during physical examinations the perceptions of adolescents and their caregivers. *Pediatr Emerg Care.* Published online December 1, 2023. PubMed doi: https://doi.org/10.1097/pec.0000000000003087
6. Alam SM, Malik M, Thompson J, Mirza M, Kowalik CG. Patient preferences regarding chaperone use for sensitive examinations. *Urol Pract.* 2022;9(5):379–388. PubMed doi: 10.1097/UPJ.0000000000000327
7. Curfman AL, Hackell JM, Herendeen NE, et al; SECTION ON TELEHEALTH CARE, COMMITTEE ON PRACTICE AND AMBULATORY MEDICINE, COMMITTEE ON PEDIATRIC WORKFORCE. Telehealth: improving access to and quality of pediatric health care. *Pediatrics.* 2021;148(3):e2021053129. PubMed doi: 10.1542/peds.2021-053129
8. Sinha S, De A, Jones N, Jones M, Williams RJ, Vaughan-Williams E. Patients' attitude towards the use of a chaperone in breast examination. *Ann R Coll Surg Engl.* 2009;91(1):46–49. PubMed doi: 10.1308/003588409X358971
9. Duffee J, Szilagyi M, Forkey H, Kelly ET; COUNCIL ON COMMUNITY PEDIATRICS, COUNCIL ON FOSTER CARE, ADOPTION, AND KINSHIP CARE, COUNCIL ON CHILD ABUSE AND NEGLECT, COMMITTEE ON PSYCHOSOCIAL ASPECTS OF CHILD AND FAMILY HEALTH. Policy statement. Trauma-informed care in child health systems. *Pediatrics.* 2021;148(2):e2021052579. PubMed doi: 10.1542/peds.2021-052579

SECTION 4

Current Policies

From the American Academy of Pediatrics

(Through December 31, 2025)

- ***Policy Statements***
  ORGANIZATIONAL PRINCIPLES TO GUIDE AND DEFINE THE CHILD HEALTH CARE SYSTEM AND TO IMPROVE THE HEALTH OF ALL CHILDREN

- ***Clinical Reports***
  GUIDANCE FOR THE CLINICIAN IN RENDERING PEDIATRIC CARE

- ***Technical Reports***
  BACKGROUND INFORMATION TO SUPPORT AMERICAN ACADEMY OF PEDIATRICS POLICY

American Academy of Pediatrics

Policy Statements, Clinical Reports, Technical Reports

Current through December 31, 2025
The companion *Pediatric Clinical Practice Guidelines & Policies* eBook
points to the full text of all titles listed herein.

2025 RECOMMENDATIONS FOR PREVENTIVE PEDIATRIC HEALTH CARE

Committee on Practice and Ambulatory Medicine

ABSTRACT. The 2025 Recommendations for Preventive Pediatric Health Care (Periodicity Schedule) has been approved by the American Academy of Pediatrics (AAP). Each child and family is unique; therefore, these recommendations are designed for the care of children who are receiving nurturing parenting, have no manifestations of any important health problems, and are growing and developing in a satisfactory fashion. Developmental, psychosocial, and chronic disease issues for children and adolescents may require more frequent counseling and treatment visits separate from preventive care visits. Additional visits also may become necessary if circumstances suggest concerns. The AAP continues to emphasize the great importance of continuity of care in comprehensive health supervision and the need to avoid fragmentation of care.

To ensure that health care professionals have the most current recommendations, the Periodicity Schedule is not published in *Pediatrics* but is posted on the American Academy of Pediatrics website (www.aap.org/periodicityschedule). This webpage includes the most recent version of the Periodicity Schedule and the full set of footnotes. The Periodicity Schedule is reviewed and revised annually to reflect current evidence and recommendations. This review process did not identify sufficient evidence to support updates to the 2025 Periodicity Schedule. The approved 2025 Periodicity Schedule remains unchanged from the 2024 Periodicity Schedule. (4/25)

See full text on page 37.

https://doi.org/10.1542/peds.2025-071066

AAP PERSPECTIVE: SUPPORTING OUR PEDIATRIC ADVOCATES

Mark Del Monte, JD

ABSTRACT. Advocacy has been, and always will be, a defining element of pediatrics. We know that so much of what determines a child's health happens outside the exam room and that the root causes of health—and health disparities—are driven as much by policy and politics than any other cause.

From vaccines to air quality, from seatbelt safety to smoking cessation, public health has been made better (or worse) by legislation, regulations, and policy choices made at the state and federal level. And the American Academy of Pediatrics (AAP) will work with lawmakers from any political party, at any time, to help improve the health of children. (2/23)

https://doi.org/10.1542/peds.2022-061032

ABUSIVE HEAD TRAUMA IN INFANTS AND CHILDREN

Sandeep K. Narang, MD, JD, FAAP; Amanda Fingarson, DO, FAAP; James Lukefahr, MD, FAAP; and Council on Child Abuse and Neglect

ABSTRACT. Abusive head trauma (AHT) remains a significant cause of morbidity and mortality in the pediatric population, especially in young infants. In the past decade, advancements in research have refined medical understanding of the epidemiological, clinical, biomechanical, and pathologic factors comprising the diagnosis, thereby enhancing clinical detection of a challenging diagnostic entity. Failure to recognize AHT and respond appropriately at any step in the process, from medical diagnosis to child protection and legal decision-making, can place children at risk. The American Academy of Pediatrics revises the 2009 policy statement on AHT to incorporate the growing body of knowledge on the topic. Although this statement incorporates some of that growing body of knowledge, it is not a comprehensive exposition of the science (https://doi.org/10.1542/peds.2024-070457). This statement aims to provide pediatric practitioners with general guidance on a complex subject. The Academy recommends that pediatric practitioners remain vigilant for the signs and symptoms of AHT, conduct thorough medical evaluations, consult with pediatric medical subspecialists when necessary, and embrace the challenges and need for strong advocacy on the subject. (3/20, reaffirmed 4/25 with reference & data updates)

https://doi.org/10.1542/peds.2020-0203

ABUSIVE HEAD TRAUMA IN INFANTS AND CHILDREN (TECHNICAL REPORT)

Sandeep K. Narang, MD, JD, FAAP; Suzanne Haney, MD, MS, FAAP; Ann-Christine Duhaime, MD, FAAP; Jonathan Martin, MD, FAANS, FACS, FAAP; Gil Binenbaum, MD, MSCE FAAP; Alejandra G. de Alba Campomanes, MD, MPH, FAAP; Rich Barth, MD, FAAP; Gina Bertocci, PhD; Margarite Care, MD; Declan McGuone, MD; Council on Child Abuse and Neglect; Section on Ophthalmology; Section on Radiology; and Section on Neurological Surgery (joint with Society for Pediatric Radiology; American Association of Certified Orthoptists; American Association for Pediatric Ophthalmology and Strabismus; and American Academy of Ophthalmology)

ABSTRACT. Abusive head trauma (AHT) in infants and children is a complex and challenging clinical diagnosis. Because of its clinical, social, and legal implications, few pediatric diagnoses evoke as much cognitive difficulty and emotional distress as AHT. Over the past several decades, considerable literature has been published on various aspects of the AHT diagnosis including epidemiology, historical features, clinical findings, biomechanics, differential diagnoses, outcomes, and prevention. The volume and critical analysis of the published literature can be daunting to even the most motivated pediatric provider.

To date, the American Academy of Pediatrics (AAP) has not promulgated, in the form of a technical report, a comprehensive review of the evidence-based literature surrounding AHT. Although the AAP has addressed the subject matter in other treatises, a scientific review in the form of a technical report offers the benefit of openly available, readily accessible, and more frequently updatable scientific information. Additionally, as the diagnosis has engendered some media and legal controversy, which then spills into a clinical venue, a technical report can assist the pediatric provider in communicating the scientific information to interdisciplinary colleagues such as child welfare agencies and courts.

With respect to the methodology used for this technical report, the authors recognize that properly conducted formal systematic review methods provide a standardized, relatively objective compilation of strength-graded evidence on a specific focused topic of inquiry. However, the broad topic of AHT, in which evidence comes from a wide variety of sources, fields, and disciplines using many different methods to approach a range of related areas of focus, is not a topic that easily lends itself to a formal systematic review process. Instead, in each area of this technical report, authors or groups of authors performed a wide review of peer-reviewed publications within each subtopic (generally limited to articles published in English), emphasizing those sources with the highest quality of evidence but not eliminating sources for which descriptive methods nonetheless provide useful and relevant information. The overall manuscript was reviewed several times by multiple participants with source documents reviewed for content when appropriate. References are provided for statements and conclusions so that the reader can access the sources directly.

Additionally, there are various medical terms utilized in this technical report that are commonly encountered in the AHT diagnosis (ie, acute subdural hematoma/hemorrhage, chronic subdural hematoma/hemorrhage, short distance fall, subdural hygroma, etc) but may have some variance in definition throughout the medical literature. For transparency and to promote a common understanding of these terms, there is an Appendix of definitions at the conclusion of this report. Many of the definitions for the pathoanatomic entities were from the National Institutes of Health Common Data Elements for Traumatic Brain Injury. Some other definitions, such as those within the biomechanics section, are described/defined in more detail in the relevant sections. (2/25)

See full text on page 41.

https://doi.org/10.1542/peds.2024-070457

ACCESS TO CRITICAL HEALTH INFORMATION FOR CHILDREN DURING EMERGENCIES: EMERGENCY INFORMATION FORMS AND BEYOND

James M. Callahan, MD, FAAP, FACEP; Steve Baldwin, MD, FACEP; Chelsea Bodnar, MD, MPhil, FAAP; Susan Fuchs, MD, FAAP, FACEP; Steven Krug, MD, FAAP; Cynthiana Lightfoot, EMT-P; Mordechai Raskas, MD, EdM, FAAP; Stuart Weinberg, MD, FAAP; Committee on Pediatric Emergency Medicine; Council on Clinical Information Technology; and Council on Children and Disasters (joint with American College of Emergency Physicians Pediatric Emergency Medicine Committee)

ABSTRACT. Children with chronic medical conditions rely on complex management plans for problems that cause them to be at increased risk for suboptimal outcomes in emergency situations. The emergency information form (EIF) is a medical summary that provides rapid access to critical information to physicians and other members of the health care team so that optimal emergency medical care can be provided. This statement describes an updated approach to EIFs and the information they contain. Essential common data elements are reviewed, integration with electronic health records is discussed, and broadening the rapid availability and use of health data for all children and youth is proposed. A broader approach to data accessibility and use could extend the benefits of rapid access to critical information for all children receiving emergency care as well as further facilitating emergency preparedness during disaster management. (2/23)

https://doi.org/10.1542/peds.2022-060970

ACCESS TO OPTIMAL EMERGENCY CARE FOR CHILDREN

Kathleen M. Brown, MD, FAAP, FACEP; Alice D. Ackerman, MD, MBA, FAAP; Timothy K. Ruttan, MD, FACEP, FAAP; Sally K. Snow, RN, BSN, CPEN, FAEN; Committee on Pediatric Emergency Medicine (joint with American College of Emergency Physicians Pediatric Emergency Medicine Committee and Emergency Nurses Association Pediatric Committee, 2018–2019)

ABSTRACT. Every year, millions of pediatric patients seek emergency care. Significant barriers limit access to optimal emergency services for large numbers of children. The American Academy of Pediatrics, American College of Emergency Physicians, and Emergency Nurses Association have a strong commitment to identifying these barriers, working to overcome them, and encouraging, through education and system changes, improved access to emergency care for all children. (4/21)

https://doi.org/10.1542/peds.2021-050787

ADDRESSING EARLY EDUCATION AND CHILD CARE EXPULSION

P. Gail Williams, MD, FAAP; Michael Yogman, MD, FAAP; Council on Early Childhood; and Committee on Psychosocial Aspects of Child and Family Health

ABSTRACT. An important goal of early childhood education is teaching emotional self-regulation within the context of a safe, stable, nurturing environment. Expulsion of young children ignores underlying emotional and behavioral concerns, disproportionately affects children of color (Black or Hispanic), males, children with disabilities, and socioeconomically disadvantaged populations, and has long-term consequences on educational and life success. Addressing implicit bias and providing child mental health consultation (psychologists, social workers, developmental behavioral pediatricians, child psychiatrists, and child neurologists) to child care providers can prevent expulsion. Pediatricians and other providers within the medical home play an important part in preventing expulsion. However, pediatricians need more training in early childhood mental health and in understanding how systemic racism and implicit bias lead to preschool expulsion in children of color. By identifying children at risk for expulsion because of poverty, racial discrimination, toxic stress, insecure attachment, or history of trauma, the pediatrician can connect families with community resources that may ameliorate these effects. Pediatricians can provide information on social-emotional development in early childhood, promote positive parent-child relationships, and model and discuss age-appropriate and developmentally appropriate behavior management. Pediatricians can also guide parents toward high-quality child care programs that use mental health consultation and developmentally appropriate activities, both of which lessen the chance of child expulsion. Furthermore, behavioral health providers integrated into the medical home can provide consultation to child care providers on managing patients. These recommendations are consistent with our knowledge of early child brain development and support the current tenets of the American Academy of Pediatrics regarding the pediatrician's role in building resilience and buffering toxic stress to promote optimal child development. (10/23)

https://doi.org/10.1542/peds.2023-064049

ADOLESCENT DRUG TESTING POLICIES IN SCHOOLS

Sharon Levy, MD, MPH, FAAP; Miriam Schizer, MD, MPH, FAAP; and Committee on Substance Abuse

ABSTRACT. School-based drug testing is a controversial approach to preventing substance use by students. Although school drug testing has hypothetical benefits, and studies have noted modest reductions in self-reported student drug use, the American Academy of Pediatrics opposes widespread imple-

mentation of these programs because of the lack of solid evidence for their effectiveness. (3/15, reaffirmed 7/21)
https://doi.org/10.1542/peds.2015-0054

ADOLESCENT DRUG TESTING POLICIES IN SCHOOLS (TECHNICAL REPORT)

Sharon Levy, MD, MPH, FAAP; Miriam Schizer, MD, MPH, FAAP; and Committee on Substance Abuse

ABSTRACT. More than a decade after the US Supreme Court established the legality of school-based drug testing, these programs remain controversial, and the evidence evaluating efficacy and risks is inconclusive. The objective of this technical report is to review the relevant literature that explores the benefits, risks, and costs of these programs. (3/15, reaffirmed 7/21)
https://doi.org/10.1542/peds.2015-0055

ADOLESCENTS AND YOUNG ADULTS: THE PEDIATRICIAN'S ROLE IN HIV TESTING AND PRE- AND POSTEXPOSURE HIV PROPHYLAXIS (CLINICAL REPORT)

Katherine K. Hsu, MD, MPH, FAAP; Natella Yurievna Rakhmanina, MD, PhD, FAAP; and Committee on Pediatric AIDS

ABSTRACT. Most sexually active youth in the United States do not believe that they are at risk for contracting HIV and have never been tested. Creating safe environments that promote confidentiality and respect, obtaining an accurate sexual and reproductive health assessment, and providing nonstigmatizing risk counseling are key components of any youth encounters. Pediatricians can play a key role in preventing and controlling HIV infection by promoting risk-reduction counseling and offering routine HIV testing and prophylaxis to adolescent and young adult (youth) patients. In light of persistently high numbers of people living with HIV in the United States and documented missed opportunities for HIV testing, the Centers for Disease Control and Prevention and the US Preventive Services Task Force recommend universal and routine HIV screening among US populations, including youth. Recent advances in HIV diagnostics, treatment, and prevention help support this recommendation. This clinical report reviews epidemiological data and recommends that routine HIV screening be offered to all youth 15 years or older, at least once, in health care settings. After initial screening, youth at increased risk, including those who are sexually active, should be rescreened at least annually, and potentially as frequently as every 3 to 6 months if at high risk (male youth reporting male sexual contact, active injection drug users, transgender youth; youth having sexual partners who are HIV-infected, of both genders, or injection drug users; youth exchanging sex for drugs or money; or youth who have had a diagnosis of or have requested testing for other sexually transmitted infections). Youth at substantial risk for HIV acquisition should be routinely offered HIV preexposure prophylaxis, and HIV postexposure prophylaxis is also indicated after high-risk exposures. This clinical report also addresses consent, confidentiality, and coverage issues that pediatricians face in promoting routine HIV testing and HIV prophylaxis for their patients. (12/21)
https://doi.org/10.1542/peds.2021-055207

THE ADOLESCENT'S RIGHT TO CONFIDENTIAL CARE WHEN CONSIDERING ABORTION

Committee on Adolescence

ABSTRACT. The American Academy of Pediatrics reaffirms its position that the rights of adolescents under 18 years of age to confidential care when considering legal medical and surgical abortion therapies should be protected. Most adolescents voluntarily involve parents and other trusted adults in decisions regarding pregnancy termination and should be encouraged to do so when safe and appropriate. The legal climate surrounding abortion law is rapidly becoming more restrictive and threatens to adversely impact adolescents. Mandatory parental involvement, the judicial bypass procedure, and general restrictive abortion policies pose risks to adolescents' health by causing delays in accessing medical care, increasing volatility within a family, and limiting their pregnancy options. These harms underscore the importance of adolescents' access to confidential abortion care. This statement presents a summary of pertinent current information related to the impact of legislation requiring mandatory parental involvement in an adolescent's decision to obtain abortion services. (8/22)
https://doi.org/10.1542/peds.2022-058780

ADVANCED PRACTICE NURSING IN NEONATOLOGY (CLINICAL REPORT)

Lisa M. Grisham, PhD, DNP, NNP-BC; Jay P. Goldsmith, MD, FAAP; Ashley M. Lucke, MD FAAP; Sheila M. Gephart, PhD, RN, FAAN; and Committee on Fetus and Newborn

ABSTRACT. The participation of advanced practice registered nurses (APRNs) in neonatal care continues to be supported by the American Academy of Pediatrics. Traditionally, neonatal nurse practitioners and neonatal clinical nurse specialists were the two roles well established within the Neonatal Intensive Care Unit (NICU). With ongoing shortages of these roles, some institutions have turned toward pediatric nurse practitioners (acute and primary care) and family nurse practitioners to meet patient care needs. This clinical report aims to review the roles, scope of practice, collaboration, and credentialling of these categories of APRNs with recommendations for the safe and effective utilization of these providers in neonatal care. This clinical report will not address other roles in the NICU, including hospitalists or physician assistants in the NICU, nor speak to the potential shortages and solutions these professions are experiencing, as those topics are well covered in the Standards for Levels of Neonatal Care: II, III, IV (https://publications.aap.org/pediatrics/article/151/6/e2023061957/191305/Standards-for-Levels-of-Neonatal-Care-II-III-and) and Neonatal Provider Workforce Technical Report. (8/25)

See full text on page 115.
https://doi.org/10.1542/peds.2025-073170

ADVOCACY FOR IMPROVING NUTRITION IN THE FIRST 1000 DAYS TO SUPPORT CHILDHOOD DEVELOPMENT AND ADULT HEALTH

Sarah Jane Schwarzenberg, MD, FAAP; Michael K. Georgieff, MD, FAAP; and Committee on Nutrition

ABSTRACT. Maternal prenatal nutrition and the child's nutrition in the first 2 years of life (1000 days) are crucial factors in a child's neurodevelopment and lifelong mental health. Child and adult health risks, including obesity, hypertension, and diabetes, may be programmed by nutritional status during this period. Calories are essential for growth of both fetus and child but are not sufficient for normal brain development. Although all nutrients are necessary for brain growth, key nutrients that support neurodevelopment include protein; zinc; iron; choline; folate; iodine; vitamins A, D, B_6, and B_{12}; and long-chain polyunsaturated fatty acids. Failure to provide key nutrients during this critical period of brain development may result in lifelong deficits in brain function despite subsequent nutrient repletion. Understanding the complex interplay of micro- and macronutrients and neurodevelopment is key to moving beyond simply recommending a "good diet" to optimizing nutrient delivery for the developing child. Leaders in pediatric health and policy makers must be aware of this research given its implications for public policy at the federal and state level. Pediatricians should refer to existing services for nutrition support for pregnant and breastfeeding women, infants, and toddlers. Finally, all providers caring for children can advocate for healthy diets for mothers, infants, and young children in the first 1000 days. Prioritizing public policies that ensure the provision of adequate nutrients

and healthy eating during this crucial time would ensure that all children have an early foundation for optimal neurodevelopment, a key factor in long-term health. (1/18, reaffirmed 10/23)
https://doi.org/10.1542/peds.2017-3716

ADVOCATING FOR LIFE SUPPORT TRAINING OF CHILDREN, PARENTS, CAREGIVERS, SCHOOL PERSONNEL, AND THE PUBLIC

James M. Callahan, MD, FAAP; Susan M. Fuchs, MD, FAAP; and Committee on Pediatric Emergency Medicine

ABSTRACT. Out-of-hospital cardiac arrest occurs frequently among people of all ages, including more than 6000 children annually. Pediatric cardiac arrest in the out-of-hospital setting is a stressful event for family, friends, caregivers, classmates, school personnel, and witnesses. Immediate bystander cardiopulmonary resuscitation and the use of automated external defibrillators are associated with improved survival in adults. There is some evidence in which improved survival in children who receive immediate bystander cardiopulmonary resuscitation is shown. Pediatricians, in their role as advocates to improve the health of all children, are uniquely positioned to strongly encourage the training of children, parents, caregivers, school personnel, and the lay public in the provision of basic life support, including pediatric basic life support, as well as the appropriate use of automated external defibrillators. (5/18, reaffirmed 12/24)
https://doi.org/10.1542/peds.2018-0704

ADVOCATING FOR LIFE SUPPORT TRAINING OF CHILDREN, PARENTS, CAREGIVERS, SCHOOL PERSONNEL, AND THE PUBLIC (TECHNICAL REPORT)

Susan M. Fuchs, MD, FAAP, and Committee on Pediatric Emergency Medicine

ABSTRACT. Pediatric cardiac arrest in the out-of-hospital setting is a traumatic event for family, friends, caregivers, classmates, and school personnel. Immediate bystander cardiopulmonary resuscitation and the use of automatic external defibrillators have been shown to improve survival in adults. There is some evidence to show improved survival in children who receive immediate bystander cardiopulmonary resuscitation. Pediatricians, in their role as advocates to improve the health of all children, are uniquely positioned to strongly encourage the training of children, parents, caregivers, school personnel, and the lay public in the provision of basic life support, including pediatric basic life support, as well as the appropriate use of automated external defibrillators. (5/18, reaffirmed 12/24)
https://doi.org/10.1542/peds.2018-0705

AGE LIMIT OF PEDIATRICS

Amy Peykoff Hardin, MD, FAAP; Jesse M. Hackell, MD, FAAP; and Committee on Practice and Ambulatory Medicine

ABSTRACT. Pediatrics is a multifaceted specialty that encompasses children's physical, psychosocial, developmental, and mental health. Pediatric care may begin periconceptionally and continues through gestation, infancy, childhood, adolescence, and young adulthood. Although adolescence and young adulthood are recognizable phases of life, an upper age limit is not easily demarcated and varies depending on the individual patient. The establishment of arbitrary age limits on pediatric care by health care providers should be discouraged. The decision to continue care with a pediatrician or pediatric medical or surgical subspecialist should be made solely by the patient (and family, when appropriate) and the physician and must take into account the physical and psychosocial needs of the patient and the abilities of the pediatric provider to meet these needs. (8/17, reaffirmed 4/23)
https://doi.org/10.1542/peds.2017-2151

AGE TERMINOLOGY DURING THE PERINATAL PERIOD

Committee on Fetus and Newborn

ABSTRACT. Consistent definitions to describe the length of gestation and age in neonates are needed to compare neurodevelopmental, medical, and growth outcomes. The purposes of this policy statement are to review conventional definitions of age during the perinatal period and to recommend use of standard terminology including gestational age, postmenstrual age, chronological age, corrected age, adjusted age, and estimated date of delivery. (11/04, reaffirmed 11/08, 7/21)
https://doi.org/10.1542/peds.2004-1915

ALUMINUM EFFECTS IN INFANTS AND CHILDREN (TECHNICAL REPORT)

Mark R. Corkins, MD, FAAP; Committee on Nutrition

ABSTRACT. Aluminum has no known biological function; however, it is a contaminant present in most foods and medications. Aluminum is excreted by the renal system, and patients with renal diseases should avoid aluminum-containing medications. Studies demonstrating long-term toxicity from the aluminum content in parenteral nutrition components led the US Food and Drug Administration to implement rules for these solutions. Large-volume ingredients were required to reduce the aluminum concentration, and small-volume components were required to be labeled with the aluminum concentration. Despite these rules, the total aluminum concentration from some components continues to be above the recommended final concentration. The concerns about toxicity from the aluminum present in infant formulas and antiperspirants have not been substantiated but require more research. Aluminum is one of the most effective adjuvants used in vaccines, and a large number of studies have documented minimal adverse effects from this use. Long-term, high-concentration exposure to aluminum has been linked in meta-analyses with the development of Alzheimer disease. (12/19, reaffirmed 10/24)
https://doi.org/10.1542/peds.2019-3148

AMBIENT AIR POLLUTION: HEALTH HAZARDS TO CHILDREN

Heather L. Brumberg, MD, MPH, FAAP; Catherine J. Karr, MD, PhD, FAAP; and Council on Environmental Health

ABSTRACT. Ambient air pollution is produced by sources including vehicular traffic, coal-fired power plants, hydraulic fracturing, agricultural production, and forest fires. It consists of primary pollutants generated by combustion and secondary pollutants formed in the atmosphere from precursor gases. Air pollution causes and exacerbates climate change, and climate change worsens health effects of air pollution. Infants and children are uniquely sensitive to air pollution, because their organs are developing and they have higher air per body weight intake. Health effects linked to air pollution include not only exacerbations of respiratory diseases but also reduced lung function development and increased asthma incidence. Additional outcomes of concern include preterm birth, low birth weight, neurodevelopmental disorders, IQ loss, pediatric cancers, and increased risks for adult chronic diseases. These effects are mediated by oxidative stress, chronic inflammation, endocrine disruption, and genetic and epigenetic mechanisms across the life span. Natural experiments demonstrate that with initiatives such as increased use of public transportation, both air quality and community health improve. Similarly, the Clean Air Act has improved air quality, although exposure inequities persist. Other effective strategies for reducing air pollution include ending reliance on coal, oil, and gas; regulating industrial emissions; reducing exposure with attention to proximity of residences, schools, and child care facilities to traffic; and a greater awareness of the

Air Quality Index. This policy reviews both short- and long-term health consequences of ambient air pollution, especially in relation to developmental exposures. It examines individual, community, and legislative strategies to mitigate air pollution. (5/21)
https://doi.org/10.1542/peds.2021-051484

AMERICAN ACADEMY OF PEDIATRICS RECOMMENDATIONS FOR THE PREVENTION OF PEDIATRIC ATV-RELATED DEATHS AND INJURIES

Charles A. Jennissen, MD, FAAP; Gerene M. Denning, PhD; Mary E. Aitken, MD, MPH, FAAP; and Council on Injury, Violence, and Poison Prevention

ABSTRACT. Since all-terrain vehicles (ATVs) were introduced in the mid-1970s, regulatory agencies, injury prevention researchers, and pediatricians have documented their dangers to youth. Major risk factors, crash mechanisms, and injury patterns for children and adolescents have been well characterized. Despite this knowledge, preventing pediatric ATV-related deaths and injuries has proven difficult and has had limited success. This policy statement broadly summarizes key background information and provides detailed recommendations based on best practices. These recommendations are designed to provide all stakeholders with strategies that can be used to reduce the number of pediatric deaths and injuries resulting from youth riding on ATVs. (9/22)
https://doi.org/10.1542/peds.2022-059279

ANTENATAL COUNSELING REGARDING RESUSCITATION AND INTENSIVE CARE BEFORE 25 WEEKS OF GESTATION (CLINICAL REPORT)

James Cummings, MD, FAAP, and Committee on Fetus and Newborn

ABSTRACT. The anticipated birth of an extremely low gestational age (<25 weeks) infant presents many difficult questions, and variations in practice continue to exist. Decisions regarding care of periviable infants should ideally be well informed, ethically sound, consistent within medical teams, and consonant with the parents' wishes. Each health care institution should consider having policies and procedures for antenatal counseling in these situations. Family counseling may be aided by the use of visual materials, which should take into consideration the intellectual, cultural, and other characteristics of the family members. Although general recommendations can guide practice, each situation is unique; thus, decision-making should be individualized. In most cases, the approach should be shared decision-making with the family, guided by considering both the likelihood of death or morbidity and the parents' desires for their unborn child. If a decision is made not to resuscitate, providing comfort care, encouraging family bonding, and palliative care support are appropriate. (8/15, reaffirmed 11/21)
https://doi.org/10.1542/peds.2015-2336

ANTERIOR CRUCIATE LIGAMENT INJURIES: DIAGNOSIS, TREATMENT, AND PREVENTION (CLINICAL REPORT)

Cynthia R. LaBella, MD, FAAP; William Hennrikus, MD, FAAP; Timothy E. Hewett, PhD, FACSM; Council on Sports Medicine and Fitness; and Section on Orthopaedics

ABSTRACT. The number of anterior cruciate ligament (ACL) injuries reported in athletes younger than 18 years has increased over the past 2 decades. Reasons for the increasing ACL injury rate include the growing number of children and adolescents participating in organized sports, intensive sports training at an earlier age, and greater rate of diagnosis because of increased awareness and greater use of advanced medical imaging. ACL injury rates are low in young children and increase sharply during puberty, especially for girls, who have higher rates of noncontact ACL injuries than boys do in similar sports. Intrinsic risk factors for ACL injury include higher BMI, subtalar joint overpronation, generalized ligamentous laxity, and decreased neuromuscular control of knee motion. ACL injuries often require surgery and/or many months of rehabilitation and substantial time lost from school and sports participation. Unfortunately, regardless of treatment, athletes with ACL injuries are up to 10 times more likely to develop degenerative arthritis of the knee. Safe and effective surgical techniques for children and adolescents continue to evolve. Neuromuscular training can reduce risk of ACL injury in adolescent girls. This report outlines the current state of knowledge on epidemiology, diagnosis, treatment, and prevention of ACL injuries in children and adolescents. (4/14, reaffirmed 12/24)
https://doi.org/10.1542/peds.2014-0623

ANTIBIOTIC STEWARDSHIP IN PEDIATRICS

Jeffrey S. Gerber, MD, PhD, FAAP; Mary Anne Jackson, MD, FAAP; Pranita D. Tamma, MD, MHS; Theoklis E. Zaoutis, MD, FAAP; Committee on Infectious Diseases (joint with Pediatric Infectious Diseases Society)

ABSTRACT. Antibiotic overuse contributes to antibiotic resistance, which is a threat to public health. Antibiotic stewardship is a practice dedicated to prescribing antibiotics only when necessary and, when antibiotics are considered necessary, promoting use of the appropriate agent(s), dose, duration, and route of therapy to optimize clinical outcomes while minimizing the unintended consequences of antibiotic use. Because there are differences in common infectious conditions, drug-specific considerations, and the evidence surrounding treatment recommendations (eg, first-line therapy, duration of therapy) between children and adults, this statement provides specific guidance for the pediatric population. This policy statement discusses the rationale for inpatient and outpatient antibiotic stewardship programs; essential personnel, infrastructure, and activities required; approaches to evaluating their effectiveness; and gaps in knowledge that require further investigation. Key guidance for both inpatient and outpatient antibiotic stewardship programs are provided. (12/20, reaffirmed 9/25)
https://doi.org/10.1542/peds.2020-040295

APPRAISAL OF CLINICAL CARE PRACTICES FOR CHILD OBESITY TREATMENT. PART I: INTERVENTIONS (TECHNICAL REPORT)

Asheley C. Skinner, PhD; Amanda E. Staiano, PhD, MPP; Sarah C. Armstrong, MD, FAAP; Shari L. Barkin, MD, MSHS; Sandra G. Hassink, MD, FAAP; Jennifer E. Moore, PhD, RN, FAAN; Jennifer S. Savage, PhD; Helene Vilme, DrPH; Ashley E. Weedn, MD, MPH, FAAP; Janice Liebhart, MS; Jeanne Lindros, MPH; Eileen M. Reilly, MSW

ABSTRACT. The objective of this technical report is to provide clinicians with evidence-based, actionable information upon which to make assessment and treatment decisions for children and adolescents with obesity. In addition, this report will provide an evidence base to inform clinical practice guidelines for the management and treatment of overweight and obesity in children and adolescents.

To this end, the goal of this report was to identify all relevant studies to answer 2 overarching key questions: (KQ1) "What are clinically based, effective treatments for obesity?" and (KQ2) "What is the risk of comorbidities among children with obesity?" See Appendix 1 for the conceptual framework and a priori key questions. (1/23)
https://doi.org/10.1542/peds.2022-060642

APPRAISAL OF CLINICAL CARE PRACTICES FOR CHILD OBESITY TREATMENT. PART II: COMORBIDITIES (TECHNICAL REPORT)

Asheley C. Skinner, PhD; Amanda E. Staiano, PhD, MPP; Sarah C. Armstrong, MD, FAAP; Shari L. Barkin, MD, MSHS; Sandra G. Hassink, MD, FAAP; Jennifer E. Moore, PhD, RN, FAAN; Jennifer S. Savage, PhD; Helene Vilme, DrPH; Ashley E. Weedn, MD, MPH, FAAP; Janice Liebhart, MS; Jeanne Lindros, MPH; Eileen M. Reilly, MSW

ABSTRACT. The objective of this technical report is to provide clinicians with actionable evidence-based information upon which to make treatment decisions. In addition, this report will provide an evidence base on which to inform clinical practice guidelines for the management and treatment of overweight and obesity in children and adolescents.

To this end, the goal of this report was to identify all relevant studies to answer 2 overarching key questions: (KQ1) "What are effective clinically based treatments for obesity?" and (KQ2) "What is the risk of comorbidities among children with obesity?" See Appendix 1 for the conceptual framework and a priori Key Questions. (1/23)

https://doi.org/10.1542/peds.2022-060643

ASSESSMENT AND MANAGEMENT OF INGUINAL HERNIAS IN CHILDREN (CLINICAL REPORT)

Faraz A. Khan, MD, FAAP; Tim Jancelewicz, MD, FAAP; Kathleen Kieran, MD, FAAP; Saleem Islam, MD, FAAP; Committee on Fetus and Newborn; Section on Surgery; and Section on Urology

ABSTRACT. Inguinal hernia repair is one of the most commonly performed surgical procedures in children. However, a number of controversial issues, such as optimal timing and approach to repair, continue to be debated. This publication reviews the available data pertaining to these controversial issues and identifies best practices in management of inguinal hernias in children. (6/23)

https://doi.org/10.1542/peds.2023-062510

ATOPIC DERMATITIS: UPDATE ON SKIN-DIRECTED MANAGEMENT (CLINICAL REPORT)

Jennifer J. Schoch, MD, FAAD, FAAP; Katelyn R. Anderson, MD, FAAP, FAAD; Amie E. Jones, MD, FAAP; Megha M. Tollefson, MD, FAAP, FAAD; and Section on Dermatology

ABSTRACT. Atopic dermatitis affects 20% to 25% of children and has significant impact on quality of life of patients and families. Recent studies of the pathogenesis of AD highlight the interplay between a defective skin barrier, immune dysfunction, and the cutaneous microbiome. Standard of care for AD treatment includes topical corticosteroids for active disease and moisturization to repair the barrier defect. Emerging treatments include dupilumab and Janus kinase (JAK) inhibitors. Reduction of triggers and proactive treatment with topical corticosteroids and/or topical calcineurin inhibitors can reduce flares. Treatment plans should be clear and as simple as possible to maximize adherence. (5/25)

See full text on page 127.

https://doi.org/10.1542/peds.2025-071812

BIOLOGICS FOR ASTHMA AND ALLERGIC SKIN DISEASES IN CHILDREN (CLINICAL REPORT)

Heather Hoch De Keyser, MD, MSCS, FAAP; Bradley Chipps, MD, FAAP; Chitra Dinakar, MD, FAAP; Section on Allergy and Immunology; and Section on Pediatric Pulmonology and Sleep Medicine

ABSTRACT. An estimated 7 million children in the United States have asthma, which causes a significant health care burden and affects quality of life. The minority of these children have asthma that does not respond to Global Initiative for Asthma steps 4 and 5 care, and biological medications are recommended at this level in the 2019 Global Initiative for Asthma recommendations. In addition, biologics have been introduced into the care of children with allergic skin diseases. Omalizumab and mepolizumab are approved for children as young as 6 years, and benralizumab and dupilumab are approved for people aged ≥12 years. Reslizumab is approved only for people aged ≥18 years. These monoclonal antibodies may be added for appropriate patients when asthma or allergic skin diseases are not well controlled. Pediatricians and pediatric subspecialists should work together and be aware of the benefits and risks of these medications for their patients, as well as the practical implications of providing these options for their patients. This clinical report serves as an evaluation of the current literature on these types of medications in the treatment of children with asthma and allergic skin disease. (10/21)

https://doi.org/10.1542/peds.2021-054270

BONE DENSITOMETRY IN CHILDREN AND ADOLESCENTS (CLINICAL REPORT)

Laura K. Bachrach, MD; Catherine M. Gordon, MD, MS; and Section on Endocrinology

ABSTRACT. Concerns about bone health and potential fragility in children and adolescents have led to a high interest in bone densitometry. Pediatric patients with genetic and acquired chronic diseases, immobility, and inadequate nutrition may fail to achieve expected gains in bone size, mass, and strength, leaving them vulnerable to fracture. In older adults, bone densitometry has been shown to predict fracture risk and reflect response to therapy. The role of densitometry in the management of children at risk of bone fragility is less clear. This clinical report summarizes current knowledge about bone densitometry in the pediatric population, including indications for its use, interpretation of results, and risks and costs. The report emphasizes updated consensus statements generated at the 2013 Pediatric Position Development Conference of the International Society of Clinical Densitometry by an international panel of bone experts. Some of these recommendations are evidence-based, whereas others reflect expert opinion, because data are sparse on many topics. The statements from this and other expert panels provide general guidance to the pediatrician, but decisions about ordering and interpreting bone densitometry still require clinical judgment. The interpretation of bone densitometry results in children differs from that in older adults. The terms "osteopenia" and "osteoporosis" based on bone densitometry findings alone should not be used in younger patients; instead, bone mineral content or density that falls >2 SDs below expected is labeled "low for age." Pediatric osteoporosis is defined by the Pediatric Position Development Conference by using 1 of the following criteria: ≥1 vertebral fractures occurring in the absence of local disease or high-energy trauma (without or with densitometry measurements) or low bone density for age and a significant fracture history (defined as ≥2 long bone fractures before 10 years of age or ≥3 long bone fractures before 19 years of age). Ongoing research will help define the indications and best methods for assessing bone strength in children and the clinical factors that contribute to fracture risk. The Pediatric Endocrine Society affirms the educational value of this publication. (9/16, reaffirmed 10/22)

https://doi.org/10.1542/peds.2016-2398

BREASTFEEDING AND THE USE OF HUMAN MILK

Joan Younger Meek, MD, MS, RD, FAAP, FABM, IBCLC; Lawrence Noble, MD, FAAP, FABM, IBCLC; and Section on Breastfeeding

ABSTRACT. Breastfeeding and human milk are the normative standards for infant feeding and nutrition. The short- and long-term medical and neurodevelopmental advantages of breastfeeding make breastfeeding, or the provision of human milk, a

public health imperative. The American Academy of Pediatrics (AAP) recommends exclusive breastfeeding for approximately 6 months after birth. Furthermore, the AAP supports continued breastfeeding, along with appropriate complementary foods introduced at about 6 months, as long as mutually desired by mother and child for 2 years or beyond. These recommendations are consistent with those of the World Health Organization (WHO). Medical contraindications to breastfeeding are rare. The AAP recommends that birth hospitals or centers implement maternity care practices shown to improve breastfeeding initiation, duration, and exclusivity. The Centers for Disease Control and Prevention (CDC) and The Joint Commission monitor breastfeeding practices in US hospitals. Pediatricians play a critical role in hospitals, their practices, and communities as advocates of breastfeeding and, thus, need to be trained about the benefits of breastfeeding for mothers and children and in managing breastfeeding. (6/22)
https://doi.org/10.1542/peds.2022-057988

BREASTFEEDING AND THE USE OF HUMAN MILK (TECHNICAL REPORT)

Joan Younger Meek, MD, MS, RD, FAAP, FABM, IBCLC; and Lawrence Noble, MD, FAAP, FABM, IBCLC

ABSTRACT. Breastfeeding and human milk are the normative standards for infant feeding and nutrition. The short- and long-term medical and neurodevelopmental advantages of breastfeeding make breastfeeding or the provision of human milk a public health imperative. The American Academy of Pediatrics (AAP) recommends exclusive breastfeeding for approximately 6 months after birth. Furthermore, the AAP supports continued breastfeeding, along with appropriate complementary foods introduced at about 6 months, as long as mutually desired by mother and child for 2 years or beyond. These recommendations are consistent with those of the World Health Organization (WHO). Medical contraindications to breastfeeding are rare. The AAP recommends that birth hospitals or centers implement maternity care practices shown to improve breastfeeding initiation, duration, and exclusivity. The Centers for Disease Control and Prevention and The Joint Commission monitor breastfeeding practices in United States hospitals. Pediatricians play a critical role in hospitals, their practices, and communities as advocates of breastfeeding and, thus, need to be trained about the benefits of breastfeeding for mothers and children and in managing breastfeeding. Efforts to improve breastfeeding rates must acknowledge existing disparities and the impact of racism in promoting equity in breastfeeding education, support, and services. (6/22)
https://doi.org/10.1542/peds.2022-057989

THE BUILT ENVIRONMENT AND PEDIATRIC HEALTH

Aparna Bole, MD, FAAP; Aaron Bernstein, MD, MPH, FAAP; Michelle J. White, MD, MPH, FAAP; Council on Environmental Health and Climate Change; and Section on Minority Health, Equity, and Inclusion

ABSTRACT. Buildings, parks, and roads are all elements of the "built environment," which can be described as the human-made structures that comprise the neighborhoods and communities where people live, work, learn, and recreate (https://www.epa.gov/smm/basic-information-about-built-environment). The design of communities where children and adolescents live, learn, and play has a profound impact on their health. Moreover, the policies and practices that determine community design and the built environment are a root cause of disparities in the social determinants of health that contribute to health inequity. An understanding of the links between the built environment and pediatric health will help to inform pediatricians' and other pediatric health care professionals' care for patients and advocacy on their behalf. This policy statement outlines community design solutions that can improve pediatric physical and mental health, and improve health equity. It describes opportunities for pediatricians and the health care sector to incorporate this knowledge in patient care, as well as to play a role in advancing a health-promoting built environment for all children and families. The accompanying technical report reviews the range of pediatric physical and mental health conditions influenced by the built environment, as well as historical and persistent effects of the built environment on health disparities. (12/23)
https://doi.org/10.1542/peds.2023-064772

THE BUILT ENVIRONMENT AND PEDIATRIC HEALTH (TECHNICAL REPORT)

Aparna Bole, MD, FAAP; Aaron Bernstein, MD, MPH, FAAP; Michelle J. White, MD, MPH, FAAP; Council on Environmental Health and Climate Change; and Section on Minority Health, Equity, and Inclusion

ABSTRACT. Buildings, parks, and roads are all elements of the "built environment," which can be described as the human-made structures that comprise the neighborhoods and communities where people live, work, learn, and recreate (https://www.epa.gov/smm/basic-information-about-built-environment). The design of communities where children and adolescents live, learn, and play has a profound impact on their health. Moreover, the policies and practices that determine community design and the built environment are a root cause of disparities in the social determinants of health that contribute to health inequity. An understanding of the links between the built environment and pediatric health will help to inform pediatricians' and other pediatric health professionals' care for patients and advocacy on their behalf. This technical report describes the range of pediatric physical and mental health conditions influenced by the built environment, as well as historical and persistent effects of the built environment on health disparities. The accompanying policy statement outlines community design solutions that can improve pediatric health and health equity, including opportunities for pediatricians and the health care sector to incorporate this knowledge in patient care, as well as to play a role in advancing a health-promoting built environment for all children and families. (12/23)
https://doi.org/10.1542/peds.2023-064773

CALCIUM AND VITAMIN D REQUIREMENTS OF ENTERALLY FED PRETERM INFANTS (CLINICAL REPORT)

Steven A. Abrams, MD; Committee on Nutrition

ABSTRACT. Bone health is a critical concern in managing preterm infants. Key nutrients of importance are calcium, vitamin D, and phosphorus. Although human milk is critical for the health of preterm infants, it is low in these nutrients relative to the needs of the infants during growth. Strategies should be in place to fortify human milk for preterm infants with birth weight <1800 to 2000 g and to ensure adequate mineral intake during hospitalization and after hospital discharge. Biochemical monitoring of very low birth weight infants should be performed during their hospitalization. Vitamin D should be provided at 200 to 400 IU/day both during hospitalization and after discharge from the hospital. Infants with radiologic evidence of rickets should have efforts made to maximize calcium and phosphorus intake by using available commercial products and, if needed, direct supplementation with these minerals. (4/13, reaffirmed 6/24 with reference & data updates)
https://doi.org/10.1542/peds.2013-0420

CARE OF ADOLESCENT PARENTS AND THEIR CHILDREN (CLINICAL REPORT)

Makia E. Powers, MD, MPH, FAAP; Jennifer Takagishi, MD, FAAP; Committee on Adolescence; and Council on Early Childhood

ABSTRACT. Teen pregnancy and parenting remain important public health issues in the United States and around the world. A significant proportion of teen parents reside with their families of origin, which may positively or negatively affect the family structure. Teen parents, defined as those 15 to 19 years of age, are at high risk for repeat births. Pediatricians can play an important role in the care of adolescent parents and their children. This clinical report updates a previous report on the care of adolescent parents and their children and addresses clinical management specific to this population, including updates on breastfeeding, prenatal management, and adjustments to parenthood. Challenges unique to teen parents and their children are reviewed, along with suggestions for the pediatrician on models for intervention and care. (4/21)

https://doi.org/10.1542/peds.2021-050919

CARE OF THE ADOLESCENT AFTER AN ACUTE SEXUAL ASSAULT (CLINICAL REPORT)

James E. Crawford-Jakubiak, MD, FAAP; Elizabeth M. Alderman, MD, FAAP, SAHM; John M. Leventhal, MD, FAAP; Committee on Child Abuse and Neglect; and Committee on Adolescence

ABSTRACT. Sexual violence is a broad term that encompasses a wide range of sexual victimizations. Since the American Academy of Pediatrics published its last policy statement on sexual assault in 2008, additional information and data have emerged about sexual violence affecting adolescents and the treatment and management of the adolescent who has been a victim of sexual assault. This report provides new information to update physicians and focuses on the acute assessment and care of adolescent victims who have experienced a recent sexual assault. Follow-up of the acute assault, as well as prevention of sexual assault, are also discussed. (2/17, reaffirmed 12/24)

https://doi.org/10.1542/peds.2016-4243

CAREGIVER-FABRICATED ILLNESS IN A CHILD: A MANIFESTATION OF CHILD MALTREATMENT (CLINICAL REPORT)

Emalee G. Flaherty, MD, FAAP; Harriet L. MacMillan, MD; and Committee on Child Abuse and Neglect

ABSTRACT. Caregiver-fabricated illness in a child is a form of child maltreatment caused by a caregiver who falsifies and/or induces a child's illness, leading to unnecessary and potentially harmful medical investigations and/or treatment. This condition can result in significant morbidity and mortality. Although caregiver-fabricated illness in a child has been widely known as Munchausen syndrome by proxy, there is ongoing discussion about alternative names, including pediatric condition falsification, factitious disorder (illness) by proxy, child abuse in the medical setting, and medical child abuse. Because it is a relatively uncommon form of maltreatment, pediatricians need to have a high index of suspicion when faced with a persistent or recurrent illness that cannot be explained and that results in multiple medical procedures or when there are discrepancies between the history, physical examination, and health of a child. This report updates the previous clinical report "Beyond Munchausen Syndrome by Proxy: Identification and Treatment of Child Abuse in the Medical Setting." The authors discuss the need to agree on appropriate terminology, provide an update on published reports of new manifestations of fabricated medical conditions, and discuss approaches to assessment, diagnosis, and management, including how best to protect the child from further harm. (8/13, reaffirmed 9/23)

https://doi.org/10.1542/peds.2013-2045

CARING FOR AMERICAN INDIAN AND ALASKA NATIVE CHILDREN AND ADOLESCENTS

Shaquita Bell, MD, FAAP; Jason F. Deen, MD, FAAP; Molly Fuentes, MD, MS; Kelly Moore, MD, FAAP; and Committee on Native American Child Health

ABSTRACT. American Indian and Alaska Native (AI/AN) populations have substantial health inequities, and most of their disease entities begin in childhood. In addition, AI/AN children and adolescents have excessive disease rates compared with the general pediatric population. Because of this, providers of pediatric care are in a unique position not only to attenuate disease incidence during childhood but also to improve the health status of this special population as a whole. This policy statement examines the inequitable disease burden observed in AI/AN youth, with a focus on toxic stress, mental health, and issues related to suicide and substance use disorder, risk of and exposure to injury and violence in childhood, obesity and obesity-related cardiovascular risk factors and disease, foster care, and the intersection of lesbian, gay, bisexual, transgender, queer, and Two-Spirit and AI/AN youth. Opportunities for advocacy in policy making also are presented. (3/21)

https://doi.org/10.1542/peds.2021-050498

CHILD FATALITY REVIEW

Erich K. Batra, MD, FAAP; Kyran Quinlan, MD, MPH, FAAP; Vincent J. Palusci, MD, MS, FAAP; Howard Needelman, MD, FAAP; Abby Collier, MS; Section on Child Death Review and Prevention; Council on Injury, Violence, and Poison Prevention; and Council on Child Abuse and Neglect

ABSTRACT. Understanding why children die is necessary to implement strategies to prevent future deaths and improve the health of any community. Child fatality review teams (CFRTs) have existed since the 1970s and provide a necessary framework to ensure that proper questions are asked about a child's death. CFRTs provide a vital function in a community to ensure that preventable causes of deaths are identified. Pediatricians are necessary members of CFRTs because they provide medical expertise and context around a child's death. All CFRTs should have pediatric physician representation, and results from team meetings should inform public policy at all levels of government. Pediatricians should be supported in their efforts to be present on CFRTs, and they should use data from team meetings to help advocate for implementing prevention strategies. (2/24)

https://doi.org/10.1542/peds.2023-065481

CHILD PEDESTRIAN SAFETY

Sadiqa Kendi, MD, FAAP; Brian D. Johnston, MD, MPH, FAAP; and Council on Injury, Violence, and Poison Prevention

ABSTRACT. The field of pedestrian safety has advanced with new evidence related to pediatric pedestrian education, the risks of distracted walking, the benefits of design and programming in safe routes to school, and the emergence of the "Vision Zero" strategy to eliminate all traffic fatalities and severe injuries while increasing safe, healthy, equitable mobility for all.

This statement is a revision of the 2009 American Academy of Pediatrics policy statement "Pedestrian Safety" and is accompanied by a technical report (www.pediatrics.org/cgi/doi/10.1542/peds.2023-062508) providing additional detail to support recommendations. This statement is intended to assist practicing pediatricians to offer evidence-based advice to families about the benefits of active transportation and the specific risks and safety precautions to consider for child pedestrians at

different ages. For community pediatricians and the American Academy of Pediatrics, the statement provides an overview of specific programs and policies that, if implemented, could foster independent mobility for children while increasing pediatric pedestrian safety. This statement identifies trends in public health and urban design relevant to pedestrian safety. (6/23)
https://doi.org/10.1542/peds.2023-062506

THE CHILD WITNESS IN THE COURTROOM

Robert H. Pantell, MD, FAAP, and Committee on Psychosocial Aspects of Child and Family Health

ABSTRACT. Beginning in the 1980s, children have increasingly served as witnesses in the criminal, civil, and family courts; currently, >100 000 children appear in court each year. This statement updates the 1992 American Academy of Pediatrics (AAP) policy statement "The Child as a Witness" and the subsequent 1999 "The Child in Court: A Subject Review." It also builds on existing AAP policy on adverse life events affecting children and resources developed to understand and address childhood trauma. The purpose of this policy statement is to provide background information on some of the legal issues involving children testifying in court, including the accuracy and psychological impact of child testimony; to provide suggestions for how pediatricians can support patients who will testify in court; and to make recommendations for policy improvements to minimize the adverse psychological consequences for child witnesses. These recommendations are, for the most part, based on studies on the psychological and physiologic consequences of children witnessing and experiencing violence, as well as appearing in court, that have emerged since the previous AAP publications on the subject. The goal is to reduce the secondary traumatization of and long-term consequences for children providing testimony about violence they have experienced or witnessed. This statement primarily addresses children appearing in court as victims of physical or sexual abuse or as witnesses of violent acts; most of the scientific literature addresses these specific situations. It may apply, in certain situations, to children required to provide testimony in custody disputes, child welfare proceedings, or immigration court. It does not address children appearing in court as offenders or as part of juvenile justice proceedings. (2/17, reaffirmed 8/23 with reference & data updates)
https://doi.org/10.1542/peds.2016-4008

CHILDREN WITH INTELLECTUAL AND DEVELOPMENTAL DISABILITIES AS ORGAN TRANSPLANTATION RECIPIENTS

Mindy B. Statter, MD, MBE; Garey Noritz, MD; Committee on Bioethics; and Council on Children With Disabilities

ABSTRACT. The demand for transplantable solid organs far exceeds the supply of deceased donor organs. Patient selection criteria are determined by individual transplant programs; given the scarcity of solid organs for transplant, allocation to those most likely to benefit takes into consideration both medical and psychosocial factors. Children with intellectual and developmental disabilities have historically been excluded as potential recipients of organ transplants. When a transplant is likely to provide significant health benefits, denying a transplant to otherwise eligible children with disabilities may constitute illegal and unjustified discrimination. Children with intellectual and developmental disabilities should not be excluded from the potential pool of recipients and should be referred for evaluation as recipients of solid organ transplants. (4/20, reaffirmed 8/24 with reference & data updates)
https://doi.org/10.1542/peds.2020-0625

CLIMATE CHANGE AND CHILDREN'S HEALTH: BUILDING A HEALTHY FUTURE FOR EVERY CHILD

Samantha Ahdoot, MD, FAAP; Carl R. Baum, MD, FACMT, FAAP; Mary Bono Cataletto, MD, FAAP, FCCP; Patrick Hogan, MD; Christina B. Wu, MD, MPH, FAAP; Aaron Bernstein, MD, MPH, FAAP; Council on Environmental Health and Climate Change; Council on Children and Disasters; Section on Pediatric Pulmonology and Sleep Medicine; and Section on Minority Health, Equity, and Inclusion

ABSTRACT. The warming of our planet matters to every child. Driven by fossil fuel-generated greenhouse gas emissions, climate conditions stable since the founding of modern pediatrics in the mid-nineteenth century have shifted, and old certainties are falling away. Children's physical and mental health are threatened by climate change through its effects on temperature, precipitation, and extreme weather; ecological disruption; and community disruption. These impacts expose and amplify existing inequities and create unprecedented intergenerational injustice. Fossil fuel extraction and combustion cause harm today and reach centuries into the future, jeopardizing the health, safety, and prosperity of today's children and future generations. Appreciating the unique vulnerability of their patients, pediatricians have become leading health advocates for climate actions necessary to protect all living and future children. Policies that reduce reliance on fossil fuels and promote cleaner air, facilitate walking and bicycling, encourage more sustainable diets, increase access to nature, and develop more connected communities lead to immediate gains in child health and equity, and build a foundation for generations of children to thrive. (2/24)
https://doi.org/10.1542/peds.2023-065504

CLIMATE CHANGE AND CHILDREN'S HEALTH: BUILDING A HEALTHY FUTURE FOR EVERY CHILD (TECHNICAL REPORT)

Samantha Ahdoot, MD, FAAP; Carl R. Baum, MD, FACMT, FAAP; Mary Bono Cataletto, MD, FAAP, FCCP; Patrick Hogan, MD; Christina B. Wu, MD, MPH, FAAP; Aaron Bernstein, MD, MPH, FAAP; Council on Environmental Health and Climate Change; Council on Children and Disasters; Section on Pediatric Pulmonology and Sleep Medicine; and Section on Minority Health, Equity, and Inclusion

ABSTRACT. Observed changes in temperature, precipitation patterns, sea level, and extreme weather are destabilizing major determinants of human health. Children are at higher risk of climate-related health burdens than adults because of their unique behavior patterns; developing organ systems and physiology; greater exposure to air, food, and water contaminants per unit of body weight; and dependence on caregivers. Climate change harms children through numerous pathways, including air pollution, heat exposure, floods and hurricanes, food insecurity and nutrition, changing epidemiology of infections, and mental health harms. As the planet continues to warm, climate change's impacts will worsen, threatening to define the health and welfare of children at every stage of their lives. Children who already bear higher burden of disease because of living in low-wealth households and communities, lack of access to high quality education, and experiencing racism and other forms of unjust discrimination bear greater risk of suffering from climate change hazards. Climate change solutions, advanced through collaborative work of pediatricians, health systems, communities, corporations, and governments lead to immediate gains in child health and equity and build a foundation for generations of children to thrive. This technical report reviews the nature of climate change and its associated child health effects and supports the recommendations in the accompanying policy statement on climate change and children's health. (2/24)
https://doi.org/10.1542/peds.2023-065505

COCHLEAR IMPLANTS IN CHILDREN: SURGICAL SITE INFECTIONS AND PREVENTION AND TREATMENT OF ACUTE OTITIS MEDIA AND MENINGITIS

Lorry G. Rubin, MD; Blake Papsin, MD; Committee on Infectious Diseases; and Section on Otolaryngology—Head and Neck Surgery

ABSTRACT. The use of cochlear implants is increasingly common, particularly in children younger than 3 years. Bacterial meningitis, often with associated acute otitis media, is more common in children with cochlear implants than in groups of control children. Children with profound deafness who are candidates for cochlear implants should receive all age-appropriate doses of pneumococcal conjugate and Haemophilus influenzae type b conjugate vaccines and appropriate annual immunization against influenza. In addition, starting at 24 months of age, a single dose of 23-valent pneumococcal polysaccharide vaccine should be administered. Before implant surgery, primary care providers and cochlear implant teams should ensure that immunizations are up-to-date, preferably with completion of indicated vaccines at least 2 weeks before implant surgery. Imaging of the temporal bone/inner ear should be performed before cochlear implantation in all children with congenital deafness and all patients with profound hearing impairment and a history of bacterial meningitis to identify those with inner-ear malformations/cerebrospinal fluid fistulas or ossification of the cochlea. During the initial months after cochlear implantation, the risk of complications of acute otitis media may be higher than during subsequent time periods. Therefore, it is recommended that acute otitis media diagnosed during the first 2 months after implantation be initially treated with a parenteral antibiotic (eg, ceftriaxone or cefotaxime). Episodes occurring 2 months or longer after implantation can be treated with a trial of an oral antimicrobial agent (eg, amoxicillin or amoxicillin/clavulanate at a dose of approximately 90 mg/kg per day of amoxicillin component), provided the child does not appear toxic and the implant does not have a spacer/positioner, a wedge that rests in the cochlea next to the electrodes present in certain implant models available between 1999 and 2002. "Watchful waiting" without antimicrobial therapy is inappropriate for children with implants with acute otitis media. If feasible, tympanocentesis should be performed for acute otitis media, and the material should be sent for culture, but performance of this procedure should not result in an undue delay in initiating antimicrobial therapy. For patients with suspected meningitis, cerebrospinal fluid as well as middle-ear fluid, if present, should be sent for culture. Empiric antimicrobial therapy for meningitis occurring within 2 months of implantation should include an agent with broad activity against Gram-negative bacilli (eg, meropenem) plus vancomycin. For meningitis occurring 2 months or longer after implantation, standard empiric antimicrobial therapy for meningitis (eg, ceftriaxone plus vancomycin) is indicated. For patients with meningitis, urgent evaluation by an otolaryngologist is indicated for consideration of imaging and surgical exploration. (7/10, reaffirmed 1/18, 5/24)

https://doi.org/10.1542/peds.2010-1427

COLLABORATIVE CARE IN THE IDENTIFICATION AND MANAGEMENT OF PSYCHOSIS IN ADOLESCENTS AND YOUNG ADULTS (CLINICAL REPORT)

Liwei L. Hua, MD, PhD, and Committee on Adolescence

ABSTRACT. Pediatricians are often the first physicians to encounter adolescents and young adults presenting with psychotic symptoms. Although pediatricians would ideally be able to refer these patients immediately into psychiatric care, the shortage of child and adolescent psychiatry services may sometimes require pediatricians to make an initial assessment or continue care after recommendations are made by a specialist. Knowing how to identify and further evaluate these symptoms in pediatric patients and how to collaborate with and refer to specialty care is critical in helping to minimize the duration of untreated psychosis and to optimize outcomes. Because not all patients presenting with psychotic-like symptoms will convert to a psychotic disorder, pediatricians should avoid prematurely assigning a diagnosis when possible. Other contributing factors, such as co-occurring substance abuse or trauma, should also be considered. This clinical report describes psychotic and psychotic-like symptoms in the pediatric age group as well as etiology, risk factors, and recommendations for pediatricians, who may be among the first health care providers to identify youth at risk. (5/21)

https://doi.org/10.1542/peds.2021-051486

COLLABORATIVE ROLE OF THE PEDIATRICIAN IN THE DIAGNOSIS AND MANAGEMENT OF BIPOLAR DISORDER IN ADOLESCENTS (CLINICAL REPORT)

Benjamin N. Shain, MD, PhD, and Committee on Adolescence

ABSTRACT. Despite the complexity of diagnosis and management, pediatricians have an important collaborative role in referring and partnering in the management of adolescents with bipolar disorder. This report presents the classification of bipolar disorder as well as interviewing and diagnostic guidelines. Treatment options are described, particularly focusing on medication management and rationale for the common practice of multiple, simultaneous medications. Medication adverse effects may be problematic and better managed with collaboration between mental health professionals and pediatricians. Case examples illustrate a number of common diagnostic and management issues. (11/12, reaffirmed 9/21)

https://doi.org/10.1542/peds.2012-2756

COMANAGEMENT OF SURGICAL PEDIATRIC PATIENTS IN THE ACUTE CARE INPATIENT SETTING (CLINICAL REPORT)

Rebecca E. Rosenberg, MD, MPH, FAAP; David M. Pressel, MD, PhD, FAAP; David I. Rappaport, MD, FAAP; Joshua M. Abzug, MD, FAAP; and Section on Hospital Medicine

ABSTRACT. The care of children with primary surgical diagnoses in acute care units often involves a shared surgical and medical model ("comanagement"). There are no formal guidelines for how such programs should be structured or care provided. We used a modified Delphi process, including national experts in pediatrics and pediatric medical subspecialties, pediatric surgical specialties, and pediatric anesthesiology, to develop recommendations for best practices for comanagement programs in community and tertiary care settings. (12/23)

https://doi.org/10.1542/peds.2023-064775

COMMUNITY PEDIATRICS: NAVIGATING THE INTERSECTION OF MEDICINE, PUBLIC HEALTH, AND SOCIAL DETERMINANTS OF CHILDREN'S HEALTH

Council on Community Pediatrics

ABSTRACT. This policy statement provides a framework for the pediatrician's role in promoting the health and well-being of all children in the context of their families and communities. It offers pediatricians a definition of community pediatrics, emphasizes the importance of recognizing social determinants of health, and delineates the need to partner with public health to address population-based child health issues. It also recognizes the importance of pediatric involvement in child advocacy at local, state, and federal levels to ensure all children have access to a high-quality medical home and to eliminate child health disparities. This statement provides a set of specific recommendations that underscore the critical nature of this dimension of pediatric practice, teaching, and research. (2/13, reaffirmed 10/16, 12/23)

https://doi.org/10.1542/peds.2012-3933

A COMPREHENSIVE REPORT ON ALL-TERRAIN VEHICLES AND YOUTH: CONTINUING CHALLENGES FOR INJURY PREVENTION (TECHNICAL REPORT)

Charles A. Jennissen, MD, FAAP; Gerene M. Denning, PhD; Mary E. Aitken, MD, MPH, FAAP; and Council on Injury, Violence, and Poison Prevention

ABSTRACT. All-terrain vehicles (ATVs) represent a serious and ongoing public health and safety concern for children and adolescents. Survey studies indicate that high proportions of youth ride ATVs in both rural and nonrural populations. The significant human and economic costs of pediatric ATV-related deaths and injuries result from a number of major risk factors that are highly common in pediatric ATV crashes: operating adult-size vehicles, riding with or as passengers, lack of protective equipment, and riding on public roads. Other less well-studied but potentially significant risk factors are speed, riding at night, alcohol use among older teenagers, and lack of training and supervision. Although potentially safer than adult ATVs, youth models present a number of safety concerns that have not been addressed with rigorous study. The most common ATV crash mechanism is a noncollision event—for example, a rollover. Common injury mechanisms include ejection from the vehicle, resulting in extremity and head injuries, and being pinned or crushed by the vehicle with resulting multiorgan trauma and/or compression asphyxia. Traumatic brain injury and multisystem trauma are the 2 most common causes of death and disabling injury. Taken together, a large multidecade body of evidence is the basis for the American Academy of Pediatrics policy statement recommendation that no child younger than 16 years of age ride on an ATV. Because children continue to be allowed to ride these vehicles, however, efforts to prevent pediatric ATV-related deaths and injuries require multipronged strategies, including education of both youth and parents, safety-based engineering, and enforcement of evidence-based safety laws. (9/22)
https://doi.org/10.1542/peds.2022-059280

CONFIDENTIALITY IN THE CARE OF ADOLESCENTS

Richard J. Chung, MD, FSAHM, FAAP; Janet B. Lee, MD, FAAP; Jesse M. Hackell, MD, FAAP; Elizabeth M. Alderman, MD, FSAHM, FAAP; Committee on Adolescence; and Committee on Practice & Ambulatory Medicine

ABSTRACT. Confidentiality is an essential component of high-quality health care for adolescents and young adults and can have an impact on the health care experiences and health outcomes of youth. Federal and state laws, professional guidelines, and ethical standards provide a core framework for guidance in the implementation of confidentiality protections in clinical practice. This policy statement provides recommendations for pediatricians and other pediatric health care professionals, clinics, health systems, payers, and electronic health record developers to optimize confidentiality practices and protections for adolescents and young adults across the spectrum of care. (4/24)
https://doi.org/10.1542/peds.2024-066326

CONFIDENTIALITY IN THE CARE OF ADOLESCENTS (TECHNICAL REPORT)

Richard J. Chung, MD, FSAHM, FAAP; Janet B. Lee, MD, FAAP; Jesse M. Hackell, MD, FAAP; Elizabeth M. Alderman, MD, FSAHM, FAAP; Committee on Adolescence; and Committee on Practice & Ambulatory Medicine

ABSTRACT. Confidentiality is a foundational element of high-quality, accessible, and equitable health care. Despite strong grounding in federal and state laws, professional guidelines, and ethical standards, health care professionals and adolescent patients face a range of complexities and barriers to seeking and providing confidential care to adolescents across different settings and circumstances. The dynamic needs of adolescents, the oftentimes competing interests of key stakeholders, the rapidly evolving technological context of care, and variable health care billing and claims requirements are all important considerations in understanding how to optimize care to focus on and meet the needs of the adolescent patient. The following assessment of the evolving evidence base offers a view of the current state and best practices while pointing to numerous unmet needs and opportunities for improvement in the care experiences of youth as well as their health outcomes. (4/24)
https://doi.org/10.1542/peds.2024-066327

CONGENITAL HYPOTHYROIDISM: SCREENING AND MANAGEMENT (CLINICAL REPORT)

Susan R. Rose, MD, FAAP; Ari J. Wassner, MD; Kupper A. Wintergerst, MD, FAAP; Nana-Hawa Yayah-Jones, MD; Robert J. Hopkin, MD, FAAP; Janet Chuang, MD; Jessica R. Smith, MD; Katherine Abell, MD; Stephen H. LaFranchi, MD, FAAP; Section on Endocrinology Executive Committee; and Council on Genetics Executive Committee

ABSTRACT. Untreated congenital hypothyroidism (CH) leads to intellectual disabilities. Newborn screening (NBS) for CH should be performed in all infants. Prompt diagnosis by NBS leading to early and adequate treatment results in grossly normal neurocognitive outcomes in adulthood. However, NBS for hypothyroidism is not yet practiced in all countries globally. Seventy percent of neonates worldwide do not undergo NBS.

The recommended initial treatment of CH is levothyroxine, 10 to 15 mcg/kg daily. The goals of treatment are to maintain consistent euthyroidism with normal thyroid-stimulating hormone and with free thyroxine in the upper half of the age-specific reference range during the first 3 years of life. Controversy remains regarding the detection of thyroid dysfunction and optimal management of special populations, including preterm or low-birth-weight infants and infants with transient or mild CH, trisomy 21, or central hypothyroidism.

NBS alone is not sufficient to prevent adverse outcomes from CH in a pediatric population. In addition to NBS, the management of CH requires timely confirmation of the diagnosis, accurate interpretation of thyroid function testing, effective treatment, and consistent follow-up. Physicians need to consider hypothyroidism in the face of clinical symptoms, even if NBS thyroid test results are normal. When clinical symptoms and signs of hypothyroidism are present (such as large posterior fontanelle, large tongue, umbilical hernia, prolonged jaundice, constipation, lethargy, and/or hypothermia), measurement of serum thyroid-stimulating hormone and free thyroxine is indicated, regardless of NBS results. (12/22)
https://doi.org/10.1542/peds.2022-060419

CONGENITAL HYPOTHYROIDISM: SCREENING AND MANAGEMENT (TECHNICAL REPORT)

Susan R. Rose, MD, FAAP; Ari J. Wassner, MD; Kupper A. Wintergerst, MD, FAAP; Nana-Hawa Yayah-Jones, MD; Robert J. Hopkin, MD, FAAP; Janet Chuang, MD; Jessica R. Smith, MD; Katherine Abell, MD; Stephen H. LaFranchi, MD, FAAP; Section on Endocrinology Executive Committee; and Council on Genetics Executive Committee

ABSTRACT. Untreated congenital hypothyroidism (CH) leads to intellectual disabilities. Prompt diagnosis by newborn screening (NBS) leading to early and adequate treatment results in grossly normal neurocognitive outcomes in adulthood. However, NBS for hypothyroidism is not yet established in all countries globally. Seventy percent of neonates worldwide do not undergo NBS.

The initial treatment of CH is levothyroxine, 10 to 15 mcg/kg daily. The goals of treatment are to maintain consistent euthyroidism with normal thyroid-stimulating hormone and free thyroxine in the upper half of the age-specific reference range during the first 3 years of life. Controversy remains regarding detection of thyroid dysfunction and optimal management of special populations, including preterm or low-birth weight infants and infants with transient or mild CH, trisomy 21, or central hypothyroidism.

Newborn screening alone is not sufficient to prevent adverse outcomes from CH in a pediatric population. In addition to NBS, the management of CH requires timely confirmation of the diagnosis, accurate interpretation of thyroid function testing, effective treatment, and consistent follow-up. Physicians need to consider hypothyroidism in the face of clinical symptoms, even if NBS thyroid test results are normal. When clinical symptoms and signs of hypothyroidism are present (such as large posterior fontanelle, large tongue, umbilical hernia, prolonged jaundice, constipation, lethargy, and/or hypothermia), measurement of serum thyroid-stimulating hormone and free thyroxine is indicated, regardless of NBS results. (12/22)
https://doi.org/10.1542/peds.2022-060420

CONSENT BY PROXY FOR NONURGENT PEDIATRIC CARE (CLINICAL REPORT)

Jonathan M. Fanaroff, MD, JD, FAAP, FCLM, and Committee on Medical Liability and Risk Management

ABSTRACT. Minor-aged patients are often brought to the pediatrician for nonurgent acute medical care, physical examinations, or health supervision visits by someone other than their legally authorized representative, which, in most situations, is a parent. These surrogates or proxies can be members of the child's extended family, such as a grandparent, adult sibling, or aunt/uncle; a noncustodial parent or stepparent in cases of divorce and remarriage; an adult who lives in the home but is not biologically or legally related to the child; or even a child care provider (eg, au pair, nanny, private-duty nurse/nurse's aide, group home supervisor). This report identifies common situations in which pediatricians may encounter "consent by proxy" for nonurgent medical care for minors, including physical examinations, and explains the potential for liability exposure associated with these circumstances. The report suggests practical steps that balance the need to minimize the physician's liability exposure with the patient's access to health care. Key issues to be considered when creating or updating office policies for obtaining and documenting consent by proxy are offered. (1/17, reaffirmed 11/24)
https://doi.org/10.1542/peds.2016-3911

CONSIDERATIONS FOR ALTERNATIVE DECISION-MAKING WHEN TRANSITIONING TO ADULTHOOD FOR YOUTH WITH INTELLECTUAL AND DEVELOPMENTAL DISABILITIES

Renee M. Turchi, MD, MPH, FAAP; Dennis Z. Kuo, MD, MHS, FAAP; John W. Rusher, MD, JD, FAAP; Rebecca R. Seltzer, MD, MHS, FAAP; Christoph U. Lehmann, MD, FAAP; Randall W. Grout, MD, MS, FAAP; Council on Children With Disabilities; and Committee on Medical Liability and Risk Management

ABSTRACT. With advances in medical care, more youth with intellectual and/or developmental disabilities (IDD) are transitioning into adulthood. Patient- and family-centered, integrated care is warranted around this time of transition. Support teams (including the youth, caregivers, teachers, and pediatricians) should engage in transition planning, ideally starting between 12 and 14 years of age, to identify and develop resources to support the maturing youth's capacity for independent decision-making. Care teams should consider the varied levels of alternative decision-making support, which may include supported decision-making, medical proxy decision-making, power of attorney, and/or establishment of legal guardianship arrangements, to support the youth's health and well-being optimally. Ultimately, if independent decision-making is not appropriate, the goal for youth with IDD should be the least restrictive alternative, while preserving human rights and human dignity and promoting their autonomy. These considerations review alternative decision-making support, concepts, and legal requirements available for youth with IDD and their care teams. Pediatricians can support youth with IDD and their families in the transition process and decision-making autonomy by actively engaging the youth in care decisions, supporting needs for augmentative communication, fostering their expression of preferences and understanding of care decisions, and linking them to resources such as the medical-legal partnership model. (5/24)
https://doi.org/10.1542/peds.2024-066841

CONSIDERATIONS IN THE DETERMINATION OF MEDICAL NECESSITY IN CHILDREN: APPLICATION TO CONTRACTUAL LANGUAGE

Angelo P. Giardino, MD, PhD, FAAP; Mark L. Hudak, MD, FAAP; Beena G. Sood, MD, MS, FAAP; Stephen A. Pearlman, MD, MSHQS, FAAP; and Committee on Child Health Financing

ABSTRACT. Through this policy statement, the American Academy of Pediatrics advocates that all health care insurers adopt consistent medical necessity definitions that reflect the needs of infants, children, adolescents, and young adults (hereafter noted as "children") as a function of developmental, epidemiologic, dependency, demographic, and cost-related factors that change over the pediatric continuum and that differ from adults. Optimally, the scope of benefits defined in health care contracts should address the complete spectrum of health care needs of children and families, but in reality, many plans offer a limited scope of benefits for children. Even if a proposed intervention falls within the scope of benefits or is not specifically excluded from coverage, the health plan may still deny the intervention. In such cases, contractual language may allow an appeal to succeed if the provider demonstrates medical necessity. With the assistance of experienced pediatric physicians and other providers with pediatric expertise, health care payers and agencies should clearly detail the processes that define, evaluate, and determine medical necessity and through which providers may appeal decisions. A basic requirement for any medical necessity process is the consideration of input from the physician(s) caring for a pediatric patient for whom a medical necessity determination is necessary. (8/22)
https://doi.org/10.1542/peds.2022-058882

CONSIDERATIONS ON THE USE OF NEONATAL AND PEDIATRIC RESUSCITATION GUIDELINES FOR HOSPITALIZED NEONATES AND INFANTS: ON BEHALF OF THE AMERICAN HEART ASSOCIATION EMERGENCY CARDIOVASCULAR CARE COMMITTEE AND THE AMERICAN ACADEMY OF PEDIATRICS

Taylor Sawyer, DO, MBA, MEd, FAAP; Mary E. McBride, MD, MEd, FAAP; Anne Ades, MD, MSEd, FAAP; Vishal S. Kapadia, MD, MSCS, FAAP; Tina A. Leone, MD, FAAP; Satyan Lakshminrusimha, MD, FAAP; Norjahan Ali, MD, MSc, FAAP; Stephanie Marshall, MD; Georg M. Schmölzer, MD, PhD; Kelly D. Kadlec, MD, MEd, FAAP; Martin V. Pusic, MD, PhD; Blair L. Bigham, MD, MS; Farhan Bhanji, MD, MSc Ed FRCPC; Aaron J. Donoghue, MD, MSCE, FAHA, FAAP; Tia Raymond, MD, FAAP, FAHA, FCCM; Beena D. Kamath-Rayne, MD, MPH, FAAP; Allan de Caen, MD, FRCPC

ABSTRACT. Between 0.25% and 3% of admissions to the NICU, PICU, and PCICU receive cardiopulmonary resuscitation (CPR). Most CPR events occur in patients <1 year old. The incidence of CPR is 10 times higher in the NICU than at birth. Therefore, optimizing the approach to CPR in hospitalized neonates and infants is important.

At birth, the resuscitation of newborns is performed according to neonatal resuscitation guidelines. In older infants and children, resuscitation is performed according to pediatric resuscitation guidelines. Neonatal and pediatric guidelines differ in several important ways. There are no published recommendations to guide the transition from neonatal to pediatric guidelines. Therefore, hospitalized neonates and infants can be resuscitated using neonatal guidelines, pediatric guidelines, or a hybrid approach.

This report summarizes the current neonatal and pediatric resuscitation guidelines, considers how to apply them to hospitalized neonates and infants, and identifies knowledge gaps and future priorities. The lack of strong scientific data makes it impossible to provide definitive recommendations on when to transition from neonatal to pediatric resuscitation guidelines. Therefore, it is up to health care teams and institutions to decide if neonatal or pediatric guidelines are the best choice in a given location or situation, considering local circumstances, health care team preferences, and resource limitations. (12/23)

https://doi.org/10.1542/peds.2023-064681

CONTRACEPTION FOR ADOLESCENTS

Mary A. Ott, MD, MA, FAAP; Andrea J. Hoopes, MD, MPH, FAAP; Gina S. Sucato, MD, MPH, FSAHM, FAAP; Maayan Leroy-Melamed, MD, MPH, FAAP; and Committee on Adolescence

ABSTRACT. The American Academy of Pediatrics recommends that pediatricians provide contraceptive care for adolescents. Contraceptive prescribing and counseling skills ensure the safety and well-being of adolescents, enabling pediatricians to help adolescents achieve optimal reproductive health. This policy statement updates the 2014 policy statement on contraception for adolescents and is designed to be used in tandem with the accompanying clinical report, "Contraceptive Counseling and Methods for Adolescents" and the series of method-specific policy statements and clinical reports from the Academy. This policy statement provides the pediatrician with evidence-informed and equity-informed practices in contraceptive care for adolescents. (6/25)

See full text on page 143.

https://doi.org/10.1542/peds.2025-072217

CONTRACEPTION FOR HIV-INFECTED ADOLESCENTS (CLINICAL REPORT)

Athena P. Kourtis, MD, PhD, MPH, FAAP; Ayesha Mirza, MD, FAAP; and Committee on Pediatric AIDS

ABSTRACT. Access to high-quality reproductive health care is important for adolescents and young adults with HIV infection to prevent unintended pregnancies, sexually transmitted infections, and secondary transmission of HIV to partners and children. As perinatally HIV-infected children mature into adolescence and adulthood and new HIV infections among adolescents and young adults continue to occur in the United States, medical providers taking care of such individuals often face issues related to sexual and reproductive health. Challenges including drug interactions between several hormonal methods and antiretroviral agents make decisions regarding contraceptive options more complex for these adolescents. Dual protection, defined as the use of an effective contraceptive along with condoms, should be central to ongoing discussions with HIV-infected young women and couples wishing to avoid pregnancy. Last, reproductive health discussions need to be integrated with discussions on HIV care, because a reduction in plasma HIV viral load below the level of detection (an "undetectable viral load") is essential for the individual's health as well as for a reduction in HIV transmission to partners and children. (8/16, reaffirmed 7/21 with reference & data updates)

https://doi.org/10.1542/peds.2016-1892

CONTRACEPTIVE COUNSELING AND METHODS FOR ADOLESCENTS (CLINICAL REPORT)

Mary A. Ott, MD, MA, FAAP; Gina S. Sucato, MD, MPH, FSAHM, FAAP; Maayan Leroy-Melamed, MD, MPH, FAAP; Andrea J. Hoopes, MD, MPH, FAAP; and Committee on Adolescence

ABSTRACT. To provide contraceptive care to adolescents, pediatricians need a working knowledge about counseling basics as well as a full range of contraceptive methods. Pediatricians may provide contraception for pregnancy prevention or for menstrual suppression and other medical indications. This clinical report is a companion to the revised policy statement "Contraception for Adolescents," and it provides updates for pediatricians on adolescent-centered counseling approaches and contraceptive methods, including long-acting reversible contraceptives, hormonal contraceptives, barrier methods, and emergency contraceptives. Together, these documents provide the pediatrician with evidence-informed and equity-informed practices in counseling and prescribing contraception for adolescents. (6/25)

See full text on page 155.

https://doi.org/10.1542/peds.2025-072218

CORPORAL PUNISHMENT IN SCHOOLS

Mandy A. Allison, MD, MSPH, MEd, FAAP; Nathaniel Beers, MD, MPA, FAAP; Jaime W. Peterson, MD, MPH, FAAP; and Council on School Health

ABSTRACT. The use of corporal punishment in schools is not an effective or ethical method for management of behavior concerns and causes harm to students. The American Academy of Pediatrics recommends that corporal punishment in all school settings be abolished in all states by law and replaced by alternative forms of student behavior management. Corporal punishment remains legal in many public and private schools in the United States and is disproportionately used among Black students and children with disabilities. The aims of this policy statement are to review the incidence of school-based corporal punishment; the negative physical, psychological, and developmental impact of corporal punishment on students; and the need for continued advocacy by pediatricians, educators, and parents to abolish corporal punishment in all schools. (8/23)

https://doi.org/10.1542/peds.2023-063284

COUNSELING PARENTS AND TEENS ABOUT MARIJUANA USE IN THE ERA OF LEGALIZATION OF MARIJUANA (CLINICAL REPORT)

Sheryl A. Ryan, MD, FAAP; Seth D. Ammerman, MD, FAAP; and Committee on Substance Use and Prevention

ABSTRACT. Many states have recently made significant changes to their legislation making recreational and/or medical marijuana use by adults legal. Although these laws, for the most part, have not targeted the adolescent population, they have created an environment in which marijuana increasingly is seen as acceptable, safe, and therapeutic. This clinical report offers guidance to the practicing pediatrician based on existing evidence and expert opinion/consensus of the American Academy of Pediatrics regarding anticipatory guidance and counseling to teenagers and their parents about marijuana and its use. The recently published technical report provides the detailed evidence and references regarding the research on which the information in this clinical report is based. (2/17, reaffirmed 1/24)

https://doi.org/10.1542/peds.2016-4069

CREATING WORK AND LEARNING ENVIRONMENTS FREE OF GENDER-BASED HARASSMENT IN PEDIATRIC HEALTH CARE

Julie Story Byerley, MD, MPH, FAAP; Nancy A. Dodson, MD, MPH, FAAP; Tiffany St. Clair, MD, FAAP; Valencia P. Walker, MD, MPH, FAAP; and Committee on Pediatric Workforce

ABSTRACT. Although gender harassment has long been a concern of the American Academy of Pediatrics, recent attention has helped to highlight the pervasive scope of the issue and identify previously under recognized harassment concerns for people of gender and sexual minorities. More subtle forms of harassment such as microaggressions have been recognized to contribute to significant negative outcomes for those who experience them. Patients and their families have also been recognized as potential perpetrators of harassment. Work and learning environments should support a clear no-tolerance policy regarding sexual harassment by employees or educators, and perpetrators should be held accountable for their actions. Sexual harassment that occurs with patients or family members as perpetrators, although more complicated given the nature of the caregiving relationship, should be stopped. Work and learning environments free of gender-based harassment support pediatric physicians, enhance vitality, advance equity, and improve patient care. (8/22)

https://doi.org/10.1542/peds.2022-058880

CRITICAL ELEMENTS FOR THE PEDIATRIC PERIOPERATIVE ANESTHESIA ENVIRONMENT

Section on Anesthesiology and Pain Medicine

ABSTRACT. The American Academy of Pediatrics proposes guidance for the pediatric perioperative anesthesia environment. Essential components are identified to optimize the perioperative environment for the anesthetic care of infants and children. Such an environment promotes the safety and well-being of infants and children by reducing the risk of adverse events. (11/15, reaffirmed 5/23)

https://doi.org/10.1542/peds.2015-3595

CROWDING IN THE EMERGENCY DEPARTMENT: CHALLENGES AND BEST PRACTICES FOR THE CARE OF CHILDREN (TECHNICAL REPORT)

Toni K. Gross, MD, MPH, FAAP; Natalie E. Lane, MD, FAAP; Nathan L. Timm, MD, FAAP; and Committee on Pediatric Emergency Medicine

ABSTRACT. Emergency department (ED) crowding has been and continues to be a national concern. ED crowding is defined as a situation in which the identified need for emergency services outstrips available resources in the ED. Crowding is associated with higher morbidity and mortality, delayed pain control, delayed time to administration of antibiotics, increased medical errors, and less-than-optimal health care. ED crowding impedes a hospital's ability to achieve national quality and patient safety goals, diminishes the effectiveness of the health care safety net, and limits the capacity of hospitals to respond to a disaster and/or sudden surge in disease. Both children and adults seeking care in emergency settings are placed at risk. Crowding negatively influences the experience for patients, families, and providers, and can impact employee turnover and well-being. No single factor is implicated in creating the issue of crowding, but elements that influence crowding can be divided into those that affect input (prehospital and outpatient care), throughput (ED), and output (hospital and outpatient care). The degree of ED crowding is difficult to quantify but has been linked to markers such as hours on ambulance diversion, hours of inpatient boarding in the emergency setting, increasing wait times, and patients who leave without being seen. A number of organizations, including the American College of Emergency Physicians, the Emergency Nurses Association, and the National Quality Forum, have convened to better define emergency metrics and definitions that help provide data for benchmarks for patient throughput performance. The Joint Commission has acknowledged that patient safety is tied to patient throughput and has developed guidance for hospitals to ensure that hospital leadership engages in the process of safe egress of the patient out of the ED and, most recently, to address efficient disposition of patients with mental health emergencies. It is important that the American Academy of Pediatrics acknowledges the potential impact on access to optimal emergency care for children in the face of ED crowding and helps guide health policy decision-makers toward effective solutions that promote the medical home and timely access to emergency care. (2/23)

https://doi.org/10.1542/peds.2022-060972

CROWDING IN THE EMERGENCY DEPARTMENT: CHALLENGES AND RECOMMENDATIONS FOR THE CARE OF CHILDREN

Toni K. Gross, MD, MPH, FAAP; Natalie E. Lane, MD, FAAP; Nathan L. Timm, MD, FAAP; and Committee on Pediatric Emergency Medicine

ABSTRACT. Emergency department (ED) crowding results when available resources cannot meet the demand for emergency services. ED crowding has negative impacts on patients, health care workers, and the community. Primary considerations for reducing ED crowding include improving the quality of care, patient safety, patient experience, and the health of populations, as well as reducing the per capita cost of health care. Evaluating causes, effects, and seeking solutions to ED crowding can be done within a conceptual framework addressing input, throughput, and output factors. ED leaders must coordinate with hospital leadership, health system planners and policy decision makers, and those who provide pediatric care to address ED crowding. Proposed solutions in this policy statement promote the medical home and timely access to emergency care for children. (2/23)

https://doi.org/10.1542/peds.2022-060971

THE CRUCIAL ROLE OF RECESS IN SCHOOL

Council on School Health

ABSTRACT. Recess is at the heart of a vigorous debate over the role of schools in promoting the optimal development of the whole child. A growing trend toward reallocating time in school to accentuate the more academic subjects has put this important facet of a child's school day at risk. Recess serves as a necessary break from the rigors of concentrated, academic challenges in the classroom. But equally important is the fact that safe and well-supervised recess offers cognitive, social, emotional, and physical benefits that may not be fully appreciated when a decision is made to diminish it. Recess is unique from, and a complement to, physical education—not a substitute for it. The American Academy of Pediatrics believes that recess is a crucial and necessary component of a child's development and, as such, it should not be withheld for punitive or academic reasons. (12/12, reaffirmed 4/23)

https://doi.org/10.1542/peds.2012-2993

DEATH OF A CHILD IN THE EMERGENCY DEPARTMENT

Committee on Pediatric Emergency Medicine (joint with American College of Emergency Physicians Pediatric Emergency Medical Committee and Emergency Nurses Association Pediatric Committee)

ABSTRACT. The American Academy of Pediatrics, American College of Emergency Physicians, and Emergency Nurses Association have collaborated to identify practices and principles to guide the care of children, families, and staff in the challenging and uncommon event of the death of a child in the

emergency department in this policy statement and in an accompanying technical report. (7/14, reaffirmed 11/24)
https://doi.org/10.1542/peds.2014-1245

DEATH OF A CHILD IN THE EMERGENCY DEPARTMENT (TECHNICAL REPORT)

Patricia O'Malley, MD; Isabel Barata, MD; Sally Snow, RN; and Committee on Pediatric Emergency Medicine (joint with American College of Emergency Physicians Pediatric Emergency Medical Committee and Emergency Nurses Association Pediatric Committee)

ABSTRACT. The death of a child in the emergency department (ED) is one of the most challenging problems facing ED clinicians. This revised technical report and accompanying policy statement reaffirm principles of patient- and family-centered care. Recent literature is examined regarding family presence, termination of resuscitation, bereavement responsibilities of ED clinicians, support of child fatality review efforts, and other issues inherent in caring for the patient, family, and staff when a child dies in the ED. Appendices are provided that offer an approach to bereavement activities in the ED, carrying out forensic responsibilities while providing compassionate care, communicating the news of the death of a child in the acute setting, providing a closing ritual at the time of terminating resuscitation efforts, and managing the child with a terminal condition who presents near death in the ED. (7/14, reaffirmed 11/24)
https://doi.org/10.1542/peds.2014-1246

DETENTION OF IMMIGRANT CHILDREN

Julie M. Linton, MD, FAAP; Marsha Griffin, MD, FAAP; Alan J. Shapiro, MD, FAAP; and Council on Community Pediatrics

ABSTRACT. Immigrant children seeking safe haven in the United States, whether arriving unaccompanied or in family units, face a complicated evaluation and legal process from the point of arrival through permanent resettlement in communities. The conditions in which children are detained and the support services that are available to them are of great concern to pediatricians and other advocates for children. In accordance with internationally accepted rights of the child, immigrant and refugee children should be treated with dignity and respect and should not be exposed to conditions that may harm or traumatize them. The Department of Homeland Security facilities do not meet the basic standards for the care of children in residential settings. The recommendations in this statement call for limited exposure of any child to current Department of Homeland Security facilities (ie, Customs and Border Protection and Immigration and Customs Enforcement facilities) and for longitudinal evaluation of the health consequences of detention of immigrant children in the United States. From the moment children are in the custody of the United States, they deserve health care that meets guideline-based standards, treatment that mitigates harm or traumatization, and services that support their health and well-being. This policy statement also provides specific recommendations regarding postrelease services once a child is released into communities across the country, including a coordinated system that facilitates access to a medical home and consistent access to education, child care, interpretation services, and legal services. (4/17, reaffirmed 11/22)
https://doi.org/10.1542/peds.2017-0483

DIAGNOSIS, TREATMENT, AND PREVENTION OF CONGENITAL TOXOPLASMOSIS IN THE UNITED STATES (TECHNICAL REPORT)

Yvonne A. Maldonado, MD, FAAP; Jennifer S. Read, MD, MS, MPH, DTM&H, FAAP; and Committee on Infectious Diseases

ABSTRACT. Congenital toxoplasmosis (CT) is a parasitic disease that can cause significant fetal and neonatal harm. Coordinated efforts by pregnant women, researchers, physicians, and health policy makers regarding potential primary and secondary preventive measures for CT and their implementation may lead to a lower incidence of CT as well as lower morbidity and mortality rates associated with CT. The purpose of this technical report is to summarize available information regarding the diagnosis, treatment, and prevention of CT. (1/17, reaffirmed 1/22 with reference & data updates)
https://doi.org/10.1542/peds.2016-3860

DIAGNOSIS AND CARE OF CHILDREN WITH CEREBRAL/CORTICAL VISUAL IMPAIRMENT (CLINICAL REPORT)

Sharon S. Lehman, MD, FAAP; Larry Yin, MD, MSPH, FAAP; Melinda Y. Chang, MD, FAAP; Section on Ophthalmology; and Council on Children With Disabilities (joint with American Association for Pediatric Ophthalmology and Strabismus; American Academy of Ophthalmology; and American Association of Certified Orthoptists)

ABSTRACT. Cerebral/cortical visual impairment (CVI) is a leading cause of pediatric visual impairment in nations with developed economies and is increasing in those with developing economies. Because vision is the predominant sense used for learning, delay in diagnosis of CVI can negatively affect education, making early detection and management important. The American Academy of Pediatrics has published the policy statement "Visual System Assessment in Infants, Children, and Young Adults by Pediatricians" and an accompanying clinical report that are based on identifying potential causes of ocular visual impairment in children. Yet, routine vision screening may not accurately identify the brain-based visual impairment in children with CVI. Moreover, children with CVI often have medical complexity with other neurocognitive impairments and serious medical conditions that can make the diagnosis of CVI more difficult. Strategies are necessary for early identification of CVI to promote early diagnosis and referral for vision services that may allow a child with CVI to engage more fully in school, activities of daily living, vocational pursuits, and recreational activities. Knowledge of the characteristics of CVI as well as risk factors for CVI will assist the pediatrician in identifying children with CVI. This clinical report is complementary to previous vision screening policies, allowing both ocular and brain-based visual impairments in children to be identified and addressed. Pediatricians, other primary care physicians, pediatric ophthalmologists, neurologists, and other specialized pediatric eye care clinicians can identify children with CVI and coordinate effective evaluation, diagnosis, and referrals for vision services for these children. (11/24)
https://doi.org/10.1542/peds.2024-068465

DIAGNOSIS AND MANAGEMENT OF HYPERBILIRUBINEMIA IN THE NEWBORN INFANT 35 OR MORE WEEKS OF GESTATION (TECHNICAL REPORT)

Jonathan L. Slaughter, MD, MPH, FAAP; Alex R. Kemper, MD, MPH, MS, FAAP; and Thomas B. Newman, MD, MPH, FAAP

ABSTRACT. The 2022 American Academy of Pediatrics publication, "Clinical Practice Guideline Revision: Diagnosis and Management of Hyperbilirubinemia in the Newborn Infant 35 or More Weeks of Gestation," builds on the previous 2004 guideline, "Management of Hyperbilirubinemia in the Newborn Infant 35 or More Weeks of Gestation," and a 2009 follow-up commentary, "Hyperbilirubinemia in the Newborn Infant ≥35 Weeks' Gestation: An Update With Clarifications." The gestational age cutoff of ≥35 weeks was chosen because it includes most newborn infants cared for by general pediatricians and other primary care clinicians in mother-baby units and well-baby nurseries. This guideline does not apply to preterm newborns born <35 weeks' gestation, who generally receive care in neonatal intensive care units (NICUs). (8/22)
https://doi.org/10.1542/peds.2022-058865

DIAGNOSIS AND TREATMENT OF IDIOPATHIC CONGENITAL CLUBFOOT (CLINICAL REPORT)

Robert Cady, MD, FAAP; Theresa A. Hennessey, MD, MHCDS, FAAP; Richard M. Schwend, MD, FAAP; and Section on Orthopedics

ABSTRACT. Idiopathic congenital clubfoot is the most common serious musculoskeletal birth defect in the United States and the world. The natural history of the deformity is to persist into adult life with a significant decrease in function and quality of life. The Ponseti method (serial casting, Achilles tenotomy, and bracing of the clubfoot) has become the most effective and accepted treatment of children born with clubfoot worldwide. The treatment is successful, particularly when the Ponseti-trained practitioner (often a pediatric orthopedic surgeon), the primary care clinician, and the family work together to facilitate success. An important factor in the ultimate success of the Ponseti method is parental understanding of the bracing phase. There is a very high rate of recurrent deformity when bracing is not done properly or is stopped prematurely. The importance of positive education and support for the parents to complete the entire treatment protocol cannot be overstated. The goal of treatment is a deformity-free, functional, comfortable foot. Ponseti clubfoot programs have been launched in most countries throughout the world, including many countries with limited resources. Ultimately, the goal is that every infant born with a clubfoot will have access to care with the Ponseti method. This clinical report is intended for medical practitioners who are involved in the care of pediatric patients with clubfoot. Understanding the standard of care will help these practitioners to care for patients and their families. (1/22)

https://doi.org/10.1542/peds.2021-055555

DIRECT ADMISSION TO HOSPITAL FOR CHILDREN IN THE UNITED STATES

JoAnna K. Leyenaar, MD, PhD, MPH, FAAP; Vanessa Hill, MD, FAAP; Vinh Lam, MD, FAAP; Rebecca Stern, MD; Kristin Williams Vaughan, MD, FAAP; and Committee on Hospital Care

ABSTRACT. One in four unscheduled hospital admissions for children and adolescents in the United States occurs via direct admission, defined as hospital admission without first receiving care in the hospital's emergency department. The purpose of this policy statement is to present recommendations to optimize the quality and safety of this hospital admission approach for children. Recommendations included in this policy statement provide guidance related to: (i) direct admission written guidelines, (ii) clear systems of communication between members of the health care team and with families of children requiring admission, (iii) triage systems to identify patient acuity and disease severity, (iv) identification of hospital resources needed to support direct admission systems of care, (v) consideration of patient populations that may be at increased risk of adverse outcomes during the hospital admission process, (vi) addressing the relevance of local factors and resources, and (vii) ongoing evaluation of direct admission processes and outcomes. The recommendations included in this policy statement are intended to support the implementation of safe direct admission processes and to foster awareness of outcomes associated with this common portal of hospital admission. (2/23)

https://doi.org/10.1542/peds.2022-060973

DISCLOSURE OF ADVERSE EVENTS IN PEDIATRICS

Laura Sigman, MD, JD, FAAP; Robert Turbow, MD, JD, FAAP; Daniel Neuspiel, MD, MPH, FAAP; Julia M. Kim, MD, MPH, FAAP; Committee on Medical Liability and Risk Management; and Council on Quality Improvement and Patient Safety

ABSTRACT. Disclosure of adverse events has become the expectation in medicine and is widely regarded as the appropriate path when medical errors occur. Although data are limited on adverse events in pediatrics, that they occur frequently is uncontested. Types and rates of errors vary depending on the care setting and patient population. Patients with complex medical conditions or from historically marginalized groups or minoritized communities likely suffer disparate health and safety outcomes. Systemic factors, including nonpunitive safety cultures and supportive environments within institutions, are essential to promoting disclosure. State laws protecting apologies from use in legal proceedings can also help to encourage open communication. Some states have adopted laws to advance disclosure, and governmental agencies provide materials encouraging open communication and early resolution after adverse events occur. Many programs emphasize the importance of supporting health care workers involved in adverse events. Shame, fear of professional and legal repercussions, and lack of training remain barriers to disclosure. Education for health care clinicians, support in health care settings, additional research on programs and disparities, and governmental and regulatory initiatives can support disclosure of adverse events. (3/25)

See full text on page 173.

https://doi.org/10.1542/peds.2025-070880

DISPENSING MEDICATIONS AT THE HOSPITAL UPON DISCHARGE FROM AN EMERGENCY DEPARTMENT (TECHNICAL REPORT)

Suzan S. Mazor, MD, FAAP; Michelle C. Barrett, PharmD, BCPS, BCPPS; Corinne Shubin, MD, FAAP; Shannon Manzi, PharmD, BCPPS, FPPA; and Committee on Pediatric Emergency Medicine

ABSTRACT. Although most health care services can be provided in the medical home, children will be referred or require visits to the emergency department (ED) for a variety of conditions ranging from nonurgent to emergent. Continuation of medical care after discharge from an ED is dependent on parents or caregivers' understanding of follow-up instructions and adherence to medication administration recommendations. Barriers to obtaining medications after ED visits include lack of access because of pharmacy hours, affordability, and lack of understanding the importance of medication as part of treatment. ED visits often occur at times when community-based pharmacies are closed. Caregivers are typically concerned with getting their ill or injured child directly home once discharged from the ED. Approximately one-third of patients fail to obtain priority medications from a pharmacy after discharge from an ED. The option of judiciously dispensing medications at ED discharge from the outpatient pharmacy within the health care facility is a major convenience that helps to overcome this obstacle, improving the likelihood of medication adherence. Emergency care encounters should routinely be followed by visits to the primary care provider medical home to ensure complete and comprehensive care. (5/23)

https://doi.org/10.1542/peds.2023-062144

DONOR HUMAN MILK FOR THE HIGH-RISK INFANT: PREPARATION, SAFETY, AND USAGE OPTIONS IN THE UNITED STATES

Committee on Nutrition; Section on Breastfeeding; and Committee on Fetus and Newborn

ABSTRACT. The use of donor human milk is increasing for high-risk infants, primarily for infants born weighing <1500 g or those who have severe intestinal disorders. Pasteurized donor milk may be considered in situations in which the supply of maternal milk is insufficient. The use of pasteurized donor milk is safe when appropriate measures are used to screen donors and collect, store, and pasteurize the milk and then distribute it through established human milk banks. The use of nonpasteurized donor milk and other forms of direct, Internet-based, or informal human milk sharing does not involve this level of safety and is not recommended. It is important that health care providers counsel

families considering milk sharing about the risks of bacterial or viral contamination of nonpasteurized human milk and about the possibilities of exposure to medications, drugs, or herbs in human milk. Currently, the use of pasteurized donor milk is limited by its availability and affordability. The development of public policy to improve and expand access to pasteurized donor milk, including policies that support improved governmental and private financial support for donor milk banks and the use of donor milk, is important. (1/17, reaffirmed 10/24)
https://doi.org/10.1542/peds.2016-3440

DRINKING WATER FROM PRIVATE WELLS AND RISKS TO CHILDREN

Alan D. Woolf, MD, MPH, FAAP; Bryan D. Stierman, MD, FAAP; Elizabeth D. Barnett, MD, FAAP; Lori G. Byron, MD, FAAP; Council on Environmental Health and Climate Change; and Committee on Infectious Diseases

ABSTRACT. Drinking water for >23 million US households is obtained from private wells. These wells can become contaminated by chemicals, naturally occurring toxic substances, or pathogenic organisms that can cause illness in children. Although the US Environmental Protection Agency and most states offer some guidance for the construction, maintenance, and testing of private wells, most states only regulate the construction of new private water wells. With few exceptions, well owners are responsible for their own wells after the initial construction. Children may also drink well water at childcare or when traveling. This policy statement provides recommendations for the inspection, testing, and remediation of private wells to provide safe drinking water for children. (1/23)
https://doi.org/10.1542/peds.2022-060644

DRINKING WATER FROM PRIVATE WELLS AND RISKS TO CHILDREN (TECHNICAL REPORT)

Alan D. Woolf, MD, MPH, FAAP; Bryan D. Stierman, MD, FAAP; Elizabeth D. Barnett, MD, FAAP; Lori G. Byron, MD, FAAP; Council on Environmental Health and Climate Change; and Committee on Infectious Diseases

ABSTRACT. Drinking water for approximately 23 million US households is obtained from private wells. These wells can become contaminated by pollutant chemicals or pathogenic organisms, leading to significant illness. Although the US Environmental Protection Agency and all states offer guidance for construction, maintenance, and testing of private wells, most states only regulate the construction of new private water wells. With a few exceptions, there is little regulation after construction. Well owners are responsible for their own wells. Children may also drink well water at child care or when traveling. Illness resulting from children's ingestion of contaminated water can be severe. This report reviews relevant aspects of groundwater and wells; describes the common chemical and microbiologic contaminants; gives an algorithm with recommendations for inspection, testing, and remediation for wells providing drinking water for children; and provides references and Internet resources for more information. (1/23)
https://doi.org/10.1542/peds.2022-060645

E-CIGARETTES AND SIMILAR DEVICES

Brian P. Jenssen, MD; Susan C. Walley, MD; Section on Tobacco Control

ABSTRACT. Electronic cigarettes (e-cigarettes) are the most commonly used tobacco product among youth. The 2016 US Surgeon General's Report on e-cigarette use among youth and young adults concluded that e-cigarettes are unsafe for children and adolescents. Furthermore, strong and consistent evidence finds that children and adolescents who use e-cigarettes are significantly more likely to go on to use traditional cigarettes—a product that kills half its long-term users. E-cigarette manufacturers target children with enticing candy and fruit flavors and use marketing strategies that have been previously successful with traditional cigarettes to attract youth to these products. Numerous toxicants and carcinogens have been found in e-cigarette solutions. Nonusers are involuntarily exposed to the emissions of these devices with secondhand and thirdhand aerosol. To prevent children, adolescents, and young adults from transitioning from e-cigarettes to traditional cigarettes and minimize the potential public health harm from e-cigarette use, there is a critical need for e-cigarette regulation, legislative action, and counterpromotion to protect youth. (1/19, reaffirmed 8/25)
https://doi.org/10.1542/peds.2018-3652

EARLY CHILDHOOD CARIES IN INDIGENOUS COMMUNITIES

Steve Holve, MD; Patricia Braun, MD, MPH; James D. Irvine, MD; Kristen Nadeau, MD, MS; Robert J. Schroth, DMD, MSc, PhD; Committee on Native American Child Health; and Section on Oral Health (joint with Canadian Paediatric Society First Nations Inuit and Métis Health Committee)

ABSTRACT. The oral health of Indigenous children of Canada (First Nations, Inuit, and Métis) and the United States (American Indian and Alaska native) is a major child health disparity when compared with the general population of both countries. Early childhood caries (ECC) occurs in Indigenous children at an earlier age, with a higher prevalence, and at much greater severity than in the general population. ECC results in adverse oral health, affecting childhood health and well-being, and may result in high rates of costly surgical treatment under general anesthesia. ECC is an infectious disease that is influenced by multiple factors, but the social determinants of health are particularly important. This policy statement includes recommendations for preventive and clinical oral health care for infants, toddlers, preschool-aged children, and pregnant women by primary health care providers. It also addresses community-based health-promotion initiatives and access to dental care for Indigenous children. This policy statement encourages oral health interventions at early ages in Indigenous children, including referral to dental care for the use of sealants, interim therapeutic restorations, and silver diamine fluoride. Further community-based research on the microbiology, epidemiology, prevention, and management of ECC in Indigenous communities is also needed to reduce the dismally high rate of caries in this population. (5/21)
https://doi.org/10.1542/peds.2021-051481

EARLY CHILDHOOD HOME VISITING

James H. Duffee, MD, MPH, FAAP; Alan L. Mendelsohn, MD, FAAP; Alice A. Kuo, MD, PhD, FAAP; Lori A. Legano, MD, FAAP; Marian F. Earls, MD, MTS, FAAP; Council on Community Pediatrics; Council on Early Childhood; and Committee on Child Abuse and Neglect

ABSTRACT. High-quality home-visiting services for infants and young children can improve family relationships, advance school readiness, reduce child maltreatment, improve maternal-infant health outcomes, and increase family economic self-sufficiency. The American Academy of Pediatrics supports unwavering federal funding of state home-visiting initiatives, the expansion of evidence-based programs, and a robust, coordinated national evaluation designed to confirm best practices and cost-efficiency. Community home visiting is most effective as a component of a comprehensive early childhood system that actively includes and enhances a family-centered medical home. (8/17, reaffirmed 10/22)
https://doi.org/10.1542/peds.2017-2150

EARLY INTERVENTION, IDEA PART C SERVICES, AND THE MEDICAL HOME: COLLABORATION FOR BEST PRACTICE AND BEST OUTCOMES (CLINICAL REPORT)

Richard C. Adams, MD; Carl Tapia, MD; and Council on Children With Disabilities

ABSTRACT. The medical home and the Individuals With Disabilities Education Act Part C Early Intervention Program share many common purposes for infants and children ages 0 to 3 years, not the least of which is a family-centered focus. Professionals in pediatric medical home practices see substantial numbers of infants and toddlers with developmental delays and/or complex chronic conditions. Economic, health, and family-focused data each underscore the critical role of timely referral for relationship-based, individualized, accessible early intervention services and the need for collaborative partnerships in care. The medical home process and Individuals With Disabilities Education Act Part C policy both support nurturing relationships and family-centered care; both offer clear value in terms of economic and health outcomes. Best practice models for early intervention services incorporate learning in the natural environment and coaching models. Proactive medical homes provide strategies for effective developmental surveillance, family-centered resources, and tools to support high-risk groups, and comanagement of infants with special health care needs, including the monitoring of services provided and outcomes achieved. (9/13, reaffirmed 4/24)

https://doi.org/10.1542/peds.2013-2305

THE EFFECTS OF ARMED CONFLICT ON CHILDREN

Sherry Shenoda, MD, FAAP; Ayesha Kadir, MD, MSc, FAAP; Shelly Pitterman, PhD; Jeffrey Goldhagen, MD, MPH, FAAP; and Section on International Child Health

ABSTRACT. Children are increasingly exposed to armed conflict and targeted by governmental and nongovernmental combatants. Armed conflict directly and indirectly affects children's physical, mental, and behavioral health. It can affect every organ system, and its impact can persist throughout the life course. In addition, children are disproportionately impacted by morbidity and mortality associated with armed conflict. A children's rights–based approach provides a framework for collaboration by the American Academy of Pediatrics, child health professionals, and national and international partners to respond in the domains of clinical care, systems development, and policy formulation. The American Academy of Pediatrics and child health professionals have critical and synergistic roles to play in the global response to the impact of armed conflict on children. (11/18, reaffirmed 12/23)

https://doi.org/10.1542/peds.2018-2585

ELIMINATING RACE-BASED MEDICINE

Joseph L. Wright, MD, MPH, FAAP; Wendy S. Davis, MD, FAAP; Madeline M. Joseph, MD, FAAP; Angela M. Ellison, MD, MSc, FAAP; Nia J. Heard-Garris, MD, MSc, FAAP; Tiffani L. Johnson, MD, MSc, FAAP; and Board Committee on Equity

ABSTRACT. Race-based medicine has been pervasively interwoven into the fabric of health care delivery in the United States for more than 400 years. Race is a historically derived social construct that has no place as a biologic proxy. In addition to valid measures of social determinants of health, the effects of racism require consideration in clinical decision-making tools in ways that are evidence informed and not inappropriately conflated with the limiting phenotype of race categorization. This policy statement addresses the elimination of race-based medicine as part of a broader commitment to dismantle the structural and systemic inequities that lead to racial health disparities. (6/22)

https://doi.org/10.1542/peds.2022-057998

ELIMINATION OF PERINATAL HEPATITIS B: PROVIDING THE FIRST VACCINE DOSE WITHIN 24 HOURS OF BIRTH

Committee on Infectious Diseases and Committee on Fetus and Newborn

ABSTRACT. After the introduction of the hepatitis B vaccine in the United States in 1982, a greater than 90% reduction in new infections was achieved. However, approximately 1000 new cases of perinatal hepatitis B infection are still identified annually in the United States. Prevention of perinatal hepatitis B relies on the proper and timely identification of infants born to mothers who are hepatitis B surface antigen positive and to mothers with unknown status to ensure administration of appropriate postexposure immunoprophylaxis with hepatitis B vaccine and immune globulin. To reduce the incidence of perinatal hepatitis B transmission further, the American Academy of Pediatrics endorses the recommendation of the Advisory Committee on Immunization Practices of the Centers for Disease Control and Prevention that all newborn infants with a birth weight of greater than or equal to 2000 g receive hepatitis B vaccine by 24 hours of age. (8/17, reaffirmed 4/22 with reference & data updates)

https://doi.org/10.1542/peds.2017-1870

ENHANCING PEDIATRIC WORKFORCE DIVERSITY AND PROVIDING CULTURALLY EFFECTIVE PEDIATRIC CARE: IMPLICATIONS FOR PRACTICE, EDUCATION, AND POLICY MAKING

Committee on Pediatric Workforce

ABSTRACT. This policy statement serves to combine and update 2 previously independent but overlapping statements from the American Academy of Pediatrics (AAP) on culturally effective health care (CEHC) and workforce diversity. The AAP has long recognized that with the ever-increasing diversity of the pediatric population in the United States, the health of all children depends on the ability of all pediatricians to practice culturally effective care. CEHC can be defined as the delivery of care within the context of appropriate physician knowledge, understanding, and appreciation of all cultural distinctions, leading to optimal health outcomes. The AAP believes that CEHC is a critical social value and that the knowledge and skills necessary for providing CEHC can be taught and acquired through focused curricula across the spectrum of lifelong learning.

This statement also addresses workforce diversity, health disparities, and affirmative action. The discussion of diversity is broadened to include not only race, ethnicity, and language but also cultural attributes such as gender, religious beliefs, sexual orientation, and disability, which may affect the quality of health care. The AAP believes that efforts must be supported through health policy and advocacy initiatives to promote the delivery of CEHC and to overcome educational, organizational, and other barriers to improving workforce diversity. (9/13, reaffirmed 10/15, 12/22)

https://doi.org/10.1542/peds.2013-2268

ENSURING COMPREHENSIVE CARE AND SUPPORT FOR TRANSGENDER AND GENDER-DIVERSE CHILDREN AND ADOLESCENTS

Jason Rafferty, MD, MPH, EdM, FAAP; Committee on Psychosocial Aspects of Child and Family Health; Committee on Adolescence; and Section on Lesbian, Gay, Bisexual, and Transgender Health and Wellness

ABSTRACT. As a traditionally underserved population that faces numerous health disparities, youth who identify as transgender and gender diverse (TGD) and their families are increasingly presenting to pediatric providers for education, care, and referrals. The need for more formal training, standardized treatment, and research on safety and medical outcomes often leaves providers feeling ill equipped to support and care for patients that

identify as TGD and families. In this policy statement, we review relevant concepts and challenges and provide suggestions for pediatric providers that are focused on promoting the health and positive development of youth that identify as TGD while eliminating discrimination and stigma. (9/18, reaffirmed 8/23)
https://doi.org/10.1542/peds.2018-2162

ENSURING THE HEALTH OF CHILDREN IN DISASTERS

Disaster Preparedness Advisory Council and Committee on Pediatric Emergency Medicine

ABSTRACT. Infants, children, adolescents, and young adults have unique physical, mental, behavioral, developmental, communication, therapeutic, and social needs that must be addressed and met in all aspects of disaster preparedness, response, and recovery. Pediatricians, including primary care pediatricians, pediatric medical subspecialists, and pediatric surgical specialists, have key roles to play in preparing and treating families in cases of disasters. Pediatricians should attend to the continuity of practice operations to provide services in time of need and stay abreast of disaster and public health developments to be active participants in community planning efforts. Federal, state, tribal, local, and regional institutions and agencies that serve children should collaborate with pediatricians to ensure the health and well-being of children in disasters. (10/15, reaffirmed 4/21)
https://doi.org/10.1542/peds.2015-3112

ENVIRONMENTAL ISSUES IN GLOBAL PEDIATRIC HEALTH

Lauren Zajac, MD, MPH, FAAP; Philip J. Landrigan, MD, MSc, FAAP; and Council on Environmental Health and Climate Change

ABSTRACT. Pediatricians and pediatric trainees in North America are increasingly involved in caring for children and adolescents in or from low- and middle-income countries (LMICs). In many LMICs, hazardous environmental exposures—notably outdoor and household air pollution, water pollution, lead, pesticides, and other manufactured chemicals—are highly prevalent and account for twice the proportion of disease and deaths among young children as in North America. Climate change will likely worsen these exposures.

It is important that pediatricians and other pediatric health professionals from high-income countries who work in LMICs be aware of the disproportionately severe impacts of toxic environmental hazards, become knowledgeable about the major local/regional environmental threats, and consider environmental factors in their differential diagnoses. Likewise, pediatricians in high-income countries who care for patients who have emigrated from LMICs need to be aware that these children may be at elevated risk of toxic environmental diseases from past exposures to toxic environmental hazards in their countries of origin as well as ongoing exposures in products imported from their home countries, including traditional foods, medications, and cosmetics.

Because diseases of toxic environmental origin seldom have unique physical signatures, pediatricians can utilize the environmental screening history, supplemented by laboratory testing, as a diagnostic tool. To prepare pediatricians to care for children in and from LMICs, pediatric organizations could increase the amount of environmental health and climate change content offered in continuing medical education (CME) credits, maintenance of certification (MOC) credits, and certification and recertification examinations. Broadly, it is important that governments and international agencies increase resources directed to pollution prevention, strengthen the environmental health workforce, and expand public health infrastructure in all countries. (1/25)

See full text on page 185.
https://doi.org/10.1542/peds.2024-070075

ENVIRONMENTAL ISSUES IN GLOBAL PEDIATRIC HEALTH (TECHNICAL REPORT)

Lauren Zajac, MD, MPH, FAAP; Philip J. Landrigan, MD, MSc, FAAP; and Council on Environmental Health and Climate Change

ABSTRACT. Pediatricians and pediatric trainees in North America are increasingly involved in caring for children and adolescents in or from low- and middle-income countries (LMICs). In many LMICs, toxic environmental exposures—notably outdoor and household air pollution, water pollution, lead, hazardous waste disposal, pesticides, and other manufactured chemicals—are highly prevalent and account for twice as great a proportion of disease and deaths among young children as in North America. Climate change will likely worsen these exposures.

It is important that pediatricians and other pediatric health professionals from high-income countries who plan to work in LMICs be aware of the disproportionately severe impacts of environmental hazards, become knowledgeable about the major toxic threats to children's health in the countries and communities where they will be working, and consider environmental factors in their differential diagnoses. Likewise, pediatricians in high-income countries who care for children and adolescents who have emigrated from LMICs need to be aware that these children may be at elevated risk of diseases caused by past exposures to toxic environmental hazards in their countries of origin as well as ongoing exposures in products such as traditional foods, medications, and cosmetics imported from their original home countries.

Because diseases of toxic environmental origin seldom have unique physical signatures, the environmental screening history, supplemented by laboratory testing, is the principal diagnostic tool. The goal of this technical report is to enhance pediatricians' ability to recognize, diagnose, and manage disease caused by hazardous environmental exposures, especially toxic chemical exposures, in all countries and especially in LMICs. (1/25)

See full text on page 199.
https://doi.org/10.1542/peds.2024-070076

EPIDEMIOLOGY AND DIAGNOSIS OF HEALTH CARE–ASSOCIATED INFECTIONS IN THE NICU (TECHNICAL REPORT)

Committee on Fetus and Newborn and Committee on Infectious Diseases

ABSTRACT. Health care–associated infections in the NICU are a major clinical problem resulting in increased morbidity and mortality, prolonged length of hospital stays, and increased medical costs. Neonates are at high risk for health care–associated infections because of impaired host defense mechanisms, limited amounts of protective endogenous flora on skin and mucosal surfaces at time of birth, reduced barrier function of neonatal skin, the use of invasive procedures and devices, and frequent exposure to broad-spectrum antibiotics. This statement will review the epidemiology and diagnosis of health care–associated infections in newborn infants. (3/12, reaffirmed 3/23)
https://doi.org/10.1542/peds.2012-0147

EPIDEMIOLOGY AND PREVENTION OF CHILD PEDESTRIAN INJURY (TECHNICAL REPORT)

Sadiqa Kendi, MD, FAAP; Brian D. Johnston, MD, MPH, FAAP; Council on Injury, Violence, and Poison Prevention

ABSTRACT. This report supports policy recommendations in the accompanying policy statement "Child Pedestrian Safety" (www.pediatrics.org/cgi/doi/10.1542/peds.2023-62506). It reviews trends in public health and urban design relevant to pedestrian safety and provides information to assist practicing pediatricians discussing the benefits of active transportation and the specific risks and safety precautions to consider for child pedestrians at different ages. The report offers the evidence base for which programs and policies that, if implemented, could foster independent mobility for children while increasing pediatric pedestrian safety.

Since the previous policy statement was published in 2009, the field of pedestrian safety has advanced with new evidence related to pediatric pedestrian education, the risks of distracted walking, the benefits of design and programming in safe routes to school, and the emergence of the "Vision Zero" public health and safety initiatives to prevent all serious and fatal transportation injuries. (6/23)

https://doi.org/10.1542/peds.2023-062508

EPINEPHRINE FOR FIRST-AID MANAGEMENT OF ANAPHYLAXIS (CLINICAL REPORT)

Scott H. Sicherer, MD, FAAP; F. Estelle R. Simons, MD, FAAP; and Section on Allergy and Immunology

ABSTRACT. Anaphylaxis is a severe, generalized allergic or hypersensitivity reaction that is rapid in onset and may cause death. Epinephrine (adrenaline) can be life-saving when administered as rapidly as possible once anaphylaxis is recognized. This clinical report from the American Academy of Pediatrics is an update of the 2007 clinical report on this topic. It provides information to help clinicians identify patients at risk of anaphylaxis and new information about epinephrine and epinephrine autoinjectors (EAs). The report also highlights the importance of patient and family education about the recognition and management of anaphylaxis in the community. Key points emphasized include the following: (1) validated clinical criteria are available to facilitate prompt diagnosis of anaphylaxis; (2) prompt intramuscular epinephrine injection in the mid-outer thigh reduces hospitalizations, morbidity, and mortality; (3) prescribing EAs facilitates timely epinephrine injection in community settings for patients with a history of anaphylaxis and, if specific circumstances warrant, for some high-risk patients who have not previously experienced anaphylaxis; (4) prescribing epinephrine for infants and young children weighing <15 kg, especially those who weigh 7.5 kg and under, currently presents a dilemma, because the lowest dose available in EAs, 0.15 mg, is a high dose for many infants and some young children; (5) effective management of anaphylaxis in the community requires a comprehensive approach involving children, families, preschools, schools, camps, and sports organizations; and (6) prevention of anaphylaxis recurrences involves confirmation of the trigger, discussion of specific allergen avoidance, allergen immunotherapy (eg, with stinging insect venom, if relevant), and a written, personalized anaphylaxis emergency action plan; and (7) the management of anaphylaxis also involves education of children and supervising adults about anaphylaxis recognition and first-aid treatment. (2/17, reaffirmed 3/24)

https://doi.org/10.1542/peds.2016-4006

ETHICAL CONSIDERATIONS IN PEDIATRICIANS' USE OF SOCIAL MEDIA (CLINICAL REPORT)

Robert Macauley, MD, FAAP; Nanette Elster, JD, MPH; Jonathan M. Fanaroff, MD, JD, FAAP; Committee on Bioethics; and Committee on Medical Liability and Risk Management

ABSTRACT. Increasing use of social media by patients and clinicians creates opportunities as well as dilemmas for pediatricians, who must recognize the inherent ethical and legal complexity of these communication platforms and maintain professionalism in all contexts. Social media can be a useful tool in the practice of medicine by educating both physicians and patients, expanding access to health care, identifying high-risk behaviors, contributing to research, promoting networking and online support, enhancing advocacy, and nurturing professional compassion. At the same time, there are confidentiality, privacy, professionalism, and boundary issues that need to be considered whenever potential interactions occur between physicians and patients via social media. This clinical report is designed to assist pediatricians in identifying and navigating ethical issues to harness the opportunities and avoid the pitfalls of social media. (2/21)

https://doi.org/10.1542/peds.2020-049685

EVALUATING FOR SUSPECTED CHILD ABUSE: CONDITIONS THAT PREDISPOSE TO BLEEDING (TECHNICAL REPORT)

Shannon L. Carpenter, MD, MS, FAAP; Thomas C. Abshire, MD; Emily Killough, MD, FAAP; James D. Anderst, MD, MS, FAAP; Section on Hematology/Oncology; and Council on Child Abuse and Neglect (joint with American Society of Pediatric Hematology/Oncology)

ABSTRACT. Child abuse might be suspected when children present with cutaneous bruising, intracranial hemorrhage, or other manifestations of bleeding. In these cases, it is necessary to consider medical conditions that predispose to easy bleeding or bruising. When evaluating for the possibility of bleeding disorders and other conditions that predispose to hemorrhage, it is important for pediatricians to consider the child's presenting history, medical history, and physical examination findings before initiating a laboratory investigation. Many medical conditions can predispose to easy bleeding. Before ordering laboratory tests for a disease, it is useful to understand the biochemical basis and clinical presentation of the disorder, condition prevalence, and test characteristics. This technical report reviews the major medical conditions that predispose to bruising or bleeding and should be considered when evaluating for abusive injury. (9/22)

https://doi.org/10.1542/peds.2022-059277

EVALUATING YOUNG CHILDREN WITH FRACTURES FOR CHILD ABUSE (CLINICAL REPORT)

Suzanne Haney, MD, FAAP; Susan Scherl, MD, FAAP; Linda DiMeglio, MD, FAAP; Jeannette Perez-Rossello, MD, FAAP; Sabah Servaes, MD, FAAP; Nadia Merchant, MD, FAAP; Council on Child Abuse and Neglect; Section on Orthopaedics; Section on Radiology; and Section on Endocrinology (joint with Society for Pediatric Radiology)

ABSTRACT. Fractures are common injuries in childhood and can be caused by unintentional injury, medical conditions, and child abuse. Although the consequences of failing to diagnose an abusive injury in a child can be grave, the consequences of incorrectly diagnosing child abuse in a child whose fractures have another etiology are also significant. This report aims to review recent advances in the understanding of fracture specificity, fracture mechanisms, and other medical conditions that predispose infants and children to fracture. This clinical report will aid pediatricians and pediatric care providers in developing an evidence-based differential diagnosis and performing appropriate evaluations when assessing a child with fractures. (1/25)

See full text on page 221.

https://doi.org/10.1542/peds.2024-070074

EVALUATION AND MANAGEMENT OF CHILDREN AND ADOLESCENTS WITH ACUTE MENTAL HEALTH OR BEHAVIORAL PROBLEMS. PART I: COMMON CLINICAL CHALLENGES OF PATIENTS WITH MENTAL HEALTH AND/ OR BEHAVIORAL EMERGENCIES (CLINICAL REPORT)

Thomas H. Chun, MD, MPH, FAAP; Sharon E. Mace, MD, FAAP, FACEP; Emily R. Katz, MD, FAAP; and Committee on Pediatric Emergency Medicine (joint with American College of Emergency Physicians Pediatric Emergency Medicine Committee)

INTRODUCTION. Mental health problems are among the leading contributors to the global burden of disease. Unfortunately, pediatric populations are not spared of mental health problems.

In the United States, 21% to 23% of children and adolescents have a diagnosable mental health or substance use disorder. Among patients of emergency departments (EDs), 70% screen positive for at least 1 mental health disorder, 23% meet criteria for 2 or more mental health concerns, 45% have a mental health problem resulting in impaired psychosocial functioning, and 10% of adolescents endorse significant levels of psychiatric distress at the time of their ED visit. In pediatric primary care settings, the reported prevalence of mental health and behavioral disorders is between 12% to 22% of children and adolescents.

Although the American Academy of Pediatrics (AAP) has published a policy statement on mental health competencies and a Mental Health Toolkit for pediatric primary care providers, no such guidelines or resources exist for clinicians who care for pediatric mental health emergencies. This clinical report supports the 2006 joint policy statement of the AAP and American College of Emergency Physicians (ACEP) on pediatric mental health emergencies, with the goal of addressing the knowledge gaps in this area. The report is written primarily from the perspective of ED clinicians, but it is intended for all clinicians who care for children and adolescents with acute mental health and behavioral problems.

Recent epidemiologic studies of mental health visits have revealed a rapid burgeoning of both ED and primary care visits. An especially problematic trend is the increase in "boarding" of psychiatric patients in the ED and inpatient pediatric beds (ie, extended stays lasting days or even weeks). Although investigation of boarding practices is still in its infancy, the ACEP and the American Medical Association have both expressed concern about it, because it significantly taxes the functioning and efficiency of both the ED and hospital, and mental health services may not be available in the ED.

In addition, compared with other pediatric care settings, ED patients are known to be at higher risk of mental health disorders, including depression, anxiety, posttraumatic stress disorder, and substance abuse. These mental health conditions may be unrecognized not only by treating clinicians but also by the child/adolescent and his or her parents. A similar phenomenon has been described with suicidal patients. Individuals who have committed suicide frequently visited a health care provider in the months preceding their death. Although a minority of suicidal patients present with some form of self-harm, many have vague somatic complaints (eg, headache, gastrointestinal tract distress, back pain, concern for a sexually transmitted infection) masking their underlying mental health condition.

Despite studies demonstrating moderate agreement between emergency physicians and psychiatrists in the assessment and management of patients with mental health problems, ED clinicians frequently cite lack of training and confidence in their abilities as barriers to caring for patients with mental health emergencies. Another study of emergency medicine and pediatric emergency medicine training programs found that formal training in psychiatric problems is not required nor offered by most programs. Pediatric primary care providers report similar barriers to caring for their patients with mental health problems.

Part I of this clinical report focuses on the issues relevant to patients presenting to the ED with a mental health chief complaint and covers the following topics:

- Medical clearance of pediatric psychiatric patients
- Suicidal ideation and suicide attempts
- Involuntary hospitalization
- Restraint of the agitated patient
  - — Verbal restraint
  - — Chemical restraint
  - — Physical restraint
- Coordination with the medical home

Part II discusses challenging patients with primarily medical or indeterminate presentations, in which the contribution of an underlying mental health condition may be unclear or a complicating factor, including:

- Somatic symptom and related disorders
- Adverse effects to psychiatric medications
  - — Antipsychotic adverse effects
  - — Neuroleptic malignant syndrome
  - — Serotonin syndrome
- Children with special needs in the ED (autism spectrum and developmental disorders)
- Mental health screening in the ED

An executive summary of this clinical report can be found at www.pediatrics.org/cgi/doi/10.1542/peds.2016-1571. (8/16, reaffirmed 2/22)

https://doi.org/10.1542/peds.2016-1570

EVALUATION AND MANAGEMENT OF CHILDREN WITH ACUTE MENTAL HEALTH OR BEHAVIORAL PROBLEMS. PART II: RECOGNITION OF CLINICALLY CHALLENGING MENTAL HEALTH RELATED CONDITIONS PRESENTING WITH MEDICAL OR UNCERTAIN SYMPTOMS (CLINICAL REPORT)

Thomas H. Chun, MD, MPH, FAAP; Sharon E. Mace, MD, FAAP, FACEP; Emily R. Katz, MD, FAAP; and Committee on Pediatric Emergency Medicine (joint with American College of Emergency Physicians Pediatric Emergency Medicine Committee)

INTRODUCTION. Part I of this clinical report (http://www.pediatrics.org/cgi/doi/10.1542/peds.2016-1570) discusses the common clinical issues that may be encountered in caring for children and adolescents presenting to the emergency department (ED) or primary care setting with a mental health condition or emergency and includes the following:

- Medical clearance of pediatric psychiatric patients
- Suicidal ideation and suicide attempts
- Involuntary hospitalization
- Restraint of the agitated patient
  - — Verbal restraint
  - — Chemical restraint
  - — Physical restraint
- Coordination with the medical home

Part II discusses the challenges a pediatric clinician may face when evaluating patients with a mental health condition, which may be contributing to or a complicating factor for a medical or indeterminate clinical presentation. Topics covered include the following:

- Somatic symptom and related disorders
- Adverse effects of psychiatric medications
  - — Antipsychotic adverse effects
  - — Neuroleptic malignant syndrome
  - — Serotonin syndrome
- Children with special needs (autism spectrum disorders [ASDs] and developmental disorders [DDs])
- Mental health screening

The report is written primarily from the perspective of ED clinicians, but it is intended for all clinicians who care for children and adolescents with acute mental health and behavioral problems. An executive summary of this clinical report can be found at http://www.pediatrics.org/cgi/doi/10.1542/peds.2016-1574. (8/16, reaffirmed 2/22)

https://doi.org/10.1542/peds.2016-1573

EVALUATION AND REFERRAL FOR DEVELOPMENTAL DYSPLASIA OF THE HIP IN INFANTS (CLINICAL REPORT)

Brian A. Shaw, MD, FAAOS, FAAP; Lee S. Segal, MD, FAAOS, FAAP; and Section on Orthopaedics

ABSTRACT. Developmental dysplasia of the hip (DDH) encompasses a wide spectrum of clinical severity, from mild developmental abnormalities to frank dislocation. Clinical hip instability occurs in 1% to 2% of full-term infants, and up to 15% have hip instability or hip immaturity detectable by imaging studies. Hip dysplasia is the most common cause of hip arthritis in women younger than 40 years and accounts for 5% to 10% of all total hip replacements in the United States. Newborn and periodic screening have been practiced for decades, because DDH is clinically silent during the first year of life, can be treated more effectively if detected early, and can have severe consequences if left untreated. However, screening programs and techniques are not uniform, and there is little evidence-based literature to support current practice, leading to controversy. Recent literature shows that many mild forms of DDH resolve without treatment, and there is a lack of agreement on ultrasonographic diagnostic criteria for DDH as a disease versus developmental variations. The American Academy of Pediatrics has not published any policy statements on DDH since its 2000 clinical practice guideline and accompanying technical report. Developments since then include a controversial US Preventive Services Task Force "inconclusive" determination regarding usefulness of DDH screening, several prospective studies supporting observation over treatment of minor ultrasonographic hip variations, and a recent evidence-based clinical practice guideline from the American Academy of Orthopaedic Surgeons on the detection and management of DDH in infants 0 to 6 months of age. The purpose of this clinical report was to provide literature-based updated direction for the clinician in screening and referral for DDH, with the primary goal of preventing and/or detecting a dislocated hip by 6 to 12 months of age in an otherwise healthy child, understanding that no screening program has eliminated late development or presentation of a dislocated hip and that the diagnosis and treatment of milder forms of hip dysplasia remain controversial. (11/16, reaffirmed 6/21)

https://doi.org/10.1542/peds.2016-3107

EVALUATION FOR BLEEDING DISORDERS IN SUSPECTED CHILD ABUSE (CLINICAL REPORT)

James Anderst, MD, MSCI, FAAP; Shannon L. Carpenter, MD, MS, FAAP; Thomas C. Abshire, MD; Emily Killough, MD, FAAP; Section on Hematology/Oncology; and Council on Child Abuse and Neglect (joint with American Society of Pediatric Hematology/Oncology)

ABSTRACT. Bruising or bleeding in a child can raise the concern for child abuse. Assessing whether the findings are the result of trauma and/or whether the child has a bleeding disorder is critical. Many bleeding disorders are rare, and not every child with bruising/bleeding that may raise a concern for abuse requires an evaluation for bleeding disorders. However, in some instances, bleeding disorders can present in a manner similar to child abuse. Bleeding disorders cannot be ruled out solely on the basis of patient and family history, no matter how extensive. The history and clinical evaluation can be used to determine the necessity of an evaluation for a possible bleeding disorder, and prevalence and known clinical presentations of individual bleeding disorders can be used to guide the extent of laboratory testing. This clinical report provides guidance to pediatricians and other clinicians regarding the evaluation for bleeding disorders when child abuse is suspected. (9/22)

https://doi.org/10.1542/peds.2022-059276

THE EVALUATION OF SEXUAL BEHAVIORS IN CHILDREN (CLINICAL REPORT)

Nancy D. Kellogg, MD, and Committee on Child Abuse and Neglect

ABSTRACT. Most children will engage in sexual behaviors at some time during childhood. These behaviors may be normal but can be confusing and concerning to parents or disruptive or intrusive to others. Knowledge of age-appropriate sexual behaviors that vary with situational and environmental factors can assist the clinician in differentiating normal sexual behaviors from sexual behavior problems. Most situations that involve sexual behaviors in young children do not require child protective services intervention; for behaviors that are age-appropriate and transient, the pediatrician may provide guidance in supervision and monitoring of the behavior. If the behavior is intrusive, hurtful, and/or age-inappropriate, a more comprehensive assessment is warranted. Some children with sexual behavior problems may reside or have resided in homes characterized by inconsistent parenting, violence, abuse, or neglect and may require more immediate intervention and referrals. (8/09, reaffirmed 3/13, 10/18, 9/24)

https://doi.org/10.1542/peds.2009-1692

THE EVALUATION OF SUSPECTED CHILD PHYSICAL ABUSE (CLINICAL REPORT)

Cindy W. Christian, MD, FAAP, and Committee on Child Abuse and Neglect

ABSTRACT. Child physical abuse is an important cause of pediatric morbidity and mortality and is associated with major physical and mental health problems that can extend into adulthood. Pediatricians are in a unique position to identify and prevent child abuse, and this clinical report provides guidance to the practitioner regarding indicators and evaluation of suspected physical abuse of children. The role of the physician may include identifying abused children with suspicious injuries who present for care, reporting suspected abuse to the child protection agency for investigation, supporting families who are affected by child abuse, coordinating with other professionals and community agencies to provide immediate and long-term treatment to victimized children, providing court testimony when necessary, providing preventive care and anticipatory guidance in the office, and advocating for policies and programs that support families and protect vulnerable children. (4/15, reaffirmed 11/21 with reference & data updates)

https://doi.org/10.1542/peds.2015-0356

EVALUATION OF THE VISUAL SYSTEM BY THE PRIMARY CARE PROVIDER FOLLOWING CONCUSSION (CLINICAL REPORT)

Christina L. Master, MD, FAAP, CAQSM, FACSM, FAMSSM; Darron Bacal, MD, FAAP; Matthew F. Grady, MD, FAAP, CAQSM, FAMSSM; Richard Hertle, MD, FAAO, FACS, FAAP; Ankoor S. Shah, MD, PhD; Mitchell Strominger, MD, FAAO, FNANOS, FAAPOS, FAAP; Sarah Whitecross, MMedSci, CO, OC(C); Geoffrey E. Bradford, MD, MS, FAAP; Flora Lum, MD; Sean P. Donahue, MD, PhD; and Section on Ophthalmology (joint with American Academy of Ophthalmology; American Association for Pediatric Ophthalmology and Strabismus; and American Association of Certified Orthoptists)

ABSTRACT. Concussion is a common injury in childhood and has the potential for substantial impact on quality of life. Visual issues have been increasingly recognized as a common problem after concussion. Many children initially seek care for concussion with their pediatrician, making it even more important for pediatricians to recognize, evaluate, and refer children with visual issues after concussion. This clinical report is intended to support the recommendations in the companion policy statement on vision and concussion and provides definitions of some of the

physiologic aspects of the visual system as they relate to concussion. A description of clinically feasible testing methodologies is provided in more detail to aid the clinician in assessing the visual system in a focused fashion after concussion. This guidance helps direct clinical management, including support for return to school, sports, and other activities, as well as potential referral for subspecialty care for the subset of those with persistent symptoms. (7/22)
https://doi.org/10.1542/peds.2021-056048

EVIDENCE BASE FOR 2022 UPDATED RECOMMENDATIONS FOR A SAFE INFANT SLEEPING ENVIRONMENT TO REDUCE THE RISK OF SLEEP-RELATED INFANT DEATHS (TECHNICAL REPORT)

Rachel Y. Moon, MD, FAAP; Rebecca F. Carlin, MD, FAAP; Ivan Hand, MD, FAAP; Task Force on Sudden Infant Death Syndrome; and Committee on Fetus and Newborn

ABSTRACT. Every year in the United States, approximately 3500 infants die of sleep-related infant deaths, including sudden infant death syndrome (SIDS) (*International Statistical Classification of Diseases and Related Health Problems 10th Revision* [ICD-10] R95), ill-defined deaths (ICD-10 R99), and accidental suffocation and strangulation in bed (ICD-10 W75). After a substantial decline in sleep-related deaths in the 1990s, the overall death rate attributable to sleep-related infant deaths have remained stagnant since 2000, and disparities persist. The triple risk model proposes that SIDS occurs when an infant with intrinsic vulnerability (often manifested by impaired arousal, cardiorespiratory, and/or autonomic responses) undergoes an exogenous trigger event (eg, exposure to an unsafe sleeping environment) during a critical developmental period. The American Academy of Pediatrics recommends a safe sleep environment to reduce the risk of all sleep-related deaths. This includes supine positioning; use of a firm, noninclined sleep surface; room sharing without bed sharing; and avoidance of soft bedding and overheating. Additional recommendations for SIDS risk reduction include human milk feeding; avoidance of exposure to nicotine, alcohol, marijuana, opioids, and illicit drugs; routine immunization; and use of a pacifier. New recommendations are presented regarding noninclined sleep surfaces, short-term emergency sleep locations, use of cardboard boxes as a sleep location, bed sharing, substance use, home cardiorespiratory monitors, and tummy time. In addition, additional information to assist parents, physicians, and nonphysician clinicians in assessing the risk of specific bed-sharing situations is included. The recommendations and strength of evidence for each recommendation are published in the accompanying policy statement, which is included in this issue. (6/22)
https://doi.org/10.1542/peds.2022-057991

EVIDENCE FOR THE USE OF OPIOID MEDICATION FOR PEDIATRIC ACUTE PAIN IN THE OUTPATIENT SETTING (TECHNICAL REPORT)

Sudha R. Raman, PhD; Michael J. Smith, MD, MSCE

ABSTRACT. This technical report summarizes the results of a systematic review designed to support the American Academy of Pediatrics' "Clinical Practice Guideline: Opioid Prescribing for Acute Pain Management in Children and Adolescents in Outpatient Settings." PubMed and Excerpta Medica Database were searched from 2010 to 2023 to identify randomized clinical trials and systematic reviews related to outpatient opioid prescribing to children. Overall, 11 randomized controlled trials were included. Although data were limited, no evidence was found that pain control by opioids is superior to nonopioid alternatives. Further, opioids are often associated with adverse events. The review also suggests that family and patient education and providing disposal methods may decrease risks associated with opioid prescription. Future studies can build on this foundation of evidence to support the appropriate use of opioids for acute pain in children treated in the outpatient setting. (10/24)
https://doi.org/10.1542/peds.2024-068753

EXAMINING PERMANENT CONTRACEPTION FOR CHILDREN, ADOLESCENTS, AND YOUNG ADULTS WITH INTELLECTUAL DEVELOPMENTAL DISORDER: ETHICAL, LEGAL, AND MEDICAL CONSIDERATIONS (CLINICAL REPORT)

Gina M. Geis, MD, MS, FAAP; Barbara S. Saunders, DO, FAAP; Paula Hillard, MD, FACOG; Committee on Bioethics; and Council on Children With Disabilities

ABSTRACT. There have been significant advances in the medical and surgical options available for contraception and management of menses for individuals, including those with intellectual developmental disorder. This new statement frames the ethical, legal, and medical issues of permanent contraception in children, adolescents, and young adults with intellectual developmental disorder, emphasizing the importance of utilizing long-acting reversible and minimally invasive treatments, whenever possible. The historical use and abuse of permanent contraception is briefly reviewed, providing the foundation for ongoing ethical and legal considerations, including issues of informed consent. The authors then discuss medical decision-making and patient preferences that should be considered and make recommendations to providers who are contemplating permanent contraception therapies in this population. (10/24)
https://doi.org/10.1542/peds.2024-068955

EXECUTIVE SUMMARY: CRITERIA FOR CRITICAL CARE OF INFANTS AND CHILDREN: PICU ADMISSION, DISCHARGE, AND TRIAGE PRACTICE STATEMENT AND LEVELS OF CARE GUIDANCE

Benson S. Hsu, MD, MBA, FAAP; Vanessa Hill, MD, FAAP; Lorry R. Frankel, MD, FCCM; Timothy S. Yeh, MD, MCCM; Shari Simone, CRNP, DNP, FCCM, FAANP, FAAN; Marjorie J. Arca, MD, FACS, FAAP; Jorge A. Coss-Bu, MD; Mary E. Fallat, MD, FACS, FAAP; Jason Foland, MD; Samir Gadepalli, MD, MBA; Michael O. Gayle, BS, MD, FCCM; Lori A. Harmon, RRT, MBA, CPHQ; Christa A. Joseph, RN, MSN; Aaron D. Kessel, BS, MD; Niranjan Kissoon, MD, MCCM; Michele Moss, MD, FCCM; Mohan R. Mysore, MD, FAAP, FCCM; Michele C. Papo, MD, MPH, FCCM; Kari L. Rajzer-Wakeham, CCRN, MSN, PCCNP, RN; Tom B. Rice, MD; David L. Rosenberg, MD, FAAP, FCCM; Martin K. Wakeham, MD; Edward E. Conway, Jr, MD, FCCM, MS; Michael S.D. Agus, MD, FAAP, FCCM

ABSTRACT. This is an executive summary of the 2019 update of the 2004 guidelines and levels of care for PICU. Since previous guidelines, there has been a tremendous transformation of Pediatric Critical Care Medicine with advancements in pediatric cardiovascular medicine, transplant, neurology, trauma, and oncology as well as improvements of care in general PICUs. This has led to the evolution of resources and training in the provision of care through the PICU. Outcome and quality research related to admission, transfer, and discharge criteria as well as literature regarding PICU levels of care to include volume, staffing, and structure were reviewed and included in this statement as appropriate. Consequently, the purposes of this significant update are to address the transformation of the field and codify a revised set of guidelines that will enable hospitals, institutions, and individuals in developing the appropriate PICU for their community needs. The target audiences of the practice statement and guidance are broad and include critical care professionals; pediatricians; pediatric subspecialists; pediatric surgeons; pediatric surgical subspecialists; pediatric imaging physicians; and

other members of the patient care team such as nurses, therapists, dieticians, pharmacists, social workers, care coordinators, and hospital administrators who make daily administrative and clinical decisions in all PICU levels of care. (10/19, reaffirmed 3/25)
https://doi.org/10.1542/peds.2019-2433

EXECUTIVE SUMMARY: IDENTIFICATION, EVALUATION, AND MANAGEMENT OF CHILDREN WITH AUTISM SPECTRUM DISORDER (CLINICAL REPORT)

Council on Children With Disabilities; Section on Developmental and Behavioral Pediatrics

INTRODUCTION. Autism spectrum disorder (ASD) is a common neurodevelopmental disorder with reported prevalence in the United States of 1 in 59 children (approximately 1.7%). ASD significantly influences the lives of affected children and families because they may need extensive behavioral, educational, health, and other services. Primary care providers play a critical role in identifying, diagnosing, and managing ASD in children and providing support for their families. This document provides a summary of the clinical report "Identification, Evaluation, and Management of Children with Autism Spectrum Disorder," published concurrently in the online version of *Pediatrics*. In the years since 2007, when the American Academy of Pediatrics published the clinical reports "Identification and Diagnosis of Children with Autism Spectrum Disorders" and "Management of Children with Autism Spectrum Disorders," reported prevalence rates of children with ASD have increased, understanding of potential risk factors has expanded, awareness of co-occurring medical and behavioral conditions and genetic contribution to etiology has improved, and the body of research supporting evidence-based interventions has grown substantially. The updated document discusses evaluation and treatment as a continuum in 1 publication with a table of contents to help the reader identify topic areas within the report. ASD is more commonly diagnosed than in the past, and the significant health, educational, and social needs of individuals with ASD and their families constitute an area of critical need for resources, research, and professional education. (1/20, reaffirmed 10/25)
https://doi.org/10.1542/peds.2019-3448

EXECUTIVE SUMMARY: PROVIDING A PRIMARY CARE MEDICAL HOME FOR CHILDREN AND YOUTH WITH CEREBRAL PALSY (CLINICAL REPORT)

Garey Noritz, MD, FAAP, FACP; Lynn Davidson, MD, FAAP; Katherine Steingass, MD, FAAP; and Council on Children With Disabilities (joint with American Academy for Cerebral Palsy and Developmental Medicine)

ABSTRACT. Cerebral palsy (CP) is the most common motor disorder of childhood, with prevalence estimates ranging from 1.5 to 4/1000 live births. This executive summary is a companion for the full clinical report "Providing a Primary Care Medical Home for Children With Cerebral Palsy" and specifically seeks to provide primary care physicians (PCPs) with guidance to detect CP in children; collaborate with specialists treating patients with CP; manage associated medical, developmental, and behavioral problems; and provide primary medical care to their patients with CP. (11/22)
https://doi.org/10.1542/peds.2022-060056

EXPERT WITNESS PARTICIPATION IN CIVIL AND CRIMINAL PROCEEDINGS

Stephan R. Paul, MD, JD, FAAP; Sandeep K. Narang, MD, JD, FAAP; and Committee on Medical Liability and Risk Management

ABSTRACT. The interests of the public and both the medical and legal professions are best served when scientifically sound and unbiased expert witness testimony is readily available in civil and criminal proceedings. As members of the medical community, patient advocates, and private citizens, pediatricians have ethical and professional obligations to assist in the civil and criminal judicial processes. This policy statement offers recommendations on advocacy, education, research, qualifications, standards, and ethical business practices all aimed at improving expert testimony. (2/17, reaffirmed 6/24)
https://doi.org/10.1542/peds.2016-3862

EXPERT WITNESS PARTICIPATION IN CIVIL AND CRIMINAL PROCEEDINGS (TECHNICAL REPORT)

Sandeep K. Narang, MD, JD, FAAP; Stephan R. Paul, MD, JD, FAAP; and Committee on Medical Liability and Risk Management

ABSTRACT. The interests of the public and both the medical and legal professions are best served when scientifically sound and unbiased expert witness testimony is readily available in civil and criminal proceedings. As members of the medical community, patient advocates, and private citizens, pediatricians have ethical and professional obligations to assist in the civil and criminal judicial processes. This technical report explains how the role of the expert witness differs in civil and criminal proceedings, legal and ethical standards for expert witnesses, and strategies that have been employed to deter unscientific and irresponsible testimony. A companion policy statement offers recommendations on advocacy, education, research, qualifications, standards, and ethical business practices all aimed at improving expert testimony. (2/17, reaffirmed 6/24)
https://doi.org/10.1542/peds.2016-4122

EXPLOITATION, LABOR AND SEX TRAFFICKING OF CHILDREN AND ADOLESCENTS: HEALTH CARE NEEDS OF PATIENTS (CLINICAL REPORT)

Jordan Greenbaum, MD; Dana Kaplan, MD, FAAP; Janine Young, MD, FAAP; Council on Child Abuse and Neglect; and Council on Immigrant Child and Family Health

ABSTRACT. Exploitation and labor and sex trafficking of children and adolescents is a major public health problem in the United States and throughout the world. Significant numbers of US and non-US–born children and adolescents (including unaccompanied immigrant minors) are affected by this growing concern and may experience a range of serious physical and mental health problems associated with human trafficking and exploitation (T/E). Despite these considerations, there is limited information available for health care providers regarding the nature and scope of T/E and how providers may help recognize and protect children and adolescents. Knowledge of risk factors, recruitment practices, possible indicators of T/E, and common medical, mental, and emotional health problems experienced by affected individuals will assist health care providers in recognizing vulnerable children and adolescents and responding appropriately. A trauma-informed, rights-based, culturally sensitive approach helps providers identify and treat patients who have experienced or are at risk for T/E. As health care providers, educators, and leaders in child advocacy and development, pediatricians play an important role in addressing the public health issues faced by children and adolescents who experience exploitation and trafficking. Working across disciplines with professionals in the community, health care providers can offer evidence-based medical screening, treatment, and holistic services to individuals who have experienced T/E and assist vulnerable patients and families in recognizing signs of T/E. (12/22)
https://doi.org/10.1542/peds.2022-060416

EXPOSURE TO NONTRADITIONAL PETS AT HOME AND TO ANIMALS IN PUBLIC SETTINGS: RISKS TO CHILDREN (CLINICAL REPORT)

Larry K. Pickering, MD; Nina Marano, DVM, MPH; Joseph A. Bocchini, MD; Frederick J. Angulo, DVM, PhD; and Committee on Infectious Diseases

ABSTRACT. Exposure to animals can provide many benefits during the growth and development of children. However, there are potential risks associated with animal exposures, including exposure to nontraditional pets in the home and animals in public settings. Educational materials, regulations, and guidelines have been developed to minimize these risks. Pediatricians, veterinarians, and other health care professionals can provide advice on selection of appropriate pets as well as prevention of disease transmission from nontraditional pets and when children contact animals in public settings. (10/08, reaffirmed 12/11, 1/15, 6/15, 5/19, 6/24 with reference & data updates)
https://doi.org/10.1542/peds.2008-1942

THE EYE EXAMINATION IN THE EVALUATION OF CHILD ABUSE (CLINICAL REPORT)

Cindy W. Christian, MD, FAAP; Alex V. Levin, MD, MHSc, FAAO, FRCSC, FAAP; Council on Child Abuse and Neglect; and Section on Ophthalmology (joint with American Association of Certified Orthoptists, American Association for Pediatric Ophthalmology and Strabismus, and American Academy of Ophthalmology)

ABSTRACT. Child abuse can cause injury to any part of the eye. The most common manifestations are retinal hemorrhages (RHs) in infants and young children with abusive head trauma (AHT). Although RHs are an important indicator of possible AHT, they are also found in other conditions. Distinguishing the number, type, location, and pattern of RHs is important in evaluating a differential diagnosis. Eye trauma can be seen in cases of physical abuse or AHT and may prompt referral for ophthalmologic assessment. Physicians have a responsibility to consider abuse in the differential diagnosis of pediatric eye trauma. Identification and documentation of inflicted ocular trauma requires a thorough examination by an ophthalmologist, including indirect ophthalmoscopy, most optimally through a dilated pupil, especially for the evaluation of possible RHs. An eye examination is helpful in detecting abnormalities that can help identify a medical or traumatic etiology for previously well young children who experience unexpected and unexplained mental status changes with no obvious cause, children with head trauma that results in significant intracranial hemorrhage and brain injury, and children with unexplained death. (7/18, reaffirmed 11/23 with reference & data updates)
https://doi.org/10.1542/peds.2018-1411

FAMILIES AFFECTED BY PARENTAL SUBSTANCE USE (CLINICAL REPORT)

Vincent C. Smith, MD, MPH, FAAP; Celeste R. Wilson, MD, FAAP; and Committee on Substance Use and Prevention

ABSTRACT. Children whose parents or caregivers use drugs or alcohol are at increased risk of short- and long-term sequelae ranging from medical problems to psychosocial and behavioral challenges. In the course of providing health care services to children, pediatricians are likely to encounter families affected by parental substance use and are in a unique position to intervene. Therefore, pediatricians need to know how to assess a child's risk in the context of a parent's substance use. The purposes of this clinical report are to review some of the short-term effects of maternal substance use during pregnancy and long-term implications of fetal exposure; describe typical medical, psychiatric, and behavioral symptoms of children and adolescents in families affected by substance use; and suggest proficiencies for pediatricians involved in the care of children and adolescents of families affected by substance use, including screening families, mandated reporting requirements, and directing families to community, regional, and state resources that can address needs and problems. (7/16, reaffirmed 9/22)
https://doi.org/10.1542/peds.2016-1575

FATHERS' ROLES IN THE CARE AND DEVELOPMENT OF THEIR CHILDREN: THE ROLE OF PEDIATRICIANS (CLINICAL REPORT)

Michael Yogman, MD, FAAP; Craig F. Garfield, MD, FAAP; and Committee on Psychosocial Aspects of Child and Family Health

ABSTRACT. Fathers' involvement in and influence on the health and development of their children have increased in a myriad of ways in the past 10 years and have been widely studied. The role of pediatricians in working with fathers has correspondingly increased in importance. This report reviews new studies of the epidemiology of father involvement, including nonresidential as well as residential fathers. The effects of father involvement on child outcomes are discussed within each phase of a child's development. Particular emphasis is placed on (1) fathers' involvement across childhood ages and (2) the influence of fathers' physical and mental health on their children. Implications and advice for all child health providers to encourage and support father involvement are outlined. (6/16, reaffirmed 4/24)
https://doi.org/10.1542/peds.2016-1128

FECAL MICROBIOTA TRANSPLANTATION: INFORMATION FOR THE PEDIATRICIAN (CLINICAL REPORT)

Maria Oliva-Hemker, MD, FAAP; Stacy A. Kahn, MD, FAAP; William J. Steinbach, MD, FAAP; Section on Gastroenterology, Hepatology, and Nutrition; and Committee on Infectious Diseases

ABSTRACT. Fecal microbiota transplantation (FMT) involves the delivery of an entire microbial community from a healthy donor to a recipient with the intention of ameliorating or curing a specific disease. Current evidence strongly supports a role for FMT in the treatment of *Clostridiodes difficile* infection, with cure rates of approximately 80% to 90%. This success has led to increasing attention for FMT as a potential therapeutic intervention for other conditions associated with disturbances of the intestinal microbiome, including inflammatory bowel diseases, autism spectrum disorder, and obesity. This clinical report endorses the joint society statement by the North American Society for Pediatric Gastroenterology, Hepatology and Nutrition, and the European Society for Pediatric Gastroenterology, Hepatology and Nutrition and is meant to provide the general pediatrician with a broad overview to enable appropriate guidance to families seeking FMT as treatment of a child's condition. (11/23)
https://doi.org/10.1542/peds.2023-062922

THE FEMALE ATHLETE TRIAD (CLINICAL REPORT)

Amanda K. Weiss Kelly, MD, FAAP; Suzanne Hecht, MD, FACSM; and Council on Sports Medicine and Fitness

ABSTRACT. The number of girls participating in sports has increased significantly since the introduction of Title XI in 1972. As a result, more girls have been able to experience the social, educational, and health-related benefits of sports participation. However, there are risks associated with sports participation, including the female athlete triad. The triad was originally recognized as the interrelationship of amenorrhea, osteoporosis, and disordered eating, but our understanding has evolved to recognize that each of the components of the triad exists on a spectrum from optimal health to disease. The triad occurs when energy intake does not adequately compensate for exercise-related energy expenditure, leading to adverse effects on reproductive, bone, and cardiovascular health. Athletes can present with a sin-

gle component or any combination of the components. The triad can have a more significant effect on the health of adolescent athletes than on adults because adolescence is a critical time for bone mass accumulation. This report outlines the current state of knowledge on the epidemiology, diagnosis, and treatment of the triad conditions. (7/16, reaffirmed 12/21)
https://doi.org/10.1542/peds.2016-0922

FETAL ALCOHOL SPECTRUM DISORDERS (CLINICAL REPORT)

Janet F. Williams, MD, FAAP; Vincent C. Smith, MD, MPH, FAAP; and Committee on Substance Abuse

ABSTRACT. Prenatal exposure to alcohol can damage the developing fetus and is the leading preventable cause of birth defects and intellectual and neurodevelopmental disabilities. In 1973, fetal alcohol syndrome was first described as a specific cluster of birth defects resulting from alcohol exposure in utero. Subsequently, research unequivocally revealed that prenatal alcohol exposure causes a broad range of adverse developmental effects. Fetal alcohol spectrum disorder (FASD) is the general term that encompasses the range of adverse effects associated with prenatal alcohol exposure. The diagnostic criteria for fetal alcohol syndrome are specific, and comprehensive efforts are ongoing to establish definitive criteria for diagnosing the other FASDs. A large and growing body of research has led to evidence-based FASD education of professionals and the public, broader prevention initiatives, and recommended treatment approaches based on the following premises:

- Alcohol-related birth defects and developmental disabilities are completely preventable when pregnant women abstain from alcohol use.
- Neurocognitive and behavioral problems resulting from prenatal alcohol exposure are lifelong.
- Early recognition, diagnosis, and therapy for any condition along the FASD continuum can result in improved outcomes.
- During pregnancy:
  - — no amount of alcohol intake should be considered safe;
  - — there is no safe trimester to drink alcohol;
  - — all forms of alcohol, such as beer, wine, and liquor, pose similar risk; and
  - — binge drinking poses dose-related risk to the developing fetus. (10/15, reaffirmed 1/21 with reference & data updates)

https://doi.org/10.1542/peds.2015-3113

FEVER AND ANTIPYRETIC USE IN CHILDREN (CLINICAL REPORT)

Janice E. Sullivan, MD; Henry C. Farrar, MD; Section on Clinical Pharmacology and Therapeutics; and Committee on Drugs

ABSTRACT. Fever in a child is one of the most common clinical symptoms managed by pediatricians and other health care providers and a frequent cause of parental concern. Many parents administer antipyretics even when there is minimal or no fever, because they are concerned that the child must maintain a "normal" temperature. Fever, however, is not the primary illness but is a physiologic mechanism that has beneficial effects in fighting infection. There is no evidence that fever itself worsens the course of an illness or that it causes long-term neurologic complications. Thus, the primary goal of treating the febrile child should be to improve the child's overall comfort rather than focus on the normalization of body temperature. When counseling the parents or caregivers of a febrile child, the general well-being of the child, the importance of monitoring activity, observing for signs of serious illness, encouraging appropriate fluid intake, and the safe storage of antipyretics should be emphasized. Current evidence suggests that there is no substantial difference in the safety and effectiveness of acetaminophen and ibuprofen in the care of a generally healthy child with fever. There is evidence that combining these 2 products is more effective than the use of a single agent alone; however, there are concerns that combined treatment may be more complicated and contribute to the unsafe use of these drugs. Pediatricians should also promote patient safety by advocating for simplified formulations, dosing instructions, and dosing devices. (2/11, reaffirmed 10/22 with reference & data updates)
https://doi.org/10.1542/peds.2010-3852

FINANCING OF PEDIATRIC HOME HEALTH CARE

Edwin Simpser, MD, FAAP; Mark L. Hudak, MD, FAAP; Section on Home Care; and Committee on Child Health Financing

ABSTRACT. Pediatric home health care is an effective and holistic venue of treatment of children with medical complexity or developmental disabilities who otherwise may experience frequent and/or prolonged hospitalizations or who may enter chronic institutional care. Demand for pediatric home health care is increasing while the provider base is eroding, primarily because of inadequate payment or restrictions on benefits. As a result, home care responsibilities assumed by family caregivers have increased and imposed financial, physical, and psychological burdens on the family. The Patient Protection and Affordable Care Act set forth 10 mandated essential health benefits. Home care should be considered as an integral component of the habilitative and rehabilitative services and devices benefit, even though it is not explicitly recognized as a specific category of service. Pediatric-specific home health care services should be defined clearly as components of pediatric services, the 10th essential benefit, and recognized by all payers. Payments for home health care services should be sufficient to maintain an adequate provider work force with the pediatric-specific expertise and skills to care for children with medical complexity or developmental disability. Furthermore, coordination of care among various providers and the necessary direct patient care from which these care coordination plans are developed should be required and enabled by adequate payment. The American Academy of Pediatrics advocates for high-quality care by calling for development of pediatric-specific home health regulations and the licensure and certification of pediatric home health providers. (2/17, reaffirmed 6/22)
https://doi.org/10.1542/peds.2016-4202

FIREARM-RELATED INJURIES AND DEATHS IN CHILDREN AND YOUTH

Lois K. Lee, MD, MPH, FAAP; Eric W. Fleegler, MD, MPH, FAAP; Monika K. Goyal, MD, MSCE, FAAP; Kiesha Fraser Doh, MD, FAAP; Danielle Laraque-Arena, MD, FAAP; Benjamin D. Hoffman, MD, FAAP; and Council on Injury, Violence, and Poison Prevention

ABSTRACT. Firearms are the leading cause of death in children and youth 0 to 24 years of age in the United States. In 2020, firearms resulted in 10 197 deaths (fatality rate 9.91 per 100 000 youth 0–24 years old). Firearms are the leading mechanism of death in pediatric suicides and homicides. Increased access to firearms is associated with increased rates of firearm deaths. Substantial disparities in firearm injuries and deaths exist by age, sex, race, ethnicity, and sexual orientation and gender identity and for deaths related to legal intervention. Barriers to firearm access can decrease the risk to youth for firearm suicide, homicide, unintentional shooting injury, and death. Given the high lethality of firearms and the impulsivity associated with suicidal ideation, removing firearms from the home or securely storing

them—referred to as lethal means restriction of firearms—is critical, especially for youth at risk for suicide. Primary care-, emergency department-, mental health-, hospital-, and community-based intervention programs can effectively screen and intervene for individuals at risk for harming themselves or others. The delivery of anticipatory guidance coupled with safety equipment provision improves firearm safer storage. Strong state-level firearm legislation is associated with decreased rates of firearm injuries and death. This includes legislation focused on comprehensive firearm licensing strategies and extreme risk protection order laws. A firm commitment to confront this public health crisis with a multipronged approach engaging all stakeholders, including individuals, families, clinicians, health systems, communities, public health advocates, firearm owners and nonowners, and policy makers, is essential to address the worsening firearm crisis facing US youth today. (11/22)
https://doi.org/10.1542/peds.2022-060071

FIREARM-RELATED INJURIES AND DEATHS IN CHILDREN AND YOUTH: INJURY PREVENTION AND HARM REDUCTION

Lois K. Lee, MD, MPH, FAAP; Eric W. Fleegler, MD, MPH, FAAP; Monika K. Goyal, MD, MSCE, FAAP; Kiesha Fraser Doh, MD, FAAP; Danielle Laraque-Arena, MD, FAAP; Benjamin D. Hoffman, MD, FAAP; and Council on Injury, Violence, and Poison Prevention

ABSTRACT. Firearms are the leading cause of death in children and youth 0 to 24 years of age in the United States. They are also an important cause of injury with long-term physical and mental health consequences. A multipronged approach with layers of protection focused on harm reduction, which has been successful in decreasing motor vehicle-related injuries, is essential to decrease firearm injuries and deaths in children and youth. Interventions should be focused on the individual, household, community, and policy levels. Strategies for harm reduction for pediatric firearm injuries include providing anticipatory guidance regarding the increased risk of firearm injuries and deaths with firearms in the home as well as the principles of safer firearm storage. In addition, lethal means counseling for patients and families with individuals at risk for self-harm and suicide is important. Community-level interventions include hospital and community-based violence intervention programs. The implementation of safety regulations for firearms as well as enacting legislation are also essential for firearm injury prevention. Increased funding for data infrastructure and research is also crucial to better understand risks and protective factors for firearm violence, which can then inform effective prevention interventions. To reverse this trend of increasing firearm violence, it is imperative for the wider community of clinicians, public health advocates, community stakeholders, researchers, funders, and policy makers to collaboratively address the growing public health crisis of firearm injuries in US youth. (11/22)
https://doi.org/10.1542/peds.2022-060070

FORGOING MEDICALLY PROVIDED NUTRITION AND HYDRATION IN CHILDREN (CLINICAL REPORT)

Douglas S. Diekema, MD, MPH; Jeffrey R. Botkin, MD, MPH; and Committee on Bioethics

ABSTRACT. There is broad consensus that withholding or withdrawing medical interventions is morally permissible when requested by competent patients or, in the case of patients without decision-making capacity, when the interventions no longer confer a benefit to the patient or when the burdens associated with the interventions outweigh the benefits received. The withdrawal or withholding of measures such as attempted resuscitation, ventilators, and critical care medications is common in the terminal care of adults and children. In the case of adults, a consensus has emerged in law and ethics that the medical administration of fluid and nutrition is not fundamentally different from other medical interventions such as use of ventilators; therefore, it can be forgone or withdrawn when a competent adult or legally authorized surrogate requests withdrawal or when the intervention no longer provides a net benefit to the patient. In pediatrics, forgoing or withdrawing medically administered fluids and nutrition has been more controversial because of the inability of children to make autonomous decisions and the emotional power of feeding as a basic element of the care of children. This statement reviews the medical, ethical, and legal issues relevant to the withholding or withdrawing of medically provided fluids and nutrition in children. The American Academy of Pediatrics concludes that the withdrawal of medically administered fluids and nutrition for pediatric patients is ethically acceptable in limited circumstances. Ethics consultation is strongly recommended when particularly difficult or controversial decisions are being considered. (7/09, reaffirmed 1/14, 6/24)
https://doi.org/10.1542/peds.2009-1299

GENETIC EVALUATION OF THE CHILD WITH INTELLECTUAL DISABILITY OR GLOBAL DEVELOPMENTAL DELAY (CLINICAL REPORT)

American Academy of Pediatrics
DEDICATED TO THE HEALTH OF ALL CHILDREN®
AAP Partnership for Policy Implementation
– See Appendix 1

Lance H. Rodan, MD; Joan Stoler, MD, FAAP; Emily Chen, MD, PhD; Timothy Geleske, MD, FAAP; and Council on Genetics

ABSTRACT. Genetic neurodevelopmental disorders are common in the pediatric population, and establishing a specific diagnosis early provides multiple benefits including prognostication, surveillance for disorder-related complications, accurate recurrence risk, and specific management. This report provides an approach to the genetic evaluation of developmental delay/intellectual disability for the general pediatrician. When possible, genetic testing should be selected by phenotype, and typical distinguishing clinical features to facilitate this are presented. If a specific disorder or group of disorders cannot be ascertained by phenotype, an agnostic (or hypothesis-free) approach is utilized. Recommendations are provided for this agnostic approach based on diagnostic yield and also practical considerations such as test complexity and impact on management. The general guidance in this report for genetic testing does not preclude further evaluation by relevant subspecialists as necessary, including neurologists, developmental pediatricians, and clinical geneticists. (6/25)

See full text on page 257.
https://doi.org/10.1542/peds.2025-072219

GUIDANCE FOR CARING FOR INFANTS AND CHILDREN WITH TRISOMY 13 AND TRISOMY 18 (CLINICAL REPORT)

Alaina K. Pyle, MD, FAAP; Thomas N. George, MD, FAAP; James J. Cummings, MD, FAAP; Naomi T. Laventhal, MD, HEC-C, FAAP; Committee on Bioethics; Section on Neonatal-Perinatal Medicine; and Committee on Fetus and Newborn

ABSTRACT. Over the last several decades, there has been a steady increase in medical and surgical interventions provided for infants and children with trisomy 13 or trisomy 18 (chromosomal syndromes associated with a range of congenital anomalies and universally severe neurodevelopmental impairment). Despite previous characterizations of these disorders as being uniformly lethal, multiple studies have demonstrated improved morbidity and mortality when indicated interventions, such as cardiac surgery, are performed, and these interventions and their potential risks and benefits can be carefully explored with parents who may wish to pursue them. Although the presence of trisomy 13 or trisomy 18 impacts prognosis for survival and long-term outcomes and cannot be disregarded in complex decision making, there are no ethical justifications for universal, principle-based differential treatment based solely on these genetic diagnoses. Thus, which medical and surgical interventions are offered, denied, or required for patients should be based on the best available evidence and appropriately tailored to the individual's clinical context, should respect the same moral principles as are applied to other children, and should not vary widely between institutions. Pediatric and obstetric clinicians participating in the care of these patients should maintain current knowledge of the literature to provide adequate counseling through a shared decision-making process and offer the broad range of support that is needed for families throughout the continuum of care from the prenatal to postnatal time period and extending throughout the child's life. (7/25)

See full text on page 271.

https://doi.org/10.1542/peds.2025-072719

GUIDANCE FOR PEDIATRIC END-OF-LIFE CARE (CLINICAL REPORT)

Jennifer S. Linebarger, MD, MPH, FAAP; Victoria Johnson, DO, FAAP; Renee D. Boss, MD, MHS, FAAP; and Section on Hospice and Palliative Care

ABSTRACT. The final hours, days, and weeks in the life of a child or adolescent with serious illness are stressful for families, pediatricians, and other pediatric caregivers. This clinical report reviews essential elements of pediatric care for these patients and their families, establishing end-of-life care goals, anticipatory counseling about the dying process (expected signs or symptoms, code status, desired location of death), and engagement with palliative and hospice resources. This report also outlines postmortem tasks for the pediatric team, including staff debriefing and bereavement. (4/22)

https://doi.org/10.1542/peds.2022-057011

GUIDANCE FOR THE PRIMARY CARE PROVIDER IN IDENTIFYING INFANTS WITH BILIARY ATRESIA BY 2–4 WEEKS OF LIFE (CLINICAL REPORT)

American Academy of Pediatrics

DEDICATED TO THE HEALTH OF ALL CHILDREN®

AAP Partnership for Policy Implementation

– See Appendix 1

Sanjiv Harpavat, MD, PhD, FAAP; Susan W. Aucott, MD, FAAP; Saul J. Karpen, MD, PhD, FAAP; Benjamin L. Shneider, MD, FAAP; Kasper Wang, MD, FAAP; Section on Gastroenterology, Hepatology, and Nutrition; Committee on Fetus and Newborn; and Section on Surgery

ABSTRACT. This report helps pediatric primary care providers quickly identify infants with biliary atresia, which has the potential to improve outcomes and reduce need for liver transplant. The strategy is intended to be used between 2 and 4 weeks of life at the "By 1 month" well-child visit in the Bright Futures/American Academy of Pediatrics "Recommendations for Preventive Pediatric Health Care." The strategy involves examining every infant's eye color, stool color, and prior laboratory results to determine whether measurement of a direct or conjugated bilirubin level is warranted. (2/25)

See full text on page 287.

https://doi.org/10.1542/peds.2024-070077

GUIDANCE FOR STRUCTURING A PEDIATRIC INTERMEDIATE CARE UNIT

Nicholas A. Ettinger, MD, PhD, CMQ, CPPS, FAAP; Vanessa L. Hill, MD, FAAP; Christiana M. Russ, MD, FAAP; Katherine J. Rakoczy, MD, FAAP; Mary E. Fallat, MD, FAAP; Tiffany N. Wright, MD; Karen Choong, MB, BCh, MSc, FRCPC; Michael S.D. Agus, MD, FAAP; Benson Hsu, MD, MBA, FAAP; Section on Critical Care; Committee on Hospital Care; and Section on Surgery

ABSTRACT. The purpose of this policy statement is to update the 2004 American Academy of Pediatrics clinical report and provide enhanced guidance for institutions, administrators, and providers in the development and operation of a pediatric intermediate care unit (IMCU). Since 2004, there have been significant advances in pediatric medical, surgical, and critical care that have resulted in an evolution in the acuity and complexity of children potentially requiring IMCU admission. A group of 9 clinical experts in pediatric critical care, hospital medicine, intermediate care, and surgery developed a consensus on priority topics requiring updates, reviewed the relevant evidence, and, through a series of virtual meetings, developed the document. The intended audience of this policy statement is broad and includes pediatric critical care professionals, pediatric hospitalists, pediatric surgeons, other pediatric medical and surgical subspecialists, general pediatricians, nurses, social workers, care coordinators, hospital administrators, health care funders, and policymakers, primarily in resource-rich settings. Key priority topics were delineation of core principles for an IMCU, clarification of target populations, staffing recommendations, and payment. (4/22)

https://doi.org/10.1542/peds.2022-057009

GUIDANCE ON COMPLETING A WRITTEN ALLERGY AND ANAPHYLAXIS EMERGENCY PLAN (CLINICAL REPORT)

Julie Wang, MD, FAAP; Scott H. Sicherer, MD, FAAP; and Section on Allergy and Immunology

ABSTRACT. Anaphylaxis is a potentially life-threatening, severe allergic reaction. The immediate assessment of patients having an allergic reaction and prompt administration of epinephrine, if criteria for anaphylaxis are met, promote optimal outcomes. National and international guidelines for the management of anaphylaxis, including those for management of allergic reactions at school, as well as several clinical reports from the American Academy of Pediatrics, recommend the provision of written emergency action plans to those at risk of anaphylaxis, in addition to the prescription of epinephrine autoinjectors. This clinical report provides information to help health care providers understand the role of a written, personalized allergy and anaphylaxis emergency plan to enhance the care of children at risk of allergic reactions, including anaphylaxis. This report offers a comprehensive written plan, with advice on individualizing instructions to suit specific patient circumstances. (2/17, reaffirmed 9/23)

https://doi.org/10.1542/peds.2016-4005

GUIDANCE ON FORGOING LIFE-SUSTAINING MEDICAL TREATMENT

Kathryn L. Weise, MD, MA, FAAP; Alexander L. Okun, MD, FAAP; Brian S. Carter, MD, FAAP; Cindy W. Christian, MD, FAAP; Committee on Bioethics; Section on Hospice and Palliative Medicine; and Committee on Child Abuse and Neglect

ABSTRACT. Pediatric health care is practiced with the goal of promoting the best interests of the child. Treatment generally is rendered under a presumption in favor of sustaining life. However, in some circumstances, the balance of benefits and burdens to the child leads to an assessment that forgoing life-sustaining medical treatment (LSMT) is ethically supportable or

advisable. Parents are given wide latitude in decision-making concerning end-of-life care for their children in most situations. Collaborative decision-making around LSMT is improved by thorough communication among all stakeholders, including medical staff, the family, and the patient, when possible, throughout the evolving course of the patient's illness. Clear communication of overall goals of care is advised to promote agreed-on plans, including resuscitation status. Perceived disagreement among the team of professionals may be stressful to families. At the same time, understanding the range of professional opinions behind treatment recommendations is critical to informing family decision-making. Input from specialists in palliative care, ethics, pastoral care, and other disciplines enhances support for families and medical staff when decisions to forgo LSMT are being considered. Understanding specific applicability of institutional, regional, state, and national regulations related to forgoing LSMT is important to practice ethically within existing legal frameworks. This guidance represents an update of the 1994 statement from the American Academy of Pediatrics on forgoing LSMT. (8/17, reaffirmed 6/23)
https://doi.org/10.1542/peds.2017-1905

GUIDING PRINCIPLES FOR MANAGED CARE ARRANGEMENTS FOR THE HEALTH OF NEWBORNS, INFANTS, CHILDREN, ADOLESCENTS AND YOUNG ADULTS

Kenneth M. Carlson, MD, FAAP; Suzanne K. Berman, MD, FAAP; Jonathan Price, MD, FAAP; and Committee on Child Health Financing

ABSTRACT. Managed care arrangements are an approach to health care delivery in which the payer or other health care entity has policies that affect where care is delivered, what services are covered, and how payment is determined. When policies are intentionally designed, transparently administered, and continuously monitored, they are more likely to improve the population's utilization of services, access to quality primary and specialty care, and access to appropriate medications. When managed care arrangements are designed well, particularly within evolving payment models, health care can be delivered in a manner that supports the goals of the Quadruple Aim: to reduce per capita costs of health care, to improve the health of populations, to improve the experience of patients receiving care, and to improve the experience of those who are providing care.

The American Academy of Pediatrics (AAP) urges payers and health care entities to use the key principles outlined in this statement when designing and implementing managed care arrangements and policies that cover newborn infants, infants, children, adolescents, and young adults to support the goal of improving the effectiveness of the health care delivery system for the pediatric population. The principles described in this statement are intended to complement those previously published in other AAP policies including "Principles of Child Health Care Financing," "Scope of Health Care Benefits for Children From Birth Through Age 26," "Patient- and Family-Centered Care and the Pediatrician's Role," and the "AAP Access Principles." (7/22)
https://doi.org/10.1542/peds.2022-058396

GUIDING PRINCIPLES FOR TEAM-BASED PEDIATRIC CARE

Julie P. Katkin, MD, FAAP; Susan J. Kressly, MD, FAAP; Anne R. Edwards, MD, FAAP; James M. Perrin, MD, FAAP; Colleen A. Kraft, MD, FAAP; Julia E. Richerson, MD, FAAP; Joel S. Tieder, MD, MPH, FAAP; Liz Wall; and Task Force on Pediatric Practice Change

ABSTRACT. The American Academy of Pediatrics (AAP) recognizes that children's unique and ever-changing needs depend on a variety of support systems. Key components of effective support systems address the needs of the child and family in the context of their home and community and are dynamic so that they reflect, monitor, and respond to changes as the needs of the child and family change. The AAP believes that team-based care involving medical providers and community partners (eg, teachers and state agencies) is a crucial and necessary component of providing high-quality care to children and their families. Team-based care builds on the foundation of the medical home by reaching out to a potentially broad array of participants in the life of a child and incorporating them into the care provided. Importantly, the AAP believes that a high-functioning team includes children and their families as essential partners. The overall goal of team-based care is to enhance communication and cooperation among the varied medical, social, and educational partners in a child's life to better meet the global needs of children and their families, helping them to achieve their best potential. In support of the team-based approach, the AAP urges stakeholders to invest in infrastructure, education, and privacy-secured technology to meet the needs of children. This statement includes limited specific examples of potential team members, including health care providers and community partners, that are meant to be illustrative and in no way represent a complete or comprehensive listing of all team members who may be of importance for a specific child and family. (7/17, reaffirmed 12/23 with reference & data updates)
https://doi.org/10.1542/peds.2017-1489

HALF CENTURY SINCE SIDS: A REAPPRAISAL OF TERMINOLOGY (CLINICAL REPORT)

Carrie K. Shapiro-Mendoza, PhD, MPH; Vincent J. Palusci, MD, MS, FAAP; Benjamin Hoffman, MD, FAAP; Erich Batra, MD, FAAP; Marc Yester, MD, FAAP; Tracey S. Corey, MD; Mary Ann Sens, MD, PhD; Task Force on Sudden Infant Death Syndrome; Council on Child Abuse and Neglect; Council on Injury, Violence, and Poison Prevention; and Section on Child Death Review and Prevention (joint with National Association of Medical Examiners)

ABSTRACT. After a sudden infant death, parents and caregivers need accurate and open communication about why their infant died. Communicating tragic news about a child's death to families and caregivers is difficult. Shared and consistent terminology is essential for pediatricians, other physicians, and nonphysician clinicians to improve communication with families and among themselves. When families do not have complete information about why their child died, pediatricians will not be able to support them through the process and make appropriate referrals for pediatric specialty and mental health care. Families can only speculate about the cause and may blame themselves or others for the infant's death. The terminology used to describe infant deaths that occur suddenly and unexpectedly includes an assortment of terms that vary across and among pediatrician, other physician, or nonphysician clinician disciplines. Having consistent terminology is critical to improve the understanding of the etiology, pathophysiology, and epidemiology of these deaths and communicate with families. A lack of consistent terminology also makes it difficult to reliably monitor trends in mortality and hampers the ability to develop effective interventions. This report describes the history of sudden infant death terminology and summarizes the debate over the terminology and the resulting diagnostic shift of these deaths. This information is to assist pediatricians, other physicians, and nonphysician clinicians in caring for families during this difficult time. The importance of consistent terminology is outlined, followed by a summary of progress toward consensus. Recommendations for pediatricians, other physicians, and nonphysician clinicians are proposed. (9/21)
https://doi.org/10.1542/peds.2021-053746

HEAD LICE (CLINICAL REPORT)

Dawn Nolt, MD, MPH, FAAP; Scot Moore, MD, FAAP; Albert C. Yan, MD, FAAP, FAAD; Laura Melnick, MD, FAAP, FAAD; Committee on Infectious Diseases; Committee on Practice and Ambulatory Medicine; and Section on Dermatology

American Academy of Pediatrics
DEDICATED TO THE HEALTH OF ALL CHILDREN®
AAP Partnership for Policy Implementation
– *See Appendix 1*

ABSTRACT. Head lice infestation is associated with limited morbidity but causes a high level of anxiety among caregivers of school-aged children and adolescents. Since the 2015 clinical report on head lice was published by the American Academy of Pediatrics, new medications have been approved, and an algorithm for management of affected patients is included. This revised clinical report clarifies current diagnosis and treatment protocols. (9/22)
https://doi.org/10.1542/peds.2022-059282

HEALTH CARE CLINICIANS AND PRODUCT PROMOTION BY INDUSTRY

Douglas S. Diekema, MD, MPH, FAAP; and Committee on Bioethics

ABSTRACT. Medical pharmaceutical and device manufacturers are essential in making products that benefit patients, and collaboration between health care providers and industry is necessary in the design, testing, and manufacture of these medical products. However, health care providers must recognize that their duties and the interests of industry may, at times, diverge. Relationships with industry, even seemingly minor ones, have the potential to shape the decisions made on behalf of patients. The marketing divisions of pharmaceutical and medical device firms view health care providers as a target of their efforts, and some of the interactions that occur between industry and health care providers have the potential to alter decision making in ways that may not necessarily benefit patients. Health care providers have an ethical duty to recognize situations and marketing strategies that are designed to influence their choice of diagnostic and therapeutic options for their patients. Health care providers should be aware of the techniques used to attempt to alter their behavior and guard against them. (3/22)
https://doi.org/10.1542/peds.2022-056548

HEALTH CARE CLINICIANS AND PRODUCT PROMOTION BY INDUSTRY (TECHNICAL REPORT)

Douglas S. Diekema, MD, MPH, FAAP

ABSTRACT. Medical pharmaceutical and device manufacturers are essential in making products that benefit patients, and collaboration between health care clinicians and the industry is necessary for the design and manufacture of these medical products. However, health care clinicians must recognize that their duties and the interests of the industry may at times diverge. Relationships with the industry, even seemingly minor ones, have the potential to shape the decisions made on behalf of patients. The marketing divisions of pharmaceutical and medical device firms view health care clinicians as targets of their efforts, and some of the interactions that occur between the industry and health care clinicians have the potential to alter decision making in ways that may not necessarily benefit patients. Health care clinicians have an ethical duty to recognize situations and marketing strategies that are designed to influence their choice of diagnostic and therapeutic options for their patients. At a minimum, health care clinicians should be aware of the techniques used to attempt to alter their behavior and guard against them. (3/22)
https://doi.org/10.1542/peds.2022-056549

HEALTH CARE OF YOUTH AGING OUT OF FOSTER CARE

Council on Foster Care, Adoption, and Kinship Care and Committee on Early Childhood

ABSTRACT. Youth transitioning out of foster care face significant medical and mental health care needs. Unfortunately, these youth rarely receive the services they need because of lack of health insurance. Through many policies and programs, the federal government has taken steps to support older youth in foster care and those aging out. The Fostering Connections to Success and Increasing Adoptions Act of 2008 (Pub L No. 110-354) requires states to work with youth to develop a transition plan that addresses issues such as health insurance. In addition, beginning in 2014, the Patient Protection and Affordable Care Act of 2010 (Pub L No. 111-148) makes youth aging out of foster care eligible for Medicaid coverage until age 26 years, regardless of income. Pediatricians can support youth aging out of foster care by working collaboratively with the child welfare agency in their state to ensure that the ongoing health needs of transitioning youth are met. (11/12, reaffirmed 7/23)
https://doi.org/10.1542/peds.2012-2603

HEALTH INFORMATION TECHNOLOGY AND THE MEDICAL HOME

Council on Clinical Information Technology

ABSTRACT. The American Academy of Pediatrics (AAP) supports development and universal implementation of a comprehensive electronic infrastructure to support pediatric information functions of the medical home. These functions include (1) timely and continuous management and tracking of health data and services over a patient's lifetime for all providers, patients, families, and guardians, (2) comprehensive organization and secure transfer of health data during patient-care transitions between providers, institutions, and practices, (3) establishment and maintenance of central coordination of a patient's health information among multiple repositories (including personal health records and information exchanges), (4) translation of evidence into actionable clinical decision support, and (5) reuse of archived clinical data for continuous quality improvement. The AAP supports universal, secure, and vendor-neutral portability of health information for all patients contained within the medical home across all care settings (ambulatory practices, inpatient settings, emergency departments, pharmacies, consultants, support service providers, and therapists) for multiple purposes including direct care, personal health records, public health, and registries. The AAP also supports financial incentives that promote the development of information tools that meet the needs of pediatric workflows and that appropriately recognize the added value of medical homes to pediatric care. (4/11, reaffirmed 3/22)
https://doi.org/10.1542/peds.2011-0454

HEALTH SUPERVISION FOR CHILDREN AND ADOLESCENTS WITH DOWN SYNDROME (CLINICAL REPORT)

American Academy of Pediatrics
DEDICATED TO THE HEALTH OF ALL CHILDREN®
AAP Partnership for Policy Implementation
– *See Appendix 1*

Marilyn J. Bull, MD, FAAP; Tracy Trotter, MD, FAAP; Stephanie L. Santoro, MD, FAAP; Celanie Christensen, MD, MS, FAAP; Randall W. Grout, MD, MS, FAAP; and Council on Genetics

ABSTRACT. This clinical report is designed to assist the pediatrician in caring for the child, adolescent, and family in whom a diagnosis of Down syndrome has been confirmed by chromosome analysis or suspected by prenatal screening. Although a pediatrician's initial contact with the child is usually during infancy, occasionally the pregnant woman who has been given a prenatal diagnosis of Down syndrome will be referred for review of the condition and genetic counseling; this report offers

guidance for this situation, as well. Age-specific guidance for the clinician is provided in Supplemental Fig 1. (4/22)
https://doi.org/10.1542/peds.2022-057010

HEALTH SUPERVISION FOR CHILDREN AND ADOLESCENTS WITH MARFAN SYNDROME (CLINICAL REPORT)

Brad T. Tinkle, MD, PhD; Ronald V. Lacro, MD; Leah W. Burke, MD, FAAP; and Council on Genetics

ABSTRACT. Marfan syndrome is a heritable connective tissue disorder that affects many different organ systems. In some cases, features of Marfan syndrome can be recognized at birth, but the majority will have manifestations that emerge throughout childhood and into adulthood. Significant morbidity and mortality are associated with this syndrome, and its features are best managed using a multidisciplinary approach. This clinical report is designed to assist the pediatrician in recognizing the features of Marfan syndrome as well as caring for the individual with Marfan syndrome to maximize their health and quality of life. (3/23)
https://doi.org/10.1542/peds.2023-061450

HEALTH SUPERVISION FOR CHILDREN AND ADOLESCENTS WITH SICKLE CELL DISEASE (CLINICAL REPORT)

American Academy of Pediatrics
DEDICATED TO THE HEALTH OF ALL CHILDREN®
AAP Partnership for Policy Implementation
– *See Appendix 1*

Amber M. Yates, MD; Banu Aygun, MD; Rachelle Nuss, MD; Zora R. Rogers, MD; Section on Hematology/Oncology (joint with American Society of Pediatric Hematology/Oncology)

ABSTRACT. Sickle cell disease (SCD) is a group of complex genetic disorders of hemoglobin with multisystem manifestations. The scope of this clinical report is such that in-depth recommendations for management of all complications is not possible. Rather, the authors present an overview focused on the practical management of children and adolescents with SCD and the complications that are of particular relevance to pediatric primary care providers. References with detailed commentary provide further information. Timely and appropriate treatment of acute illness is critical, because life-threatening complications may develop rapidly. Specialized comprehensive medical care decreases morbidity and mortality during childhood. The provision of comprehensive care is a time-intensive endeavor that includes ongoing patient and family education, periodic comprehensive evaluations and other disease-specific health maintenance services, nursing support, psychosocial care, and genetic counseling. Ideally, this care includes comanagement by the pediatrician or other pediatric primary care provider and a team of specialist SCD experts: Hematologist, other pediatric specialists, advanced practice providers, nurse specialists, social workers, patient navigators, and educational liaisons. (7/24)
https://doi.org/10.1542/peds.2024-066842

HEALTH SUPERVISION FOR CHILDREN WITH 22q11.2 DELETION SYNDROME (CLINICAL REPORT)

American Academy of Pediatrics
DEDICATED TO THE HEALTH OF ALL CHILDREN®
AAP Partnership for Policy Implementation
– *See Appendix 1*

Angela E. Scheuerle, MD, FAAP; Timothy A. Geleske, MD, FAAP; Nadia Merchant, MD, FAAP; Paula C. Goldenberg, MD, FAAP; and Council on Genetics

ABSTRACT. 22q11.2 deletion syndrome is the most frequent chromosomal microdeletion syndrome, with an estimated frequency of about 1/4000 in children younger than 1 year. Associated features in neonates and infants are conotruncal heart defects, interrupted aortic arch type B, cleft palate, hypocalcemia (which can present as seizures), feeding problems, developmental delay, and immune system abnormalities. Older children, adolescents, and adults may have neurocognitive impairments and/or speech disorders. Psychiatric diagnoses are more common than in the general population. Newborn infants may have a positive newborn screening for severe combined immunodeficiency (SCID). Genetic diagnosis is confirmed by chromosome microarray. This document is intended to provide guidance for health care providers to help identify individual patients at high risk of developing serious sequelae and to enable intervention before complications develop. (7/25)

See full text on page 297.
https://doi.org/10.1542/peds.2025-072717

HEARING ASSESSMENT IN INFANTS, CHILDREN, AND ADOLESCENTS: RECOMMENDATIONS BEYOND NEONATAL SCREENING (CLINICAL REPORT)

American Academy of Pediatrics
DEDICATED TO THE HEALTH OF ALL CHILDREN®
AAP Partnership for Policy Implementation
– *See Appendix 1*

Charles Bower, MD, FAAP; Brian Kip Reilly, MD, FAAP; Julia Richerson, MD, FAAP; Julia L. Hecht, MD, FAAP; Committee on Practice and Ambulatory Medicine; and Section on Otolaryngology-Head and Neck Surgery

ABSTRACT. Children who are deaf or hard of hearing (D/HH) are at high risk for permanent deficits in language acquisition and downstream effects such as poor academic performance, personal–social maladjustments, and emotional difficulties. Identification of children born D/HH through newborn hearing screening and subsequent timely early intervention can prevent or reduce many of these adverse consequences. Ongoing surveillance for changes in hearing thresholds after infancy is also important and should be accomplished by subjective assessment for signs of atypical hearing and with objective screening tests. Scheduled hearing screening may take place in the primary care setting, or via referral to an audiologist according to the Bright Futures/American Academy of Pediatrics "Recommendations for Preventive Pediatric Health Care" (also known as the periodicity schedule). This report covers hearing assessment beyond the newborn period, reviews risk factors for hearing level change, and provides guidance for providers of pediatric primary care on the assessment and care of children who are D/HH. (8/23)
https://doi.org/10.1542/peds.2023-063288

HELMET USE IN PREVENTING HEAD INJURIES IN BICYCLING, SNOW SPORTS, AND OTHER RECREATIONAL ACTIVITIES AND SPORTS

Lois K. Lee, MD, MPH, FAAP; Michael R. Flaherty, DO; Ashley M. Blanchard, MD, MSc, FAAP; Maneesha Agarwal, MD, FAAP; and Council on Injury, Violence, and Poison Prevention

ABSTRACT. Recreational activities and sports are a common and popular way for youth to enjoy physical activity; however, there are risks related to physical injury. Injuries can potentially result in death and long-term disability, especially from traumatic brain injury. Helmet use can significantly decrease the risk of fatal and nonfatal head injury, including severe traumatic brain injury and facial injuries when participating in recreational sports. The most robust evidence of helmet effectiveness has been demonstrated with bicycling and snow sports (eg, skiing, snowboarding). Despite this evidence, helmets are not worn consistently with all recreational sports. A multipronged approach is necessary to increase helmet use by children and youth participating in recreational sports. This approach includes legislation and enforcement, public educational campaigns, child education programs, and anticipatory guidance from clinicians. This policy statement guides clinicians, public health advocates, and policymakers on

best practices for increasing helmet use in recreational sports, including bicycling and snow sports. (8/22)
https://doi.org/10.1542/peds.2022-058877

HELMET USE IN PREVENTING HEAD INJURIES IN BICYCLING, SNOW SPORTS, AND OTHER RECREATIONAL ACTIVITIES AND SPORTS (TECHNICAL REPORT)

Lois K. Lee, MD, MPH, FAAP; Michael R. Flaherty, DO; Ashley M. Blanchard, MD, MSc, FAAP; Maneesha Agarwal, MD, FAAP; and Council on Injury, Violence, and Poison Prevention

ABSTRACT. Bicycling, snow sports, and other recreational activities and sports are important activities to keep children and youth active as part of a healthy lifestyle. These activities can be associated with serious and fatal head and facial injuries. Helmets, when worn correctly, are effective in decreasing head injuries and fatalities related to these activities. Legislation for helmet use is effective in increasing helmet use in children and, ultimately, in decreasing deaths and head and facial injuries. A multipronged strategy employing legislation, enforcement of laws, and medical clinicians and community programs is important for increasing helmet use to decrease deaths and injuries from recreational sports. (8/22)
https://doi.org/10.1542/peds.2022-058878

HELPING CHILDREN AND FAMILIES DEAL WITH DIVORCE AND SEPARATION (CLINICAL REPORT)

George J. Cohen, MD, FAAP; Carol C. Weitzman, MD, FAAP; Committee on Psychosocial Aspects of Child and Family Health; and Section on Developmental and Behavioral Pediatrics

ABSTRACT. For the past several years in the United States, there have been more than 800 000 divorces and parent separations annually, with over 1 million children affected. Children and their parents can experience emotional trauma before, during, and after a separation or divorce. Pediatricians can be aware of their patients' behavior and parental attitudes and behaviors that may indicate family dysfunction and that can indicate need for intervention. Age-appropriate explanation and counseling for the child and advice and guidance for the parents, as well as recommendation of reading material, may help reduce the potential negative effects of divorce. Often, referral to professionals with expertise in the social, emotional, and legal aspects of the separation and its aftermath may be helpful for these families. (11/16, reaffirmed 6/22)
https://doi.org/10.1542/peds.2016-3020

HOME HEALTH CARE OF CHILDREN, ADOLESCENTS AND YOUNG ADULTS WITH COMPLEX MEDICAL NEEDS (CLINICAL REPORT)

Elaine Lin, MD, FAAP; Garey Noritz, MD, FAAP, FACP; Council on Children With Disabilities; and Section on Home Care

ABSTRACT. The majority of children, adolescents, and young adults with complex medical needs, especially those who use life-sustaining equipment, are cared for at home by their families and community. Home health care is an essential service that supports families to be able to safely care for their children outside of the hospital, and the medical home serves as the hub to help coordinate and communicate between providers and families. It is essential that pediatric health care providers develop and implement an interdisciplinary and coordinated plan of care that addresses the child's ongoing health care needs. The goal is to ensure that each child remains healthy, thrives, and obtains optimal medical home and developmental supports that promote ongoing care at home. Discharge planning from long-term hospitalizations and rehabilitation for this population can be a complicated process that requires a deliberate, multistep approach. This clinical report presents an approach to addressing the needs of children with complex medical needs and their families in the home environment and supporting the transitions between hospital and home. (8/25)

See full text on page 317.
https://doi.org/10.1542/peds.2025-073171

HONORING DO-NOT-ATTEMPT-RESUSCITATION REQUESTS IN SCHOOLS

Council on School Health; Committee on Bioethics

ABSTRACT. Increasingly, children and adolescents with complex chronic conditions are living in the community. Federal legislation and regulations facilitate their participation in school. Some of these children and adolescents and their families may wish to forego life-sustaining medical treatment, including cardiopulmonary resuscitation, because they would be ineffective or because the risks outweigh the benefits. Honoring these requests in the school environment is complex because of the limited availability of school nurses and the frequent lack of supporting state legislation and regulations. Understanding and collaboration on the part of all parties is essential. Pediatricians have an important role in helping school nurses incorporate a specific action plan into the student's individualized health care plan. The action plan should include both communication and comfort-care plans. Pediatricians who work directly with schools can also help implement policies, and professional organizations can advocate for regulations and legislation that enable students and their families to effectuate their preferences. (5/10, reaffirmed 12/24)
https://doi.org/10.1542/peds.2010-0452

THE HOSPITALIZED ADOLESCENT

Cora C. Breuner, MD, MPH, FAAP; Elizabeth M. Alderman, MD, FSAHM, FAAP; Jennifer A. Jewell, MD, MS, FAAP; Committee on Adolescence; and Committee on Hospital Care

ABSTRACT. This policy statement is the first published statement in the United States on this topic and the authors aim to provide pediatricians with evidence-based information on the unique aspects required to care for hospitalized adolescents. Included in this policy statement is a description of the possible effects hospitalization may have on the developmental and emotional progress of adolescence, the role of the hospital setting, the importance of confidentiality, and issues related to legal/ethical matters and bias and institutional and systemic racism that may occur during hospitalization. (1/23)
https://doi.org/10.1542/peds.2022-060646

THE HOSPITALIZED ADOLESCENT (CLINICAL REPORT)

Cora C. Breuner, MD, MPH, FAAP; Elizabeth M. Alderman, MD, FSAHM, FAAP; Jennifer A. Jewell, MD, MS, FAAP; Committee on Adolescence; and Committee on Hospital Care

ABSTRACT. This clinical report provides pediatricians evidence-based information on the developmentally appropriate, comprehensive clinical care for hospitalized adolescents. Included in this report are opportunities and challenges facing pediatricians when caring for specific hospitalized adolescent populations. The companion policy statement, "The Hospitalized Adolescent," includes detailed descriptions of adolescent hospital admission demographics, personnel recommendations, and hospital setting and design advice, as well as sections on educational services, legal and ethical matters, and transitions to adult facilities. (1/23)
https://doi.org/10.1542/peds.2022-060647

HUMAN TRAFFICKING AND EXPLOITATION OF CHILDREN AND ADOLESCENTS

Jordan Greenbaum, MD; Dana Kaplan, MD; Nia Bodrick, MD, MPH; Council on Child Abuse and Neglect; and Section on Global Health

ABSTRACT. Trafficking of children and adolescents for labor and sexual exploitation is associated with significant adverse physical and mental health implications. Pediatricians and other health care professionals may encounter affected patients who present with infections, injuries, posttraumatic stress disorder, suicidality, or a variety of other health and mental health conditions. The health sector response requires a public health approach based on scientific research using an equity and social justice lens, community participatory strategies, and rigorous study designs, including implementation science, which build a solid evidence base. It should include training for pediatric clinicians (eg, pediatricians, other physicians, and nonphysician clinicians treating children and adolescents) to recognize possible signs of exploitation and to intervene using a culturally responsive, community-centered, sensitive, trauma-informed, rights-based, and patient-centered approach. The health sector response should include a multidisciplinary approach to the provision of service, with clinicians working with a diverse group of professionals in the community to assist children and adolescents at risk for trafficking and exploitation. Advocacy is needed for legislation and policies that promote child rights and victim/survivor services for all children and adolescents, regardless of immigration status. The health sector should support policies that address the social drivers of health, which influence the vulnerability to human trafficking. This policy statement outlines major issues regarding public policy, medical education, research, and collaboration in the area of child labor and sex trafficking/exploitation and provides recommendations for future work. (6/25)

See full text on page 337.

https://doi.org/10.1542/peds.2025-072214

HYPOTHERMIA AND NEONATAL ENCEPHALOPATHY (CLINICAL REPORT)

Committee on Fetus and Newborn

ABSTRACT. Data from large randomized clinical trials indicate that therapeutic hypothermia, using either selective head cooling or systemic cooling, is an effective therapy for neonatal encephalopathy. Infants selected for cooling must meet the criteria outlined in published clinical trials. The implementation of cooling needs to be performed at centers that have the capability to manage medically complex infants. Because the majority of infants who have neonatal encephalopathy are born at community hospitals, centers that perform cooling should work with their referring hospitals to implement education programs focused on increasing the awareness and identification of infants at risk for encephalopathy, and the initial clinical management of affected infants. (5/14, reaffirmed 9/21)

https://doi.org/10.1542/peds.2014-0899

IDENTIFICATION, EVALUATION, AND MANAGEMENT OF CHILDREN WITH AUTISM SPECTRUM DISORDER (CLINICAL REPORT)

Susan L. Hyman, MD, FAAP; Susan E. Levy, MD, MPH, FAAP; Scott M. Myers, MD, FAAP; Council on Children With Disabilities; Section on Developmental and Behavioral Pediatrics

ABSTRACT. Autism spectrum disorder (ASD) is a common neurodevelopmental disorder with reported prevalence in the United States of 1 in 59 children (approximately 1.7%). Core deficits are identified in 2 domains: social communication/interaction and restrictive, repetitive patterns of behavior. Children and youth with ASD have service needs in behavioral, educational, health, leisure, family support, and other areas. Standardized screening for ASD at 18 and 24 months of age with ongoing developmental surveillance continues to be recommended in primary care (although it may be performed in other settings), because ASD is common, can be diagnosed as young as 18 months of age, and has evidenced-based interventions that may improve function. More accurate and culturally sensitive screening approaches are needed. Primary care providers should be familiar with the diagnostic criteria for ASD, appropriate etiologic evaluation, and co-occurring medical and behavioral conditions (such as disorders of sleep and feeding, gastrointestinal tract symptoms, obesity, seizures, attention-deficit/hyperactivity disorder, anxiety, and wandering) that affect the child's function and quality of life. There is an increasing evidence base to support behavioral and other interventions to address specific skills and symptoms. Shared decision making calls for collaboration with families in evaluation and choice of interventions. This single clinical report updates the 2007 American Academy of Pediatrics clinical reports on the evaluation and treatment of ASD in one publication with an online table of contents and section view available through the American Academy of Pediatrics Gateway to help the reader identify topic areas within the report. (1/20, reaffirmed 10/25)

https://doi.org/10.1542/peds.2019-3447

IDENTIFICATION AND MANAGEMENT OF ANKYLOGLOSSIA AND ITS EFFECT ON BREASTFEEDING IN INFANTS (CLINICAL REPORT)

Jennifer Thomas, MD, MPH, FAAP; Maya Bunik, MD, MPH, FAAP; Alison Holmes, MD, MPH, FAAP; Martha Ann Keels, DDS, PhD; Brenda Poindexter, MD, MS, FAAP; Anna Meyer, MD, FAAP; Alison Gilliland, MD, FAAP; Section on Breastfeeding; Section on Oral Health; Council on Quality Improvement and Patient Safety; Committee on Fetus and Newborn; and Section on Otolaryngology-Head and Neck Surgery

ABSTRACT. Ankyloglossia refers to a congenitally tight lingual frenulum that limits the motion of the tongue. Whether the release of a tight lingual frenulum in neonates improves breastfeeding is not clear. Because many of the symptoms of ankyloglossia overlap those of other breastfeeding difficulties, a team partnership is necessary. (7/24)

https://doi.org/10.1542/peds.2024-067605

IMMUNIZATION INFORMATION SYSTEMS

Jesse M. Hackell, MD, FAAP; Sheila L. Palevsky, MD, MPH, FAAP; Micah Resnick, MD, FAAP; Committee on Practice and Ambulatory Medicine; Council on Clinical Information Technology; and Section on Early Career Physicians

ABSTRACT. Immunization (IZ) information systems (IISs) are confidential, computerized, population-based systems that collect and consolidate IZ data from vaccination providers. The American Academy of Pediatrics continues to support the development and implementation of IISs as a beneficial tool to provide quality health care for children. Since the last revision of the American Academy of Pediatrics policy statement on IISs in 2006, numerous public health events and new data demonstrate the importance and value of these systems in society and expand the functionality and benefits of IISs beyond the basic IZ database intended to improve childhood IZ rates. This policy statement update will describe additional functions and benefits of IISs, as well as persistent and novel challenges and barriers that these systems face and pose to practicing pediatricians. Pediatricians and other pediatric health care practitioners should be aware of the value of IISs to society, the incentives and barriers involved in incorporating IIS access into a medical practice, and the opportunities to improve IISs and their functionality and usability in daily pediatric practice. (9/22)

https://doi.org/10.1542/peds.2022-059281

IMMUNIZING AGAINST HATE: OVERCOMING ASIAN AMERICAN AND PACIFIC ISLANDER RACISM

Lee Savio Beers, MD, FAAP; Moira Szilagyi, MD, PhD, FAAP; Warren M. Seigel, MD, MBA, FAAP; Wendy S. Davis, MD, FAAP; Yasuko Fukuda, MD, FAAP; Madeline Joseph, MD, FAAP; Joseph L. Wright, MD, MPH, FAAP; Sara H. Goza, MD, FAAP; Board of Directors Executive Committee; and Board Committee on Equity

ABSTRACT. It has been more than a year since Immediate Past President of the American Academy of Pediatrics (AAP), Sally Goza, MD, FAAP, warned against the threat severe acute respiratory syndrome-coronavirus 2 (SARS-CoV-2) posed to children and families, including the harm coronavirus disease 2019 (COVID-19)–fueled racism and xenophobia could cause the Asian American community. Sadly, as the COVID-19 pandemic spread, racism and violent attacks on Asian Americans spread along with it. (6/21)

https://doi.org/10.1542/peds.2021-051836

IMMUNIZING PARENTS AND OTHER CLOSE FAMILY CONTACTS IN THE PEDIATRIC OFFICE SETTING

Herschel R. Lessin, MD; Kathryn M. Edwards, MD; Committee on Practice and Ambulatory Medicine; Committee on Infectious Diseases

ABSTRACT. Additional strategies are needed to protect children from vaccine-preventable diseases. In particular, very young infants, as well as children who are immunocompromised, are at especially high risk for developing the serious consequences of vaccine-preventable diseases and cannot be immunized completely. There is some evidence that children who become infected with these diseases are exposed to pathogens through household contacts, particularly from parents or other close family contacts. Such infections likely are attributable to adults who are not fully protected from these diseases, either because their immunity to vaccine-preventable diseases has waned over time or because they have not received a vaccine. There are many challenges that have added to low adult immunization rates in the United States. One option to increase immunization coverage for parents and close family contacts of infants and vulnerable children is to provide alternative locations for these adults to be immunized, such as the pediatric office setting. Ideally, adults should receive immunizations in their medical homes; however, to provide greater protection to these adults and reduce the exposure of children to pathogens, immunizing parents or other adult family contacts in the pediatric office setting could increase immunization coverage for this population to protect themselves as well as children to whom they provide care. (1/12, reaffirmed 11/24)

https://doi.org/10.1542/peds.2011-2937

THE IMPACT OF MARIJUANA POLICIES ON YOUTH: CLINICAL, RESEARCH, AND LEGAL UPDATE

Committee on Substance Abuse and Committee on Adolescence

ABSTRACT. This policy statement is an update of the American Academy of Pediatrics policy statement "Legalization of Marijuana: Potential Impact on Youth," published in 2004. Pediatricians have special expertise in the care of children and adolescents and may be called on to advise legislators about the potential impact of changes in the legal status of marijuana on adolescents. Parents also may look to pediatricians for advice as they consider whether to support state-level initiatives that propose to legalize the use of marijuana for medical and nonmedical purposes or to decriminalize the possession of small amounts of marijuana. This policy statement provides the position of the American Academy of Pediatrics on the issue of marijuana legalization. The accompanying technical report reviews what is currently known about the relationships of marijuana use with health and the developing brain and the legal status of marijuana and adolescents' use of marijuana to better understand how change in legal status might influence the degree of marijuana use by adolescents in the future. (2/15, reaffirmed 1/24)

https://doi.org/10.1542/peds.2014-4146

THE IMPACT OF MARIJUANA POLICIES ON YOUTH: CLINICAL, RESEARCH, AND LEGAL UPDATE (TECHNICAL REPORT)

Seth Ammerman, MD, FAAP; Sheryl Ryan, MD, FAAP; William P. Adelman, MD, FAAP; Committee on Substance Abuse; and Committee on Adolescence

ABSTRACT. This technical report updates the 2004 American Academy of Pediatrics technical report on the legalization of marijuana. Current epidemiology of marijuana use is presented, as are definitions and biology of marijuana compounds, side effects of marijuana use, and effects of use on adolescent brain development. Issues concerning medical marijuana specifically are also addressed. Concerning legalization of marijuana, 4 different approaches in the United States are discussed: legalization of marijuana solely for medical purposes, decriminalization of recreational use of marijuana, legalization of recreational use of marijuana, and criminal prosecution of recreational (and medical) use of marijuana. These approaches are compared, and the latest available data are presented to aid in forming public policy. The effects on youth of criminal penalties for marijuana use and possession are also addressed, as are the effects or potential effects of the other 3 policy approaches on adolescent marijuana use. Recommendations are included in the accompanying policy statement. (2/15, reaffirmed 1/24)

https://doi.org/10.1542/peds.2014-4147

IMPROVING HEALTH AND SAFETY AT CAMP

Michael J. Ambrose, MD, FAAP; Edward A. Walton, MD, FAAP; and Council on School Health

ABSTRACT. The American Academy of Pediatrics has created recommendations for health appraisal and preparation of young people before participation in day, resident, or family camps and to guide health and safety practices at camp. These recommendations are intended for parents and families, primary health care providers, and camp administration and health center staff. Although camps have diverse environments, there are general guidelines that apply to all situations and specific recommendations that are appropriate under special conditions. This policy statement has been reviewed and is supported by the American Camp Association and Association of Camp Nursing. (6/19, reaffirmed 10/24)

https://doi.org/10.1542/peds.2019-1355

IMPROVING SUBSTANCE USE PREVENTION, ASSESSMENT, AND TREATMENT FINANCING TO ENHANCE EQUITY AND IMPROVE OUTCOMES AMONG CHILDREN, ADOLESCENTS, AND YOUNG ADULTS

Deepa R. Camenga, MD, MHS, FAAP; Lawrence D. Hammer, MD, FAAP; Committee on Substance Use and Prevention; and Committee on Child Health Financing

ABSTRACT. Access to timely prevention and treatment services remains challenging for many children, adolescents, young adults, and families affected by substance use. The American Academy of Pediatrics recognizes the scope and urgency of this problem and has developed this policy statement for consideration by Congress, federal and state policy makers, and public and private payers. This policy statement updates the 2001 policy statement "Improving Substance Abuse Prevention, Assessment, and Treatment Financing for Children and Adolescents" and provides recommendations for financing substance use prevention, assessment, and treatment of children, adolescents, and young adults. (6/22)

https://doi.org/10.1542/peds.2022-057992

INCORPORATING RECOGNITION AND MANAGEMENT OF PERINATAL DEPRESSION INTO PEDIATRIC PRACTICE

Marian F. Earls, MD; Michael W. Yogman, MD; Gerri Mattson, MD; Jason Rafferty, MD; Committee on Psychosocial Aspects of Child and Family Health

ABSTRACT. Perinatal depression (PND) is the most common obstetric complication in the United States. Even when screening results are positive, mothers often do not receive further evaluation, and even when PND is diagnosed, mothers do not receive evidence-based treatments. Studies reveal that postpartum depression (PPD), a subset of PND, leads to increased costs of medical care, inappropriate medical treatment of the infant, discontinuation of breastfeeding, family dysfunction, and an increased risk of abuse and neglect. PPD, specifically, adversely affects this critical early period of infant brain development. PND is an example of an adverse childhood experience that has potential long-term adverse health complications for the mother, her partner, the infant, and the mother-infant dyad. However, PND can be treated effectively, and the stress on the infant can be buffered. Pediatric medical homes should coordinate care more effectively with prenatal providers for women with prenatally diagnosed maternal depression; establish a system to implement PPD screening at the 1-, 2-, 4-, and 6-month well-child visits; use community resources for the treatment and referral of the mother with depression; and provide support for the maternal-child (dyad) relationship, including breastfeeding support. State chapters of the American Academy of Pediatrics, working with state departments of public health, public and private payers, and maternal and child health programs, should advocate for payment and for increased training for PND screening and treatment. American Academy of Pediatrics recommends advocacy for workforce development for mental health professionals who care for young children and mother-infant dyads, and for promotion of evidence-based interventions focused on healthy attachment and parent-child relationships. (1/19, reaffirmed 4/25 with reference & data updates)

https://doi.org/10.1542/peds.2018-3259

INCORPORATING RECOGNITION AND MANAGEMENT OF PERINATAL DEPRESSION INTO PEDIATRIC PRACTICE (TECHNICAL REPORT)

Jason Rafferty, MD; Gerri Mattson, MD; Marian F. Earls, MD; Michael W. Yogman, MD; Committee on Psychosocial Aspects of Child and Family Health

ABSTRACT. Perinatal depression is the most common obstetric complication in the United States, with prevalence rates of 15% to 20% among new mothers. Untreated, it can adversely affect the well-being of children and families through increasing the risk for costly complications during birth and lead to deterioration of core supports, including partner relationships and social networks. Perinatal depression contributes to long-lasting, and even permanent, consequences for the physical and mental health of parents and children, including poor family functioning, increased risk of child abuse and neglect, delayed infant development, perinatal obstetric complications, challenges with breastfeeding, and costly increases in health care use. Perinatal depression can interfere with early parent-infant interaction and attachment, leading to potentially long-term disturbances in the child's physical, emotional, cognitive, and social development. Fortunately, perinatal depression is identifiable and treatable. The US Preventive Services Task Force, Centers for Medicare and Medicaid Services, and many professional organizations recommend routine universal screening for perinatal depression in women to facilitate early evidence-based treatment and referrals, if necessary. Despite significant gains in screening rates from 2004 to 2013, a minority of pediatricians routinely screen for postpartum depression, and many mothers are still not identified or treated. Pediatric primary care clinicians, with a core mission of promoting child and family health, are in an ideal position to implement routine postpartum depression screens at several well-child visits throughout infancy and to provide mental health support through referrals and/or the interdisciplinary services of a pediatric patient-centered medical home model. (1/19, reaffirmed 4/25)

https://doi.org/10.1542/peds.2018-3260

INCREASING ACCESS TO ANTIRETROVIRAL THERAPY FOR THE PREVENTION AND TREATMENT OF HIV IN INFANTS, CHILDREN, AND YOUTH IN THE UNITED STATES

Rosemary Olivero, MD, FAAP, FPIDS; Susan Gillespie, MD, PHD, FAAP; and Committee on Pediatric and Adolescent HIV

ABSTRACT. Although significant progress has been made in prevention and treatment of HIV in the United States, nationally and globally, infants and children younger than 13 years have less access to optimal antiretroviral therapy compared with youth (13–24 years) and adults, which can negatively affect health outcomes for those with HIV. Despite youth having nearly as many antiretroviral options for HIV management as adults, optimal HIV management in youth is challenged by psychosocial and structural barriers that result in poor access to HIV prevention and care. Significant barriers remain in providing equitable access to optimal HIV treatment and prevention services in the pediatric population. (7/25)

See full text on page 355.

https://doi.org/10.1542/peds.2025-072718

INDIVIDUAL MEDICAL EMERGENCIES OCCURRING AT SCHOOL

Rani S. Gereige, MD, MPH, FAAP; Toni Gross, MD, MPH, FAAP; Ebaa Jastaniah, MD, MPH, MBA, FAAP; Council on School Health; and Committee on Pediatric Emergency Medicine

ABSTRACT. Children and adults may face emergency medical situations because of injuries, complications of chronic health conditions, or unexpected major illnesses that occur in schools. The American Academy of Pediatrics published a policy statement in 2001 titled "Guidelines for Emergency Medical Care in Schools," and in 2008, published its revision, "Medical Emergencies Occurring at School." Those statements focused on the preparedness of schools to address individual student emergencies. The increase in the number of children with special health care needs and chronic medical conditions attending schools, together with the added challenges faced by school districts to ensure that schools have access to on-site, licensed health care professionals on an ongoing basis, have contributed to added risks that medical and nonmedical personnel face in dealing with medical emergencies in schools. This newly revised policy statement serves as an update of the statement published in 2008 and reaffirmed in 2017, and intends to increase pediatricians' awareness of schools' roles in preparing for individual student emergencies and provide recommendations for the medical home and school physicians on how to assist and support school personnel. This statement does not address schoolwide or communitywide emergencies that might occur as a result of natural or man-made disasters. (6/22)

https://doi.org/10.1542/peds.2022-057987

INDOOR ENVIRONMENTAL CONTROL PRACTICES AND ASTHMA MANAGEMENT (CLINICAL REPORT)

Elizabeth C. Matsui, MD, MHS, FAAP; Stuart L. Abramson, MD, PhD, AE-C, FAAP; Megan T. Sandel, MD, MPH, FAAP; Section on Allergy and Immunology; and Council on Environmental Health

ABSTRACT. Indoor environmental exposures, particularly allergens and pollutants, are major contributors to asthma morbidity in children; environmental control practices aimed at reducing these exposures are an integral component of asthma manage-

ment. Some individually tailored environmental control practices that have been shown to reduce asthma symptoms and exacerbations are similar in efficacy and cost to controller medications. As a part of developing tailored strategies regarding environmental control measures, an environmental history can be obtained to evaluate the key indoor environmental exposures that are known to trigger asthma symptoms and exacerbations, including both indoor pollutants and allergens. An environmental history includes questions regarding the presence of pets or pests or evidence of pests in the home, as well as knowledge regarding whether the climatic characteristics in the community favor dust mites. In addition, the history focuses on sources of indoor air pollution, including the presence of smokers who live in the home or care for children and the use of gas stoves and appliances in the home. Serum allergen-specific immunoglobulin E antibody tests can be performed or the patient can be referred for allergy skin testing to identify indoor allergens that are most likely to be clinically relevant. Environmental control strategies are tailored to each potentially relevant indoor exposure and are based on knowledge of the sources and underlying characteristics of the exposure. Strategies include source removal, source control, and mitigation strategies, such as high-efficiency particulate air purifiers and allergen-proof mattress and pillow encasements, as well as education, which can be delivered by primary care pediatricians, allergists, pediatric pulmonologists, other health care workers, or community health workers trained in asthma environmental control and asthma education. (10/16, reaffirmed 2/24)
https://doi.org/10.1542/peds.2016-2589

INFANT FEEDING FOR PERSONS LIVING WITH AND AT RISK FOR HIV IN THE UNITED STATES (CLINICAL REPORT)

Lisa Abuogi, MD, MS, FAAP; Lawrence Noble, MD, FAAP; Christiana Smith, MD, MS, FAAP; Committee on Pediatric and Adolescent HIV; and Section on Breastfeeding

ABSTRACT. Pediatricians and pediatric health care professionals caring for infants born to people living with and at risk for HIV infection are likely to be involved in providing guidance on recommended infant feeding practices. Care team members need to be aware of the HIV transmission risk from breastfeeding and the recommendations for feeding infants with perinatal HIV exposure in the United States. The risk of HIV transmission via breastfeeding from a parent with HIV who is receiving antiretroviral treatment (ART) and is virally suppressed is estimated to be less than 1%. The American Academy of Pediatrics recommends that for people with HIV in the United States, avoidance of breastfeeding is the only infant feeding option with 0% risk of HIV transmission. However, people with HIV may express a desire to breastfeed, and pediatricians should be prepared to offer a family-centered, nonjudgmental, harm reduction approach to support people with HIV on ART with sustained viral suppression below 50 copies per mL who desire to breastfeed. Pediatric health care professionals who counsel people with HIV who are not on ART or who are on ART but without viral suppression should recommend against breastfeeding. Pediatric health care professionals should recommend HIV testing for all pregnant persons and HIV preexposure prophylaxis to pregnant or breastfeeding persons who test negative for HIV but are at high risk of HIV acquisition. (5/24)
https://doi.org/10.1542/peds.2024-066843

INFECTION PREVENTION AND CONTROL IN PEDIATRIC AMBULATORY SETTINGS

Mobeen H. Rathore, MD, FAAP; Mary Anne Jackson, MD, FAAP; and Committee on Infectious Diseases

ABSTRACT. Since the American Academy of Pediatrics published its statement titled "Infection Prevention and Control in Pediatric Ambulatory Settings" in 2007, there have been significant changes that prompted this updated statement. Infection prevention and control is an integral part of pediatric practice in ambulatory medical settings as well as in hospitals. Infection prevention and control practices should begin at the time the ambulatory visit is scheduled. All health care personnel should be educated regarding the routes of transmission and techniques used to prevent the transmission of infectious agents. Policies for infection prevention and control should be written, readily available, updated every 2 years, and enforced. Many of the recommendations for infection control and prevention from the Centers for Disease Control and Prevention for hospitalized patients are also applicable in the ambulatory setting. These recommendations include requirements for pediatricians to take precautions to identify and protect employees likely to be exposed to blood or other potentially infectious materials while on the job. In addition to emphasizing the key principles of infection prevention and control in this policy, we update those that are relevant to the ambulatory care patient. These guidelines emphasize the role of hand hygiene and the implementation of diagnosis- and syndrome-specific isolation precautions, with the exemption of the use of gloves for routine diaper changes and wiping a well child's nose or tears for most patient encounters. Additional topics include respiratory hygiene and cough etiquette strategies for patients with a respiratory tract infection, including those relevant for special populations like patients with cystic fibrosis or those in short-term residential facilities; separation of infected, contagious children from uninfected children when feasible; safe handling and disposal of needles and other sharp medical devices; appropriate use of personal protective equipment, such as gloves, gowns, masks, and eye protection; and appropriate use of sterilization, disinfection, and antisepsis. Lastly, in this policy, we emphasize the importance of public health interventions, including vaccination for patients and health care personnel, and outline the responsibilities of the health care provider related to prompt public health notification for specific reportable diseases and communication with colleagues who may be providing subsequent care of an infected patient to optimize the use of isolation precautions and limit the spread of contagions. (10/17, reaffirmed 12/22)
https://doi.org/10.1542/peds.2017-2857

INFECTIOUS COMPLICATIONS WITH THE USE OF BIOLOGIC RESPONSE MODIFIERS IN INFANTS AND CHILDREN (CLINICAL REPORT)

H. Dele Davies, MD, FAAP, and Committee on Infectious Diseases

ABSTRACT. Biologic response modifiers (BRMs) are substances that interact with and modify the host immune system. BRMs that dampen the immune system are used to treat conditions such as juvenile idiopathic arthritis, psoriatic arthritis, or inflammatory bowel disease and often in combination with other immunosuppressive agents, such as methotrexate and corticosteroids. Cytokines that are targeted include tumor necrosis factor α; interleukins (ILs) 6, 12, and 23; and the receptors for IL-1α (IL-1A) and IL-1β (IL-1B) as well as other molecules. Although the risk varies with the class of BRM, patients receiving immune-dampening BRMs generally are at increased risk of infection or reactivation with mycobacterial infections (*Mycobacterium tuberculosis* and nontuberculous mycobacteria), some viral (herpes simplex virus, varicella-zoster virus, Epstein-Barr virus, hepatitis B) and fungal (histoplasmosis, coccidioidomycosis) infections, as well as other opportunistic infections. The use of BRMs warrants careful determination of infectious risk on the basis of history (including exposure, residence, and travel and immunization history) and selected baseline screening test results. Routine immunizations should be given at least 2 weeks (inactivated or subunit vaccines) or 4 weeks (live vaccines) before initiation of BRMs whenever feasible, and inactivated influenza vaccine should be given annually. Inactivated and subunit vaccines

should be given when needed while taking BRMs, but live vaccines should be avoided unless under special circumstances in consultation with an infectious diseases specialist. If the patient develops a febrile or serious respiratory illness during BRM therapy, consideration should be given to stopping the BRM while actively searching for and treating possible infectious causes. (7/16, reaffirmed 3/21)
https://doi.org/10.1542/peds.2016-1209

INFLUENZA IMMUNIZATION FOR ALL HEALTH CARE PERSONNEL: KEEP IT MANDATORY

Committee on Infectious Diseases

ABSTRACT. The purpose of this statement is to reaffirm the American Academy of Pediatrics' support for a mandatory influenza immunization policy for all health care personnel. With an increasing number of organizations requiring influenza vaccination, coverage among health care personnel has risen to 75% in the 2013 to 2014 influenza season but still remains below the Healthy People 2020 objective of 90%. Mandatory influenza immunization for all health care personnel is ethical, just, and necessary to improve patient safety. It is a crucial step in efforts to reduce health care–associated influenza infections. (9/15, reaffirmed 9/25)
https://doi.org/10.1542/peds.2015-2922

INFORMED CONSENT IN DECISION-MAKING IN PEDIATRIC PRACTICE

Committee on Bioethics

ABSTRACT. Informed consent should be seen as an essential part of health care practice; parental permission and childhood assent is an active process that engages patients, both adults and children, in health care. Pediatric practice is unique in that developmental maturation allows, over time, for increasing inclusion of the child's and adolescent's opinion in medical decision-making in clinical practice and research. (7/16, reaffirmed 1/23)
https://doi.org/10.1542/peds.2016-1484

INFORMED CONSENT IN DECISION-MAKING IN PEDIATRIC PRACTICE (TECHNICAL REPORT)

Aviva L. Katz, MD, FAAP; Sally A. Webb, MD, FAAP; and Committee on Bioethics

ABSTRACT. Informed consent should be seen as an essential part of health care practice; parental permission and childhood assent is an active process that engages patients, both adults and children, in their health care. Pediatric practice is unique in that developmental maturation allows, over time, for increasing inclusion of the child's and adolescent's opinion in medical decision-making in clinical practice and research. This technical report, which accompanies the policy statement "Informed Consent in Decision-Making in Pediatric Practice," was written to provide a broader background on the nature of informed consent, surrogate decision-making in pediatric practice, information on child and adolescent decision-making, and special issues in adolescent informed consent, assent, and refusal. It is anticipated that this information will help provide support for the recommendations included in the policy statement. (7/16, reaffirmed 1/23)
https://doi.org/10.1542/peds.2016-1485

INSTITUTIONAL ETHICS COMMITTEES

Margaret Moon, MD, MPH, FAAP, and Committee on Bioethics

ABSTRACT. In hospitals throughout the United States, institutional ethics committees (IECs) have become a standard vehicle for the education of health professionals about biomedical ethics, for the drafting and review of hospital policy, and for clinical ethics case consultation. In addition, there is increasing interest in a role for the IEC in organizational ethics. Recommendations are made about the membership and structure of an IEC, and guidance is provided for those serving on an IEC. (4/19, reaffirmed 6/23)
https://doi.org/10.1542/peds.2019-0659

INTEGRATING WEB SERVICES/APPLICATIONS TO IMPROVE PEDIATRIC FUNCTIONALITIES IN ELECTRONIC HEALTH RECORDS

Stuart T. Weinberg, MD, FAAP, FAMIA; Craig Monsen, MD, MS; Christoph U. Lehmann, MD, FAAP, FACMI, FIAHSI; Michael G. Leu, MD, MS, MHS, FAAP, FAMIA; and Council on Clinical Information Technology

ABSTRACT. The past decade has seen a substantial increase in the use of electronic health records (EHRs) by health care providers caring for children. However, gaps in pediatric-specific functionalities continue to exist in some EHR systems, including population-specific growth curves, immunization clinical decision support, weight-based medication dosing with rounding, calculation of pediatric hypertension percentiles, age-specific developmental assessment, newborn bilirubin nomograms, anticipatory guidance reminders, and other functionalities described elsewhere. Implementing pediatric functionalities into EHRs is critical to the provision of safe pediatric care. As an alternative to direct implementation in EHRs, EHR vendor agnostic Web applications, Web services, and application programming interfaces offer an opportunity to provide pediatric functionalities and eliminate the need for each vendor to develop these functionalities. Successful implementation of Web services and related technologies requires responsible attention from both EHR vendors and developers of Web services, Web applications, and application programming interfaces to the use of data terminology standards, adherence to privacy and security requirements, rigorous testing, change management processes, and robust system support and maintenance. Education of health care providers about opportunities to improve pediatric functionalities in EHRs by using these services can facilitate discussions in EHR user groups in which vendors can be lobbied to implement them. This policy statement emphasizes the need to address pediatric-specific functionalities in EHRs by providing insight and recommendations into the development, maintenance, integration, and support of these novel solutions. (6/21)
https://doi.org/10.1542/peds.2021-052047

INTERPRETATION OF DO NOT ATTEMPT RESUSCITATION ORDERS FOR CHILDREN REQUIRING ANESTHESIA AND SURGERY (CLINICAL REPORT)

Mary E. Fallat, MD, FAAP; Courtney Hardy, MD, MBA, FAAP; Section on Surgery; Section on Anesthesiology and Pain Medicine; and Committee on Bioethics

ABSTRACT. This clinical report addresses the topic of preexisting do not attempt resuscitation or limited resuscitation orders for children and adolescents undergoing anesthesia and surgery. Pertinent considerations for the clinician include the rights of children, decision-making by parents or legally approved representatives, the process of informed consent, and the roles of surgeon and anesthesiologist. A process of re-evaluation of the do not attempt resuscitation orders, called "required reconsideration," should be incorporated into the process of informed consent for surgery and anesthesia, distinguishing between goal-directed and procedure-directed approaches. The child's individual needs are best served by allowing the parent or legally approved representative and involved clinicians to consider whether full resuscitation, limitations based on procedures, or limitations based on goals is most appropriate. (4/18, reaffirmed 11/24)
https://doi.org/10.1542/peds.2018-0598

INTIMATE PARTNER VIOLENCE: ROLE OF THE PEDIATRICIAN (CLINICAL REPORT)

Jonathan Thackeray, MD, FAAP; Nina Livingston, MD, FAAP; Maya I. Ragavan, MD, MPH, FAAP; Judy Schaechter, MD, MBA, FAAP; Eric Sigel, MD, FAAP; Council on Child Abuse and Neglect; and Council on Injury, Violence, and Poison Prevention

ABSTRACT. The American Academy of Pediatrics and its members recognize the importance of improving the physician's ability to recognize intimate partner violence (IPV) and understand its effects on child health and development and its role in the continuum of family violence. Pediatricians are in a unique position to identify IPV survivors in pediatric settings, to evaluate and treat children exposed to IPV, and to connect families with available local and national resources. Children exposed to IPV are at increased risk of being abused and neglected and are more likely to develop adverse health, behavioral, psychological, and social disorders later in life. Pediatricians should be aware of these profound effects of exposure to IPV on children and how best to support and advocate for IPV survivors and their children. (6/23)
https://doi.org/10.1542/peds.2023-062509

LACTOSE INTOLERANCE IN INFANTS, CHILDREN, AND ADOLESCENTS (CLINICAL REPORT)

Melvin B. Heyman, MD, MPH; Committee on Nutrition

ABSTRACT. The American Academy of Pediatrics Committee on Nutrition presents an updated review of lactose intolerance in infants, children, and adolescents. Differences between primary, secondary, congenital, and developmental lactase deficiency that may result in lactose intolerance are discussed. Children with suspected lactose intolerance can be assessed clinically by dietary lactose elimination or by tests including noninvasive hydrogen breath testing or invasive intestinal biopsy determination of lactase (and other disaccharidase) concentrations. Treatment consists of use of lactase-treated dairy products or oral lactase supplementation, limitation of lactose-containing foods, or dairy elimination. The American Academy of Pediatrics supports use of dairy foods as an important source of calcium for bone mineral health and of other nutrients that facilitate growth in children and adolescents. If dairy products are eliminated, other dietary sources of calcium or calcium supplements need to be provided. (9/06, reaffirmed 11/24)
https://doi.org/10.1542/peds.2006-1721

LEUKODYSTROPHIES IN CHILDREN: DIAGNOSIS, CARE, AND TREATMENT (CLINICAL REPORT)

Joshua L. Bonkowsky, MD, PhD, FAAP; Stephanie Keller, MD, FAAP; Section on Neurology; and Council on Genetics

ABSTRACT. Leukodystrophies are a group of genetically determined disorders that affect development or maintenance of central nervous system myelin. Leukodystrophies have an incidence of at least 1 in 4700 live births and significant morbidity and elevated risk of early death. This report includes a discussion of the types of leukodystrophies; their prevalence, clinical presentation, symptoms, and diagnosis; and current and future treatments. Leukodystrophies can present at any age from infancy to adulthood, with variability in disease progression and clinical presentation, ranging from developmental delay to seizures to spasticity. Diagnosis is based on a combination of history, examination, and radiologic and laboratory findings, including genetic testing. Although there are few cures, there are significant opportunities for care and improvements in patient well-being. Rapid advances in imaging and diagnosis, the emergence of and requirement for timely treatments, and the addition of leukodystrophy screening to newborn screening, make an understanding of the leukodystrophies necessary for pediatricians and other care providers for children. (8/21)
https://doi.org/10.1542/peds.2021-053126

LEVELS OF NEONATAL CARE

Committee on Fetus and Newborn

ABSTRACT. Provision of risk-appropriate care for newborn infants and mothers was first proposed in 1976. This updated policy statement provides a review of data supporting evidence for a tiered provision of care and reaffirms the need for uniform, nationally applicable definitions and consistent standards of service for public health to improve neonatal outcomes. Facilities that provide hospital care for newborn infants should be classified on the basis of functional capabilities, and these facilities should be organized within a regionalized system of perinatal care. (8/12, reaffirmed 12/21)
https://doi.org/10.1542/peds.2012-1999

THE LINK BETWEEN SCHOOL ATTENDANCE AND GOOD HEALTH

Mandy A. Allison, MD, MSPH, FAAP; Elliott Attisha, DO, FAAP; and Council on School Health

ABSTRACT. More than 6.5 million children in the United States, approximately 13% of all students, miss 15 or more days of school each year. The rates of chronic absenteeism vary between states, communities, and schools, with significant disparities based on income, race, and ethnicity. Chronic school absenteeism, starting as early as preschool and kindergarten, puts students at risk for poor school performance and school dropout, which in turn, put them at risk for unhealthy behaviors as adolescents and young adults as well as poor long-term health outcomes. Pediatricians and their colleagues caring for children in the medical setting have opportunities at the individual patient and/or family, practice, and population levels to promote school attendance and reduce chronic absenteeism and resulting health disparities. Although this policy statement is primarily focused on absenteeism related to students' physical and mental health, pediatricians may play a role in addressing absenteeism attributable to a wide range of factors through individual interactions with patients and their parents and through community-, state-, and federal-level advocacy. (1/19, reaffirmed 2/24)
https://doi.org/10.1542/peds.2018-3648

LITERACY PROMOTION: AN ESSENTIAL COMPONENT OF PRIMARY CARE PEDIATRIC PRACTICE

Perri Klass, MD, FAAP; Anna Miller-Fitzwater, MD, MPH, FAAP; Pamela C. High, MD, MS, FAAP; and Council on Early Childhood

ABSTRACT. Reading together often with infants and young children strengthens their relationships with parents and caregivers at a critical time in child development, stimulating brain circuitry and early attachment. A positive parenting practice, shared reading helps build the foundation for healthy social-emotional, cognitive, language, and literacy development, setting the stage for school readiness and providing enduring benefits across the life course.

Pediatric physicians and advanced care providers have a unique opportunity to encourage parents and caregivers to establish routines and enjoy conversations around books and stories with their children beginning in infancy. Research has demonstrated that parents read and children learn when pediatricians offer literacy promotion as a practical and evidence-based primary prevention strategy in primary care practice to support early brain and child development. This supports families with a strengths-based approach, shaping a child's life trajectory and helping mitigate stress and adverse experiences.

The American Academy of Pediatrics (AAP) recommends that pediatricians encourage shared reading, beginning at birth and continuing at least through kindergarten, as a strategy for supporting parents and caregivers, enhancing foundational relationships, promoting positive language-rich interactions, and helping families create nurturing and stimulating home envi-

ronments. The integration of literacy promotion into pediatric resident education is crucial to achieve that goal and thus is also essential. The AAP supports advocacy toward establishing public and private funding for diverse high-quality, developmentally appropriate children's books in the languages preferred by the family to be provided at pediatric health supervision visits to all children but especially to children living in underresourced communities. This statement is supported by multiple AAP policies and implementation resources, including the accompanying "Literacy Promotion: An Essential Component of Primary Care Pediatric Practice: Technical Report." (11/24)
https://doi.org/10.1542/peds.2024-069090

LITERACY PROMOTION: AN ESSENTIAL COMPONENT OF PRIMARY CARE PEDIATRIC PRACTICE (TECHNICAL REPORT)

Perri Klass, MD, FAAP; Alan L. Mendelsohn, MD, FAAP; John S. Hutton, MD, MS, FAAP; Marny Dunlap, MD, FAAP; Ashaunta T. Anderson, MD, MPH, MSHS, FAAP; Pamela C. High, MD, MS, FAAP; Dipesh Navsaria, MD, MPH, MSLIS, FAAP; and Council on Early Childhood

ABSTRACT. Early literacy promotion in pediatric primary care supports parents and caregivers in reading with their children from birth, offering counseling in interactive, developmentally appropriate strategies and providing developmentally and culturally appropriate and appealing children's books. This technical report reviews the evidence that reading with young children supports language, cognitive, and social-emotional development. Promoting early literacy in pediatric primary care offers a strengths-based strategy to support families in creating positive childhood experiences, which strengthen early relational health. An increasing body of evidence, reviewed in this report, shows that clinic-based literacy promotion, provided with fidelity to an evidence-based model, has benefits for children, for parents and caregivers, and for pediatric physicians and advanced care providers as well. Reading with young children supports early brain development and the neural "reading network," and improves school readiness. High-quality literacy promotion is especially essential for children who face disparities and inequities because of social factors, systemic racism, and socioeconomic risk. All families benefit from high-quality and diverse books and from developmentally appropriate guidance supporting interactions around books and stories. Thus, literacy promotion can be a universal primary prevention strategy to strengthen families and support healthy development. Partnerships at community, local, and state levels offer opportunities for integration with other programs, services, and platforms. Literacy promotion in primary care pediatric practice, recognized by the American Academy of Pediatrics as an essential component since 2014, has become increasingly common. There are successful models for public funding at federal, state, county, and municipal levels, but sustainable funding, including payment to pediatric physicians and advanced care providers, remains a need so that the benefits of pediatric early literacy promotion and the joys of books and shared reading can truly be offered on a population level. (11/24)
https://doi.org/10.1542/peds.2024-069091

LONG-TERM FOLLOW-UP CARE FOR CHILDHOOD, ADOLESCENT, AND YOUNG ADULT CANCER SURVIVORS (CLINICAL REPORT)

Melissa M. Hudson, MD; Smita Bhatia, MD, MPH; Jacqueline Casillas, MD, MSHS; Wendy Landier, PhD, RN, CPNP; and Section on Hematology/Oncology (joint with Children's Oncology Group and American Society of Pediatric Hematology/Oncology)

ABSTRACT. Progress in therapy has made survival into adulthood a reality for most children, adolescents, and young adults with a cancer diagnosis today. Notably, this growing population remains vulnerable to a variety of long-term therapy-related sequelae. Systematic ongoing follow-up of these patients is, therefore, important to provide for early detection of and intervention for potentially serious late-onset complications. In addition, health counseling and promotion of healthy lifestyles are important aspects of long-term follow-up care to promote risk reduction for physical and emotional health problems that commonly present during adulthood. Both general and subspecialty health care providers are playing an increasingly important role in the ongoing care of childhood cancer survivors, beyond the routine preventive care, health supervision, and anticipatory guidance provided to all patients. This report is based on the guidelines that have been developed by the Children's Oncology Group to facilitate comprehensive long-term follow-up of childhood, adolescent, and young adult cancer survivors (www.survivorshipguidelines.org). (8/21)
https://doi.org/10.1542/peds.2021-053127

LOW-CARBOHYDRATE DIETS IN CHILDREN AND ADOLESCENTS WITH OR AT RISK FOR DIABETES (CLINICAL REPORT)

Anna Neyman, MD, FAAP; Tamara S. Hannon, MD, FAAP; and Committee on Nutrition

ABSTRACT. Carbohydrate restriction is increasingly popular as a weight loss strategy and for achieving better glycemic control in people with diabetes, including type 1 and type 2 diabetes. However, evidence to support low-carbohydrate diets in youth (children and adolescents 2–18 years of age) with obesity or diabetes is limited. There are no guidelines for restricting dietary carbohydrate consumption to reduce risk for diabetes or improve diabetes outcomes in youth. Thus, there is a need to provide practical recommendations for pediatricians regarding the use of low-carbohydrate diets in patients who elect to follow these diets, including those with type 1 diabetes and for patients with obesity, prediabetes, and type 2 diabetes.

This clinical report will:

- Provide background on current dietary patterns in youth, describe how moderate-, low-, and very low-carbohydrate diets differ, and review safety concerns associated with the use of these dietary patterns
- Review the physiologic rationale for carbohydrate reduction in youth with type 1 diabetes and for youth with obesity, prediabetes, and type 2 diabetes
- Review the evidence for low-carbohydrate diets in the management of youth with type 1 diabetes
- Review the evidence for low-carbohydrate diets in the management of youth with obesity, prediabetes, and type 2 diabetes
- Provide practical information for pediatricians counseling families and youth on carbohydrate recommendations for type 1 diabetes and for obesity, prediabetes, and type 2 diabetes (9/23)

https://doi.org/10.1542/peds.2023-063755

MAINTAINING AND IMPROVING THE ORAL HEALTH OF YOUNG CHILDREN (CLINICAL REPORT)

David M. Krol, MD, MPH, FAAP; Kaitlin Whelan, MD, FAAP; and Section on Oral Health

ABSTRACT. Oral health is an integral part of the overall health of children. Dental caries is a common and chronic disease process with significant short- and long-term consequences. The prevalence of dental caries remains greater than 40% among children 2 to 19 years of age. Although dental visits have increased in all age, race, and geographic categories in the United States, disparities continue to exist, and a significant portion of children have difficulty accessing dental care. As health care professionals responsible for the overall health of children, pediatricians frequently confront morbidity associated with dental caries.

Because the youngest children visit the pediatrician more often than they visit the dentist, it is important that pediatricians be knowledgeable about the disease process of dental caries, prevention of disease, interventions to maintain and restore health, and the social determinants of children's oral health. (12/22)
https://doi.org/10.1542/peds.2022-060417

MALTREATMENT OF CHILDREN WITH DISABILITIES (CLINICAL REPORT)

Lori A. Legano, MD, FAAP; Larry W. Desch, MD, FAAP; Stephen A. Messner, MD, FAAP; Sheila Idzerda, MD, FAAP; Emalee G. Flaherty, MD, FAAP; Council on Child Abuse and Neglect; and Council on Children With Disabilities

ABSTRACT. Over the past decade, there have been widespread efforts to raise awareness about maltreatment of children. Pediatric providers have received education about factors that make a child more vulnerable to being abused and neglected. The purpose of this clinical report is to ensure that children with disabilities are recognized as a population at increased risk for maltreatment. This report updates the 2007 American Academy of Pediatrics clinical report "Maltreatment of Children With Disabilities." Since 2007, new information has expanded our understanding of the incidence of abuse in this vulnerable population. There is now information about which children with disabilities are at greatest risk for maltreatment because not all disabling conditions confer the same risks of abuse or neglect. This updated report will serve as a resource for pediatricians and others who care for children with disabilities and offers guidance on risks for subpopulations of children with disabilities who are at particularly high risk of abuse and neglect. The report will also discuss ways in which the medical home can aid in early identification and intervene when abuse and neglect are suspected. It will also describe community resources and preventive strategies that may reduce the risk of abuse and neglect. (4/21)
https://doi.org/10.1542/peds.2021-050920

THE MANAGEMENT OF CHILDREN AND YOUTH WITH PEDIATRIC MENTAL AND BEHAVIORAL HEALTH EMERGENCIES

Mohsen Saidinejad, MD, MS, MBA, FAAP, FACEP; Susan Duffy, MD, MPH, FAAP; Dina Wallin, MD; Jennifer A. Hoffmann, MD, FAAP; Madeline M. Joseph, MD, FAAP, FACEP; Jennifer Schieferle Uhlenbrock, DNP, MBA, RN, TCRN; Kathleen Brown, MD, FAAP; Muhammad Waseem, MD, MS, FAAP, FACEP, CHSE-A; Sally Snow, BSN, RN, CPEN, FAEN; Madeline Andrew, MD; Alice A. Kuo, MD, PhD, MBA, FAAP; Carmen Sulton, MD, FAAP; Thomas Chun, MD, MPH, FAAP; Lois K. Lee, MD, MPH, FAAP, FACEP; and Committee on Pediatric Emergency Medicine (joint with American College of Emergency Physicians Pediatric Emergency Medicine Committee and Emergency Nurses Association Pediatric Committee)

ABSTRACT. Mental and behavioral health (MBH) emergencies in children and youth continue to increasingly affect not only the emergency department (ED), but the entire spectrum of emergency medical services for children, from prehospital services to the community. Inadequate community and institutional infrastructure to care for children and youth with MBH conditions makes the ED an essential part of the health care safety net for these patients. As a result, an increasing number of children and youth are referred to the ED for evaluation of a broad spectrum of MBH emergencies, from depression and suicidality to disruptive and aggressive behavior. However, challenges in providing optimal care to these patients include lack of personnel, capacity, and infrastructure; challenges with timely access to a mental health professional; the nature of a busy ED environment; and paucity of outpatient post-ED discharge resources. These factors contribute to prolonged ED stays and boarding, which negatively affect patient care and ED operations. Strategies to improve care for MBH emergencies, including systems-level coordination of care, are therefore essential. The goal of this policy statement and its companion technical report is to highlight strategies, resources, and recommendations for improving emergency care delivery for pediatric MBH. (8/23)
https://doi.org/10.1542/peds.2023-063255

THE MANAGEMENT OF CHILDREN AND YOUTH WITH PEDIATRIC MENTAL AND BEHAVIORAL HEALTH EMERGENCIES (TECHNICAL REPORT)

Mohsen Saidinejad, MD, MS, MBA, FAAP, FACEP; Susan Duffy, MD, MPH, FAAP; Dina Wallin, MD; Jennifer A. Hoffmann, MD, FAAP; Madeline M. Joseph, MD, FAAP, FACEP; Jennifer Schieferle Uhlenbrock, DNP, MBA, RN, TCRN; Kathleen Brown, MD, FAAP; Muhammad Waseem, MD, MS, FAAP, FACEP, CHSE-A; Sally Snow, BSN, RN, CPEN, FAEN; Madeline Andrew, MD; Alice A. Kuo, MD, PhD, MBA, FAAP; Carmen Sulton, MD, FAAP; Thomas Chun, MD, MPH, FAAP; Lois K. Lee, MD, MPH, FAAP, FACEP; and Committee on Pediatric Emergency Medicine (joint with American College of Emergency Physicians Pediatric Emergency Medicine Committee and Emergency Nurses Association Pediatric Committee)

ABSTRACT. Mental and behavioral health (MBH) visits of children and youth to emergency departments are increasing in the United States. Reasons for these visits range from suicidal ideation, self-harm, and eating and substance use disorders to behavioral outbursts, aggression, and psychosis. Despite the increase in prevalence of these conditions, the capacity of the health care system to screen, diagnose, and manage these patients continues to decline. Several social determinants also contribute to great disparities in child and adolescent (youth) health, which affect MBH outcomes. In addition, resources and space for emergency physicians, physician assistants, nurse practitioners, and prehospital practitioners to manage these patients remain limited and inconsistent throughout the United States, as is financial compensation and payment for such services. This technical report discusses the role of physicians, physician assistants, and nurse practitioners, and provides guidance for the management of acute MBH emergencies in children and youth. Unintentional ingestions and substance use disorder are not within the scope of this report and are not specifically discussed. (8/23)
https://doi.org/10.1542/peds.2023-063256

MANAGEMENT OF DENTAL TRAUMA IN A PRIMARY CARE SETTING (CLINICAL REPORT)

Martha Ann Keels, DDS, PhD, and Section on Oral Health

ABSTRACT. The American Academy of Pediatrics and its Section on Oral Health have developed this clinical report for pediatricians and primary care physicians regarding the diagnosis, evaluation, and management of dental trauma in children aged 1 to 21 years. This report was developed through a comprehensive search and analysis of the medical and dental literature and expert consensus. Guidelines published and updated by the International Association of Dental Traumatology (www.dentaltraumaguide.com) are an excellent resource for both dental and nondental health care providers. (1/14, reaffirmed 9/21 with reference & data updates)
https://doi.org/10.1542/peds.2013-3792

MANAGEMENT OF FOOD ALLERGY IN SCHOOLS (CLINICAL REPORT)

Scott H. Sicherer, MD, FAAP; Sonja O'Leary, MD, FAAP; Michael Pistiner, MD, MMSc, FAAP; Julie Wang, MD, FAAP; Section on Allergy and Immunology; Council on School Health

ABSTRACT. This clinical report updates and replaces a 2010 clinical report from the American Academy of Pediatrics that addressed food allergy management in schools. Food allergy affects up to 10% of children, and anaphylaxis is estimated to occur in 1 in 15 schools per year. School food allergy management requires strategies to reduce the risk of ingestion of the allergen as well as procedures to recognize and treat allergic reactions and anaphylaxis. The role of the pediatrician or pediatric primary care clinician may include diagnosing and documenting a potentially life-threatening food allergy; prescribing self-administered epinephrine to individual patients or for general use in a school (stock/unassigned epinephrine); educating children, parents, and school personnel on prevention, recognition, and management of allergic reactions to food; and working with schools in developing plans to reduce the risk of anaphylaxis and to implement emergency treatment in the event of a reaction. This clinical report highlights the role of the pediatrician and primary care clinician in managing students with food allergies. (11/25)

See full text on page 367.

https://doi.org/10.1542/peds.2025-073168

MEDIA AND YOUNG MINDS

Council on Communications and Media

ABSTRACT. Infants, toddlers, and preschoolers are now growing up in environments saturated with a variety of traditional and new technologies, which they are adopting at increasing rates. Although there has been much hope for the educational potential of interactive media for young children, accompanied by fears about their overuse during this crucial period of rapid brain development, research in this area still remains limited. This policy statement reviews the existing literature on television, videos, and mobile/interactive technologies; their potential for educational benefit; and related health concerns for young children (0 to 5 years of age). The statement also highlights areas in which pediatric providers can offer specific guidance to families in managing their young children's media use, not only in terms of content or time limits, but also emphasizing the importance of parent-child shared media use and allowing the child time to take part in other developmentally healthy activities. (10/16, reaffirmed 7/22)

https://doi.org/10.1542/peds.2016-2591

MEDIA USE IN SCHOOL-AGED CHILDREN AND ADOLESCENTS

Council on Communications and Media

ABSTRACT. This policy statement focuses on children and adolescents 5 through 18 years of age. Research suggests both benefits and risks of media use for the health of children and teenagers. Benefits include exposure to new ideas and knowledge acquisition, increased opportunities for social contact and support, and new opportunities to access health-promotion messages and information. Risks include negative health effects on weight and sleep; exposure to inaccurate, inappropriate, or unsafe content and contacts; and compromised privacy and confidentiality. Parents face challenges in monitoring their children's and their own media use and in serving as positive role models. In this new era, evidence regarding healthy media use does not support a one-size-fits-all approach. Parents and pediatricians can work together to develop a Family Media Use Plan (www.healthychildren.org/MediaUsePlan) that considers their children's developmental stages to individualize an appropriate balance for media time and consistent rules about media use, to mentor their children, to set boundaries for accessing content and displaying personal information, and to implement open family communication about media. (10/16, reaffirmed 7/22 with reference & data updates)

https://doi.org/10.1542/peds.2016-2592

MEDIATORS AND ADVERSE EFFECTS OF CHILD POVERTY IN THE UNITED STATES (TECHNICAL REPORT)

John M. Pascoe, MD, MPH, FAAP; David L. Wood, MD, MPH, FAAP; James H. Duffee, MD, MPH, FAAP; Alice Kuo, MD, PhD, MEd, FAAP; Committee on Psychosocial Aspects of Child and Family Health; and Council on Community Pediatrics

ABSTRACT. The link between poverty and children's health is well recognized. Even temporary poverty may have an adverse effect on children's health, and data consistently support the observation that poverty in childhood continues to have a negative effect on health into adulthood. In addition to childhood morbidity being related to child poverty, epidemiologic studies have documented a mortality gradient for children aged 1 to 15 years (and adults), with poor children experiencing a higher mortality rate than children from higher-income families. The global great recession is only now very slowly abating for millions of America's children and their families. At this difficult time in the history of our nation's families and immediately after the 50th anniversary year of President Lyndon Johnson's War on Poverty, it is particularly germane for the American Academy of Pediatrics, which is "dedicated to the health of all children," to publish a research-supported technical report that examines the mediators associated with the long-recognized adverse effects of child poverty on children and their families. This technical report draws on research from a number of disciplines, including physiology, sociology, psychology, economics, and epidemiology, to describe the present state of knowledge regarding poverty's negative impact on children's health and development. Children inherit not only their parents' genes but also the family ecology and its social milieu. Thus, parenting skills, housing, neighborhood, schools, and other factors (eg, medical care) all have complex relations to each other and influence how each child's genetic canvas is expressed. Accompanying this technical report is a policy statement that describes specific actions that pediatricians and other child advocates can take to attenuate the negative effects of the mediators identified in this technical report and improve the well-being of our nation's children and their families. (3/16, reaffirmed 4/21)

https://doi.org/10.1542/peds.2016-0340

MEDICAID AND THE CHILDREN'S HEALTH INSURANCE PROGRAM: OPTIMIZATION TO PROMOTE EQUITY IN CHILD AND YOUNG ADULT HEALTH

Jennifer D. Kusma, MD, MS, FAAP; Jean L. Raphael, MD, MPH, FAAP; James M. Perrin, MD, FAAP; Mark L. Hudak, MD, FAAP; and Committee on Child Health Financing

ABSTRACT. The American Academy of Pediatrics envisions a child and adolescent health care system that provides individualized, family-centered, equitable, and comprehensive care that integrates with community resources to help each child and family achieve optimal growth, development, and well-being. All infants, children, adolescents, and young adults should have access to this system. Medicaid and the Children's Health Insurance Program (CHIP) provide critical support and foundation for this vision. Together, the programs currently serve about half of all children, many of whom are members of racial

and ethnic minoritized populations or have complex medical conditions. Medicaid and CHIP have greatly improved the health and well-being of US infants, children, adolescents, and young adults. This statement reviews key program aspects and proposes both program reforms and enhancements to support a higher-quality, more comprehensive, family-oriented, and equitable system of care that increases access to services, reduces disparities, and improves health outcomes into adulthood. This statement recommends foundational changes in Medicaid and CHIP that can improve child health, achieve greater equity in health and health care, further dismantle structural racism within the programs, and reduce major state-by-state variations. The recommendations focus on (1) eligibility and duration of coverage; (2) standardization of covered services and quality of care; and (3) program financing and payment. In addition to proposed foundational changes in the Medicaid and CHIP program structure, the statement indicates stepwise, coordinated actions that regulation from the Centers for Medicare and Medicaid Services or federal legislation can accomplish in the shorter term. A separate technical report will address the origins and intents of the Medicaid and CHIP programs; the current state of the program including variations across states and payment structures; Medicaid for special populations; program innovations and waivers; and special Medicaid coverage and initiatives. (10/23)
https://doi.org/10.1542/peds.2023-064088

MEDICAL COUNTERMEASURES FOR CHILDREN IN PUBLIC HEALTH EMERGENCIES, DISASTERS, OR TERRORISM

Disaster Preparedness Advisory Council

ABSTRACT. Significant strides have been made over the past 10 to 15 years to develop medical countermeasures (MCMs) to address potential disaster hazards, including chemical, biological, radiologic, and nuclear threats. Significant and effective collaboration between the pediatric health community, including the American Academy of Pediatrics, and federal partners, such as the Office of the Assistant Secretary for Preparedness and Response, Centers for Disease Control and Prevention, Federal Emergency Management Agency, National Institutes of Health, Food and Drug Administration, and other federal agencies, over the past 5 years has resulted in substantial gains in addressing the needs of children related to disaster preparedness in general and MCMs in particular. Yet, major gaps still remain related to MCMs for children, a population highly vulnerable to the effects of exposure to such threats, because many vaccines and pharmaceuticals approved for use by adults as MCMs do not yet have pediatric formulations, dosing information, or safety information. As a result, the nation's stockpiles and other caches (designated supply of MCMs) where pharmacotherapeutic and other MCMs are stored are less prepared to address the needs of children compared with those of adults in the event of a disaster. This policy statement provides recommendations to close the remaining gaps for the development and use of MCMs in children during public health emergencies or disasters. The progress made by federal agencies to date to address the needs of children and the shared commitment of collaboration that characterizes the current relationship between the pediatric health community and the federal agencies responsible for MCMs should encourage all child advocates to invest the necessary energy and resources now to complete the process of remedying the remaining significant gaps in preparedness. (1/16, reaffirmed 5/22)
https://doi.org/10.1542/peds.2015-4273

MEDICAL VS NONMEDICAL IMMUNIZATION EXEMPTIONS FOR CHILD CARE AND SCHOOL ATTENDANCE

Jesse M. Hackell, MD, FAAP; Kyle Brothers, MD, PhD, FAAP; Sara Bode, MD, FAAP; Lisa M. Costello, MD, MPH, FAAP; Lisa M. Kafer, MD, FAAP; Sean T. O'Leary, MD, MPH, FAAP; Committee on Practice and Ambulatory Medicine; Committee on Infectious Diseases; Committee on State Government Affairs; and Council on School Health

ABSTRACT. Routine childhood immunizations against infectious diseases are an integral part of our public health infrastructure. They provide direct protection to the immunized individual and indirect protection to children and adults unable to be immunized by reducing spread of vaccine-preventable diseases in the community. All 50 states, the District of Columbia, and Puerto Rico have regulations requiring proof of immunization as a condition for child care and school attendance as a public health strategy to protect children in these settings and to secondarily serve as a mechanism to promote timely immunization of children by their caregivers. Although all states and the District of Columbia have mechanisms to exempt school attendees from specific immunizations for medical reasons, the majority also have a heterogeneous collection of regulations and laws that allow nonmedical reasons for exemption. The American Academy of Pediatrics (AAP) supports certification of immunization to attend child care and school as a sound means of providing a safe environment for attendees and employees of these settings. The AAP also supports medically indicated exemptions to specific immunizations as determined for each individual child. The AAP advocates for the elimination of nonmedical exemptions from immunizations as contrary to optimal individual and public health. (7/25)

See full text on page 381.

https://doi.org/10.1542/peds.2025-072714

METRIC UNITS AND THE PREFERRED DOSING OF ORALLY ADMINISTERED LIQUID MEDICATIONS

Committee on Drugs

ABSTRACT. Medication overdoses are a common, but preventable, problem among children. Volumetric dosing errors and the use of incorrect dosing delivery devices are 2 common sources of these preventable errors for orally administered liquid medications. To reduce errors and increase precision of drug administration, milliliter-based dosing should be used exclusively when prescribing and administering liquid medications. Teaspoon- and tablespoon-based dosing should not be used. Devices that allow for precise dose administration (preferably syringes with metric markings) should be used instead of household spoons and should be distributed with the medication. (3/15, reaffirmed 5/25 with reference & data updates)
https://doi.org/10.1542/peds.2015-0072

MOTOR DELAYS: EARLY IDENTIFICATION AND EVALUATION (CLINICAL REPORT)

Garey H. Noritz, MD; Nancy A. Murphy, MD; and Neuromotor Screening Expert Panel

ABSTRACT. Pediatricians often encounter children with delays of motor development in their clinical practices. Earlier identification of motor delays allows for timely referral for developmental interventions as well as diagnostic evaluations and treatment planning. A multidisciplinary expert panel developed an algorithm for the surveillance and screening of children for motor delays within the medical home, offering guidance for the initial workup and referral of the child with possible delays in motor development. Highlights of this clinical report include suggestions for formal developmental screening at the 9-, 18-, 30-, and 48-month well-child visits; approaches to the neurologic

examination, with emphasis on the assessment of muscle tone; and initial diagnostic approaches for medical home providers. Use of diagnostic tests to evaluate children with motor delays are described, including brain MRI for children with high muscle tone, and measuring serum creatine kinase concentration of those with decreased muscle tone. The importance of pursuing diagnostic tests while concurrently referring patients to early intervention programs is emphasized. (5/13, reaffirmed 5/17, 11/22)
https://doi.org/10.1542/peds.2013-1056

NEEDS OF KINSHIP CARE FAMILIES AND PEDIATRIC PRACTICE

David Rubin, MD, FAAP; Sarah H. Springer, MD, FAAP; Sarah Zlotnik, MSW, MSPH; Christina D. Kang-Yi, PhD; and Council on Foster Care, Adoption, and Kinship Care

ABSTRACT. As many as 3% of children in the United States live in kinship care arrangements with caregivers who are relatives but not the biological parents of the child. A growing body of evidence suggests that children who cannot live with their biological parents fare better, overall, when living with extended family than with nonrelated foster parents. Acknowledging this, federal laws and public policies increasingly favor kinship care over nonrelative foster care when children are unable to live with their biological parents. Despite overall better outcomes, families providing kinship care experience many hardships, and the children experience many of the same adversities of children in traditional foster care. This policy statement reviews both the strengths and vulnerabilities of kinship families and suggests strategies for pediatricians to use to address the needs of individual patients and families. Strategies are also outlined for community, state, and federal advocacy on behalf of these children and their families. (3/17, reaffirmed 6/22)
https://doi.org/10.1542/peds.2017-0099

NEONATAL PROVIDER WORKFORCE (TECHNICAL REPORT)

Erin L. Keels, DNP, APRN-CNP, NNP-BC; Jay P. Goldsmith, MD, FAAP; Committee on Fetus and Newborn

ABSTRACT. This technical report reviews education, training, competency requirements, and scopes of practice of the different neonatal care providers who work to meet the special needs of neonatal patients and their families in the NICU. Additionally, this report examines the current workforce issues of NICU providers, offers suggestions for establishing and monitoring quality and safety of care, and suggests potential solutions to the NICU provider workforce shortages now and in the future. (12/19, reaffirmed 3/25)
https://doi.org/10.1542/peds.2019-3147

NEW AND EVOLVING DIMENSIONS IN THE PEDIATRICIAN-FAMILY-PATIENT RELATIONSHIP: MAINTAINING AND MANAGING BOUNDARIES (CLINICAL REPORT)

Douglas J. Opel, MD, MPH, FAAP; Douglas S. Diekema, MD, MPH, FAAP; and Committee on Bioethics

ABSTRACT. Maintaining and managing boundaries in relationships with patients and their family members remains extremely important for the practicing pediatrician. Technological innovations that facilitate communication and information sharing, such as social media, have created new dimensions within the pediatrician-family-patient relationship. Shifts in patient and family expectations of the medical profession that have occurred over time, such as a greater desire among patients and families to have increased access to their pediatrician, also present novel challenges to traditional professional boundaries. Further, social and political issues that have bearing on the practice of medicine have raised questions about pediatricians' role as advocates for individual patients and child health within the pediatrician-family-patient relationship. The 2009 AAP policy statement, "Pediatrician-Family-Patient Relationships: Managing the Boundaries," offers guidance for pediatricians in navigating several key scenarios regarding professional boundaries, including accepting gifts, dual relationships, and romantic relationships with patients or caregivers. Since the content in this 2009 policy statement remains relevant, the intent of this clinical report is to complement the 2009 statement and provide guidance for navigating new and evolving dimensions of the traditional pediatrician-family-patient relationship, including advocacy within the pediatric clinical encounter, self-disclosure, and social media relationships with patients or caregivers. (6/25)
See full text on page 391.
https://doi.org/10.1542/peds.2025-072215

NEWBORN SCREENING FOR CRITICAL CONGENITAL HEART DISEASE: A NEW ALGORITHM AND OTHER UPDATED RECOMMENDATIONS (CLINICAL REPORT)

American Academy of Pediatrics
DEDICATED TO THE HEALTH OF ALL CHILDREN®
AAP Partnership for Policy Implementation
– *See Appendix 1*

Matthew E. Oster, MD, MPH, FAAP; Nelangi M. Pinto, MD; Arun K. Pramanik, MD, FAAP; Allison Markowsky, MD, MSHS, FAAP; Bryanna N. Schwartz, MD, MPH, FAAP; Alex R. Kemper, MD, MPH, MS, FAAP; Lisa A. Hom, RN, Esq; Gerard R. Martin, MD, FAAP; Section on Cardiology and Cardiac Surgery; Section on Hospital Medicine; and Committee on Fetus and Newborn

ABSTRACT. Critical congenital heart disease (CCHD) screening was added to the US Recommended Uniform Screening Panel in 2011 and adopted by all US states and territories by 2018. In addition to reviewing key developments in CCHD screening since the initial American Academy of Pediatrics (AAP) endorsement in 2011, this clinical report provides 3 updated recommendations. First, a new AAP algorithm has been endorsed for use in CCHD screening. Compared with the original AAP algorithm from 2011, this new algorithm a) has a passing oxygen saturation threshold of ≥95% in both pre- and post-ductal measurements; and b) has only 1 retest instead of 2 for infants who did not pass the first screen. Second, to continue to improve screening, state newborn screening programs should collect a recommended minimum uniform dataset to aid in surveillance and monitoring of the program. Finally, stakeholders should be educated on the limitations of screening, the significance of non-CCHD conditions, and the importance of protocol adherence. Future directions of CCHD screening include improving overall sensitivity and implementing methods to reduce health inequities. It will remain critical that the AAP and its chapters and members work with health departments and hospitals to achieve awareness and implementation of these recommendations. (12/24)
See full text on page 401.
https://doi.org/10.1542/peds.2024-069667

NONDISCRIMINATION IN PEDIATRIC HEALTH CARE

Committee on Pediatric Workforce

ABSTRACT. This policy statement is a revision of a 2001 statement and articulates the positions of the American Academy of Pediatrics on nondiscrimination in pediatric health care. It addresses both pediatricians who provide health care and the infants, children, adolescents, and young adults whom they serve. (10/07, reaffirmed 6/11, 5/21)
https://doi.org/10.1542/peds.2007-2334

NONEMERGENCY ACUTE CARE: WHEN IT'S NOT THE MEDICAL HOME

Gregory P. Conners, MD, MPH, MBA, FAAP; Susan J. Kressly, MD, FAAP; James M. Perrin, MD, FAAP; Julia E. Richerson, MD, FAAP; Usha M. Sankrithi, MBBS, MPH, FAAP; Committee on Practice and Ambulatory Medicine; Committee on Pediatric Emergency Medicine; Section on Telehealth Care; Section on Emergency Medicine; Subcommittee on Urgent Care; and Task Force on Pediatric Practice Change

ABSTRACT. The American Academy of Pediatrics (AAP) affirms that the optimal location for children to receive care for acute, nonemergency health concerns is the medical home. The medical home is characterized by the AAP as a care model that "must be accessible, family centered, continuous, comprehensive, coordinated, compassionate, and culturally effective." However, some children and families use acute care services outside the medical home because there is a perceived or real benefit related to accessibility, convenience, or cost of care. Examples of such acute care entities include urgent care facilities, retail-based clinics, and commercial telemedicine services. Children deserve high-quality, appropriate, and safe acute care services wherever they access the health care system, with timely and complete communication with the medical home, to ensure coordinated and continuous care. Treatment of children under established, new, and evolving practice arrangements in acute care entities should adhere to the core principles of continuity of care and communication, best practices within a defined scope of services, pediatric-trained staff, safe transitions of care, and continuous improvement. In support of the medical home, the AAP urges stakeholders, including payers, to avoid any incentives (eg, reduced copays) that encourage visits to external entities for acute issues as a preference over the medical home. (4/17, reaffirmed 4/24)

https://doi.org/10.1542/peds.2017-0629

NONMEDICAL USE OF CONTROLLED MEDICATIONS BY ADOLESCENTS AND YOUNG ADULTS (CLINICAL REPORT)

Nicholas Chadi, MD, MPH, FAAP, FRCPC; Leslie Walker-Harding, MD, FAAP; and Committee on Substance Use and Prevention

ABSTRACT. Nonmedical prescription drug use (NMPDU), the use of controlled prescription medications for purposes other than initially intended by the prescriber, is common among adolescents and young adults (AYAs). Prescription stimulants, sedatives, and opioid medications are the 3 main categories of controlled medications nonmedically used by AYAs. The intent of this clinical report is to provide an overview of the epidemiology, motives, sources, and risk factors of NMPDU among AYAs. This report also describes acute and long-term morbidity and mortality associated with NMPDU and discusses the importance of primary and secondary prevention to reduce the burden of NMPDU among AYAs. This report concludes with a series of recommendations on how pediatricians can address NMPDU with patients and their families. (11/24)

https://doi.org/10.1542/peds.2024-069298

NONORAL FEEDING FOR CHILDREN AND YOUTH WITH DEVELOPMENTAL OR ACQUIRED DISABILITIES (CLINICAL REPORT)

Richard C. Adams, MD, FAAP; Ellen Roy Elias, MD, FAAP; Council on Children With Disabilities

ABSTRACT. The decision to initiate enteral feedings is multifaceted, involving medical, financial, cultural, and emotional considerations. Children who have developmental or acquired disabilities are at risk for having primary and secondary conditions that affect growth and nutritional well-being. This clinical report provides (1) an overview of clinical issues in children who have developmental or acquired disabilities that may prompt a need to consider nonoral feedings, (2) a systematic way to support the child and family in clinical decisions related to initiating nonoral feeding, (3) information on surgical options that the family may need to consider in that decision-making process, and (4) pediatric guidance for ongoing care after initiation of nonoral feeding intervention, including care of the gastrostomy tube and skin site. Ongoing medical and psychosocial support is needed after initiation of nonoral feedings and is best provided through the collaborative efforts of the family and a team of professionals that may include the pediatrician, dietitian, social worker, and/or therapists. (12/14, reaffirmed 6/19, 8/25)

https://doi.org/10.1542/peds.2014-2829

OFFICE-BASED CARE FOR LESBIAN, GAY, BISEXUAL, TRANSGENDER, AND QUESTIONING YOUTH

Committee on Adolescence

ABSTRACT. The American Academy of Pediatrics issued its last statement on homosexuality and adolescents in 2004. Although most lesbian, gay, bisexual, transgender, and questioning (LGBTQ) youth are quite resilient and emerge from adolescence as healthy adults, the effects of homophobia and heterosexism can contribute to health disparities in mental health with higher rates of depression and suicidal ideation, higher rates of substance abuse, and more sexually transmitted and HIV infections. Pediatricians should have offices that are teen-friendly and welcoming to sexual minority youth. Obtaining a comprehensive, confidential, developmentally appropriate adolescent psychosocial history allows for the discovery of strengths and assets as well as risks. Referrals for mental health or substance abuse may be warranted. Sexually active LGBTQ youth should have sexually transmitted infection/HIV testing according to recommendations of the Sexually Transmitted Diseases Treatment Guidelines of the Centers for Disease Control and Prevention based on sexual behaviors. With appropriate assistance and care, sexual minority youth should live healthy, productive lives while transitioning through adolescence and young adulthood. (6/13, reaffirmed 4/21)

https://doi.org/10.1542/peds.2013-1282

OFFICE-BASED CARE FOR LESBIAN, GAY, BISEXUAL, TRANSGENDER, AND QUESTIONING YOUTH (TECHNICAL REPORT)

David A. Levine, MD, and Committee on Adolescence

ABSTRACT. The American Academy of Pediatrics issued its last statement on homosexuality and adolescents in 2004. This technical report reflects the rapidly expanding medical and psychosocial literature about sexual minority youth. Pediatricians should be aware that some youth in their care may have concerns or questions about their sexual orientation or that of siblings, friends, parents, relatives, or others and should provide factual, current, nonjudgmental information in a confidential manner. Although most lesbian, gay, bisexual, transgender, and questioning (LGBTQ) youth are quite resilient and emerge from adolescence as healthy adults, the effects of homophobia and heterosexism can contribute to increased mental health issues for sexual minority youth. LGBTQ and MSM/WSW (men having sex with men and women having sex with women) adolescents, in comparison with heterosexual adolescents, have higher rates of depression and suicidal ideation, higher rates of substance abuse, and more risky sexual behaviors. Obtaining a comprehensive, confidential, developmentally appropriate adolescent psychosocial history allows for the discovery of strengths and assets as well as risks. Pediatricians should have offices that are teen-friendly and welcoming to sexual minority youth. This includes having supportive, engaging office staff members who ensure that there are no barriers to care. For transgender youth, pediatricians should provide the opportunity to acknowledge and affirm their feelings of gender dysphoria and desires to transition to the opposite gender. Referral of transgender youth

to a qualified mental health professional is critical to assist with the dysphoria, to educate them, and to assess their readiness for transition. With appropriate assistance and care, sexual minority youth should live healthy, productive lives while transitioning through adolescence and young adulthood. (6/13, reaffirmed 4/21)
https://doi.org/10.1542/peds.2013-1283

OLDER INFANT-YOUNG CHILD "FORMULAS" (CLINICAL REPORT)

George J. Fuchs, III, MD, FAAP; Steven A. Abrams, MD, FAAP; A. Adjowa Amevor, MD, FAAP; and Committee on Nutrition

ABSTRACT. The category of "formulas" directed at older infants and toddlers 6 to 36 months of age has increased in prominence over the last years but is characterized by lack of standardization in nomenclature and composition as well as questionable marketing practices. There has been uncertainty and misperception regarding some of the roles of these beverages in ensuring adequate childhood nutrition. The aim of this clinical report is to review the context, evidence, and rationale for older infant-young child formulas, followed by recommendations. (10/23)
https://doi.org/10.1542/peds.2023-064050

OPTIMIZING ADVANCED IMAGING OF THE PEDIATRIC PATIENT IN THE EMERGENCY DEPARTMENT

Jennifer R. Marin, MD, MSc, FAAP, FACEP; Todd W. Lyons, MD, MPH, FAAP; Ilene Claudius, MD, FACEP; Mary E. Fallat, MD, FAAP, FACS; Michael Aquino, MD; Timothy Ruttan, MD, FACEP, FAAP; Reza J. Daugherty, MD, FAAP; Committee on Pediatric Emergency Medicine; and Section on Radiology (joint with American College of Radiology and American College of Emergency Physicians Pediatric Emergency Medicine Committee)

ABSTRACT. Advanced imaging, including ultrasonography, computed tomography, and magnetic resonance imaging, is an integral component to the evaluation and management of ill and injured children in the emergency department. As with any test or intervention, the benefits and potential impacts on management must be weighed against the risks to ensure that high-value care is being delivered. There are important considerations specific to the pediatric patient related to the ordering and interpretation of advanced imaging. This policy statement provides guidelines for institutions and those who care for children to optimize the use of advanced imaging in the emergency department setting and was coauthored by experts in pediatric and general emergency medicine, pediatric radiology, and pediatric surgery. The intent is to guide decision-making where children may access care. (6/24)
https://doi.org/10.1542/peds.2024-066854

OPTIMIZING ADVANCED IMAGING OF THE PEDIATRIC PATIENT IN THE EMERGENCY DEPARTMENT (TECHNICAL REPORT)

Jennifer R. Marin, MD, MSc, FAAP, FACEP; Todd W. Lyons, MD, MPH, FAAP; Ilene Claudius, MD, FACEP; Mary E. Fallat, MD, FAAP, FACS; Michael Aquino, MD; Timothy Ruttan, MD, FACEP, FAAP; Reza J. Daugherty, MD, FAAP; Committee on Pediatric Emergency Medicine; and Section on Radiology (joint with American College of Radiology and American College of Emergency Physicians Pediatric Emergency Medicine Committee)

ABSTRACT. Advanced diagnostic imaging modalities, including ultrasonography, computed tomography, and magnetic resonance imaging, are key components in the evaluation and management of pediatric patients presenting to the emergency department. Advances in imaging technology have led to the availability of faster and more accurate tools to improve patient care. Notwithstanding these advances, it is important for physicians, physician assistants, and nurse practitioners to understand the risks and limitations associated with advanced imaging in children and to limit imaging studies that are considered low value, when possible. This technical report provides a summary of imaging strategies for specific conditions where advanced imaging is commonly considered in the emergency department. As an accompaniment to the policy statement, this document provides resources and strategies to optimize advanced imaging, including clinical decision support mechanisms, teleradiology, shared decision-making, and rationale for deferred imaging for patients who will be transferred for definitive care. (6/24)
https://doi.org/10.1542/peds.2024-066855

OPTIMIZING PEDIATRIC PATIENT SAFETY IN THE EMERGENCY CARE SETTING

Madeline M. Joseph, MD, FAAP, FACEP; Prashant Mahajan, MD, MPH, MBA; Sally K. Snow, BSN, RN, CPEN, FAEN; Brandon C. Ku, MD; Mohsen Saidinejad, MD, MS, MBA; and Committee on Pediatric Emergency Medicine (joint with American College of Emergency Physicians Pediatric Emergency Medicine Committee and Emergency Nurses Association Pediatric Committee)

ABSTRACT. This is a revision of the previous American Academy of Pediatrics policy statement titled "Patient Safety in the Emergency Care Setting," and is the first joint policy statement by the American Academy of Pediatrics, the American College of Emergency Physicians, and the Emergency Nurses Association to address pediatric patient safety in the emergency care setting. Caring for children in the emergency setting can be prone to medical errors because of a number of environmental and human factors. The emergency department (ED) has frequent workflow interruptions, multiple care transitions, and barriers to effective communication. In addition, the high volume of patients, high-decision density under time pressure, diagnostic uncertainty, and limited knowledge of patients' history and preexisting conditions make the safe care of critically ill and injured patients even more challenging. It is critical that all EDs, including general EDs who care for the majority of ill and injured children, understand the unique safety issues related to children. Furthermore, it is imperative that all EDs practice patient safety principles, support a culture of safety, and adopt best practices to improve safety for all children seeking emergency care. This policy statement outlines the recommendations necessary for EDs to minimize pediatric medical errors and to provide safe care for children of all ages. (10/22)
https://doi.org/10.1542/peds.2022-059673

OPTIMIZING PEDIATRIC PATIENT SAFETY IN THE EMERGENCY CARE SETTING (TECHNICAL REPORT)

Madeline M. Joseph, MD, FAAP, FACEP; Prashant Mahajan, MD, MPH, MBA; Sally K. Snow, BSN, RN, CPEN, FAEN; Brandon C. Ku, MD; Mohsen Saidinejad, MD, MS, MBA; and Committee on Pediatric Emergency Medicine (joint with American College of Emergency Physicians Pediatric Emergency Medicine Committee and Emergency Nurses Association Pediatric Committee)

ABSTRACT. Patient safety is the foundation of high-quality health care and remains a critical priority for all clinicians caring for children. There are numerous aspects of pediatric care that increase the risk of patient harm, including but not limited to risk from medication errors attributable to weight-dependent dosing and need for appropriate equipment and training. Of note, the majority of children who are ill and injured are brought to community hospital emergency departments. It is, therefore, imperative that all emergency departments practice patient safety principles, support a culture of safety, and adopt best practices to improve safety for all children seeking emergency care. This technical report outlined the challenges and resources necessary to minimize pediatric medical errors and to provide safe medical care for children of all ages in emergency care settings. (10/22)
https://doi.org/10.1542/peds.2022-059674

OPTIONS COUNSELING FOR THE PREGNANT ADOLESCENT PATIENT

Committee on Adolescence

ABSTRACT. Although teenage pregnancy rates have decreased over the past 30 years, many adolescents become pregnant every year. It is important for pediatricians to have the ability and the resources to make a timely pregnancy diagnosis in their adolescent patients and provide them with nonjudgmental counseling that includes the full range of pregnancy options. Counseling includes an unbiased discussion of the adolescent's options to continue or terminate the pregnancy, supporting the adolescent in the decision-making process, and referring the adolescent to appropriate resources and services. It is important for pediatricians to be familiar with laws and policies impacting access to abortion care, especially for minor adolescents, as well as laws that seek to limit health care professionals' provision of unbiased pregnancy options counseling and referrals, either for abortion care or continuation of pregnancy in accordance with the adolescent's choice. Pediatricians who choose not to provide such discussions should promptly refer pregnant adolescent patients to a health care professional who will offer developmentally appropriate pregnancy options counseling that includes the full range of pregnancy options. Pediatricians should be aware of and oppose policies that restrict their ability to provide pregnant adolescents with unbiased counseling that includes the full range of pregnancy options. This approach to pregnancy options counseling has not changed since the original 1989 American Academy of Pediatrics statement on this issue. (8/22)

https://doi.org/10.1542/peds.2022-058781

ORAL AND DENTAL ASPECTS OF CHILD ABUSE AND NEGLECT (CLINICAL REPORT)

Anupama Rao Tate, DMD, MPH; Susan A. Fisher-Owens, MD, MPH, FAAP; Lora Spiller, MD, FAAP; Jillian Muhlbauer, DMD; James L. Lukefahr, MD, FAAP; Section on Oral Health; and Council on Child Abuse and Neglect

ABSTRACT. In all 50 states, the District of Columbia, and the Commonwealth of Puerto Rico, pediatricians, dental professionals, and other physicians are mandated to report suspected cases of abuse and neglect to social service or law enforcement agencies. The purpose of this clinical report is to review the oral aspects of abuse and dental neglect in children and the role of pediatricians, dental professionals, and other physicians in evaluating such conditions. This clinical report addresses recommendations on the evaluation of bite marks, as well as perioral and intraoral injuries, infections, and diseases that may raise suspicion for child abuse or neglect. Some physicians may have received less education pertaining to oral health, dental injury, and oral disease. These physicians may not detect the mouth and gum findings possibly related to abuse or neglect as readily as abuse injuries involving other areas of the body. Therefore, pediatricians, dental professionals, and other physicians are encouraged to collaborate to increase the prevention, detection, and treatment of these conditions in children. (8/24)

https://doi.org/10.1542/peds.2024-068024

ORAL HEALTH CARE FOR CHILDREN AND YOUTH WITH DEVELOPMENTAL DISABILITIES (CLINICAL REPORT)

Elise Sarvas, DDS, MSD, MPH; Jessica Webb, DDS, MSD, MA, MSRT; Mary Landrigan-Ossar, MD, PhD, FAAP; Larry Yin, MD, MSPH, FAAP; Section on Oral Health; Council on Children With Disabilities; and Section on Anesthesiology and Pain Medicine

ABSTRACT. Oral health is an essential component of overall health for all individuals. The oral health of children and youth with developmental disabilities (CYDD) involves unique characteristics and needs of which pediatricians and pediatric clinicians can be aware. Risk for oral disease in CYDD is multifactorial and includes underlying medical conditions, medications, and ability to participate in preventive oral health care and treatment, and lack of access to providers is common for this population despite being eligible for Medicaid. Pediatric clinicians are uniquely positioned to support the oral health needs of CYDD and their families through the medical home. This clinical report aims to inform pediatric clinicians about the unique oral health needs of CYDD. It provides guidance on assessing caries risk and periodontal status using structured screening instruments; understanding dental trauma, the role of diet and caries risk, trauma prevention, and malocclusion; and providing anticipatory guidance on oral hygiene that includes tooth brushing, use of fluoridated toothpaste, assessing community water fluoridation, advocating for a dental home by 1 year of age, and transition to adult dental care as part of adolescent health care. It also highlights special considerations for dental treatment rendered under sedation or general anesthesia that CYDD may need. Pediatric clinicians can help reduce risk of CYDD developing dental disease by understanding the unique needs of their patients and their barriers to accessing oral health care in their community, communicating with the child's dental home, and advocating for safe and accessible dental procedures. (7/24)

https://doi.org/10.1542/peds.2024-067603

ORGANIZED SPORTS FOR CHILDREN, PREADOLESCENTS, AND ADOLESCENTS (CLINICAL REPORT)

Kelsey Logan, MD, MPH, FAAP; Steven Cuff, MD, FAAP; and Council on Sports Medicine and Fitness

ABSTRACT. Interest and participation in organized sports for children, preadolescents, and adolescents continue to grow. Because of increased participation, and younger entry age, in organized sports, appropriate practice, game schedules, and content become more important, taking into account athlete developmental stage and skills. Parental support for organized sports in general, with focus on development and fun instead of winning, has emerged as a key factor in the athlete's enjoyment of sports. Schools and community sports organizations who support multiple levels of sport (eg, recreational, competitive, elite) can include more youth who want to play sports and combat sport dropout. This report reviews the benefits and risks of organized sports as well as the roles of schools, community organizations, parents, and coaches in organized sports. It is designed to complement the American Academy of Pediatrics clinical reports "Physical Activity Assessment and Counseling in Pediatric Clinical Settings" and "Sports Specialization and Intensive Training in Young Athletes" by reviewing relevant literature on healthy organized sports for youth and providing guidance on organized sport readiness and entry. The report also provides guidance for pediatricians on counseling parents and advocating for healthy organized sports participation. (5/19, reaffirmed 7/23)

https://doi.org/10.1542/peds.2019-0997

OUT-OF-HOME PLACEMENT FOR CHILDREN AND ADOLESCENTS WITH DISABILITIES (CLINICAL REPORT)

Sandra L. Friedman, MD, MPH, FAAP; Miriam A. Kalichman, MD, FAAP; and Council on Children With Disabilities

ABSTRACT. The vast majority of children and youth with chronic and complex health conditions who also have intellectual and developmental disabilities are cared for in their homes. Social, legal, policy, and medical changes through the years have allowed for an increase in needed support within the community. However, there continues to be a relatively small group of children who live in various types of congregate care settings. This clinical report describes these settings and the care and services that are provided in them. The report also discusses rea-

sons families choose out-of-home placement for their children, barriers to placement, and potential effects of this decision on family members. We examine the pediatrician's role in caring for children with severe intellectual and developmental disabilities and complex medical problems in the context of responding to parental inquiries about out-of-home placement and understanding factors affecting these types of decisions. Common medical problems and care issues for children residing outside the family home are reviewed. Variations in state and federal regulations, challenges in understanding local systems, and access to services are also discussed. (9/14, reaffirmed 2/19, 11/24)
https://doi.org/10.1542/peds.2014-2279

OUT-OF-HOME PLACEMENT FOR CHILDREN AND ADOLESCENTS WITH DISABILITIES—ADDENDUM: CARE OPTIONS FOR CHILDREN AND ADOLESCENTS WITH DISABILITIES AND MEDICAL COMPLEXITY (CLINICAL REPORT)

Sandra L. Friedman, MD, MPH, FAAP; Kenneth W. Norwood Jr, MD, FAAP; and Council on Children With Disabilities

ABSTRACT. Children and adolescents with significant intellectual and developmental disabilities and complex medical problems require safe and comprehensive care to meet their medical and psychosocial needs. Ideally, such children and youth should be cared for by their families in their home environments. When this type of arrangement is not possible, there should be exploration of appropriate, alternative noncongregate community-based settings, especially alternative family homes. Government funding sources exist to support care in the community, although there is variability among states with regard to the availability of community programs and resources. It is important that families are supported in learning about options of care. Pediatricians can serve as advocates for their patients and their families to access community-based services and to increase the availability of resources to ensure that the option to live in a family home is available to all children with complex medical needs. (11/16, reaffirmed 2/19, 11/24)
https://doi.org/10.1542/peds.2016-3216

OVERUSE INJURIES, OVERTRAINING, AND BURNOUT IN YOUNG ATHLETES (CLINICAL REPORT)

Joel S. Brenner, MD, MPH, FAAP; Andrew Watson, MD, MS, FAAP; and Council on Sports Medicine and Fitness

ABSTRACT. Sports participation can have tremendous physical and mental health benefits for children. Properly implemented progressive training programs can yield a broad range of beneficial physiologic adaptations, but imbalances of training load and recovery can have important negative consequences. Overuse injuries, for example, can result from repetitive stress without sufficient recovery that leads to accumulated musculoskeletal damage. In addition, extended periods of increased training loads that exceed the intervening recovery can have systemic consequences such as overtraining syndrome, which results in decreased performance, increased injury and illness risk, and derangement of endocrine, neurologic, cardiovascular, and psychological systems. Burnout represents one of the primary reasons for attrition in youth sports. Broadly defined as physical or mental exhaustion and a reduced sense of accomplishment that leads to devaluation of sport, burnout represents a direct threat to the goal of lifelong physical activity and the wide-ranging health benefits that it provides. This clinical report is intended to provide pediatricians with information regarding the risk factors, diagnosis, management, and prevention of these conditions to assist in the identification of at-risk children, the treatment of young athletes, and the guidance of families in the promotion of safe and healthy sport participation. (1/24)
https://doi.org/10.1542/peds.2023-065129

OXYGEN TARGETING IN EXTREMELY LOW BIRTH WEIGHT INFANTS (CLINICAL REPORT)

James J. Cummings, MD; Richard A. Polin, MD; Committee on Fetus and Newborn

ABSTRACT. The use of supplemental oxygen plays a vital role in the care of the critically ill preterm infant, but the unrestricted use of oxygen can lead to unintended harms, such as chronic lung disease and retinopathy of prematurity. An overly restricted use of supplemental oxygen may have adverse effects as well. Ideally, continuous monitoring of tissue and cellular oxygen delivery would allow clinicians to better titrate the use of supplemental oxygen, but such monitoring is not currently feasible in the clinical setting. The introduction of pulse oximetry has greatly aided the clinician by providing a relatively easy and continuous estimate of arterial oxygen saturation, but pulse oximetry has several practical, technical, and physiologic limitations. Recent randomized clinical trials comparing different pulse oximetry targets have been conducted to better inform the practice of supplemental oxygen use. This clinical report discusses the benefits and limitations of pulse oximetry for assessing oxygenation, summarizes randomized clinical trials of oxygen saturation targeting, and addresses implications for practice. (8/16, reaffirmed 9/23)
https://doi.org/10.1542/peds.2016-1576

PAID FAMILY AND MEDICAL LEAVE

Christiane E. L. Dammann, MD; Kimberly Montez, MD, MPH; Mala Mathur, MD, MPH; Sherri L. Alderman, MD, MPH, IMHM-E; Maya Bunik, MD, MPH; Council on Community Pediatrics; Council on Early Childhood; Section on Breastfeeding; and Section on Neonatal Perinatal Medicine

ABSTRACT. Paid family and medical leave (PFML) helps parents balance the competing obligations of work, personal illness, and family. PFML is needed when adding a new member of the family or when a family member or individual becomes acutely or chronically ill. The United States lacks universally available PFML, despite the benefits for child and family health and well-being. Universally available PFML is a key component of improving the health of children and families and is critically needed in the United States. (10/24)
https://doi.org/10.1542/peds.2024-068958

PAIN ASSESSMENT AND TREATMENT IN CHILDREN WITH SIGNIFICANT IMPAIRMENT OF THE CENTRAL NERVOUS SYSTEM (CLINICAL REPORT)

Julie Hauer, MD, FAAP; Amy J. Houtrow, MD, PhD, MPH, FAAP; Section on Hospice and Palliative Medicine; and Council on Children With Disabilities

ABSTRACT. Pain is a frequent and significant problem for children with impairment of the central nervous system, with the highest frequency and severity occurring in children with the greatest impairment. Despite the significance of the problem, this population remains vulnerable to underrecognition and undertreatment of pain. Barriers to treatment may include uncertainty in identifying pain along with limited experience and fear with the use of medications for pain treatment. Behavioral pain-assessment tools are reviewed in this clinical report, along with other strategies for monitoring pain after an intervention. Sources of pain in this population include acute-onset pain attributable to tissue injury or inflammation resulting in nociceptive pain, with pain then expected to resolve after treatment directed at the source. Other sources can result in chronic intermittent pain that, for many, occurs on a weekly to daily basis, commonly attributed to gastroesophageal reflux, spasticity, and hip subluxation. Most challenging are pain sources attributable to the impaired central nervous system, requiring empirical medication trials directed at causes that cannot be identified by

diagnostic tests, such as central neuropathic pain. Interventions reviewed include integrative therapies and medications, such as gabapentinoids, tricyclic antidepressants, α-agonists, and opioids. This clinical report aims to address, with evidence-based guidance, the inherent challenges with the goal to improve comfort throughout life in this vulnerable group of children. (5/17, reaffirmed 11/21 with reference & data updates)
https://doi.org/10.1542/peds.2017-1002

PARENTAL LEAVE FOR RESIDENTS AND PEDIATRIC TRAINING PROGRAMS

Jennifer Takagishi, MD, FAAP; Katiana Garagozlo, MD; Council on Early Childhood; and Section on Pediatric Trainees

ABSTRACT. Residency and fellowship are unique occupational time periods for many early career physicians, generally consisting of long duty hours. Many early career physicians have or are in the process of building their families during this time period. The literature suggests many medical and psychosocial benefits of protected parental leave for both parents and children, which necessitates parental leaves of absence. The Institutional Requirements of the Accreditation Council for Graduate Medical Education require training programs to provide written policies regarding leaves of absence, including parental leave, and these policies must comply with current legislation such as the Family Medical Leave Act. The length of leave has considerable variability among residency programs. This policy statement aims to navigate and outline the challenges of parental leave policies in training programs and to put forth recommendations to protect trainees and their families. The definition of families should also be expanded to include all types of families. (2/22)
https://doi.org/10.1542/peds.2021-055988

PATENT DUCTUS ARTERIOSUS IN PRETERM INFANTS (CLINICAL REPORT)

Namasivayam Ambalavanan, MD; Susan W. Aucott, MD; Arash Salavitabar, MD; Victor Y. Levy, MD; Committee on Fetus and Newborn; and Section on Cardiology and Cardiac Surgery

ABSTRACT. Despite extensive research in basic science and in clinical settings with thousands of infants over decades, uncertainty and controversy persist regarding the significance, assessment, and management of the patent ductus arteriosus (PDA) in preterm infants, resulting in substantial variability in clinical approach. This clinical report aims to succinctly review the available evidence to guide evaluation and treatment of preterm infants with prolonged ductal patency. Delayed closure of the PDA is common in preterm infants, particularly at more extreme immaturity. Echocardiography is essential for confirming the presence of a PDA and assessing hemodynamic significance. Medical closure of a PDA using ibuprofen or acetaminophen is an option for a hemodynamically significant PDA (hsPDA). Recent data from multiple clinical trials indicate the lack of benefits of prophylactic or early (<2 weeks of age) medical closure of PDA as compared with expectant management, and they are, therefore, not recommended. There are insufficient data to support firm recommendations on management of infants with an hsPDA beyond 2 weeks of age as relative benefits and risks of expectant management with close monitoring, attempted pharmacologic closure, or procedural (transcatheter/surgical) closure have not been adequately defined. Many clinicians attempt medical closure of an hsPDA beyond 2 weeks of age. If the hsPDA persists despite medical therapy (or if medical therapy is contraindicated), such infants may be considered for either transcatheter closure or surgical ligation. In recent years, surgical closure of the PDA has become less frequent, and transcatheter closure is more common in many centers. Although there are known adverse effects of an hsPDA, there is a lack of evidence to guide management, necessitating equipoise regarding treatment options and timing and a need for trials that can expand the available body of evidence, especially regarding long-term cardiopulmonary and neurodevelopmental outcomes. (4/25)
See full text on page 413.
https://doi.org/10.1542/peds.2025-071425

PATIENT- AND FAMILY-CENTERED CARE COORDINATION: A FRAMEWORK FOR INTEGRATING CARE FOR CHILDREN AND YOUTH ACROSS MULTIPLE SYSTEMS

Council on Children With Disabilities and Medical Home Implementation Project Advisory Committee

ABSTRACT. Understanding a care coordination framework, its functions, and its effects on children and families is critical for patients and families themselves, as well as for pediatricians, pediatric medical subspecialists/surgical specialists, and anyone providing services to children and families. Care coordination is an essential element of a transformed American health care delivery system that emphasizes optimal quality and cost outcomes, addresses family-centered care, and calls for partnership across various settings and communities. High-quality, cost-effective health care requires that the delivery system include elements for the provision of services supporting the coordination of care across settings and professionals. This requirement of supporting coordination of care is generally true for health systems providing care for all children and youth but especially for those with special health care needs. At the foundation of an efficient and effective system of care delivery is the patient-/family-centered medical home. From its inception, the medical home has had care coordination as a core element. In general, optimal outcomes for children and youth, especially those with special health care needs, require interfacing among multiple care systems and individuals, including the following: medical, social, and behavioral professionals; the educational system; payers; medical equipment providers; home care agencies; advocacy groups; needed supportive therapies/services; and families. Coordination of care across settings permits an integration of services that is centered on the comprehensive needs of the patient and family, leading to decreased health care costs, reduction in fragmented care, and improvement in the patient/family experience of care. (4/14, reaffirmed 4/23)
https://doi.org/10.1542/peds.2014-0318

PEDIATRIC ACUTE-ONSET NEUROPSYCHIATRIC SYNDROME (PANS) (CLINICAL REPORT)

American Academy of Pediatrics

INTRODUCTION AND BACKGROUND. The sudden onset of severe behavioral and neuropsychiatric symptoms in children is a frightening and potentially life-changing situation. The pediatric health care providers and clinicians to whom families turn need guidance on how to accurately diagnose and treat new-onset neuropsychiatric symptoms in children. They need expert guidance about whether these symptoms indicate a diagnosis compatible with pediatric acute-onset neuropsychiatric syndrome (PANS). The cause of PANS is unknown, but it is theorized to be triggered, in some cases, by a recent infection and/or autoimmunity issues (similar to Sydenham chorea, autoimmune encephalitis [AE], and Guillain-Barré syndrome). The condition is challenging from a clinical perspective, because it lacks disease-specific biomarkers, strong evidence for pathogenic causes, and consensus on treatment of clinical symptoms. Further, the evidence base for PANS encompasses multiple subspecialties, including child and adolescent psychiatry, pediatric rheumatology, pediatric neurology, pediatric infectious diseases, pediatric immunology, and developmental-behavioral pediatrics.

Given this complexity, there is a clear need for guidance and advice for pediatric clinicians and the families they serve and support. To that end, with the encouragement of the Board of Directors, the American Academy of Pediatrics (AAP) has developed this clinical report. It focuses primarily on PANS, an umbrella condition that encompasses pediatric autoimmune neuropsychiatric disorders associated with streptococcal infections (PANDAS). Although PANDAS is, by definition, associated with streptococcal infection, it is now considered by many to represent a subset of the larger spectrum of infection-induced acute-onset neuropsychiatric symptoms. This clinical report was developed after a comprehensive literature review and analysis of the findings. Because they are limited by the present level of evidence on the topic, the findings are presented as a report rather than a clinical practice guideline. The contents are intended to aid the pediatric health care provider in evaluating, diagnosing, and treating sudden-onset and severe behavioral changes in children that could indicate potential PANS and in supporting these children and their families. (2/25)

See full text on page 429.

https://doi.org/10.1542/peds.2024-070334

PEDIATRIC MEDICATION SAFETY IN THE EMERGENCY DEPARTMENT

Lee Benjamin, MD, FAAP, FACEP; Karen Frush, MD, FAAP; Kathy Shaw, MD, MSCE, FAAP; Joan E. Shook, MD, MBA, FAAP; Sally K. Snow, BSN, RN, CPEN, FAEN; and Committee on Pediatric Emergency Medicine (joint with American College of Emergency Physicians Pediatric Emergency Medicine Committee and Emergency Nurses Association Pediatric Emergency Medicine Committee)

ABSTRACT. Pediatric patients cared for in emergency departments (EDs) are at high risk of medication errors for a variety of reasons. A multidisciplinary panel was convened by the Emergency Medical Services for Children program and the American Academy of Pediatrics Committee on Pediatric Emergency Medicine to initiate a discussion on medication safety in the ED. Top opportunities identified to improve medication safety include using kilogram-only weight-based dosing, optimizing computerized physician order entry by using clinical decision support, developing a standard formulary for pediatric patients while limiting variability of medication concentrations, using pharmacist support within EDs, enhancing training of medical professionals, systematizing the dispensing and administration of medications within the ED, and addressing challenges for home medication administration before discharge. (2/18, reaffirmed 9/23 with reference & data updates)

https://doi.org/10.1542/peds.2017-4066

PEDIATRIC METABOLIC AND BARIATRIC SURGERY: EVIDENCE, BARRIERS, AND BEST PRACTICES

Sarah C. Armstrong, MD, FAAP; Christopher F. Bolling, MD, FAAP; Marc P. Michalsky, MD, FACS, FAAP, FASMBS; Kirk W. Reichard, MD, MBA, FAAP, FACS; Section on Obesity; Section on Surgery

ABSTRACT. Severe obesity among youth is an "epidemic within an epidemic" and portends a shortened life expectancy for today's children compared with those of their parents' generation. Severe obesity has outpaced less severe forms of childhood obesity in prevalence, and it disproportionately affects adolescents. Emerging evidence has linked severe obesity to the development and progression of multiple comorbid states, including increased cardiometabolic risk resulting in end-organ damage in adulthood. Lifestyle modification treatment has achieved moderate short-term success among young children and those with less severe forms of obesity, but no studies to date demonstrate significant and durable weight loss among youth with severe obesity. Metabolic and bariatric surgery has emerged as an important treatment for adults with severe obesity and, more recently, has been shown to be a safe and effective strategy for groups of youth with severe obesity. However, current data suggest that youth with severe obesity may not have adequate access to metabolic and bariatric surgery, especially among underserved populations. This report outlines the current evidence regarding adolescent bariatric surgery, provides recommendations for practitioners and policy makers, and serves as a companion to an accompanying technical report, "Metabolic and Bariatric Surgery for Pediatric Patients With Severe Obesity," which provides details and supporting evidence. (11/19, reaffirmed 8/25 with reference & data updates)

https://doi.org/10.1542/peds.2019-3223

PEDIATRIC ORGAN DONATION AND TRANSPLANTATION: ACROSS THE CARE CONTINUUM

Benson Hsu, MD, MBA, FAAP, FCCM; Alexander Bondoc, MD, FAAP; Alex G. Cuenca, MD, PhD; Kristin Hittle Gigli, PhD, RN, CPNP-AC; Naomi Laventhal, MD, MA, HEC-C, FAAP; Thomas Nakagawa, MD, FAAP, FCCM; Committee on Hospital Care; Section on Critical Care; and Committee on Bioethics

ABSTRACT. This policy statement aims to enhance comfort and increase knowledge of pediatric organ donation and transplantation to the general pediatric community, specifically focusing on the pediatric health care professional and the medical home. The pediatric health care professional will care for neonates, infants, children, and adolescents who may become donors or transplant recipients and, thus, is a crucial member of the pediatric patient's care team. Understanding donation, transplantation, and follow-up care are important to primary care engagement. Furthermore, the pediatric health care professional may play a role in shaping public policies related to the process of organ donation and access to organ transplantation. (7/23)

https://doi.org/10.1542/peds.2023-062923

PEDIATRIC PRIMARY HEALTH CARE: THE CENTRAL ROLE OF PEDIATRICIANS IN MAINTAINING CHILDREN'S HEALTH IN EVOLVING HEALTH CARE MODELS

Alexy Boudreau, MD, FAAP; Alex Hamling, MD, FAAP; Edward Pont, MD, FAAP; Thomas W. Pendergrass, MD, MSPH, FAAP; Julia Richerson, MD, FAAP; Committee on Pediatric Workforce; and Committee on Practice and Ambulatory Medicine

ABSTRACT. Pediatric primary health care (PPHC) is of principal importance to the health and development of all children, helping them reach their true potential. Pediatricians, as the clinicians most intensively trained and experienced in child health, are the natural leaders of PPHC within the context of the medical home. Given the rapidly evolving models of pediatric health care delivery, including the explosion of telehealth in the wake of the COVID-19 pandemic, pediatricians, together with their representative national organizations such as the American Academy of Pediatrics (AAP), are the most capable clinicians to guide policy innovations on both the local and national stage. (1/22)

https://doi.org/10.1542/peds.2021-055553

PEDIATRIC READINESS IN THE EMERGENCY DEPARTMENT

Katherine Remick, MD, FAAP, FACEP, FAEMS; Marianne Gausche-Hill, MD, FAAP, FACEP, FAEMS; Madeline M. Joseph, MD, FAAP, FACEP; Kathleen Brown, MD, FAAP, FACEP; Sally K. Snow, BSN, RN, CPEN, FAEN; Joseph L. Wright, MD, MPH, FAAP; Committee on Pediatric Emergency Medicine; and Section on Surgery (joint with American College of Emergency Physicians Pediatric Emergency Medicine Committee and Emergency Nurses Association Pediatric Committee)

ABSTRACT. This is a revision of the previous joint Policy Statement titled "Guidelines for Care of Children in the Emergency Department." Children have unique physical and psychosocial needs that are heightened in the setting of serious

or life-threatening emergencies. The majority of children who are ill and injured are brought to community hospital emergency departments (EDs) by virtue of proximity. It is therefore imperative that all EDs have the appropriate resources (medications, equipment, policies, and education) and capable staff to provide effective emergency care for children. In this Policy Statement, we outline the resources necessary for EDs to stand ready to care for children of all ages. These recommendations are consistent with the recommendations of the Institute of Medicine (now called the National Academy of Medicine) in its report "The Future of Emergency Care in the US Health System." Although resources within emergency and trauma care systems vary locally, regionally, and nationally, it is essential that ED staff, administrators, and medical directors seek to meet or exceed these recommendations to ensure that high-quality emergency care is available for all children. These updated recommendations are intended to serve as a resource for clinical and administrative leadership in EDs as they strive to improve their readiness for children of all ages. (10/18, reaffirmed 1/24)
https://doi.org/10.1542/peds.2018-2459

THE PEDIATRICIAN'S ROLE IN PREVENTING CHILD MALTREATMENT (CLINICAL REPORT)

John Stirling, MD, FAAP; Amy Gavril, MD, MSCI, FAAP; Brian Brennan, MD, FAAP; Robert D. Sege, MD, PhD, FAAP; Howard Dubowitz, MD, MS, FAAP; and Council on Child Abuse and Neglect

ABSTRACT. Pediatricians have always seen the value of preventing health harms; this should be no less true for child maltreatment than for disease or unintentional injuries. Research continues to demonstrate that maltreatment can be prevented, underscoring the vital roles of both the family and society in healthy childhood development and the importance of strong, stable, nurturing relationships in preventing maltreatment and building the child's resilience to adversity. This clinical report elaborates the pediatrician's multitiered role in supporting relational health from infancy through adolescence, from universal interventions assessing for maltreatment risks and protective factors to targeted interventions addressing identified needs and building on strengths. When maltreatment has already occurred, interventions can prevent further victimization and mitigate long-term sequelae. Advice is provided on engaging community resources, including those that provide food, shelter, or financial support for families in need. (7/24)
https://doi.org/10.1542/peds.2024-067608

THE PEDIATRICIAN'S ROLE IN THE EVALUATION AND PREPARATION OF PEDIATRIC PATIENTS UNDERGOING ANESTHESIA

Section on Anesthesiology and Pain Medicine

ABSTRACT. Pediatricians play a key role in helping prepare patients and families for anesthesia and surgery. The questions to be answered by the pediatrician fall into 2 categories. The first involves preparation: is the patient in optimal medical condition for surgery, and are the patient and family emotionally and cognitively ready for surgery? The second category concerns logistics: what communication and organizational needs are necessary to enable safe passage through the perioperative process? This revised statement updates the recommendations for the pediatrician's role in the preoperative preparation of patients. (8/14, reaffirmed 2/21)
https://doi.org/10.1542/peds.2014-1840

PERINATAL URINARY TRACT DILATION: RECOMMENDATIONS ON PRE-/POSTNATAL IMAGING, PROPHYLACTIC ANTIBIOTICS, AND FOLLOW-UP (CLINICAL REPORT)

American Academy of Pediatrics
DEDICATED TO THE HEALTH OF ALL CHILDREN®

AAP Partnership for Policy Implementation

– *See Appendix 1*

C. D. Anthony Herndon, MD, FAAP; Hansel J. Otero, MD, FAAP; David Hains, MD, FAAP; Rebecca M. Sweeney, MD, FAAP; Gina M. Lockwood, MD, MS, FAAP; Section on Urology; Section on Nephrology; Section on Radiology; and Section on Hospital Medicine

ABSTRACT. Perinatal urinary tract dilation (UTD) occurs in approximately 1% of all pregnancies and represents the second most common congenital anomaly detected prenatally, second only to cardiac defects. Causes of UTD include transient dilation, vesicoureteral reflux (VUR) and genitourinary obstruction. A vast majority of these conditions will never require surgical intervention. However, a subset of patients will be at increased risk of urologic and kidney disease. The purpose of this clinical report will be to review the current imaging modalities used for the evaluation of perinatal UTD and discuss the risk stratification for UTD, the indications for prophylactic antibiotics, and the use of lower tract imaging and renal scintigraphy (RS). Ultimately, the management of these children is individualized and should involve a shared-decision making process between the physician and parent/guardian that is evidence based.

The evaluation and management of more severe forms of bilateral UTD in boys who are at high risk for bladder outlet obstruction is outside of the scope of this document. Any concern for this entity should prompt an immediate consultation with a nephrology/urology specialist. (6/25)

See full text on page 445.
https://doi.org/10.1542/peds.2025-071814

PHOTOTHERAPY TO PREVENT SEVERE NEONATAL HYPERBILIRUBINEMIA IN THE NEWBORN INFANT 35 OR MORE WEEKS OF GESTATION (TECHNICAL REPORT)

Vinod K. Bhutani, MD, FAAP; Ronald J. Wong, PhD; David Turkewitz, MD, FAAP; Daniel A. Rauch, MD, FAAP; Meredith E. Mowitz, MD, MS, FAAP; Wanda D. Barfield, MD, MPH, FAAP; and Committee on Fetus and Newborn

OBJECTIVE. To summarize the principles and application of phototherapy consistent with the current 2022 American Academy of Pediatrics "Clinical Practice Guideline Revision for the Management of Hyperbilirubinemia in the Newborn Infant 35 or More Weeks of Gestation." (8/24)
https://doi.org/10.1542/peds.2024-068026

PHYSICAL ACTIVITY ASSESSMENT AND COUNSELING IN PEDIATRIC CLINICAL SETTINGS (CLINICAL REPORT)

Felipe Lobelo, MD, PhD; Natalie D. Muth, MD, MPH, FAAP, FACSM; Sara Hanson, PhD; Blaise A. Nemeth, MD, FAAP; Council on Sports Medicine and Fitness; and Section on Obesity

ABSTRACT. Physical activity plays an important role in children's cardiovascular health, musculoskeletal health, mental and behavioral health, and physical, social, and cognitive development. Despite the importance in children's lives, pediatricians are unfamiliar with assessment and guidance regarding physical activity in children. With the release of the 2018 Physical Activity Guidelines by the US Department of Health and Human Services, pediatricians play a critical role in encouraging physical activity in children through assessing physical activity and physical literacy; providing guidance toward meeting recommendations by children and their families; advocating for opportunities for physical activity for all children in schools, communities, and hospitals; setting an example and remaining physically active personally; advocating for the use of assessment tools and insurance coverage of physical activity

and physical literacy screening; and incorporating physical activity assessment and prescription in medical school curricula. (2/20, reaffirmed 11/24 with reference & data updates)
https://doi.org/10.1542/peds.2019-3992

PHYSICIAN HEALTH AND WELLNESS (CLINICAL REPORT)

Hilary H. McClafferty, MD, FAAP; Dena K. Hubbard, MD, FAAP; Dana Foradori, MD, MEd, FAAP; Melanie L. Brown, MD, MSE, FAAP; Jochen Profit, MD, MPH, FAAP; Daniel S. Tawfik, MD, MS, FAAP; and Section on Integrative Medicine

ABSTRACT. Physician health and wellness is a complex topic relevant to all pediatricians. Survey studies have established that pediatricians experience burnout at comparable rates to colleagues across medical specialties. Prevalence of burnout increased for all pediatric disciplines from 2011 to 2014. During that time, general pediatricians experienced a more than 10% increase in burnout, from 35.3% to 46.3%. Pediatric medical subspecialists and pediatric surgical specialists experienced slightly higher baseline rates of burnout in 2011 and similarly increased to just under 50%. Women currently constitute a majority of pediatricians, and surveys report a 20% to 60% higher prevalence of burnout in women physicians compared with their male counterparts. The purpose of this report is to update the reader and explore approaches to pediatrician well-being and reduction of occupational burnout risk throughout the stages of training and practice. Topics covered include burnout prevalence and diagnosis; overview of national progress in physician wellness; update on physician wellness initiatives at the American Academy of Pediatrics; an update on pediatric-specific burnout and well-being; recognized drivers of burnout (organizational and individual); a review of the intersection of race, ethnicity, gender, and burnout; protective factors; and components of wellness (organizational and individual). The development of this clinical report has inevitably been shaped by the social, cultural, public health, and economic factors currently affecting our communities. The coronavirus disease 2019 (COVID-19) pandemic has layered new and significant stressors onto medical practice with physical, mental, and logistical challenges and effects that cannot be ignored. (10/22)
https://doi.org/10.1542/peds.2022-059665

POSTNATAL CORD BLOOD SAMPLING (CLINICAL REPORT)

David A. Kaufman, MD, FAAP; Ashley M. Lucke, MD, FAAP; James J. Cummings, MD, FAAP; and Committee on Fetus and Newborn

ABSTRACT. Blood contained in the umbilical cord after placental separation originates from the infant and can be used for neonatal blood sampling and testing after birth. The most common indications for phlebotomy after birth include care processes for any infant admitted to the neonatal intensive care unit, early-onset sepsis evaluations, and congenital anomalies. Postnatal umbilical cord blood sampling (PCBS), rather than obtaining blood from the neonate, avoids significant neonatal blood loss at a critical time of extrauterine transition and prevents phlebotomy pain in infants without a catheter for blood drawing. Studies of PCBS in very low birth weight infants have demonstrated additional benefits including stable blood pressure, less need for vasopressors and erythrocyte transfusions in the first week, and a potentially decreased risk for intracranial hemorrhage.

PCBS can be used for any full-term or preterm infant when the need for phlebotomy is known at or shorty after delivery. PCBS can be the first option and reliably used for complete blood cell counts, blood cultures, blood typing and crossmatching, newborn screening and metabolic tests, genetic testing, blood chemistries, and coagulation studies. Additionally, PCBS allows the collection of larger blood volumes for blood culture, thereby improving positivity rate. Finally, PCBS can be performed after delayed cord clamping or cord milking and in conjunction with research studies and/or cord blood banking. This report describes the evidence, safety, and methods for collecting cord blood after delivery. (5/25)

See full text on page 467.
https://doi.org/10.1542/peds.2025-071811

POVERTY AND CHILD HEALTH IN THE UNITED STATES

Council on Community Pediatrics

ABSTRACT. Almost half of young children in the United States live in poverty or near poverty. The American Academy of Pediatrics is committed to reducing and ultimately eliminating child poverty in the United States. Poverty and related social determinants of health can lead to adverse health outcomes in childhood and across the life course, negatively affecting physical health, socioemotional development, and educational achievement. The American Academy of Pediatrics advocates for programs and policies that have been shown to improve the quality of life and health outcomes for children and families living in poverty. With an awareness and understanding of the effects of poverty on children, pediatricians and other pediatric health practitioners in a family-centered medical home can assess the financial stability of families, link families to resources, and coordinate care with community partners. Further research, advocacy, and continuing education will improve the ability of pediatricians to address the social determinants of health when caring for children who live in poverty. Accompanying this policy statement is a technical report that describes current knowledge on child poverty and the mechanisms by which poverty influences the health and well-being of children. (3/16, reaffirmed 4/21)
https://doi.org/10.1542/peds.2016-0339

THE POWER OF PLAY: A PEDIATRIC ROLE IN ENHANCING DEVELOPMENT IN YOUNG CHILDREN (CLINICAL REPORT)

Michael Yogman, MD, FAAP; Andrew Garner, MD, PhD, FAAP; Jeffrey Hutchinson, MD, FAAP; Kathy Hirsh-Pasek, PhD; Roberta Michnick Golinkoff, PhD; Committee on Psychosocial Aspects of Child and Family Health; and Council on Communications and Media

ABSTRACT. Children need to develop a variety of skill sets to optimize their development and manage toxic stress. Research demonstrates that developmentally appropriate play with parents and peers is a singular opportunity to promote the social-emotional, cognitive, language, and self-regulation skills that build executive function and a prosocial brain. Furthermore, play supports the formation of the safe, stable, and nurturing relationships with all caregivers that children need to thrive.

Play is not frivolous: it enhances brain structure and function and promotes executive function (ie, the process of learning, rather than the content), which allow us to pursue goals and ignore distractions.

When play and safe, stable, nurturing relationships are missing in a child's life, toxic stress can disrupt the development of executive function and the learning of prosocial behavior; in the presence of childhood adversity, play becomes even more important. The mutual joy and shared communication and attunement (harmonious serve and return interactions) that parents and children can experience during play regulate the body's stress response. This clinical report provides pediatric providers with the information they need to promote the benefits of play and to write a prescription for play at well visits to complement reach out and read. At a time when early childhood programs are pressured to add more didactic components and less playful learning, pediatricians can play an important role in emphasizing the role of a balanced curriculum that includes the importance of

playful learning for the promotion of healthy child development. (8/18, reaffirmed 1/25)
https://doi.org/10.1542/peds.2018-2058

PRESCRIBING ASSISTIVE TECHNOLOGY: FOCUS ON CHILDREN WITH COMPLEX COMMUNICATION NEEDS (CLINICAL REPORT)

Larry W. Desch, MD, FAAP; Laura J. Hobart-Porter, DO, FAAP, FAAPMR; Amy Houtrow, MD, PhD, MPH, FAAP; and Council on Children With Disabilities

ABSTRACT. The primary care pediatrician and other pediatric physicians play a critical role in the interdisciplinary team effort to provide appropriate augmentative and alternative communication (AAC) technology to children with absent or severely impaired verbal communication, recently recategorized as a complex communication need. This clinical report describes the different types of AAC technology, the device assessment process, and the training required for successful integration into a child's communication. The report further describes the role of the pediatrician in acquisition and appropriate utilization of this technology with a focus on key specialists and funding sources. Decades of research confirm that use of AAC promotes language development; therefore, primary care physicians can reassure families that AAC will likely help their child to learn to communicate more effectively. There is an important need for key resources for AAC to be identified in every community; the majority of relevant professional organizations, including the American Academy of Pediatrics, recognize that these resources are a shared medical, educational, therapeutic, and family responsibility. (6/25)

See full text on page 477.
https://doi.org/10.1542/peds.2025-072216

PRESCRIBING PHYSICAL, OCCUPATIONAL, AND SPEECH THERAPY SERVICES FOR CHILDREN WITH DISABILITIES (CLINICAL REPORT)

Amy Houtrow, MD, PhD, MPH, FAAP, FAAPMR; Nancy Murphy, MD, FAAP, FAAPMR; and Council on Children With Disabilities

ABSTRACT. Pediatric health care providers are frequently responsible for prescribing physical, occupational, and speech therapies and monitoring therapeutic progress for children with temporary or permanent disabilities in their practices. This clinical report will provide pediatricians and other pediatric health care providers with information about how best to manage the therapeutic needs of their patients in the medical home by reviewing the International Classification of Functioning, Disability and Health; describing the general goals of habilitative and rehabilitative therapies; delineating the types, locations, and benefits of therapy services; and detailing how to write a therapy prescription and include therapists in the medical home neighborhood. (3/19, reaffirmed 7/23 with reference & data updates)
https://doi.org/10.1542/peds.2019-0285

PREVENTING CHILDHOOD TOXIC STRESS: PARTNERING WITH FAMILIES AND COMMUNITIES TO PROMOTE RELATIONAL HEALTH

Andrew Garner, MD, PhD, FAAP; Michael Yogman, MD, FAAP; Committee on Psychosocial Aspects of Child and Family Health; Section on Developmental and Behavioral Pediatrics; and Council on Early Childhood

ABSTRACT. By focusing on the safe, stable, and nurturing relationships (SSNRs) that buffer adversity and build resilience, pediatric care is on the cusp of a paradigm shift that could reprioritize clinical activities, rewrite research agendas, and realign our collective advocacy. Driving this transformation are advances in developmental sciences as they inform a deeper understanding of how early life experiences, both nurturing and adverse, are biologically embedded and influence outcomes in health, education, and economic stability across the life span. This revised policy statement on childhood toxic stress acknowledges a spectrum of potential adversities and reaffirms the benefits of an ecobiodevelopmental model for understanding the childhood origins of adult-manifested disease and wellness. It also endorses a paradigm shift toward relational health because SSNRs not only buffer childhood adversity when it occurs but also promote the capacities needed to be resilient in the future. To translate this relational health framework into clinical practice, generative research, and public policy, the entire pediatric community needs to adopt a public health approach that builds relational health by partnering with families and communities. This public health approach to relational health needs to be integrated both vertically (by including primary, secondary, and tertiary preventions) and horizontally (by including public service sectors beyond health care). The American Academy of Pediatrics asserts that SSNRs are biological necessities for all children because they mitigate childhood toxic stress responses and proactively build resilience by fostering the adaptive skills needed to cope with future adversity in a healthy manner. (7/21)
https://doi.org/10.1542/peds.2021-052582

PREVENTING EXCESSIVE NOISE EXPOSURE IN INFANTS, CHILDREN, AND ADOLESCENTS

Sophie J. Balk, MD, FAAP; Risa E. Bochner, MD, FAAP; Mahindra A. Ramdhanie, AuD, FAAA, CCC-A; Brian K. Reilly, MD, FAAP, FACS; Council on Environmental Health and Climate Change, and Section on Otolaryngology-Head and Neck Surgery

ABSTRACT. Noise affects people of all ages. Noise-induced hearing loss, a major problem for adults, is also a problem for young people. Sensorineural hearing loss is usually irreversible. Environmental noise, such as traffic noise, can affect learning, physiologic parameters, sleep, and quality of life. Children and adolescents have unique vulnerabilities. Infants and young children must rely on adults to remove them from noisy situations; children may not recognize hazardous noise exposures; teenagers often do not understand consequences of high exposure to music from personal listening devices or attending concerts and dances. Personal listening devices are increasingly used, even by small children. Environmental noise has disproportionate effects on underserved communities. This statement and its accompanying technical report review common sources and effects of noise as well as specific pediatric exposures. Because noise exposure often starts in infancy and effects are cumulative, more attention to noise in everyday activities is needed starting early in life. Pediatricians can potentially lessen harms by raising awareness of children's specific vulnerabilities to noise. Safer listening is possible. Noise exposure is underrecognized as a serious public health issue in the United States. Greater awareness of noise hazards is needed at a societal level. (10/23)
https://doi.org/10.1542/peds.2023-063752

PREVENTING EXCESSIVE NOISE EXPOSURE IN INFANTS, CHILDREN, AND ADOLESCENTS (TECHNICAL REPORT)

Sophie J. Balk, MD, FAAP; Risa E. Bochner, MD, FAAP; Mahindra A. Ramdhanie, AuD, FAAA, CCC-A; Brian K. Reilly, MD, FAAP, FACS; Council on Environmental Health and Climate Change, and Section on Otolaryngology-Head and Neck Surgery

ABSTRACT. Noise exposure is a major cause of hearing loss in adults. Yet, noise affects people of all ages, and noise-induced hearing loss is also a problem for young people. Sensorineural hearing loss caused by noise and other toxic exposures is usually irreversible. Environmental noise, such as traffic noise, can affect learning, physiologic parameters, and quality of life. Children and adolescents have unique vulnerabilities to noise. Children

may be exposed beginning in NICUs and well-baby nurseries, at home, at school, in their neighborhoods, and in recreational settings. Personal listening devices are increasingly used, even by small children. Infants and young children cannot remove themselves from noisy situations and must rely on adults to do so, children may not recognize hazardous noise exposures, and teenagers generally do not understand the consequences of high exposure to music from personal listening devices or attending concerts and dances. Environmental noise exposure has disproportionate effects on underserved communities. In this report and the accompanying policy statement, common sources of noise and effects on hearing at different life stages are reviewed. Noise-abatement interventions in various settings are discussed. Because noise exposure often starts in infancy and its effects result mainly from cumulative exposure to loud noise over long periods of time, more attention is needed to its presence in everyday activities starting early in life. Listening to music and attending dances, concerts, and celebratory and other events are sources of joy, pleasure, and relaxation for many people. These situations, however, often result in potentially harmful noise exposures. Pediatricians can potentially lessen exposures, including promotion of safer listening, by raising awareness in parents, children, and teenagers. Noise exposure is underrecognized as a serious public health issue in the United States, with exposure limits enforceable only in workplaces and not for the general public, including children and adolescents. Greater awareness of noise hazards is needed at a societal level. (10/23)
https://doi.org/10.1542/peds.2023-063753

PREVENTING HOME MEDICATION ADMINISTRATION ERRORS

H. Shonna Yin, MD, MSc, FAAP; Daniel R. Neuspiel, MD, MPH, FAAP; Ian M. Paul, MD, MSc, FAAP; Council on Quality Improvement and Patient Safety; and Committee on Drugs

ABSTRACT. Medication administration errors that take place in the home are common, especially when liquid preparations are used and complex medication schedules with multiple medications are involved; children with chronic conditions are disproportionately affected. Parents and other caregivers with low health literacy and/or limited English proficiency are at higher risk for making errors in administering medications to children in their care. Recommended strategies to reduce home medication errors relate to provider prescribing practices; health literacy–informed verbal counseling strategies (eg, teachback and showback) and written patient education materials (eg, pictographic information) for patients and/or caregivers across settings (inpatient, outpatient, emergency care, pharmacy); dosing-tool provision for liquid medication measurement; review of medication lists with patients and/or caregivers (medication reconciliation) that includes prescription and over-the-counter medications, as well as vitamins and supplements; leveraging the medical home; engaging adolescents and their adult caregivers; training of providers; safe disposal of medications; regulations related to medication dosing tools, labeling, packaging, and informational materials; use of electronic health records and other technologies; and research to identify novel ways to support safe home medication administration. (11/21)
https://doi.org/10.1542/peds.2021-054666

PREVENTING OBESITY AND EATING DISORDERS IN ADOLESCENTS (CLINICAL REPORT)

Neville H. Golden, MD, FAAP; Marcie Schneider, MD, FAAP; Christine Wood, MD, FAAP; Committee on Nutrition; Committee on Adolescence; and Section on Obesity

ABSTRACT. Obesity and eating disorders (EDs) are both prevalent in adolescents. There are concerns that obesity prevention efforts may lead to the development of an ED. Most adolescents who develop an ED did not have obesity previously, but some teenagers, in an attempt to lose weight, may develop an ED. This clinical report addresses the interaction between obesity prevention and EDs in teenagers, provides the pediatrician with evidence-informed tools to identify behaviors that predispose to both obesity and EDs, and provides guidance about obesity and ED prevention messages. The focus should be on a healthy lifestyle rather than on weight. Evidence suggests that obesity prevention and treatment, if conducted correctly, do not predispose to EDs. (8/16, reaffirmed 6/22)
https://doi.org/10.1542/peds.2016-1649

PREVENTION AND MANAGEMENT OF PROCEDURAL PAIN IN THE NEONATE: AN UPDATE

Committee on Fetus and Newborn and Section on Anesthesiology and Pain Medicine

ABSTRACT. The prevention of pain in neonates should be the goal of all pediatricians and health care professionals who work with neonates, not only because it is ethical but also because repeated painful exposures have the potential for deleterious consequences. Neonates at greatest risk of neurodevelopmental impairment as a result of preterm birth (ie, the smallest and sickest) are also those most likely to be exposed to the greatest number of painful stimuli in the NICU. Although there are major gaps in knowledge regarding the most effective way to prevent and relieve pain in neonates, proven and safe therapies are currently underused for routine minor, yet painful procedures. Therefore, every health care facility caring for neonates should implement (1) a pain-prevention program that includes strategies for minimizing the number of painful procedures performed and (2) a pain assessment and management plan that includes routine assessment of pain, pharmacologic and nonpharmacologic therapies for the prevention of pain associated with routine minor procedures, and measures for minimizing pain associated with surgery and other major procedures. (1/16, reaffirmed 7/20, 4/25)
https://doi.org/10.1542/peds.2015-4271

PREVENTION OF CHILDHOOD LEAD TOXICITY

Council on Environmental Health

ABSTRACT. Blood lead concentrations have decreased dramatically in US children over the past 4 decades, but too many children still live in housing with deteriorated lead-based paint and are at risk for lead exposure with resulting lead-associated cognitive impairment and behavioral problems. Evidence continues to accrue that commonly encountered blood lead concentrations, even those below 5 µg/dL (50 ppb), impair cognition; there is no identified threshold or safe level of lead in blood. From 2007 to 2010, approximately 2.6% of preschool children in the United States had a blood lead concentration ≥5 µg/dL (≥50 ppb), which represents about 535 000 US children 1 to 5 years of age. Evidence-based guidance is available for managing increased lead exposure in children, and reducing sources of lead in the environment, including lead in housing, soil, water, and consumer products, has been shown to be cost-beneficial. Primary prevention should be the focus of policy on childhood lead toxicity. (6/16, reaffirmed 4/21)
https://doi.org/10.1542/peds.2016-1493

PREVENTION OF DROWNING (TECHNICAL REPORT)

Sarah A. Denny, MD, FAAP; Linda Quan, MD, FAAP; Julie Gilchrist, MD, FAAP; Tracy McCallin, MD, FAAP; Rohit Shenoi, MD, FAAP; Shabana Yusuf, MD, Med, FAAP; Jeffrey Weiss, MD, FAAP; Benjamin Hoffman, MD, FAAP; and Council on Injury, Violence, and Poison Prevention

ABSTRACT. Drowning is a leading cause of injury-related death in children. In 2018, almost 900 US children younger than 20 years died of drowning. A number of strategies are available to prevent these tragedies. As educators and advocates, pediatri-

cians can play an important role in prevention of drowning. (7/21)
https://doi.org/10.1542/peds.2021-052227

PRIMARY CARE FRAMEWORK TO MONITOR PRETERM INFANTS FOR NEURO-DEVELOPMENTAL OUTCOMES IN EARLY CHILDHOOD (CLINICAL REPORT)

American Academy of Pediatrics
DEDICATED TO THE HEALTH OF ALL CHILDREN®
AAP Partnership for Policy Implementation
– *See Appendix 1*

Beth Ellen Davis, MD, MPH, FAAP; Mary O'Connor Leppert, MD, FAAP; Kendell German, MD, FAAP; Christoph U. Lehmann, MD, FAAP; Ira Adams-Chapman, MD, MPH, FAAP; Council on Children With Disabilities; and Committee on Fetus and Newborn

ABSTRACT. To support decision-making in the primary care medical home, this clinical report links preterm birth and perinatal complications to early childhood developmental disability risks. It consolidates extensive contemporary outcome research from 2005 onward into an easy-to-use framework and stratifies prematurity and NICU experiences by degree of risk for developmental impairments. This framework informs and prioritizes point-of-care screening and surveillance strategies for pediatricians caring for children born preterm, guides additional assessment and referral for appropriate therapies, and offers opportunities for reassurance (when applicable) in office settings. (6/23)
https://doi.org/10.1542/peds.2023-062511

PRINCIPLES OF CHILD HEALTH CARE FINANCING

Alison A. Galbraith, MD, MPH, FAAP; Jonathan Price, MD, FAAP; Claire Abraham, MD, FAAP; Angelo P. Giardino, MD, MPH, PhD, FAAP; and Committee on Child Health Financing

ABSTRACT. The American Academy of Pediatrics believes that the United States can and should ensure that all children, adolescents, and young adults from birth through the age of 26 years who reside within its borders have affordable access to high-quality comprehensive health care. Comprehensive, high-quality care addresses issues, challenges, and opportunities unique to children and young adults and addresses the effects of historic and present inequities. All families should have equitable access to professionals and facilities with expertise in the care of children within a reasonable distance of their residence. Payment methodologies should be structured to guarantee the economic viability of the pediatric medical home and of pediatric specialty and subspecialty practices. The recent increase in child uninsurance over the last several years is a threat to the well-being of children and families in the short- and long-term. Deficiencies in plans currently covering insured children pose similar threats. The AAP believes that the United States must not sacrifice recent hard-won gains for our children and that child health care financing should be based on the following guiding principles: (1) coverage with quality, affordable health insurance should be universal; (2) comprehensive pediatric services should be covered; (3) cost sharing should be affordable and should not negatively affect care; (4) payment should be adequate to strengthen family- and patient-centered medical homes; (5) child health financing policy should promote equity and address longstanding health and health care disparities; and (6) the unique characteristics and needs of children should be reflected. (8/23)
https://doi.org/10.1542/peds.2023-063283

PROBIOTICS AND PREBIOTICS IN PEDIATRICS (CLINICAL REPORT)

Dan W. Thomas, MD; Frank R. Greer, MD; Committee on Nutrition; and Section on Gastroenterology, Hepatology, and Nutrition

ABSTRACT. This clinical report reviews the currently known health benefits of probiotic and prebiotic products, including those added to commercially available infant formula and other food products for use in children. Probiotics are supplements or foods that contain viable microorganisms that cause alterations of the microflora of the host. Use of probiotics has been shown to be modestly effective in randomized clinical trials (RCTs) in (1) treating acute viral gastroenteritis in healthy children; and (2) preventing antibiotic-associated diarrhea in healthy children. There is some evidence that probiotics prevent necrotizing enterocolitis in very low birth weight infants (birth weight between 1000 and 1500 g), but more studies are needed. The results of RCTs in which probiotics were used to treat childhood *Helicobacter pylori* gastritis, irritable bowel syndrome, chronic ulcerative colitis, and infantile colic, as well as in preventing childhood atopy, although encouraging, are preliminary and require further confirmation. Probiotics have not been proven to be beneficial in treating or preventing human cancers or in treating children with Crohn disease. There are also safety concerns with the use of probiotics in infants and children who are immunocompromised, chronically debilitated, or seriously ill with indwelling medical devices.

Prebiotics are supplements or foods that contain a nondigestible food ingredient that selectively stimulates the favorable growth and/or activity of indigenous probiotic bacteria. Human milk contains substantial quantities of prebiotics. There is a paucity of RCTs examining prebiotics in children, although there may be some long-term benefit of prebiotics for the prevention of atopic eczema and common infections in healthy infants. Confirmatory well-designed clinical research studies are necessary. (11/10, reaffirmed 3/21)
https://doi.org/10.1542/peds.2010-2548

PROCEDURES FOR THE EVALUATION OF THE VISUAL SYSTEM BY PEDIATRICIANS (CLINICAL REPORT)

Sean P. Donahue, MD, PhD, FAAP; Cynthia N. Baker, MD, FAAP; Committee on Practice and Ambulatory Medicine; and Section on Ophthalmology (joint with American Association of Certified Orthoptists, American Association for Pediatric Ophthalmology and Strabismus, and American Academy of Ophthalmology)

ABSTRACT. Vision screening is crucial for the detection of visual and systemic disorders. It should begin in the newborn nursery and continue throughout childhood. This clinical report provides details regarding methods for pediatricians to use for screening. (12/15, reaffirmed 2/22)
https://doi.org/10.1542/peds.2015-3597

PROMOTING EDUCATION, MENTORSHIP, AND SUPPORT FOR PEDIATRIC RESEARCH

Committee on Pediatric Research

ABSTRACT. Pediatricians play a key role in advancing child health research to best attain and improve the physical, mental, and social health and well-being of all infants, children, adolescents, and young adults. Child health presents unique issues that require investigators who specialize in pediatric research. In addition, the scope of the pediatric research enterprise is transdisciplinary and includes the full spectrum of basic science, translational, community-based, health services, and child health policy research. Although most pediatricians do not directly engage in research, knowledge of research methodologies and approaches promotes critical evaluation of scientific literature, the practice of evidence-based medicine, and advocacy for evidence-based child health policy. This statement includes

specific recommendations to promote further research education and support at all levels of pediatric training, from premedical to continuing medical education, as well as recommendations to increase support and mentorship for research activities. Pediatric research is crucial to the American Academy of Pediatrics' goal of improving the health of all children. The American Academy of Pediatrics continues to promote and encourage efforts to facilitate the creation of new knowledge and ways to reduce barriers experienced by trainees, practitioners, and academic faculty pursuing research. (4/14, reaffirmed 11/23)
https://doi.org/10.1542/peds.2014-0448

PROMOTING FOOD SECURITY FOR ALL CHILDREN

Council on Community Pediatrics and Committee on Nutrition

ABSTRACT. Sixteen million US children (21%) live in households without consistent access to adequate food. After multiple risk factors are considered, children who live in households that are food insecure, even at the lowest levels, are likely to be sick more often, recover from illness more slowly, and be hospitalized more frequently. Lack of adequate healthy food can impair a child's ability to concentrate and perform well in school and is linked to higher levels of behavioral and emotional problems from preschool through adolescence. Food insecurity can affect children in any community, not only traditionally underserved ones. Pediatricians can play a central role in screening and identifying children at risk for food insecurity and in connecting families with needed community resources. Pediatricians should also advocate for federal and local policies that support access to adequate healthy food for an active and healthy life for all children and their families. (10/15, reaffirmed 3/21)
https://doi.org/10.1542/peds.2015-3301

PROMOTING HEALTHY SEXUALITY FOR CHILDREN AND ADOLESCENTS WITH DISABILITIES

Amy Houtrow, MD, PhD, MPH, FAAP; Ellen Roy Elias, MD, FAAP, FACMG; Beth Ellen Davis, MD, MPH, FAAP; and Council on Children With Disabilities

ABSTRACT. This clinical report updates a 2006 report from the American Academy of Pediatrics titled "Sexuality of Children and Adolescents With Developmental Disabilities." The development of a healthy sexuality best occurs through appropriate education, absence of coercion and violence, and developmental acquisition of skills to navigate feelings, desires, relationships, and social pressures. Pediatric health care providers are important resources for anticipatory guidance and education for all children and youth as they understand their changing bodies, feelings, and behaviors. Yet, youth with disabilities and their families report inadequate education and guidance from pediatricians regarding sexual health development. In the decade since the original clinical report was published, there have been many advancements in the understanding and care of children and youth with disabilities, in part because of an increased prevalence and breadth of autism spectrum disorder as well as an increased longevity of individuals with medically complex and severely disabling conditions. During this same time frame, sexual education in US public schools has diminished, and there is emerging evidence that the attitudes and beliefs of all youth (with and without disability) about sex and sexuality are being formed through media rather than formal education or parent and/or health care provider sources. This report aims to provide the pediatric health care provider with resources and tools for clinical practice to address the sexual development of children and youth with disabilities. The report emphasizes strategies to promote competence in achieving a healthy sexuality regardless of physical, cognitive, or socioemotional limitations. (6/21, reaffirmed 4/25 with reference & data updates)
https://doi.org/10.1542/peds.2021-052043

PROMOTING HUMAN MILK AND BREASTFEEDING FOR THE VERY LOW BIRTH WEIGHT INFANT (CLINICAL REPORT)

Margaret G. Parker, MD, MPH; Lisa M. Stellwagen, MD; Lawrence Noble, MD; Jae H. Kim, MD, PhD; Brenda B. Poindexter, MD; Karen M. Puopolo, MD, PhD; AAP Section on Breastfeeding; Committee on Nutrition; and Committee on Fetus and Newborn

ABSTRACT. Provision of mother's own milk for hospitalized very low birth weight (VLBW) (≤1500 g) infants in the NICU provides short- and long-term health benefits. Mother's own milk, appropriately fortified, is the optimal nutrition source for VLBW infants. Every mother should receive information about the critical importance of mother's own milk to the health of a VLBW infant. Pasteurized human donor milk is recommended when mother's own milk is not available or sufficient. Neonatal health care providers can support lactation in the NICU and potentially reduce disparities in the provision of mother's own milk by providing institutional supports for early and frequent milk expression and by promoting skin-to-skin contact and direct breastfeeding, when appropriate. Promotion of human milk and breastfeeding for VLBW infants requires multidisciplinary and system-wide adoption of lactation support practices. (10/21)
https://doi.org/10.1542/peds.2021-054272

PROMOTING OPTIMAL DEVELOPMENT: IDENTIFYING INFANTS AND YOUNG CHILDREN WITH DEVELOPMENTAL DISORDERS THROUGH DEVELOPMENTAL SURVEILLANCE AND SCREENING (CLINICAL REPORT)

Paul H. Lipkin, MD, FAAP; Michelle M. Macias, MD, FAAP; Council on Children With Disabilities; and Section on Developmental and Behavioral Pediatrics

ABSTRACT. Early identification and intervention for developmental disorders are critical to the well-being of children and are the responsibility of pediatric professionals as an integral function of the medical home. This report models a universal system of developmental surveillance and screening for the early identification of conditions that affect children's early and long-term development and achievement, followed by ongoing care. These conditions include autism, deafness/hard-of-hearing, intellectual and motor disabilities, behavioral conditions, and those seen in other medical conditions. Developmental surveillance is supported at every health supervision visit, as is as the administration of standardized screening tests at the 9-, 18-, and 30-month visits. Developmental concerns elicited on surveillance at any visit should be followed by standardized developmental screening testing or direct referral to intervention and specialty medical care. Special attention to surveillance is recommended at the 4- to 5-year well-child visit, prior to entry into elementary education, with screening completed if there are any concerns. Developmental surveillance includes bidirectional communication with early childhood professionals in child care, preschools, Head Start, and other programs, including home visitation and parenting, particularly around developmental screening. The identification of problems should lead to developmental and medical evaluations, diagnosis, counseling, and treatment, in addition to early developmental intervention. Children with diagnosed developmental disorders are identified as having special health care needs, with initiation of chronic condition management in the pediatric medical home. (1/19, reaffirmed 4/24 with reference & data updates)
https://doi.org/10.1542/peds.2019-3449

PROMOTING OPTIMAL DEVELOPMENT: SCREENING FOR MENTAL HEALTH, EMOTIONAL, AND BEHAVIORAL PROBLEMS (CLINICAL REPORT)

Carol Weitzman, MD, FAAP; James Guevara, MD, MPH, FAAP; Michelle Curtin, DO, FAAP; Michelle Macias, MD, FAAP; Section on Developmental and Behavioral Pediatrics; Council on Early Childhood; and Committee on Psychosocial Aspects of Child and Family Health (joint with Society for Developmental and Behavioral Pediatrics)

ABSTRACT. Rates of mental health, emotional, and behavioral (MEB) problems in the United States continue to rise, with current estimates of 13% to 20% of children having an MEB disorder and an additional 19% with problems causing impairment or distress that do not meet diagnostic criteria for a specific disorder. This clinical report incorporates and expands on recommendations from the 2019 American Academy of Pediatrics policy statement "Mental Health Competencies for Pediatric Practice" as well as "Recommendations for Preventive Pediatric Health Care." It addresses the rising MEB needs of youth since the previous clinical report, "Promoting Optimal Development: Screening for Behavioral and Emotional Problems," was published in 2015. This report outlines specific guidance for MEB screening, identification, and care of children in pediatric primary care. Screening, as part of regular health supervision visits and surveillance, begins within the first month of life to identify postpartum depression in caregivers. Child-focused screening for MEB problems begins at 6 months of age and continues at 12-, 24-, and 36-month health supervision visits, alternating with recommended developmental and autism spectrum disorder screenings at every visit in the Bright Futures Periodicity schedule and additionally when clinically indicated. After age 3, MEB screening continues annually. This report also 1) reviews updated information on prevalence of MEB problems; 2) articulates the current state of detection of these problems in pediatric primary care; 3) addresses how to manage a positive screen; 4) describes barriers to screening, including special population needs, and potential models to address those barriers; and 5) discusses potential changes at a practice and systems level that facilitate successful MEB screening. (8/25)

See full text on page 497.

https://doi.org/10.1542/peds.2025-073172

PROMOTING THE PARTICIPATION OF CHILDREN AND ADOLESCENTS WITH DISABILITIES IN SPORTS, RECREATION, AND PHYSICAL ACTIVITY (CLINICAL REPORT)

Paul S. Carbone, MD, FAAP; Peter J. Smith, MD, MA, FAAP; Charron Lewis, MD, FAAP; Claire LeBlanc, MD, FAAP; Council on Children With Disabilities; and Council on Sports Medicine and Fitness

ABSTRACT. The benefits of physical activity are likely universal for all children, including children and adolescents with disabilities (CWD). The participation of CWD in physical activity, including adaptive or therapeutic sports and recreation, promotes inclusion, minimizes deconditioning, optimizes physical functioning, improves mental health as well as academic achievement, and enhances overall well-being. Despite these benefits, CWD face barriers to participation and have lower levels of fitness, reduced rates of participation, and a higher prevalence of overweight and obesity compared with typically developing peers. Pediatricians and caregivers may overestimate the risks or overlook the benefits of physical activity in CWD, which further limits participation. Preparticipation evaluations often include assessment of health status, functional capacity, individual activity preferences, availability of appropriate programs, and safety precautions. Given the complexity, the preparticipation evaluation for CWD may not occur in the context of a single office visit but rather over a period of time with input from the child's multidisciplinary team (physicians, coaches, physical education teachers, school nurses, adaptive recreation specialists, physical and occupational therapists, and others). Some CWD may desire to participate in organized sports to experience the challenge of competition, and others may prefer recreational activities for enjoyment. To reach the goal of inclusion in appropriate physical activities for all children with disabilities, child, family, financial, and societal barriers to participation need to be identified and addressed. Health care providers can facilitate participation by encouraging physical activity among CWD and their families during visits. Health care providers can create "physical activity prescriptions" for CWD on the basis of the child's preferred activities, functional status, need for adaptation of the activity and the recreational opportunities available in the community. This clinical report discusses the importance of participation in sports, recreation, and physical activity for CWD and offers practical suggestions to health care providers. (11/21, reaffirmed 8/25 with reference & data updates)

https://doi.org/10.1542/peds.2021-054664

PROMOTING THE WELL-BEING OF CHILDREN WHOSE PARENTS ARE GAY OR LESBIAN

Committee on Psychosocial Aspects of Child and Family Health

ABSTRACT. To promote optimal health and well-being of all children, the American Academy of Pediatrics (AAP) supports access for all children to (1) civil marriage rights for their parents and (2) willing and capable foster and adoptive parents, regardless of the parents' sexual orientation. The AAP has always been an advocate for, and has developed policies to support, the optimal physical, mental, and social health and well-being of all infants, children, adolescents, and young adults. In so doing, the AAP has supported families in all their diversity, because the family has always been the basic social unit in which children develop the supporting and nurturing relationships with adults that they need to thrive. Children may be born to, adopted by, or cared for temporarily by married couples, nonmarried couples, single parents, grandparents, or legal guardians, and any of these may be heterosexual, gay or lesbian, or of another orientation. Children need secure and enduring relationships with committed and nurturing adults to enhance their life experiences for optimal social-emotional and cognitive development. Scientific evidence affirms that children have similar developmental and emotional needs and receive similar parenting whether they are raised by parents of the same or different genders. If a child has 2 living and capable parents who choose to create a permanent bond by way of civil marriage, it is in the best interests of their child(ren) that legal and social institutions allow and support them to do so, irrespective of their sexual orientation. If 2 parents are not available to the child, adoption or foster parenting remain acceptable options to provide a loving home for a child and should be available without regard to the sexual orientation of the parent(s). (3/13, reaffirmed 9/22)

https://doi.org/10.1542/peds.2013-0376

PROMOTING THE WELL-BEING OF CHILDREN WHOSE PARENTS ARE GAY OR LESBIAN (TECHNICAL REPORT)

Ellen C. Perrin, MD, MA; Benjamin S. Siegel, MD; and Committee on Psychosocial Aspects of Child and Family Health

ABSTRACT. Extensive data available from more than 30 years of research reveal that children raised by gay and lesbian parents have demonstrated resilience with regard to social, psychological, and sexual health despite economic and legal disparities and social stigma. Many studies have demonstrated that children's well-being is affected much more by their relationships with their parents, their parents' sense of competence and security, and the presence of social and economic support for the family than by the gender or the sexual orientation of their parents. Lack of opportunity for same-gender couples to marry adds

to families' stress, which affects the health and welfare of all household members. Because marriage strengthens families and, in so doing, benefits children's development, children should not be deprived of the opportunity for their parents to be married. Paths to parenthood that include assisted reproductive techniques, adoption, and foster parenting should focus on competency of the parents rather than their sexual orientation. (3/13, reaffirmed 9/22)
https://doi.org/10.1542/peds.2013-0377

PROMOTION OF HEALTHY WEIGHT-CONTROL PRACTICES IN YOUNG ATHLETES (CLINICAL REPORT)

Rebecca L. Carl, MD, MS, FAAP; Miriam D. Johnson, MD, FAAP; Thomas J. Martin, MD, FAAP; and Council on Sports Medicine and Fitness

ABSTRACT. Children and adolescents may participate in sports that favor a particular body type. Some sports, such as gymnastics, dance, and distance running, emphasize a slim or lean physique for aesthetic or performance reasons. Participants in weight-class sports, such as wrestling and martial arts, may attempt weight loss so they can compete at a lower weight class. Other sports, such as football and bodybuilding, highlight a muscular physique; young athletes engaged in these sports may desire to gain weight and muscle mass. This clinical report describes unhealthy methods of weight loss and gain as well as policies and approaches used to curb these practices. The report also reviews healthy strategies for weight loss and weight gain and provides recommendations for pediatricians on how to promote healthy weight control in young athletes. (8/17, reaffirmed 7/21)
https://doi.org/10.1542/peds.2017-1871

PROTECTING CHILDREN AND ADOLESCENTS FROM TOBACCO AND NICOTINE

Brian P. Jenssen, MD, FAAP; Susan C. Walley, MD, FAAP; Rachel Boykan, MD, FAAP; Alice Little Caldwell, MD, MPH, IBCLC, FAAP; Deepa Camenga, MD, FAAP; Section on Nicotine and Tobacco Prevention and Treatment; and Committee on Substance Use and Prevention

ABSTRACT. Tobacco use remains the leading preventable cause of disease and death for adults in the United States. Significant strides have been made in reducing rates of cigarette smoking among adolescents in the United States. However, rates of e-cigarette and similar device use among youth are high, and rates of other tobacco product use, such as cigars and hookahs, have not declined. Public policy actions to protect children and adolescents from tobacco and nicotine use, as well as tobacco smoke and aerosol exposure, have proven effective in reducing harm. Effective public health approaches need to be both extended to include e-cigarettes, similar devices, and other and emerging tobacco products and expanded to reduce the toll that the tobacco epidemic takes on children and adolescents. (4/23)
https://doi.org/10.1542/peds.2023-061804

PROTECTING CHILDREN AND ADOLESCENTS FROM TOBACCO AND NICOTINE (CLINICAL REPORT)

Brian P. Jenssen, MD, FAAP; Susan C. Walley, MD, FAAP; Rachel Boykan, MD, FAAP; Alice Little Caldwell, MD, MPH, IBCLC, FAAP; Deepa Camenga, MD, FAAP; Section on Nicotine and Tobacco Prevention and Treatment; and Committee on Substance Use and Prevention

ABSTRACT. Significant strides have been made in reducing rates of cigarette smoking among adolescents in the United States. However, rates of e-cigarette and similar device use among youth are high, and rates of other tobacco product use, such as cigars and hookahs, have not declined. In addition, almost 40% of children 3 to 11 years of age are regularly exposed to secondhand tobacco smoke, and rates of secondhand exposure to e-cigarette aerosol have increased over the last decade. Pediatricians are uniquely positioned to help children, adolescents, and their families live tobacco-free lives. Actions by pediatricians can help reduce children's risk of developing tobacco and nicotine use disorder and reduce children's tobacco smoke and/or aerosol exposure. (4/23)
https://doi.org/10.1542/peds.2023-061805

PROTECTING CHILDREN AND ADOLESCENTS FROM TOBACCO AND NICOTINE (TECHNICAL REPORT)

Brian P. Jenssen, MD, FAAP; Susan C. Walley, MD, FAAP; Rachel Boykan, MD, FAAP; Alice Little Caldwell, MD, MPH, IBCLC, FAAP; Deepa Camenga, MD, FAAP; Section on Nicotine and Tobacco Prevention and Treatment; and Committee on Substance Use and Prevention

ABSTRACT. This technical report provides the evidence base for the accompanying tobacco clinical report and policy statement. It builds on, strengthens, and expands AAP recommendations from the previous version in 2015. Tobacco use remains the leading preventable cause of disease and death for adults in the United States. The tobacco epidemic takes a substantial toll on children's and adolescent's health, including harms because of prenatal exposure during pregnancy, secondhand and thirdhand exposure during infancy and childhood, and/or direct use during adolescence. Tobacco and nicotine use almost always starts in childhood or adolescence. Almost 40% of children aged 3 to 11 years are regularly exposed to secondhand tobacco smoke, and rates of secondhand exposure to e-cigarette aerosol have increased over the last decade. (4/23)
https://doi.org/10.1542/peds.2023-061806

PROTECTING CHILDREN AND CONDEMNING HATE DURING A TIME OF WAR

American Academy of Pediatrics Board of Directors

The violence, suffering, and death from the terrorist attack on Israel and the Israel-Hamas War weigh on us all. Pediatricians—who are called to care for children and keep them safe and healthy—have been reaching out to the American Academy of Pediatrics expressing anguish, outrage, and a deep desire to help stop the killing, ease the suffering, and protect all children from harm. (2/24)
https://doi.org/10.1542/peds.2023-065582

PROTECTING CHILDREN FROM SEXUAL ABUSE BY HEALTH CARE PROFESSIONALS AND IN THE HEALTH CARE SETTING

Antoinette Laskey, MD, MPH, MBA, FAAP; Suzanne Haney, MD, MS, FAAP; Sarah Northrop, MD, FAAP; and Council on Child Abuse and Neglect

ABSTRACT. Sexual abuse or exploitation of children is never acceptable. Such behavior by pediatricians and health care professionals is particularly concerning because of the trust that children and their families place on adults in the health care profession. The American Academy of Pediatrics stands strongly behind the social and moral prohibition against sexual abuse or exploitation of children by health care professionals.

Pediatricians and health care professionals should be trained to recognize and abide by appropriate provider-patient boundaries. Medical institutions should screen staff members for a history of child abuse issues, train them to respect and maintain appropriate boundaries, and establish policies and procedures to receive and investigate concerns about patient abuse. Everyone has a responsibility to ensure the safety of children in health care settings and to scrupulously follow appropriate legal and ethical reporting and investigation procedures. (8/22)
https://doi.org/10.1542/peds.2022-058879

PROVIDING A PRIMARY CARE MEDICAL HOME FOR CHILDREN AND YOUTH WITH CEREBRAL PALSY (CLINICAL REPORT)

Garey Noritz, MD, FAAP, FACP; Lynn Davidson, MD, FAAP; Katherine Steingass, MD, FAAP; and Council on Children with Disabilities (joint with American Academy for Cerebral Palsy and Developmental Medicine)

ABSTRACT. Cerebral palsy (CP) is the most common motor disorder of childhood, with prevalence estimates ranging from 1.5 to 4 in 1000 live births. This clinical report seeks to provide primary care physicians with guidance to detect children with CP; collaborate with specialists in treating the patient; manage associated medical, developmental, and behavioral problems; and provide general medical care to their patients with CP. (11/22)

https://doi.org/10.1542/peds.2022-060055

PROVIDING CARE FOR CHILDREN AND ADOLESCENTS FACING HOMELESSNESS AND HOUSING INSECURITY

Council on Community Pediatrics

ABSTRACT. Child health and housing security are closely intertwined, and children without homes are more likely to suffer from chronic disease, hunger, and malnutrition than are children with homes. Homeless children and youth often have significant psychosocial development issues, and their education is frequently interrupted. Given the overall effects that homelessness can have on a child's health and potential, it is important for pediatricians to recognize the factors that lead to homelessness, understand the ways that homelessness and its causes can lead to poor health outcomes, and when possible, help children and families mitigate some of the effects of homelessness. Through practice change, partnership with community resources, awareness, and advocacy, pediatricians can help optimize the health and well-being of children affected by homelessness. (5/13, reaffirmed 10/16, 2/22)

https://doi.org/10.1542/peds.2013-0645

PROVIDING CARE FOR INFANTS BORN AT HOME

Kristi Watterberg, MD, FAAP, and Committee on Fetus and Newborn

ABSTRACT. The American Academy of Pediatrics (AAP) believes that current data show that hospitals and accredited birth centers are the safest settings for birth in the United States. The AAP does not recommend planned home birth, which has been reported to be associated with a twofold to threefold increase in infant mortality in the United States. The AAP recognizes that women may choose to plan a home birth. This statement is intended to help pediatricians provide constructive, informed counsel to women considering home birth while retaining their role as child advocates and to summarize appropriate care for newborn infants born at home that is consistent with care provided for infants born in a medical care facility. Regardless of the circumstances of his or her birth, including location, every newborn infant deserves health care consistent with that highlighted in this statement, which is more completely described in other publications from the AAP, including *Guidelines for Perinatal Care* and the *Textbook of Neonatal Resuscitation*. All health care clinicians and institutions should promote communications and understanding on the basis of professional interaction and mutual respect. (4/20, reaffirmed 9/25)

https://doi.org/10.1542/peds.2020-0626

PSYCHOLOGICAL MALTREATMENT (CLINICAL REPORT)

Roberta Hibbard, MD; Jane Barlow, DPhil; Harriet MacMillan, MD; Committee on Child Abuse and Neglect (joint with American Academy of Child and Adolescent Psychiatry Child Maltreatment and Violence Committee)

ABSTRACT. Psychological or emotional maltreatment of children may be the most challenging and prevalent form of child abuse and neglect. Caregiver behaviors include acts of omission (ignoring need for social interactions) or commission (spurning, terrorizing); may be verbal or nonverbal, active or passive, and with or without intent to harm; and negatively affect the child's cognitive, social, emotional, and/or physical development. Psychological maltreatment has been linked with disorders of attachment, developmental and educational problems, socialization problems, disruptive behavior, and later psychopathology. Although no evidence-based interventions that can prevent psychological maltreatment have been identified to date, it is possible that interventions shown to be effective in reducing overall types of child maltreatment, such as the Nurse Family Partnership, may have a role to play. Furthermore, prevention before occurrence will require both the use of universal interventions aimed at promoting the type of parenting that is now recognized to be necessary for optimal child development, alongside the use of targeted interventions directed at improving parental sensitivity to a child's cues during infancy and later parent-child interactions. Intervention should, first and foremost, focus on a thorough assessment and ensuring the child's safety. Potentially effective treatments include cognitive behavioral parenting programs and other psychotherapeutic interventions. The high prevalence of psychological abuse in advanced Western societies, along with the serious consequences, point to the importance of effective management. Pediatricians should be alert to the occurrence of psychological maltreatment and identify ways to support families who have risk indicators for, or evidence of, this problem. (8/12, reaffirmed 9/23)

https://doi.org/10.1542/peds.2012-1552

PSYCHOSOCIAL SUPPORT FOR YOUTH LIVING WITH HIV (CLINICAL REPORT)

Jaime Martinez, MD, FAAP; Rana Chakraborty, MD, FAAP; and Committee on Pediatric AIDS

ABSTRACT. This clinical report provides guidance for the pediatrician in addressing the psychosocial needs of adolescents and young adults living with HIV, which can improve linkage to care and adherence to life-saving antiretroviral (ARV) therapy. Recent national case surveillance data for youth (defined here as adolescents and young adults 13 to 24 years of age) revealed that the burden of HIV/AIDS fell most heavily and disproportionately on African American youth, particularly males having sex with males. To effectively increase linkage to care and sustain adherence to therapy, interventions should address the immediate drivers of ARV compliance and also address factors that provide broader social and structural support for HIV-infected adolescents and young adults. Interventions should address psychosocial development, including lack of future orientation, inadequate educational attainment and limited health literacy, failure to focus on the long-term consequences of near-term risk behaviors, and coping ability. Associated challenges are closely linked to the structural environment. Individual case management is essential to linkage to and retention in care, ARV adherence, and management of associated comorbidities. Integrating these skills into pediatric and adolescent HIV practice in a medical home setting is critical, given the alarming increase in new HIV infections in youth in the United States. (2/14, reaffirmed 7/21)

https://doi.org/10.1542/peds.2013-4061

RACE, ETHNICITY, AND SOCIOECONOMIC STATUS IN RESEARCH ON CHILD HEALTH

Tina L. Cheng, MD, MPH, FAAP; Elizabeth Goodman, MD, FAAP; and Committee on Pediatric Research

ABSTRACT. An extensive literature documents the existence of pervasive and persistent child health, development, and health care disparities by race, ethnicity, and socioeconomic status (SES). Disparities experienced during childhood can result in a wide variety of health and health care outcomes, including adult

morbidity and mortality, indicating that it is crucial to examine the influence of disparities across the life course. Studies often collect data on the race, ethnicity, and SES of research participants to be used as covariates or explanatory factors. In the past, these variables have often been assumed to exert their effects through individual or genetically determined biologic mechanisms. However, it is now widely accepted that these variables have important social dimensions that influence health. SES, a multidimensional construct, interacts with and confounds analyses of race and ethnicity. Because SES, race, and ethnicity are often difficult to measure accurately, leading to the potential for misattribution of causality, thoughtful consideration should be given to appropriate measurement, analysis, and interpretation of such factors. Scientists who study child and adolescent health and development should understand the multiple measures used to assess race, ethnicity, and SES, including their validity and shortcomings and potential confounding of race and ethnicity with SES. The American Academy of Pediatrics (AAP) recommends that research on eliminating health and health care disparities related to race, ethnicity, and SES be a priority. Data on race, ethnicity, and SES should be collected in research on child health to improve their definitions and increase understanding of how these factors and their complex interrelationships affect child health. Furthermore, the AAP believes that researchers should consider both biological and social mechanisms of action of race, ethnicity, and SES as they relate to the aims and hypothesis of the specific area of investigation. It is important to measure these variables, but it is not sufficient to use these variables alone as explanatory for differences in disease, morbidity, and outcomes without attention to the social and biologic influences they have on health throughout the life course. The AAP recommends more research, both in the United States and internationally, on measures of race, ethnicity, and SES and how these complex constructs affect health care and health outcomes throughout the life course. (12/14, reaffirmed 9/22)
https://doi.org/10.1542/peds.2014-3109

RECOGNITION AND MANAGEMENT OF CARDIOVASCULAR INSUFFICIENCY IN THE VERY LOW BIRTH WEIGHT NEWBORN (CLINICAL REPORT)

Jay P. Goldsmith, MD, FAAP; Erin Keels, DNP, APRN-CNP, NNP-BC; and Committee on Fetus and Newborn (joint with National Association of Neonatal Nurses)

ABSTRACT. The measurement of blood pressure in the very low birth weight newborn infant is not simple and may be erroneous because of numerous factors. Assessment of cardiovascular insufficiency in this population should be based on multiple parameters and not only on numeric blood pressure readings. The decision to treat cardiovascular insufficiency should be made after considering the potential complications of such treatment. There are numerous potential strategies to avoid or mitigate hypoperfusion states in the very low birth weight infant. (2/22)
https://doi.org/10.1542/peds.2021-056051

RECOGNITION AND MANAGEMENT OF IATROGENICALLY INDUCED OPIOID DEPENDENCE AND WITHDRAWAL IN CHILDREN (CLINICAL REPORT)

Adam C. Adler, MD, MS, FAAP, FASE; Linda B. Siegel, MD, FAAP, FAAHPM; Robert T. Wilder, MD, PhD, FAAP; Julie Good, MD, FAAP; Committee on Drugs; Section on Critical Care; and Section on Anesthesiology and Pain Medicine

ABSTRACT. Opioids are often prescribed to children for pain relief related to procedures, acute injuries, and chronic conditions. Around-the-clock dosing of opioids can produce physiologic opioid dependence within 5 days. According to a 2001 consensus paper from the American Academy of Pain Medicine, American Pain Society, and American Society of Addiction Medicine, dependence is defined as "a state of adaptation that is manifested by a drug class specific withdrawal syndrome that can be produced by abrupt cessation, rapid dose reduction, decreasing blood level of the drug, or administration of an antagonist." The experience of children undergoing iatrogenic withdrawal symptoms is variable and may be mild and go unreported or can be severe and even life threatening. Guidance on opioid withdrawal is available only for adults and primarily for adults with substance use disorders. This report will summarize existing literature and provide readers with information on how to screen for symptoms of iatrogenic opioid withdrawal as well as mechanisms for opioid withdrawal prevention. (8/25)
See full text on page 517.
https://doi.org/10.1542/peds.2025-073169

RECOGNITION AND MANAGEMENT OF MEDICAL COMPLEXITY (CLINICAL REPORT)

Dennis Z. Kuo, MD, MHS, FAAP; Amy J. Houtrow, MD, PhD, MPH, FAAP; and Council on Children With Disabilities

ABSTRACT. Children with medical complexity have extensive needs for health services, experience functional limitations, and are high resource utilizers. Addressing the needs of this population to achieve high-value health care requires optimizing care within the medical home and medical neighborhood. Opportunities exist for health care providers, payers, and policy makers to develop strategies to enhance care delivery and to decrease costs. Important outcomes include decreasing unplanned hospital admissions, decreasing emergency department use, ensuring access to health services, limiting out-of-pocket expenses for families, and improving patient and family experiences, quality of life, and satisfaction with care. This report describes the population of children with medical complexity and provides strategies to optimize medical and health outcomes. (11/16, reaffirmed 6/21 with reference & data updates)
https://doi.org/10.1542/peds.2016-3021

RECOMMENDATIONS FOR COVID-19 VACCINES IN INFANTS, CHILDREN, AND ADOLESCENTS

Committee on Infectious Diseases

INTRODUCTION. This policy statement updates the recommendations of the American Academy of Pediatrics (AAP) for the use of coronavirus disease 2019 (COVID-19) vaccines in the prevention of severe COVID-19 in children. These COVID-19 vaccine recommendations may change in future seasons or as additional variants emerge.

COVID-19 continues to be a cause of hospitalization and death in the pediatric population. COVID-19 vaccines are safe and effective in protecting individuals and populations against serious outcomes associated with severe acute respiratory syndrome coronavirus 2 (SARS-CoV-2) infection, including post-acute sequelae of SARS-CoV-2 infection (PASC) and multisystem inflammatory syndrome in children (MIS-C). (10/25)
See full text on page 527.
https://doi.org/10.1542/peds.2025-073924

RECOMMENDATIONS FOR PREVENTION AND CONTROL OF INFLUENZA IN CHILDREN, 2025–2026

American Academy of Pediatrics
DEDICATED TO THE HEALTH OF ALL CHILDREN®

AAP Partnership for Policy Implementation
– See Appendix 1

Committee on Infectious Diseases

ABSTRACT. This statement updates the recommendations of the American Academy of Pediatrics (AAP) for the use of influenza vaccines and antiviral medications in the prevention and treatment of influenza in children during the 2025–2026 influenza season. A review of the evidence supporting these recommendations is in the accompanying technical report (https://doi.org/10.1542/peds.2025-073622).

The AAP recommends annual influenza vaccination of all children without medical contraindications starting at 6 months of age. Influenza vaccination is an important strategy for protecting children and the broader community as well as reducing the overall burden of respiratory illnesses when other viruses are cocirculating. Any licensed influenza vaccine appropriate for age and health status can be administered, as soon as possible in the season, without preference for one product or formulation.

Antiviral treatment of influenza is recommended for children with suspected or confirmed influenza who are hospitalized or have severe or progressive disease or have underlying conditions that increase their risk of complications of influenza. In this situation, antiviral treatment should be started as soon as possible regardless of duration of illness. Antiviral treatment is an option in the outpatient setting for other children with suspected or confirmed influenza in some circumstances.

Antiviral chemoprophylaxis is an option in certain individuals, especially exposed children who are asymptomatic and are at high risk for influenza complications but have not yet been immunized or those who are not expected to mount an effective immune response. (9/25)

https://doi.org/10.1542/peds.2025-073620

RECOMMENDATIONS FOR PREVENTION AND CONTROL OF INFLUENZA IN CHILDREN, 2025–2026 (TECHNICAL REPORT)

American Academy of Pediatrics
DEDICATED TO THE HEALTH OF ALL CHILDREN®

AAP Partnership for Policy Implementation
– *See Appendix 1*

Committee on Infectious Diseases

ABSTRACT. This technical report accompanies the recommendations of the American Academy of Pediatrics for the routine use of influenza vaccine and antiviral medications in the prevention and treatment of influenza in children during the 2025–2026 influenza season. The rationale for the American Academy of Pediatrics recommendation for annual influenza vaccination of all children without medical contraindications starting at 6 months of age is provided. Influenza vaccination is an important strategy for protecting children and the broader community against influenza. This technical report summarizes recent influenza seasons, morbidity and mortality in children, vaccine effectiveness, and vaccination coverage and provides detailed guidance on vaccine storage, administration, and implementation. The report also provides a brief background on inactivated (non-live) and live attenuated influenza vaccines, available vaccines for the 2025–2026 influenza season, vaccination during pregnancy and breastfeeding, diagnostic testing for influenza, and antiviral medications for treatment and chemoprophylaxis. Strategies to promote vaccine uptake are emphasized. (9/25)

https://doi.org/10.1542/peds.2025-073622

RECOMMENDATIONS FOR THE PREVENTION OF RSV DISEASE IN INFANTS AND CHILDREN

Committee on Infectious Diseases (10/25)

See full text on page 587.

https://doi.org/10.1542/peds.2025-073923

RECOMMENDED CHILDHOOD AND ADOLESCENT IMMUNIZATION SCHEDULE: UNITED STATES, 2026

Sean T. O'Leary, MD, MPH, FAAP, and Committee on Infectious Diseases

See full text on page 593.

https://doi.org/10.1542/peds.2025-075754

RECOMMENDED ESSENTIAL EQUIPMENT FOR BASIC LIFE SUPPORT AND ADVANCED LIFE SUPPORT GROUND AMBULANCES 2020: A JOINT POSITION STATEMENT

John Lyng, MD, NRP; Kathleen Adelgais, MD, MPH; Rachael Alter, BA; Justin Beal, RN; Bruce Chung, MD; Toni Gross, MD; Marc Minkler, NRP; Brian Moore, MD; Tim Stebbins, MD; Sam Vance, NRP; Ken Williams, MD; and Allen Yee, MD

ABSTRACT. The National Association of EMS Physicians, along with these coauthoring associations: American Academy of Pediatrics, American College of Surgeons Committee on Trauma, EMS for Children Innovation and Improvement Center, Emergency Nurses Association, and National Association of State EMS Officials and as also endorsed by the National Association of Emergency Medical Technicians, believes that the delivery of high-quality and effective EMS care is dependent on several factors, including but not limited to the presence of the following:

— providers who have been credentialed to ensure they demonstrate appropriate cognitive knowledge, affective ability, psychomotor skills, and critical thinking;
— clinical protocols or guidelines that are supported by the best available scientific evidence; and
— equipment and supplies necessary to deliver appropriate care as directed by clinical protocols and/or guidelines for patients of all ages.

Several documents, including previous versions of this joint position statement, the National Model EMS Clinical Guidelines Version 2.2, the 2018 National EMS Scope of Practice Model, the Clinical Credentialing of EMS Providers, Physician Oversight of Pediatric Care in Emergency Medical Services, Pediatric Readiness in Emergency Medical Services Systems, and core performance measures from the US Department of Health and Human Services Health Resources and Services Administration EMS for Children (EMSC) Program have been developed to lay the foundation of several of the concepts noted above. (5/21)

https://doi.org/10.1542/peds.2021-051508

RECOMMENDED TERMINOLOGY FOR SUBSTANCE USE DISORDERS IN THE CARE OF CHILDREN, ADOLESCENTS, YOUNG ADULTS, AND FAMILIES

Rachel H. Alinsky, MD, MPH, FAAP; Scott E. Hadland, MD, MPH, MS, FAAP; Joanna Quigley, MD, FAAP; Stephen W. Patrick, MD, MPH, MS, FAAP; and Committee on Substance Use and Prevention

ABSTRACT. Pediatricians across the United States encounter infants, children, adolescents, young adults, and families affected by substance use disorders in their daily practice. For much of history, substance use has been viewed as a moral failing for which individuals themselves are to blame; however, as addiction became understood as a medical disorder, clinical terminology has shifted along with a growing awareness of harm of stigmatizing language in medicine. In issuing this policy statement, the American Academy of Pediatrics (AAP) joins other large organizations in providing recommendations regarding medically accurate, person-first, and nonstigmatizing terminology. As the first pediatric society to offer guidance on preferred language regarding substance use to be used among pediatricians, media, policymakers, and government agencies and in its own peer-reviewed publications, the AAP aims to promote child health by highlighting the specific context of infants, children, adolescents, young adults, and families. In this policy statement, the AAP provides 3 specific recommendations, accompanied by a table that presents a summary of problematic language to be avoided, paired with the recommended more appropriate language and explanations for each. Pediatricians have an important role in advocating for the health of children and adolescents in the context of families affected by substance use and are optimally empowered to do so by avoiding the use

of stigmatizing language in favor of medically accurate terminology that respects the dignity and personhood of individuals with substance use disorders and the children and adolescents raised in families affected by substance use. (5/22)
https://doi.org/10.1542/peds.2022-057529

REDUCING INJURY RISK FROM BODY CHECKING IN BOYS' YOUTH ICE HOCKEY

Council on Sports Medicine and Fitness

ABSTRACT. Ice hockey is an increasingly popular sport that allows intentional collision in the form of body checking for males but not for females. There is a two- to threefold increased risk of all injury, severe injury, and concussion related to body checking at all levels of boys' youth ice hockey. The American Academy of Pediatrics reinforces the importance of stringent enforcement of rules to protect player safety as well as educational interventions to decrease unsafe tactics. To promote ice hockey as a lifelong recreational pursuit for boys, the American Academy of Pediatrics recommends the expansion of nonchecking programs and the restriction of body checking to elite levels of boys' youth ice hockey, starting no earlier than 15 years of age. (5/14, reaffirmed 11/24)
https://doi.org/10.1542/peds.2014-0692

RESCUE MEDICINE FOR EPILEPSY IN EDUCATION SETTINGS (CLINICAL REPORT)

Adam L. Hartman, MD; Cynthia Di Laura Devore, MD; Section on Neurology; Council on School Health

ABSTRACT. Children and adolescents with epilepsy may experience prolonged seizures in school-associated settings (eg, during transportation, in the classroom, or during sports activities). Prolonged seizures may evolve into status epilepticus. Administering a seizure rescue medication can abort the seizure and may obviate the need for emergency medical services and subsequent care in an emergency department. In turn, this may save patients from the morbidity of more invasive interventions and the cost of escalated care. There are significant variations in prescribing practices for seizure rescue medications, partly because of inconsistencies between jurisdictions in legislation and professional practice guidelines among potential first responders (including school staff). There also are potential liability issues for prescribers, school districts, and unlicensed assistive personnel who might administer the seizure rescue medications. This clinical report highlights issues that providers may consider when prescribing seizure rescue medications and creating school medical orders and/or action plans for students with epilepsy. Collaboration among prescribing providers, families, and schools may be useful in developing plans for the use of seizure rescue medications. (1/16, reaffirmed 10/24)
https://doi.org/10.1542/peds.2015-3876

RESISTANCE TRAINING FOR CHILDREN AND ADOLESCENTS (CLINICAL REPORT)

Paul R. Stricker, MD, FAAP; Avery D. Faigenbaum, EdD, FACSM, FNSCA; Teri M. McCambridge, MD, FAAP; and Council on Sports Medicine and Fitness

ABSTRACT. Resistance training is becoming more important as an integral part of comprehensive sport training regimens, school physical education classes, and after-school fitness programs. The increasing number of youth who are involved in sport activities, coupled with the health problems of inactivity and being overweight, have resulted in increased interest in resistance training. Secular declines in measures of muscular fitness in modern-day youth highlight the need for participation in youth resistance training for nonathletes as well as athletes. Parents often ask pediatricians to offer advice regarding the safety, benefits, and implementation of an effective resistance-training program. This report is a revision of the 2008 American Academy of Pediatrics policy statement and reviews current information and research on the benefits and risks of resistance training for children and adolescents. (5/20, reaffirmed 11/24)
https://doi.org/10.1542/peds.2020-1011

RESPONDING TO PARENTAL REQUESTS FOR NONDISCLOSURE TO PATIENTS OF DIAGNOSTIC AND PROGNOSTIC INFORMATION IN THE SETTING OF SERIOUS DISEASE (CLINICAL REPORT)

Sara Taub, MD, FAAP; Robert Macauley, MD, MDiv, FAAP; and Committee on Bioethics

ABSTRACT. Learning that one's child is seriously ill can be devastating, requiring families to decide when and how to share information about diagnosis and prognosis with their child. In most cases, this disclosure is made thoughtfully and collaboratively with the medical team. Some parents, however, may be concerned that disclosure will take away their child's hope, cause emotional pain, or exceed the child's capacity for understanding. Faced with competing obligations of truth-telling to their patient and respect for parental wishes, pediatricians may be unsure how to proceed. This clinical report examines ethical duties and legal considerations, providing practical and culturally sensitive case-based guidance for clinicians to approach parental requests for nondisclosure of diagnostic or prognostic information. (9/23)
https://doi.org/10.1542/peds.2023-063754

RESPONSIBLE INNOVATION IN CHILDREN'S SURGICAL CARE

Section on Surgery and Committee on Bioethics (joint with American Pediatric Surgical Association New Technology Committee)

ABSTRACT. Advances in medical care may occur when a change in practice incorporates a new treatment or methodology. In surgery, this may involve the translation of a completely novel concept into a new procedure or device or the adaptation of existing treatment approaches or technology to a new clinical application. Regardless of the specifics, innovation should have, as its primary goal, the enhancement of care leading to improved outcomes from the patient's perspective. This policy statement examines innovation as it pertains to surgical care, focusing on some of the definitions that help differentiate applied innovation or innovative therapy from research. The ethical challenges and the potential for conflict of interest for surgeons or institutions seeking to offer innovative surgical therapy are examined. The importance of engaging patients and families as "innovation partners" to ensure complete transparency of expectations from the patient's and provider's perspectives is also examined, with specific emphasis on cultural competence and mutually respectful approaches. A framework for identifying, evaluating, and safely implementing innovative surgical therapy in children is provided. (12/16, reaffirmed 9/23)
https://doi.org/10.1542/peds.2016-3437

RETURNING TO LEARNING FOLLOWING A CONCUSSION (CLINICAL REPORT)

Mark E. Halstead, MD, FAAP; Karen McAvoy, PsyD; Cynthia D. Devore, MD, FAAP; Rebecca Carl, MD, FAAP; Michael Lee, MD, FAAP; Kelsey Logan, MD, FAAP; Council on Sports Medicine and Fitness; and Council on School Health

ABSTRACT. Following a concussion, it is common for children and adolescents to experience difficulties in the school setting. Cognitive difficulties, such as learning new tasks or remembering previously learned material, may pose challenges in the classroom. The school environment may also increase symptoms with exposure to bright lights and screens or noisy cafeterias and hallways. Unfortunately, because most children and adolescents look physically normal after a concussion, school officials often fail to recognize the need for academic or environmental adjust-

ments. Appropriate guidance and recommendations from the pediatrician may ease the transition back to the school environment and facilitate the recovery of the child or adolescent. This report serves to provide a better understanding of possible factors that may contribute to difficulties in a school environment after a concussion and serves as a framework for the medical home, the educational home, and the family home to guide the student to a successful and safe return to learning. (10/13, reaffirmed 4/23)
https://doi.org/10.1542/peds.2013-2867

RISKS OF INFECTIOUS DISEASES IN NEWBORNS EXPOSED TO ALTERNATIVE PERINATAL PRACTICES (CLINICAL REPORT)

Susan W. Aucott, MD, FAAP; Committee on Infectious Diseases; and Committee on Fetus and Newborn

ABSTRACT. The purpose of this report is to educate providers about the risk of infectious diseases associated with emerging alternative peripartum and neonatal practices. This report will provide information pediatricians may use to counsel families before birth and to appropriately evaluate and treat neonates who have been exposed to these practices. (1/22)
https://doi.org/10.1542/peds.2021-055554

THE ROLE OF THE PEDIATRICIAN IN THE PROMOTION OF HEALTHY, ACTIVE LIVING (CLINICAL REPORT)

Natalie D. Muth, MD, RDN, MPH, FAAP, FACSM; Christopher Bolling, MD, FAAP; Tamara Hannon, MD, MS, FAAP; Mona Sharifi, MD, MPH, FAAP; Section on Obesity; and Committee on Nutrition

ABSTRACT. Few children and adolescents meet federal nutrition or physical activity recommendations, and many experience poor or inadequate sleep and negative health effects from screen use and social media. These lifestyle factors exacerbate physical and mental health risks for children and adolescents. This clinical report provides guidance to help pediatricians address the nutritional, physical activity, sleep, media and screen use, and social-emotional factors that affect child and adolescent health and wellness. The recommendations in this clinical report aim to promote health and wellness practices for infants, children, and adolescents across several domains of influence, including the individual, interpersonal, institutional, community, and public policy levels. (2/24)
https://doi.org/10.1542/peds.2023-065480

ROLE OF THE SCHOOL NURSE IN PROVIDING SCHOOL HEALTH SERVICES

Council on School Health

ABSTRACT. The American Academy of Pediatrics recognizes the important role school nurses play in promoting the optimal biopsychosocial health and well-being of school-aged children in the school setting. Although the concept of a school nurse has existed for more than a century, uniformity among states and school districts regarding the role of a registered professional nurse in schools and the laws governing it are lacking. By understanding the benefits, roles, and responsibilities of school nurses working as a team with the school physician, as well as their contributions to school-aged children, pediatricians can collaborate with, support, and promote school nurses in their own communities, thus improving the health, wellness, and safety of children and adolescents. (5/16, reaffirmed 7/23)
https://doi.org/10.1542/peds.2016-0852

SAFE ADMINISTRATION OF MEDICATION IN SCHOOL

Mary Beth Miotto, MD, MPH, FAAP; Brooke Balchan, DO, FAAP; Laurie Combe, MN, RN, NCSN, FNASN; Council on School Health (joint with National Association of School Nurses)

ABSTRACT. Many youth with acute and chronic health conditions require medication to be administered during the school day. This policy statement offers guidance to school physicians, community prescribers, school nurses, other school health professionals, and groups providing oversight to school health activities and ensures patient safety and equity lenses are applied to administration of medications during school and for school-related activities. The American Academy of Pediatrics supports a robust collaborative model that allows all those involved in student health, including the student and family, to communicate, participate in effective medication management, inform delegated medication responsibilities, and promote safe medication storage and administration. School medication administration protocols are developed to help prevent medication administration errors specific to potential risks in the school setting and are responsive to the maturing students' evolving understanding of their health needs, growing autonomy, and responsibility. All protocols involving school nurses, unlicensed assistive personnel, and prescribers must be consistent with state and federal regulations on scope of practice, student privacy laws, and professional nursing organization guidelines. Consistent policies and messaging on safety of the patient and the entire school community enable school health teams to ensure equitable treatment of students prescribed therapeutic agents newly regulated by the US Food and Drug Administration, over-the-counter medications, or products that are currently not regulated by the US Food and Drug Administration. (5/24)
https://doi.org/10.1542/peds.2024-066839

SAFE SLEEP AND SKIN-TO-SKIN CARE IN THE NEONATAL PERIOD FOR HEALTHY TERM NEWBORNS (CLINICAL REPORT)

Lori Feldman-Winter, MD, MPH, FAAP; Jay P. Goldsmith, MD, FAAP; Committee on Fetus and Newborn; and Task Force on Sudden Infant Death Syndrome

ABSTRACT. Skin-to-skin care (SSC) and rooming-in have become common practice in the newborn period for healthy newborns with the implementation of maternity care practices that support breastfeeding as delineated in the World Health Organization's "Ten Steps to Successful Breastfeeding." SSC and rooming-in are supported by evidence that indicates that the implementation of these practices increases overall and exclusive breastfeeding, safer and healthier transitions, and improved maternal-infant bonding. In some cases, however, the practice of SSC and rooming-in may pose safety concerns, particularly with regard to sleep. There have been several recent case reports and case series of severe and sudden unexpected postnatal collapse in the neonatal period among otherwise healthy newborns and near fatal or fatal events related to sleep, suffocation, and falls from adult hospital beds. Although these are largely case reports, there are potential dangers of unobserved SSC immediately after birth and throughout the postpartum hospital period as well as with unobserved rooming-in for at-risk situations. Moreover, behaviors that are modeled in the hospital after birth, such as sleep position, are likely to influence sleeping practices after discharge. Hospitals and birthing centers have found it difficult to develop policies that will allow SSC and rooming-in to continue in a safe manner. This clinical report is intended for birthing centers and delivery hospitals caring for healthy newborns to assist in the establishment of appropriate SSC and safe sleep policies. (8/16, reaffirmed 6/22 with reference & data updates)
https://doi.org/10.1542/peds.2016-1889

SAFETY IN CHEERLEADING: EPIDEMIOLOGY AND RECOMMENDATIONS

Greg Canty, MD, FAAP; Jennifer King, DO, FAAP; and Council on Sports Medicine and Fitness

ABSTRACT. Participation in cheerleading has continued to increase over the last decade, and the sport has evolved to require a higher level of athleticism. More than 3.5 million youth currently participate, with the vast majority being females between the ages of 6 and 17 years. Cheer occurs in both scholastic and nonscholastic settings; participants may perform to support other interscholastic teams or engage in competitions to showcase their skills against other squads. With the increased athletic demands of the sport and the year-round nature of competition, the number of injuries, including concussions, has risen. The overall injury rate for cheer is fairly low, but average time away from sport after injury is lengthy suggesting injuries can be severe. This policy statement reviews the epidemiology of cheerleading injuries and offers recommendations on how to improve the safety of cheerleading for all youth. (10/24)
https://doi.org/10.1542/peds.2024-068956

SCHOOL SUSPENSION AND EXPULSION

Susanna K. Jain, MD, FAAP; Nathaniel Beers, MD, FAAP; Ryan Padrez, MD, FAAP; and Council on School Health

ABSTRACT. Exclusionary school discipline practices—ie, suspension and expulsion—represent some of the most severe consequences a school district can implement for unacceptable student behavior. Suspension and expulsion were traditionally used for student behaviors that caused serious harm, such as bringing a weapon to school. Currently, the most common indications for exclusionary school discipline are for behaviors that are neither violent nor criminal. There is little evidence that exclusionary school discipline practices make schools safer or deter future misbehavior. American Indian/Alaska Native students, Black students, students whose caregivers have low socioeconomic status, male students, lesbian, gay, bisexual, transgender, and queer or questioning students, and students with disabilities are disproportionately disciplined with suspension and expulsion. In addition, exclusionary school discipline in the preschool period can be harmful to early childhood development. Children and adolescents affected by exclusionary school discipline are at higher risk for dropping out of high school and for involvement with the juvenile justice system. Both of those experiences are associated with a worse profile of physical and mental health outcomes. A multidisciplinary and trauma-informed approach to reducing exclusionary school discipline practices is described. Recommendations are provided at both the practice level for pediatric health care providers and at the systems level for both pediatric health care providers and educators. (9/24)
https://doi.org/10.1542/peds.2024-068466

SCHOOL-BASED HEALTH CENTERS AND PEDIATRIC PRACTICE

Chris Kjolhede, MD, MPH, FAAP; April C. Lee, MD, FAAP; and Council on School Health

ABSTRACT. School-based health centers (SBHCs) are unique health care settings for our nation's school-aged children and adolescents. SBHCs represent the collaboration between the health and school communities to support the health and mental health needs and the academic achievements of children and adolescents, particularly students with health disparities or poor access to health care. SBHCs improve access to health care services for students by decreasing financial, geographic, age, and cultural barriers. This policy statement provides an overview of SBHCs, including the scope of services as well as some of the documented benefits and challenges. This policy statement also reviews the role of SBHCs in working with the pediatric medical home and provides recommendations that support the coordination of SBHCs with pediatric primary care providers and the pediatric medical home. (9/21)
https://doi.org/10.1542/peds.2021-053758

SCOPE OF HEALTH CARE BENEFITS FOR NEONATES, INFANTS, CHILDREN, ADOLESCENTS, AND YOUNG ADULTS THROUGH AGE 26

Mark L. Hudak, MD, FAAP; and Committee on Child Health Financing

ABSTRACT. Timely access to appropriate health care from the prenatal period onward is one of several pillars essential to optimize the health of a child preparing to become an adult. In 1967, Congress passed legislation that specified an Early and Periodic Screening, Diagnostic and Treatment standard as the mandatory child health component of Medicaid. Subsequent legislative amendments have generally strengthened this standard. In particular, state Medicaid programs must provide any health care service for children that is covered by the federal Medicaid program even if the state does not cover that service for adults. An initial set of detailed recommendations concerning the best preventive care services for children, adolescents, and young adults was published in 1994 based on deliberations of a large group of expert pediatric health care providers and family representatives. The most recent updated recommendations are available in the 2017 fourth edition of *Bright Futures: Guidelines for Health Supervision of Infants, Children, and Adolescents.* The Patient Protection and Affordable Care Act of 2010 (Pub L No. 114-148) referenced Bright Futures recommendations as a standard for access to and design of age-appropriate health insurance benefits for neonates, infants, children, adolescents, and young adults. This policy statement summarizes recent developments pertaining to the scope of health care benefits offered for children by public and private payers. The statement identifies barriers that impede achievement of a uniform standard that all payers can adopt. Finally, the statement refreshes a recommended set of health insurance benefits for neonates, infants, children, adolescents, and young adults through age 26. (8/22)
https://doi.org/10.1542/peds.2022-058881

SEXUALITY EDUCATION FOR CHILDREN AND ADOLESCENTS (CLINICAL REPORT)

Cora C. Breuner, MD, MPH, FAAP; Gerri Mattson, MD, MSPH, FAAP; Committee on Adolescence; and Committee on Psychosocial Aspects of Child and Family Health

ABSTRACT. The purpose of this clinical report is to provide pediatricians updated research on evidence-based sexual and reproductive health education conducted since the original clinical report on the subject was published by the American Academy of Pediatrics in 2001. Sexuality education is defined as teaching about human sexuality, including intimate relationships, human sexual anatomy, sexual reproduction, sexually transmitted infections, sexual activity, sexual orientation, gender identity, abstinence, contraception, and reproductive rights and responsibilities. Developmentally appropriate and evidence-based education about human sexuality and sexual reproduction over time provided by pediatricians, schools, other professionals, and parents is important to help children and adolescents make informed, positive, and safe choices about healthy relationships, responsible sexual activity, and their reproductive health. Sexuality education has been shown to help to prevent and reduce the risks of adolescent pregnancy, HIV, and sexually transmitted infections for children and adolescents with and without chronic health conditions and disabilities in the United States. (7/16, reaffirmed 1/22)
https://doi.org/10.1542/peds.2016-1348

SHARED DECISION-MAKING AND CHILDREN WITH DISABILITIES: PATHWAYS TO CONSENSUS (CLINICAL REPORT)

Richard C. Adams, MD, FAAP; Susan E. Levy, MD, MPH, FAAP; and Council on Children With Disabilities

ABSTRACT. Shared decision-making (SDM) promotes family and clinician collaboration, with ultimate goals of improved health and satisfaction. This clinical report provides a basis for a systematic approach to the implementation of SDM by clinicians for children with disabilities. Often in the discussion of treatment plans, there are gaps between the child's/family's values, priorities, and understanding of perceived "best choices" and those of the clinician. When conducted well, SDM affords an appropriate balance incorporating voices of all stakeholders, ultimately supporting both the child/family and clinician. With increasing knowledge of and functional use of SDM skills, the clinician will become an effective partner in the decision-making process with families, providing family-centered care. The outcome of the process will support the beneficence of the physician, the authority of the family, and the autonomy and well-being of the child. (5/17, reaffirmed 9/21 with reference & data updates)

https://doi.org/10.1542/peds.2017-0956

SLEEP-RELATED INFANT DEATHS: UPDATED 2022 RECOMMENDATIONS FOR REDUCING INFANT DEATHS IN THE SLEEP ENVIRONMENT

Rachel Y. Moon, MD, FAAP; Rebecca F. Carlin, MD, FAAP; Ivan Hand, MD, FAAP; Task Force on Sudden Infant Death Syndrome; and Committee on Fetus and Newborn

ABSTRACT. Each year in the United States, ~3500 infants die of sleep-related infant deaths, including sudden infant death syndrome (SIDS) (International Classification of Diseases, 10th Revision [ICD-10] R95), ill-defined deaths (ICD-10 R99), and accidental suffocation and strangulation in bed (ICD-10 W75). After a substantial decline in sleep-related deaths in the 1990s, the overall death rate attributable to sleep-related infant deaths has remained stagnant since 2000, and disparities persist. The triple risk model proposes that SIDS occurs when an infant with intrinsic vulnerability (often manifested by impaired arousal, cardiorespiratory, and/or autonomic responses) undergoes an exogenous trigger event (eg, exposure to an unsafe sleeping environment) during a critical developmental period. The American Academy of Pediatrics recommends a safe sleep environment to reduce the risk of all sleep-related deaths. This includes supine positioning; use of a firm, noninclined sleep surface; room sharing without bed sharing; and avoidance of soft bedding and overheating. Additional recommendations for SIDS risk reduction include human milk feeding; avoidance of exposure to nicotine, alcohol, marijuana, opioids, and illicit drugs; routine immunization; and use of a pacifier. New recommendations are presented regarding noninclined sleep surfaces, short-term emergency sleep locations, use of cardboard boxes as a sleep location, bed sharing, substance use, home cardiorespiratory monitors, and tummy time. Additional information to assist parents, physicians, and nonphysician clinicians in assessing the risk of specific bed-sharing situations is also included. The recommendations and strength of evidence for each recommendation are included in this policy statement. The rationale for these recommendations is discussed in detail in the accompanying technical report. (6/22)

https://doi.org/10.1542/peds.2022-057990

SNACKS, SWEETENED BEVERAGES, ADDED SUGARS, AND SCHOOLS

Council on School Health and Committee on Nutrition

ABSTRACT. Concern over childhood obesity has generated a decade-long reformation of school nutrition policies. Food is available in school in 3 venues: federally sponsored school meal programs; items sold in competition to school meals, such as a la carte, vending machines, and school stores; and foods available in myriad informal settings, including packed meals and snacks, bake sales, fundraisers, sports booster sales, in-class parties, or other school celebrations. High-energy, low-nutrient beverages, in particular, contribute substantial calories, but little nutrient content, to a student's diet. In 2004, the American Academy of Pediatrics recommended that sweetened drinks be replaced in school by water, white and flavored milks, or 100% fruit and vegetable beverages. Since then, school nutrition has undergone a significant transformation. Federal, state, and local regulations and policies, along with alternative products developed by industry, have helped decrease the availability of nutrient-poor foods and beverages in school. However, regular access to foods of high energy and low quality remains a school issue, much of it attributable to students, parents, and staff. Pediatricians, aligning with experts on child nutrition, are in a position to offer a perspective promoting nutrient-rich foods within calorie guidelines to improve those foods brought into or sold in schools. A positive emphasis on nutritional value, variety, appropriate portion, and encouragement for a steady improvement in quality will be a more effective approach for improving nutrition and health than simply advocating for the elimination of added sugars. (2/15, reaffirmed 4/23)

https://doi.org/10.1542/peds.2014-3902

SOCCER INJURIES IN CHILDREN AND ADOLESCENTS (CLINICAL REPORT)

Andrew Watson, MD, MS, FAAP; Jeffrey M. Mjaanes, MD, FAAP; Council on Sports Medicine and Fitness

ABSTRACT. Participation in youth soccer in the United States continues to increase steadily, with a greater percentage of preadolescent participants than perhaps any other youth sport. Despite the wide-ranging health benefits of participation in organized sports, injuries occur and represent a threat to the health and performance of young athletes. Youth soccer has a greater reported injury rate than many other contact sports, and recent studies suggest that injury rates are increasing. Large increases in the incidence of concussions in youth soccer have been reported, and anterior cruciate ligament injuries remain a significant problem in this sport, particularly among female athletes. Considerable new research has identified a number of modifiable risk factors for lower-extremity injuries and concussion, and several prevention programs have been identified to reduce the risk of injury. Rule enforcement and fair play also serve an important role in reducing the risk of injury among youth soccer participants. This report provides an updated review of the relevant literature as well as recommendations to promote the safe participation of children and adolescents in soccer. (10/19, reaffirmed 7/23)

https://doi.org/10.1542/peds.2019-2759

SPECIAL REQUIREMENTS OF ELECTRONIC HEALTH RECORD SYSTEMS IN PEDIATRICS (CLINICAL REPORT)

Kevin R. Dufendach, MD, MS, FAAP; Christoph U. Lehmann, MD, FAAP, FACMI; S. Andrew Spooner, MD, MS, FAAP; and Council on Clinical Information Technology

ABSTRACT. Pediatricians' use of electronic health record (EHR) systems has become nearly ubiquitous in the United States, yet many systems lack full functionality to deliver effective and efficient pediatric care. This clinical report seeks to provide a compendium of core pediatric functionality of importance to child health care providers that may serve as the focus for EHR developers and clinicians as they evaluate their EHR needs. Also reviewed are important but less critical functions, any of which might be of importance in a specific pediatric context. The major

areas described here are immunization management, growth and development, social drivers of health tracking, decision support for orders, patient identification, data normalization, privacy, and system functionality standards in pediatric contexts. (9/24)
https://doi.org/10.1542/peds.2024-068509

SPORT-RELATED CONCUSSION IN CHILDREN AND ADOLESCENTS (CLINICAL REPORT)

Mark E. Halstead, MD, FAAP; Kevin D. Walter, MD, FAAP; Kody Moffatt, MD, FAAP; and Council on Sports Medicine and Fitness

ABSTRACT. Sport-related concussion is an important topic in nearly all sports and at all levels of sport for children and adolescents. Concussion knowledge and approaches to management have progressed since the American Academy of Pediatrics published its first clinical report on the subject in 2010. Concussion's definition, signs, and symptoms must be understood to diagnose it and rule out more severe intracranial injury. Pediatric health care providers should have a good understanding of diagnostic evaluation and initial management strategies. Effective management can aid recovery and potentially reduce the risk of long-term symptoms and complications. Because concussion symptoms often interfere with school, social life, family relationships, and athletics, a concussion may affect the emotional well-being of the injured athlete. Because every concussion has its own unique spectrum and severity of symptoms, individualized management is appropriate. The reduction, not necessarily elimination, of physical and cognitive activity is the mainstay of treatment. A full return to activity and/or sport is accomplished by using a stepwise program while evaluating for a return of symptoms. An understanding of prolonged symptoms and complications will help the pediatric health care provider know when to refer to a specialist. Additional research is needed in nearly all aspects of concussion in the young athlete. This report provides education on the current state of sport-related concussion knowledge, diagnosis, and management in children and adolescents. (11/18, reaffirmed 4/24)
https://doi.org/10.1542/peds.2018-3074

SPORTS SPECIALIZATION AND INTENSIVE TRAINING IN YOUNG ATHLETES (CLINICAL REPORT)

Joel S. Brenner, MD, MPH, FAAP, and Council on Sports Medicine and Fitness

ABSTRACT. Sports specialization is becoming the norm in youth sports for a variety of reasons. When sports specialization occurs too early, detrimental effects may occur, both physically and psychologically. If the timing is correct and sports specialization is performed under the correct conditions, the athlete may be successful in reaching specific goals. Young athletes who train intensively, whether specialized or not, can also be at risk of adverse effects on the mind and body. The purpose of this clinical report is to assist pediatricians in counseling their young athlete patients and their parents regarding sports specialization and intensive training. This report supports the American Academy of Pediatrics clinical report "Overuse Injuries, Overtraining, and Burnout in Child and Adolescent Athletes." (8/16, reaffirmed 2/21 with reference & data updates)
https://doi.org/10.1542/peds.2016-2148

STANDARD TERMINOLOGY FOR FETAL, INFANT, AND PERINATAL DEATHS (CLINICAL REPORT)

Wanda D. Barfield, MD; Committee on Fetus and Newborn

ABSTRACT. Accurately defining and reporting perinatal deaths (ie, fetal and infant deaths) is a critical first step in understanding the magnitude and causes of these important events. In addition to obstetric health care providers, neonatologists and pediatricians should have easy access to current and updated resources that clearly provide US definitions and reporting requirements for live births, fetal deaths, and infant deaths. Correct identification of these vital events will improve local, state, and national data so that these deaths can be better addressed and prevented. (5/16, reaffirmed 12/24)
https://doi.org/10.1542/peds.2016-0551

STANDARDS FOR HEALTH INFORMATION TECHNOLOGY TO ENSURE ADOLESCENT PRIVACY

Committee on Adolescence and Council on Clinical Information Technology

ABSTRACT. Privacy and security of health information is a basic expectation of patients. Despite the existence of federal and state laws safeguarding the privacy of health information, health information systems currently lack the capability to allow for protection of this information for minors. This policy statement reviews the challenges to privacy for adolescents posed by commercial health information technology systems and recommends basic principles for ideal electronic health record systems. This policy statement has been endorsed by the Society for Adolescent Health and Medicine. (10/12, reaffirmed 12/18, 12/21)
https://doi.org/10.1542/peds.2012-2580

STRATEGIES FOR IMPROVING VACCINE COMMUNICATION AND UPTAKE (CLINICAL REPORT)

Sean T. O'Leary, MD, MPH, FAAP; Douglas J. Opel, MD, MPH; Jessica R. Cataldi, MD, FAAP; Jesse M. Hackell, MD, FAAP; Committee on Infectious Diseases; Committee on Practice and Ambulatory Medicine; and Committee on Bioethics

ABSTRACT. Vaccines have led to a significant decrease in rates of vaccine-preventable diseases and have made a significant impact on the health of children. However, some parents express concerns about vaccine safety and the necessity of vaccines. The concerns of parents range from hesitancy about some immunizations to refusal of all vaccines. This clinical report provides information about the scope and impact of the problem, the facts surrounding common vaccination concerns, and the latest evidence regarding effective communication techniques for the vaccine conversation.

After reading this clinical report, readers can expect to:

1. Understand concepts and underlying determinants of vaccine uptake and vaccine hesitancy.
2. Understand the relationship between vaccine hesitancy and costs of preventable medical care.
3. Recognize and address specific concerns (eg, vaccine safety) with caregivers when hesitancy is present. (2/24)

https://doi.org/10.1542/peds.2023-065483

STRATEGIES FOR PREVENTION OF HEALTH CARE–ASSOCIATED INFECTIONS IN THE NICU (CLINICAL REPORT)

Richard A. Polin, MD; Susan Denson, MD; Michael T. Brady, MD; Committee on Fetus and Newborn; and Committee on Infectious Diseases

ABSTRACT. Health care–associated infections in the NICU result in increased morbidity and mortality, prolonged lengths of stay, and increased medical costs. Neonates are at high risk of acquiring health care–associated infections because of impaired host-defense mechanisms, limited amounts of protective endogenous flora on skin and mucosal surfaces at time of birth, reduced barrier function of their skin, use of invasive procedures and devices, and frequent exposure to broad-spectrum antibiotic agents. This clinical report reviews management and prevention of health care–associated infections in newborn infants. (3/12, reaffirmed 3/23)
https://doi.org/10.1542/peds.2012-0145

SUBSTANCE USE SCREENING, BRIEF INTERVENTION, AND REFERRAL TO TREATMENT (CLINICAL REPORT)

Sharon J. L. Levy, MD, MPH, FAAP; Janet F. Williams, MD, FAAP; and Committee on Substance Use and Prevention

ABSTRACT. The enormous public health impact of adolescent substance use and its preventable morbidity and mortality highlight the need for the health care sector, including pediatricians and the medical home, to increase its capacity regarding adolescent substance use screening, brief intervention, and referral to treatment (SBIRT). The American Academy of Pediatrics first published a policy statement on SBIRT and adolescents in 2011 to introduce SBIRT concepts and terminology and to offer clinical guidance about available substance use screening tools and intervention procedures. This clinical report provides a simplified adolescent SBIRT clinical approach that, in combination with the accompanying updated policy statement, guides pediatricians in implementing substance use prevention, detection, assessment, and intervention practices across the varied clinical settings in which adolescents receive health care. (6/16, reaffirmed 11/23)

https://doi.org/10.1542/peds.2016-1211

SUCCESSES AND LESSONS LEARNED IN RESPONDING TO THE NEEDS OF PEDIATRICIANS, CHILDREN, AND FAMILIES DURING THE COVID-19 PANDEMIC

COVID-19 Working Group

ABSTRACT. The coronavirus disease 2019 pandemic has presented tremendous challenges to the United States health care system, as well as to individual physicians, communities, and families. Throughout the pandemic, the American Academy of Pediatrics (AAP) has striven to elevate the needs of infants, children, and adolescents, as well as the pediatricians who care for this population. Historically, these communities have often been overlooked and deprioritized in health care systems, and these deficits persisted into the pandemic. To fill this gap, the AAP took on an essential role in leading the national response for pediatrics. This article details the AAP pandemic response and includes the perspectives of multiple AAP leaders involved in the response and details on Academy advocacy with high-level staff and officials at federal agencies and the executive branch. The AAP provided initial guidance to pediatricians that predated the World Health Organization's declaration of a public health emergency. The Academy then developed entirely new approaches to meet the unprecedented needs of its practicing members and families by providing timely, rigorous information endorsed by pediatric experts. When coronavirus disease 2019 vaccines were developed, the AAP strongly advised the inclusion of those younger than 18 years in vaccine trials and advocated for equitable distribution plans. The AAP provided its members with strategies for combating misinformation. The Academy was at the forefront of advocating for the safe return to in-person schooling, recognizing that social isolation was contributing to the growing mental health crisis among youth. In 2021, the AAP, the American Academy of Child and Adolescent Psychiatry, and the Children's Hospital Association declared a national emergency in child and adolescent mental health. In addition, the AAP implemented educational and training opportunities for clinicians and developed resources for youth and their families. After the end of the public health emergency, AAP members continue to use innovations and efficiencies developed as part of their pandemic response. The successes of the AAP pandemic response, alongside lessons learned, help define an important model for responding to future pandemics and public health emergencies in ways that support children, families, and the pediatric workforce. (5/24)

https://doi.org/10.1542/peds.2024-066634

SUDDEN DEATH IN THE YOUNG: INFORMATION FOR THE PRIMARY CARE PROVIDER

Christopher C. Erickson, MD, FAAP; Jack C. Salerno, MD; Stuart Berger, MD, FAAP; Robert Campbell, MD, FAAP; Bryan Cannon, MD; James Christiansen, MD; Kody Moffatt, MD, MS, FAAP; Andreas Pflaumer, MD; Christopher S. Snyder, MD, FAAP; Chandra Srinivasan, MD; Santiago O. Valdes, MD, FAAP; Victoria L. Vetter, MD, MPH, FAAP; Frank Zimmerman, MD; and Section on Cardiology and Cardiac Surgery (joint with Pediatric and Congenital Electrophysiology Society [PACES] Task Force on Prevention of Sudden Death in the Young)

ABSTRACT. There are multiple conditions that can make children prone to having a sudden cardiac arrest (SCA) or sudden cardiac death (SCD). Efforts have been made by multiple organizations to screen children for cardiac conditions, but the emphasis has been on screening before athletic competition. This article is an update of the previous American Academy of Pediatrics policy statement of 2012 that addresses prevention of SCA and SCD. This update includes a comprehensive review of conditions that should prompt more attention and cardiology evaluation. The role of the primary care provider is of paramount importance in the evaluation of children, particularly as they enter middle school or junior high. There is discussion about whether screening should find any cardiac condition or just those that are associated with SCA and SCD. This update reviews the 4 main screening questions that are recommended, not just for athletes, but for all children. There is also discussion about how to handle post-SCA and SCD situations as well as discussion about genetic testing. It is the goal of this policy statement update to provide the primary care provider more assistance in how to screen for life-threatening conditions, regardless of athletic status. (6/21)

https://doi.org/10.1542/peds.2021-052044

SUICIDE AND SUICIDE RISK IN ADOLESCENTS (CLINICAL REPORT)

Liwei L. Hua, MD, PhD; Janet Lee, MD, FAAP; Maria H. Rahmandar, MD, FAAP; Eric J. Sigel, MD, FAAP; Committee on Adolescence; and Council on Injury, Violence, and Poison Prevention

ABSTRACT. Suicide is the second leading cause of death for 10- to 24-year-olds in the United States and is a global public health issue, with a recent declaration of a National State of Emergency in Children's Mental Health by the American Academy of Pediatrics, American Academy of Child and Adolescent Psychiatry, and Children's Hospital Association. This clinical report is an update to the previous American Academy of Pediatrics clinical report, "Suicide and Suicide Attempts in Adolescents." Because pediatricians and pediatric health care providers are at the front line of care for adolescents amid a child and adolescent mental health crisis, and because of the chronic and severe shortage of mental health specialists, it is important that pediatric health care providers become facile with recognizing risk factors associated with suicidality and at-risk populations, screening and further assessment of suicidality as indicated, and evidence-based interventions for patients with suicidal ideation and associated behaviors. Suicide risk can be mitigated by appropriate screening, bolstering of protective factors, indicated treatment, community resources, and referrals to mental health providers when available. (12/23)

https://doi.org/10.1542/peds.2023-064800

SUPPLEMENTAL SECURITY INCOME (SSI) FOR CHILDREN AND YOUTH WITH DISABILITIES

Council on Children With Disabilities

ABSTRACT. The Supplemental Security Income (SSI) program remains an important source of financial support for low-income families of children with special health care needs and

disabling conditions. In most states, SSI eligibility also qualifies children for the state Medicaid program, providing access to health care services. The Social Security Administration (SSA), which administers the SSI program, considers a child disabled under SSI if there is a medically determinable physical or mental impairment or combination of impairments that results in marked and severe functional limitations. The impairment(s) must be expected to result in death or have lasted or be expected to last for a continuous period of at least 12 months. The income and assets of families of children with disabilities are also considered when determining financial eligibility. When an individual with a disability becomes an adult at 18 years of age, the SSA considers only the individual's income and assets. The SSA considers an adult to be disabled if there is a medically determinable impairment (or combination of impairments) that prevents substantial gainful activity for at least 12 continuous months. SSI benefits are important for youth with chronic conditions who are transitioning to adulthood. The purpose of this statement is to provide updated information about the SSI medical and financial eligibility criteria and the disability-determination process. This statement also discusses how pediatricians can help children and youth when they apply for SSI benefits. (11/09, reaffirmed 2/15, 8/21)
https://doi.org/10.1542/peds.2009-2557

SUPPORTING THE FAMILY AFTER THE DEATH OF A CHILD OR ADOLESCENT (CLINICAL REPORT)

Meaghann S. Weaver, MD, PhD, MPH, FAAP; Arwa Nasir, MBBS, MSc, MPH, FAAP; Blyth T. Lord, EdM; Amy Starin, PhD, LCSW; Jennifer S. Linebarger, MD, MPH, FAAP; Committee on Psychosocial Aspects of Child and Family Health; and Section on Hospice and Palliative Medicine

ABSTRACT. Whether death occurs in the context of a chronic illness or as the sudden loss of a previously healthy infant, child, or adolescent, the death of a child is a highly stressful and traumatic event. Psychosocial support for families after the death of a child embodies core medical values of professional fidelity, compassion, respect for human dignity, and promotion of the best interests of a grieving family. The pediatrician has an important role in supporting the family unit after the death of a child through a family-centered, culturally humble, trauma-informed approach. This clinical report aims to provide the pediatrician with a review of the current evidence on grief, bereavement, and mourning after the loss of a child and with practical guidance to support family caregivers, siblings, and the child's community. Pediatricians have an important role in helping siblings and helping families understand sibling needs during grief. Ways for pediatricians to support family members with cultural sensitivity are suggested and other helpful resources in the community are described. (11/23)
https://doi.org/10.1542/peds.2023-064426

SUPPORTING THE GRIEVING CHILD AND FAMILY (CLINICAL REPORT)

David J. Schonfeld, MD, FAAP; Thomas Demaria, PhD; Arwa Nasir, MBBS, MSc, MPH, FAAP; Sairam Kumar, MD, FAAP; Committee on Psychosocial Aspects of Child and Family Health; and Council on Children and Disasters

ABSTRACT. The death of someone close to a child often has a profound and lifelong effect on the child and results in a range of both short- and long-term reactions. Pediatricians, within a patient-centered medical home, are in an excellent position to provide guidance to caregivers and to offer assistance and support to grieving children of all ages and their families. This clinical report offers practical suggestions on how to talk with grieving children to help them better understand what has happened and its implications. An understanding of guilt, shame, and other common reactions as well as an appreciation of the role of secondary losses and the unique challenges facing children in communities characterized by chronic trauma and cumulative loss will help the pediatrician to address factors that may impair children's adjustment and to identify complicated mourning and situations when professional counseling is indicated. Advice on how to support children's participation in funerals and other memorial services and to anticipate and address grief triggers and anniversary reactions is provided so that pediatricians are in a better position to advise caregivers and to offer consultation to and collaborate with professionals in schools, early education and child care facilities, and other child congregate care sites. Pediatricians often enter their profession out of a profound desire to minimize the suffering of children and may find it personally challenging to bear witness to the distress of children who are acutely grieving. The importance of professional preparation and self-care is, therefore, emphasized, and resources are recommended. (6/24)
https://doi.org/10.1542/peds.2024-067212

SUPPORTING THE HEALTH CARE TRANSITION FROM ADOLESCENCE TO ADULTHOOD IN THE MEDICAL HOME (CLINICAL REPORT)

Patience H. White, MD, MA, FAAP, FACP; W. Carl Cooley, MD, FAAP; American Academy of Pediatrics (joint with Transitions Clinical Report Authoring Group, American Academy of Family Physicians, and American College of Physicians)

ABSTRACT. Risk and vulnerability encompass many dimensions of the transition from adolescence to adulthood. Transition from pediatric, parent-supervised health care to more independent, patient-centered adult health care is no exception. The tenets and algorithm of the original 2011 clinical report, "Supporting the Health Care Transition from Adolescence to Adulthood in the Medical Home," are unchanged. This updated clinical report provides more practice-based quality improvement guidance on key elements of transition planning, transfer, and integration into adult care for all youth and young adults. It also includes new and updated sections on definition and guiding principles, the status of health care transition preparation among youth, barriers, outcome evidence, recommended health care transition processes and implementation strategies using quality improvement methods, special populations, education and training in pediatric onset conditions, and payment options. The clinical report also includes new recommendations pertaining to infrastructure, education and training, payment, and research. (10/18, reaffirmed 7/23 with reference & data updates)
https://doi.org/10.1542/peds.2018-2587

SYSTEMS-BASED CARE OF THE INJURED CHILD

Katherine T. Flynn-O'Brien, MD, MPH, FAAP, FACS; Vijay Srinivasan, MBBS, MD, FCCM, FAAP; Mary E. Fallat, MD, FAAP, FACS; Committee on Pediatric Emergency Medicine; Council on Injury, Violence, and Poison Prevention; Section on Critical Care; Section on Surgery; and Section on Transport Medicine (joint with Pediatric Trauma Society and Society of Trauma Nurses Pediatric Committee)

ABSTRACT. Injury is the leading cause of death and a frequent cause of disability in children and negatively affects physical health, mental health, and quality of life in both the short- and long-term. The goal of a pediatric trauma system is to optimize the care for children within a state or region encompassing the entire continuum of care regardless of where children live or where traumatic events occur. This continuum includes injury prevention, prehospital care, emergency department care, interfacility transport, acute and critical inpatient care, inpatient and outpatient rehabilitation, and reintegration into the community and primary care medical home. A systems-based approach requires distinct elements of structure and function to perform together in an interrelated and cohesive manner to improve care quality. In this case, it represents a sequential practice of evidence-based evaluation and management along the continuum of care. To improve outcomes after injury, a cohesive system must effectively provide optimal care for the "right child, at the right place, at the right time" across this continuum. (8/25)

See full text on page 601.

https://doi.org/10.1542/peds.2025-072720

SYSTEMS-BASED CARE OF THE INJURED CHILD (TECHNICAL REPORT)

Katherine T. Flynn-O'Brien, MD, MPH, FAAP, FACS; Vijay Srinivasan, MBBS, MD, FCCM, FAAP; Mary E. Fallat, MD, FAAP, FACS; Committee on Pediatric Emergency Medicine; Council on Injury, Violence, and Poison Prevention; Section on Critical Care; Section on Surgery; Section on Transport Medicine (joint with Pediatric Trauma Society and Society of Trauma Nurses Pediatric Committee)

ABSTRACT. Injury is the leading cause of death and a cause of disability in children and negatively affects physical health, mental health, and quality of life in both the short- and long-term. The goal of a pediatric trauma system is to optimize the care for children within a state, regional, or national trauma system across the entire continuum of care regardless of where they live or where the traumatic event occurs. This continuum includes injury prevention, prehospital care, interfacility transport between hospitals providing different levels of care, acute and critical inpatient care, inpatient and outpatient rehabilitation, and reintegration into the community and primary care medical home. A systems-based approach, one that requires distinct elements of structure and function to perform together in an interrelated and cohesive manner to improve care quality, is essential. To improve outcomes after injury, a cohesive system must effectively provide optimal care for the "right child, at the right place, at the right time" across this continuum. (8/25)

See full text on page 613.

https://doi.org/10.1542/peds.2025-072721

TELEHEALTH: IMPROVING ACCESS TO AND QUALITY OF PEDIATRIC HEALTH CARE

Alison L. Curfman, MD, MBA, FAAP; Jesse M. Hackell, MD, FAAP; Neil E. Herendeen, MD, MS, FAAP; Joshua J. Alexander, MD, FAAP; James P. Marcin, MD, MPH, FAAP; William B. Moskowitz, MD, FAAP; Chelsea E. F. Bodnar, MD, MPhil, FAAP; Harold K. Simon, MD, MBA, FAAP; S. David McSwain, MD, FAAP; Section on Telehealth Care; Committee on Practice and Ambulatory Medicine; and Committee on Pediatric Workforce

ABSTRACT. All children and adolescents deserve access to quality health care regardless of their race/ethnicity, health conditions, financial resources, or geographic location. Despite improvements over the past decades, severe disparities in the availability and access to high-quality health care for children and adolescents continue to exist throughout the United States. Economic and racial factors, geographic maldistribution of primary care pediatricians, and limited availability of pediatric medical subspecialists and pediatric surgical specialists all contribute to inequitable access to pediatric care. Robust, comprehensive telehealth coverage is critical to improving pediatric access and quality of care and services, particularly for under-resourced populations. (8/21)

https://doi.org/10.1542/peds.2021-053129

TELEHEALTH: OPPORTUNITIES TO IMPROVE ACCESS, QUALITY, AND COST IN PEDIATRIC CARE (TECHNICAL REPORT)

Alison Curfman, MD, MBA, FAAP; Jesse M. Hackell, MD, FAAP; Neil E. Herendeen, MD, MS, FAAP; Joshua Alexander, MD, FAAP; James P. Marcin, MD, MPH, FAAP; William B. Moskowitz, MD, FAAP; Chelsea E. F. Bodnar, MD, MPhil, FAAP; Harold K. Simon, MD, MBA, FAAP; S. David McSwain, MD, FAAP; Section on Telehealth Care; Committee on Practice and Ambulatory Medicine; and Committee on Pediatric Workforce

ABSTRACT. The use of telehealth technology to connect with patients has expanded significantly over the past several years, particularly in response to the global coronavirus disease 2019 pandemic. This technical report describes the present state of telehealth and its current and potential applications. Telehealth has the potential to transform the way care is delivered to pediatric patients, expanding access to pediatric care across geographic distances, leveraging the pediatric workforce for care delivery, and improving disparities in access to care. However, implementation will require significant efforts to address the digital divide to ensure that telehealth does not inadvertently exacerbate inequities in care. The medical home model will continue to evolve to use telehealth to provide high-quality care for children, particularly for children and youth with special health care needs, in accordance with current and evolving quality standards. Research and metric development are critical for the development of evidence-based best practices and policies in these new models of care. Finally, as pediatric care transitions from traditional fee-for-service payment to alternative payment methods, telehealth offers unique opportunities to establish value-based population health models that are financed in a sustainable manner. (2/22)

https://doi.org/10.1542/peds.2021-056035

TELEMEDICINE FOR EVALUATION OF RETINOPATHY OF PREMATURITY (TECHNICAL REPORT)

Walter M. Fierson, MD, FAAP; Antonio Capone Jr, MD; and Section on Ophthalmology (joint with American Academy of Ophthalmology and American Association of Certified Orthoptists)

ABSTRACT. Retinopathy of prematurity (ROP) remains a significant threat to vision for extremely premature infants despite the availability of therapeutic modalities capable, in most cases, of managing this disorder. It has been shown in many controlled trials that application of therapies at the appropriate time is essential to successful outcomes in premature infants affected by ROP. Bedside binocular indirect ophthalmoscopy has been the standard technique for diagnosis and monitoring of ROP in these patients. However, implementation of routine use of this screening method for at-risk premature infants has presented challenges within our existing care systems, including relative local scarcity of qualified ophthalmologist examiners in some locations and the remote location of some NICUs. Modern technology, including the development of wide-angle ocular digital fundus photography, coupled with the ability to send digital images electronically to remote locations, has led to the development of telemedicine-based remote digital fundus imaging (RDFI-TM) evaluation techniques. These techniques have the potential to allow the diagnosis and monitoring of ROP to occur in lieu of the necessity for some repeated on-site examinations in NICUs. This report reviews the currently available literature on RDFI-TM evaluations for ROP and outlines pertinent practical and risk management considerations that should be used when including RDFI-TM in any new or existing ROP care structure. (12/14, reaffirmed 2/21)

https://doi.org/10.1542/peds.2014-0978

TOPICAL NASAL DECONGESTANT OXYMETAZOLINE: SAFETY CONSIDERATIONS FOR PERIOPERATIVE PEDIATRIC USE (CLINICAL REPORT)

Richard Cartabuke, MD, FAAP; Joseph D. Tobias, MD, FAAP; Kris R. Jatana, MD, FAAP; Section on Anesthesiology and Pain Medicine; and Section on Otolaryngology—Head and Neck Surgery

ABSTRACT. The over-the-counter nasal decongestant oxymetazoline (eg, Afrin) is used in the pediatric population for a variety of conditions in the operating room setting. Given its vasoconstrictive properties, it can have cardiovascular adverse effects when systemically absorbed. There have been several reports of cardiac and respiratory complications related to use of oxymetazoline in the pediatric population. Current US Food and Drug Administration approval for oxymetazoline is for patients ≥6 years of age, but medical professionals may elect to use it short-term and off label for younger children in particular clinical scenarios in which the potential benefit may outweigh risks (eg, active bleeding, acute respiratory distress from nasal obstruction, acute complicated sinusitis, improved surgical visualization, nasal decongestion for scope examination, other conditions, etc). To date, there have not been adequate pediatric pharmacokinetic studies of oxymetazoline, so caution should be exercised with both the quantity of dosing and the technique of administration. In the urgent care setting, emergency department, or inpatient setting, to avoid excessive administration of the medication, medical professionals should use the spray bottle in an upright position with the child upright. In addition, in the operating room setting, both monitoring the quantity used and effective communication between the surgeon and anesthesia team are important. Further studies are needed to understand the systemic absorption and effects in children in both nonsurgical and surgical nasal use of oxymetazoline. (10/21)
https://doi.org/10.1542/peds.2021-054271

TRAMPOLINE SAFETY IN CHILDHOOD AND ADOLESCENCE

Council on Sports Medicine and Fitness

ABSTRACT. Despite previous recommendations from the American Academy of Pediatrics discouraging home use of trampolines, recreational use of trampolines in the home setting continues to be a popular activity among children and adolescents. This policy statement is an update to previous statements, reflecting the current literature on prevalence, patterns, and mechanisms of trampoline-related injuries. Most trampoline injuries occur with multiple simultaneous users on the mat. Cervical spine injuries often occur with falls off the trampoline or with attempts at somersaults or flips. Studies on the efficacy of trampoline safety measures are reviewed, and although there is a paucity of data, current implementation of safety measures have not appeared to mitigate risk substantially. Therefore, the home use of trampolines is strongly discouraged. The role of trampoline as a competitive sport and in structured training settings is reviewed, and recommendations for enhancing safety in these environments are made. (9/12, reaffirmed 3/25 with reference & data updates)
https://doi.org/10.1542/peds.2012-2082

TRANSITION TO A SAFE HOME SLEEP ENVIRONMENT FOR THE NICU PATIENT

Michael H. Goodstein, MD, FAAP; Dan L. Stewart, MD, FAAP; Erin L. Keels, DNP, APRN-CNP, NNP-BC; Rachel Y. Moon, MD, FAAP; Committee on Fetus and Newborn; and Task Force on Sudden Infant Death Syndrome

ABSTRACT. Of the nearly 3.8 million infants born in the United States in 2018, 8.3% had low birth weight (ie, weight <2500 g) and 10% were born preterm (ie, gestational age of <37 weeks). Ten to fifteen percent of infants (approximately 500000 annually), including low birth weight and preterm infants and others with congenital anomalies, perinatally acquired infections, and other diseases, require admission to a NICU. Every year, approximately 3600 infants in the United States die of sudden unexpected infant death (SUID), including sudden infant death syndrome (SIDS), unknown and undetermined causes, and accidental suffocation and strangulation in an unsafe sleep environment. Preterm and low birth weight infants are 2 to 3 times more likely than healthy term infants to die suddenly and unexpectedly. Thus, it is important that health care professionals prepare families to maintain their infant in a safe home sleep environment as per recommendations of the American Academy of Pediatrics. Medical needs of the NICU infant often require practices such as nonsupine positioning, which should be transitioned as soon as medically possible and well before hospital discharge to sleep practices that are safe and appropriate for the home environment. This clinical report outlines the establishment of appropriate NICU protocols for the timely transition of these infants to a safe home sleep environment. The rationale for these recommendations is discussed in the accompanying technical report "Transition to a Safe Home Sleep Environment for the NICU Patient," included in this issue of *Pediatrics*. (6/21)
https://doi.org/10.1542/peds.2021-052045

TRANSITION TO A SAFE HOME SLEEP ENVIRONMENT FOR THE NICU PATIENT (TECHNICAL REPORT)

Michael H. Goodstein, MD, FAAP; Dan L. Stewart, MD, FAAP; Erin L. Keels, DNP, APRN-CNP, NNP-BC; Rachel Y. Moon, MD, FAAP; Committee on Fetus and Newborn; and Task Force on Sudden Infant Death Syndrome

ABSTRACT. Of the nearly 3.8 million infants born in the United States in 2018, 8.3% had low birth weight (<2500 g [5.5 lb]) and 10% were born preterm (gestational age of <37 completed weeks). Many of these infants and others with congenital anomalies, perinatally acquired infections, and other disease require admission to a NICU. In the past decade, admission rates to NICUs have been increasing; it is estimated that between 10% and 15% of infants will spend time in a NICU, representing approximately 500 000 neonates annually. Approximately 3600 infants die annually in the United States from sleep-related deaths, including sudden infant death syndrome *International Classification of Diseases, 10th Revision* (R95), ill-defined deaths (R99), and accidental suffocation and strangulation in bed (W75). Preterm and low birth weight infants are particularly vulnerable, with an incidence of death 2 to 3 times greater than healthy term infants. Thus, it is important for health care professionals to prepare families to maintain their infant in a safe sleep environment, as per the recommendations of the American Academy of Pediatrics. However, infants in the NICU setting commonly require care that is inconsistent with infant sleep safety recommendations. The conflicting needs of the NICU infant with the necessity to provide a safe sleep environment before hospital discharge can create confusion for providers and distress for families. This technical report is intended to assist in the establishment of appropriate NICU protocols to achieve a consistent approach to transitioning NICU infants to a safe sleep environment as soon as medically possible, well before hospital discharge. (6/21)
https://doi.org/10.1542/peds.2021-052046

TRAUMA-INFORMED CARE (CLINICAL REPORT)

Heather Forkey, MD, FAAP; Moira Szilagyi, MD, PhD, FAAP; Erin T. Kelly, MD, FAAP, FACP; James Duffee, MD, MPH, FAAP; Council on Foster Care, Adoption, and Kinship Care; Council on Community Pediatrics; Council on Child Abuse and Neglect; and Committee on Psychosocial Aspects of Child and Family Health

ABSTRACT. Most children will experience some type of trauma during childhood, and many children suffer from significant adversities. Research in genetics, neuroscience, and epidemiol-

ogy all provide evidence that these experiences have effects at the molecular, cellular, and organ level, with consequences on physical, emotional, developmental, and behavioral health across the life span. Trauma-informed care translates that science to inform and improve pediatric care and outcomes. To practically address trauma and promote resilience, pediatric clinicians need tools to assess childhood trauma and adversity experiences as well as practical guidance, resources, and interventions. In this clinical report, we summarize current, practical advice for rendering trauma-informed care across varied medical settings. (7/21)
https://doi.org/10.1542/peds.2021-052580

TRAUMA-INFORMED CARE IN CHILD HEALTH SYSTEMS

James Duffee, MD, MPH, FAAP; Moira Szilagyi, MD, PhD, FAAP; Heather Forkey, MD, FAAP; Erin T. Kelly, MD, FAAP, FACP; Council on Community Pediatrics; Council on Foster Care, Adoption, and Kinship Care; Council on Child Abuse and Neglect; and Committee on Psychosocial Aspects of Child and Family Health

ABSTRACT. Recent progress in understanding the lifelong effects of early childhood adversities has clarified the need for an organized strategy to identify and intervene with children, adolescents, and families who may be at risk for maladaptive responses. Trauma-informed care (TIC) in child health care operationalizes the biological evidence of toxic stress with the insights of attachment and resilience to enhance health care delivery to mitigate the effects of trauma. The resulting pediatric health care delivery strategy promotes and restores resilience in children and adolescents, partners with families to support relational health, and reduces secondary trauma among pediatric health care clinicians. This policy statement summarizes what policy makers, legislators, and health care organizations need to consider in terms of infrastructure, resources, and financial support to facilitate the integration of TIC principles into all pediatric points of care. The accompanying clinical report describes the elements of TIC in the direct care of children, adolescents, and families and covers the spectrum from prevention to treatment. The recommendations in this statement and the clinical report build on other American Academy of Pediatrics policies that address the needs of special populations (such as children and adolescents in foster or kinship care, in immigrant and refugee families, or in poor or homeless families) and are congruent with American Academy of Pediatrics policies and technical reports concerning the role of pediatric clinicians in the promotion of lifelong health. (7/21)
https://doi.org/10.1542/peds.2021-052579

TUBERCULOSIS INFECTION IN CHILDREN AND ADOLESCENTS: TESTING AND TREATMENT (CLINICAL REPORT)

Dawn Nolt, MD, MPH, FAAP; Jeffrey R. Starke, MD, FAAP; and Committee on Infectious Diseases

ABSTRACT. Tuberculosis (TB) remains an important problem among children in the United States and throughout the world. There is no diagnostic reference standard for latent tuberculosis infection (also referred to as tuberculosis infection [TBI]). The tuberculin skin test (TST) has many limitations, including difficulty in administration and interpretation, the need for a return visit by the patient, and false-positive results caused by cross-reaction with Mycobacterium bovis–bacille Calmette-Guerin vaccines and many nontuberculous mycobacteria. Interferon-gamma release assays (IGRAs) are blood tests that use antigens specific for M tuberculosis; as a result, IGRAs yield fewer false-positive results than the TST. Both IGRAs and the TST have reduced sensitivity in immunocompromised children, including children with severe TB disease. Both methods have high positive predictive value when applied to children with risk factors for TBI, especially recent contact with a person who has TB disease. The advantages of using IGRAs and diminished experience with the placement and interpretation of the TST favor expanded use of IGRAs in children in the United States. There are now several effective and safe regimens for the treatment of TBI in children. For improved adherence to therapy, the 3 rifamycin-based regimens are preferred because of their short duration. Daily isoniazid can be used if there is intolerance or drug interactions with rifamycins. A TB specialist should be involved when there are questions regarding testing interpretation, selection of an appropriate treatment regimen, or management of adverse effects. (11/21)
https://doi.org/10.1542/peds.2021-054663

UNDERSTANDING LIABILITY RISKS AND PROTECTIONS FOR PEDIATRIC PROVIDERS DURING DISASTERS

Robin L. Altman, MD; Karen A. Santucci, MD; Michael R. Anderson, MD; William M. McDonnell, MD; Committee on Medical Liability and Risk Management

ABSTRACT. Although most health care providers will go through their careers without experiencing a major disaster in their local communities, if one does occur, it can be life and career altering. The American Academy of Pediatrics has been at the forefront of providing education and advocacy on the critical importance of disaster preparedness. From experiences over the past decade, new evidence and analysis have broadened our understanding that the concept of preparedness is also applicable to addressing the unique professional liability risks that can occur when caring for patients and families during a disaster. In our recommendations in this policy statement, we target pediatric health care providers, advocates, and policy makers and address how individuals, institutions, and government can work together to strengthen the system of liability protections during disasters so that appropriate and timely care can be delivered with minimal fear of legal reprisal or confusion. (3/19, reaffirmed 1/25)
https://doi.org/10.1542/peds.2018-3892

UNDERSTANDING LIABILITY RISKS AND PROTECTIONS FOR PEDIATRIC PROVIDERS DURING DISASTERS (TECHNICAL REPORT)

Robin L. Altman, MD; Karen A. Santucci, MD; Michael R. Anderson, MD; William M. McDonnell, MD; Committee on Medical Liability and Risk Management

ABSTRACT. Although most health care providers will go through their careers without experiencing a major disaster in their local communities, if one does occur, it can be life and career altering. The American Academy of Pediatrics has been in the forefront of providing education and advocacy on the critical importance of disaster preparedness. From experiences over the past decade, new evidence and analysis have broadened our understanding that the concept of preparedness is also applicable to addressing the unique professional liability risks that can occur when caring for patients and families during a disaster. Concepts explored in this technical report will help to inform pediatric health care providers, advocates, and policy makers about the complexities of how providers are currently protected, with a focus on areas of unappreciated liability. The timeliness of this technical report is emphasized by the fact that during the time of its development (ie, late summer and early fall of 2017), the United States went through an extraordinary period of multiple, successive, and overlapping disasters within a concentrated period of time of both natural and man-made causes. In a companion policy statement (http://www.pediatrics.org/cgi/doi/10.1542/peds.2018-3892), recommendations are offered on how individuals, institutions, and governments can work together to strengthen the system of liability protections during disasters so

that appropriate and timely care can be delivered with minimal fear of legal reprisal or confusion. (3/19, reaffirmed 1/25)
https://doi.org/10.1542/peds.2018-3893

THE UNIQUE VALUE PROPOSITION OF PEDIATRIC HEALTH CARE

James M. Perrin, MD, FAAP; Patricia Flanagan, MD, FAAP; Julie Katkin, MD, FAAP; Greg Barabell, MD, FAAP; Jonathan Price, MD, FAAP; and Committee on Child Health Financing

ABSTRACT. This document provides a framework for the value proposition of pediatric health care. It is intended to provide a succinct set of principles for establishing this proposition that demonstrates the short- and long-term value to the child and family, the health care system, and society as a whole. (1/23)
https://doi.org/10.1542/peds.2022-060681

USE OF ANTIBIOTICS IN ANIMAL AGRICULTURE: IMPLICATIONS FOR PEDIATRICS (TECHNICAL REPORT)

Sophie E. Katz, MD, FAAP; Ritu Banerjee, MD, PhD, FAAP; Committee on Infectious Diseases; and Council on Environmental Health and Climate Change

ABSTRACT. Antimicrobial resistance is a global public health threat. Antimicrobial-resistant infections are on the rise and are associated with increased morbidity, mortality, and health care costs. Infants and children are affected by transmission of antimicrobial-resistant zoonotic pathogens through the food supply, direct contact with animals, environmental pathways, and contact with infected or colonized humans. Although the judicious use of antimicrobial agents is necessary for maintaining the health and welfare of humans and animals, it must be recognized that all use of antimicrobial agents exerts selective pressure that increases the risk of development of resistance. This report describes historical and recent use of antibiotics in animal agriculture, reviews the mechanisms of how such use contributes to development of resistance and can adversely affect child health, and discusses US initiatives to curb unnecessary use of antimicrobial agents in agriculture. (9/24)
https://doi.org/10.1542/peds.2024-068467

USE OF CHAPERONES FOR THE PEDIATRIC AND ADOLESCENT ENCOUNTER

Abeba Berhane, MD, FAAP; Jesse M. Hackell, MD, FAAP; Stephenie Wallace, MD, FAAP; Committee on Practice and Ambulatory Medicine; and Committee on Adolescence

ABSTRACT. Pediatric inpatient and outpatient encounters often include examinations that may be perceived as intrusive or uncomfortable by patients because of examination of sensitive body areas. The presence of a chaperone during these examinations can serve to optimize the patient's sense of comfort and safety, as well as protecting the physician. Chaperones should usually be clinical staff members, although providing adequate staffing may not be feasible for many small practices. Thus, the decision to use a chaperone and the specific choice of chaperone should be made jointly by the patient, parent and clinician providing care, considering the wishes of all parties to the encounter. Certain situations, including telemedicine encounters, unaccompanied minors, patients with intellectual disability, those suffering from abuse, exploitation or trafficking and those who are otherwise unable to assent to care or participate in shared decision making require special consideration for sensitive examinations, with attention paid to principles of trauma-informed care. All outpatient practices and inpatient services should develop policies addressing the situations which might prompt the need for a chaperone, and address their ability to provide one, and be prepared to involve the patient and family in the decision-making process. (5/25)
See full text on page 641.
https://doi.org/10.1542/peds.2025-071810

USE OF GENETICALLY MODIFIED ORGANISM (GMO)-CONTAINING FOOD PRODUCTS IN CHILDREN (CLINICAL REPORT)

Steven A. Abrams, MD, FAAP; Jaclyn Lewis Albin, MD, FAAP; Philip J. Landrigan, MD, FAAP; Committee on Nutrition; and Council on Environmental Health and Climate Change

ABSTRACT. Families increasingly raise questions about the use of genetically modified organism (GMO)-containing food products. These products are widely found in the US food supply but originate from a narrow list of crops. Although GMO technology could be used to increase the micronutrient content of foods, this does not occur in the United States; instead, GMO technology has been used to make crops resistant to chemical herbicides. As a result, herbicide use has increased exponentially. The World Health Organization's International Agency on Research for Cancer has determined that glyphosate, an herbicide widely used in producing GMO food crops, is a probable human carcinogen. Measurable quantities of glyphosate are detected in some GMO foods. Families who wish to minimize GMO food products can do so by focusing on a dietary pattern of primarily whole, plant-based foods while minimizing ultra-processed foods. Pediatricians play a vital role in their efforts to minimize fear-based messaging and support families through shared decision-making. Pediatrician awareness of GMO labeling can guide individualized conversations, particularly that non-GMO labeling does not indicate organic status and that increased cost of some non-GMO foods, especially if also organic, may limit this choice for many families. (12/23)
https://doi.org/10.1542/peds.2023-064774

USE OF INHALED NITRIC OXIDE IN PRETERM INFANTS (CLINICAL REPORT)

Praveen Kumar, MD; Committee on Fetus and Newborn

ABSTRACT. Nitric oxide, an important signaling molecule with multiple regulatory effects throughout the body, is an important tool for the treatment of full-term and late-preterm infants with persistent pulmonary hypertension of the newborn and hypoxemic respiratory failure. Several randomized controlled trials have evaluated its role in the management of preterm infants ≤34 weeks' gestational age with varying results. The purpose of this clinical report is to summarize the existing evidence for the use of inhaled nitric oxide in preterm infants and provide guidance regarding its use in this population. (1/14, reaffirmed 8/25)
https://doi.org/10.1542/peds.2013-3444

THE USE OF NONNUTRITIVE SWEETENERS IN CHILDREN

Carissa M. Baker-Smith, MD, MPH, FAAP; Sarah D. de Ferranti, MD, MPH, FAAP; William J. Cochran, MD, FAAP; Committee on Nutrition; Section on Gastroenterology, Hepatology, and Nutrition

ABSTRACT. The prevalence of nonnutritive sweeteners (NNSs) in the food supply has increased over time. Not only are more children and adolescents consuming NNSs, but they are also consuming a larger quantity of NNSs in the absence of strong scientific evidence to refute or support the safety of these agents. This policy statement from the American Academy of Pediatrics is intended to provide the pediatric provider with a review of (1) previous steps taken for approved use of NNSs, (2) existing data regarding the safety of NNS use in the general pediatric population, (3) what is known regarding the potential benefits and/or adverse effects of NNS use in children and adolescents, (4) identified gaps in existing knowledge and potential areas of future research, and (5) suggested talking points that pediatricians may use when discussing NNS use with families. (11/19, reaffirmed 8/25)
https://doi.org/10.1542/peds.2019-2765

USE OF POINT-OF-CARE ULTRASONOGRAPHY IN THE NICU FOR DIAGNOSTIC AND PROCEDURAL PURPOSES (CLINICAL REPORT)

Dan L. Stewart, MD, FAAP; Yasser Elsayed, MD, FRCPC; María V. Fraga, MD; Brian D. Coley, MD, FAAP, FACR; Aparna Annam, DO, FAAP; Sarah Sarvis Milla, MD, FAAP; Committee on Fetus and Newborn; and Section on Radiology

ABSTRACT. Point-of-care ultrasonography (POCUS) refers to the use of portable imaging performed by the treating clinician at the bedside for diagnostic, therapeutic, and procedural purposes. POCUS may be considered an extension of the physical examination but not a substitute for diagnostic imaging. Use of POCUS in emergency situations can be lifesaving in the NICU if performed in a timely fashion for cardiac tamponade, pleural effusions, pneumothorax, etc, with potential for enhancing the quality of care and improving outcomes. In the past 2 decades, POCUS has gained significant acceptance in clinical medicine in many parts of the world and in many subspecialties. Formal accredited training and certification programs are available for neonatology trainees, as well as for many other subspecialties in Canada, Australia, and New Zealand. Although no formal training program or certification is available to neonatologists in Europe, POCUS is also widely available to providers in NICUs. A formal institutional POCUS fellowship is now available in Canada, and recently, the Royal College of Physicians and Surgeons (Canada) recognized targeted neonatal echocardiography performed by the neonatologist as area of focus competency for certification. In the United States, many clinicians have the skills to perform POCUS and have incorporated it in their daily clinical practice. However, appropriate equipment remains limited, and many barriers exist to POCUS program implementation. Recently, the first international, evidence-based POCUS guidelines for the use in neonatology and pediatric critical care were published. Considering the potential benefits, a recent national survey of neonatologists confirmed that the majority of clinicians were inclined to adopt POCUS in their clinical practice if the barriers could be resolved. This clinical report describes the current landscape of neonatal POCUS, outlines barriers for implementation, and provides a suggested educational framework and overall strategy for successful implementation of a POCUS program. Diagnostic and procedural applications of POCUS in the NICU will be explored in detail in the accompanying technical report, which can be found in this issue of *Pediatrics*. (11/22)

https://doi.org/10.1542/peds.2022-060052

USE OF POINT-OF-CARE ULTRASONOGRAPHY IN THE NICU FOR DIAGNOSTIC AND PROCEDURAL PURPOSES (TECHNICAL REPORT)

Dan L. Stewart, MD, FAAP; Yasser Elsayed, MD, FRCPC; Maria V. Fraga, MD; Brian D. Coley, MD, FAAP, FACR; Aparna Annam, DO, FAAP; Sarah Sarvis Milla, MD, FAAP; Committee on Fetus and Newborn; and Section on Radiology

ABSTRACT. Point-of-care ultrasonography (POCUS) refers to the use of portable imaging performed by the provider clinician at the bedside for diagnostic, therapeutic, and procedural purposes. POCUS could be considered an extension of the physical examination but not a substitute for diagnostic imaging. Use of POCUS in emergency situations can be lifesaving in the NICU if performed in a timely fashion for cardiac tamponade, pleural effusions, pneumothorax, etc, with potential for enhancing quality of care and improving outcomes.

In the past 2 decades, POCUS has gained significant acceptance in clinical medicine in many parts of the world and in many subspecialties. Formal accredited training and certification programs are available for neonatology trainees as well as for many other subspecialties in Canada, Australia, and New Zealand. Although no formal training program or certification is available to neonatologists in Europe, POCUS is widely available to providers in NICUs. A formal institutional POCUS fellowship is now available in Canada. In the United States, many clinicians have the skills to perform POCUS and have incorporated it in their daily clinical practice. However, appropriate equipment remains limited, and many barriers exist to POCUS program implementation.

Recently, the first international evidence-based POCUS guidelines for use in neonatology and pediatric critical care were published. Considering the potential benefits, a recent national survey of neonatologists confirmed that the majority of clinicians were inclined to adopt POCUS in their clinical practice if the barriers could be resolved.

This technical report describes many potential POCUS applications in the NICU for diagnostic and procedural purposes. (11/22)

https://doi.org/10.1542/peds.2022-060053

USE OF PROBIOTICS IN PRETERM INFANTS (CLINICAL REPORT)

Brenda Poindexter, MD, MS, FAAP, and Committee on Fetus and Newborn

ABSTRACT. Probiotic products in the United States are available for use in the general category of dietary supplements, bypassing the rigor of the US Food and Drug Administration (FDA) approval process in safety, efficacy, and manufacturing standards. As a result, currently available probiotics lack FDA-approved drug labeling and cannot be marketed to treat or prevent disease in preterm infants, including necrotizing enterocolitis and late-onset sepsis. Despite lack of availability of a pharmaceutical-grade product, the number of preterm infants receiving probiotics in the United States and Canada is steadily increasing. According to recent reports from large collaborative databases in the United States, approximately 10% of extremely low gestational age neonates receive a probiotic preparation during their stay in the NICU, with wide variation in practice among units. In sum, more than 10 000 preterm infants have been enrolled in randomized clinical trials of probiotic supplementation worldwide. Methodologic differences among study protocols included different strains and combinations of therapy, masking of trials, and a priori definitions of the primary outcome measure. Large meta-analyses of these trials have demonstrated the efficacy of multiple-strain probiotics in reducing necrotizing enterocolitis and all-cause mortality, whereas the efficacy of single-strain probiotic preparations is less certain. In the absence of an appropriate medical-grade product in the United States, dietary supplement–grade probiotics, some of which have been the subject of recent recalls for contamination, are being prescribed. Given the lack of FDA-regulated pharmaceutical-grade products in the United States, conflicting data on safety and efficacy, and potential for harm in a highly vulnerable population, current evidence does not support the routine, universal administration of probiotics to preterm infants, particularly those with a birth weight of <1000 g. (5/21)

https://doi.org/10.1542/peds.2021-051485

VENTRICULAR FIBRILLATION AND THE USE OF AUTOMATED EXTERNAL DEFIBRILLATORS ON CHILDREN

Committee on Pediatric Emergency Medicine and Section on Cardiology and Cardiac Surgery

ABSTRACT. The use of automated external defibrillators (AEDs) has been advocated in recent years as one part of the chain of survival to improve outcomes for adult cardiac arrest victims. When AEDs first entered the market, they had not been tested for pediatric usage and rhythm interpretation. In addition, the presumption was that children do not experience ventricular fibrillation, so they would not benefit from the use of AEDs.

Recent literature has shown that children do experience ventricular fibrillation, which has a better outcome than do other cardiac arrest rhythms. At the same time, the arrhythmia software on AEDs has become more extensive and validated for children, and attenuation devices have become available to downregulate the energy delivered by AEDs to allow their use on children. Pediatricians are now being asked whether AED programs should be implemented, and where they are being implemented, pediatricians are being asked to provide guidance on the use of them on children. As AED programs expand, pediatricians must advocate on behalf of children so that their needs are accounted for. For pediatricians to be able to provide guidance and ensure that children are included in AED programs, it is important for pediatricians to know how AEDs work, be up-to-date on the literature regarding pediatric fibrillation and energy delivery, and understand the role of AEDs as life-saving interventions for children. (11/07, reaffirmed 7/25)
https://doi.org/10.1542/peds.2007-2676

VISION AND CONCUSSION: SYMPTOMS, SIGNS, EVALUATION, AND TREATMENT

Christina L. Master, MD, FAAP; Darron Bacal, MD, FAAP; Matthew F. Grady, MD, FAAP; Richard Hertle, MD, FAAP; Ankoor S. Shah, MD, PhD; Mitchell Strominger, MD, FAAP; Sarah Whitecross, MMedSci, CO; Geoffrey E. Bradford, MD, MS, FAAP; Flora Lum, MD; Sean P. Donahue, MD, PhD; and Section on Ophthalmology (joint with American Academy of Ophthalmology; American Association for Pediatric Ophthalmology and Strabismus; and American Association of Certified Orthoptists)

ABSTRACT. Visual symptoms are common after concussion in children and adolescents, making it essential for clinicians to understand how to screen, identify, and initiate clinical management of visual symptoms in pediatric patients after this common childhood injury. Although most children and adolescents with visual symptoms after concussion will recover on their own by 4 weeks, for a subset who do not have spontaneous recovery, referral to a specialist with experience in comprehensive concussion management (eg, sports medicine, neurology, neuropsychology, physiatry, ophthalmology, otorhinolaryngology) for additional assessment and treatment may be necessary. A vision-specific history and a thorough visual system examination are warranted, including an assessment of visual acuity, ocular alignment in all positions of gaze, smooth pursuit (visual tracking of a moving object), saccades (visual fixation shifting between stationary targets), vestibulo-ocular reflex (maintaining image focus during movement), near point of convergence (focusing with both eyes at near and accommodation (focusing with one eye at near because any of these functions may be disturbed after concussion. These deficits may contribute to difficulty with returning to both play and the learning setting at school, making the identification of these problems early after injury important for the clinician to provide relevant learning accommodations, such as larger font, preprinted notes, and temporary use of audio books. Early identification and appropriate management of visual symptoms, such as convergence insufficiency or accommodative insufficiency, may mitigate the negative effects of concussion on children and adolescents and their quality of life. (7/22)
https://doi.org/10.1542/peds.2021-056047

VISUAL SYSTEM ASSESSMENT IN INFANTS, CHILDREN, AND YOUNG ADULTS BY PEDIATRICIANS

Committee on Practice and Ambulatory Medicine and Section on Ophthalmology (joint with American Association of Certified Orthoptists, American Association for Pediatric Ophthalmology and Strabismus, and American Academy of Ophthalmology)

ABSTRACT. Appropriate visual assessments help identify children who may benefit from early interventions to correct or improve vision. Examination of the eyes and visual system should begin in the nursery and continue throughout both childhood and adolescence during routine well-child visits in the medical home. Newborn infants should be examined using inspection and red reflex testing to detect structural ocular abnormalities, such as cataract, corneal opacity, and ptosis. Instrument-based screening, if available, should be first attempted between 12 months and 3 years of age and at annual well-child visits until acuity can be tested directly. Direct testing of visual acuity can often begin by 4 years of age, using age-appropriate symbols (optotypes). Children found to have an ocular abnormality or who fail a vision assessment should be referred to a pediatric ophthalmologist or an eye care specialist appropriately trained to treat pediatric patients. (12/15, reaffirmed 10/21)
https://doi.org/10.1542/peds.2015-3596

VITAMIN K AND THE NEWBORN INFANT

Ivan Hand, MD, FAAP; Lawrence Noble, MD, FAAP; Steven A. Abrams, MD, FAAP; Committee on Fetus and Newborn; Section on Breastfeeding; and Committee on Nutrition

ABSTRACT. Intramuscular administration of vitamin K for prevention of vitamin K deficiency bleeding (VKDB) has been a standard of care since the American Academy of Pediatrics recommended it in 1961. Despite the success of prevention of VKDB with vitamin K administration, the incidence of VKDB appears to be on the rise. This increase in incidence of VKDB is attributable to parental refusal as well as lowered efficacy of alternate methods of administration. The aim of this statement is to discuss the current knowledge of prevention of VKDB with respect to the term and preterm infant and address parental concerns regarding vitamin K administration. (2/22)
https://doi.org/10.1542/peds.2021-056036

WEB SERVICES AND CLOUD COMPUTING IN PEDIATRIC CARE (TECHNICAL REPORT)

Michael G. Leu, MD, MS, MHS, FAAP, FAMIA; Stuart T. Weinberg, MD, FAAP, FAMIA; Craig Monsen, MD, MS; Christoph U. Lehmann, MD, FAAP, FACMI, FIAHSI; and Council on Clinical Information Technology

ABSTRACT. Electronic health record (EHR) systems do not uniformly implement pediatric-supportive functionalities. One method of adding these capabilities across EHR platforms is to integrate Web services and Web applications that may perform decision support and store data in the cloud when the EHR platform is able to integrate Web services. Specific examples of these services are described, such as immunization clinical decision support services, consumer health resources, and bilirubin nomograms. Health care providers, EHR vendors, and developers share responsibilities in the appropriate development, integration, and use of Web services and Web applications as they relate to best practices in the areas of data security and confidentiality, technical availability, audit trails, terminology and messaging standards, compliance with the Health Insurance Portability and Accountability Act, testing, usability, and other considerations. It is desirable for health care providers to have knowledge of Web services and Web applications that can improve pediatric capabilities in their own EHRs because this will naturally inform discussions concerning EHR features and facilitate implementation and subsequent use of these capabilities by clinicians caring for children. (6/21)
https://doi.org/10.1542/peds.2021-052048

SECTION 5

Endorsed Policies

The American Academy of Pediatrics endorses and accepts as its policy the following documents from other organizations.

AMERICAN ACADEMY OF PEDIATRICS

Endorsed Policies

THE 21ST CENTURY CURES ACT & ADOLESCENT CONFIDENTIALITY

North American Society for Pediatric and Adolescent Gynecology and Society for Adolescent Health and Medicine

INTRODUCTION. In 2020 the Office of the National Coordinator for Heath Information Technology (ONC) issued a Final Rule to implement specific requirements of the 21st Century Cures Act. The goal of the Final Rule is to increase access, use, and exchange of electronic health information. The North American Society for Pediatric and Adolescent Gynecology (NASPAG) and the Society for Adolescent Health and Medicine (SAHM) agree that sharing health information with patients and families allows for improved medical care. We believe it is equally important to recognize the right of adolescent minors to access confidential care, which is protected to some degree in every U.S. state. As experts in the care of adolescents, NASPAG and SAHM are in a unique position to inform institutional policies around release of information for this population. (2/21)

ANAPHYLAXIS DEFINITION, OVERVIEW, AND CLINICAL SUPPORT TOOL: 2024 CONSENSUS REPORT—A GA²LEN PROJECT*

Timothy E. Dribin, MD; Antonella Muraro, MD, PhD; Carlos A. Camargo, Jr, MD, DrPH; Paul J. Turner, FRCPCH, PhD; Julie Wang, MD; Graham Roberts, DM; Aikaterini Anagnostou, MD, PhD; Susanne Halken, DM, DMSc; Jay Liebermann, MD; Margitta Worm, MD; Torsten Zuberbier, MD; Hugh A. Sampson, MD; on behalf of the GA₂LEN Anaphylaxis Study Team

ABSTRACT. *Background.* The 2006 National Institute of Allergy and Infectious Disease/Food Allergy and Anaphylaxis Network anaphylaxis criteria are widely used in clinical care and research. In 2020, the World Allergy Organization published modified criteria that have not been uniformly adopted. Different criteria contribute to inconsistent care and research outcomes.

Objective. We sought to develop a consensus anaphylaxis definition, overview, and clinical support tool.

Methods. A 12-member writing group developed draft outputs modified with input from a 46-member international expert panel, 31 medical stakeholder organizations, and 15 patient advocacy organizations. The expert panel participated in a modified Delphi process to seek consensus for the outputs using a ≥80% consensus threshold.

Results. The first sentence of the definition reads, "Anaphylaxis is a serious allergic (hypersensitivity) reaction that can progress rapidly and may cause death." The definition also describes organ systems that may be involved and signs of life-threatening reactions. The overview includes details of anaphylaxis recognition and management. The clinical support tool incorporates new clinical criteria to help determine the likelihood that patients are having anaphylaxis, intramuscular epinephrine indications and dosing, and common findings from the anaphylaxis organ systems. In addition, 93.5% (43/46), 97.8% (45/46), and 93.5% (43/46) of experts agreed with the definition, overview, and clinical support tool, respectively.

Conclusion. The anaphylaxis overview is a novel educational tool conveying key elements of anaphylaxis recognition and management. We propose that the definition and clinical support tool should replace previous definitions and clinical criteria. The clinical support tool should facilitate improved anaphylaxis recognition and management across different clinical settings and standardize research outcomes. (8/25)

*The American Academy of Pediatrics endorsed the following 3 items in this publication: (1) the anaphylaxis definition; (2) clinical support tool; and (3) the clinical support legend.

CRITERIA FOR PLACENTAL EXAMINATION FOR OBSTETRICAL AND NEONATAL PROVIDERS

Drucilla J. Roberts, MD; Rebecca N. Baergen, MD; Theonia K. Boyd, MD; Chrystalle Katte Carreon, MD; Virginia E. Duncan, MD; Linda M. Ernst, MD; Ona M. Faye-Petersen, MD; Ann K. Folkins, MD; Jonathon L. Hecht, MD, PhD; Amy Heerema-McKenney, MD; Debra S. Heller, MD; Rebecca L. Linn, MD; Carolyn Polizzano, MHS, PA (ASCP); Sanjita Ravishankar, MD; Raymond W. Redline, MD; Carolyn M. Salafia, MD, MPH; Vanda F. Torous, MD; Eumenia C. Castro, MD

ABSTRACT. Pathologic examination of the placenta can provide insight into likely (and unlikely) causes of antepartum and intrapartum events, diagnoses with urgent clinical relevance, prognostic information for mother and infant, support for practice evaluation and improvement, and insight into advancing the sciences of obstetrics and neonatology. Although it is true that not all placentas require pathologic examination (although alternative opinions have been expressed), prioritization of placentas for pathologic examination should be based on vetted indications such as maternal comorbidities or pregnancy complications in which placental pathology is thought to be useful for maternal or infant care, understanding pathophysiology, or practice modifications. Herein we provide placental triage criteria for the obstetrical and neonatal provider based on publications and expert opinion of 16 placental pathologists and a pathologists' assistant, formulated using a modified Delphi approach. These criteria include indications in which placental pathology has clinical relevance, such as pregnancy loss, maternal infection, suspected abruption, fetal growth restriction, preterm birth, nonreassuring fetal heart testing requiring urgent delivery, preeclampsia with severe features, or neonates with early evidence of multiorgan system failure including neurologic compromise. We encourage a focused gross examination by the provider or an attendant at delivery for all placentas and provide guidance for this examination. We recommend that any placenta that is abnormal on gross examination undergo a complete pathology examination. In addition, we suggest practice criteria for placental pathology services, including a list of critical values to be used by the relevant provider. We hope that these sets of triage indications, criteria, and practice suggestions will facilitate appropriate submission of placentas for pathologic examination and improve its relevance to clinical care. (5/23)

INITIAL RESUSCITATION ALGORITHM FOR CHILDREN

Society of Critical Care Medicine (2020)

NASPAG POSITION STATEMENT: ELIMINATING PERIOD POVERTY IN ADOLESCENTS AND YOUNG ADULTS LIVING IN NORTH AMERICA

Megan E. Harrison, Shelby Davies, Nichole Tyson, Andrea Swartzendruber, Laura K. Grubb, Elizabeth M. Alderman (12/22)

RECOMMENDATIONS FOR CENTERS PERFORMING PEDIATRIC HEART SURGERY IN THE UNITED STATES

Carl L. Backer, MD; David M. Overman, MD; Joseph A. Dearani, MD; Jennifer C. Romano, MD, MS; James S. Tweddell, MD; S. Ram Kumar, MD, PhD; Bradley S. Marino, MD, MPP, MSCE, MBA; Emile A. Bacha, MD; Robert D.B. Jaquiss, MD; Ali N. Zaidi, MD; Michelle Gurvitz, MD; John M. Costello, MD, MPH; Trudy A. Pierick, MSN, ARNP, CPNP-PC; William J. Ravekes, MD; James A. Reagor, MPS, CCP, FPP; James D. St. Louis, MD; James Spaeth, MD; William T. Mahle, MD; Andrew Y. Shin, MD; Keila N. Lopez, MD, MPH; Tara Karamlou, MD, MSc; Karl F. Welke, MD, MS; Roosevelt Bryant, MD; S. Adil Husain, MD; Jonathan M. Chen, MD; Aditya Kaza, MD, MBA; Winfield J. Wells, MD; Andrew C. Glatz, MD, MSCE; Mitchell I. Cohen, MD; Doff B. McElhinney, MD; David A. Parra, MD; Sara K. Pasquali, MD, MHS

ABSTRACT. Care and outcomes for the more than 40,000 patients undergoing pediatric and congenital heart surgery in the United States annually are known to vary widely. While consensus recommendations have been published across numerous fields as one mechanism to promote a high level of care delivery across centers, it has been more than two decades since the last pediatric heart surgery recommendations were published in the United States. More recent guidance is lacking, and collaborative efforts involving the many disciplines engaged in caring for these children have not been undertaken to date. The present initiative brings together professional societies spanning numerous care domains and congenital cardiac surgeons, pediatric cardiologists, nursing, and other healthcare professionals from diverse programs around the country to develop consensus recommendations for United States centers. The focus of this initial work is on pediatric heart surgery, and it is recommended that future efforts focus in detail on the adult congenital population. We describe the background, rationale, and methodology related to this collaborative effort, and recommendations put forth for Essential Care Centers (essential services necessary for any program), and Comprehensive Care Centers (services to optimize comprehensive and high-complexity care), encompassing structure, process, and outcome metrics across 14 domains. (12/23)

REDUCING TOPICAL DRUG WASTE IN OPHTHALMIC SURGERY: MULTISOCIETY POSITION PAPER

David J. Palmer, MD; Alan L. Robin, MD; Cathleen M. McCabe, MD; David F. Chang, MD; for the Ophthalmic Instrument Cleaning and Sterilization Task Force

ABSTRACT. This position article on reducing topical drug waste with ophthalmic surgery was written by the Ophthalmic Instrument Cleaning and Sterilization Task Force, comprising representatives of the ASCRS, American Academy of Ophthalmology, American Glaucoma Society, and Outpatient Ophthalmic Surgery Society. Drug waste significantly increases the costs and carbon footprint of ophthalmic surgery. Surgical facilities should be permitted to use topical drugs in multidose containers on multiple patients until the manufacturer's labeled date of expiration, if proper guidelines are followed. Surgical patients requiring a topical medication not used for other patients should be allowed to bring that partially used medication home for postoperative use. These recommendations are based on published evidence and clarification of policies from multiple regulatory and accrediting agencies with jurisdiction over surgical facilities. Surveys suggest that most ambulatory surgery centers and hospitals performing cataract surgery are wasting topical drugs unnecessarily. (9/22)

RESTRICTIVE HOUSING IN JUVENILE CORRECTIONAL SETTINGS

National Commission on Correctional Health Care

INTRODUCTION. NCCHC asserts that "juveniles, mentally ill individuals, and pregnant women should be excluded from solitary confinement of any duration" (NCCHC, 2016). However, the practice of juvenile solitary confinement and broader forms of restrictive housing still occurs today. A 2015 survey of solitary confinement rules in juvenile justice systems revealed that 47% of juvenile detention centers reported locking youth in some type of isolation for more than 4 hours at a time (Lowenstein Center, 2016). Given the widespread use of restrictive housing and the well-understood negative health impacts of these practices, it is imperative that juvenile correctional facilities work to reduce or eliminate the use of restrictive housing and establish clear protocols for the rare instances when isolation is deemed essential (e.g., medical necessity) to ensure safety for youth. (2/21)

WEIGHING ALL PATIENTS IN KILOGRAMS

Emergency Nurses Association (2021)

Appendix 1

PPI: AAP Partnership for Policy Implementation

BACKGROUND

The American Academy of Pediatrics (AAP) develops policies that promote optimal physical, mental, and social health and well-being for all infants, children, adolescents, and young adults. These documents are valued highly not only by clinicians who provide direct health care to children but by members of organizations who share similar goals and by parents, payers, public health officials, and legislators. To increase clarity and actionability of AAP clinical guidance and recommendations for providers at the point of care, the AAP formed the Partnership for Policy Implementation (PPI). The PPI is a group of clinical informaticians who partner with authors of AAP clinical practice guidelines and clinical reports to ensure that clinical recommendations are stated with the precision needed to implement them in an electronic health record (EHR) system.[1] This process also makes recommendations easier for humans to follow and apply. Partnership for Policy Implementation volunteers focus on helping content experts develop clinical guidance that specifies exactly who is to do what, for whom, and under what circumstances.

VISION

The vision of the PPI is that all AAP clinical recommendations include clear, unambiguous guidance on how pediatricians can implement those recommendations into their patient care and that AAP clinical guidance can be easily incorporated within EHR decision-support systems.

MISSION

The mission of the PPI is to facilitate implementation of AAP recommendations at the point of care by ensuring that AAP documents are written in a practical, action-oriented fashion with unambiguous recommendations.

WHAT THE PPI IS

The PPI is a network of pediatric informaticians who work with AAP authors and clinical practice guideline subcommittees throughout the writing process.

Contributions of the PPI to the AAP writing process include disambiguation and specification; development of clear definitions; clearly defined logic; implementation techniques; action-oriented recommendations, including clinical algorithms; transparency of the evidence base for recommendations; and use of health information technology (HIT) standards.

WHAT THE PPI HAS ACCOMPLISHED

Since the PPI's inception, more than 30 statements have been published using the PPI process, covering a wide variety of child health topics, including perinatal urinary tract dilation (*Pediatrics*. 2025;156[1]:e2025071814), influenza prevention and control (*Pediatrics*. 2025;156[6]:e2025073620), healthy, active living (*Pediatrics*. 2024;153[3]:e2023065480), opioid prescribing (*Pediatrics*. 2024;154[5]:e2024068752), obesity (*Pediatrics*. 2023;151[2]:e2022060640).

One example of how a statement developed using the PPI process has gained broader acceptance is the AAP annual influenza statement. Since 2007, the Centers for Disease Control and Prevention has adopted components of the PPI statement (specifically, the clinical algorithm) within its own statement on the same topic.

WHAT THE PPI IS DOING NOW

In addition to creating and shaping practical, action-oriented guidance that pediatricians can use at the point of care, the PPI works to make it easier for these recommendations to be incorporated into electronic systems. To date, the PPI has focused its involvement on the statement development process. Involvement of the PPI during the writing process produces a clear, more concise document. As these standards of care become well documented, the PPI can begin to focus on building or mapping pediatric vocabulary; once solidified, this vocabulary can be built into EHR systems. The standards of care can also be matched to various logical and functional HIT standards that already exist today. Through this work, the PPI improves AAP policy documents by providing specific guidance to pediatricians at the point of care, ensuring that EHRs are designed to assist pediatricians in providing optimal care for children. The PPI developed a short video that provides an overview of its mission and process. This video is available on the AAP YouTube channel at www.youtube.com/watch?v=woTfeoNcxn4.

The PPI continues to expand and mentor new members. For more information on the application process and about the PPI, please contact Lisa Krams, MS (lkrams@aap.org).

[1]Lehmann CU, Adams WG, Chaparro JD, et al. Better guidelines and policies: AAP's Partnership for Policy Implementation. *Pediatrics*. 2024;154(1):e2023061360. doi: 10.1542/peds.2023-061360. PMID: 38864111

APPENDIX 2

American Academy of Pediatrics Acronyms

AACAP American Academy of Child and Adolescent Psychiatry
AAFP American Academy of Family Physicians
AAMC Association of American Medical Colleges
AAOS American Academy of Orthopaedic Surgeons
AAP American Academy of Pediatrics
AAPD American Academy of Pediatric Dentistry
ABM Academy of Breastfeeding Medicine
ABMS American Board of Medical Specialties
ABP American Board of Pediatrics
ACCME Accreditation Council for Continuing Medical Education
ACEP American College of Emergency Physicians
ACGME Accreditation Council for Graduate Medical Education
ACIP Advisory Committee on Immunization Practices
ACMG American College of Medical Genetics
ACO Accountable Care Organization
ACOG American College of Obstetricians and Gynecologists
ACOP American College of Osteopathic Pediatricians
ACP American College of Physicians
ADAMHA Alcohol, Drug Abuse, and Mental Health Administration
AG-M Action Group—Multidisciplinary (Section Forum)
AG-M1 Action Group—Medical 1 (Section Forum)
AG-M2 Action Group—Medical 2 (Section Forum)
AG-S Action Group—Surgical (Section Forum)
AHA American Heart Association
AHA American Hospital Association
AHRQ Agency for Healthcare Research and Quality
ALF Annual Leadership Forum
AMA American Medical Association
AMCHP Association of Maternal and Child Health Programs
AMSA American Medical Student Association
AMSPDC Association of Medical School Pediatric Department Chairs
AMWA American Medical Women's Association
APA Academic Pediatric Association
APHA American Public Health Association
APLS Advanced Pediatric Life Support
APPD Association of Pediatric Program Directors
APQ Alliance for Pediatric Quality
APS American Pediatric Society
AQA Ambulatory Care Quality Alliance
ASHG American Society of Human Genetics
ASPHO American Society of Pediatric Hematology/Oncology
ASPN American Society of Pediatric Nephrology
ASTM American Society of Testing and Materials
BHP Bureau of Health Professions
BIA Bureau of Indian Affairs
BLAST Babysitter Lessons and Safety Training
BOD Board of Directors
BPC Breastfeeding Promotion Consortium
CAG Corporate Advisory Group
CAMLWG Children, Adolescents, and Media Leadership Workgroup
CAP College of American Pathologists
CAQI Chapter Alliance for Quality Improvement
CATCH Community Access to Child Health
CDC Centers for Disease Control and Prevention
CESP Confederation of European Specialty Pediatrics
CFMC Chapter Forum Management Committee
CFT Cross Functional Team
CHA Children's Hospital Association
CHIC Child Health Informatics Center
CHIP Children's Health Insurance Program
CMC Council Management Committee
CME Continuing Medical Education
CMS Centers for Medicare & Medicaid Services
CMSS Council of Medical Specialty Societies
CnF Council Forum
COAYA Council on Adolescents and Young Adults
COA Committee on Adolescence
COB Committee on Bioethics
COCAN Council on Child Abuse and Neglect
COCD Council on Children and Disasters
COCHF Committee on Child Health Financing
COCIT Council on Clinical Information Technology
COCM Council on Communications and Media
COCME Committee on Continuing Medical Education
COCN Committee on Coding and Nomenclature
COCP Council on Community Pediatrics
COCWD Council on Children With Disabilities
COD Committee on Drugs
COEC Council on Early Childhood
COEHCC Council on Environmental Health and Climate Change
CoF Committee Forum
COFCAKC Council on Foster Care, Adoption, and Kinship Care
COFN Committee on Fetus and Newborn
COG Committee on Genetics
COGME Council on Graduate Medical Education (DHHS/HRSA)
COHC Committee on Hospital Care
COHE Council on Health Equity
COHMED Council on Healthy Mental and Emotional Development
COICFH Council on Immigrant Child and Family Health
COID Committee on Infectious Diseases

COIVPP	Council on Injury, Violence, and Poison Prevention
COMLRM	Committee on Medical Liability and Risk Management
COMSEP	Council on Medical Student Education in Pediatrics (AMSPDC)
CON	Committee on Nutrition
CONACH	Committee on Native American Child Health
COPACFH	Committee on Psychosocial Aspects of Child and Family Health
COPAH	Committee on Pediatric and Adolescent HIV
COPAM	Committee on Practice and Ambulatory Medicine
COPE	Committee on Pediatric Education
COPEM	Committee on Pediatric Emergency Medicine
COPHiL	Committee on Philanthropy
COPR	Committee on Pediatric Research
COPW	Committee on Pediatric Workforce
COQIPS	Council on Quality Improvement and Patient Safety
COSGA	Committee on State Government Affairs
COSH	Council on School Health
COSMF	Council on Sports Medicine and Fitness
COSUP	Committee on Substance Use and Prevention
CPS	Canadian Paediatric Society
CPTI	Community Pediatrics Training Initiatives
CQN	Chapter Quality Network
CSHCN	Children With Special Health Care Needs
DHHS	Department of Health and Human Services
DOD	Department of Defense
DVC	District Vice Chairpersons Committee
EBCDLWG	Early Brain and Child Development Leadership Workgroup
EC	Executive Committee
ECHO	Expanding Capacity for Health Outcomes
EHDI	Early Hearing Detection and Intervention
ELWG	Epigenetics Leadership Workgroup
EMSC	Emergency Medical Services for Children
EPA	Environmental Protection Agency
EQIPP	Education in Quality Improvement for Pediatric Practice
eTACC	Electronic Translation of Academy Clinical Content
FAAN	Federal Advocacy Action Network
FASD	Fetal Alcohol Spectrum Disorders
FCF	Friends of Children Fund
FDA	Food and Drug Administration
FERPA	Family Educational Rights and Privacy Act
FOPE II	Future of Pediatric Education II
FOPO	Federation of Pediatric Organizations
FPN	Family Partnerships Network
FTC	Federal Trade Commission
Glo-NAC	Global Neonatal Advisory Committee
GME	Graduate Medical Education
HAAC	Historical Archives Advisory Committee
HBB	Helping Babies Breathe
HCCA	Healthy Child Care America
HEDIS	Healthcare Effectiveness Data and Information Set
HHS	Health and Human Services
HIPAA	Health Insurance Portability and Accountability Act of 1996
HMO	Health Maintenance Organization
HOF	Headquarters of the Future
HQA	Hospital Quality Alliance
HRSA	Health Resources and Services Administration
HTC	Help the Children
HTPCP	Healthy Tomorrows Partnership for Children Program
IHS	Indian Health Service
IMG	International Medical Graduate
IPA	International Pediatric Association
IPC	International Pediatric Congress
IRB	Institutional Review Board
LLLI	La Leche League International
LWG	Leadership Workgroup
MCAN	Merck Childhood Asthma Network
MCH	Maternal and Child Health
MCHB	Maternal and Child Health Bureau
MCN	Migrant Clinicians Network
MHICSN-PAC	Medical Home Initiatives for Children With Special Needs Project Advisory Committee
MHLWG	Mental Health Leadership Work Group
MOC	Maintenance of Certification
MRT	Media Resource Team
NACHC	National Association of Community Health Centers
NAEMSP	National Association of EMS Physicians
NAEPP	National Asthma Education and Prevention Program
NAM	National Academy of Medicine
NAPNAP	National Association of Pediatric Nurse Practitioners
NASPGHAN	North American Society for Pediatric Gastroenterology, Hepatology, and Nutrition
NAWD	National Association of WIC Directors
NBME	National Board of Medical Examiners
NCBDDD	National Center on Birth Defects and Developmental Disabilities
NCE	National Conference & Exhibition
NCEPG	National Conference & Exhibition Planning Group
NCQA	National Committee for Quality Assurance
NHLBI	National Heart, Lung, and Blood Institute
NHMA	National Hispanic Medical Association
NHTSA	National Highway Traffic Safety Administration
NIAAA	National Institute on Alcohol Abuse and Alcoholism
NICHD	National Institute of Child Health and Human Development
NICHQ	National Initiative for Children's Health Quality
NIDA	National Institute on Drug Abuse
NIH	National Institutes of Health
NIMH	National Institute of Mental Health
NMA	National Medical Association
NNC	National Nominating Committee
NQF	National Quality Forum
NRHA	National Rural Health Association
NRMP	National Resident Matching Program
NRP	Neonatal Resuscitation Program
NSC	National Safety Council
NVAC	National Vaccine Advisory Committee
ODPHP	Office of Disease Prevention and Health Promotion
OED	Office of the Executive Director
OHISC	Oral Health Initiative Steering Committee
OLWG	Obesity Leadership Workgroup
P4P	Pay for Performance
PAAC	Payer Advocacy Advisory Committee
PAC	Project Advisory Committee
PACC	Pediatric Acute and Critical Care Quality Network
PAHO	Pan American Health Organization

PALS	Pediatric Advanced Life Support
PAS	Pediatric Academic Societies
PCO	*Pediatric Care Online*™
PCOC	Primary Care Organizations Consortium
PCPCC	Patient-Centered Primary Care Collaborative
PCPI	Physician Consortium on Performance Improvement
PEAC	Practice Expense Advisory Committee
PECOS	Pediatric Education in Community and Office Settings
PECS	Pediatric Education in Community Settings
PEPP	Pediatric Education for Prehospital Professionals
PIR	*Pediatrics in Review*
PLA	Pediatric Leadership Alliance
PPAAC	Private Payer Advocacy Advisory Committee (COCHF Subcommittee)
PPAC	Past President's Advisory Committee
PPC	Pediatric Primary Care Quality Network
PPC-PCMH	Physician Practice Connections—Patient-Centered Medical Home (NCQA)
PPI	Partnership for Policy Implementation
PPMA	Pediatric Practice Management Alliance
PREP	Pediatric Review and Education Program
PROS	Pediatric Research in Office Settings
PUPVS	Project Universal Preschool Vision Screening
QA	Quality Assurance
QI	Quality Improvement
QuIIN	Quality Improvement Innovation Network
RBPE	Resource-Based Practice Expense
RBRVS	Resource-Based Relative Value Scale
RCE	Richmond Center of Excellence
RRC	Residency Review Committee (ACGME)
RUC	AMA/Specialty Society Relative Value Scale Update Committee
RVU	Relative Value Unit
SAM	Society for Adolescent Medicine
SAMHSA	Substance Abuse and Mental Health Services Administration
SCHIP	State Children's Health Insurance Program
SDBP	Society for Developmental and Behavioral Pediatrics
SF	Section Forum
SFMC	Section Forum Management Committee
SLGBTHW	Section on Lesbian, Gay, Bisexual, and Transgender Health and Wellness
SOA	Section on Anesthesiology and Pain Medicine
SOAI	Section on Allergy and Immunology
SOAPM	Section on Administration and Practice Management
SOATT	Section on Advances in Therapeutics and Technology
SOB	Section on Bioethics
SOBr	Section on Breastfeeding
SOCC	Section on Critical Care
SOCCS	Section on Cardiology and Cardiac Surgery
SOCDRP	Section on Child Death Review and Prevention
SOCPT	Section on Clinical Pharmacology and Therapeutics
SOD	Section on Dermatology
SODBP	Section on Developmental and Behavioral Pediatrics
SOECP	Section on Early Career Physicians
SOEM	Section on Emergency Medicine
SOEn	Section on Endocrinology
SOEPHE	Section on Epidemiology, Public Health, and Evidence
SOGH	Section on Global Health
SOGHN	Section on Gastroenterology, Hepatology, and Nutrition
SOHCa	Section on Home Care
SOHM	Section on Hospital Medicine
SOHO	Section on Hematology/Oncology
SOHPM	Section on Hospice and Palliative Medicine
SOID	Section on Infectious Diseases
SOIM	Section on Integrative Medicine
SOIMG	Section on International Medical Graduates
SOMP	Section on Medicine-Pediatrics
SONp	Section on Nephrology
SONPM	Section on Neonatal-Perinatal Medicine
SONs	Section on Neurological Surgery
SONTPT	Section on Nicotine and Tobacco Prevention and Treatment
SONu	Section on Neurology
SOOb	Section on Obesity
SOOH	Section on Oral Health
SOOHNS	Section on Otolaryngology—Head and Neck Surgery
SOOp	Section on Ophthalmology
SOOPe	Section on Osteopathic Pediatricians
SOOr	Section on Orthopaedics
SOPPSM	Section on Pediatric Pulmonology and Sleep Medicine
SOPS	Section on Plastic Surgery
SOPT	Section on Pediatric Trainees
SORa	Section on Radiology
SORh	Section on Rheumatology
SOSILM	Section on Simulation and Innovative Learning Methods
SOSM	Section on Senior Members
SOSu	Section on Surgery
SOTC	Section on Telehealth Care
SOTCo	Section on Tobacco Control
SOTM	Section on Transport Medicine
SOU	Section on Urology
SOUCM	Section on Urgent Care Medicine
SOUS	Section on Uniformed Services
SPR	Society for Pediatric Research
SPWG	Strategic Planning Work Group
TA	Technical Assistance
TA	Technology Assessment
TFOA	Task Force on Access (also known as Task Force on Health Insurance Coverage and Access to Care)
TFOC	Task Force on Circumcision
TFOSIDS	Task Force on Sudden Infant Death Syndrome
TIPP	The Injury Prevention Program
TJC	The Joint Commission
UNICEF	United Nations Children's Fund
UNOS	United Network for Organ Sharing
USDA	US Department of Agriculture
VIP	Value in Inpatient Pediatrics
WHO	World Health Organization
WIC	Special Supplemental Nutrition Program for Women, Infants, and Children

Subject Index

Page numbers followed by *f* denote figures and *t* denote tables.

A

B

C

D

E

F

G

J

K

L

M

N

O

P

R

S

T

U

V